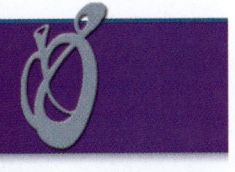

Mechanical Circulatory Support

A Companion to Braunwald's Heart Disease

Mechanical Circulatory Support

A Companion to Braunwald's Heart Disease

Robert L. Kormos, MD, FRCS(C), FACS, FAHA
Professor of Surgery
Co-Director, Heart Transplantation
Director, Artificial Heart Program
Heart and Vascular Institute
University of Pittsburgh Medical Center
Pittsburgh, Pennsylvania

Leslie W. Miller, MD
Edward C. Wright Professor of Cardiovascular Medicine
Chair, Department of Cardiovascular Sciences
CEO of Cardiovascular Clinical Research
University of South Florida Health
Tampa, Florida

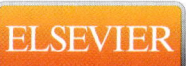

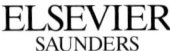

1600 John F. Kennedy Blvd.
Ste. 1800
Philadelphia, PA 19103-2899

Mechanical Circulatory Support: A Companion to
Braunwald's Heart Disease,

ISBN: 978-1-4160-6001-7

Notice

Knowledge and best practice in this field are constantly changing. As new research and
experience broaden our knowledge, changes in practice, treatment and drug therapy may
become necessary or appropriate. Readers are advised to check the most current information
provided (i) on procedures featured or (ii) by the manufacturer of each product to be
administered, to verify the recommended dose or formula, the method and duration of
administration, and contraindications. It is the responsibility of the practitioner, relying
on their own experience and knowledge of the patient, to make diagnoses, to determine
dosages and the best treatment for each individual patient, and to take all appropriate safety
precautions. To the fullest extent of the law, neither the Publisher nor the [Editors/Authors]
[delete as appropriate] assumes any liability for any injury and/or damage to persons or
property arising out of or related to any use of the material contained in this book.

The Publisher

Library of Congress Cataloging-in-Publication Data
Mechanical circulatory support : a companion to Braunwald's heart disease / [edited by] Robert L. Kormos,
Leslie W. Miller. – 1st ed.
    p. ; cm.
  A companion to: Braunwald's heart disease / edited by Robert O. Bonow . . . [et al.]. 9th ed. c2012.
  Includes bibliographical references and index.
  ISBN 978-1-4160-6001-7 (hardback : alk. paper)   1. Blood, Circulation, Artificial – Instruments.
2. Heart failure – Treatment.   I. Kormos, Robert L.   II. Miller, Leslie W. (Leslie William), 1946-
III. Braunwald's heart disease.
  [DNLM: 1. Heart-Assist Devices. 2. Heart Failure – surgery. 3. Heart Failure – therapy. WG 169.5]
  RD598.35.A77M443 2012
  616.1'2 – dc23

2011024585

ISBN: 978-1-4160-6001-7

Acquisitions Editor: Natasha Andjelkovic
Developmental Editor: Brad McIlwain
Publishing Services Manager: Patricia Tannian
Project Managers: John Casey and Vijay Vincent
Designer: Steven Stave

Printed in United States of America

Last digit is the print number: 9 8 7 6 5 4 3 2 1

Contributors

Keith D. Aaronson, MD, MS
Professor of Internal Medicine
Division of Cardiovascular Medicine
Medical Director, Heart Transplantation and Center
  for Circulatory Support
Co-Director, Heart Failure and Transplant Management Program
University of Michigan
Ann Arbor, Michigan

Shahab A. Akhter, MD
Associate Professor of Surgery
Section of Cardiac and Thoracic Surgery
The University of Chicago Medical Center
Chicago, Illinois

James F. Antaki, PhD
Professor, Biomedical Engineering and Computer Science
Carnegie Mellon University
Pittsburgh, Pennsylvania

Deborah D. Ascheim, M.D.
Associate Professor of Health Evidence & Policy and Medicine
Clinical Director of Research, International Center for Health
  Outcomes and Innovation Research (InCHOIR)
Department of Health Evidence & Policy
Cardiovascular Institute
Mount Sinai School of Medicine
New York, New York

J. Timothy Baldwin, PhD
Deputy Chief, Advanced Technologies and Surgery Branch
Division of Cardiovascular Sciences
  National Heart Lung and Blood Institute
National Institutes of Health
Bethesda, Maryland

Christian A. Bermudez, MD
Assistant Professor of Surgery
Associate Director, Heart Transplantation Program
Medical Director, ECMO Program
University of Pittsburgh Medical Center
Pittsburgh, Pennsylvania

Emma J. Birks, MRCP, PhD
Professor of Medicine
Cardiovascular Medicine
University of Louisville;
Medical Director, Heart Failure, Transplantation, and
  Mechanical Support
Jewish Hospital
Louisville, Kentucky

Elizabeth D. Blume, MD
Medical Director, Heart Failure / Transplant Program
Department of Cardiology
Children's Hospital Boston
Associate Professor of Pediatrics
Harvard Medical School
Boston, Massachusetts

Robin Roberts Bostic
Corporate Vice President Health Policy/Economics and
  Government Affairs
Thoratec Corporation
Pleasanton, California

Andrew Boyle, MD
Clinical Associate Professor of Medicine
Medical Director of Heart Failure, Cardiac Transplantation
  and Mechanical Circulatory Support
Aurora St. Luke's Medical Center
Milwaukee, Wisconsin

Eric A. Chen, MS
Director, Humanitarian Use Device
  Designation Program
Office of Orphan Products Development
Food and Drug Administration
Silver Spring, Maryland

Walter Dembitsky, MD
Program Director
Mechanical Circulatory Support
Chair, Department of Cardiac Thoracic Surgery
Sharp Memorial Hospital
San Diego, California

Mary Amanda Dew, PhD
Professor of Psychiatry, Psychology, Epidemiology, and
  Biostatistics
Department of Psychiatry
University of Pittsburgh School of Medicine and
  Medical Center
Pittsburgh, Pennsylvania

Annetine C. Gelijns, PhD
Professor of Health Evidence & Policy
Co-Chair, Department of Health Evidence & Policy
Co-Director, International Center for Health Outcomes and
  Innovation Research (InCHOIR)
Mount Sinai School of Medicine
New York, New York

Theresa Gelzinis, MD
Assistant Professor
Department of Anesthesiology
University of Pittsburgh
Presbyterian Hospital
Pittsburgh, Pennsylvania

Eiran Z. Gorodeski, MD, MPH
Assistant Professor of Medicine
Section of Heart Failure and Cardiac
  Transplantation
Department of Cardiovascular Medicine
Heart and Vascular Institute
Cleveland Clinic
Cleveland, Ohio

Kathleen L. Grady, PhD, APN, FAAN
Associate Professor of Surgery
Division of Cardiac Surgery
Department of Surgery
Northwestern University
Administrative Director, Center for Heart Failure
Bluhm Cardiovascular Institute
Northwestern Memorial Hospital
Chicago, Illinois

Igor Gregoric, MD
Director of Cardiac Support
Texas Heart Institute at St. Luke's Episcopal
Houston, Texas

Jennifer L. Hall, PhD
University of Minnesota, Lillehei Heart Institute
Associate Professor of Medicine
Director, Program in Translation Cardiovascular
    Genomics
Medicine / Cardiovascular Division
University of Minnesota
Minneapolis, Minnesota

J. Thomas Heywood, MD
Director, Heart Failure Recovery & Research Program
Scripps Clinic
La Jolla, California

William L. Holman, MD
Professor of Surgery
Division of Cardiothoracic Surgery
University of Alabama at Birmingham
Birmingham, Alabama

Tina Ommaya Ivovic
Corporate Director of Reimbursement Services
Thoratec Corporation
Pleasanton, California

Brian Jaski, MD
Medical Director
Advanced Heart Failure and Cardiac
    Transplant Programs
Sharp Memorial Hospital
San Diego, California

Valluvan Jeevanandam, MD
Professor of Surgery
Chief, Section of Cardiac and Thoracic Surgery
University of Chicago
Chicago, Illinois

Ranjit John
Associate Professor
Department of Surgery
University of Minnesota;
Director, Mechanical Circulatory
    Support Program
University of Minnesota Medical Center
Minneapolis, Minnesota

Francesca Joseph, MD
Medical Officer
Office of Orphan Products Development
Food and Drug Administration
Silver Spring, Maryland

Robert L. Kormos, MD, FRCS(C), FACS, FAHA
Professor of Surgery
Co-Director, Heart Transplantation
Director, Artificial Heart Program
Heart and Vascular Institute
University of Pittsburg Medical Center
Pittsburg, Pennsylvania

Kathleen L. Lockard, RN, BSN, MBA, CCTC
University of Pittsburgh Medical Center
Artificial Heart Program
Pittsburgh, Pennsylvania

Donna Mancini, MD
Choudhrie Professor of Medicine
Director, Center for Advanced Cardiac Care
Department of Medicine
Columbia University
New York, New York

Leslie W. Miller, MD
Edward G. Wright Professor of Cardiovascular Medicine
Chair, Department of Cardiovascular Sciences
CEO of Cardiovascular Clinical Research
University of South Florida Health
Tampa, Florida

Alan Moskowitz, MD, FACP
Professor of Health Evidence and Policy and Medicine
Vice Chair, Department of Health Evidence and Policy
Co-Director, InCHOIR
Mount Sinai School of Medicine
New York, New York

Yoshifumi Naka, MD, PhD
Associate Professor of Surgery
Department of Surgery
Columbia University College of Physicians and Surgeons
New York, New York

Francis D. Pagani, MD, PhD
Otto Gago, M.D. Professor in Cardiac Surgery
Surgical Director, Heart Transplant Program
Surgical Director, Center for Circulatory Support
University of Michigan
Ann Arbor, Michigan

Michael K. Parides, PhD
Professor of Biostatistics
Department of Health Evidence & Policy
Director of Biostatistics, InCHOIR
Mount Sinai School of Medicine
New York, New York

Sonna M. Patel-Raman, PhD
Center for Devices and Radiological Health
Food and Drug Administration
Silver Spring, Maryland

Marc S. Penn, MD, PhD
Director of Research
Summa Cardiovascular Institute
Summa Health System
Akron, Ohio
Skirball Laboratory of Cardiovascular Cellular Therapeutics
Department of Integrated Medical Sciences
Northeast Ohio Medical University
Rootstown, Ohio

Shradha Rathi, MD
Cardiology Fellow
University of California, San Francisco
Fresno, California

Joseph G. Rogers, MD
Associate Professor of Medicine
Medical Director, Cardiac Transplant and Mechanical
    Circulatory Support Program
Duke University Medical Center
Durham, North Carolina

Stuart D. Russell, MD
Associate Professor of Medicine
Clinical Chief, Heart Failure and Transplantation
Johns Hopkins Hospital
Baltimore, Maryland

Mark S. Slaughter, MD
Professor of Surgery
Chief, Division of Thoracic and Cardiovascular Surgery
Director, Mechanical Assist Device Program
University of Louisville
Louisville, Kentucky

Randall C. Starling, MD, MPH
Professor of Medicine
Vice Chairman, Department of Cardiovascular Medicine
Section Head, Heart Failure and Cardiovascular Medicine
Kaufman Center for Heart Failure
Heart and Vascular Institute
Cleveland Clinic
Cleveland, Ohio

Lynne Warner Stevenson, MD
Director, Heart Failure Program
Cardiovascular Division
Brigham and Women's Hospital
Professor of Medicine
Harvard Medical School
Boston, Massachusetts

Jeffrey Teuteberg, MD
Assistant Professor of Medicine
Medical Director, Mechanical Circulatory Support
Heart and Vascular Institute
University of Pittsburgh
Pittsburgh, Pennsylvania

Guillermo Torre-Amione, MD, PhD, FACC
Associate Professor of Medicine
Wells Medical College of Cornell University
Medical Director, Heart Transplant Program
Methodist DeBakey Heart Center at the Methodist Hospital
Houston, Texas

William R. Wagner, PhD
Deputy Director, McGowan Institute for Regenerative
    Medicine
Professor of Surgery, Bioengineering, and Chemical
    Engineering
University of Pittsburgh
Pittsburgh, Pennsylvania

Richard K. Wampler, MD
Independent Consultant
Loomis, California

John T. Watson, PhD
Professor and Galletti Scholar
Bioengineering Department
UC San Diego
La Jolla, California

Peter D. Wearden, MD, PhD
Assistant Professor of Cardiothoracic Surgery
Division of Pediatric Cardiothoracic Surgery
University of Pittsburgh School of Medicine
Pittsburgh, Pennsylvania

Joshua R. Woolley, PhD
Department of Bioengineering
McGowan Institute for Regenerative Medicine
University of Pittsburgh
Pittsburgh, Pennsylvania

James B. Young, MD
Professor of Medicine and Executive Dean
George and Linda Kaufman Chair
Cleveland Clinic Lerner College of Medicine of Case
    Western Reserve University
Cleveland, Ohio

**To Mary Anne, Katherine, Mary Ellen,
Alexandra, and Michael**
My stars and my strength
—RLK

To Liz and Graham
*whose love and support inspire me
and helped bring this book to completion*
—LWM

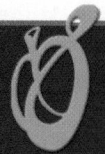

The information in this textbook represents the most contemporary thinking in the field of mechanical circulatory support. However, a short historical perspective is important in understanding how quickly we moved to rapid adoption of this technology. The therapy of mechanical circulatory support began only 60 years ago, rooted in the concept of capitalizing on the augmentative abilities of the skeletal muscle of the hemi-diaphragm to support cardiac contractility. In 1959, the pioneer, Adrian Kantrowicz, wrote extensively about using the diaphragm in a counter pulsation mode long before his development of the intra-aortic balloon pump. But limitations caused by the challenges of chronic phrenic nerve stimulation turned his team toward utilizing a mechanical prosthesis as an auxiliary ventricle. A recently arrived Japanese research partner, Yuki Nose, discovered that this prosthesis worked more effectively the closer it was placed to the native heart. Simultaneously, John Gibbon, Clarence Dennis, and Walt Lillihei were developing the pump oxygenator while Willem Kolff, Frank Hastings, and Bret Kusserow pursued the total artificial heart. Interestingly many of the early systems were based on the concept of counterpulsation with blood being removed via one femoral artery and returned to the next. This led Moulopoulis and others to further explore counterpulsation using an intra-aortic balloon pump in 1962. In 1960 in a second family of approaches, Salisbury showed the value of left ventricular bypass, demonstrating its theoretical applications in experimental heart failure. Dennis et al. reported a technique for acute left heart failure, using a large-bore cannula for transjugular/transseptal drainage of the left atrium, which made left ventricular bypass possible without thoracotomy. By 1964 they had used the procedure in 12 patients. Potential application of left ventricular bypass for prolonged left ventricular support began with Kusserow's report in 1961 of a paracorporeal pump located in juxtaposition to the outer surface of the thoracic cage. Further experimentation was carried out by Domingo Liotta, Michael DeBakey, and their colleagues. This led in 1966 to DeBakey's first clinical use of such a pump in a 37-year-old woman who could not be weaned from the pump oxygenator. The patient was supported on the bypass pump for 10 days; she recovered and was discharged from the hospital. In 1962, applying the principle of diastolic augmentation, Kolff and Clauss had reported mock circulation and canine studies with an intra-aortic balloon pump, inflating the balloon with carbon dioxide and synchronizing it to the electrocardiogram. But it was up to Kantrowicz and his team in 1966 to design and fabricate balloon pumps in the laboratory. They quickly learned the advantage of using helium as the driving gas and by 1968, human studies were being reported

Dr. Benjamin Eiseman, who was interested in organ failure, chaired a conference in the fall of 1964 that focused on mechanical devices to assist the failing heart. It was co-sponsored by the Committee on Trauma, the Division of Medical Sciences, the National Academy of Sciences, and the National Research Council along with experts and pioneers in the fields of engineering and surgery who had an interest in circulatory support. Dr Eiseman's opening comment was that, "The heart is a set of pumps. Therefore there is no logical reason why it cannot be replaced by a mechanical equivalent." The challenges for this development, although intimidating in their engineering hurdles, he considered "mere details of design." Even at this early stage Dr. Eiseman had identified two principle uses for such devices: reversible failure where temporary use could lead to recovery and irreversible damage where a more permanent substitute would be required for one or both sides of the heart. The primary challenge Eiseman identified was to have engineers and surgeons work closely together to solve the issues of design.

An active participant in this meeting was Peter Salisbury, mentioned above, who first introduced the concept of left heart bypass for heart failure. But he also elaborated on the characteristics of heart failure defined by Roy and Adam in 1888 as a syndrome of abnormally high left-sided diastolic filling pressures, pulmonary hypertension, and a vicious cycle of progressive hemodynamic and clinical deterioration manifested by organ failure. He recommended, therefore, that assisted circulation could have a major role when self-perpetuating cardiac abnormalities due to low cardiac output exists and when these are accompanied by ventricular dilatation due to excess diastolic pressure and dilatation in a failing ventricle and cannot be reversed by any other therapy. These concepts for the indications for left ventricular support have remained essentially unchanged in clinical practice until 10 years ago when knowledge of patient selection was modified. This will be explored later in the book. In his presentation at this meeting in 1964, Salisbury goes on to distinguish the acute hemodynamic collapse that occurs with acute cardiogenic shock and its profound effects on the body and how this situation may be less effectively corrected with assisted circulation as compared to more chronic heart failure. (Prophetic insight, given the struggles modern clinicians have in accomplishing success with assisted circulation even with more advanced and exotic technology in their hands.) On a last note of interest, Salisbury predicts the current interest in myocardial recovery using left ventricular assist devices when he states, "A popular notion has it that 'tired' hearts should be helped by 'rest' and what could be more reposing for the heart than having its 'work' taken over by an auxiliary pump?"

The participants in this early meeting discussed in a rather animated fashion their concerns with future pump designs; the shortcomings and challenges of biocompatibility, the effects of shear on the blood components, and ongoing debate between proponents of pulsatile vs. non-pulsatile pump designs. It was at this meeting that Michael DeBakey and Domingo Liotta set forth their requirements for an ideal implantable heart pump: (1) it should be capable of long-term support (weeks or months); (2) it should be useable with or without anticoagulants; (3) it should cause minimal blood trauma; (4) it should make it possible to reduce mean left atrial pressure to near normal; (5) it should maintain normal aortic perfusion pressure; (6) it should enable function to be discontinued for long intervals with normal resumption of function (without the need for general heparinization and without danger of pump thrombosis); (7) it should enable synchronized pumping during any preselected time of the cardiac cycle; and (8) it should be easy to implant. These principles are interesting as the reader will see when outcomes with devices and design principles of modern pumps are reviewed.

At the conclusion of this meeting, the participants agreed that certain challenges faced the field: (1) the engineers and clinicians needed to work more closely together; (2) there was a need to move from case reports to more population-based studies; (3) the need for pulsatile flow had not been well-studied; (4) the field of biomaterials was not well-developed; (5) there were no clear guidelines or criteria for the implementation of assisted circulation; and (6) the utility of assisted circulation for congenital heart disease in the setting of pulmonary artery hypertension was yet to be defined.

From an historical perspective, the field of mechanical circulatory support has gone through several more recent decades of change. The decade of the 1960's defined the problem and cardiac assistance was limited to aortic counterpulsation, direct cardiac compression, extensions of cardiopulmonary bypass, left atrial to femoral bypass techniques, and primitive pulsatile systems. The research goals during the 1970's focused on myocardial recovery following post-cardiotomy failure and shock and techniques of cannulation with further refinement of timing of support. Research in the 1980's led to the recognition and development of a need for more chronic pulsatile devices. The optimal testing field for this new technology would be those patients awaiting cardiac transplantation. Again, patient selection and timing of implantation issues were paramount. A large focus was on the determination of the role of the total artificial heart in contrast to that of the left ventricular assist device. This fact drove clinicians to better define the role of the right ventricle during left ventricular support. During the 1990's the use of a left ventricular assist device as an alternative to cardiac transplantation drove a number of clinical trials that were to be landmark in their conclusions for long-term support. During this decade clinicians moved to define the requirements for outpatient LVAD management and began to acknowledge certain instances of myocardial recovery on the LVAD. Perhaps the strongest advances at this time came from the broader utilization of the technology by more surgeons in more centers resulting in more defined and structured protocols for device implantation, early surgical management, and standards for training.

In the past decade there has been a quantum change in technology accompanied by major changes in clinical implementation. From the technology perspective, there has been a gradual reduction in size, making applicability wider and reducing the invasiveness and complications of surgery. In addition, we have seen the introduction and acceptance of rotary blood pumps based first on axial flow technology and soon followed by centrifugal designs. These devices have virtually replaced the use of pulsatile systems except for the more acute post-cardiotomy settings. There has been an introduction of smaller and more portable peripheral components such as the wearable controllers and batteries along with smaller and more flexible external drivelines. Finally, a new line of devices has been introduced as ultra-short term LVADs for acute cardiogenic shock and even smaller devices for neonatal and pediatric uses. We have seen evolution not only in technology but also in utilization. Devices are now approved or on the threshold of being approved for not only bridge to transplantation but also for destination or permanent therapy. Patient selection is now based on earlier risk assessment scales that aim to identify those patients at risk who stand to benefit from device utilization before the onset of preoperative risks that further drive postoperative morbidity and mortality. Thus the device application is seen to be moving to earlier indications, in particular for those patients who are looking at these devices as permanent solutions. Indeed there is a gradual acceptance by clinicians that the intended use of a LVAD device for chronic support may change during the period of support from one indication to another. Recovery of function after ventricular assist device support is being considered more often for cases not only presenting acutely, but also in some instances following chronic support. Finally the care of patients after implantation has moved from strictly inpatient care to exclusively outpatient care, raising even more challenges for the paradigms of care. Along with this has been the gradual development of the specialty of advanced heart failure cardiology that encompassed the understanding and chronic management of ventricular assist devices. It is for this reason that we have attempted to represent both surgical and cardiologic perspectives in this textbook as the field of mechanical circulatory support moves forward as a true medical and surgical collaboration.

There has been enormous progress in the field of MCS in the past 5 years, including significant growth in the development of a number of systems designed for temporary support of severe HF and shock. Their use has been associated with increasing success in reversing shock and improving end organ and neurologic function in critically ill patients, and has led to the concept of "Bridge to a Bridge or Bridge to Decision,"

While the early days of pulsatile MCS were not based on many controlled trials, especially randomized against medical therapy (due to the critical nature of the HF/shock in these patients who were largely awaiting a heart transplant), the recent near total transition from pulsatile to rotary pumps has been driven by large clinical controlled trial evidence. The durability of the devices now in use or in clinical trials has allowed a conversion from emergent to near totally elective implantation. This change has been aided by development of risk scores and profiles that help identify the highest risk patient by co-morbidities associated with high risk of poor outcome during the index hospitalization. There remains a critical need to develop similar contemporary risk models for predicting the outcome of HF patients with medical therapy alone.

The future of MCS seems very promising based on the progress of the last decade. With increased manufacturers in the field, continued improvements and progressive miniaturization of the devices is expected. This will then lead to expanded indications into patients with less severe heart failure. The new pumps will need to be free of an external drive line and some type of transcutaneous energy transfer that will greatly enhance patient satisfaction and reduce long-term risk of infection. The number of patients, especially over 65 years of age, with advanced heart failure will continue to increase, leading to the overwhelming use as a long-term alternative to heart transplantation. This expanded use in patients with less critical heart failure will hopefully lead to reduction in cost that will be associated with greater adoption of their use.

Finally, we salute not only the courageous pioneers mentioned above, along with the engineers, surgeons, heart failure cardiologists, and other clinicians and coordinators that now make up the VAD team, but also the amazing patients whose courage and sacrifices have helped to bring this technology to its current state. They inspire all in the field to continue the progress seen in the past 60 years and help them enjoy prolonged life with markedly improved function and quality of life.

ROBERT L. KORMOS

LESLIE W. MILLER

Contents

Historical Aspects of Mechanical Circulatory Support

J. Timothy Baldwin and John T. Watson

INTRODUCTION

"If one could substitute for the heart a kind of injection ... of arterial blood, either natural or artificially made ... one would succeed easily in maintaining alive indefinitely any part of the body."

Julien-Jean-Cesar
Legallois (1770-1814)

Legallois recognized the "magical nature" of human physiology. However, an organized test of his hypothesis would not commence until the 21st century with the origins of mechanical circulatory support (MCS). To duplicate partially the control and function of a single human organ would require a measured stepwise effort of the collaborative clinical, scientific, and engineering expertise of academia, industry, and government. The development of the needed intellectual capacity discussed in this historical account was possible only by mandate from the U.S. Congress. In many respects, providing MCS for several years has been found to be more challenging than landing on the moon.

This account of events focuses on the Artificial Heart Program (AHP) of the National Heart, Lung and Blood Institute (NHLBI). The AHP was carefully monitored by ad hoc and standing advisory committees, and all funding decisions included standard National Institutes of Health (NIH) peer-review processes. Although the AHP was centered in the United States, contributors around the world, without reservation, generously shared their laboratory and clinical results for the common goal of improving survival and quality of life for patients with heart failure (HF). Notable among these contributors, but certainly not all-inclusive, are research teams in Japan, Germany, Russia, Korea, Austria, and the former Republic of Czechoslovakia.[1] Industrial leadership and expertise have also been essential ingredients for the successes of the program. Without a strong and respectful collaboration between academia, industry, and government, the MCS field as we know it today would not exist.

Establishing the Concept

In the 1930s, Carrel and Lindbergh developed an in vitro artificial heart–like apparatus for keeping organs alive outside the body. They removed hearts, kidneys, ovaries, adrenal glands, thyroid glands, and spleens of small animals to watch them develop and function over the course of several days.[2] Acute animal studies in Russia and the United States followed in the 1940s. However, the meaningful origin of the modern era of MCS can be traced to the development of the heart-lung machine by Gibbon and its first successful clinical use in 1953.[3] The device was developed for cardiopulmonary bypass so that surgical cardiac procedures that require hours of circulatory support could be performed. The success of the device and the need for prolonged circulatory support for patients who could not be weaned from the heart-lung machine or whose hearts could recover with longer durations of support provided the initial impetus for developing devices that could provide long-term circulatory support. The optimism in the 1950s and 1960s that the circulation could be successfully supported for extended periods by an artificial heart spurred its development by pioneers such as Kolff, Akutsu, DeBakey, Liotta, and Kantrowitz.[4] In 1963, DeBakey and Lederberg testified before the U.S. Congress on the need for an artificial heart in very different domains: for patients otherwise healthy except for their failed heart and for isolated travelers on long space journeys.[5] These hearings coincided with the debate about the implications of the Russian Sputnik Program and unbridled national enthusiasm for taking on large technologic challenges such as the program to put the first man on the moon, which had begun just a few years earlier.

In 1964, with special congressional approval, the National Heart Advisory Council established the mission-oriented AHP to design and develop devices to assist a failing heart and to rehabilitate HF patients.[6] After reviewing the relevant science and engineering base, the NIH Director concluded that in addition to the artificial heart, there was also a need for a targeted program to improve acute coronary care for heart attacks. This decision resulted in appropriations by the U.S. Congress for the Artificial Heart–Myocardial Infarction Program and the support for the Myocardial Infarction Research Units.

The original AHP plan included emergency devices, temporary devices and instrumentation, physiology and implantable materials, fabrication and testing, short-term circulatory assist devices, long-term ventricular assist devices (VADs), and long-term replacement devices. Initially, all projects were supported by 1-year contracts, and many involved coinvestigators from industry. Progress on biomaterials and devices for emergency and temporary use was rapid. Consequently, circulatory support for days to a few weeks proved to be quickly successful. However, the technology at that time was inadequate to use MCS successfully for a period of a few months. The early years of the program reaffirmed the importance of strengthening the underlying science of the human environment and using engineering first principles to design implantable systems with the expected "mission" of 5 to 10 years of circulatory support.

The limited heart transplantation experience in the United States in the late 1960s emphasized both the lack of understanding of organ transplantation and the need and potential for alternative therapies such as MCS. From the beginning, the AHP underwent external assessment by medical, technical, ethical, psychological, and economic advisers. In addition to the NHLBI Advisory Council, other Institute Advisory Committees and five special technical and five nontechnical panels provided oversight and recommendations for the program.[6] Based on measurable progress, the consensus of these review groups was to focus on VADs and encourage more basic and engineering research on the total artificial heart (TAH) supported by research grants. Administratively, 1-year contracts proved inefficient to advance elements of the AHP, and the contracts were subsequently planned for 3 to 5 years in coordination with investigator-initiated and program project grants.

Since the inception of the AHP, many technical and clinical challenges have been encountered and successfully addressed. As a result, MCS devices are smaller and more reliable and provide patients with advanced HF a needed option for improved survival, functional capacity, and quality of life. The progress made in MCS devices is important because the need for the devices continues to grow. In 1968, the time at which many of initial MCS developments were taking place, the annual number of deaths in the United States for which HF was the primary cause was 10,000.[7] That number has steadily increased over the past 40 years and surpassed 60,000 in 2006. The impact of HF on mortality in the United States is much greater, however, as evidenced by the listing of HF on more than 282,000 death certificates in 2006, although not identified as the primary cause.[8]

With HF patients in the United States numbering 5.8 million with half having primarily reduced systolic function and the superior clinical outcomes in patients supported using the latest-generation of MCS devices, MCS therapy is becoming more widely used to treat patients with advanced HF. (Chapter 2 discusses the current and expanding need for MCS in detail.) The level of clinical use of MCS support today and the projected plans for its use have resulted from the many developments in technology, clinical sciences, and the devices themselves. This chapter describes the milestones and accomplishments that have occurred over the past 6 decades in the development of MCS devices (Table 1-1).

TABLE 1-1	Mechanical Circulatory Support Milestones*			
Year	Event	TAH	PVAD	RVAD
1953	1st use of heart-lung machine for cardiopulmonary bypass (Gibbon)	X	X	X
1958	1st successful use of TAH in dog (Kolff and Akutso)	X		
1963	1st use of LVAD in human (DeBakey)		X	
1964	Artificial Heart Program established at NIH	X	X	X
	Six contracts awarded to analyze issues and needs for program	X	X	X
1966	1st successful use of LVAD in humans (DeBakey)		X	
1968	1st clinical use of intra-aortic balloon pump (Kantrowitz)		X	
1969	1st artificial heart implant in humans	X		
1977	NHLBI RFPs for blood pumps, energy converters, and energy transmission		X	X
	NHLBI RFA on blood-materials interactions	X	X	X
1980	NHLBI RFP for integration of blood pumps designed for 2-yr use		X	
1982	Barney Clark received first TAH implant for destination therapy	X		
1984	NHLBI RFP for 2-yr reliability studies		X	
	1st use of Pierce-Donachy VAD (Thoratec PVAD) as BTT		X	
	1st implant of Novacor VAD (1st use of electromechanical VAD)		X	
1985	1st use of CardioWest TAH as BTT	X		
1986	1st implant of Thoratec HeartMate IP VAD		X	
1988	1st use in humans of Hemopump (Rich Wampler)—1st rotary blood pump used			X
	NHLBI awards four contracts to develop portable, durable TAHs	X		
1989	Manual of operations for Novacor VAD NHLBI clinical trial completed		X	
1991	1st HeartMate VE (and XVE) implants		X	
1994	FDA approval for pneumatic HeartMate VE as BTT		X	
1996	NHLBI IVAS contracts awarded for Jarvik 2000, HeartMate II, CorAide VADs			X
	Pilot trial (PREMATCH) for destination therapy begins		X	
	NHLBI awards two contracts for TAH Clinical Readiness Program (Abiomed, Penn State)	X		

TABLE 1-1	Mechanical Circulatory Support Milestones*—Cont'd			
Year	Event	TAH	PVAD	RVAD
1998	FDA approval for HeartMate XVE as BTT		X	
	FDA approval for Novacor as BTT		X	
	REMATCH trial begins		X	
	1st DeBakey VAD implant			X
1999	1st human implant of Arrow LionHeart VAD (1st use of TETS)		X	
2000	1st HeartMate II implant (July 27, 2000)			X
	1st Jarvik 2000 implant (June 20, 2000)			X
2001	REMATCH trial completed		X	
	1st implant of the AbioCor TAH	X		
2002	FDA approval of HeartMate XVE as destination therapy		X	
2003	CMS coverage decision for destination therapy		X	
2004	NHLBI pediatric mechanical circulatory support program launched		X	X
	1st implant of DuraHeart VAD (January 19, 2004)		X	X
2006	1st implant of HeartWare HVAD (March 22, 2006)			X
	1st implant of Levacor VAD (March 8, 2006)			X
	FDA approval of AbioCor TAH	X		
	INTERMACS registry launched (June 23, 2006)	X	X	X
2007	1st implant of Circulite Synergy device; advent of miniature VADs (August 8, 2007)			X
	Peter Houghton dies after a record 2714 days of VAD support			X
2008	HeartMate II BTT clinical trial completed			X
2009	FDA approval of HeartMate II for BTT			X
	HeartMate II destination therapy clinical trial completed			X
	850th implant of the CardioWest TAH	X		
2010	FDA approval of HeartMate II for destination therapy			X

*Relevance to development of total artificial heart (TAH), pulsatile ventricular assist devices (PVADs), and rotary ventricular assist devices (RVADs) are noted.
BTT, bridge to transplant; CMS, Centers for Medicare and Medicaid services; FDA, U.S. Food and Drug Administration; INTERMACS, Interagency Registry for Mechanically Assisted Circulatory Support; IVAS, Innovative Ventricular Assist System; LVAD, left ventricular assist device; NHLBI, National Heart, Lung and Blood Institute; NIH, National Institutes of Health; REMATCH, Randomized Evaluation of Mechanical Assistance for the Treatment of Congestive Heart Failure; RFA, request for application; RFP, request for proposal; TETS, transcutaneous energy transmission system; VAD, ventricular assist device.

EVOLUTION OF PULSATILE FLOW VENTRICULAR ASSIST DEVICES

After the establishment of the AHP, the NIH focused on facilitating and funding research to develop technologies that would improve the performance and, ultimately, the clinical outcomes of patients supported by MCS devices. This focus resulted from a plan developed through a group of contracts awarded in 1964 to assess the needs of the AHP. The plan called for the development of a group of devices, and to help accomplish this goal, contracts were awarded for the study and development of "blood pumps, energy converters, physiological effects, instrumentation, fabrication, energy transmission, blood compatible materials, energy storage, blood flow control, endogenous heat transfer, oxygenators, and test and evaluation."[9] Between fiscal years 1970 and 1972, 27 NIH contracts for the program were active. These included contracts to evaluate intra-aortic balloon pumps and design membrane oxygenators; develop, test, and evaluate new materials; study device fluid mechanics; and develop and perform in vivo tests of prototype nuclear and electrically powered VADs.[10]

In the 1960s, the prevalence of myocardial infarctions (MIs) was growing rapidly in the United States, and the novel therapy of cardiac transplantation to treat patients who experienced HF after MI was limited to a very few patients by the end of the decade. Consequently, clinical experts, realizing the potential needed therapy to be provided by MCS devices, defined the design objectives for the first generation of implantable ventricular assist and cardiac replacement systems for treating patients with advanced HF. The ideal system at that time needed to be capable of a cardiac output of 10 L/min at a mean arterial pressure of 120 mm Hg with a filling pressure of 20 mm Hg and a beat rate that did not exceed 120 beats/min. Considering all the technical and quality-of-life factors at the time, the initial mission goal for ventricular assist systems was set at 2 years of maintenance-free operation. With an average of 40 to 50 million natural heartbeats per year, the NHLBI required testing the first pulsatile systems out to at least 100 million real-time cycles.

Since the beginning of the AHP, the system specifications of MCS systems have been demanding. To simulate the natural heart in a pulsatile pump, the blood must be rapidly accelerated and decelerated between essentially 0 and 25 L/min. The material composition and geometry of the pump and connections must not damage or compromise the function of the delicate blood components, particularly red blood cells and platelets. Controls must adapt automatically to meet metabolic demands of the patient. The implant configuration needs to conform to quite variable human anatomy. Components must be structurally sound in the corrosive warm saline environment of the body. The design of the rigid structure needs to have acceptability joined to anatomy with age-related viscoelasticity. System movement, vibration, and waste heat production need to be below threshold levels that would damage surrounding tissues. Blood-contacting surfaces need to be biocompatible to minimize the risks of thrombosis and stroke. Meeting these specifications far exceeded expectations of any existing energized, implantable medical device at that time. Blood-contacting surfaces proved to be exceptionally challenging. For pulsatile systems with large and reciprocating surfaces, counterintuitive textured surfaces, which encouraged cellular deposition, resulted in good biocompatibility. Consequently, the resulting devices were the first to enter clinical trials.

After years of tradeoff design evaluations, animal studies, and fatigue testing, Biomer (Dupont, Wilmington, DE) was selected as the biomaterial of choice by the leading investigative teams. However, in the late 1980s, after more than 15 years of testing, Dupont informed the NHLBI that Biomer would be withdrawn from potential human use for fear of litigation. This fallout originated from the breast implant litigation against Dow Corning and forced the field to create new biomaterials and validate them for long-term use in patients. The U.S. Congress, after considering the impact of the Dow Corning litigation, passed the Biomaterials Access Assurance Act of 1997 to ensure that patients received properly designed implants in a timely manner.

Before beginning clinical trials, the NHLBI required assessment of the "readiness" of the devices and processes for surgical procedures. The first NHLBI clinical readiness program required consecutive successful bovine implants for twice the intended period of use and analysis of thousands of hours of mock loop testing.

Clinical studies and trials of pneumatic pulsatile flow VADs began in the 1970s and showed the clinical utility of MCS devices and the progress that had been made in the devices since the initial experiences in the 1960s. The first NHLBI-coordinated clinical trial employed an axisymmetric pulsatile flow blood pump that could be used either paracorporeally or intra-abdominally in postcardiotomy patients with cardiogenic shock.[11,12] The devices had both smooth and textured surfaces. From the mid-1970s, 41 patients were studied over a 5-year period. The patients improved, and six patients were long-term survivors. These patients had recovery of cardiac function after removal of the device even with coagulation or contraction band necrosis. In parallel, in the 1970s, Pierce worked with faculty and students from the Colleges of Engineering and Medicine at Penn State to develop what later became the Thoratec pulsatile ventricular assist device (PVAD) (Fig. 1-1) through an NIH grant.[13] The device was initially known as the Pierce-Donachy VAD and received approval from the U.S. Food and Drug Administration (FDA) for postcardiotomy recovery and as a bridge to transplantation (BTT). It continues to be used to provide left ventricular, right ventricular, and biventricular support.

IMPLANTABLE ELECTROMECHANICAL VENTRICULAR ASSIST DEVICES

The program plan for completely implantable ventricular assist systems (VAS) was formulated in 1977. This program was the first effort directed at an integrated system designed for at least 2 years of human use. The system included a blood pump, energy converter, electrical power source, percutaneous or transcutaneous energy transmission mechanisms, and an automatic controller in a hermetically sealed configuration (i.e., unvented). Also in 1977, the NHLBI Devices and Technology Branch (DTB) established an annual contractors' meeting to provide a public forum for reporting the progress on all the funded contracts and to exchange information among the project teams. Based on the success of the first conference and grantee requests, the annual conference was opened to all DTB grantees and contractors. Held each December in Bethesda, Maryland, the conference was enthusiastically attended for several years until moving to Louisville, Kentucky (Jack Norman), and then to Washington, D.C. (Hank Edmunds), and by mutual agreement added to the cardiovascular section of the annual meeting of the American Society for Artificial Internal Organs.

Better fundamental understanding of biomaterials was clearly needed so that they could be developed and used to meet the biologic and engineering requirements for long-term MCS. The dawn of the modern field of cardiovascular biomaterials research grants can probably be traced to release of the Request for Application (RFA) for "Blood Materials Interactions." Subsequently, the DTB formed working groups and published guidelines for characterizing biomaterials and investigating interactions with tissue to enhance the comparability between laboratories and accelerate the pace of research findings.[14] The NHLBI also supported efforts to develop the specialized materials fabrication methods that were needed for the VADs under development.

Over a 15-year period, 10 separate NHLBI-directed VAS research subprograms of 3 to 5 years each were planned and implemented. The initial 3-year projects were proof-of-concept for blood pumps, energy converters, and energy transmission methods. Based on the progress on these systems components, the follow-on 4-year program integrated the most promising approaches into completely implantable VAD systems. These activities involved creating new knowledge and technologies while developing the manufacturing and quality assurance procedures for medical grade systems.

By 1984, system concept feasibility was shown, and five different VASs emerged in this vanguard project. The four system concepts of highest merit received contracts; these were awarded to Abiomed (Danvers, MA), Nimbus (Rancho Cordova, CA), Novacor (Oakland, CA), and Thermo Cardiosystems (Woburn, MA), and each concept entered device readiness testing to measure their actual 2-year reliability and to test biocompatibility in animals. This was the first NIH program to undertake the formal requirements of a device reliability assessment. Rigorous test protocols were followed in the program, and the function of each device was continuously monitored remotely at the NHLBI for physiologic cardiac output and blood pressure. Devices were mounted close to the surgical implant position. Saline at 37° C was the perfusion fluid. Filters, ultraviolet light, and hand cleaning helped to minimize microorganism fouling of the system. The systems emulated a patient at rest and undertaking normal activities, moderate exercise, and short periods requiring maximum flow and pressure. No maintenance was allowed on the systems, and the entire bank of test systems was quarantined with controlled access. The Novacor VAD had an early failure. After restart, however, no failures occurred in any of the 12 required systems at 2 years, and two systems remained on test for 3 years. The Novacor VAD was the only system to complete the rigorous testing. Readiness testing was the first and only program that exceeded the time and costs of the master plan.

With the successful testing of the Novacor system, a clinical trial was organized with three clinical centers, a production center, and a data coordinating center.[15–17] There were 30 VASs planned: 20 for the randomized clinical trial and 10 for backup and testing. The steering committee, comprising

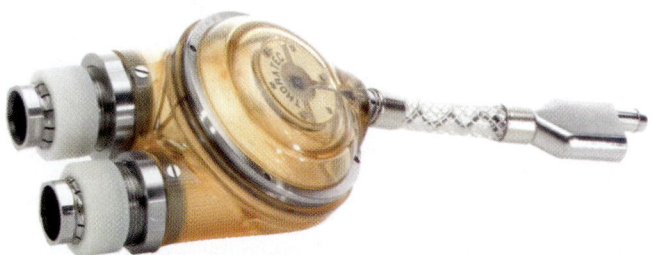

FIGURE 1-1 The Pierce-Donachy VAD (later known as the Thoratec PVAD) is a pneumatic VAD developed in the 1970s that continues to be used for left ventricular, right ventricular, and biventricular support. *(Courtesy of Thoratec, Inc., Pleasanton, CA.)*

investigators and ad hoc FDA and NHLBI members, developed protocols for patient and device endpoints, patient selection, patient and device management, quality of life, and follow-up. A Data and Safety Monitoring Board was established for added expertise and oversight. Beyond this 3-year start-up period, discussions were under way between Baxter Healthcare Company (Deerfield, IL) and the NHLBI to cost-share the clinical trial. Baxter, parent company of Novacor, made a business decision to withdraw from the trial. Although no human subjects were enrolled in the trial, the VAS program resulted in the HeartMate XVE (Fig. 1-2) and the Novacor VAD (Fig. 1-3), both of which later proved to be safe and effective in clinical trials.

Thermo Cardiosystems continued the reliability testing of the Heartmate XVE and planning a clinical trial for support of patients with end-stage HF awaiting cardiac transplantation. The effort took 9 years and cost approximately $42 million. The FDA approved the pneumatic Heartmate VE in 1994 as a BTT. The FDA approved the Novacor VAD and electric-powered Heartmate XVE 4 years later to be used as bridges to cardiac transplantation. During this period Penn State, in conjunction with Arrow International, Inc. (Reading, PA), developed a fully implantable left ventricular assist device by using a novel transcutaneous energy transmission system (TETS). The first implantation of the device, known as the LionHeart LVD 2000 (Fig. 1-4), was performed in 1999; although the device seemed to provide good clinical outcomes, Arrow decided to end development and sales of the device for financial reasons.[18] Nevertheless, it was the first and only one of two devices to date to show the success and benefits of TETS for MCS devices.

The approved devices were increasingly being considered as the forerunners of the systems that might serve as an alternative to biologic cardiac transplantation. To address this question, the Randomized Evaluation of Mechanical Assistance for the Treatment of Congestive Heart Failure (REMATCH) trial was submitted to the NIH as an investigator-initiated clinical trial.[19,20] The manual of operations and the published papers from the clinical trial developed for the Novacor VAD became the foundation for the design of the pilot REMATCH (PreMATCH) trial and ultimately the REMATCH trial. Following considerable revision of protocols, the REMATCH study design was approved by peer review, and funding was provided by the NHLBI as a cooperative agreement between Columbia University, Thoratec Corporation, and the NHLBI. The multicenter study compared long-term implantation of left ventricular assist devices with optimal medical management for patients with end-stage HF who require but who do not qualify to receive cardiac transplantation. The investigators randomly assigned 129 patients with end-stage HF who were ineligible for cardiac transplantation to receive optimal medical management or the HeartMate XVE left ventricular assist device. Kaplan-Meier survival curves showed reduction of all-cause deaths by 48% for the patients receiving the

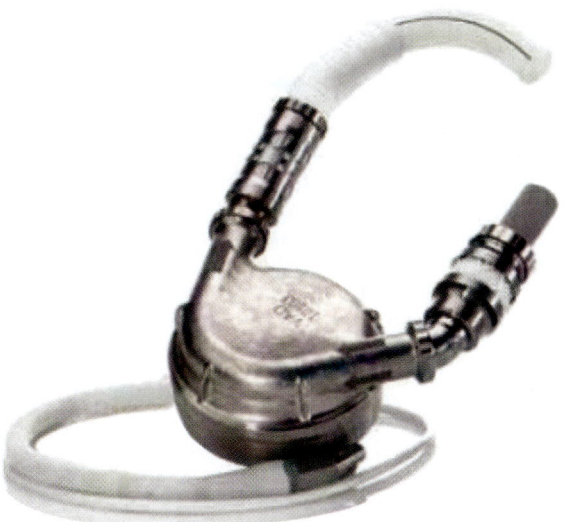

FIGURE 1-2 The Thoratec HeartMate XVE uses a textured blood-contacting surface. The device was used in the landmark REMATCH trial and became the first device approved by the U.S. Food and Drug Administration (FDA) for destination therapy. *(Courtesy of Thoratec, Inc., Pleasanton, CA. Note: Thoratec acquired Thermo Cardiosystems in 2001.)*

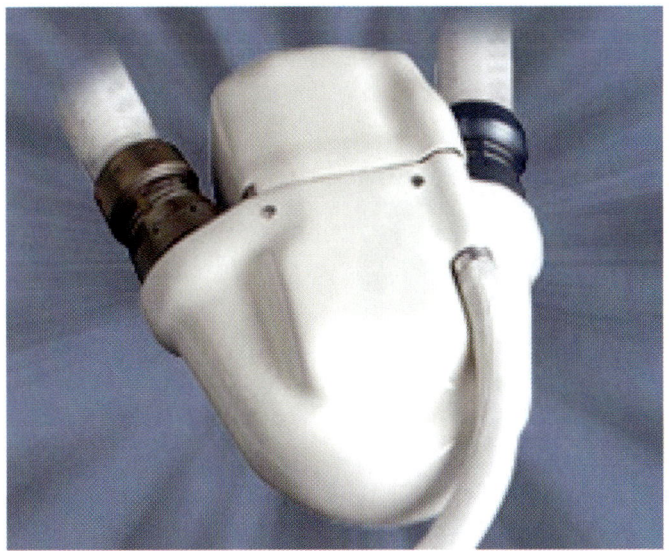

FIGURE 1-3 The Novacor VAD was the only device to complete the rigorous readiness testing of the 1980s. *(Courtesy of WorldHeart, Inc., Salt Lake City, UT.)*

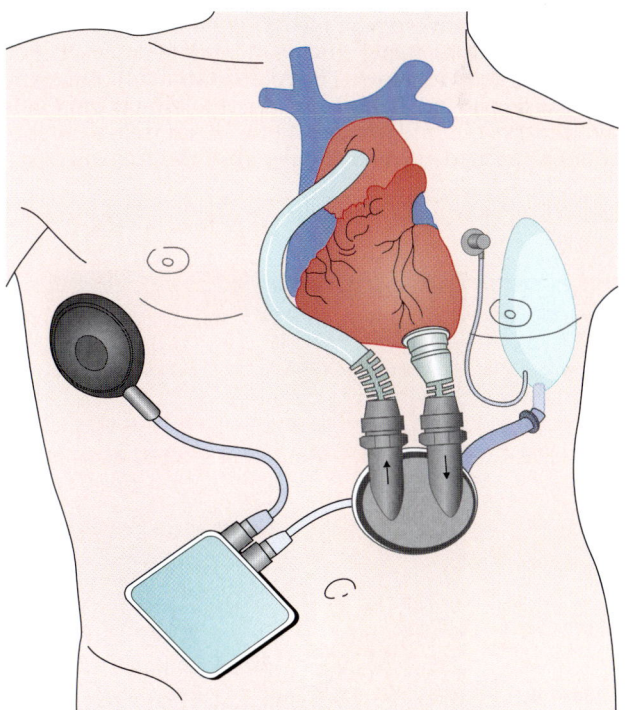

Left Ventricular Assist System (LVAS)

FIGURE 1-4 The LionHeart LVD 2000 was a completely implantable system that was the first to use a transcutaneous energy transmission system (TETS). The implanted TETS coil is shown in the upper left. *(Courtesy of Arrow International, Inc., Reading, PA.)*

VAD at 1 year. Although adverse events were increased in the device group, quality of life was significantly improved at 1 year for the device group. The survival of the patients receiving optimal medical management was much poorer than predicted. This potential was difficult to predict because the technology in the HeartMate XVE was conceived 26 years earlier without previous clinical experience.

The landmark REMATCH trial showed that MCS can successfully provide long-term permanent circulatory support while improving quality of life in patients with late-stage HF. The REMATCH trial led to FDA approval in 2002 of the HeartMate XVE for use as destination therapy in patients with end-stage HF who were ineligible for transplant. Coverage by the Centers for Medicare and Medicaid Services (CMS) for destination therapy followed 1 year later.

EVOLUTION OF TOTAL ARTIFICIAL HEARTS

The early development efforts and first reports of successfully using a TAH in animal studies were by Akutsu and Kolff in the 1950s at the Cleveland Clinic.[1,4] While the work continued there, in Houston, Liotta and the Baylor-Rice research team were developing an artificial heart that would provide total biventricular support by bypassing both left and right ventricles. The first-in-human artificial heart implant was performed by Cooley in 1969 using the Liotta TAH. The device was used for 64 hours and bridged the patient to a heart transplant, which, at that time, was a new therapy itself.[4,21,22]

Also in 1969, a National Heart Institute Ad Hoc Task Force on Cardiac Replacement concluded that the most serious technical problem for MCS devices was biocompatible materials and recommended that the AHP consider the promising research and development of VADs.[6] Efforts became focused on further development of TAH devices over the next decade through individual and program project grants. Kolff, Nose, and Pierce led major programs and formed a critical mass of investigators working on the myriad daunting research tasks using pneumatic implantable artificial hearts designed for calves. The Akutsu Model III pneumatic TAH was developed at the Texas Heart Institute, and Cooley used it in 1981 to bridge a patient to a heart transplantation, although the patient died 7 days after the transplant as a

result of multiple organ failure.[23] At the University of Utah, Kolff worked with a team on what became the Jarvik-7 TAH; in 1982, the device was first used as permanent destination therapy when DeVries implanted the device in Barney Clark.[24] Clark, a retired dentist, survived 112 days with the device, and subsequent permanent TAH implants provided support for up to 620 days. Despite the ability of the TAH to provide long-term support, the adverse events and compromised quality of life that the patients experienced while on the devices, including strokes caused by either emboli out of the pump or the high flows used at that time, soon redirected the use of the TAH to bridge patients to heart transplant rather than as destination therapy, at least until a more suitable device was developed.

The first use of the Jarvik-7 model TAH as BTT was performed by Copeland in 1985.[25] A pneumatic TAH developed at Penn State was also implanted shortly afterward in 2 patients as BTT.[26] Since 1985, the Jarvik-7 TAH has been renamed the SynCardia temporary TAH (Fig. 1-5) and has been implanted more than 850 times. The development of a portable Freedom driver now provides patients with the Syncardia TAH device much greater mobility. To date, no controlled clinical trials of the Syncardia TAH have been reported. Only a summary of the clinical experience with the first 100 patients was published in 1989.[27]

In 1988, the NHLBI awarded contracts to Penn State/3M, Abiomed/Texas Heart Institute, the University of Utah, and Nimbus/Cleveland Clinic to develop integrated and completely implantable TAHs.[28] This program resulted in the AbioCor TAH, which was initially implanted in 2001 (Fig. 1-6). The system achieved the initial goal of being completely implantable and received FDA approval under a Humanitarian Device Exemption in 2006. The device is intended for patients with end-stage HF, with a life expectancy of less than 30 days, who are ineligible for a heart transplant, and who have no other treatment options.[29] To date, less than 20 patients have received the device, with the longest reported survival of 17 months.[30,31] The longest survivor was able to return to his home in a small city, live a relatively normal life, and see the birth of his last grandchild. An increased rate of thromboembolism for the AbioCor TAH, which was attributed to thrombus that formed on the support struts, resulted in a design change to the sewing cuff and the postimplantation anticoagulation strategy.[30]

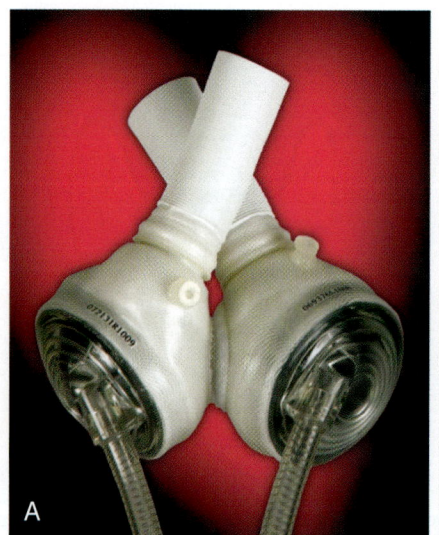 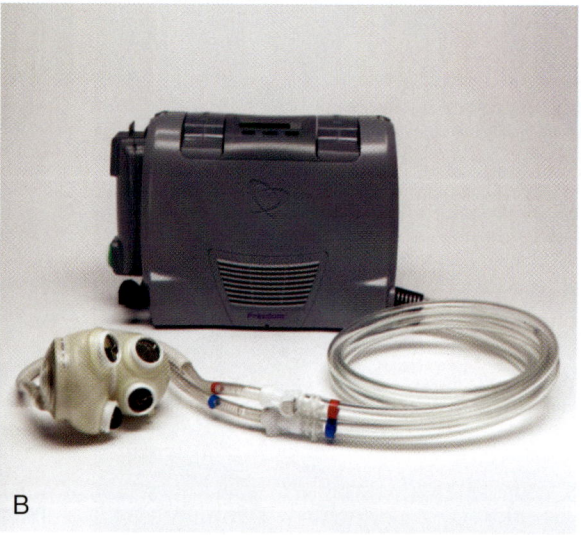

FIGURE 1-5 The SynCardia Temporary Total Artificial Heart **(A)** shown with the wearable driver system **(B)**. *(Courtesy of Syncardia. Systems, Inc., Tucson, AZ.)*

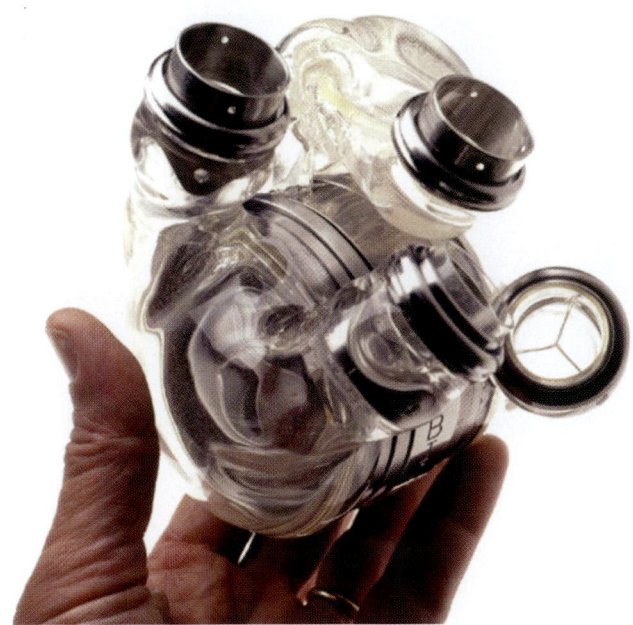

FIGURE 1-6 The AbioCor TAH is a completely implantable device and relies on a transcutaneous energy transmission system. *(Courtesy of Discovery Communications, LLC.)*

REVOLUTION OF ROTARY VENTRICULAR ASSIST DEVICES

A revolution in the development of VADs began in 1988 when the first rotary pump was used to support the circulation in patients who were experiencing cardiogenic shock.[32] The device, known as the Hemopump (Fig. 1-7), was a catheter-mounted VAD for short-term support designed and developed by Wampler. The device used a drive shaft to power turbine blades at 17,500 to 44,000 revolutions per minute to supply 2 to 4 L/min of blood. The Hemopump revealed that red

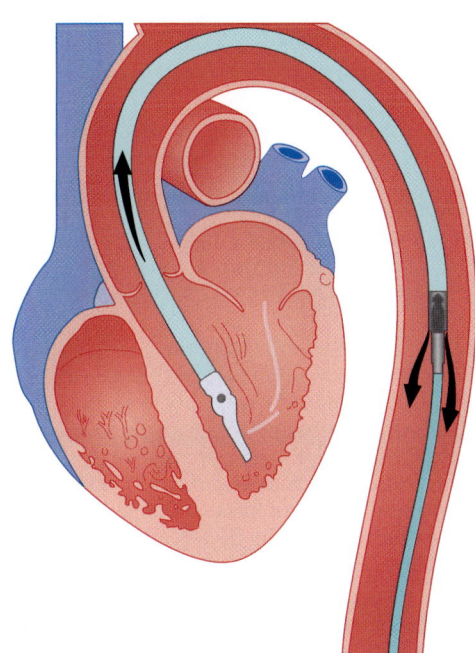

FIGURE 1-7 The Hemopump was a catheter-mounted VAD that used a drive shaft to power turbine blades. The device was the first used that revealed rotary devices could successfully pump blood despite the high speed of the blades. *(Courtesy of Medtronic, Inc., Grand Rapids, MI.)*

blood cells would have minimal damage when exposed to a high shear environment if the residence time was carefully controlled.

In contrast to electromechanical and pneumatic VADs, which pumped blood using positive-displacement methods that provided a pulse mimicking the action of the natural heart, the Hemopump pumped blood continuously.[32,33] These devices soon became known synonymously as "rotary" or "continuous flow" VADs. With the revelation that the device did not cause hemolysis or damage to other formed blood elements despite the high revolutions per minute at which it operated and because rotary pumps could be made quite small and provide ample cardiac support, MCS research focus shifted in the late 1980s to the development of continuous flow VADs. Early work on this generation of devices was supported by various means including NHLBI-funded Small Business Innovation Research (SBIR) grants.

Based on the progress with the pulsatile devices and limited but promising results with alternative devices (including rotary VADs), the NHLBI implemented the Innovative Ventricular Assist System (IVAS) program in 1996. The IVAS program led to research and development activities on numerous rotary devices, which eventually became the HeartMate II, Jarvik 2000, and CorAide VADs.

The first implants of a continuous flow VAD intended for long-term support were performed using a DeBakey VAD. This device, which is now known as the HeartAssist 5, was developed outside of the IVAS program through a long-standing association between MicroMed, Inc., and the National Aeronautics and Space Administration (NASA). DeBakey VADs were implanted in two patients who were experiencing end-stage HF in 1998 in Vienna, Austria.[34] The first implants of the Jarvik 2000 VAD (Fig. 1-8) and the HeartMate II VAD (Fig. 1-9) occurred in 2000. Since then, first-in-human implants and clinical trials have begun on other continuous flow VADs, such as the Circulite Synergy Pocket micropump (Fig. 1-10), which is placed using a minimally invasive procedure; the HeartWare HVAD (Fig. 1-11); the WorldHeart Levacor VAD (Fig. 1-12); and the Terumo DuraHeart VAD (Fig. 1-13).[35-38] Table 1-1 includes the date of the first implant of each of these devices. A milestone involving the Jarvik 2000 is the 2714 days of circulatory support that the VAD provided to the first recipient, Peter Houghton, who died of acute renal failure in December 2007. To date, this is the record for support on a single VAD.

The Thoratec HeartMate II VAD is the first continuous flow VAD to receive FDA approval for treating adult HF. The device received approval for BTT in 2009 and for destination

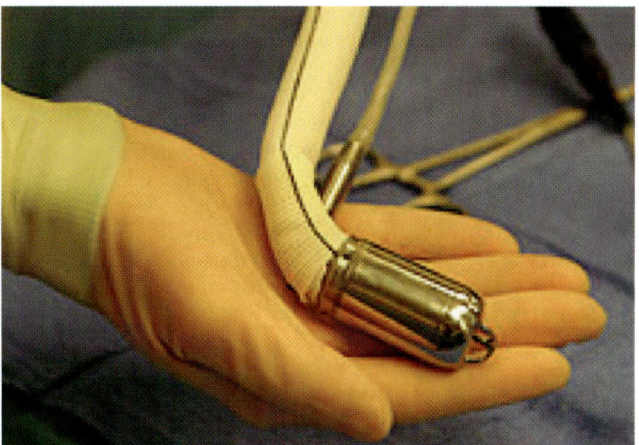

FIGURE 1-8 The Jarvik 2000 Flowmaker is placed in the left ventricle so that no inlet cannula is needed. The longest living patient on a single device was supported with the Jarvik 2000 Flowmaker for more than 7 years. *(Courtesy of University of Maryland Medical System, Baltimore, MD.)*

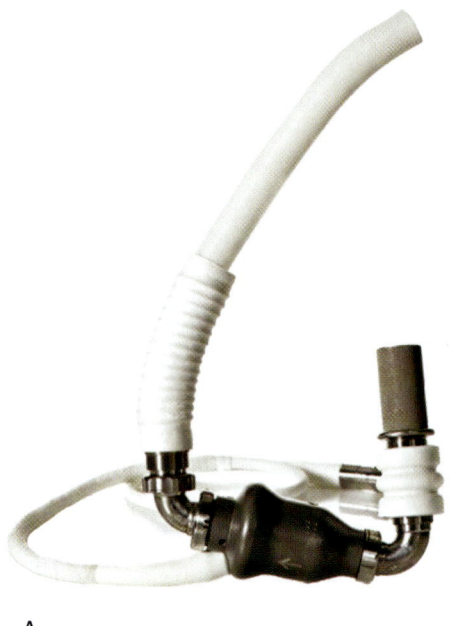

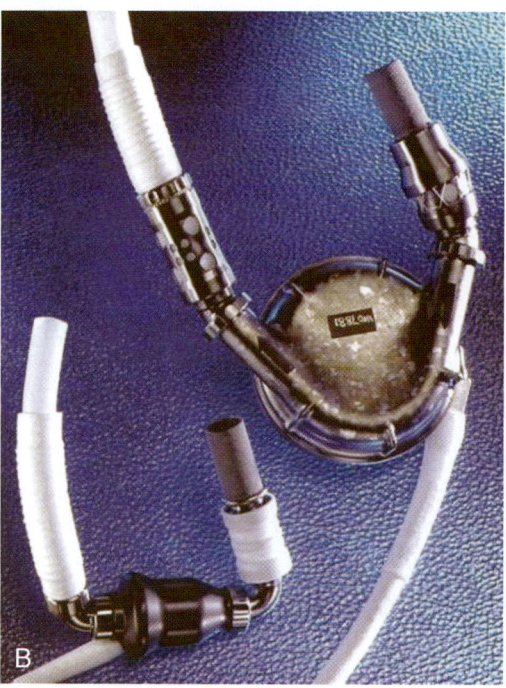

A

B

FIGURE 1-9 The HeartMate II (**A** and **B,** lower left) compared with the Heartmate XVE (**B**). The HeartMate II was the first rotary VAD to receive U.S. Food and Drug Administration (FDA) approval for bridge to transplant and destination therapy. *(Courtesy of Thoratec, Inc., Pleasanton, CA.)*

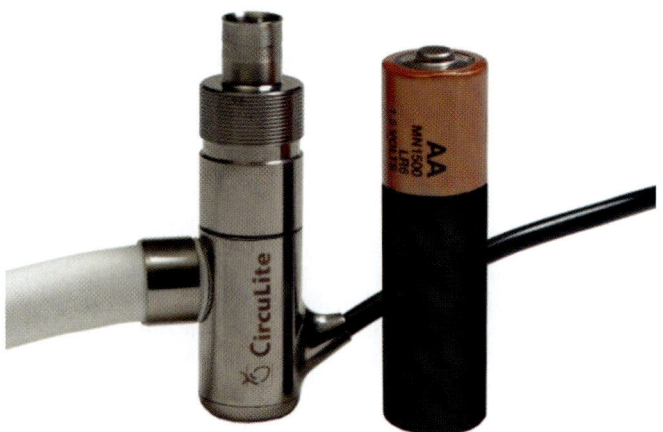

FIGURE 1-10 The Circulite Synergy Pocket Micro-Pump. The device is designed to be implanted without cardiopulmonary bypass or a sternotomy. Blood is drawn from the left atrium through the inflow cannula and pumped back through the outflow graft to the subclavian artery. *(Courtesy of Circulite, Inc., Saddle Brook, NJ.)*

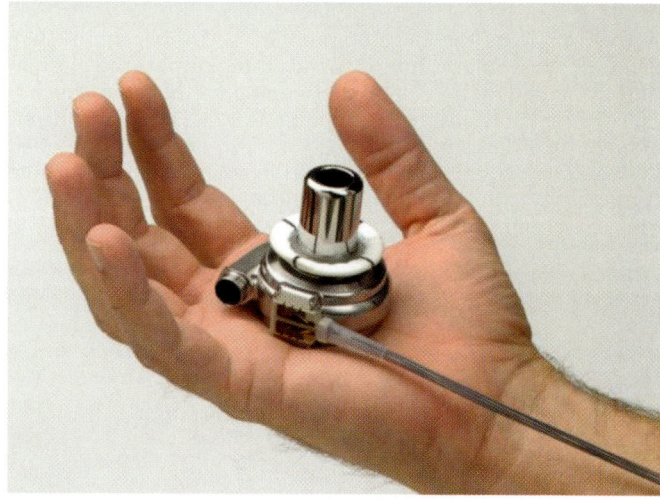

FIGURE 1-11 The HeartWare HVAD is a centrifugal pump that uses hydrodynamic bearings. Its small size and design allow it to be implanted above the diaphragm in all patients. *(Courtesy HeartWare, Inc., Framingham, MA.)*

therapy in 2010 and has received rapid adoption with more than 4000 implants reported to date. The outcomes and success with the new continuous flow VADs have led to almost total cessation of use of the pulsatile design devices.[39] With the availability of this continuous flow VAD in the United States, new options became available for those smaller patients, especially women, in whom the implantable positive displacement VADs, such as the HeartMate XVE, would not fit well or at all. Also, because its durability well exceeded that of the 2-year design life of the HeartMate XVE, the HeartMate II provides reliability better suited for use in patients receiving destination therapy.

With the advent and clinical performance of continuous flow VADs, equipoise has developed within the HF community that the outcomes may now equal if not exceed that for medical therapy alone. These devices have been considered to be a potentially viable therapy in patients with moderately advanced, rather than late-stage, HF. To this end, the

NHLBI released an RFP for the Randomized Evaluation of VAD InterVEntion before Inotropic Therapy (REVIVE-IT) pilot trial in July 2009.[42] The objective of the trial is to explore the potential benefit of MCS therapy using VADs in functionally impaired patients with advanced HF who have not yet developed serious consequences from their disease and have yet to reach the stage of being managed with use of intravenous inotropic agents. The trial is expected to begin in the first quarter of 2012.

LOOKING TOWARD THE FUTURE

It is exciting to reflect on the creation and growth of clinical, laboratory, and engineering capacity in the MCS field. As we look to the future, it is important to remember Frank Hastings' admonition of the importance of sustaining a "biomedical capacity" in the field. Although great progress has been made in the engineering and physiology of MCS over the past 5 decades,

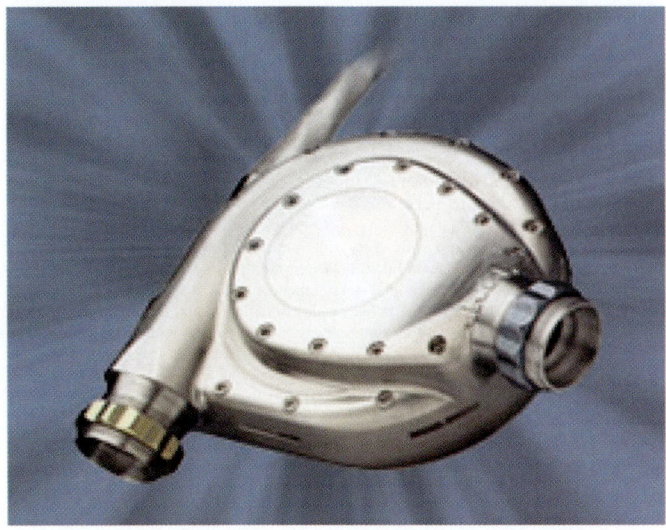

FIGURE 1-12 The WorldHeart Levacor VAD uses a magnetically levitated impeller to improve durability. *(Courtesy of WorldHeart, Inc., Salt Lake City, UT.)*

DuraHeart Pump

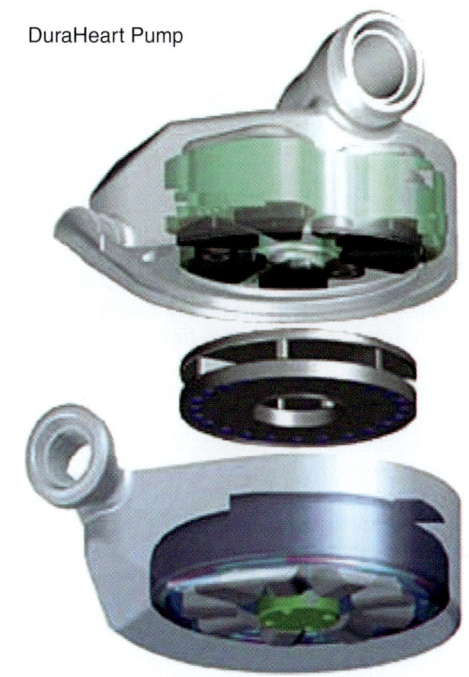

FIGURE 1-13 The Terumo Heart DuraHeart is a centrifugal pump that uses a magnetically levitated impeller. *(Courtesy of Terumo Corporation, Tokyo.)*

there is considerable room for improvement. For patients and their loved ones, it is crucial to optimize the implants, the procedures, the peripherals (e.g., external controllers and batteries), the medical management, and the costs. A new cadre of fully informed and committed clinicians, engineers, and scientists is needed to fulfill the potential of the field.

Progress is likely for the prevalent population of patients with HF in need of MCS, and one of the tools that will facilitate that progress is the NHLBI-funded Interagency Registry for Mechanically Assisted Circulatory Support (INTERMACS).[40] This national registry was launched in 2006 through a joint effort of the NHLBI, the CMS, the FDA, clinicians, scientists, and industry representatives. It has been organized, run, and maintained by the University of Alabama at Birmingham in conjunction with the United Network for Organ Sharing (UNOS) since initially launched and is used specifically to collect data on patients who receive MCS devices for long-term treatment of advanced HF. Analysis and outcomes from the INTERMACS data are expected to improve patient selection and clinical management and to help identify opportunities for device improvements and enhancements. Scientific investigation and long-term follow-up of these patients will provide new insights and understanding HF's basic mechanisms. By using these tools, our hope is also to identify patients who would respond to MCS and adjunctive therapies with recovery of native cardiac function that would allow removal of the MCS device.[42] This would provide the very best quality of life for these patients.[43]

The current therapy would benefit if adverse events such as stroke, bleeding, and infections were addressed sufficiently; if the implantation procedures were less invasive; and the interfaces between the patients and the devices were more conducive to leading normal lives. Some current research and development activities may help achieve these goals. One example is the NHLBI-sponsored Pumps for Kids, Infants, and Neonates (PumpKIN) program, which supports four programs that have the ultimate goals of obtaining FDA approval for MCS devices for very small children with severe HF.[44,45] VADs being developed in this program are small enough that they could potentially be delivered via minimally invasive procedures in adults to augment cardiac output. Two of the devices developed through the program are the Infant Jarvik 2000 VAD and the PediaFlow VAD shown in Figure 1-14. The Infant Jarvik device is the size of a "double A" battery and contains a novel hydrodynamic bearing design to reduce the potential for thrombosis. Some of the newer generations of VADs, such as the WorldHeart Levacor VAD, the Berlin Heart INCOR LVAD, and the Terumo DuraHeart, use magnetically levitated bearings; further development and use of this technology are expected given its potential to help improve biocompatibility and energy efficiency in MCS devices.

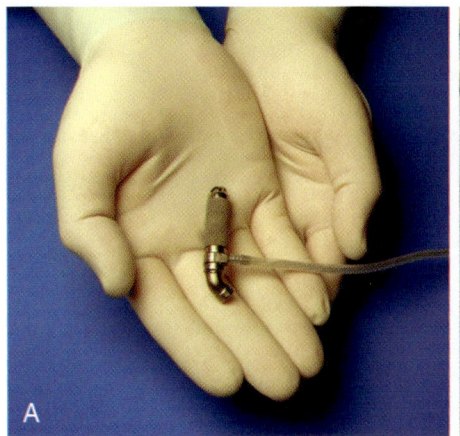
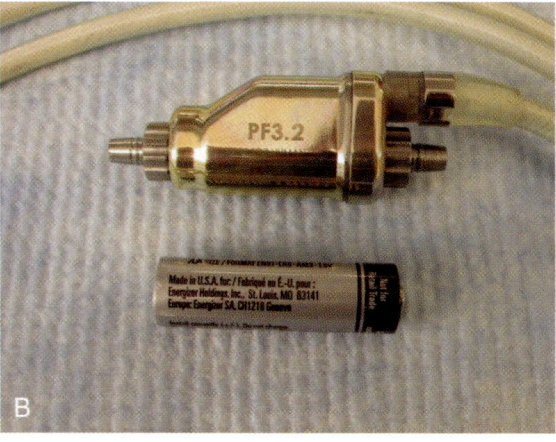

FIGURE 1-14 The Infant Jarvik 2000 VAD **(A)** and the PediaFlow VAD **(B)** are being developed for neonates, infants, and small children but may be adapted for adults in the future. *(Courtesy of Jarvik Heart Inc., New York.)*

Ongoing challenges for MCS devices include the power sources and power delivery to the implanted devices. Although battery sizes for the devices have decreased and battery life has improved over the years, the batteries that are used today are still burdensome for the patient because of their weight and need for frequent recharging and change out. Batteries are an area of research that needs focus to improve the quality of life for patients with MCS devices. The delivery of the power to the device is a related challenge. Although the LionHeart VAD and the AbioCor TAH showed years ago that power can be delivered successfully across the skin via TETS, all other electrically powered devices have relied on percutaneous lines for energy delivery and venting. Percutaneous lines provide pathways for infection, increase the burden on the patients and their caregivers to keep the percutaneous access sites clean, and limit patient mobility and activities. Greater efforts by the MCS industry are needed to adapt the already proven TETS technology to these existing MCS systems to address these issues. In addition to this straightforward goal, alternative energy sources should be investigated and developed potentially to replace the conventional cumbersome battery systems used today.

One of the other ongoing challenges related to MCS devices is the development of devices to treat right HF. Most of the VADs available today were developed to support the failing left ventricle. The only viable independent options today for providing support for the right ventricle are the Thoratec PVAD and extracorporeal MCS devices. Although some research is being done to develop right ventricular assist devices, more concerted efforts are needed to provide viable options in the future to treat right HF using MCS devices.[41]

The promise of implantable, internally activated TAH systems remains unfulfilled. Pneumatically powered TAH systems have outstanding clinical results. The limited results for completing implanted systems suggest the potential for similar outcomes. Novel promising TAH research continues. Groups at the Texas Heart Institute and the Cleveland Clinic are investigating the use of dual continuous flow devices to replace the function of the left and right ventricles. Such TAH devices may offer similar advantages as the continuous flow VADs have over the pulsatile flow VADs, such as greater reliability and smaller size.

Because patients with MCS devices continue to experience adverse events, more research is needed to understand their underlying causes in relation to the device itself. Although improvements in the devices will continue and will help to improve further the morbidity and mortality associated with the devices, understanding the physiology and biology of the complications and development of adjunctive therapies to treat or prevent them may prove to be the needed solution.

We would be remiss not to recognize the tireless efforts, devotion, and collegiality of the workers in the MCS field. Without their openness and intellectual generosity to share information—both the progress and the problems—MCS would still be in the speculation stage. HF remains a nemesis, but MCS has made huge inroads toward treating it effectively, and the future holds great potential for more progress.

REFERENCES

1. Nose Y. The birth of the artificial heart programs in the world: a special tribute to Tetsuo Akutsu and Valery Shumakov. *Artif Organs*. 2008;32:667–683.
2. Carrel A, Lindbergh CA. The culture of whole organs. *Science*. 1935;81:621–623.
3. Stoney WS. Evolution of cardiopulmonary bypass. *Circulation*. 2009;119:2844–2853.
4. Frazier OH, Kirklin JK. *Mechanical Circulatory Support*. Philadelphia: Elsevier; 2006.
5. DeBakey ME. Development of mechanical heart devices. *Ann Thorac Surg*. 2005; 79:S2228–S2231.
6. U.S. Institute of Medicine Committee to Evaluate the Artificial Heart Program of the National Heart, Lung and Blood Institute, Hogness JR, VanAntwerp M, National Heart Lung and Blood Institute. *The Artificial Heart: Prototypes, Policies, and Patients*. Washington, D.C.: National Academy Press; 1991.
7. Ho K, Anderson K, Kannel W, et al. Survival after the onset of congestive heart failure in Framingham Heart Study subjects. *Circulation*. 1993;88:107–115.
8. Writing Group Members, Lloyd-Jones D, Adams RJ, et al. Heart disease and stroke statistics—2010 update: a report from the American Heart Association. *Circulation*. 2010;121:e46–e215.
9. Vancitters RL, Bauer CB, Christopherson LK, et al. Artificial-heart and assist devices—directions, needs, costs, societal and ethical issues. *Artif Organs*. 1985;9:375–415.
10. Altieri FD, Powell RS, Hanks JB. *The Artificial Heart Program: 1964–1975*. Washington, D.C.: National Heart and Lung Institute; 1975.
11. Schoen FJ, Palmer DC, Bernhard WF, et al. Clinical temporary ventricular assist: pathologic findings and their implications in a multi-institutional study of 41 patients. *J Thorac Cardiovasc Surg*. 1986;92:1071–1081.
12. Pennington DG, Bernhard WF, Golding LR, et al. Long-term follow-up of postcardiotomy patients with profound cardiogenic shock treated with ventricular assist devices. *Circulation*. 1985;72:II216–II226.
13. Pierce WS, Brighton JA, O'Bannon W, et al. Complete left ventricular bypass with a paracorporeal pump: design and evaluation. *Ann Surg*. 1974;180:418–426.
14. National Heart, Lung and Blood Institute Writers Group. *Guidelines for Blood Materials Interactions*. Bethesda, MD: National Heart, Lung and Blood Institute; 1985.
15. Pennington DG, Griffith BP, Swartz MT, et al. Evaluation of an implantable ventricular assist system for humans with chronic refractory heart failure: patient selection. LVAS Study Group. Left Ventricular Assist System. *ASAIO J*. 1995;41:23–26.
16. Pennington DG, Griffith BP, McKinlay SM, et al. Evaluation of an implantable ventricular assist system for humans with chronic refractory heart failure: study overview. LVAS Study Group. Left Ventricular Assist System. *ASAIO J*. 1995;41:11–15.
17. Swartz MT, Borovetz HS, Miller PJ, et al. Evaluation of an implantable ventricular assist system for humans with chronic refractory heart failure: technical considerations. LVAS Study Group. Left Ventricular Assist System. *ASAIO J*. 1995;41:27–31.
18. El-Banayosy A, Arusoglu L, Kizner L, et al. Preliminary experience with the LionHeart left ventricular assist device in patients with end-stage heart failure. *Ann Thorac Surg*. 2003;75:1469–1475.
19. Rose EA, Moskowitz AJ, Packer M, et al. The REMATCH trial: rationale, design, and end points. Randomized Evaluation of Mechanical Assistance for the Treatment of Congestive Heart Failure. *Ann Thorac Surg*. 1999;67:723–730.
20. Rose EA, Gelijns AC, Moskowitz AJ, et al. Long-term use of a left ventricular assist device for end-stage heart failure. *N Engl J Med*. 2001;345:1435–1443.
21. Cooley DA, Liotta D, Hallman GL, et al. Orthotopic cardiac prosthesis for two-staged cardiac replacement. *Am J Cardiol*. 1969;24:723–730.
22. DeBakey ME. The odyssey of the artificial heart. *Artif Organs*. 2000;24:405–411.
23. Cooley DA, Akutsu T, Norman JC, et al. Total artificial heart in two-staged cardiac transplantation. *Cardiovasc Dis*. 1981;8:305–319.
24. DeVries WC, Anderson JL, Joyce LD, et al. Clinical use of the total artificial heart. *N Engl J Med*. 1984;310:273–278.
25. Copeland JG, Smith R, Icenogle T, et al. Orthotopic total artificial heart bridge to transplantation: preliminary results. *J Heart Transplant*. 1989;8:124–137.
26. Magovern JA, Pennock JL, Campbell DB, et al. Bridge to heart transplantation: the Penn State experience. *J Heart Transplant*. 1986;5:196–202.
27. Joyce LD, Johnson KE, Toninato CJ, et al. Results of the first 100 patients who received Symbion Total Artificial Hearts as a bridge to cardiac transplantation. *Circulation*. 1989;80:III192–III201.
28. Gray JNA, Selzman CH. Current status of the total artificial heart. *Am Heart J*. 2006;152:4–10.
29. AbioCor FAQs. 2010. Available at http://www.abiomed.com/products/faqs.cfm. Accessed June 1, 2010.
30. Frazier OH, Dowling RD, Gray Jr LA, et al. The total artificial heart: where we stand. *Cardiology*. 2004;101:117–121.
31. Gemmato CJ, Forrester MD, Myers TJ, et al. Thirty-five years of mechanical circulatory support at the Texas Heart Institute: an updated overview. *Tex Heart Inst J*. 2005;32:168–177.
32. Frazier OH, Wampler RK, Duncan JM, et al. First human use of the Hemopump, a catheter-mounted ventricular assist device. *Ann Thorac Surg*. 1990;49:299–304.
33. Cooper GJ, Loisance DY, Miyama M, et al. Direct mechanical assistance of the right ventricle with the Hemopump in a porcine model. *Ann Thorac Surg*. 1995;59:443–447.
34. Wieselthaler GM, Schima H, Hiesmayr M, et al. First clinical experience with the DeBakey VAD continuous-axial-flow pump for bridge to transplantation. *Circulation*. 2000;101:356–359.
35. Griffith K, Jenkins E, Pagani FD. First American experience with the Terumo DuraHeart left ventricular assist system. *Perfusion*. 2009;24:83–89.
36. Meyns B, Ector J, Rega F, et al. First human use of partial left ventricular heart support with the Circulite synergy micro-pump as a bridge to cardiac transplantation. *Eur Heart J*. 2008;29:2582.
37. Pitsis AA, Visouli AN, Vassilikos V, et al. First human implantation of a new rotary blood pump: design of the clinical feasibility study. *Hellenic J Cardiol*. 2006;47:368–376.
38. Strueber M, Meyer AL, Malehsa D, et al. Successful use of the HeartWare HVAD rotary blood pump for biventricular support. *J Thorac Cardiovasc Surg*. 2010;140:936–937.
39. Kirklin JK, Naftel DC, Kormos RL, et al. Second INTERMACS annual report: more than 1,000 primary left ventricular assist device implants. *J Heart Lung Transplant*. 2010;29:1–10.
40. Kirklin JK, Naftel DC, Stevenson LW, et al. INTERMACS database for durable devices for circulatory support: first annual report. *J Heart Lung Transplant*. 2008;27:1065–1072.
41. Fukamachi K, Saeed D, Massiello AL, et al. Development of DexAide right ventricular assist device: update II. *ASAIO J*. 2008;54:589–593.
42. National Heart, Lung, and Blood Institute: Request for Proposals for the Randomized Evaluation of VAD InterVEntion before Inotropic Therapy Pilot Trial Bethesda, MD, National Heart, Lung, and Blood Institute, 2009, RFP NHLBI-HV-10-14.
43. Watson JT. Innovative ventricular assist systems. *ASAIO Journal*. 1994; 40:M902.
44. National Heart, Lung, and Blood Institute: Request for Proposals for the Pumps for Kids, Infants, and Neonates (PumpKIN) Pre-Clinical Program. Bethesda, MD, National Heart, Lung, and Blood Institute, 2008, RFP NHLBI-HV-09-14(2).
45. National Heart, Lung, and Blood Institute: Request for Proposals for the Pumps for Kids, Infants, and Neonates (PumpKIN) Clinical Trial. Bethesda, MD, National Heart, Lung, and Blood Institute, 2010, RFP NHLBI-HV-12-03.

CHAPTER 2

Potential Population for Long-Term Use of Left Ventricular Assist Devices

Randall C. Starling and Eiran Z. Gorodeski

INTRODUCTION

Heart transplantation, although highly successful for most recipients,[1] is "epidemiologically trivial"[2] with currently only approximately 2200 transplants done yearly in the United States and 3300 done worldwide.[1] The donor supply has not changed in the past decade (Fig. 2-1), and although new preservation techniques offer hope of increasing the recovery of some marginal heart donors, the overall impact is likely to be negligible. Life expectancy after heart transplantation is estimated at 50% at 10 years.[1] Further improvement in survival after transplantation is unlikely to be achieved. New adjunctive therapies, such as stem cell and gene therapies, offer hope of improving native ventricular function and avoidance of transplant, but progress is slow.

The use of left ventricular assist devices (LVADs) was limited until more recent years, when it increased significantly with the introduction of the new design of continuous flow devices. These devices are much smaller and have been shown to provide significantly superior survival, functional capacity, and quality of life in patients implanted for both bridge to transplantation and long-term or destination therapy indications.[3-6] Patients implanted to date have largely been in cardiogenic shock or deteriorating on intravenous therapy with inotropes (see Chapter 24). As use of continuous flow LVADs continues to increase in light of positive results from clinical trials, improved real-world outcomes showing survival outcomes comparable to transplantation continue suggesting equipoise between these therapies (Fig. 2-2).[6] This possibility has raised the question of how many patients with advanced systolic heart failure (HF) might be candidates for LVAD therapy now and in the future. This chapter reviews data available to address this important question and provides some predictions and estimates for the next several decades.

CURRENT ESTIMATES OF LEFT VENTRICULAR ASSIST DEVICE POPULATION

Specific estimates of prevalence of advanced symptomatic HF, in particular, among patients who may be LVAD candidates, are controversial and based on limited data. The U.S. Bureau of the Census estimates the current U.S. population to be 310 million,[7] with 75%[8] being 20 years old or older—yielding approximately 240 million adults. The most recent American Heart Association (AHA) statistics estimate the prevalence of HF at 2.6%,[9] yielding an approximate absolute prevalence of adult HF of 6.24 million in the United States in 2010. This estimate does not take into account the pediatric population. Additional worldwide estimates are shown in Table 2-1.

Ammar and colleagues[10] published the only community-based study to date evaluating the prevalence of HF stages. In a randomly selected sample from Olmsted County, Minnesota, approximately two-thirds of the population were classified as having risk factors for HF (stage A), asymptomatic HF (stage B), or symptomatic HF (stages C and D). Of people who had HF, approximately 17% were classified as having HF symptoms (stage C), and approximately 0.4% were classified as having severe HF (stage D). Among people with stage C HF, 3.2% were further classified as "advanced" stage C. However, these estimates are from a very homogeneous population of largely whites in a rural setting and are likely quite different from large urban centers. Such centers have a high prevalence of African Americans and individuals with hypertension and tend to see more patients with stage D HF (≥5%). Several studies from Europe and Japan suggest a prevalence of advanced HF ranging from 5% to 6%.[11,12] Making valid projections from such varying estimates of prevalence (up to a 10-fold difference) is difficult.

Our estimates of current theoretical adult candidates for LVAD therapy are presented in Figure 2-3. As mentioned previously we estimate that the current population of adult-only patients with HF in the United States is 6.24 million. Based on various population studies, it is believed that half of patients with HF have preserved systolic function,[13,14] leaving 3.12 million with systolic HF. Based on estimates of advanced HF prevalence from Olmsted County (as described earlier) and prevalence of New York Heart Association (NYHA) class IV patients from international population studies,[11,12] we estimate that current prevalence of advanced-stage C or NYHA class IIIb patients ranges from

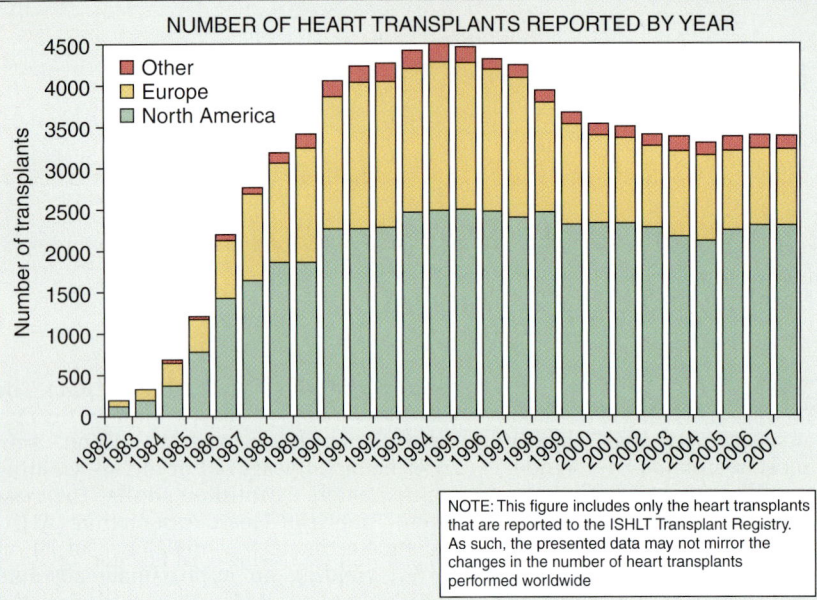

FIGURE 2-1 Number of heart transplants, stratified by year. ISHLT, International Society for Heart and Lung Transplantation. *(From Taylor DO, Stehlik J, Edwards LB, et al. Registry of the International Society for Heart and Lung Transplantation: Twenty-sixth Official Adult Heart Transplant Report—2009.* J Heart Lung Transplant. *2009;28:1007-1022.)*

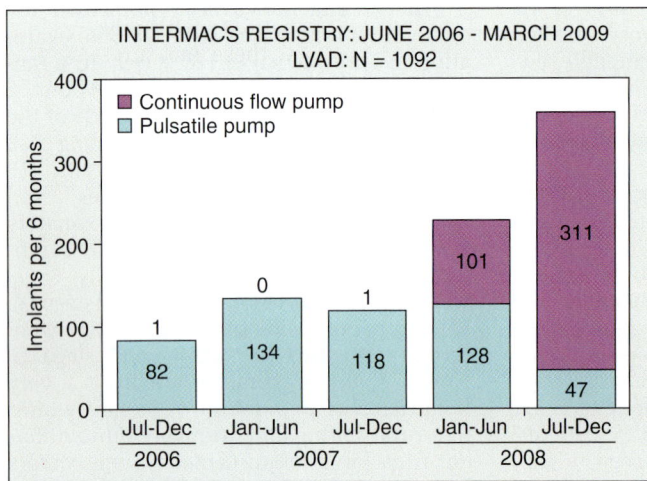

FIGURE 2-2 Use of approved left ventricular assist devices (LVADs) in the United States, 2006-2009. INTERMACS, Interagency Registry for Mechanically Assisted Circulatory Support. *(From Starling RC. Improved quantity and quality of life: a winning combination to treat advanced heart failure.* J Am Coll Cardiol. *2010;55:1835-1836.)*

TABLE 2-1	Estimated Worldwide Prevalence of Advanced Heart Failure (HF)			
	Estimated Total Population	Estimated HF Prevalence	Estimated ACCF/AHA Stage C Prevalence*	Estimated ACCF/AHA Stage D Prevalence*
Europe	>900,000,000[35]	15,000,000[34]	2,550,000	60,000
Australia	20,230,000[36]	263,000[35]	44,710	1,050
Soweto, South Africa	1,100,000[37]	1960[36]	330	10

ACCF/AHA, American College of Cardiology Foundation/American Heart Association.
*Extrapolated from estimates published by Ammar et al.[10]

93,600 to 124,800 and that current prevalence of stage D or NYHA class IV patients ranges from 15,600 to 156,000. This process yields a theoretical current adult U.S. population of 109,200 to 280,800 who may be candidates for LVAD therapy.

Our estimates are liberal because they do not account for various medical and psychosocial comorbidities that may make patients ineligible for LVAD. Actual absolute numbers are lower. Since LVAD therapy was approved in the United States in 2002, the adoption of this therapy has been far below projections until the more recent rapid growth. The following sections address how issues related to definitions of HF severity, age, sex, race, fluctuating condition, less ill patients, and accessibility to LVAD centers affect population estimates.

DEFINITIONS OF HEART FAILURE SEVERITY AND THEIR IMPACT ON POPULATION ESTIMATES

Despite advances in pharmacologic and nonpharmacologic therapies, HF commonly progresses to a state refractory to current treatments.[4,9,15] Patients with highly symptomatic refractory HF are symptomatic with dyspnea at rest or very limited activity and do not improve or experience rapid recurrence of symptoms with current guideline-directed comprehensive HF therapies. These patients characteristically have symptoms at rest or on minimal exertion, including profound fatigue; cannot perform most activities of daily living; frequently have evidence of cardiac cachexia; and typically require repeated or prolonged hospitalizations for HF management.[15] These patients may become dependent on inotropes or intolerant of usual neurohormonal antagonists (hypotension and renal deterioration), portending an ominous prognosis. Identification and careful evaluation of these patients is important because they may be candidates for advanced treatment strategies including LVAD therapy.

The current criteria used by Centers for Medicare and Medicaid Services (CMS) for candidates for LVAD destination therapy depend heavily on a mixture of subjective and

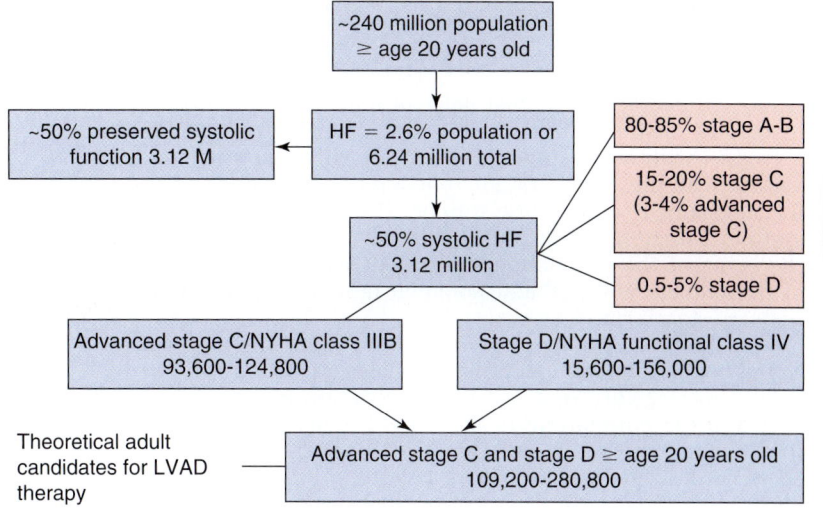

FIGURE 2-3 Current estimates of adult patients with advanced heart failure (HF) in the United States, with projected left ventricular assist device (LVAD) candidates. U.S. population estimate is derived from U.S. Census data.[7,8] Estimate of HF prevalence is derived from latest American Heart Association (AHA) statistics.[9] Estimates of HF with reduced ejection fraction and preserved ejection fraction based on population studies.[13,14] Estimates of prevalence of HF stages and New York Heart Association (NYHA) class derived from Ammar et al,[10] Goda et al,[12] and Ceia et al.[11]

objective definitions of functional capacity, as follows (http://www.cms.gov/mcd/):

VADs are reimbursed for patients who have chronic end-stage heart failure (New York Heart Association class IV end-stage left ventricular failure for at least 90 days with a life expectancy of less than 2 years), are not candidates for heart transplantation, and meet all of the following conditions:

a. The patient's class IV heart failure symptoms have failed to respond to optimal medical management, including dietary salt restriction, diuretics, digitalis, beta-blockers, and ACE inhibitors (if tolerated) for at least 60 of the last 90 days;
b. The patient has a left ventricular ejection fraction (LVEF) <25%;
c. The patient has demonstrated functional limitation with a peak oxygen consumption of <12 ml/kg/min; or the patient has a continued need for intravenous inotropic therapy owing to

symptomatic hypotension, decreasing renal function, or worsening pulmonary congestion; and
d. The patient has the appropriate body size (>1.5 m²) to support the VAD implantation.

Reliance on subjective measures of functional capacity, including NYHA class and American College of Cardiology Foundation (ACCF)/AHA stage, does not adequately capture nuanced differences among patients with advanced HF.[16] Because of their subjectivity, these measures have not been regularly incorporated into population studies of patients with HF, leading to uncertainty in population estimates. For this purpose, we encourage future use of Interagency Registry for Mechanically Assisted Circulatory Support (INTERMACS) profiles in population studies (Table 2-2).

TABLE 2-2	Functional Capacity Schemes for Advanced Heart Failure					
	NYHA Functional Class[38]	Specific Activity Scale Classification[39]	INTERMACS Levels	Time Course (Derived from RALES Study[40])	ACCF/AHA Stage	Continuous Flow LVAD Approval Status in United States
NYHA functional class IIIa	Patients with cardiac disease resulting in marked limitation of physical activity. Patients are comfortable at rest. Less than ordinary physical activity causes fatigue, palpitations, dyspnea, or angina pain. NYHA IIIb if symptoms at rest in past 6 mo	Patient can perform to completion any activity requiring ≥2 metabolic equivalents but cannot or does not perform to completion any activities requiring ≥5 metabolic equivalents	Level 7	Currently NYHA functional class III	Stage C	No current approval
NYHA functional class IIIb			Level 6	Currently NYHA functional class III, but experienced NYHA class IV symptoms in last 6 mo	Stage C	No current approval
NYHA functional class IV	Patients with cardiac disease resulting in inability to carry on any physical activity without discomfort. Symptoms of heart failure or of angina syndrome may be present even at rest. If any physical activity is undertaken, discomfort increases	Patient cannot or does not perform to completion activities requiring ≥2 metabolic equivalents	Levels 1-5		Stage C-D	Currently approved

ACCF/AHA, American College of Cardiology Foundation/American Heart Association; INTERMACS, Interagency Registry for Mechanically Assisted Circulatory Support; LVAD, left ventricular assist device; NYHA, New York Heart Association.

IMPACT OF AGE ON POPULATION ESTIMATES

Of all the demographics that have an impact on the prevalence and incidence of HF, age is the leading variable. HF increases with advancing age and likely shifts more to the variant with preserved systolic function (i.e., not candidates for mechanical circulatory support [MCS]) than reduced systolic function. Epidemiologic trends predict that with the aging of the population the prevalence and incidence of individuals with HF and potential need for LVADs will increase significantly.

The number of older Americans (≥65 years old) is projected to double from current estimates of 40 million to 80 million by 2030 (Fig. 2-4).[16] The age structure (distribution of age in the population) of the United States is projected to change most significantly among Americans older than 50 years old (Fig. 2-5). In the past century, life expectancy has increased for both American men and women 65 years old and older and 85 years old and older (Fig. 2-6). Similar trends have been seen in other industrialized countries (Fig. 2-7).

Figure 2-8 shows the dramatic increase in the prevalence of HF beginning in the fifth decade of life and affecting between 5% (women) and 9% (men) of the U.S. population after age 60. The burden of HF is especially large among older individuals. According to the most recent U.S. and European statistics, annual incidence per 1000 population of new HF events increases by decade of age regardless of sex and race (Figs. 2-9 and 2-10).[9,17] No current statistics are available on the proportion of stages C and D HF in older individuals with HF. Because the burden of HF is heaviest in elderly adults, we expect that future LVAD candidates will be disproportionately older adults.

At the present time, age 65 years or older is considered a relative contraindication in patient selection for cardiac transplantation at many U.S. centers. Patients older than 65 years warrant more extensive evaluation for comorbidities, and more conservative criteria are needed to identify patients who would have a long-term benefit from LVAD therapy. Advancing age adds risk to all conventional cardiac surgical procedures.

The average age in more recent destination therapy LVAD clinical trials for patients considered ineligible for transplant, presumably based largely on age, was 63 years. However, a significant percentage of patients were older than 65 years, and 20% were older than 70 years.[18,19] This age distribution stems from the prior practice of restricting ventricular assist device (VAD) use for patients who are candidates for heart transplantation[18] and retrospective associations between older age and worse outcomes.[20,21] More recent destination therapy VAD clinical trials enrolled patients with mean ages ranging from 50 years[3] to 62 years,[4] limiting experience and insight into VAD therapy in older individuals. Despite this limitation, clinicians have used VADs for well-selected older individuals.[22] The upper range of age in INTERMACS is 79.9 years.[23] Investigators assessing risk-adjusted associations between age and outcome found that in the absence of high-risk comorbid factors, older age alone was not a significant risk factor for mortality.[24]

IMPACT OF SEX ON POPULATION ESTIMATES

There are marked differences in the prevalence, incidence, and presentation of HF in women compared with men.[9,25] According to the latest AHA published statistics, prevalence of HF in the United States is greater in men (3.1%) than women (2.1%) (Table 2-3; see Fig. 2-8).[9] Incidence of HF is greater in men in the United States (see Fig. 2-9) and internationally (see Fig. 2-10). Morbidity associated with HF seems to be worse in women than in men with "a lower quality of life than men, more functional capacity impairment, more HF hospital stays, and depression" (Fig. 2-11).[25] Nonetheless, women with HF seem to have better survival than men, although the explanation of this difference is unknown.[25]

Estimation of prevalence of advanced HF among women, in particular, prevalence of which women may be LVAD candidates, is difficult. There is now a greater recognition that women with HF tend to have preserved systolic function (Fig. 2-12),[25,26] suggesting that on a population level fewer women would be LVAD candidates.

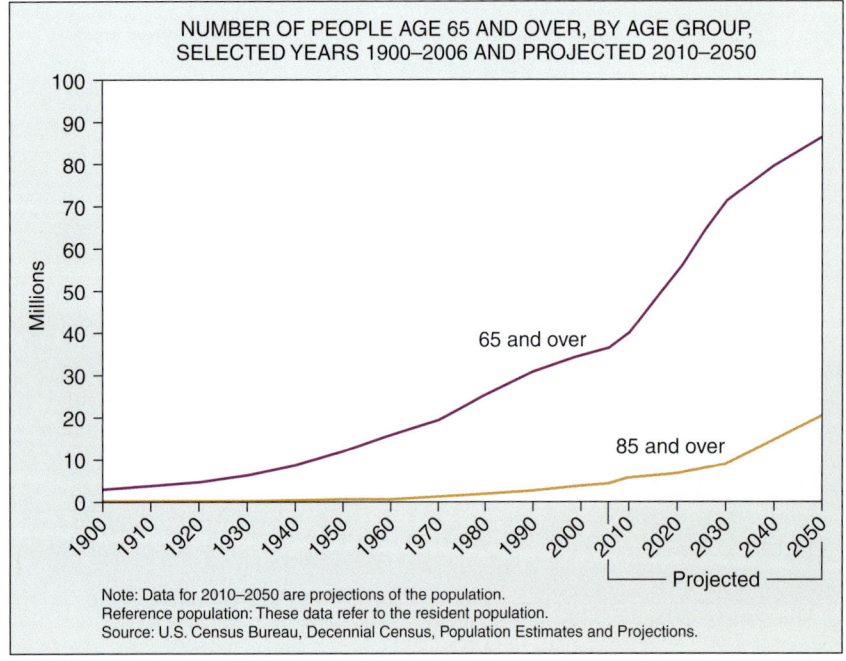

FIGURE 2-4 Number of older Americans, past and future. *(Adapted from Federal Interagency Forum on Aging-Related Statistics: Older Americans 2008: Key Indicators of Well-Being. Washington, DC: U.S. Government Printing Office; 2008. Available at http://www.aoa.gov/agingstatsdotnet/(S(oygvtrmrl5u1me55ji3t3g55))/Main_Site/Data/2008_Documents/Population.aspx.)*

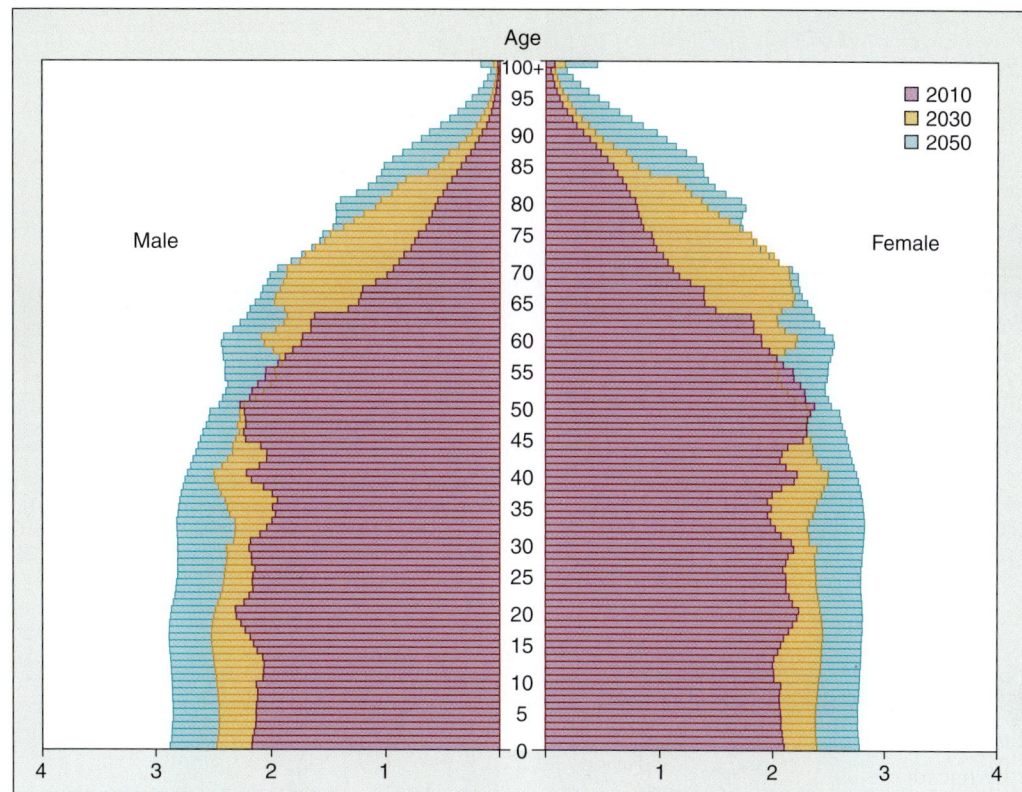

FIGURE 2-5 Age and sex structure of the U.S. population: 2010, 2030, and 2050 (2008 national projections [in millions]). *(Adapted from Ortman JM, Guarneri CE. United States Population Projections: 2000–2050. http://www. census.gov/population/www/projections/analytical-document09.pdf; p 11.)*

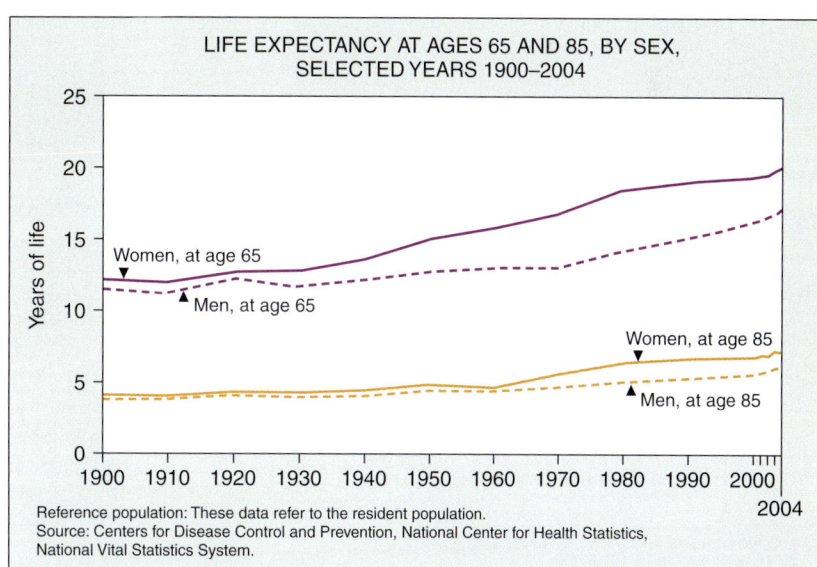

FIGURE 2-6 Life expectancy at ages 65 and 85 in the 20th century. *(Adapted from Federal Interagency Forum on Aging-Related Statistics. Older Americans 2008: Key Indicators of Well-Being. Federal Interagency Forum on Aging-Related Statistics. Washington, DC: U.S. Government Printing Office; 2008.) Available at http:// www.aoa.gov/agingstatsdotnet/(S(oygvtrmrl5u1me55ji3t3g55))/ Main_Site/Data/2008_Documents/Population.aspx.)*

Although there is no sex difference in surgical technique for implanting LVADs in women,[25] the large size of first-generation pulsatile LVADs limited their use in most women. Early trials included less than 10% women. The introduction of much smaller continuous flow LVADs has been associated with an increase in the percentage of women in trials to nearly 25% and represents a substantial potential increase in the number of candidates for LVAD therapy.[4] There were no significant survival differences between men and women in early LVAD clinical trials.

IMPACT OF RACE ON POPULATION ESTIMATES

The demographics of the U.S. population are changing, and it is projected that minorities will become the majority by 2050.[27] Current U.S. federal standards describe five racial categories (white, black or African American, American Indian or Alaska native, Asian, and native Hawaiian or other Pacific islander) and two ethnic categories ("Hispanic or Latino" or

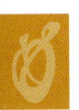

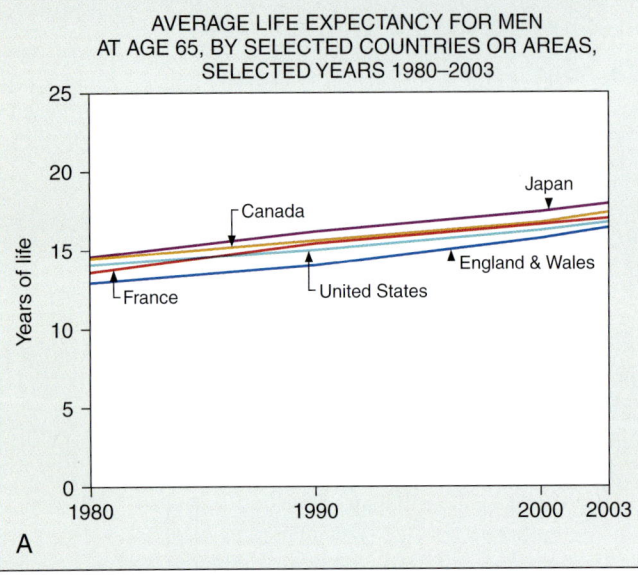

AVERAGE LIFE EXPECTANCY FOR MEN AT AGE 65, BY SELECTED COUNTRIES OR AREAS, SELECTED YEARS 1980–2003

A

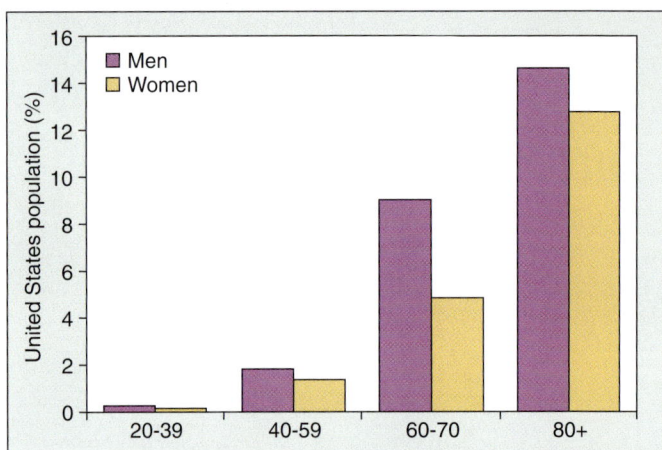

FIGURE 2-8 Prevalence of heart failure by sex and age (National Health and Nutrition Examination Survey [NHANES, 2003-2006]). *(Adapted from Lloyd-Jones D, Adams RJ, Brown TM, et al. Heart disease and stroke statistics—2010 update: a report from the American Heart Association. Circulation. 2010;121:e46-e215.)*

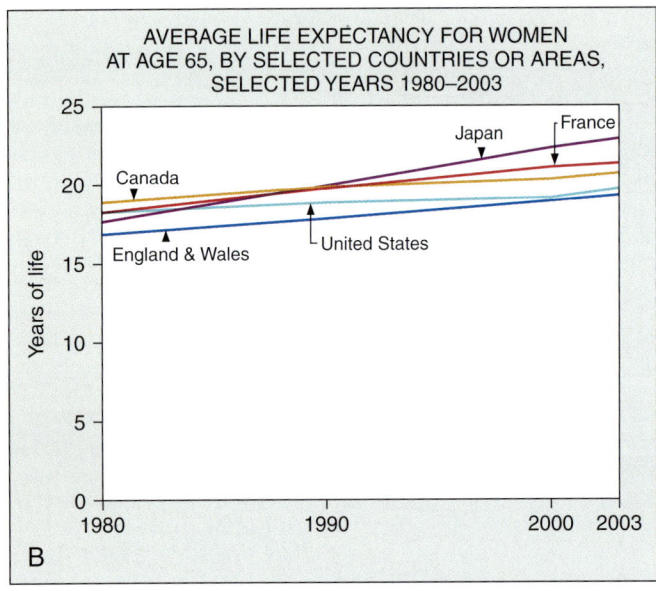

AVERAGE LIFE EXPECTANCY FOR WOMEN AT AGE 65, BY SELECTED COUNTRIES OR AREAS, SELECTED YEARS 1980–2003

B

FIGURE 2-7 Average life expectancy for men **(A)** and women **(B)** at age 65 in the last 3 decades. *(From Centers for Disease Control and Prevention, National Center for Health Statistics, Health, United States, 2007.)*

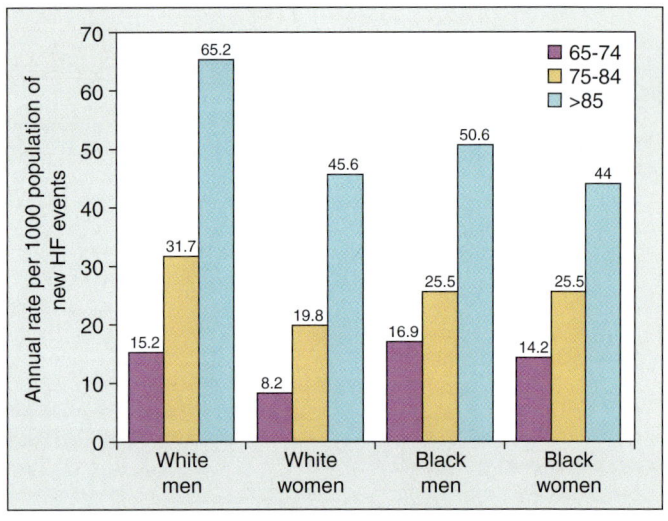

FIGURE 2-9 Annual incidence per 1000 population of new heart failure (HF) events in the United States, stratified by age, sex, and race. *(Adapted from Lloyd-Jones D, Adams RJ, Brown TM, et al. Heart disease and stroke statistics—2010 update: a report from the American Heart Association. Circulation. 2010;121:e46-e215.)*

"not Hispanic or Latino").[27] The discussion focuses specifically on African Americans and Hispanics.

African Americans

African Americans currently constitute approximately 13% of the U.S. population. This proportion is expected to remain (Fig. 2-13) the same through 2050.[28]

According to the most recent AHA statistics African American women had a higher prevalence of HF (3.6%) than white women (2.1%), whereas African American men and white men had a similar prevalence (3.0% and 3.2%).[9] The proportion of African Americans with advanced HF is unknown. Estimates of HF incidence rates among African Americans vary. In the National Heart, Lung and Blood Institute Atherosclerosis Risk in Communities (ARIC) study, the age-adjusted incidence rate per 1000 person-

years were 3.4 for white women, 6.0 for white men, 8.1 for African American women, and 9.1 for African American men.[9,29] Authors of the study hypothesized that the greater HF incidence in African Americans was explained by the greater levels of atherosclerotic risk factors in this population.[9,29] African Americans with HF tend to have a greater burden of systolic dysfunction, higher HF hospitalization rates, and higher HF case fatality than whites of both sexes.[30] Perhaps because African Americans generally have higher poverty levels and worse access to health care, they tend to present later and with more advanced disease.

African Americans make up 21%[23] of the INTERMACS registry; their short-term survival outcomes did not differ compared with whites in the registry (Fig. 2-14).[31] It has been observed that in the setting of optimal care, African Americans had similar survival outcomes with cardiac transplantation.[32] Because African Americans have a high prevalence and incidence of HF, we anticipate that LVAD use will increase in

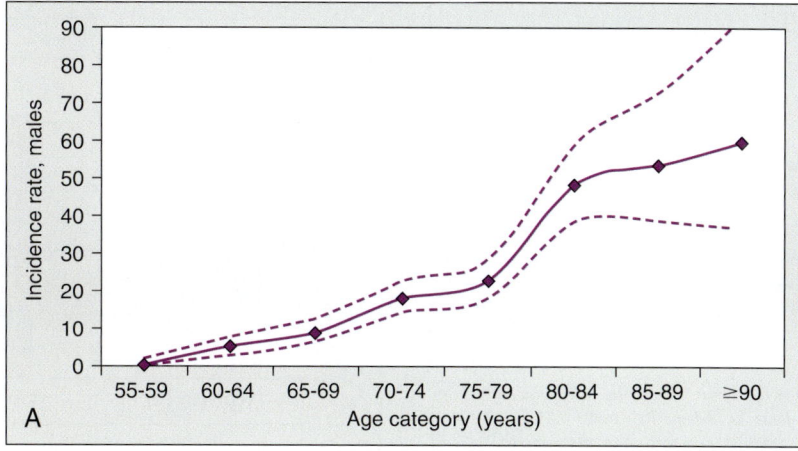

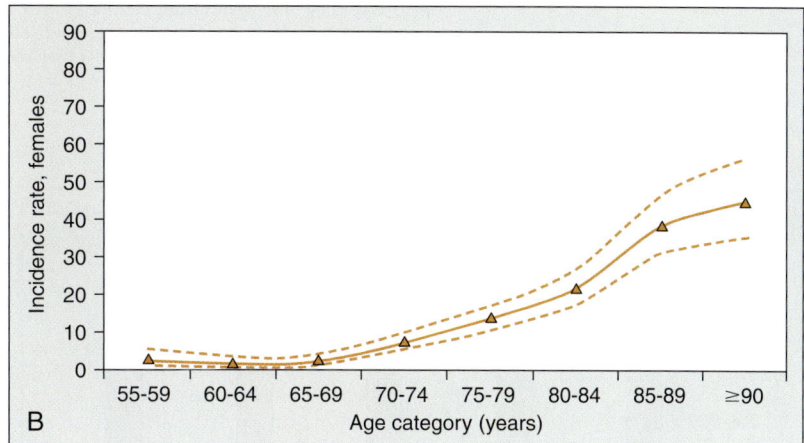

FIGURE 2-10 **A** and **B,** Age-specific incidence rates (per 1000 man years) in Rotterdam Study, stratified by sex. *(From Bleumink GS, Knetsch AM, Sturkenboom MCa, et al. Quantifying the heart failure epidemic: prevalence, incidence rate, lifetime risk and prognosis of heart failure. The Rotterdam Study. Eur Heart J. 2004;25:1614-1619.)*

TABLE 2-3	United States Statistics Regarding Heart Failure Prevalence, Incidence, Mortality, Hospital Discharges, and Cost				
Population Group	**Prevalence, 2006, Age ≥20 yr**	**Incidence (New Cases), Age ≥45 yr**	**Mortality (Any Mention), 2006, All Ages***	**Hospital Discharges, 2006, All Ages**	**Cost, 2010**
Both sexes	5,800,000 (2.6%)	670,000	282,754	1,106,000	$39.2 billion
Men	3,100,000 (3.1%)	350,000	123,600 (43.7%)†	523,000	—‡
Women	2,700,000 (2.1%)	320,000	159,167 (56.3%)†	583,000	—
Non-Hispanic white men	3.2%	—	110,250	—	—
Non-Hispanic white women	2.1%	—	142,378	—	—
Non-Hispanic black men	3.0%	—	10,926	—	—
Non-Hispanic black women	3.6%	—	14,151	—	—
Mexican American men	1.7%	—	—	—	—
Mexican American women	1.8%	—	—	—	—

*Mortality data are for whites and blacks and include Hispanics.
†These percentages represent the portion of total heart failure mortality that is for men versus women.
‡Data unavailable.
Sources: Prevalence: National Health and Nutrition Examination Survey (NHANES) 2003-2006 (National Center for Health Statistics [NCHS]) and National Heart, Lung and Blood Institute (NHLBI). Percentages are age adjusted for Americans ≥20years old. Age-specific percentages are extrapolated to the 2006 U.S. population estimates. These data are based on self-reports. Incidence: Framingham Heart Study (FHS), 1980-2003 from NHLBI Incidence and Prevalence Chart Book, 2006. Mortality: NCHS. Heart failure as an underlying cause of death accounted for 60,337 of the any-mention deaths in 2006: 23,918 men and 36,419 women. Hospital discharges: National Hospital Discharge Survey (NHDS), NCHS. Data include inpatients discharged alive, dead, or "status unknown." Cost: NHLBI. Data include estimated direct and indirect costs for 2010.
From Lloyd-Jones D, Adams RJ, Brown TM, et al. Heart disease and stroke statistics—2010 update: a report from the American Heart Association. *Circulation.* 2010;121:e46-e215.

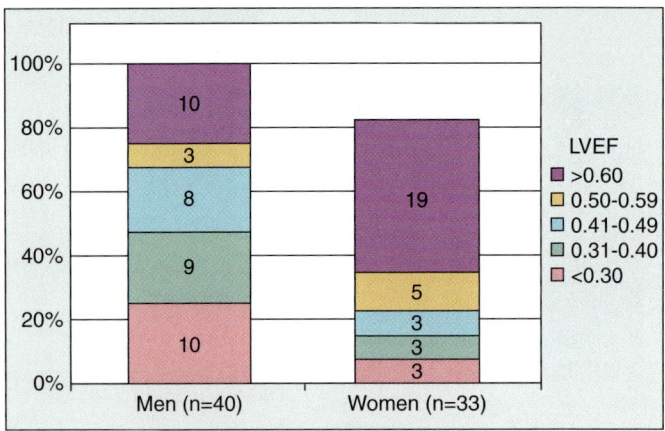

FIGURE 2-11 Hospital discharges for heart failure by sex (United States, 1979-2006). *(Adapted from Lloyd-Jones D, Adams RJ, Brown TM, et al. Heart disease and stroke statistics—2010 update: a report from the American Heart Association. Circulation. 2010;121:e46-e215.)*

FIGURE 2-12 The distribution of left ventricular ejection fraction (LVEF) in patients with congestive heart failure, stratified by sex. *(From Vasan RS, Larson MG, Benjamin EJ, et al. Congestive heart failure in subjects with normal versus reduced left ventricular ejection fraction: prevalence and mortality in a population-based cohort. J Am Coll Cardiol. 1999;33:1948-1955.)*

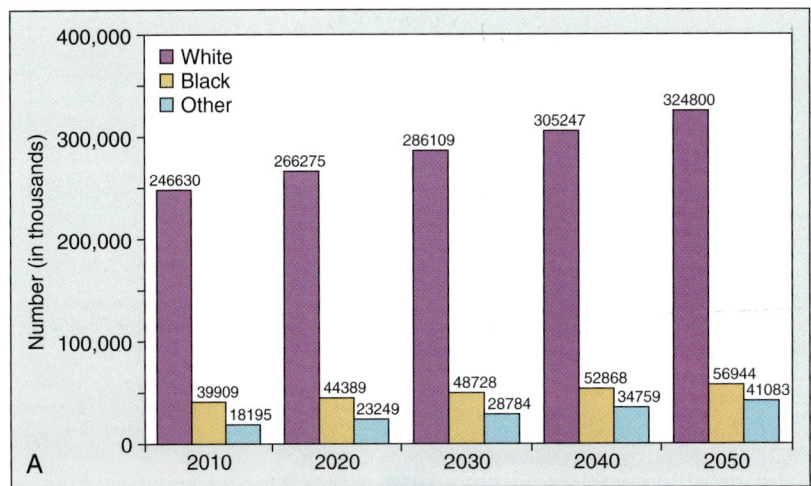

"Other" is a combination of American Indian, Alaska Native, Native Hawaiian, and other Pacific Islander. Hispanics may be of any race.

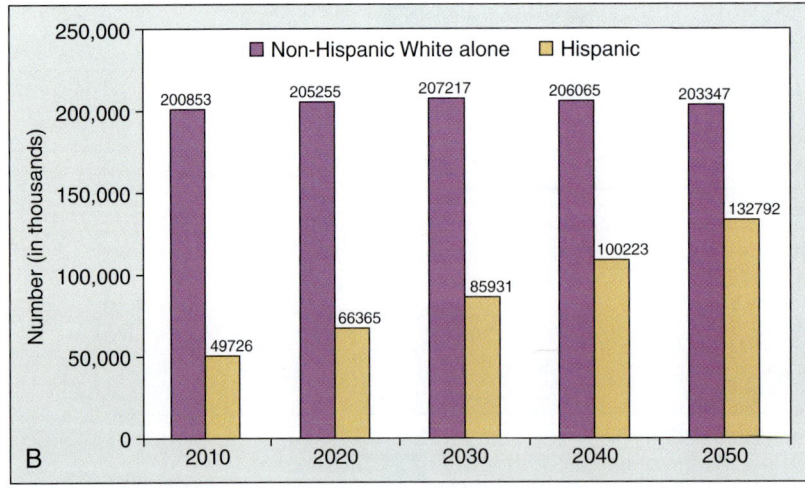

Hispanics may be of any race.

FIGURE 2-13 A, Projections and distribution of the U.S. population by race. **B,** Projections and distribution of the U.S. population by ethnic origin. *(Adapted from Ortman JM, Guarneri CE. United States Population Projections: 2000 to 2050. U.S. Census Bureau. Available at http://www.census.gov/population/www/projections/analytical-document09.pdf. Accessed July 19, 2010.)*

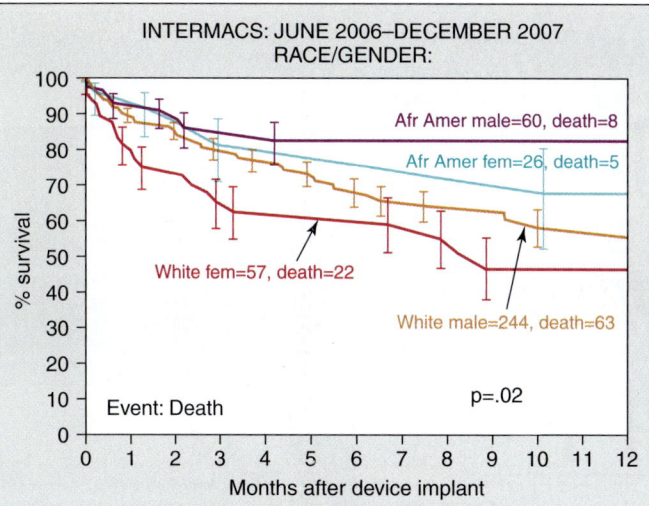

FIGURE 2-14 Interagency Registry for Mechanically Assisted Circulatory Support (INTERMACS): Survival stratified by sex and race. *(From Kirklin JK, Naftel DC, Stevenson LW, et al. INTERMACS database for durable devices for circulatory support: first annual report.* J Heart Lung Transplant. 2008;27: 1065-1072.)

this population, and we anticipate similar survival outcomes compared with whites.

Hispanics

There are approximately 45.5 million Hispanic Americans in the United States, constituting approximately 15% of the population.[27] This population has the highest rate of growth (see Fig. 2-13B) and is expected to reach more than 130 million by 2050, representing 1 in 3 U.S. residents.[27] The prevalence of HF and advanced HF in the Hispanic population is largely unknown and has been investigated in only a few studies. The incidence of HF in the Multi-Ethnic Study of Atherosclerosis was 3.5 per 1000 person-years compared with 4.6 in African Americans and 2.4 in whites.[27,33]

Because Hispanics have a "disproportionate cardio-metabolic risk burden"[27] and a higher than average incidence of HF, we estimate that the prevalence of advanced HF among this population is high. Hispanics are the fastest-growing population group in the United States and are likely to have proportionally larger needs for LVAD therapy compared with whites.

FLUCTUATING CONDITION

HF is not a static condition. Patients often fluctuate between NYHA class III and IV, or stage C and D. Patients may be hospitalized for volume overload and respond to increases in doses of medications and become class III or deteriorate and become less responsive to diuretics and other medications and require additional hospitalizations and become class IV. Corroborating this are HF hospital discharge rates. The most recent published statistics indicate there were 1,106,000 HF discharges in 2006 in the United States (see Fig. 2-11)[9]; this is likely an underestimation of the total burden of HF hospitalizations because these estimates are based on coding of only the primary diagnosis and leave out patients with HF as a secondary diagnosis. Assuming HF hospitalizations represent patients who are fluctuating between NYHA class, the difficulty in quantifying prevalence of advanced HF is underscored further.

NYHA classification is very subjective and often subdivided further into class IIIA and IIIB. The newly endorsed classification of HF into stages A through D is helpful to encourage practitioners to focus on risk factors for the development of HF, such as hypertension and diabetes, and to treat patients with documented structural disease even without symptoms, but condensing symptomatic patients into only stage C and D further compounds the problem of estimating prevalence of advanced HF. The newly created INTERMACS classification of severity of HF of patients now undergoing LVAD therapy includes five levels that are well within the definition of class IV or stage D HF, including cardiogenic shock, inotrope-dependent, or intolerance to standard medications owing to hypotension and worsening renal function (see Table 2-2). This variability in the interpretation of class IV or stage D HF is evident in published clinical trials in patients described as class IV HF, in whom the 1-year mortality can vary between 22% and 76%.[34] A pitfall of selecting patients for clinical trials and selecting candidates for LVADs is the variability in patients who are classified as NYHA IV owing to lack of standardized and validated risk stratification techniques.

Mechanical Circulatory Support for Less Ill Patients

To date, LVAD therapy has been used almost exclusively in patients with class IV or stage D disease who have very advanced disease with 65% to 100% of all patients enrolled in clinical LVAD trials in the last decade being inotrope-dependent at the time of implant, including bridge to transplantation and destination therapy indications. The impressive improvement in device durability and outcomes reported from clinical trials more recently has increased interest in use of LVADs in class IIIB or less severe HF. Data have shown that patients who undergo LVAD implantation as an elective procedure have significantly reduced length of stay and higher survival than patients who are inotrope-dependent. How many patients would be added if the indication for LVAD was extended into this population is hard to estimate because there is little subclassification of the age of patients in any NYHA class of HF stage C and D. However, it is likely that the total estimate could increase by a factor of 1.5 to 2.0; this would have a marked impact on the estimates.

Accessibility to Centers Performing Left Ventricular Assist Device Implants

Government and payers have moved more and more toward selecting centers with best outcomes, which is typically paired with the highest volumes. CMS-approved VAD centers are updated online (https://www.cms.gov/MedicareApprovedFacilitie/VAD/). The number of sites that perform LVAD implants must grow to accommodate the projected significant increase in the number of potential candidates. Typically, and with few exceptions, LVAD therapy has been tied to a heart transplant program. Although vendors would like to see this therapy extended into hospitals with moderate or greater cardiac surgical volume to manage the potential growth, there is concern that rapid and unsupervised expansion would lead to inappropriate patient selection and potentially suboptimal outcomes. Ideally, HF centers should be adequately staffed by an experienced, well-trained multidisciplinary team dedicated to short-term and long-term management of patients with advanced HF and able to provide multiple treatment options.

TABLE 2-4	Future Projections of Advanced Heart Failure Prevalence in United States, as It Relates to Potential Left Ventricular Assist Device Candidates							
Years	Average Annual % Change in Population*	U.S. Population ≥20 yr	Advanced Stage C/NYHA Class IIIB		Stage D/NYHA Class IV		Combined	
			Low	High	Low	High	Low	High
2010	—	240,000,000	93,600	124,800	15,600	156,000	109,200	280,800
2010–2020	0.81	241,944,000	94,358	125,811	15,726	157,264	110,085	283,074
2020–2030	0.72	243,686,000	95,038	126,717	15,840	158,396	110,877	285,113
2030–2040	0.64	245,246,000	95,646	127,528	15,941	159,410	111,587	286,937
2040–2050	0.63	246,791,000	96,248	128,331	16,041	160,414	112,290	288,745

*Obtained from U.S. census projections (p. 7, Table D, "Middle series").[8]

CONCLUSIONS AND ESTIMATES FOR THE FUTURE

Our current and future estimates are presented in Table 2-4 and Figure 2-3. Many factors complicate an accurate assessment, including unknown prevalence of disease in various groups including minorities, differences in urban and rural estimates of prevalence, and changes in life expectancy. Other than one report,[10] prevalence data on advanced HF as defined by stage or class are lacking.

With a rapidly aging population in the United States and industrialized world, we expect that prevalence and incidence of HF and advanced HF will increase. Demand for MCS among older patients will increase, and MCS should not remain a therapy for younger adults. Elderly patients typically have more comorbidities and higher mortality rates with cardiac surgery, and the challenge will be to refine LVAD therapy to meet the needs of this rapidly growing population. Future investigation should focus on liberalizing use of MCS among older individuals.

The number of patients who may be reasonable or good candidates for LVAD therapy is difficult to define based on current evidence. There are many factors to consider, such as expansion into women and smaller adults or pediatric patients and more appropriate use in underserved groups with advanced HF, suggesting that any estimate is likely to change significantly in the next decade. This change will be perhaps twofold if the results of clinical trials in patients with less severe HF are confirmed to show these patients to be well served by earlier use of LVAD therapy. There is a pressing need to obtain accurate estimates of the number of people with advanced systolic HF who might be candidates for VAD therapy.

REFERENCES

1. Taylor DO, Stehlik J, Edwards LB, et al. Registry of the International Society for Heart and Lung Transplantation: Twenty-sixth Official Adult Heart Transplant Report—2009. *J Heart Lung Transplant.* 2009;28:1007–1022.
2. Lund LH, Matthews J, Aaronson K. Patient selection for left ventricular assist devices. *Eur J Heart Fail.* 2010;12:434–443.
3. Miller LW, Pagani FD, Russell SD, et al. Use of a continuous-flow device in patients awaiting heart transplantation. *N Engl J Med.* 2007;357:885–896.
4. Slaughter MS, Rogers JG, Milano CA, et al. Advanced heart failure treated with continuous-flow left ventricular assist device. *N Engl J Med.* 2009;361:2241–2251.
5. Rogers JG, Aaronson KD, Boyle AJ, et al. Continuous flow left ventricular assist device improves functional capacity and quality of life of advanced heart failure patients. *J Am Coll Cardiol.* 2010;55:1826–1834.
6. Starling RC. Improved quantity and quality of life: a winning combination to treat advanced heart failure. *J Am Coll Cardiol.* 2010;55:1835–1836.
7. U.S. POPClock Projection. *U.S. Census Bureau.* Available at: http://www.census.gov/population/www/popclockus.html. Accessed 14.07.10.
8. Cheeseman JD. *Population Projections of the United States by Age, Sex, Race, and Hispanic Origin: 1995 to 2050,* U.S. Bureau of the Census, Current Population Reports, P25-1130, Washington, DC: U.S. Government Printing Office; Available at: http://www.census.gov/prod/1/pop/p25-1130.pdf; 1996 Accessed 14.07.10.
9. Lloyd-Jones D, Adams RJ, Brown TM, et al. Heart disease and stroke statistics—2010 update: a report from the American Heart Association. *Circulation.* 2010;121:e46–e215.
10. Ammar KA, Jacobsen SJ, Mahoney DW, et al. Prevalence and prognostic significance of heart failure stages: application of the American College of Cardiology/American Heart Association heart failure staging criteria in the community. *Circulation.* 2007;115:1563–1570.
11. Ceia F, Fonseca C, Mota T, et al. Prevalence of chronic heart failure in Southwestern Europe: the EPICA study. *Eur J Heart Fail.* 2002;4:531–539.
12. Goda A, Yamashita T, Suzuki S, et al. Prevalence and prognosis of patients with heart failure in Tokyo: a prospective cohort of Shinken Database 2004-5. *Int Heart J.* 2009;50:609–625.
13. Owan TE, Redfield MM. Epidemiology of diastolic heart failure. *Prog Cardiovasc Dis.* 2005;47:320–332.
14. Owan TE, Hodge DO, Herges RM, et al. Trends in prevalence and outcome of heart failure with preserved ejection fraction. *N Engl J Med.* 2006;355:251–259.
15. Hunt SA, Abraham WT, Chin MH, et al. 2009 focused update incorporated into the ACC/AHA 2005 Guidelines for the Diagnosis and Management of Heart Failure in Adults: a report of the American College of Cardiology Foundation/American Heart Association Task Force on Practice Guidelines: developed in collaboration with the International Society for Heart and Lung Transplantation. *Circulation.* 2009;119:e391–e479.
16. Stevenson LW, Pagani FD, Young JB, et al. INTERMACS profiles of advanced heart failure: the current picture. *J Heart Lung Transplant.* 2009;28:535–541.
17. Bleumink GS, Knetsch AM, Sturkenboom MC, et al. Quantifying the heart failure epidemic: prevalence, incidence rate, lifetime risk and prognosis of heart failure The Rotterdam Study. *Eur Heart J.* 2004;25:1614–1619.
18. Miller LW. Patient selection for the use of ventricular assist devices as a bridge to transplantation. *Ann Thorac Surg.* 2003;75(6 suppl):S66–S71.
19. Wilson SR, Mudge Jr GH, Stewart GC, et al. Evaluation for a ventricular assist device: selecting the appropriate candidate. *Circulation.* 2009;119:2225–2232.
20. Holman WL, Kormos RL, Naftel DC, et al. Predictors of death and transplant in patients with a mechanical circulatory support device: a multi-institutional study. *J Heart Lung Transplant.* 2009;28:44–50.
21. Klotz S, Vahlhaus C, Riehl C, et al. Pre-operative prediction of post-VAD implant mortality using easily accessible clinical parameters. *J Heart Lung Transplant.* 2010;29:45–52.
22. Adamson RM, Stahovich M, Chillcott S, et al. Critical strategies and outcomes in advanced heart failure patients older than 70 years of age receiving the HeartMate II left ventricular assist device. A community hospital experience. *J Am coll Cardiol.* 2011;57:2487–2495.
23. Kirklin JK, Naftel DC, Kormos RL, et al. Second INTERMACS annual report: more than 1,000 primary left ventricular assist device implants. *J Heart Lung Transplant.* 2010;29:1–10.
24. Huang R, Deng M, Rogers JG, et al. Effect of age on outcomes after left ventricular assist device placement. *Transplant Proc.* 2006;38:1496–1498.
25. Hsich EM, Pina IL. Heart failure in women: a need for prospective data. *J Am Coll Cardiol.* 2009;54:491–498.
26. Vasan RS, Larson MG, Benjamin EJ, et al. Congestive heart failure in subjects with normal versus reduced left ventricular ejection fraction: prevalence and mortality in a population-based cohort. *J Am Coll Cardiol.* 1999;33:1948–1955.
27. Vivo RP, Krim SR, Cevik C, et al. Heart failure in Hispanics. *J Am Coll Cardiol.* 2009;53:1167–1175.
28. Ortman JM, Guarneri CE. *United States Population Projections: 2000 to 2050.* U.S. Census Bureau; Available at: http://www.census.gov/population/www/projections/analytical-document09.pdf Accessed 19.07.10.
29. Loehr LR, Rosamond WD, Chang PP, et al. Heart failure incidence and survival (from the Atherosclerosis Risk in Communities study). *Am J Cardiol.* 2008;101:1016–1022.
30. Yancy CW. Heart failure in African Americans. *Am J Cardiol.* 2005;96:3i–12i.
31. Kirklin JK, Naftel DC. Mechanical circulatory support: registering a therapy in evolution. *Circ Heart Fail.* 2008;1:200–205.
32. Pamboukian SV, Costanzo MR, Meyer P, et al. Influence of race in heart failure and cardiac transplantation: mortality differences are eliminated by specialized, comprehensive care. *J Card Fail.* 2003;9:80–86.
33. Bahrami H, Kronmal R, Bluemke DA, et al. Differences in the incidence of congestive heart failure by ethnicity: the multi-ethnic study of atherosclerosis. *Arch Intern Med.* 2008;168:2138–2145.

34. Lindenfeld J, Feldman AM, Saxon L, et al. Effects of cardiac resynchronization therapy with or without a defibrillator on survival and hospitalizations in patients with New York Heart Association class IV heart failure. *Circulation.* 2007;115:204–212.

35. Dickstein K, Cohen-Solal A, Filippatos G, et al. ESC Guidelines for the diagnosis and treatment of acute and chronic heart failure 2008: the Task Force for the Diagnosis and Treatment of Acute and Chronic Heart Failure 2008 of the European Society of Cardiology. Developed in collaboration with the Heart Failure Association of the ESC (HFA) and endorsed by the European Society of Intensive Care Medicine (ESICM). *Eur Heart J.* 2008;29:2388–2442.

36. *Australia's health 2008.* Australian Institute of Health and Welfare; Available at: http://www.aihw.gov.au. Accessed 01.06.10.

37. Stewart S, Wilkinson D, Hansen C, et al. Predominance of heart failure in the Heart of Soweto Study cohort: emerging challenges for urban African communities. *Circulation.* 2008;118:2360–2367.

38. AHA medical/scientific statement. 1994 revisions to classification of functional capacity and objective assessment of patients with diseases of the heart. *Circulation.* 1994;90:644–645.

39. Goldman L, Hashimoto B, Cook EF, et al. Comparative reproducibility and validity of systems for assessing cardiovascular functional class: advantages of a new specific activity scale. *Circulation.* 1981;64:1227–1234.

40. Pitt B, Zannad F, Remme WJ, et al. The effect of spironolactone on morbidity and mortality in patients with severe heart failure. Randomized Aldactone Evaluation Study Investigators. *N Engl J Med.* 1999;341:709–717.

Acute Decompensated Heart Failure

James B. Young and Leslie W. Miller

INTRODUCTION

The definition of heart failure (HF) has evolved from the simplistic concept of reduced stroke volume ("... failure to adequately discharge the contents of the left ventricle"), as noted in the seminal 1933 textbook *Diseases of the Heart* by Lewis,[1] to the more complete and pathophysiologically oriented definition by Katz, which was summarized in the 2000 textbook *Heart Failure*.[2] Katz moved from solely a hemodynamic definition to a definition encompassing molecular biodynamics, cell repair, and cell death. Acute decompensated heart failure (ADHF) represents arguably the most dramatic presentation of impaired heart function. Various substantive fluid retention states were generally how patients presented and were recognized to have HF decades ago. ADHF syndromes are heterogeneous states ranging from the de novo presentation of a patient in extremis with respiratory distress secondary to acute pulmonary edema to the presentation of a patient with chronic congestion who more slowly (although rates can vary) develops intolerable edema or dyspnea. Patients can have a reduced left ventricular ejection fraction (left ventricular systolic dysfunction), or they can have more "preserved" systolic ventricular function (generally a left ventricular ejection fraction >.40) but still have substantive congestive heart failure (CHF) signs and symptoms develop. The diagnosis of ADHF is primarily a clinical one based on symptoms and findings noted at physical examination.[3]

The pathophysiology of ADHF has much to do with fluid retention and volume overload, but it is more complex than just that.[4,5] A reduction in ventricular performance, regardless of cause, leads to multiple compensatory mechanisms including local flow-mediated renal stimulation signals that cause salt and water reabsorption and sympathetic and parasympathetic nervous system stimulation, which results in increased peripheral vascular resistance and higher aortic impedance. The blood pressure often increases, sometimes quickly, and left ventricular filling pressures increase. The adrenergic state shifts from a predominantly parasympathetic modulating tone to one characterized by a more stimulating sympathetic state, with concomitant increases in epinephrine, norepinephrine, renin, and aldosterone. This altered sympathetic nervous system and circulating humoral state can precipitate arrhythmias such as ventricular tachycardia and atrial fibrillation, which contribute further to ADHF decompensation. As blood volume and pulmonary pressures increase (driven primarily by salt and water retention and accumulation), there is further fluid redistribution from the peripheral circulation to the pulmonary beds. Progression of the syndrome causes further volume overload to develop with subsequent mesenteric congestion attenuating normal function of the liver, kidneys, and gastrointestinal tract. Peripheral edema also develops.

SIGNS AND SYMPTOMS OF ACUTE DECOMPENSATED HEART FAILURE

The most common symptoms reported when patients present with ADHF are dyspnea and edema (Fig. 3-1). Box 3-1 lists the most common signs and symptoms associated with ADHF noted in the ADHERE (Acute Decompensated Heart Failure National Registry) and OPTIMIZE-HF (Organized Program to Initiate Lifesaving Treatment in Hospitalized patients with Heart Failure) databases.[6,7] Breathlessness syndromes include dyspnea on exertion, orthopnea, and paroxysmal nocturnal dyspnea. More recently, sleep apnea syndromes with periodic respirations and nocturnal oxygen desaturation have been frequently identified in patients with ADHF. Other systemic signs include edema (usually focused on the ankle and leg), abdominal swelling or discomfort, early satiety, and anorexia. Pulmonary signs of congestion and ADHF generally focus on the ravages of volume overload and pulmonary congestion. Rales, wheezing, pleural effusions, periodic respirations, S_3 gallop, worsening mitral regurgitation murmur, and hypoxia or oxygen desaturation all can be noted. Systemic signs include peripheral edema, an elevated jugular venous pulse, hepatomegaly, splenomegaly, positive hepatojugular reflux, ascites, worsening tricuspid regurgitation murmur or mitral regurgitation murmur, and anasarca. Different combinations of symptoms and signs appear, and there is a high variability of combinations.

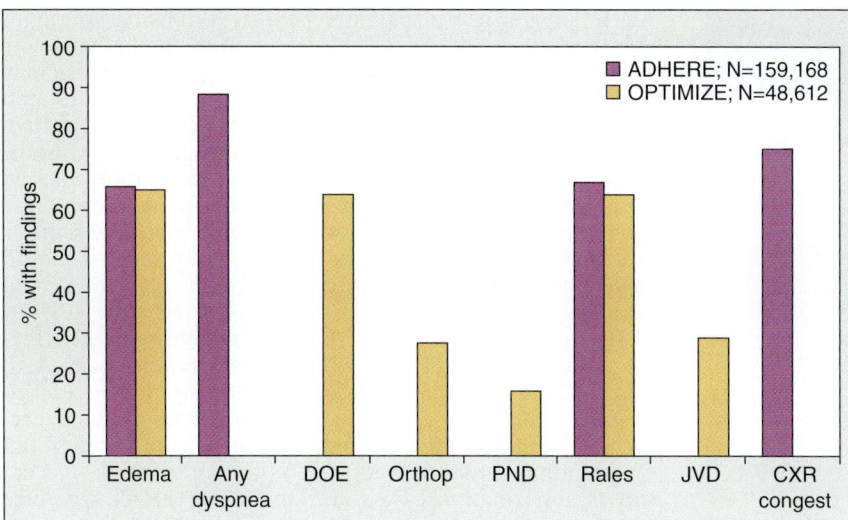

FIGURE 3-1 Presenting symptoms of patients admitted with heart failure (HF) from the ADHERE and OPTIMIZE databases. ADHF, acute decompensated heart failure; CXR, chest x-ray; DOE, dyspnea on exertion; JVD, jugular venous distention; Orthop, orthopnea; PND, paroxysmal nocturnal dyspnea. *(Data from Fonarow GC, Heywood JT, Heidenreich PA, et al. Temporal trends in clinical characteristics, treatments, and outcomes for heart failure hospitalizations, 2002 to 2004: findings from Acute Decompensated Heart Failure National Registry (ADHERE). Am Heart J. 2007;153:1021-1028; and Gheorghiade M, Abraham WT, Albert NM, et al. Systolic blood pressure at admission, clinical characteristics, and outcomes in patients hospitalized with acute heart failure. JAMA. 2006;296:2217-2226.)*

BOX 3-1 Signs and Symptoms of Congestion

Symptoms
Pulmonary
   Dyspnea
      Dyspnea on exertion
      Orthopnea
      Paroxysmal nocturnal dyspnea
Systemic
   Edema (usually ankle or leg)
   Abdominal swelling or discomfort
   Early satiety
   Anorexia

Signs
Pulmonary
   Rales
   Wheezing
   Pleural effusions
   Periodic respirations
   Sleep apnea
   Hypoxia or oxygen desaturation
   S3 gallop
   Worsening mitral regurgitation murmur
Systemic
   Peripheral edema
   Elevated jugular venous pressure
   Hepatomegaly
   Splenomegaly
   Hepatojugular reflux
   Ascites
   S3 gallop
   Worsening tricuspid regurgitation murmur
   Anasarca

Modified from Lindenfeld J, Albert NM, Boehmer JP, et al. Executive summary: HFSA 2010 comprehensive heart failure practice guideline. *J Card Fail*. 2010;16:475-506.

As might be suspected based on the primary symptoms of ADHF, physical findings are mostly related to volume overload and include obvious shortness of breath and congestion manifesting commonly as peripheral edema, pulmonary vascular congestion, pleural effusions, ascites, or central venous congestion with jugular venous distention, hepatojugular reflux, and S₃ gallop (see Box 3-1). Other conditions such as pneumonia, chronic obstructive pulmonary disease (COPD), pulmonary embolism, pulmonary hypertension, nephrotic syndrome, and hepatic cirrhosis may be difficult to differentiate from both chronic CHF and ADHF syndromes.

INDICATIONS FOR HOSPITALIZATION OF PATIENTS WITH ACUTE DECOMPENSATED HEART FAILURE

Taking these observations into account and juxtaposing outcomes noted in outpatients with ADHF, recommendations can be made for when to hospitalize a patient with ADHF. Data from one registry showed that 80% of all admissions to the hospital are through the emergency department and that 80% of patients who present in the emergency department with signs or symptoms of HF are admitted.[8] Hospital admission is suggested (Box 3-2) when severe decompensation is present, which may manifest simply as increasing peripheral edema or weight gain and increasing dyspnea or with more serious symptoms such as hypotension, worsening renal function, or altered mental status. Dyspnea at rest is troubling, and patients with tachypnea or significant oxygen desaturation should likely be admitted to the hospital. Also, hemodynamically significant arrhythmias such as atrial fibrillation with a rapid heart rate especially if newly documented, symptomatic ventricular tachycardia, and symptomatic bradycardia are best managed with an acute admission. Clear parallels exist between ADHF and acute coronary syndromes. Hospitalization should be considered when severe systemic congestion is noted; the patient has significant electrolyte disturbances; or certain comorbidities are present, such as pneumonia, pulmonary embolism, diabetic ketoacidosis, or transient ischemic attack or cerebrovascular accident. Many clinicians would suggest admitting a patient with newly diagnosed ADHF to the hospital.

When patients are admitted to the hospital, generally three ADHF subgroups can be identified (Table 3-1): normotensive patients, hypertensive patients, and hypotensive patients.[9] Most patients have significant congestion as has been shown, and this remains the major therapeutic target.[10]

BOX 3-2 Hospitalization of Patients with Acute Decompensated Heart Failure

Hospitalization Suggested
Severe Decompensation
  Hypotension
  Worsening renal function
  Altered mental status

Dyspnea at Rest
  Tachypnea
  Oxygen saturation <90%

Hemodynamically Significant Arrhythmias
  Atrial fibrillation with rapid ventricular rate
  Symptomatic ventricular tachycardia
  Symptomatic bradycardia
  Symptomatic sinus tachycardia

Acute Coronary Syndromes

Hospitalization Considered
Severe congestion
  Anasarca

Significant Electrolyte Disturbance
Presence of Certain Comorbidities
  Pneumonia
  Pulmonary embolism
  Diabetic ketoacidosis
  Transient ischemic attack or cerebrovascular accident

New-onset Acute Decompensated Heart Failure (ADHF)

Modified from Lindenfeld J, Albert NM, Boehmer JP, et al. Executive summary: HFSA 2010 comprehensive heart failure practice guideline. *J Card Fail.* 2010;16:475-506.

A few patients are in cardiogenic shock with an even distribution of normotensive and hypertensive patients. Table 3-1 summarizes the characteristics of these three main ADHF subgroups.[9] In patients with hypertension and arguably patients with normal blood pressure or perhaps low blood pressure, intravenous vasodilating medications may be helpful. In the absence of symptomatic hypotension and generally when the systolic blood pressure is greater than 90 mm Hg, intravenous nitroglycerin, nitroprusside, or nesiritide may be considered as an addition to diuretic therapy for rapid improvement of congestive symptoms. When these agents are given, monitoring the systemic blood pressure is crucial, and the drugs should be stopped or dosages should be reduced if symptomatic hypotension or worsening renal function develops.

Driving immediate concerns for a patient with ADHF is the degree of congestion, which most patients have, and this leads to the recommendation that diuretics be administered at doses necessary to produce a substantive diuresis that would achieve optimal volume status with relief of symptoms without producing volume depletion or electrolyte abnormalities. Data are lacking on which sequence of agents used is related to desirable or undesirable outcomes, and there is no consensus about the best algorithm to employ during management of HF patients who are not doing well after diuretics and whatever other first-line agent was chosen.

When congestion fails to improve after diuretic therapies, re-evaluation should include confirmation of the diagnosis of ADHF; consideration of more stringent sodium and fluid restriction; increasing the doses of the loop diuretic; using continuous infusion of a loop diuretic instead of pulsed infusions; or adding a second diuretic acting in a different fashion on the kidney such as metolazone, spironolactone, or chlorothiazide. In addition, use of a pulmonary artery catheter to confirm hemodynamics and determine better to which ADHF subgroup a patient belongs can be helpful (see Table 3-1). The routine administration of supplemental oxygen is recommended only in the presence of hypoxia or oxygen desaturation. In severely dyspneic patients with pulmonary edema, a noninvasive positive-pressure ventilation mask might be helpful.

TABLE 3-1	Three Types of Presentation of Acute Decompensated Heart Failure (ADHF)		
ADHF Subgroups	**Frequency**	**Typical Signs and Symptoms**	**Typical Hemodynamic Characteristics**
Normotensive ADHF (cardiac failure)	Common; ~47% of patients	Dyspnea	SBP 90-140 mm Hg
		Pulmonary edema (±)	Normal or mildly increased heart rate
		Rales (±)	Mild PCWP elevation
		Peripheral edema	Normal or mildly decreased CI
		Gradual symptom onset (days/weeks)	Killip class II-III
		Weight gain	LV dysfunction
Hypertensive ADHF (vascular failure)	Common; ~50% of patients	Dyspnea	SBP >140 mm Hg
		Pulmonary edema	Increased heart rate
		Rales	Moderate to severe PCWP elevation
		Minimal weight gain	Normal or mildly decreased CI
		Signs of end-organ hypoperfusion	Killip class II-IV
		CNS symptoms	Preserved LV function
		Rapid onset	
Hypotensive ADHF (low cardiac output/cardiogenic shock)	Uncommon; ~3% of patients	Dyspnea	SBP <90 mm Hg
		Pulmonary edema	Increased heart rate
		Narrow pulse pressure	Moderate to severe decrease in CI
		Signs of end-organ hypoperfusion	Mild to moderate PCWP elevation
		Altered mental status	Killip class III-IV
		Cool extremities	Severe LV dysfunction
		Decreased urine output	
		Diuretic resistance	

CI, cardiac index; CNS, central nervous system; LV, left ventricular; PCWP, pulmonary capillary wedge pressure; SBP, systolic blood pressure.

HOSPITALIZATIONS AND SURVIVAL

Because ADHF is usually recognized when patients present with substantive difficulties to hospital emergency departments or after an unscheduled visit to an outpatient clinic, the clinical and economic burden of this diagnosis is great, with 80% of hospital admissions coming from the emergency department (Fig. 3-2).[3,11-15] Box 3-3 lists many components of this burden; ADHF drives most of the observations listed. ADHF is the most common reason for hospitalization of an adult older than 65 years. There are more than 1 million hospital admissions annually primarily for ADHF, and the average hospital length of stay is 6 days, with one-third of patients staying 5 days or longer. More hospital days are spent on the care of HF patients than any other diagnosis-related group (DRG). As might be anticipated from these data, more Medicare dollars are spent on the diagnosis and treatment of HF than any other DRG. In 2005, the total combined direct and indirect cost for caring for HF patients (mainly ADHF patients admitted to the hospital) was approximately $28 billion, with about $3 billion being expended solely for medications and two-thirds being expended for inpatient care.

Reflecting the limited success with current therapies for ADHF is the fact that HF has the highest readmission rate of any DRG. Readmission rates for ADHF are also the highest of any other diagnosis: 20% at 1 month, 40% at 3 months, and greater than 50% at 6 months. The average mortality after an admission for HF at 1 year is 33% (Fig. 3-3), and survival declines significantly after each subsequent admission for HF (Fig. 3-4) emphasizing the importance of this event in prognostication of mortality with HF (see Chapter 2). Deaths from HF overall exceed deaths caused by acquired immunodeficiency syndrome (AIDS) and lung, prostate, and breast cancer combined.[14]

Although the largest part of the economic burden is driven by hospitalization, most patients die outside of the

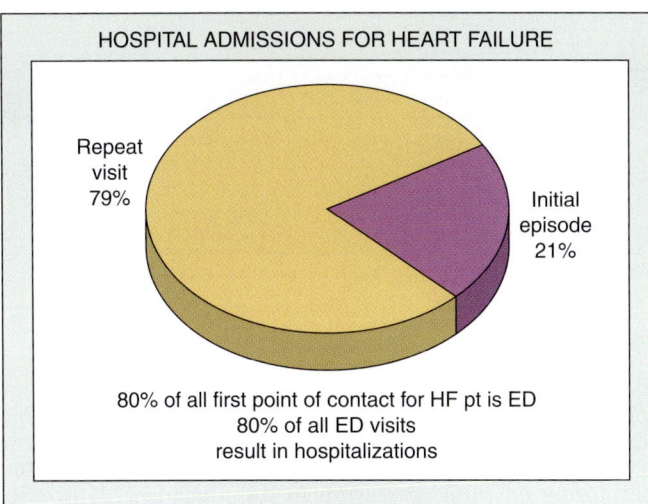

FIGURE 3-2 Initial point of contact for patients admitted with heart failure (HF) from ADHERE database. ED, emergency department.

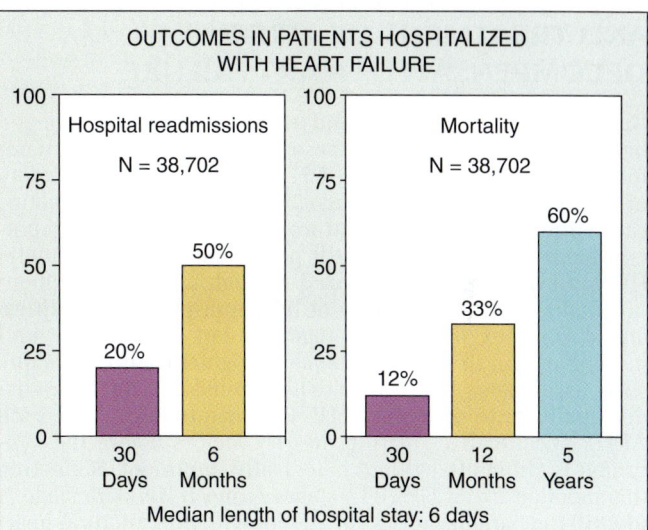

FIGURE 3-3 Likelihood of readmission for the same diagnosis after an admission for heart failure (HF) and mortality at 1 year after an admission for HF, from Canadian HF study. (*Data from Aghababian RV. Acutely decompensated heart failure: opportunities to improve care and outcomes in the emergency department.* Rev Cardiovasc Med. *2002;3[Suppl 4]:S3-S9; and Jong P, Vowinckel E, Liu PP, et al. Prognosis and determinants of survival in patients newly hospitalized for heart failure: a population-based study.* Arch Intern Med. *2002;162:1689-1694.*)

BOX 3-3 Burden of Heart Failure

- Most common reason for hospitalization of adults >65 years old
- Approximately 1 million hospital admissions annually for heart failure (HF)
- Average hospital length of stay 6 days with 33% >5 days
- More Medicare dollars spent on HF than any other diagnosis-related group (DRG)
- Readmit rates for acute decompensated heart failure (ADHF) up to 40% at 3 months and can be >50% at 6 months
- Direct and indirect costs in 2005 approximately $28 billion (about $3 billion for drugs)
- HF deaths exceed deaths caused by acquired immunodeficiency syndrome (AIDS) and lung, prostate, and breast cancer combined
- Median survival after diagnosis of congestive heart failure (CHF) 2.1 years
- After initial diagnosis of CHF, 1-year mortality 25%-40%
- Advanced American College of Cardiology Foundation (ACCF)/ American Heart Association (AHA) HF 5%

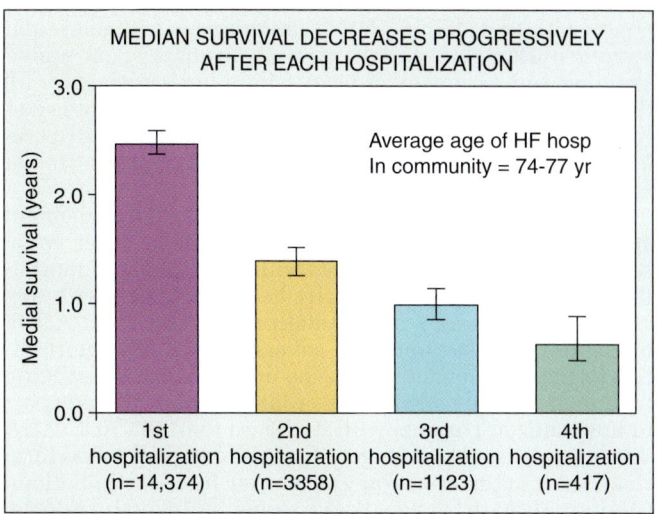

FIGURE 3-4 Median survival after each recurrent hospitalization for heart failure (HF). (*Data from Setoguchi S, Stevenson LW, Schneeweiss S, et al. Repeated hospitalizations predict mortality in the community population with heart failure.* Am Heart J. *2007;154:260-266.*)

hospital.[16] The median survival after diagnosis of CHF has been reported to be 2.1 years, and the 1-year mortality is 25% to 80%. The HF syndrome is heterogeneous, and major morbidity outcomes vary extensively. It is estimated that 5% of patients have advanced, or American College of Cardiology Foundation (ACCF)/American Heart Association (AHA) stage D, HF (see Chapter 2 and Box 3-2). The burden of HF is likely underestimated because most undiagnosed patients with HF syndrome have no symptoms or physical findings of congestion or substantive physical limitation by the broad Katz definition of HF or the definition used by professional society guidelines.[3,11–15]

GUIDELINES FOR DIAGNOSIS AND TREATMENT OF ACUTE DECOMPENSATED HEART FAILURE

Guidelines for the diagnosis and treatment of HF have emerged over the last 2 decades, but these guidelines largely have not focused on patients with ADHF. The Heart Failure Society of America 2010 Comprehensive Heart Failure Practice Guideline is a striking departure with ADHF a very important focus.[3] The document still points out that symptomatic HF is a syndrome characterized by high mortality, frequent hospitalization, poor quality of life, multiple comorbidities, and a complex therapeutic regimen, but it pays new and more attention to the importance of high-risk impact factors such as diabetes mellitus and hypertension, which predispose patients to developing HF in general and in triggering ADHF specifically. Treating the risk factors before the syndrome is clinically evident is logically important. Reflecting this practice are ACCF/AHA stages A and B HF, with stage A identifying patients at risk for HF but without structural heart disease or symptoms of the syndrome and stage B encompassing patients with structural heart disease but without symptoms of HF (Table 3-2).[8,10–14]

When the ACCF/AHA staging classification was proposed in 2005, it was a radical departure from the original ACC/AHA HF diagnosis and treatment guideline, which approached the definition of the HF syndrome in a very traditional fashion and dealt almost exclusively with symptomatic patients with CHF having left ventricular systolic dysfunction and did not address hospitalized patients with ADHF. The original guideline document in 1995 stated that the decision to focus on this cohort "… was based on the fact that the great majority of adults with heart failure in this country have left ventricular systolic dysfunction, and the greatest advances in our understanding and treatment of heart failure are associated with this disorder." Perhaps the latter part of this statement is correct, but about 50% of hospitalized patients with ADHF actually have CHF in the setting of "preserved" left ventricular systolic function.

Little could be developed in 2005 about best management strategies for ADHF; this is driven by the fact that large-scale randomized clinical trials with morbidity and mortality outcomes have not generally been performed with any significant frequency in hospitalized patients with ADHF owing to the high number of adverse events or comorbidities in these patients that may be unrelated to any specific treatment or clinical trial drug or intervention. With respect to hospitalized patients with ADHF, in the 1995 ACC/AHA document, discussion largely focused on when to perform right heart catheterization and use an intra-aortic balloon counterpulsation device.[12] For acute pulmonary edema, drug therapy with 40 to 80 mg of intravenous furosemide and 2 to 4 mg of intravenous morphine sulfate was suggested. As might be expected, and as opposed to more stable patients with chronic HF, patients with ADHF admitted

TABLE 3-2	American College of Cardiology Foundation (ACCF)/American Heart Association (AHA) Stages and Definitions of Heart Failure
Stage A	*Definition:* At high risk for HF but without structural heart disease or symptoms of HF and structural heart disease not present
	Examples: Patients with hypertension and diabetes mellitus or patients using cardiotoxins (cancer therapies) or with a family history of cardiomyopathy
Stage B	*Definition:* Structural heart disease appears including changes in chamber size or shape, valvular lesions, LVH, and frank systolic or diastolic dysfunction but no symptoms of HF
	Examples: Patients with prior myocardial infarction, hypertension with LVH, asymptomatic valvular heart disease, or asymptomatic depression of LV ejection fraction
Stage C	*Definition:* Structural heart disease with prior or current symptoms of HF
	Examples: Patients with known systolic or diastolic LV dysfunction and dyspnea syndromes or reduced exercise tolerance; most ADHF patients are at least stage C HF
Stage D	*Definition:* Refractory HF requiring specialized interventions
	Examples: Patients who have symptoms at rest despite maximal medical therapy such as patients recurrently hospitalized or who cannot safely be discharged from the hospital with interventions such as heart transplant or ventricular assist devices

ADHF, acute decompensated heart failure; HF, heart failure; LV, left ventricular; LVH, left ventricular hypertrophy.

to the hospital generally receive multiple treatments that include individual or combinations of intravenous drugs including diuretics, arterial and venous vasodilators, and positive inotropic agents noted to ameliorate the symptoms prompting hospital admission in the first place. However, the large ADHERE database of greater than 100,000 hospitalized HF patients across the United States showed that although 90% of patients received intravenous diuretics during hospitalization, there was no consensus regarding the most common second-line agent with nearly equal use of each additional agent, seemingly influenced most by culture and practice at individual sites rather than comparative data (Fig. 3-5).[16–33]

There is debate about whether or not any of these therapies translate into what some authors have termed "meaningful clinical benefits," which usually is defined by a reduction in morbidity and mortality rather than symptomatic improvement. In the future, the more important targeted outcome may be reduction in readmission combined with mortality within 30 to 60 days that can be associated with any intervention or drug. Particularly important is the dissociation between hemodynamic effects of intravenous drugs, the relief of symptoms, and morbidity. Long-term intravenous infusion of inotropes has been fraught with controversy because although some can generally increase cardiac output and reduce cardiac filling pressures, the benefits of this activity can be offset by the more frequent appearance of atrial fibrillation or malignant ventricular arrhythmias.[34] Table 3-3 compares the inotrope dobutamine (a synthetic catecholamine) and milrinone (a phosphodiesterase inhibitor), and Table 3-4 presents an overview of the outcomes of the OPTIME-CHF trial on milrinone in HF progression.[34]

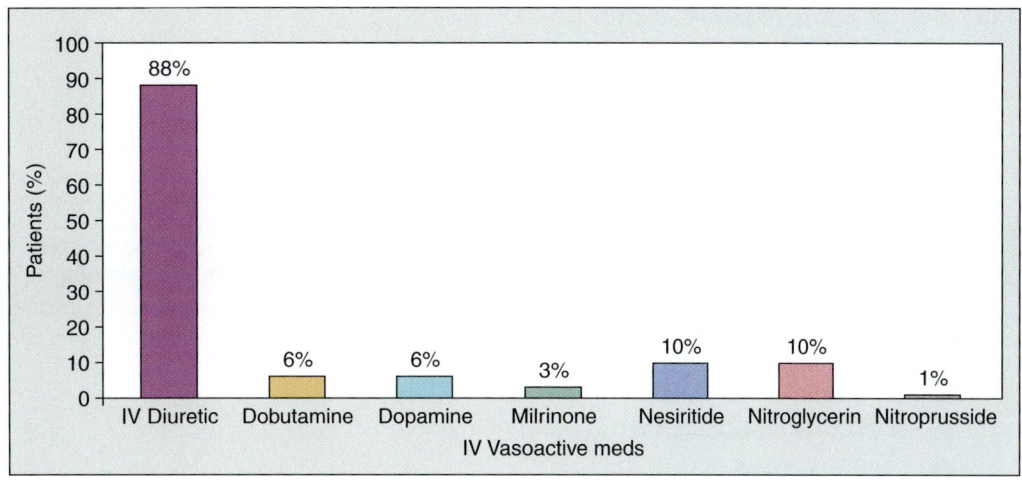

FIGURE 3-5 Most commonly prescribed intravenous (IV) medications for treatment of patients with acute decompensated heart failure (ADHF) in the ADHERE Registry database. All enrolled discharges (n=105,388), October 2001–January 2004.

TABLE 3-3	Comparison of the Inotropes Dobutamine and Milrinone*	
Parameters	**Dobutamine**	**Milrinone**
Inotropy	+	+
Proarrhythmia	++	++
Chronotropy	++	+/–
Vasodilator	+	+
Short half-life	+	–
Use with beta blockers	No	No
Diuretic effect	No	No
Beneficial effects on RAAS	No	No

*+ or – represents the presence and strength of positive or negative effects.
RAAS, renin aldosterone angiotensin system.

TABLE 3-4	OPTIME-CHF Trial: Short-Term Intravenous Milrinone for Acute Exacerbation of Chronic Heart Failure Outcomes		
Outcome	**Milrinone**	**Placebo**	**P Value**
Reduction in treatment failure	7.9%	6.6%	.536
Complications	12.6%	2.1%	< .001
New atrial fibrillation	4.6%	1.5%	.004
Sustained hypotension	10.7%	3.2%	< .001
Myocardial infarction	1.5%	0.4%	.178

Data from Cuffe MS, Califf RM, Adams KF Jr, et al; Outcomes of a Prospective Trial of Intravenous Milrinone for Exacerbations of Chronic Heart Failure (OPTIME-CHF) Investigators. Short-term intravenous milrinone for acute exacerbation of chronic heart failure: a randomized controlled trial. *JAMA.* 2002;287:1541-1547.

The complex pathophysiology of ADHF with its numerous and subjective symptoms that are difficult to measure and quantify makes it a challenging syndrome. Particularly vexing is the issue of dyspnea, a common driver of ADHF hospital admission. Randomized clinical trials have used various tools to quantify dyspnea and the response to treatments, as assessed by both patients and physicians, but these tools are subjective and have proved difficult to use with reliability. Interventions focusing on ameliorating dyspnea have been disappointing. Because of the urgency associated with treating hospitalized patients with ADHF, there is an imperative to start therapies, particularly intravenous therapies, quickly, and when clinical improvement is not seen or emerges slowly, treatments are usually intensified or changed. An algorithm of current practice for treatment of ADHF is detailed in more recent guidelines (Fig. 3-6). The level of evidence is very limited, and there are almost no randomized trials evaluating a single agent and no trials comparing therapeutic options. As a result, there is little consensus, and practices are often based solely on regional preferences.

With few exceptions, trials in hospitalized patients with ADHF have not focused on discharge events after discharge. Only the ESCAPE (Evaluation Study of Congestive Heart Failure and Pulmonary Artery Catheterization Effectiveness) trial examined outcomes at 2 months after discharge and compared laboratory results such as BNP levels and renal function at hospital discharge compared with results at 1 month after discharge. The study showed a significant adverse prognosis for patients who deteriorate in that short time interval after discharge.[8]

Despite the fact that the study of ADHF has been challenging and incomplete, with a lack of consensus in many areas, clinical decisions must be made when patients present for treatment. Multiple pharmacologic and nonpharmacologic (including mechanical circulatory support devices) treatments are available with a great deal of anecdotal information that has accrued, and "expert" opinion regarding treatment strategies is readily available. There are data beyond classic randomized clinical trials that are important and useful in guiding the clinician to greater understanding of the HF syndrome and appropriate treatments. There are few clinical trials comparing common treatment strategies, however.[3]

REGISTRY DATA: ADHERE AND OPTIMIZE

Two large-scale registries characterizing the presentation, treatment, and clinical course of patients with ADHF have been completed, and much data from these registries have been published (Table 3-5). ADHERE is a large (now having information on >100,000 patients), multicenter North American registry that was designed to collect data prospectively on

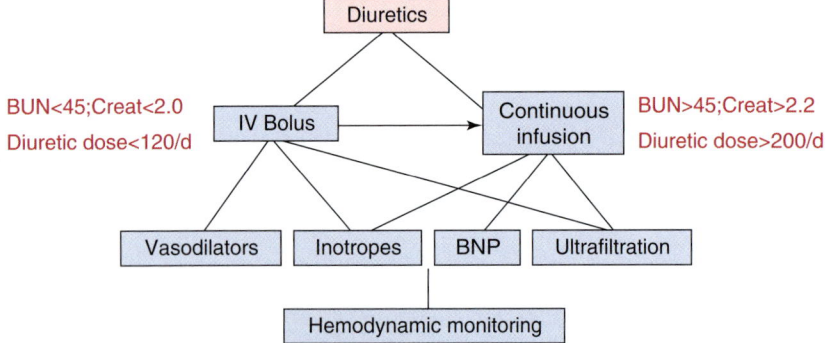

FIGURE 3-6 Suggested approach to diuretic use based on renal function and preadmission dose of diuretics in patients with acute decompensated heart failure (ADHF). BNP, brain natriuretic peptide; BUN, blood urea nitrogen; Creat, creatinine; IV, intravenous.

TABLE 3-5	ADHERE versus OPTIMIZE-HF Registries of Acute Decompensated Heart Failure
ADHERE	**OPTIMIZE-HF**
Enrollment began: July 2004	Enrollment began: March 2003
281 acute care hospital sites Large and small academic and community hospitals	259 acute care hospital sites Large and small academic and community hospitals
Entry criteria: Adults with discharge DRG 127—CHF	Entry criteria: Adults with discharge DRG 127—CHF
LV systolic and diastolic dysfunction patients included	LV systolic and diastolic dysfunction patients included
N in primary report = 65,275*	*N* in primary report = 48,612†
No out-of-hospital patient follow-up	10% of population followed for outpatient mortality or rehospitalization at 90 days
Financially supported by Scios, Inc, Fremont, CA	Financially supported by GlaxoSmithKline, Inc, Research Park Triangle, NC

*Fonarow GC, Adams KF, Abraham WT, et al. Risk stratification for in-hospital mortality in acutely decompensated heart failure: classification and regression tree analysis. *JAMA.* 2005;293:572-580.
†Gheorghiade M, Abraham WT, Albert NM, et al. Systolic blood pressure at admission, clinical characteristics, and outcomes in patients hospitalized with acute heart failure. *JAMA.* 2006;296:2217-2226.
CHF, congestive heart failure; DRG, diagnosis-related group; LV, left ventricular.

HF or if they developed significant HF symptoms during their hospitalization. Nearly 50,000 patients are included in this effort.

Figure 3-7 summarizes the presenting characteristics of hospitalized patients in the ADHERE and OPTIMIZE-HF registries. The mean age of patients was older than 70 years with an even distribution of men and women. African Americans account for about 20% of patients hospitalized. About half of the patients have "preserved" left ventricular function and ADHF, with this being defined usually as a left ventricular ejection fraction of 40% or greater. Most patients have had a prior HF history (>75%) with hypertension being present by history in at least 70% and coronary artery disease syndromes present in about 50% of patients. Greater than 40% of hospitalized patients have diabetes, about one-quarter have chronic renal insufficiency, one-third have atrial fibrillation, and almost one-third have COPD and asthma. Findings at presentation suggest almost 90% of patients have a dyspnea syndrome with more than 60% having pulmonary rales and more than 70% have some type of congestion on a chest x-ray.

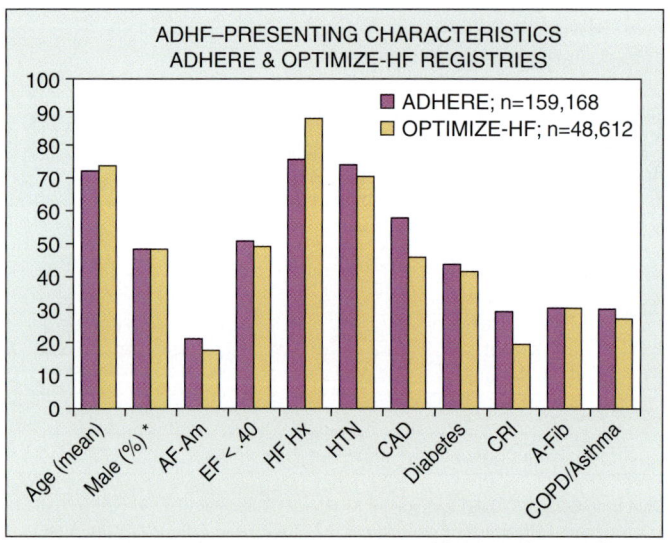

FIGURE 3-7 Presenting demographics of patients admitted with acute decompensated heart failure (ADHF) in the ADHERE and OPTIMIZE registries. AF-Am, African-American; EF, ejection fraction; HF Hx, heart failure history; HTN, hypertension; CAD, coronary artery disease; CRI, chronic renal insufficiency; A-Fib, atrial fibrillation; COPD, chronic obstructive pulmonary disease. (Data from Aghababian RV. Acutely decompensated heart failure: opportunities to improve care and outcomes in the emergency department. Rev Cardiovasc Med. 2002;3[Suppl 4]:S3-S9; and Jong P, Vowinckel E, Liu PP, et al. Prognosis and determinants of survival in patients newly hospitalized for heart failure: a population-based study. Arch Intern Med. 2002;162:1689-1694.)

ADHF hospitalization beginning with the point of initial care in the emergency department or hospital and ending with the patient's discharge, transfer out of the hospital, or inpatient death.[6,8,16–22] No out-of-hospital data were collected. More than 275 community, tertiary, and academic medical centers from all regions of the United States were representative of the nation's hospital distribution as a whole. This registry provided a unique opportunity to determine the characteristics of patients admitted with ADHF and managed in a "real-world" clinical environment.

OPTIMIZE-HF was also a national hospital-based registry in 59 hospitals across the United States, but it included a quality improvement program and 60- to 90-day follow-up in a selected representative cohort and provides valuable data regarding short-term out-of-hospital morbid events.[7,23–33] The primary objective of OPTIMIZE-HF was to improve medical care and education given to HF patients by accelerating the initiation of evidence-based guideline–recommended HF therapies. Adult patients were eligible for this registry if the primary reason for hospital admission was new or worsening

TABLE 3-6	Predictors of Heart Failure Hospital Mortality (Higher and Lower Risk)			
Cohort	N	Mortality (%)	Higher	Lower
CQ Improvement (1992-1993)	4606	19	Age Mg⁺⁺ Nitrate	ACEI Warfarin ASA Beta blocker Ca⁺⁺ block
OPTIME-CHF (1997-1999)	942	9.6	Age NYHA IV	Higher BP Higher Na⁺ Higher BUN
ADHERE (2001-2003)	33,046	4.2	BUN >43 mg/dL SCr >2.75 mg/dL	Systolic BP >115 mm Hg
OPTIMIZE-HF (2003-2004)	48,612	3.8	High SCr Low Na⁺ Age High HR CVA/TIA PVD	Higher BP Higher Na⁺ Higher cholesterol Smoking Higher BMI No HF history White race LVSD COPD

ACEI, angiotensin-converting enzyme inhibitor; ASA, acetylsalicylic acid (aspirin); BMI, body mass index; BP, blood pressure; BUN, blood urea nitrogen; COPD, chronic obstructive pulmonary disease; CVA, cerebrovascular accident; HF, heart failure; HR, heart rate; LVSD, left ventricular systolic dysfunction; NYHA, New York Heart Association; PVD, peripheral vascular disease; TIA, transient ischemic attack.

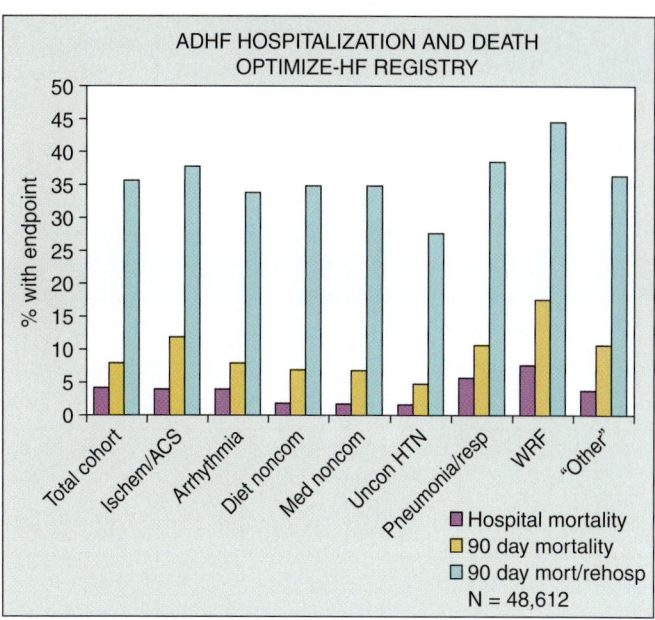

FIGURE 3-8 Comorbidities and mortality of patients admitted with acute decompensated heart failure (ADHF) in the OPTIMIZE registry database. ACS, acute coronary syndrome; noncom, noncompliance; Uncon HTN, uncontrolled hypertension; WRF, worse renal function. (Data from Fonarow GC, Abraham WT, Labert NM, et al. Factors identified as precipitating hospital admissions for heart failure and clinical outcomes: findings from the OPTIMIZE-HF. Arch Intern Med. 2008;168:847-854.)

Hospital mortality rates for patients admitted with decompensated HF have substantially decreased over the last 2 decades. Table 3-6 lists four large data repositories that assessed inpatient mortality. The decrease from 19% to the most recent observation of 3.8% likely reflects improvements in overall care of patients with HF. When a decade-by-decade analysis of HF mortality has been done using Framingham data, a steady mortality improvement has been noted. Depending on the cohort evaluated, a variety of predictors of higher and lower risk for dying in the hospital has emerged. Figure 3-8 shows the overall hospital mortality noted in the OPTIMIZE-HF registry and relationship to some precipitating factors and other clinical observations. In this cohort, the inpatient death rate was 3.8%. The highest mortality rate was seen in patients with worsening renal function. Particularly concerning is the fact that the death rates within 90 days coupled to rehospitalization rates were 45% in the cohort with worsening renal function.

The significant impact of renal dysfunction was also shown in the ADHERE database, where two of the three factors most associated with in-hospital mortality were a blood urea nitrogen value greater than 40 mg/dL and a creatinine value greater than 2.7 mg/dL on admission. The in-hospital mortality was 22% compared with mortality of 1.5% in patients with normal renal function and blood pressure (Table 3-7).

Figure 3-9, also using data abstracted from the OPTIMIZE-HF registry, shows that deaths were significantly more common in older patients, white patients, patients with ischemic heart disease, patients with COPD, patients with atrial fibrillation, patients with left ventricular systolic dysfunction, and patients with substantive evidence of congestion. Perhaps paradoxically, patients with higher blood pressure and smokers had better inpatient

survival rates. The higher blood pressure observation is likely explained by the fact that generation of higher systolic pressures requires a significant degree of ventricular function integrity. Why smoking seemingly "protects" patients with ADHF admitted to the hospital is unknown, however. Not shown in Figure 3-9 is the fact that a biphasic relationship exists with body mass and mortality. Patients with very low and very high body mass index are at greatest risk. Observations suggest that "protection" from inpatient deaths is seen in patients who are obese but not morbidly obese. "Small" patients (possibly representing early or frank cachexia) seem to have the greater hazard of death when body mass index is considered.

Figure 3-10 emphasizes the relationship between blood pressure and renal function in OPTIMIZE-HF. The highest inpatient mortality was slightly greater than 16% in patients having a systolic blood pressure less than 100 mm Hg and a serum creatinine value greater than 2.0 mg/dL.

PRECIPITATING FACTORS AND CAUSES OF ACUTE DECOMPENSATED HEART FAILURE

Modulating issues that can accelerate or exacerbate ADHF include arrhythmias, myocardial ischemia and necrosis, right HF from pulmonary hypertension, respiratory failure, alveolar-capillary membrane leakage, and renal insufficiency or frank failure. Figure 3-11 and Box 3-4 summarize precipitating factors for ADHF when they could be identified. As Figure 3-11 shows, almost 40% of patients in the OPTIMIZE-HF registry had no precipitating factor readily identified. Dietary and medication-related issues include excessive salt and water ingestion, medication nonadherence, and iatrogenic volume expansion of patients who are hospitalized for other diagnoses. Progression of underlying heart disease can occur with worsening ventricular

TABLE 3-7	Multivariate Analysis of Factors Associated with Risk of In-Hospital Mortality in Patients Admitted with Acute Decompensated Heart Failure in the ADHERE Registry Database				
		Derivation Data Set		Validation Data Set	
Risk Stratification	Clinical Characteristics	No./Risk Group (N = 32,324)	Mortality Rate (%)	No./Risk Group (N = 32,230)	Mortality Rate (%)
High risk	BUN ≥43 mg/dL SBP <115 mm Hg Cr ≥2.75 mg/dL	620	21.94	592	19.76
Intermediate I risk	BUN ≥43 mg/dL SBP <115 mm Hg Cr <2.75 mg/dL	1425	12.42	1270	13.23
Intermediate II risk	BUN ≥43 mg/dL SBP ≥115 mm Hg	5102	6.41	4834	5.63
Intermediate III risk	BUN <43 mg/dL SBP <115 mm Hg	4099	5.49	3882	5.67
Low risk	BUN <43 mg/dL SBP ≥115 mm Hg	20,834	2.14	20,820	2.31

BUN, blood urea nitrogen; Cr, creatinine; SBP, systolic blood pressure.

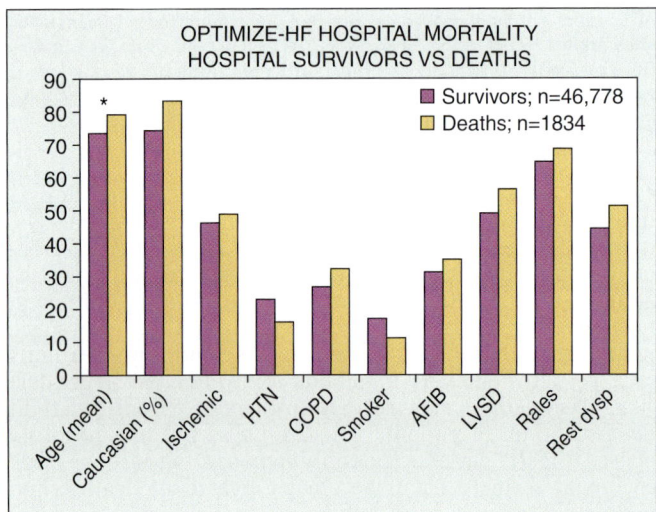

* All observations p<.001

FIGURE 3-9 Comorbidities between survivors and nonsurvivors among patients admitted with acute decompensated heart failure (ADHF) in the OPTIMIZE registry database. HTN, hypertension; COPD, chronic obstructive pulmonary disease; AFIB, atrial fibrillation; LVSD, left ventricular systolic dysfunction; Rest dysp, resting dyspnea. (Data from Abraham WT, Fonarow GC, Albert NM, et al. Predictors of in-hospital mortality in patients hospitalized for heart failure. J Am Coll Cardiol. 2008;52:347-356.)

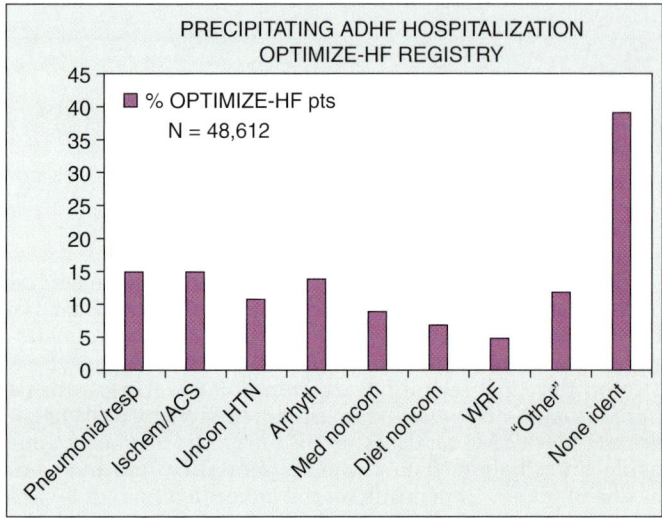

FIGURE 3-11 Factors contributing to admission for acute decompensated heart failure (ADHF) in the OPTIMIZE registry database. ACS, acute coronary syndrome; Uncon HTN, uncontrolled hypertension; WRF, worse renal function. (Data from Fonarow GC, Abraham WT, Labert NM, et al. Factors identified as precipitating hospital admissions for heart failure and clinical outcomes: findings from the OPTIMIZE-HF. Arch Intern Med. 2008;168:847-854.)

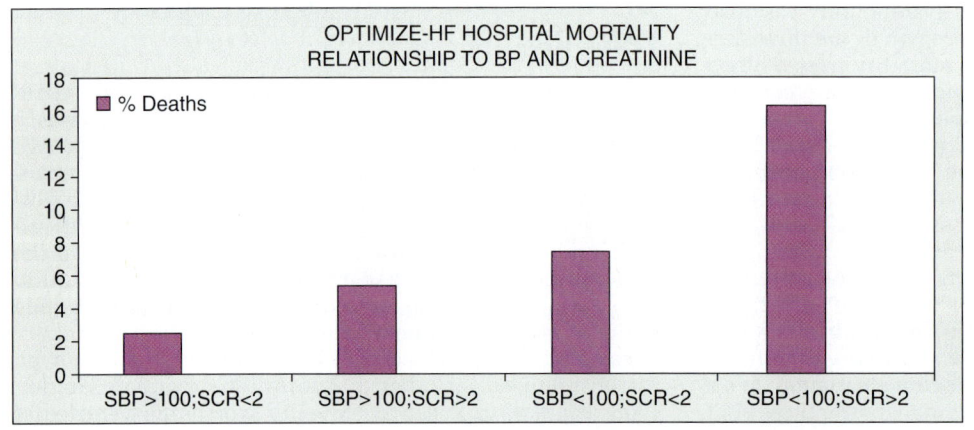

FIGURE 3-10 Impact of systolic blood pressure (SBP) and serum creatinine (SCR) and survival in patients admitted with acute decompensated heart failure (ADHF) in the OPTIMIZE registry database. (Data from Abraham WT, Fonarow GC, Albert NM, et al. Predictors of in-hospital mortality in patients hospitalized for heart failure. J Am Coll Cardiol. 2008;52:347-356.)

BOX 3-4 Precipitating Factors for Acute Decompensated Heart Failure

Dietary and medication issues
  Excessive salt and water ingestion
  Medication nonadherence
  Iatrogenic volume expansion
Progression of underlying heart disease
  Worsening ventricular performance or hemodynamics
  Effects of physical, emotional, or environmental stress
  Cardiac toxin exposure (alcohol, cocaine, cancer therapies)
  Right ventricular pacing
Cardiac arrhythmias
  Atrial fibrillation (particularly with rapid ventricular rates)
  Ventricular tachycardia
  Marked bradycardia
  Marked tachycardia
New ventricular dyssynergy
  Development of intraventricular cardiac conduction defects
Poorly controlled or uncontrolled hypertension
Myocardial ischemia or infarction
Progression of valvular heart disease
Pulmonary disease
  Pulmonary embolism
  Chronic obstructive pulmonary disease (COPD) exacerbation
  Pneumonia
  Isolated pulmonary hypertension
  Interstitial lung disease
Anemia
Systemic infection
  Sepsis
Thyroid disorders
Adverse effects of medications
  Type Ia/Ic antiarrhythmics
  Steroids
  Nonsteroidal anti-inflammatory drugs
  Cyclooxygenase-2 inhibitors
  Thiazolidinediones
  Pregabalin
  Anthracyclines
  "Targeted" chemotherapy agents
  Immunologically based rheumatologic therapies

Modified from Lindenfeld J, Albert NM, Boehmer JP, et al. Executive summary: HFSA 2010 comprehensive heart failure practice guideline. *J Card Fail.* 2010;16:475-506.

performance and, as a result, hemodynamics. Physical, emotional, and environmental stresses all have been shown to worsen ventricular function and prompt ADHF in an otherwise stable individual with no known heart disease or in someone with underlying cardiac dysfunction.

Nonetheless, as Box 3-4 details, many problems can cause clinical deterioration. Knowing these might allow subsequent interventions to prevent repeat deterioration and readmissions. Some more recent data suggest that preemptive outpatient management, such as protocol-driven routine telephone calls to patients after hospital discharge and other similar interventions, may be beneficial. One study by the Robert Wood Johnson Institute[35] examined the potential benefit of having case managers assigned to patients with frequent readmissions to go beyond routine care and go to the patient's home and learn about problems with diet and medication compliance and provide help organizing transportation to follow-up clinic visits. Despite the targeted, more intense, and more expensive model of follow-up care, the study was unable to document significant reduction in readmission.

OTHER CAUSES OF ACUTE DECOMPENSATED HEART FAILURE

A great deal of attention has been given more recently to the so-called *tako subo* cardiomyopathy, or "broken-heart syndrome," in which a life-threatening ADHF episode can be triggered by emotional distress and the electrocardiogram (ECG) mimics an acute anterior wall myocardial infarction. The injury is apparently due to high catecholamine–induced coronary vasospasm because the coronary angiogram is typically normal, but the ischemia results in an "apical ballooning" of the left ventricle that during ventriculography resembles a Japanese octopus trap (*tako subu*).[36]

It is well known that exposure to cardiac toxins such as alcohol, cocaine, and certain cancer therapies can worsen cardiac performance, as can isolated right ventricular pacing. Frequently, patients present with ADHF related to atrial fibrillation (particularly when a rapid ventricular response rate is present), symptomatic ventricular tachycardia, or marked bradycardia. More recently, it has been observed that new intraventricular dyssynergy caused by intraventricular cardiac conduction defects (and evidenced particularly by left bundle branch block on ECG) is poorly tolerated in some patients.

A more traditional presentation for ADHF has been an individual with severe, uncontrolled hypertension. Also, myocardial ischemia or infarction can precipitate decompensation in many patients. Worsening valvular heart disease, particularly aortic insufficiency and mitral regurgitation, places an increasing burden on the left ventricle, which leads to increased symptoms of dyspnea and worsening HF. Several pulmonary diseases can lead to decompensation, including pulmonary embolism, exacerbation of COPD, and pneumonia. Anemia, systemic infection, and thyroid disorders (both hyperthyroidism and hypothyroidism) can precipitate ADHF. In addition, many medications can produce cardiovascular difficulties placing patients at risk for ADHF. Antiarrhythmics, steroids, nonsteroidal anti-inflammatory drugs, cyclooxygenase-2 inhibitors, thiazolidinediones, immunologically based rheumatologic therapies, and certain cancer treatments (including mediastinal irradiation) should be sought when patients are being evaluated for ADHF.

ACUTE DECOMPENSATED HEART FAILURE WITH PRESERVED VERSUS REDUCED SYSTOLIC FUNCTION

A very important more recent observation is that about half of all ADHF patients have relatively "preserved" left ventricular systolic function.[37] Figure 3-12 compares patients with ADHF who have ejection fractions less than 40% with patients whose ejection fractions are greater than 40%. Patients with significant reduced left ventricular systolic function associated with ADHF are generally younger, are more often male and African American, and have ischemic heart disease more often than patients with "preserved" left ventricular function. Hypertension is a more frequent underlying diagnosis, and a significant hypertensive event more often accounts for ADHF than in patients with lower ejection fraction.

As might be anticipated, there is a difference in how these two cohorts are treated. Patients with left ventricular systolic dysfunction are more often treated with agents targeted at reducing systolic blood pressure, including angiotensin-converting enzyme inhibitors, aldosterone antagonists, beta blockers, loop diuretics, digoxin, aspirin, and antiarrhythmic agents. The difference in treatment is

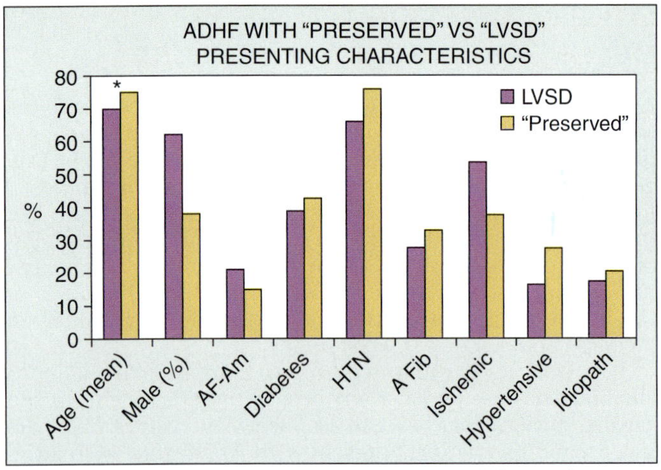

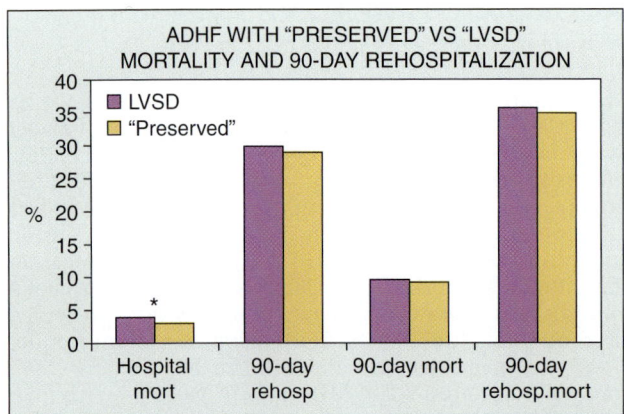

FIGURE 3-12 Differences in presenting symptoms between patients admitted with acute decompensated heart failure (ADHF) with preserved systolic function versus reduced systolic function in the OPTIMIZE registry database. AF-Am, African-American; HTN, hypertension; A Fib, atrial fibrillation. *(Data from Fonarow GC, Gattis Stough W, Abraham WT, et al. Characteristics, treatments, and outcomes of patients with preserved systolic function hospitalized for heart failure: a report from the OPTIMIZE-HF Registry.* J Am Coll Cardiol. *2007;50:768-777.)*

influenced by the type of underlying difficulties these two groups of patients have as well as the fact that no therapies have been determined definitively to benefit the cohort with "preserved" left ventricular function. Angiotensin receptor blockers (particularly candesartan) have come the closest when put to the test of large-scale randomized clinical trials.[38] When in-hospital and 90-day mortality and mortality and rehospitalization rates are observed and compared between the "preserved" and left ventricular systolic dysfunction patients, only the in-hospital mortality was significantly different (3.9% vs. 2.9%, *P* < .0001) (Fig. 3-13). The 90-day rehospitalization rate was about 30%, with 90-day rehospitalization and mortality rate increasing to about 35% for both groups.

TREATMENT GOALS FOR ACUTE DECOMPENSATED HEART FAILURE

Treatment goals for hospitalized patients with ADHF are included in Box 3-5. Symptomatic improvement is paramount. Generally, this improvement can be obtained by optimizing volume status, which largely means treating the patient's congestion and reducing the pulmonary capillary wedge pressure. Optimizing hemodynamics often means improving a low cardiac output state by increasing the cardiac index, although not at the expense of or due primarily to increase in heart rate rather than stroke volume, but the most important focus generally is the left ventricular filling pressure.

It is also essential to identify the etiology of HF and any ADHF precipitating factors. While treating the patient's congestion and improving hemodynamics with intravenous therapies, long-term oral therapy should be optimized and guideline driven. Polypharmacy protocols should be skillfully designed to minimize therapeutic side effects or adverse effects. Patients who have indications for revascularization, implantable cardioverter-defibrillator, or cardiac resynchronization therapy (or the combination of cardiac resynchronization therapy and implantable cardioverter-defibrillator) should be identified, and decisions regarding proper timing of these procedures should be made. Clinicians should determine thromboembolism risk and the need for anticoagulation. Education of the patient, family, and caregivers about self-management of HF is essential, as is consideration of disease management programs and referral for hospice or palliative care.

USE OF RIGHT HEART CATHETERIZATION IN ACUTE DECOMPENSATED HEART FAILURE

Routine right heart catheterization is likely unnecessary in most patients presenting with ADHF; however, this procedure can be very helpful in patients with confusing presentations or extreme low output HF. ESCAPE suggested that therapies to reduce volume overload during ADHF hospitalization

FIGURE 3-13 Acute decompensated heart failure (ADHF) with preserved systolic function versus left ventricular systolic dysfunction (LVSD) mortality and 90-day rehospitalization. *(Data from Fonarow GC, Gattis Stough W, Abraham WT, et al. Characteristics, treatments, and outcomes of patients with preserved systolic function hospitalized for heart failure: a report from the OPTIMIZE-HF Registry.* J Am Coll Cardiol. *2007;50:768-777.)*

> **BOX 3-5   Treatment Goals for Hospitalized Patients with Acute Decompensated Heart Failure**
>
> Improve symptoms
>   Optimize volume status (decongest, reduce pulmonary capillary wedge pressure)
>   Optimize hemodynamics (improve low output state, increase cardiac index)
> Identify etiology
>   Cause of heart failure (HF)
>   Cause of acute decompensated heart failure (ADHF)
> Optimize long-term oral therapy
> Minimize therapeutic side effects and adverse treatment effects
> Identify indications for revascularization
> Identify indications for cardiac resynchronization therapy or implantable cardioverter-defibrillator or both
> Identify thromboembolism risk and need for anticoagulation
> Educate patient, family members, and caregivers about self-management
> Consider using disease management programs
> Consider referral for hospice or palliative care

Modified from Lindenfeld J, Albert NM, Boehmer JP, et al. Executive summary: HFSA 2010 comprehensive heart failure practice guideline. *J Card Fail.* 2010;16:475-506.

lead to marked improvements in signs and symptoms of elevated filling pressures with or without the use of a pulmonary artery catheter.[37] The baseline hemodynamics showed that the patients were in quite severe HF (Table 3-8). The study also confirmed the lack of sensitivity and specificity of physical examination compared with measured hemodynamics, particularly in the estimation of central venous or right atrial pressure (Fig. 3-14 and Table 3-9). The addition of this diagnostic tool to careful clinical assessment increased adverse events but did not overall affect mortality and subsequent hospitalization (in either a positive or a negative fashion) (Fig. 3-15).

The study did not include all consecutive patients managed at each site during the enrollment period because many physicians may not have enrolled the sickest patients owing to a 50% chance of randomization to no pulmonary artery catheter use. This situation may have significantly influenced the findings of the study, which has been interpreted by many

TABLE 3-9	Utility of History and Physical Examination Components in Detecting Pulmonary Capillary Wedge Pressure Greater than 22 mm Hg		
Findings		Sensitivity (%)	Specificity (%)
Jugular venous pressure >12 cm		67	74
Rales		15	85
Ascites		21	88
Pedal edema		48	69
Orthopnea (>3 pillows)		40	60
Hepatomegaly (>4 fingerbreadths)		15	92

Data from Binanay C, Califf RM, Hasselblad V, et al; ESCAPE investigators. Evaluation study of congestive heart failure and pulmonary artery catheterization effectiveness: the ESCAPE trial. *JAMA*. 2005;294:1625-1633.

CH 3

Acute Decompensated Heart Failure

TABLE 3-8	ESCAPE Trial Patient Baseline Characteristics
Median age (25th, 75th percentile)	57 yr (47, 66)
White	61%
Ischemic etiology	49%
Measured PCWP (mm Hg)	
<12	5%
12-22	32%
23-30	37%
>30	27%
Measured CI (L/min/m²)	
<0.8	33%
1.8-2.2	40%
2.3-2.5	15%
>2.5	12%

CI, cardiac index; PCWP, pulmonary capillary wedge pressure.
Data from Binanay C, Califf RM, Hasselblad V, et al; ESCAPE investigators. Evaluation study of congestive heart failure and pulmonary artery catheterization effectiveness: the ESCAPE trial. *JAMA*. 2005;294:1625-1633.

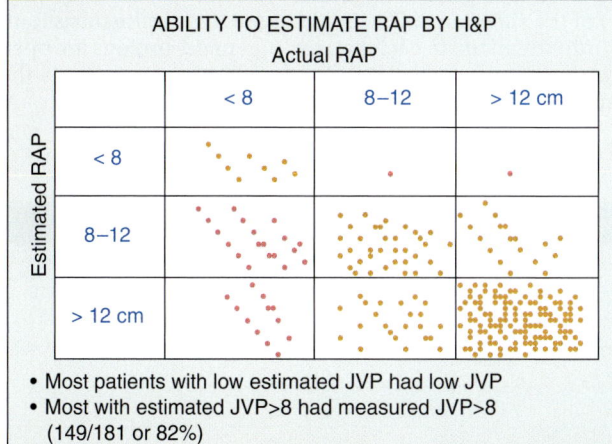

FIGURE 3-14 Ability to estimate right atrial pressure (RAP) by history and physical examination (H&P). JVP, jugular venous pressure. *Data from Binanay C, Califf RM, Hasselblad V, et al; ESCAPE investigators. Evaluation study of congestive heart failure and pulmonary artery catheterization effectiveness: the ESCAPE trial. JAMA. 2005;294:1625-1633.*

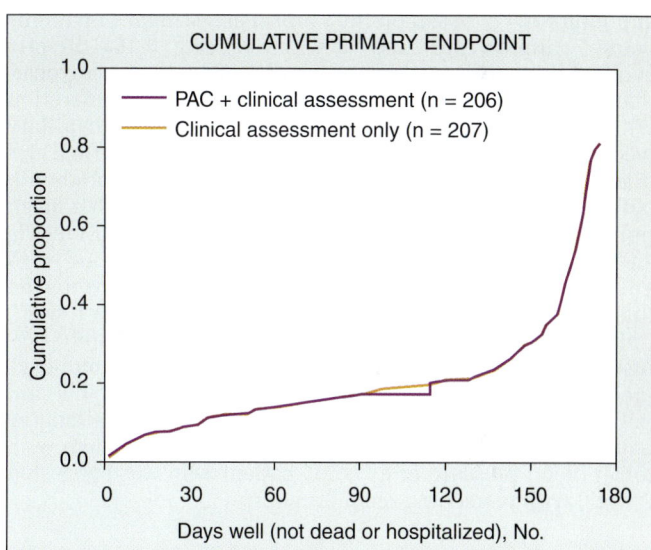

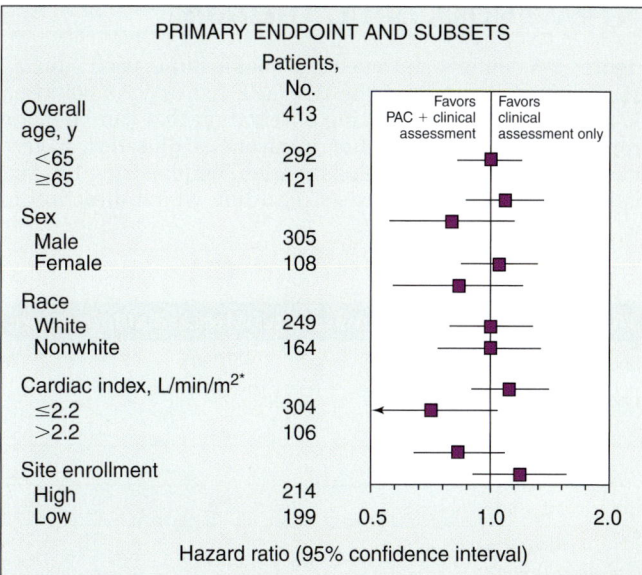

FIGURE 3-15 ESCAPE trial of pulmonary artery catheterization (PAC). *(Data from Binanay C, Califf RM, Hasselblad V, et al; ESCAPE investigators. Evaluation study of congestive heart failure and pulmonary artery catheterization effectiveness: the ESCAPE trial. JAMA. 2005;294:1625-1633.)*

authors as suggesting pulmonary artery catheter use had little impact on outcomes measured over clinical assessment alone. Invasive hemodynamic monitoring can be useful for certain patients with ADHF who have persistent symptoms despite empiric adjustment of standard therapies and uncertain fluid status or systemic hypoperfusion. These patients generally have persistently low systolic blood pressure that is associated with marked symptoms, worsening renal function, requirement of parenteral vasoactive agents, or consideration of mechanical circulatory support devices or heart transplant therapies.

DRUG TREATMENT OPTIONS FOR ACUTE DECOMPENSATED HEART FAILURE

With respect to pharmacotherapeutic management of hospitalized patients with ADHF, Table 3-10 is of historic importance and sets the stage for discussion of the current approach to these patients. Forrester, Diamond, and Swan[39] published a report in 1977 detailing the hemodynamics noted in 200 patients hospitalized for acute myocardial infarction. Our current approach to ADHF patients, popularized by Stevenson and Fonorow[40,41] based on the clinical assessment of patients being "warm or cold" and "dry or wet" (Fig. 3-16), directly evolved from this classification of patients with myocardial infarction. In patients with acute myocardial infarction with no pulmonary congestion (normal pulmonary capillary wedge pressure) and no systemic hypoperfusion (normal cardiac index), the in-hospital mortality was 3% compared with patients who manifested pulmonary congestion with a mean pulmonary capillary wedge pressure of 27 ± 8 (SD) mm Hg and a mean cardiac index of 1.6 ± 0.6 (SD) L/min/m² with a 51% in-hospital mortality rate. Figure 3-16 expands on this concept by segregating patients with congestion ("wet") linked to whether or not they are "warm" (adequately perfused) or "cold" (hypoperfused). Generally, a "warm and dry" (no congestion and no hypoperfusion) patient is stable and not usually admitted to the hospital. The most challenging patient and the highest mortality risk would be a patient with lower blood pressure or a "cold" patient who was congested ("wet") with worsening renal function.

INTRAVENOUS DRUG THERAPY

Figure 3-5 details intravenous medication used during ADHF hospitalization in the ADHERE registry. As has been pointed out, the most striking observation that can be made from this figure is that after intravenous diuretics, a very wide spectrum of medications is used, emphasizing the fact that minimal consensus exists regarding which direction to

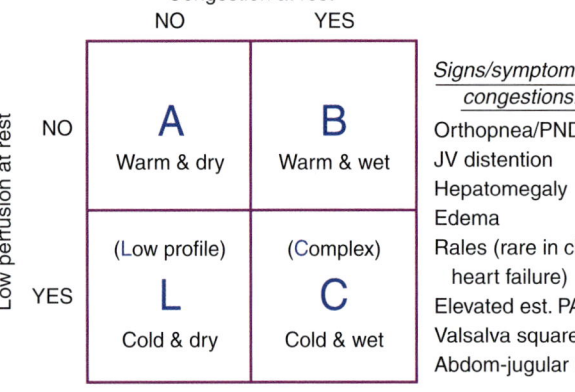

FIGURE 3-16 Assessment of patients with acute decompensated heart failure (ADHF). PND, paroxysmal nocturnal dyspnea; JV, jugular venous.

take after diuretics have been given. Approximately 90% of patients hospitalized with ADHF receive intravenous diuretics during hospitalization with about 10% being exposed to any inotrope and 20% being exposed to any intravenous vasodilator.

Intravenous Diuretics

Despite being the most commonly prescribed therapy for patients with ADHF, the choice of high-dose or low-dose diuretics and pulsed versus continuous infusion remains controversial because until more recently there have been almost no clinical trials addressing this issue. One small trial showed a 17% reduction in glomerular filtration rate in response to a bolus dose of 80 mg of furosemide compared with placebo (Fig. 3-17). The DOSE (Diuretic Optimization Strategies Evaluation) trial was a factorial designed randomized study of high-dose versus low-dose and continuous infusion versus every-12-hour pulses of intravenous diuretics.[42] This was a National Institutes of Health study performed by the Heart Failure Network investigators, and observations suggested that there was no difference in outcomes between any of the subgroups. One could argue that treatments should be individualized to each patient, and many options are open. A meta-analysis of the results of eight studies suggests that continuous infusion of a loop diuretic is overall less toxic and

TABLE 3-10	Hemodynamics after Myocardial Infarction: Forrester-Diamond-Swan Classification			
Subset	N (200)	MCI	PCWP	Mortality (%)
I (no pulmonary congestion or hypoperfusion)	75	2.7 (SD 0.5)	12 (SD 7)	3
II (isolated pulmonary congestion)	36	2.3 (SD 0.4)	23 (SD 5)	9
III (isolated hypoperfusion)	22	1.9 (SD 0.4)	12 (SD 5)	23
IV (pulmonary congestion or hypoperfusion)	67	1.6 (SD 0.6)	27 (SD 8)	51

MCI, mean cardiac index; PCWP, pulmonary capillary wedge pressure.
After Forrester JS, Diamond GA, Swan HJC. Correlative classification of clinical and hemodynamic function after acute myocardial infarction. *Am J Cardiol.* 1977;39:137-145. From Krumholz HM, Chen YT, Vaccarino V, et al. Correlates and impact on outcomes of worsening renal function in patients > or = 65 years of age with heart failure. *Am J Cardiol.* 2000;85:1110-1113.

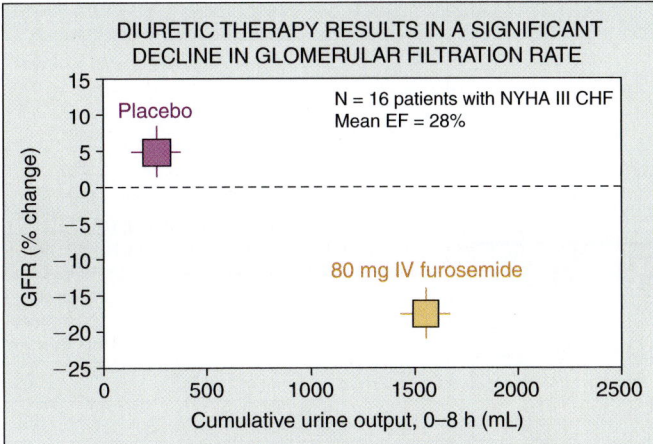

Glomerular filtration rate (GFR) was estimated using a 7-hour creatinine clearance

FIGURE 3-17 Diuretic therapy results in a significant decline in glomerular filtration rate (GFR). Reduction in renal function as measured by GFR in response to an intravenous bolus of 80 mg of furosemide compared with placebo. CHF, congestive heart failure; EF, ejection fraction; NYHA, New York Heart Association. *(Data from Gottleib SS, Brater DC, Thomas I, et al. BG9719 (CVT-124), an A1 adenosine receptor antagonist, protects against the decline in renal function observed with diuretic therapy. Circulation. 2002;105:1348-1353.)*

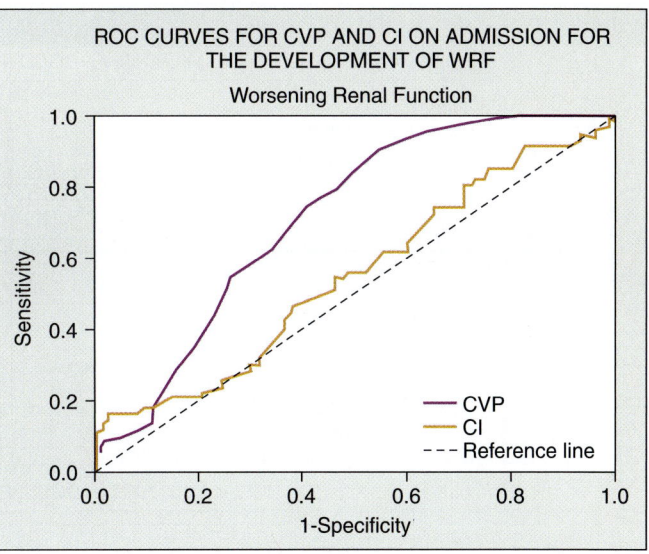

FIGURE 3-19 ROC curves for CVP and CI on admission for the development of worsening renal function (WRF). ROC, receiver operating characteristic; CVP, central venous pressure; CI, cardiac index. *(Data from Mullens W, Abrahams Z, Francis GS, et al. Importance of venous congestion for worsening of renal function in advanced decompensated heart failure. J Am Coll Cardiol. 2009;53:589-596.)*

more effective than treatment with intravenous bolus, but the level of evidence was insufficient to meet criteria for inclusion in guideline recommendations.[42]

Several factors may lead to relative diuretic resistance. One underappreciated factor is significant elevation of right atrial pressure, which is transmitted back through the venous system to cause an increase in renal vein pressure, which reduces the perfusion gradient across the glomerulus. The point at which right atrial pressure significantly and independently reduces renal function is approximately greater than 18 to 20 mm Hg (Fig. 3-18). A high central venous pressure is more likely to be associated with worsening renal function in hospitalized ADHF patients than is the cardiac index (Fig. 3-19).[43,44]

Inotropes versus Vasodilators

There is significant controversy among clinicians who believe that either inotropes or vasodilators are the most effective strategy to treat patients who remain symptomatic after treatment with intravenous diuretics. Figure 3-20 explores the hospital mortality in the ADHERE registry by creating odds ratios in pair-wise comparisons of nitroglycerin, nesiritide, milrinone, and dobutamine. In this analysis, an odds ratio of greater than 1.00 suggests increasing morbid events, whereas an odds ratio of less than 1.00 suggests a reduction in the event among the comparators. All 95% confidence intervals were either above or below 1.0 for each of the odds ratios calculated and statistically significant. This analysis shows that vasodilators such as nitroglycerin and nesiritide are superior to inotropes with respect to survival. Whether or not this superiority is due to the fact that the patient population receiving an inotrope was different than that receiving a vasodilator is unknown. The odds ratios have been presented as unadjusted ratios and have been adjusted as well for covariants and propensity scores. When nesiritide was compared with nitroglycerin, the unadjusted odds ratio was greater than 1, but the adjusted observations were less than 1. Perhaps the fairest statement to make regarding nesiritide versus nitroglycerin is that neither vasodilator produced significantly positive or negative outcomes. In the dobutamine versus milrinone comparison, the odds ratios clearly suggest increasing morbid events in the hospital.

There are two basic types of inotropes: catecholamines and phosphodiesterase inhibitors. Catecholamines rely on surface binding of norepinephrine to the beta receptor on the surface of the myocyte, which triggers intracellular signaling to increase cyclic adenosine monophosphate (cAMP) (Fig. 3-21). Phosphodiesterase inhibitors work by blocking the degradation of cAMP to AMP and does not involve the beta-adrenergic signaling (Fig. 3-22). Both types work by increasing cAMP, which leads to increased calcium mobilization and availability to the contractile proteins for increased contractility.

The data comparing the hemodynamic effects of dobutamine versus milrinone suggest that milrinone, which has significant and independent vasodilating properties beyond the inotropic action, typically reduces filling pressures more

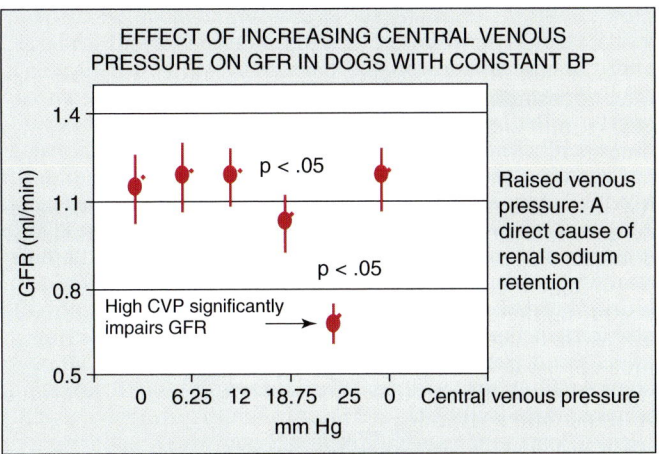

FIGURE 3-18 Adverse impact of increasing right atrial pressure on renal function as measured by glomerular filtration rate (GFR) in an animal model. BP, blood pressure; CVP, central venous pressure. *(Data from Firth JD, Raine AE, Ledingham JG: Raised venous pressure: a direct cause of renal sodium retention in oedema? Lancet. 1988;1:1033-1035.)*

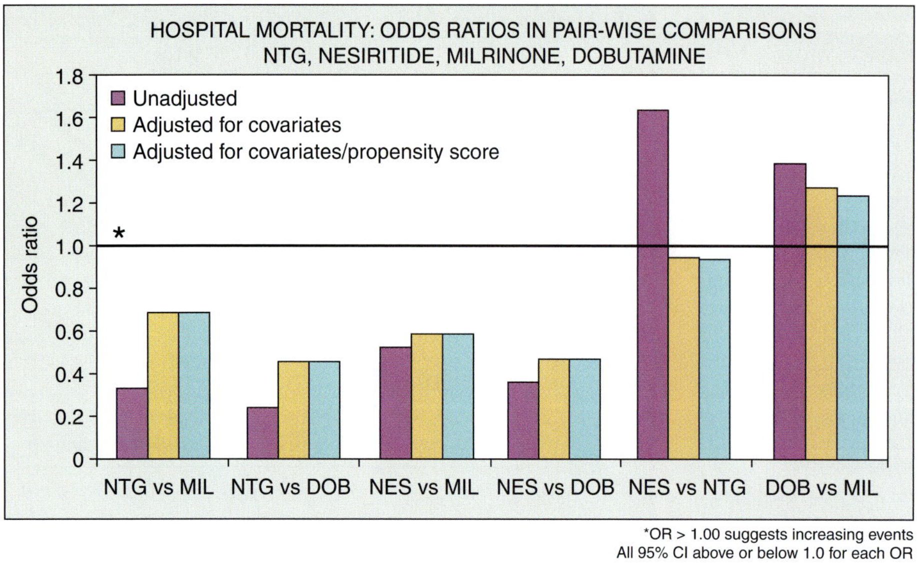

HOSPITAL MORTALITY: ODDS RATIOS IN PAIR-WISE COMPARISONS
NTG, NESIRITIDE, MILRINONE, DOBUTAMINE

Legend:
- Unadjusted
- Adjusted for covariates
- Adjusted for covariates/propensity score

Y-axis: Odds ratio (0 to 1.8)

X-axis categories: NTG vs MIL, NTG vs DOB, NES vs MIL, NES vs DOB, NES vs NTG, DOB vs MIL

*OR > 1.00 suggests increasing events
All 95% CI above or below 1.0 for each OR

FIGURE 3-20 Hospital mortality: Odds ratios in pair-wise comparisons of nitroglycerin (NTG), nesiritide (NES), milrinone (MIL), and dobutamine (DOB). *(Data from Abraham WT, Adams KF, Fonarow GC, et al. In-hospital mortality in patients with acute decompensated heart failure requiring intravenous vasoactive medications. J Am Coll Cardiol. 2005;46:56.)*

BETA ACTIVITY CASCADE

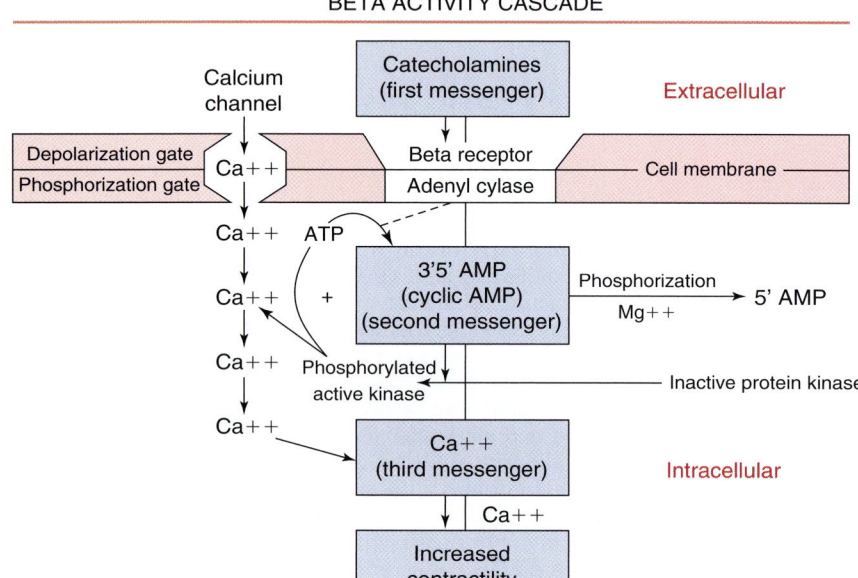

FIGURE 3-21 Myocyte intracellular signaling cascade in response to sympathetic nervous system activation in acute decompensated heart failure (ADHF) leading to calcium mobilization and increased contractility.

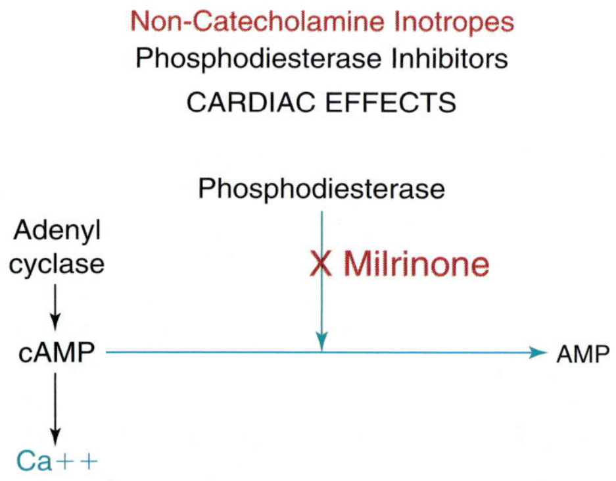

Non-Catecholamine Inotropes
Phosphodiesterase Inhibitors
CARDIAC EFFECTS

Phosphodiesterase

Adenyl cyclase → cAMP → AMP

X Milrinone

cAMP → Ca++

FIGURE 3-22 Mechanism of action of phosphodiesterase inhibitor–type inotropic agents, which increases cyclic adenosine monophosphate (AMP) activation independent of adrenergic signaling or receptors.

than dobutamine (Fig. 3-23; see Table 3-3). The major advantage of milrinone is that in contrast to the catecholamines, there is no stimulation of heart rate, and increases in cardiac output are primarily driven by direct increase in contractility. In addition, because milrinone does not involve beta-adrenergic signaling, which is the primary mechanism of dobutamine and all catecholamines, it can be used in patients receiving a beta blocker. This attribute is more important in beginning therapy with beta blockers and in titrating dosage up, as their use in patients who require intravenous inotropic support is limited because they suppress one of the primary physiologic responses to reduced contractility, which is to increase heart rate.

Intravenous Inotropes

Intravenous inotropes (generally milrinone or dobutamine; see Table 3-3) may be considered to relieve symptoms and improve end-organ function in patients with ADHF in a setting

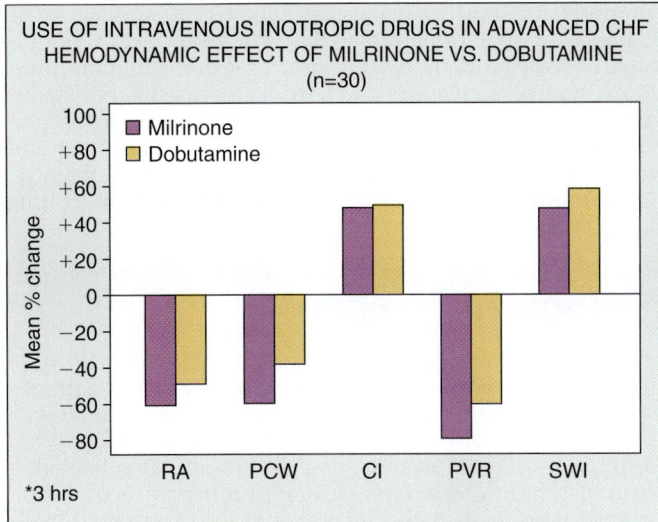

FIGURE 3-23 Comparison of hemodynamic responses to infusion of dobutamine or milrinone. CI, cardiac index; PCW, pulmonary capillary wedge pressure; RA, right atrial pressure; SWI, stroke work index expressed as a percent change from baseline to end of infusion. *(Data from Karlsberg RP, DeWood MA, DeMaria AN, et al. Comparative efficacy of short-term intravenous infusions of milrinone and dobutamine in acute congestive heart failure following acute myocardial infarction. Milrinone-Dobutamine Study Group. Clin Cardiol. 1996;19:21-30.)*

of diminished peripheral perfusion and end-organ dysfunction (low output syndrome). In particular, intravenous inotropes may be considered in a patient who presents with relative hypotension, generally considered a systolic blood pressure of less than 90 mm Hg. These patients frequently have symptomatic hypotension despite adequate filling pressures and are generally unresponsive to, or intolerant of, intravenous vasodilating medications such as nesiritide or nitroglycerin. Intravenous inotropes also should be considered in patients presenting with peripheral hypoperfusion and evidence of fluid overload that is not responding to intravenous diuretics or patients who are noted to have worsening renal function.

Because of the data presented linking inotropes to worsening morbidity, administration of vasodilators is usually considered instead of intravenous inotropes. However, use

of vasodilators as a first-line agent may be very challenging in patients with hypotension, and these agents need to be used in conjunction with a catecholamine agent to offset the direct vasodilation. Also, intravenous inotropes are not recommended unless left heart filling pressures are known to be elevated or cardiac index is severely impaired based on right heart catheterization data or clear-cut clinical signs of hypoperfusion (generally the "wet and cold" patient)

Brain Natriuretic Peptide

One vasodilating agent, brain natriuretic peptide (BNP), has received a great deal of attention, initially very positive and then negative owing to a meta-analysis suggesting substantive worsening renal function with the drug (the results of which have been largely refuted by clinical trial data) (Fig. 3-24).[45–50] This synthetic vasodilator is a mimic of one of the naturally occurring family of natriuretic peptides, which are intrinsic regulators of salt and water balance in the body (Fig. 3-25).

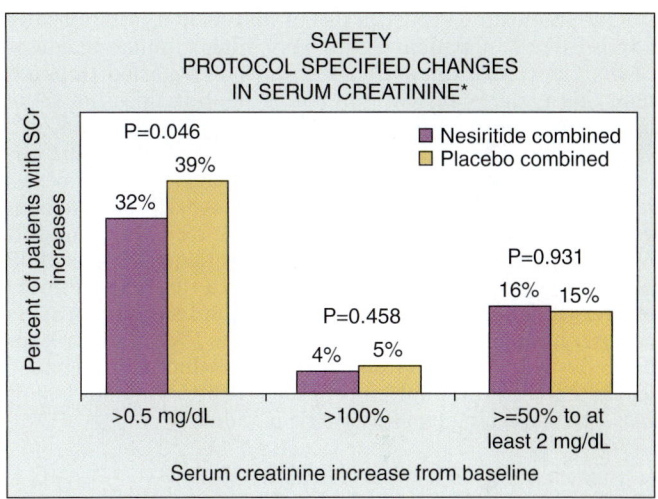

*Outpatient clinic visit values only

FIGURE 3-24 Results of FUSION 3 trial comparing change in renal function in patients treated with either intermittent infusions of brain natriuretic peptide (BNP) or placebo, showing no adverse impact with BNP in a controlled trial. SCr, serum creatinine.

PHYSIOLOGY OF NATRIURETIC PEPTIDES

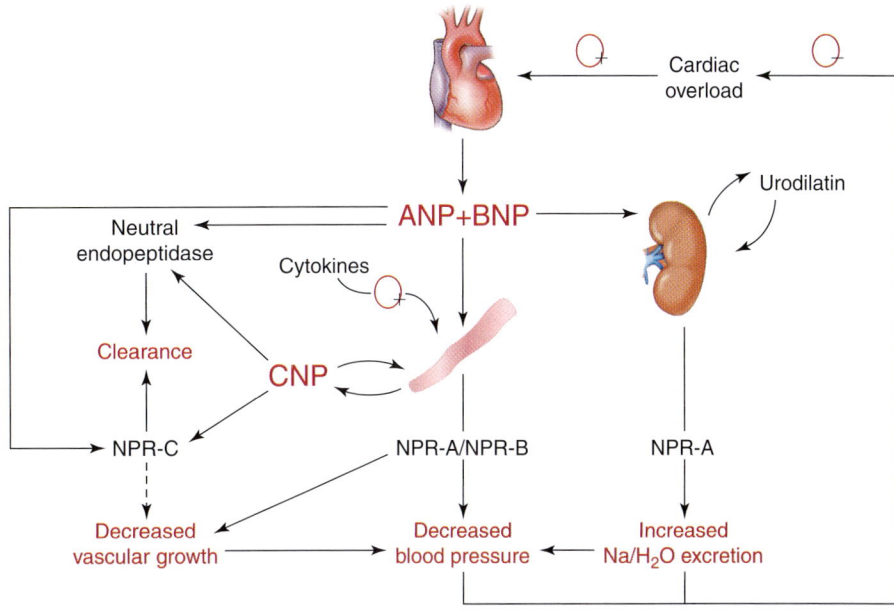

FIGURE 3-25 Physiology of natriuretic peptides. ANP, A-type natriuretic peptide; BNP, B-type natriuretic peptide; NPR, natriuretic peptide receptor A, B, C. *(Adapted from Wilkins MR, Redondo J, Brown LA. The natriuretic-peptide family. Lancet. 1997;349:1307-1310.)*

One of the early and few prospective placebo-controlled randomized trials in ADHF was the VMAC (Vasodilator Management of Heart Failure Trial),[45] which compared BNP with intravenous nitroglycerin and placebo. The primary endpoint was reduction of pulmonary capillary wedge pressure and subjective relief of dyspnea. Both of these endpoints were positive in favor of BNP (Fig. 3-26). The potency of the effect of BNP to increase diuresis and salt excretion is also controversial, but when used within the doses prescribed in the package insert, BNP may be beneficial. Timing of the use of these agents remains controversial.

The potential benefit of BNP in the treatment of ADHF is expected to be clarified with the release of the results of the very large ASCEND trial, which involves greater than 7000 patients who were randomly assigned to BNP infusion or placebo.[49] The trial went to completion without stoppage by the Data Safety Monitoring Board for concerns regarding adverse effects, perhaps showing, at the least, the prior meta-analyses concluding nesiritide was associated with substantive problems with renal dysfunction were flawed by the very nature of such studies.[50]

One interesting aspect of use of BNP is that it is typically administered in patients with very high circulating levels of BNP. Several explanations have been suggested to elucidate this paradox of why the native peptide does not seem to work (i.e., high levels in the blood, despite advanced HF). One attractive hypothesis is that the BNP protein in the circulation has undergone a "folding" or confirmational change induced by the hypoxic stress of advanced HF and no longer can bind or occupy the unique BNP receptors. Support for this hypothesis is that when the synthetic form of BNP (nesiritide) is given intravenously, often a response in terms of lowering of cardiac filling pressures and some diuresis is seen within minutes, as was shown in the VMAC trial. Other hypotheses include a mutant form is produced in response to HF that also does not bind to the receptor. A good deal of research is ongoing to address this paradox.

Intravenous Vasopressors

The use of catecholamines in doses where there is significant vasoconstriction is usually reserved for patients in shock in whom mean coronary and renal artery pressures are compromised and an increase in blood pressure cannot be achieved by increasing blood flow via inotropes or vasodilators. However, their routine use, especially in significant doses, typically increases the peripheral vascular resistance (afterload) in both the systemic and the pulmonary vascular beds and can be associated with a decline in function and increased filling pressures. An intra-aortic balloon counterpulsation pump (see Chapter 8) often is preferable in treating these patients.

CARDIORENAL SYNDROME

Patients hospitalized for ADHF and undergoing aggressive therapies to relieve congestion and ameliorate symptoms are at high risk for the development of worsening renal dysfunction, or the cardiorenal syndrome.[51-55] Careful follow-up for the development of renal dysfunction in patients treated particularly with aggressive dosing of diuretics is essential. Patients with moderate to severe renal dysfunction and volume overload should continue to receive diuretics when there is continued severe fluid overload noting that renal dysfunction may improve with diuresis as the mesentery becomes decongested and perfusion pressures improve across the renal beds. Table 3-11 presents a composite overview of the impact of worsening renal function on clinical outcomes and resource consumption when worsening renal failure manifests in hospitalized patients. In-hospital mortality is double in patients with worsening renal function with hospital length of stay being about 9.1 days versus 6.9 days in patients without cardiorenal syndrome. Hospital costs are also dramatically increased in these patients.

Table 3-12 presents an evolving classification of cardiorenal syndrome.[53] Type I refers to acute cardiorenal syndrome or an abrupt worsening of cardiac function leading to acute kidney injury and generally includes patients with acute cardiogenic shock or severely decompensated HF. Type II or chronic cardiorenal syndrome includes patients with chronic CHF. In these patients, chronic abnormalities in cardiac function cause an aggressive and potentially permanent chronic kidney injury. Type III or acute cardiorenal syndrome includes patients with acute kidney ischemia or glomerulonephritis and results in abrupt worsening of renal function

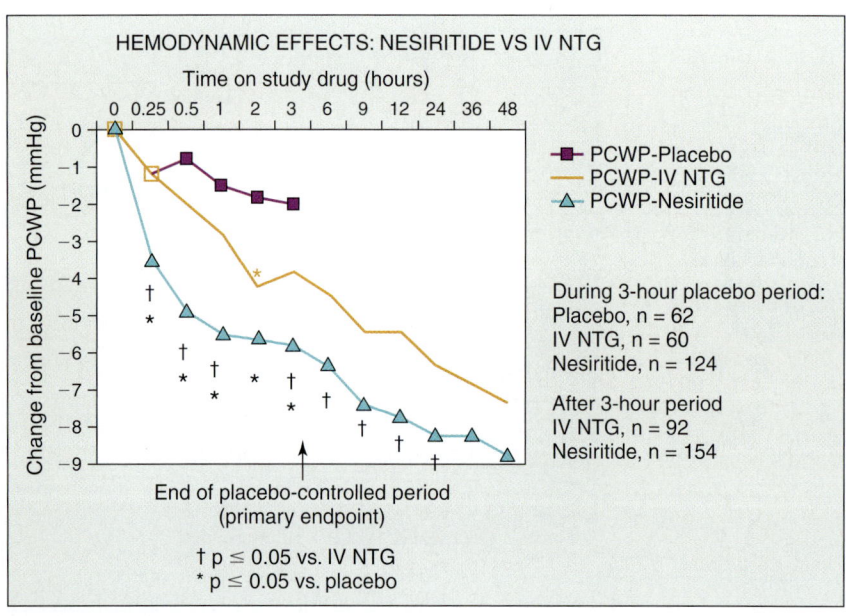

FIGURE 3-26 Results of OPTIME study comparing changes in pulmonary capillary wedge pressure (PCWP) over time with infusion of brain natriuretic peptide, intravenous nitroglycerin (IV NTG), and placebo. *(Data from Publication Committee for the VMAC Investigators [Vasodilatation in the Management of Acute CHF]. Intravenous nesiritide vs nitroglycerin for treatment of decompensated congestive heart failure: a randomized controlled trial. JAMA 2002;287:1531-1540.)*

TABLE 3-11	Impact of Worsening Renal Function on Patient Clinical Outcomes and Resource Consumption			
Outcomes	%	WRF Absent	WRF Present	Adjusted Odds Ratios (95% Confidence Intervals)
In-hospital mortality	4	3	7	2.72 (1.6-4.6)
30-day mortality	7	6	10	1.87 (1.2-2.8)
30-day readmission (all-cause)	18	17	20	1.29 (1.0-1.7)
30-day readmission (HF)	7	7	8	1.17 (0.8-1.8)
6-mo mortality	21	19	25	1.56 (1.2-2.0)
6-mo readmission (all-cause)	47	46	50	1.16 (0.9-1.4)
6-mo readmission (HF)	23	22	25	1.07 (0.8-1.4)
LOS (days)	7.5 ± 4.7	6.9 ± 3.9	9.1 ± 6.0	2.28 (0.25)
Hospital cost ($)	6823 ± 5175	6327 ± 4874	8085 ± 5665	1758 ± 287.2

HF, heart failure; LOS, length of stay; WRF, worsening renal function.
From Krumholz HM, Chen YT, Vaccarino V, et al. Correlates and impact on outcomes of worsening renal function in patients > or = 65 years of age with heart failure. *Am J Cardiol.* 2000;85:1110-1113.

TABLE 3-12	Cardiorenal Syndromes
Type I	Acute cardiorenal syndrome; acute cardiogenic shock or ADHF; abrupt worsening of cardiac function leading to acute kidney injury
Type II	Chronic cardiorenal syndrome; chronic cardiac failure; chronic abnormalities in cardiac function causing progressive and potentially permanent chronic kidney disease
Type III	Acute cardiorenal syndrome; acute kidney ischemia or glomerulonephritis; abrupt worsening of renal function causing acute cardiac disorder
Type IV	Chronic cardiorenal syndrome; chronic glomerular or interstitial disease; chronic kidney disease contributing to decreased cardiac function, cardiac hypertrophy, or increased risk of adverse cardiovascular events
Type V	Secondary cardiorenal syndrome; diabetes mellitus; sepsis; systemic condition causing both cardiac and renal dysfunction

ADHF, acute decompensated heart failure.
Data from Ronco C, Haapio M, House AA, et al. Cardiorenal syndrome. *J Am Coll Cardiol.* 2008;52:1527-1539.

that causes congestion and ADHF. Type IV is chronic cardiorenal syndrome and generally includes patients with chronic glomerular or interstitial disease (chronic kidney disease) that contributes to decreased cardiac function, cardiac hypertrophy, or increased risk of adverse cardiac events. Type V cardiorenal syndrome is seen in patients with underlying conditions such as diabetes mellitus, sepsis, or other systemic conditions causing both cardiac and renal dysfunction.

The pathophysiology of cardiorenal syndrome is complicated, and controversy exists regarding the most important underlying features. Drug toxicity and side effects of diuretics can precipitate renal dysfunction in patients with ADHF. However, hypoperfusion of the mesentery, particularly the renal parenchyma, is important.[43,44] Generally, hypoperfusion is seen with a low cardiac index, but perfusion across the mesentery bed is related to afferent pressure and flow juxtaposed to efferent pressure and flow, as alluded to earlier. A patient with ADHF frequently has substantial mesenteric congestion that causes a decline in perfusion pressure across the renal beds and contributes to worsening renal function. The central venous pressure is arguably the most important

factor in ADHF patients who develop worsening renal function (see Fig. 3-18). Cardiac index, although undoubtedly important, plays less of a role. Addressing mesenteric congestion with diuretics and optimization of intravascular volume seems crucial to preventing, and possibly treating, cardiorenal syndrome.

ULTRAFILTRATION

Because of the toxicities associated with diuretics and morbidity of congestion, techniques to "unload" mechanically or decongest patients by reducing venous congestion have been explored, including hemofiltration, hemodialysis, and more recently ultrafiltration. Although it does not decrease serum creatinine, ultrafiltration removes an ultrafiltrate that does not cause significant electrolyte disturbances and can remove 22 to 25 L of fluid per day (Fig. 3-27). Ultrafiltration was shown to be superior to aggressive doses of intravenous diuretics in the UNLOAD (Ultrafiltration versus Intravenous Diuretics for Patients Hospitalized with Acute Decompensated Heart

FLUID REMOVAL BY ULTRAFILTRATION

- Ultrafiltration can remove fluid from the blood at the same rate that fluid can be naturally recruited from the tissue

- The transient removal of blood elicits compensatory mechanisms, termed *plasma* or *intravascular refill* (PR), aimed at minimizing this reduction

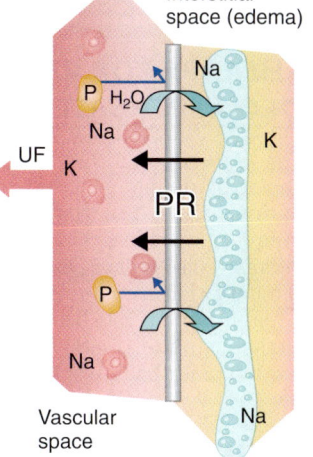

FIGURE 3-27 Fluid removal by ultrafiltration (UF). *(Data from Lauer A, Saccaggi A, Ronco C, et al. Continuous arteriovenous hemofiltration in the critically ill patient: clinical use and operational characteristics.* Ann Intern Med. *1983;99:455-460; and Marenzi G, Lauri G, Grazi M, et al. Circulatory response to fluid overload removal by extracorporeal ultrafiltration in refractory congestive heart failure.* J Am Coll Cardiol. *2001;38:963-968.)*

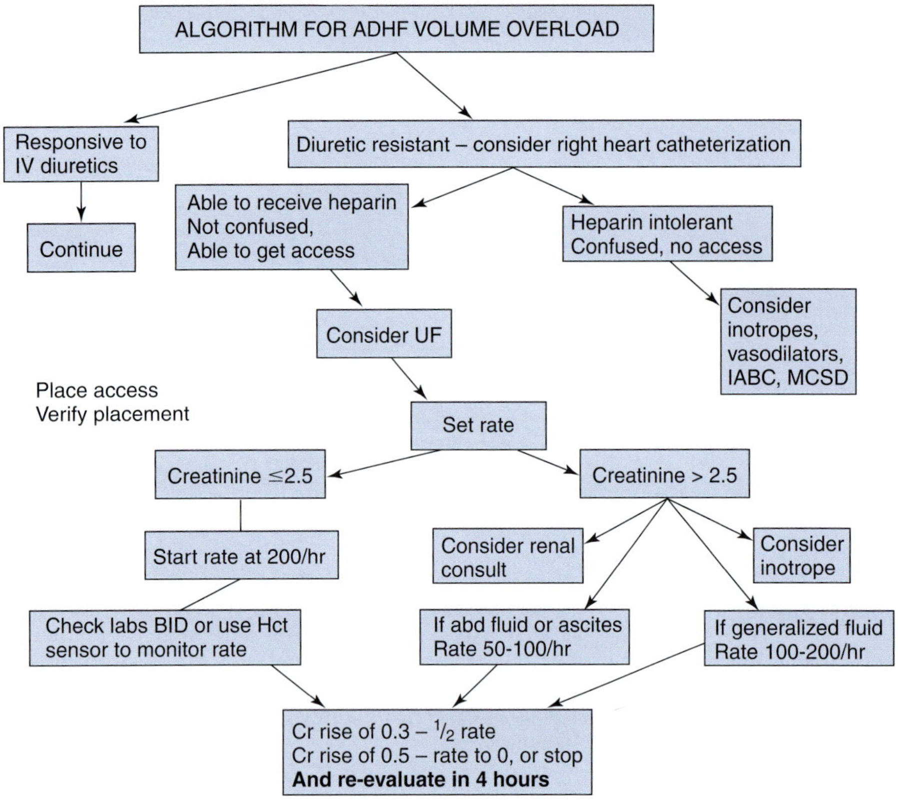

CH 3

FIGURE 3-28 Suggested algorithm for management of patients admitted with acute decompensated heart failure (ADHF). ADHF, acute decompensated heart failure; IABC, intraaortic balloon counterpulsation; MCSD, mechanical circulatory support device; UF, ultrafiltration; Cr, creatnine.

Failure) trial, which evaluated mechanical strategies for fluid removal that used a simple machine to achieve ultrafiltration.[54] The percentage of patients free from recurrent hospitalization was greater among patients undergoing ultrafiltration versus standard care, an increasingly important goal of any therapy for ADHF.[55] The ultrafiltration arm had higher cardiac index during the treatments; this gives rise to the consideration of this approach to unstable patients with ADHF who have mesenteric congestion. Diuretics are typically withheld during ultrafiltration, and serum creatinine often decreases and remains low for a period of time. However, similar to any of the options for treatment of patients with cardiorenal syndrome this therapy can be associated with worsening renal function, especially if the removal rate per hour is too high.

THERAPY FOR REFRACTORY ACUTE DECOMPENSATED HEART FAILURE

For patients admitted with ADHF who are in cardiogenic shock or do not respond to the aforementioned treatment options (Fig. 3-28), there is an increasing use of temporary or long-term mechanical circulatory support (see Chapter 8 for details). The criteria used to determine when a patient has refractory HF are evolving, but strategies that employ their use when a patient has been shown to be deteriorating or unresponsive to the aforementioned therapies seem to offer a better outcome. Trials are under way to examine this question.

SUMMARY

Despite more days spent for the care of HF patients than any other diagnosis, there is a very limited evidence base to guide management of hospitalized patients with ADHF. Nonetheless, there has been progress.[55] Two registries have helped define the demographics of patients hospitalized with ADHF. Patients

hospitalized with ADHF are elderly with an average age of 73 years; prevalence is equal between men and women; and ADHF has the highest readmission rate of any other diagnosis, which confirms the ineffectiveness of current therapeutic options. Risk factors have been identified for mortality with ADHF and emphasize the importance of cardiorenal syndrome. There are a host of reasons for worsening HF requiring admission to the hospital, and compliance with complex, multidrug regimens and salt and water use lead the list. The increasing number of hospitalizations warrants new approaches to disease management, including strategies such as increased patient education, use of telemedicine, and early and frequent office visits to intervene early before readmission is required.

REFERENCES

1. Krikler DM. Thomas Lewis, a father of modern cardiology. *Heart.* 1997;77:102–103.
2. Katz AM. The "modern" view of heart failure: how did we get here? *Circ Heart Fail.* 2008;1:63–67.
3. Lindenfeld J, Albert NM, Boehmer JP, et al. Executive summary: HFSA 2010 comprehensive heart failure practice guideline. *J Card Fail.* 2010;16:475–506.
4. Cotter G, Felker M, Adams KF, et al. The pathophysiology of acute heart failure—is it all about fluid accumulation? *Am Heart J.* 2008;155:9–18.
5. Metra M, Dei Cas L, Bristow MR. The pathophysiology of acute heart failure—it is a lot about fluid accumulation. *Am Heart J.* 2008;155:1–5.
6. Fonarow GC, Heywood JT, Heidenreich PA, et al. Temporal trends in clinical characteristics, treatments, and outcomes for heart failure hospitalizations, 2002 to 2004: findings from Acute Decompensated Heart Failure National Registry (ADHERE). *Am Heart J.* 2007;153:1021–1028.
7. Fonarow GC, Abraham WT, Albert NM, et al. Organized Program to Initiate Lifesaving Treatment in Hospitalized Patients with Heart Failure (OPTIMIZE-HF): rationale and design. *Am Heart J.* 2004;148:43–51.
8. Adams KF, Fonarow GC, Emerman CL, et al. Characteristics and outcomes of patients hospitalized for heart failure in the United States: rationale, design, and preliminary observations from the first 100,000 cases in the Acute Decompensated Heart Failure National Registry (ADHERE). *Am Heart J.* 2005;149:209–216.
9. Chatti R, Fradj NB, Travelsi W, et al. Algorithm for therapeutic management of acute heart failure syndromes. *Heart Fail Rev.* 2007;12:113–117.
10. Goldsmith SR, Brandimarte F, Gheorghiade M. Congestion as a therapeutic target in acute heart failure syndromes. *Prog Cardiovasc Dis.* 2010;52:383–392.
11. Jessup M, Abraham WT, Casey DE, et al. 2009 focused update: ACC/AHA guidelines for the diagnosis and management of heart failure. *Circulation.* 2009;119:1977–2016.

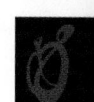

12. Hunt SA, Abraham W, Chin MH, et al. ACC/AHA 2005 guideline update for the diagnosis and management of chronic heart failure in the adult. *Circulation.* 2005;112:1825–1852.

13. Dickstein K, Cohen-Solal A, Filippatos G, et al. ESC guidelines for the diagnosis and treatment of acute and chronic heart failure 2008. *Eur Heart J.* 2008;29:2388–2442.

14. Thom T, Haase N, Rosamond W, et al. Heart disease and stroke statistics. *Circulation.* 2006;113:e85–e151.

15. Williams JF, Bristow MR, Fowler MB. Guidelines for the evaluation and management of heart failure. *Circulation.* 1995;92:2764–2784.

16. Fonarow GC. Overview of acutely decompensated congestive heart failure (ADHF): a report from the ADHERE Registry. *Heart Fail Rev.* 2004;9:179–185.

17. Abraham WT, Kirkwood KF, Fonarow GC, et al. In-hospital mortality in patients with acute decompensated heart failure requiring intravenous vasoactive medications: an analysis from the Acute Decompensated Heart Failure National Registry (ADHERE). *J Am Coll Cardiol.* 2005;46:57–64.

18. Fonarow GC, Adams KF, Abraham WT, et al. Risk stratification for in-hospital mortality in acutely decompensated heart failure: classification and regression tree analysis. *JAMA.* 2005;293:572–580.

19. Yancy CW, Lopatin M, Stevenson LW, et al. Clinical presentation, management, and in-hospital outcomes of patients admitted with acute decompensated heart failure with preserved systolic function: a report from the Acute Decompensated Heart Failure National Registry (ADHERE) database. *J Am Coll Cardiol.* 2006;47:76–84.

20. Peacock WF, Fonarow GC, Emerman CL, et al. Impact of early initiation of intravenous therapy for acute decompensated heart failure on outcomes in ADHERE. *Cardiology.* 2007;107:44–51.

21. Costanzo MR, Mills RM, Wynne J. Characteristics of "stage D" heart failure: insights from the Acute Decompensated Heart Failure National Registry Longitudinal Module (ADHERE LM). *Am Heart J.* 2008;155:339–347.

22. Maisel AS, Peacock WF, McMullin N, et al. Timing of immunoreactive B-type natriuretic peptide levels and treatment delay in acute decompensated heart failure: an ADHERE analysis. *J Am Coll Cardiol.* 2008;52:534–540.

23. Gheorghiade M, Abraham WT, Albert NM, et al. Systolic blood pressure at admission, clinical characteristics, and outcomes in patients hospitalized with acute heart failure. *JAMA.* 2006;296:2217–2226.

24. Fonarow GC, Gattis Stough W, Abraham WT, et al. Characteristics, treatments, and outcomes of patients with preserved systolic function hospitalized for heart failure: a report from the OPTIMIZE-HF Registry. *J Am Coll Cardiol.* 2007;50:768–777.

25. Fonarow GC, Abraham WT, Albert NM, et al. Prospective evaluation of beta-blocker use at the time of hospital discharge as a heart failure performance measure: results from OPTIMIZE-HF. *J Card Fail.* 2007;13:722–731.

26. Fonarow GC, Peacock WF, Phillips CO, et al. Admission B-type natriuretic peptide levels and in-hospital mortality in acute decompensated heart failure. *J Am Coll Cardiol.* 2007;49:1943–1950.

27. Fonarow GC, Stough WG, Abraham WT, et al. Characteristics, treatments and outcomes of patients with preserved systolic function hospitalized for heart failure: a report from the OPTIMIZE-HF Registry. *J Am Coll Cardiol.* 2007;50:768–777.

28. Fonarow GC, Abraham WT, Labert NM, et al. Factors identified as precipitating hospital admissions for heart failure and clinical outcomes: findings from the OPTIMIZE-HF. *Arch Intern Med.* 2008;168:847–854.

29. Fonarow GC, Abraham WT, Albert NM, et al. A smoker's paradox in patients hospitalized for heart failure: findings from OPTIMIZE-HF. *Eur Heart J.* 2008;29:1983–1991.

30. Fonarow GC, Abraham WT, Albert NM, et al. Influence of beta-blocker continuation or withdrawal on outcomes in patients hospitalized with heart failure: findings from the OPTIMIZE-HF program. *J Am Coll Cardiol.* 2008;52:190–199.

31. Abraham WT, Fonarow GC, Albert NM, et al. Predictors of in-hospital mortality in patients hospitalized for heart failure. *J Am Coll Cardiol.* 2008;52:347–356.

32. Curtis LH, Greiner MA, Hammill BG, et al. Representativeness of a national heart failure quality-of-care registry: comparison of OPTIMIZE-HF and non-OPTIMIZE-HF Medicare patients. *Circ Cardiovasc Qual Outcomes.* 2009;2:377–384.

33. O'Connor CM, Abraham WT, Albert NM, et al. Predictors of mortality after discharge in patients hospitalized with heart failure: an analysis from the Organized Program to Initiate Lifesaving Treatment in Hospitalized Patients with Heart Failure (OPTIMIZE-HF). *Am Heart J.* 2008;156:662–673.

34. Cuffe MS, Califf RM, Adams KF, et al. Short-term intravenous milrinone for acute exacerbation of chronic heart failure: a randomized controlled trial (OPTIME-CHF). *JAMA.* 2002;287:1578–1580.

35. Wagner EH. Deconstructing heart failure disease management. Robert Wood Johnson Foundation. *Ann Intern Med.* 2004;141:644–646.

36. Akashi YJ, Nef HM, Mollman H, et al. Stress cardiomyopathy. *Annu Rev Med.* 2010;61:271–286.

37. Binanay C, Califf RM, Hasselblad V, et al, ESCAPE investigators. Evaluation study of congestive heart failure and pulmonary artery catheterization effectiveness: the ESCAPE trial. *JAMA.* 2005;294:1625–1633.

38. Yusuf S, Pfeffer MA, Swedberg K, et al, CHARM Investigators and Committees. Effects of candesartan in patients with chronic heart failure and preserved left-ventricular ejection the CHARM-Preserved trial. *Lancet.* 2003;362:777–781.

39. Forrester JS, Diamond GA, Swan HJC. Correlative classification of clinical and hemodynamic function after acute myocardial infarction. *Am J Cardiol.* 1977;39:137–145.

40. Steimle AE, Stevenson LW, Chelimsky-Fallick C, et al. Sustained hemodynamic efficacy of therapy tailored to reduce filling pressures in survivors with advanced heart failure. *Circulation.* 1997;96:1165–1172.

41. Lucas C, Johnson W, Hamilton MA, et al. Freedom from congestion predicts good survival despite previous class IV symptoms of heart failure. *Am Heart J.* 2000;140:840–847.

42. Felker GM, O'Conner CM, Braunwald E Heart Failure Clinical Network investigators. Loop diuretics in acute decompensated heart failure. Necessary? Evil? A necessary Evil? *Circ Heart Fail.* 2009;2:56–62 Presented at the American College of Cardiology Scientific Sessions, Atlanta GA, March 2010.

43. Mullens W, Abrahams Z, Skouri HN, et al. Elevated intra-abdominal pressure in acute decompensated heart failure: a potential contributor to worsening renal function? *J Am Coll Cardiol.* 2008;51:300–306.

44. Mullens W, Abrahams Z, Francis GS, et al. Importance of venous congestion for worsening of renal function in advanced decompensated heart failure. *J Am Coll Cardiol.* 2009;53:589–596.

45. Publication Committee for the VMAC Investigators. Intravenous nesiritide vs nitroglycerin for treatment of decompensated congestive heart failure. *JAMA.* 2002;287:1531–1540.

46. Sackner-Bernstein JD, Skopicki HA, Aaronson KD. Risk of worsening renal function with nesiritide in patients with acutely decompensated heart failure. *Circulation.* 2005;111:1487–1491.

47. Sackner-Bernstein JD, Kowalski M, Fox M, et al. Short term risk of death after treatment with nesiritide for decompensated heart failure: a pooled analysis of randomized controlled trials. *JAMA.* 2005;293:1900–1905.

48. Burnett JC, Korinek J. The tumultuous journey of nesiritide: past, present and future. *Circ Heart Fail.* 2008;1:1–6.

49. Hernandez AF, O'Conner CM, Starling RC, et al. Rationale and design of the Acute Study of Clinical Effectiveness of Nesiritide in Decompensated Heart Failure Trial (ASCEND-HF). *Am Heart J.* 2009;157:271–277.

50. Heywood JT. The cardiorenal syndrome: lessons from the ADHERE database and treatment options. *Heart Fail Rev.* 2004;9:195–201.

51. Krumholz HM, Chen YT, Vaccarino V, et al. Correlates and impact on outcomes of worsening renal function in patients > or = 65 years of age with heart failure. *Am J Cardiol.* 2000;85:1110–1113.

52. Jessup M, Costanzo MR. The cardiorenal syndrome: do we need a change of strategy or a change of tactics? *J Am Coll Cardiol.* 2009;53:597–599.

53. Ronco C, Haapio M, House AA, et al. Cardiorenal syndrome. *J Am Coll Cardiol.* 2008;52:1527–1539.

54. Costanzo MR, Guglin ME, Saltzberg MT, et al. Ultrafiltration versus intravenous diuretics for patients hospitalized for acute decompensated heart failure. *J Am Coll Cardiol.* 2007;49:675–683.

55. Bueno H, Ross JS, Wang Y, et al. Trends in length of stay and short-term outcomes among Medicare patients hospitalized for heart failure 1993–2006. *JAMA.* 2010;303:2141–2147.

CHAPTER **4**

Pathophysiology of Stage D Heart Failure

J. Thomas Heywood, Shradha Rathi, and Brian Jaski

INTRODUCTION

The syndrome of congestive heart failure (CHF) represents a profound derangement of otherwise finely tuned physiologic mechanisms to maintain blood pressure and fluid balance. These mechanisms evolved over many millions of years to overcome the hemodynamic effects of gravity and at the same time protect an internal fluid and electrolyte balance reflective of the oceans from which the first humans emerged. Multiple systems are required to ensure homeostasis in an often hostile environment where salt and water, previously ubiquitous, were often in life-threateningly short supply. Trauma was common, and fast-acting physiologic responses were necessary to ensure survival.

The multiple, interlocking neurohormonal processes that evolved over the millennia were not designed to cope with the unaccustomed dangers imposed by an industrial society awash in salt, overabundant nutrients, and much longer life expectancies. For centuries, physicians confronted by the undeniable features of the heart failure (HF) syndrome tried to relieve their patients' suffering by developing models based on their contemporaneous worldview to explain the disease process and propose therapy, ranging across time from bloodletting to surgical replacement of the heart itself.

Understanding of the HF syndrome has evolved over time and can best be divided into four eras, as follows:

1. The *descriptive era,* beginning with Egyptian, Greek, and Arab physicians and extending to the clinicians of the 19th century, slowly developed a catalog of signs and symptoms of CHF.
2. The *hemodynamic era* largely began in the 20th century but with roots established by Harvey in the 16th century and Hales in the 18th century and ushered in quantitative measurement of cardiac function and exposed the hemodynamic basis for the HF syndrome (Figs. 4-1 and 4-2).
3. The *neurohormonal era* built on deepening understanding of biochemical processes and produced an extensive catalogue of neurohormonal alterations associated with HF. The most important development from this time was a

medical armamentarium with proven efficacy in reducing morbidity and mortality (Fig. 4-3). Over the last 30 years, this model has been spectacular and powerful, although more recent attempts to create medical therapies have been repeatedly disappointing.

4. The *biomechanical era* has combined advances in medicine and engineering to devise mechanical solutions for HF ranging from valves, to pacemaker/defibrillators, to replacements for the entire heart. More recently, mechanical platforms have provided a means of monitoring hemodynamic parameters to help modify dysfunctional physiologic mechanisms (Fig. 4-4).

Great strides have been made in understanding the pathophysiology of CHF. However, just as each generation has the good fortune to benefit from the work and insight of its predecessors, our worldview and still imperfect tools limit our vision to "understand" HF completely. Younger clinicians still have much work to do correct the incomplete picture of a disease that continues to affect millions.

CAUSES OF HEART FAILURE SYNDROME

Ischemic Myocardial Injury

Ischemic myocardial injury results from severe impairment of coronary blood supply to the heart. The primary cause is the formation of a thrombus in the coronary artery; other causes include arterial spasm and embolism. With interruption of cardiac blood flow, muscle damage extends rapidly from endocardium to epicardium. Myocardial necrosis induces complement activation and free radical generation, triggering a cytokine cascade. Studies have shown the relationship of myocardial ischemic injury to the major modes of cell death—oncosis and apoptosis.[1] Numerous processes can influence profoundly the evolution of myocardial ischemic injury. Timely reperfusion produces major effects on ischemic myocardium, including a component of reperfusion injury and a greater amount of salvage of myocardium.[2,3] Most of the treatments and interventions for

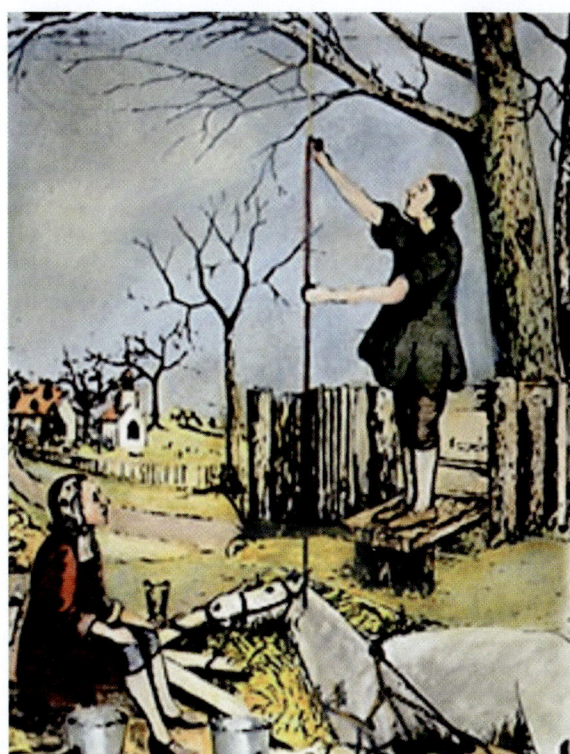

FIGURE 4-1 Stephan Kales measuring arterial blood pressure in a horse via the carotid artery in 1727. *(From Stephen Hates carotid artery cannulation. Encyclopaedia Britannica Online. The Granger Collection, New York.)*

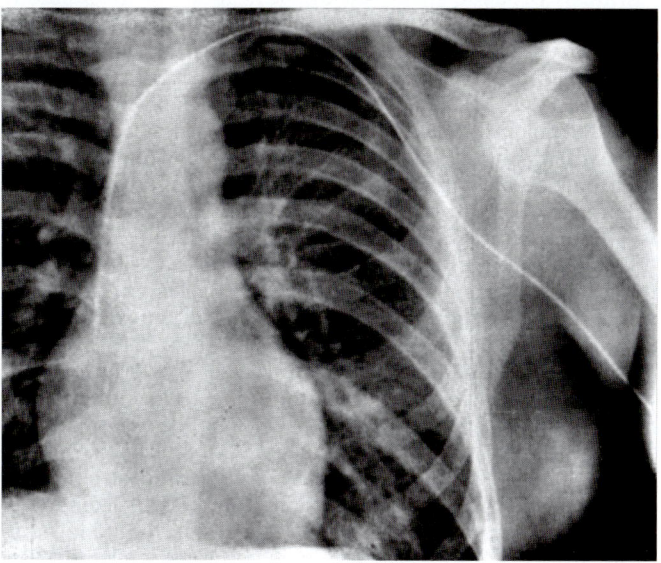

FIGURE 4-2 Chest x-ray of Werner Forssmann demonstrating the first central venous catheterization in a human (himself) from the brachial vein in 1929. *(From Forssmann W. Die Sondierung der Recten Herzens. Klim Wochensch 1929;45:2085–2086.)*

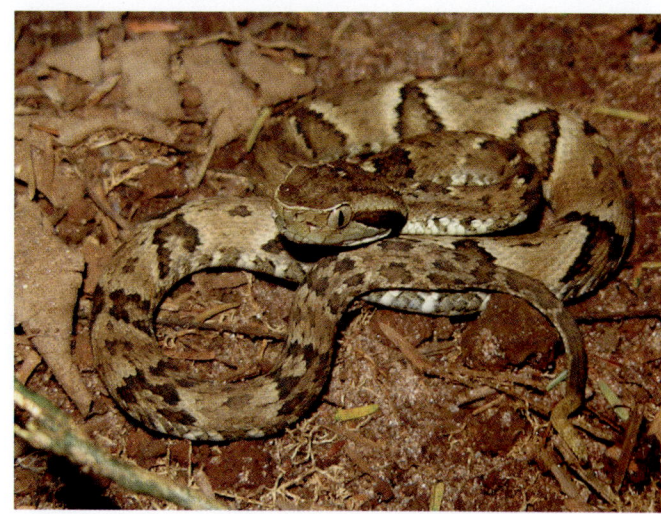

FIGURE 4-3 Sergio Ferraria isolated a component from the venom of the Brazilian viper *Bothrops jararaca* that potentiated the effects of bradykinin, most likely by inhibiting the action of angiotensin-converting enzyme. This led to the development of captopril, the first angiotensin-converting enzyme inhibitor (ACEI). *(From http://commons.wikimedia.org/wiki/File:Jararaca-verdadeira.jpg.)*

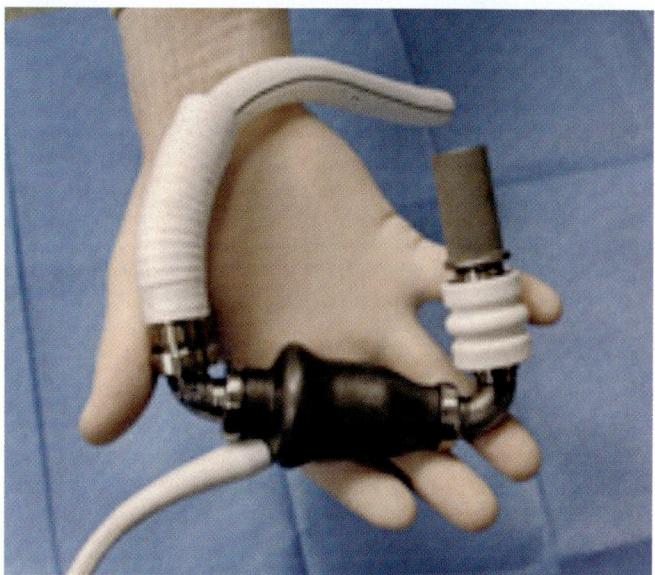

FIGURE 4-4 HeartMate II was approved for destination therapy in 2010.

acute myocardial infarction are targeted toward restoring blood flow, reducing the risk of reinfarction, reducing oxygen demands on the injured ventricle, and altering dynamics to limit ventricular remodeling and development of HF.[4]

After an acute myocardial infarction, early and successful myocardial reperfusion with the use of thrombolytic therapy or primary percutaneous coronary intervention is the most effective strategy for reducing the size of a myocardial infarct and improving the clinical outcome. However, the process of restoring blood flow to the ischemic myocardium can paradoxically induce irreversible tissue injury and cell necrosis, known as *myocardial reperfusion injury*.[5] Although early reperfusion of the heart is essential in preventing further tissue damage secondary to ischemia, reintroduction of blood flow can expedite the death of vulnerable but still viable myocardial tissue, by initiating a series of events involving both intracellular and extracellular mechanisms. In the last decade, extensive efforts have focused on the role of cytotoxic reactive oxygen species, complement activation, neutrophil adhesion, and the interactions between complement and neutrophils during myocardial reperfusion injury (Box 4-1).[6]

Inflammatory Myocardial Injury

The cause of myocarditis often remains unknown; various infections, systemic diseases, drugs, and toxins have been associated with this disease. Viruses, bacteria, and protozoa have been implicated as infectious agents. There is a consensus that viruses are a frequent cause of myocarditis in North America and Europe.

BOX 4-1 Causes of Myocardial Injury Leading to Cardiomyopathy and Heart Failure

Secondary to other cardiovascular disease
  Ischemia
  Reperfusion ischemic injury
  Hypertension
  Valvular disease
  Tachycardia-induced
Infectious
  Viral—coxsackieviruses (A and B), influenza virus (A and B),
    adenovirus, echovirus, rabies, hepatitis, yellow fever, small-
    pox, lymphocytic choriomeningitis, epidemic hemorrhagic
    fever, chikungunya, dengue fever, cytomegalovirus, Epstein-
    Barr virus, rubeola, rubella, mumps, respiratory syncytial
    virus, varicella-zoster virus, human immunodeficiency virus
  Rickettsial
  Bacterial
  Metazoal
  Protozoal
  Probable infectious—Whipple disease, Lyme disease
Metabolic
  Endocrine diseases—hyperthyroidism, hypothyroidism, acromeg-
    aly, myxedema, hypoparathyroidism, hyperparathyroidism
  Diabetes mellitus
  Electrolyte imbalance—potassium, phosphate, magnesium, other
  Nutritional—thiamine deficiency (beriberi), protein deficiency,
    starvation, carnitine deficiency
Toxic
  Drugs
  Alcohol
  Foods
  Anesthetic gases
  Heavy metals
  Poisons
Collagen-vascular disease
  Systemic lupus erythematosus
  Rheumatoid arthritis
  Progressive systemic sclerosis
  Polymyositis
  HLA-B12–associated cardiac disease
Infiltrative
  Hemochromatosis
  Amyloidosis
  Glycogen storage disease
Granulomatous (sarcoidosis)
Physical agents
  Extreme temperatures
  Ionizing radiation
  Electric shock
  Nonpenetrating thoracic injury (myocardial contusion)
Neuromuscular disorders
  Muscular dystrophy—limb-girdle (Erb dystrophy), Duchenne dys-
    trophy, fascioscapulohumeral (Landouzy-Dejerine dystrophy)
  Friedreich disease
  Myotonic dystrophy
Primary cardiac tumor (myxoma)
Peripartum
Immunologic
  Postvaccination
  Serum sickness
  Transplant rejection
Idiopathic

Viral Myocarditis

Viral myocarditis is one of the main causes of dilated cardiomyopathy and severe CHF. Initially, coxsackieviruses
(A and B) were thought to be the most common cause of
myocarditis because increasing antibody titers could be
shown in patients during acute myocarditis and convales-
cence. Later, other enteroviruses and adenoviruses were identified in endomyocardial biopsy specimens from patients
with clinically suspected myocarditis and from patients with
idiopathic dilated cardiomyopathy. For a long time, enteroviruses and adenoviruses have been considered the most common causes of viral myocarditis with possible transition to
dilated cardiomyopathy.

Viral myocarditis can produce variable degrees of illness, ranging from focal disease to diffuse pancarditis
involving myocardium, pericardium, and valve structures.
Many patients experience a flulike prodrome. Viral myocarditis is usually a self-limited, acute to subacute disease of the heart muscle that most often leads to dilated
cardiomyopathy and HF. Acute myocarditis is one of the
most challenging diagnoses in cardiology. At the present
time, no diagnostic "gold standard" is generally accepted,
owing to the insensitivity of traditional diagnostic tests.
In the past, percutaneous transvenous right ventricular
endomyocardial biopsy was used, but the Myocarditis
Treatment Trial[7] revealed no advantage for immunosuppressive therapy in biopsy-proven myocarditis, so biopsy
is not routinely performed in most cases. The need for new
diagnostic approaches resulted in the emergence of new
molecular tests and a more detailed immunohistochemical analysis of endomyocardial biopsy specimens. More
recent findings using these new diagnostic tests resulted in
increased interest in inflammatory cardiomyopathies and a
better understanding of its pathophysiology and the recognition of overlap of virus-mediated damage, inflammation,
and autoimmune dysregulation. Novel results also pointed
toward a broader spectrum of viral genomes responsible
for acute myocarditis, indicating a shift of enterovirus and
adenovirus to parvovirus B19 and human herpesvirus 6.[8]

The pathophysiology of myocardial injury in viral cardiomyopathy is that viruses affect myocardiocytes by direct cytotoxic effects and by cell-mediated (T-helper cells) destruction
of myofibers. Other mechanisms include disturbances in cellular metabolism, vascular supply of myocytes, and other
immunologic mechanisms. Because of an immunologic mechanism of myocyte destruction, several trials have investigated
the use of immunomodulatory medications. (Other trials are
currently being conducted.) According to Hahn and associates
in 1995,[7] the Myocarditis Treatment Trial showed no survival
benefit with prednisone plus cyclosporine or azathioprine in
patients with viral (lymphocytic) myocarditis. Randomized
trials are under way to evaluate intravenous immunoglobulin
as treatment for viral myocarditis.

Toxic Cardiomyopathy

Causes of toxic cardiomyopathy include certain drugs, poisons, foods, anesthetic gases, heavy metals, and alcohol.

Alcoholic Cardiomyopathy

Chronic alcoholism leads to the onset and progression of
alcoholic cardiomyopathy through toxic mechanisms of etha-
nol and its metabolite acetaldehyde. This toxic effect of alcohol on the heart affects the global left ventricular contractile
function leading to HF. The severity of the clinical symptoms is directly related to the amount and duration of alcohol
consumption.[9]

Cardiomyopathy Associated with Collagen-Vascular Disease

Several collagen-vascular diseases have been implicated in
the development of cardiomyopathies, including rheumatoid
arthritis, systemic lupus erythematosus, progressive systemic
sclerosis, and polymyositis. Diagnosis is based on identification of the underlying disease in conjunction with appropriate clinical findings of heart failure.

Granulomatous Cardiomyopathy (Sarcoidosis)

Cardiac involvement in sarcoidosis reportedly occurs in approximately 20% of cases. Endomyocardial biopsy is the most helpful diagnostic examination but has low sensitivity and low specificity because the involvement may be patchy, resulting in a negative biopsy finding. Noninvasive examination of microvolt T wave alternans is being studied as a useful diagnostic tool for detecting cardiac involvement in patients with sarcoidosis.[10] Noncaseating granulomatous infiltration of the myocardium occurs as with other organs affected by this disease. The sarcoid granulomas particularly affect the conduction system of the heart, left ventricular free wall, septum, papillary muscles, and, infrequently, heart valves.

Fibrosis and thinning of the myocardium occur as a result of the infiltrative process affecting the normal function of the myocardium. The diagnosis can also be made if some other tissue diagnosis is possible or available in conjunction with the appropriate clinical picture for HF. Patients often present with conduction disturbances or ventricular arrhythmias. In patients with normal left ventricular function, these conduction disturbances may be the primary clinical feature. Treatment of cardiac sarcoidosis with low-dose steroids may be beneficial, especially in patients with progressive disease, conduction defects, or ventricular arrhythmias.

Peripartum Cardiomyopathy

Peripartum cardiomyopathy (PPCM) is a rare form of cardiomyopathy of uncertain etiology that is defined as development of cardiac failure in the last month of pregnancy or within 5 months after delivery, absence of a demonstrable cause for the cardiac failure, absence of demonstrable heart disease before the last month of pregnancy, and documented systolic dysfunction. PPCM is more common in multiparous women. It has been reported more often in twin gestations and in women with preeclampsia, but both of these conditions are associated with a lower serum oncotic pressure that can predispose to noncardiogenic pulmonary edema in the setting of other stressors. Many cases of PPCM improve or resolve completely, but others progress to HF; an early diagnosis and medical treatment may affect the patient's long-term prognosis. The causes and pathogenesis are poorly understood. Multiple studies have focused on inflammatory, immunologic, and environmental causes; a novel hypothesis is a genetic cause.[11] Incidence in the United States ranges from 1 case per 1300, to 4000, to up to 15,000 live births. African American women have significantly higher odds of having PPCM[12]; 75% are diagnosed within the first month postpartum, and 45% present in the first week. Effective treatment reduces mortality rates and increases the number of women who fully recover left ventricular systolic function. Outcomes for subsequent pregnancy after PPCM are better in women who have first fully recovered heart function.[13]

Tachycardia-Induced Cardiomyopathy

Tachycardia-induced cardiomyopathy is a reversible cause of HF with improvement in ventricular function with rate or rhythm control. Rhythms causing tachycardia-induced cardiomyopathy include atrial fibrillation, atrial flutter, supraventricular tachycardia, ventricular tachycardia, fascicular tachycardia, ventricular ectopy, and persistent rapid DDD pacing. Persistent tachycardia is known to lead to myocyte dysfunction and cardiomyopathy.[14] The exact mechanisms by which tachycardia affects cell function are poorly understood. The possible mechanisms are depletion of energy stores, abnormal calcium channel activity, and abnormal

subendocardial oxygen delivery secondary to abnormalities in blood flow or reduced responsiveness to beta-adrenergic stimulation.

CARDIAC RESPONSE TO INJURY

In the absence of injury, the normal adult heart appears as a stable mechanical tissue pump adjusting performance to changes in loading conditions or inotropic state. Actually, the heart is a dynamic biologic structure with constant turnover of its intracellular contracting components associated with the continuous assembly and degradation of specific sarcomere proteins. The in vivo half-life of a protein is the time it takes for half of the amount of protein in a cell to break down after its synthesis in the cell. Troponin subunits (T/I/C) have half-lives of approximately 3 to 5 days; actin and tropomyosin, 7 to 10 days; and myosin, approximately 5 to 8 days.[15] The heart is an organ with potential for great plasticity primed for cellular modulation when changes in mechanical and molecular signals occur.

Myocardial injury alters the loading and biochemical environment of both impaired and uninjured cardiac cells. Endocrine, paracrine (on neighboring cells), autocrine (on the same cell), or intracrine (internally on the same cell without extracellular secretion) mechanisms all can contribute to a subsequent net biologic response.[16] As in other tissues, these signals potentially reinitiate a fetal growth repertoire of transcription and translation.[17,18] Over time, characteristic patterns of heart morphology emerge associated with progression of ventricular systolic or diastolic impairment (Fig. 4-5).

Shifts in the physical characteristics of the heart require an orchestrated sequence of cell proliferation, apoptosis, hypertrophy, and atrophy—a process referred to as *ventricular remodeling*.[17] Although remodeling may represent a reparative response to abnormal myocardial conditions, it generally contributes to ventricular dysfunction when fully manifest. This paradox may be explained partly by a limited set of mechanisms available to respond to cellular stress that evolved before current major causes of adult cardiac disability—coronary artery disease and hypertension—were prevalent.

In 1975, Grossman and coworkers[19] proposed the hypothesis that increased wall stress initiates concentric or dilated (eccentric) hypertrophy until regional wall stress returns to normal (Fig. 4-6). Since then, despite incomplete understanding, possible molecular bases of two essential components of this control circuit have been identified: (1) a mechanotransducer for detecting systolic versus diastolic stress and strain with a deformable enzymatic protein associated with the sarcomere (Fig. 4-7); (2) specific pathways to increased myofibril width (parallel sarcomere number) or length (series sarcomere number) during continuous myocyte contraction and relaxation.[20] Other components triggering hypertrophy could include stretch of the sarcomere-spanning protein titin[21] and modulation of other growth factors.

The extracellular environment provides scaffolding for and participates in differentiation of cardiac muscle and nonmuscle cells.[22] Extracellular matrix modifications[23] also are important components of ventricular remodeling. After ischemic or nonischemic insults, increased deposition of fibrous proteins including collagen[24] and fibronectin[25] contribute to the mechanical properties of the remodeled left ventricle.

Compared with a normal ventricle, a failing left ventricle may be characterized by systolic or diastolic dysfunction, or both, graphically represented by alterations in pressure volume characteristics of the left ventricular chamber (Fig. 4-8). Typically, a primary decrease in systolic function is associated with a small initial increase in heart size. Subsequently, secondary ventricular remodeling can lead to marked changes in heart size and function.

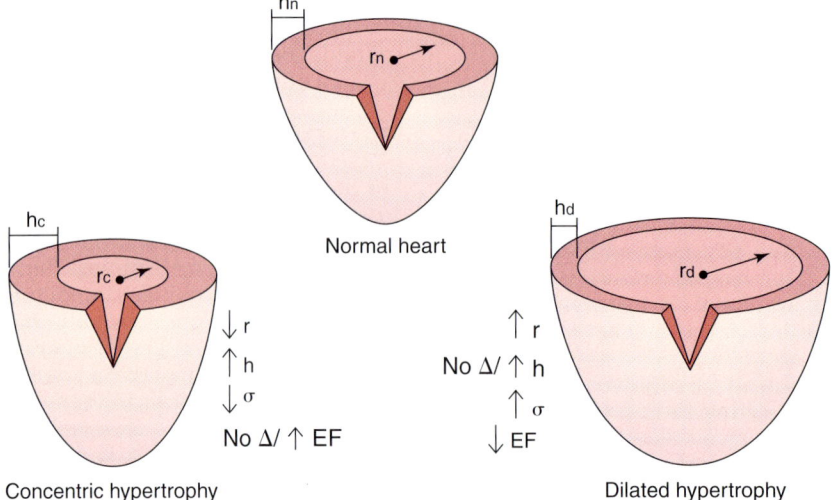

Normal heart

Concentric hypertrophy

Dilated hypertrophy

FIGURE 4-5 The normal left ventricle *(upper)* with end-diastolic wall thickness less than or equal to 11 mm surrounds a chamber diameter less than or equal to 56 mm. Concentric hypertrophy *(lower left)* can develop in response to a sustained increase in left ventricular systolic pressure. End-diastolic wall thickness, *h,* increases, and the chamber radius, *r,* and volume decrease. Because by the LaPlace relationship, wall stress, σ, at end systole is reduced, ejection fraction (EF) may initially increase to maintain a constant stroke volume. This morphologic change is typically associated with impaired filling or diastolic dysfunction. A left ventricle subjected to long-standing pressure overload can progress to a dilated ventricle. Dilated (eccentric) hypertrophy *(lower right)* can follow myocardial injury (infarction, myocarditis) or a chronic volume overload (e.g., aortic or mitral valve regurgitation). Initially, an increase in heart size achieved by passive stretch maintains a forward stroke volume via the Frank-Starling mechanism. Remodeling increases chamber size further over time. Increased heart size ultimately decreases ventricular ejection (systolic dysfunction) when systolic wall stress contributes to an excessive afterload for contracting myocytes.

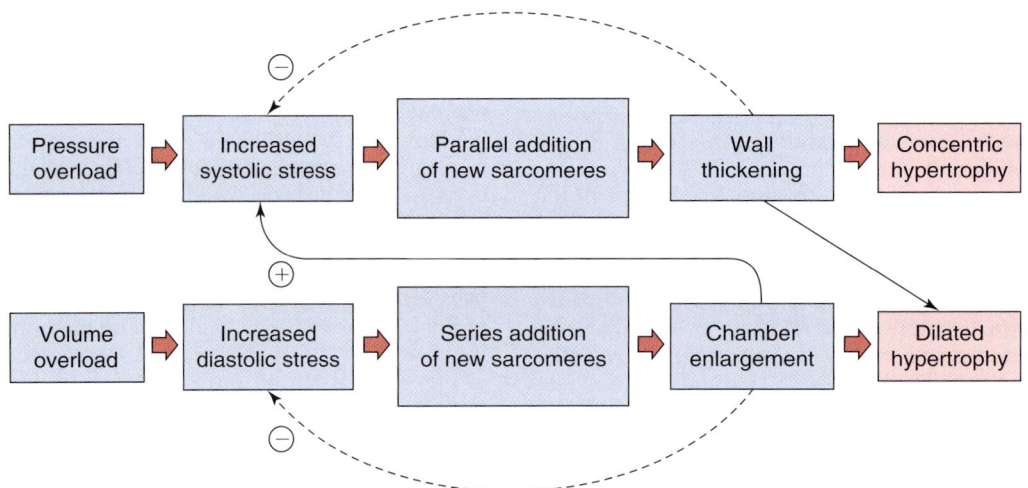

FIGURE 4-6 Proposed mechanism by which increased wall stress initiates concentric and dilated hypertrophy. This hypothesis requires that the heart can "detect" systolic and diastolic wall stress occurring with pressure and volume overload. In addition, a control mechanism is necessary to add new sarcomeres selectively and appropriately in either a parallel or series position to return wall stress toward normal. Chronic volume overload (*), chamber enlargement (r), and the LaPlace relationship ($\sigma = P \bullet r/h$) result in an increased systolic and diastolic wall stress so that both chamber enlargement and wall thickening can occur. *(Adapted from Grossman W, Jones D, McLaurin LP. Wall stress and pattens of hypertrophy in the human left ventricle. J Clin Invest. 1975; 56:61; by copyright permission of The American Society for Clinical Investigation.)*

Right ventricular dysfunction can contribute to the HF syndrome. The most common cause of right HF is left HF.[26] If right HF appears out of proportion to left HF, primary myocardial disorders, including systemic diseases such as sarcoidosis or amyloidosis, should be considered.[27]

It is often difficult to ascertain in individual patients when primary injury and secondary adverse myocardial remodeling (Fig. 4-9)[28] have progressed to a state refractory to medical intervention. Systemic factors may be as important as measurable cardiac parameters.[29] With chronic unloading in patients after left ventricular assist device implantation, reverse remodeling can return diastolic pressure volume relationships to normal (Fig. 4-10).[30] Nevertheless, improvement of systolic function adequate to permit device explantation is uncommon.[31] With left ventricular assist device placement in patients with nonischemic HF, the potential for recovery of left ventricular systolic function appears progressively reduced as diastolic dimension[32] and histologic myocyte hypertrophy and fibrosis increase.[33]

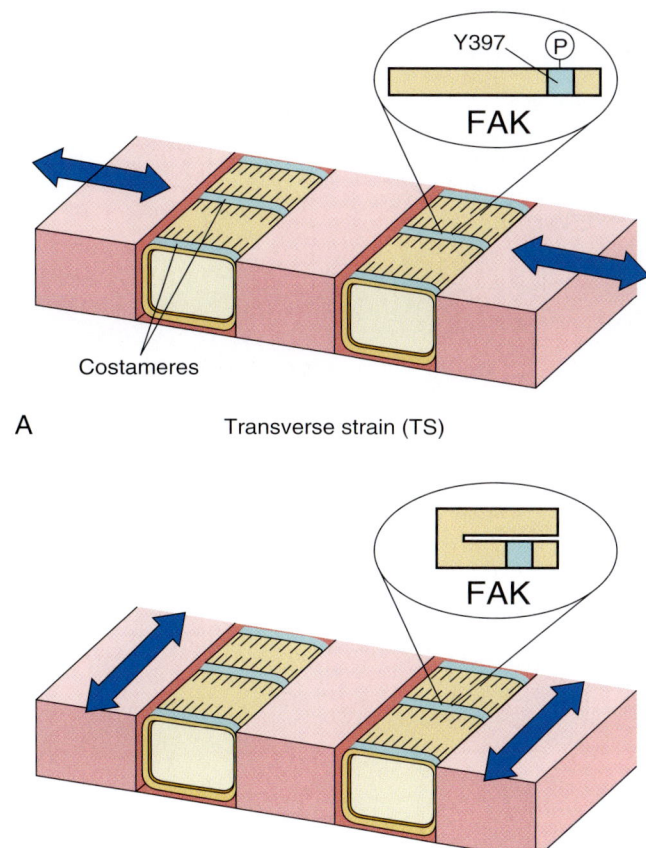

A   Transverse strain (TS)

B   Longitudinal strain (LS)

FIGURE 4-7 In aligned three-dimensional culture systems, differential stretching of myocytes allows simulation of transverse stress in pressure overload and longitudinal strain in volume overload. **A** and **B**, A proposed model of folding of focal adhesion kinase (FAK) located within protein complexes associated with the anchoring Z-disk site of thin myofilaments. Phosphorylation of residue Y397 in unfolded FAK is promoted by transverse strain that could contribute to activation of FAK and parallel versus series addition of new sarcomeres. *(From Russell B, Curtis MW, Koshman YE, Samarel AM. Mechanical stress-induced sarcomere assembly for cardiac muscle growth in length and width. J Mol Cell Cardiol. 2010;48:817-823.)*

NEUROHORMONAL RESPONSE TO MYOCARDIAL INJURY

Renin-Angiotensin-Aldosterone System

The renin-angiotensin-aldosterone system plays a key role in regulating electrolyte levels and fluid balance in normal mammalian physiology. Increased renin production by the kidney in patients with HF was shown in the 1940s.[34] It is now known that decreased stretch of the juxtaglomerular apparatus or its stimulation by the sympathetic nervous system increases renin release.[35] Higher renin levels begin the cascade via angiotensinogen and angiotensin I that result in angiotensin II formation, which plays a central role in producing the HF syndrome. Angiotensin II is an 8-amino acid peptide with diverse effects throughout the cardiovascular system. In the circulation, it acts as a powerful vasoconstrictor of vascular smooth muscle in both the arterial and the venous beds so that afterload and preload are augmented.[36]

In the kidney, angiotensin II causes vasoconstriction in the large-bore muscular renal arteries but predominantly in the efferent (postglomerular) arterioles.[37] The vasoconstriction produces higher pressure in the glomerulus and filtration of fluid and electrolytes, which pass into the proximal tubule. The lower hydrostatic pressure and increased oncotic pressure in the postglomerular vessels surrounding the proximal tubule promote reabsorption of sodium and water. Urea is passively reabsorbed along with water, whereas creatinine is not reabsorbed, leading to the high blood urea nitrogen-to-creatinine ratios seen in some patients with HF. Increased circulating levels of angiotensin II promote the release of aldosterone from the zona glomerulosa of the adrenal gland, which also results in sodium reabsorption in the distal nephron and potassium excretion.[38] Finally, angiotensin II may increase the release of arginine vasopressin via a mechanism that does not rely on changes in osmolality.[39] This nonosmotic release of vasopressin is partly responsible for hyponatremia seen with severe HF.

A tissue-based renin-angiotensin system (RAS) has also been discovered, which contributes both positively and negatively to the HF syndrome.[40] Locally produced angiotensin II increases cardiac contractility, which may help to compensate initially for myocardial injury. This effect may be mediated by increased norepinephrine release from the presynaptic nerve endings.[41] Local angiotensin II initiates the production of growth factors and has been shown to cause myocyte hypertrophy and ultimately left ventricular hypertrophy.[42] Collagen production is increased as well, which along with sodium retention and venoconstriction caused by angiotensin II brings about increased filling pressures that are responsible for many features of CHF. High aldosterone levels are associated with myocardial fibrosis as well.[43] Locally produced angiotensin II is produced within the vascular bed and by cytokine-stimulated monocytes. Monocytes via the angiotensin II receptor produce metalloproteases, which may lead to atherosclerotic plaque instability and thrombosis causing further myocardial injury.[44]

Although the use of angiotensin-converting enzyme inhibitors (ACEIs) reduces the production of angiotensin II, there are alternative pathways for its formation so that angiotensin II levels are not suppressed completely with ACEIs. This

FIGURE 4-8 A, Pressure-volume loop in systolic dysfunction. When ventricular *systolic* dysfunction occurs, the end-systolic pressure-volume curve moves from 1 to 2; this can lead to a decrease in systolic pressure, stroke volume, and ejection fraction despite a compensatory increase in the operating point on the diastolic pressure-volume curve. **B,** When ventricular *diastolic* dysfunction occurs, the diastolic pressure-volume curve shifts from 1 to 2; this can lead to an increase in diastolic pressure, a decrease in end-diastolic volume, and a decrease in ventricular stroke volume. Diastolic dysfunction can occur with or without associated systolic dysfunction. A patient with hypertensive heart disease can have diastolic dysfunction resulting in pulmonary edema with a normal or increased ejection fraction.

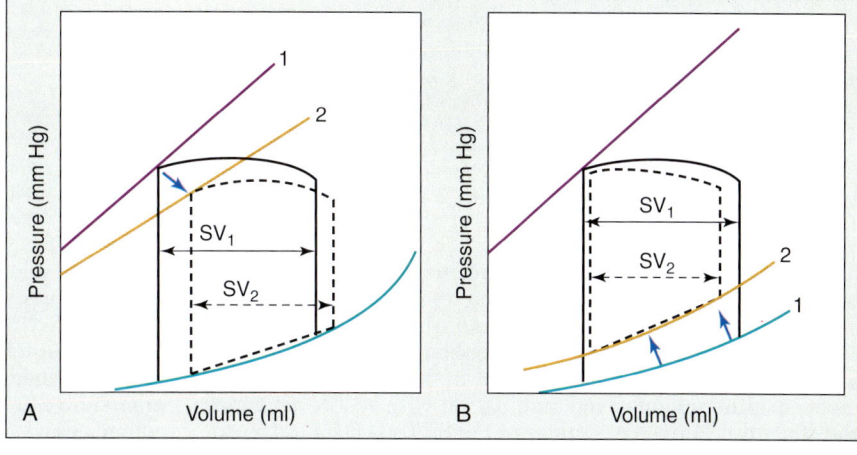

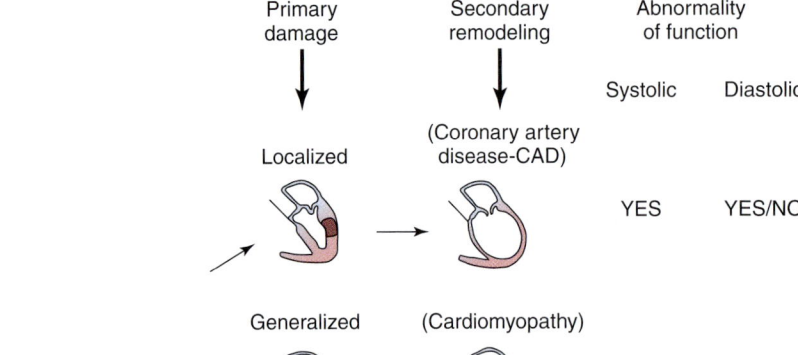

	Primary damage	Secondary remodeling	Abnormality of function	
			Systolic	Diastolic
	Localized	(Coronary artery disease-CAD)	YES	YES/NO
Pre-disease	Generalized	(Cardiomyopathy)	YES	NO
	Volume	(Valvular regurgitation)	YES	NO
	Pressure	(Hypertension)	YES/NO	YES

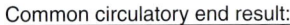

Common circulatory end result:

Low cardiac output / High filling pressure → Heart failure

FIGURE 4-9 Stages of cardiac disease versus diastolic dysfunction. Clinical heart failure may result from various causes that produce a primary insult that progresses with secondary remodeling. The clinical syndrome of heart failure (HF) (circulatory congestion or inadequate tissue perfusion) may be similar regardless of the etiology of primary damage or mechanism of systolic versus diastolic dysfunction. *(From Gorlin R. Treatment of congestive heart failure: where are we going? Circulation. 1987;75:IV109.)*

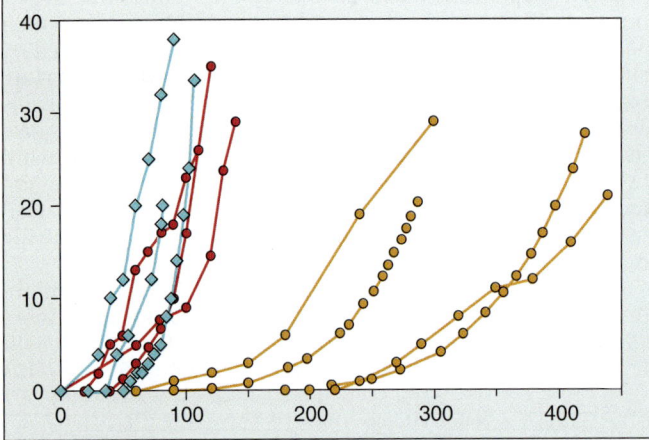

FIGURE 4-10 Graph showing end-diastolic pressure-volume relationships (EDPVRs) of hearts from four medically treated patients with end-stage idiopathic cardiomyopathy *(gold circles)*, three patients with heart failure (HF) after prolonged left ventricular assist device (LVAD) support *(red circles)*, and three normal subjects *(blue boxes)*. EDPVRs of hearts from medically treated patients are shifted far to the right of the normal hearts, whereas EDPVRs from the LVAD patients were close to normal. *x* axis, volume in milliliters; *y* axis, pressure in mm Hg.

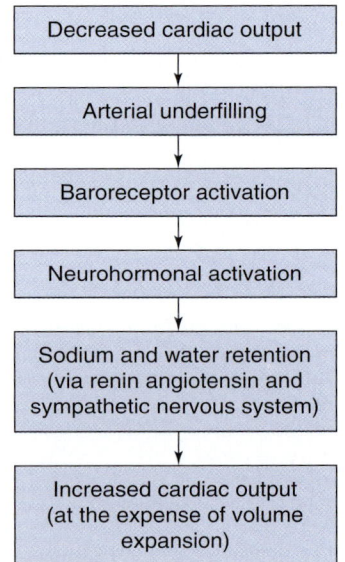

FIGURE 4-11 Role of arterial underfilling in the pathogenesis of congestive heart failure (CHF) via activation of systemic baroreceptors and activation of the renin-angiotensin system (RAS) with compensatory salt and water retention.

has been termed "ACEI escape" and may permit continued production of angiotensin II despite angiotensin-converting enzyme inhibition. Although angiotensin receptor blockers can theoretically overcome this problem by blockade of the angiotensin I receptor directly, use of angiotensin receptor blockers either alone or in combination with ACEIs have not significantly changed outcomes in HF (Fig. 4-11).[45,46]

Sympathetic Nervous System

The sympathetic nervous system is an important component in the pathogenesis of the HF syndrome, in many ways complementary to the RAS system and amplifying the effects discussed previously. Baroreceptor stimulation by low blood pressure or reduced stroke volume results in the sympathetic nervous system activation. Leimbach and colleagues[47] employed microneurography of the peroneal nerve in patients with moderate to severe HF and showed increased sympathetic nerve impulses along this nerve to the peripheral musculature. The major marker of sympathetic nervous system activity is increased norepinephrine levels; epinephrine levels are not significantly elevated in HF. Coronary sinus norepinephrine levels are many times higher than arterial levels, and increased levels are seen in renal veins as well.[48]

Stimulation of the sympathetic nervous system with release of norepinephrine has widespread physiologic effects. In normal individuals or patients in the early stages of HF, norepinephrine increases heart rate and contractility and may support cardiac function. However, in later stages of cardiac decompensation, cardiac response to norepinephrine is blunted, partly because of the decreased B receptor density seen in patients with chronic severe HF.[49] There is a shift from the normal adrenergic beta receptor density of 70% to 80%/20% to 30% beta-1-to-beta-2 ratio to a more even distribution of 60%/40%.[50]

Alpha receptors increase in the failing heart so that the end result is a more balanced distribution of alpha, beta-1, and beta-2 receptors. Decreased beta receptor density could conceivably contribute to reduced cardiac function in HF, but in an animal model of beta-1 receptor overexpression, HF actually developed.[51] In a transgenic model of alpha receptor excess, cardiac hypertrophy was produced, underscoring the role of this receptor in cellular hypertrophy.[52]

Genetic variations in beta receptor subtypes also are related to the risk of developing HF. African Americans who are homozygous for a variant of the alpha-2 receptor are five times more likely to develop HF.[53]

Peripheral arteriolar tone is increased, producing an elevation of blood pressure and cardiac afterload via alpha receptor activation. In the kidney, however, activation of the sympathetic nervous system causes significant sodium retention via disproportionate vasoconstriction of the efferent arterioles.[54] The resulting increased pressure in the glomerulus helps to maintain glomerular filtration rate (GFR) but favors the reabsorption of sodium and water in the proximal tubule.[55] In addition, sympathetic stimulation increases production of renin and angiotensin II, promoting even further sodium reabsorption.[56]

Beyond the detrimental hemodynamic effects of the sympathetic nervous system, there is evidence that norepinephrine itself produces direct detrimental effects at the cardiac level. High circulating levels of norepinephrine strongly correlate with left ventricular dysfunction and mortality.[57,58] Direct exposure to myocytes in tissue culture to levels of norepinephrine that are seen in HF results in cell death with increased intracellular calcium levels.[59] Communal and associates[60] showed norepinephrine induced cardiac apoptosis in rat adult myocytes acting through protein kinase, which was not dependent on beta receptor activation. Cardiac fibrosis is also promoted by norepinephrine acting via transforming growth factor beta-1.[61]

Endothelin

Isolated for the first time in 1988, endothelin is the most powerful vasoconstrictor discovered so far.[62] It consists of a group of peptides produced by vascular endothelial cells including endothelin-1, endothelin-2, and endothelin-3.[63] Although measurable levels are found in venous blood, endothelin acts primarily as a paracrine hormone causing powerful smooth muscle contraction via activation of endothelin A receptors.[64] Endothelin-1, a 21-amino acid peptide, has been the most widely studied and plays a wide-ranging role in vascular physiology.[63] Production has been shown in cardiac tissue, and increased levels increase contractility and heart rate.[65,66]

In myocardial cell preparations, it stimulates expression of proto-oncogenes with proliferation of myocytes.[67] Infusion of endothelin increases blood pressure and reduces forearm blood flow. Renal effects have also been shown with vasoconstriction of both glomerular afferent and efferent arterioles so that GFR is reduced.[68] Cellular transport mechanisms are inhibited in the proximal tubule and the loop of Henle so that sodium excretion is enhanced.[69,70]

Endothelin brings about the release of aldosterone from the adrenal medulla, which causes sodium retention.[71] Exposure of monocytes to endothelin increased production and release of the cytokine tumor necrosis factor-alpha (see subsequently).[72] Endothelin levels are elevated in HF, with higher levels seen with more advanced symptoms.[73,74] However, blockade of endothelin receptors has not been shown to be beneficial in systolic left ventricular dysfunction, although these agents are quite beneficial in pulmonary hypertension.[75]

Cytokines and Heart Failure

In addition to the crucial role of the RAS and sympathetic nervous system in the development and progression of the HF syndrome, cytokine inflammatory mediators such as TNF-alpha and the interleukins seem to have important effects.[76] Current understanding suggests that cytokines are elevated not only when myocardial injury occurs owing to viral or other infectious etiology, but also in hemodynamic overloading. Numerous signaling modulators mediated through cytokine release influence gene expression, apoptosis, and growth factor signaling.[77] TNF-alpha or cachexin is produced by macrophages and is an important mediator of the inflammatory response by stimulating acute phase reactants, increasing body temperature and suppressing appetite. It is postulated to be partially responsible for cachexia in advanced HF, and very elevated levels are seen in such patients. Infusion of TNF-alpha in animals reduces contractility and left ventricular systolic dysfunction. Transgenic murine models with overproduction of the molecule develop left ventricular chamber enlargement. Detailed cardiac analysis in these models shows a loss of fibrillar collagen and increased metalloprotease activity.[78,79] With continued exposure, however, fibrillar collagen increases, perhaps mediated by transforming growth factor-beta. Finally, TNF-alpha has been shown to promote apoptosis in an animal model of dilated cardiomyopathy. The peripheral levels of TNF-alpha found in HF patients reduce nitric oxide production from endothelial cells.[80]

Cardiac hypertrophy represents an adaptive response of the myocardium to mechanical and neurohormonal stimuli; ultimately, it often progresses to ventricular dilation and HF.[81] Prolonged stress overwhelms this protective response and leads to apoptosis of cardiomyocytes. This balance between the protective and apoptotic mechanisms is determined by a network of signal transduction pathways called the JAK/STAT pathway[82,83] that effects the expression of either cardioprotective or proapoptotic genes. The activated STATs move to the nucleus where they bind to the regulatory regions of the DNA to modify gene expression. Activation of STAT3 is involved in cardioprotection, whereas activation of STAT1 is associated with apoptosis.[83] Serine/threonine kinase, a collateral signaling pathway, is responsible for activation of either pathway. These pathways are activated by cytokines such as TNF-alpha, Fas ligand, and G protein–coupled receptor ligands released by the injured myocardium.[84]

Natriuretic Peptides

Discovered slightly more than 50 years ago as secretory granules in the atria, the natriuretic peptides have been the object of intense scientific study.[85] However, their role in the development or amelioration of the HF syndrome has not been fully elucidated. The natriuretic peptides (atrial natriuretic peptide [ANP] and B-type natriuretic peptide [BNP]) bind to a specific transmembrane receptor called NPR-A that results in the production of guanosine monophosphate.[86] Synthesis and release of BNP correlates with increased ventricular wall stress.[87] Infusion of BNP produces prompt reduction of right atrial, pulmonary artery, and pulmonary artery wedge pressures.[88] In addition, systemic vascular resistance declines and cardiac output improves with increased natriuretic peptide levels.[89,90] In acute infusion studies, BNP is associated with reduced circulating aldosterone and decreases norepinephrine levels in the coronary sinus of individuals with systolic dysfunction (Figs. 4-12 and 4-13).[90,91]

The data on renal effects are less consistent in HF. In animal models and in individuals without cardiac dysfunction, BNP produces natriuresis and an increase in GFR.[92,93] These effects have been shown in some studies in patients with HF but not in others.[93,94] A meta-analysis of early BNP infusion trials showed an increased risk of worsening renal function at 30 days.[95]

Despite high circulating levels of natriuretic peptides that have been consistently shown in HF and their antagonistic effects on deleterious neurohormonal activation, the syndrome persists. The reasons are unclear, but several potential explanations have been suggested. The profound activation of the RAS and sympathetic nervous system may overcome the ability of natriuretic peptides to increase sodium excretion or reduce afterload.[96] An alternative explanation for which there are new data from mass spectroscopy is that circulating natriuretic peptides are not biologically active.[97]

PATHOPHYSIOLOGY OF END-STAGE HEART FAILURE

Current therapy for systolic dysfunction, despite its limitations, has made considerable progress in the last several decades so that not all patients progress to end-stage HF. Similar to patients with prostate cancer, many individuals may die with HF but not primarily because of HF. Nonetheless, greater than 50,000 individuals die each year primarily of HF with more than 1,100,000 hospitalizations for decompensation in the United States alone.[98] The most recent American College of Cardiology Foundation (ACCF)/American Heart Association (AHA) guidelines have termed end-stage HF as *stage D HF,* in which transplant, mechanical assist devices, and hospice have the most meaningful role for patient management.[99] For these patients, medical therapy is palliative at best and fails to produce any long-term stability for the patient.[100,101]

Clinical Features of End-Stage Heart Failure

Reduction in Cardiac Output

A common misconception is that all patients with HF have a significantly reduced cardiac output. Although most patients with HF do not have a significantly reduced cardiac

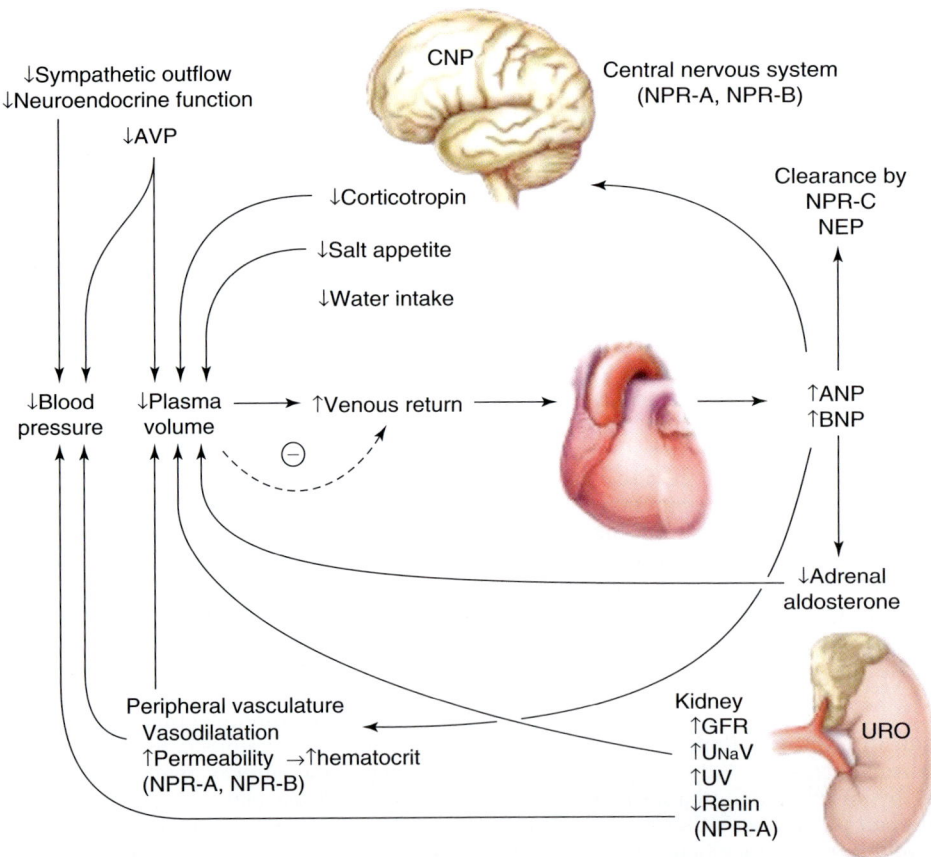

FIGURE 4-12 Natriuretic peptides counterbalance the effects of the renin-angiotensin system (RAS) by reducing blood pressure and promoting sodium excretion via effects on the kidney, adrenal glands, and vascular smooth muscle. The minus sign indicates that a decrease in venous pressure reduces the secretion of the natriuretic peptides. ANP, atrial natriuretic peptide; AVP, arginine vasopressin; BNP, B-type natriuretic peptide; BP, blood pressure; CNP, C-type natriuretic peptide; GFR, glomerular filtration rate; NEP, neutral endopeptidase; NPR-A, NPR-B, and NPR-C, natriuretic peptide receptors A, B, and C; UNaV, urinary sodium excretion; URO, urodilatin; UV, urinary volume. *(From Levin ER, Gardner DG, Samson WK. Natriuretic peptides. N Engl J Med. 1998;339:321-328.)*

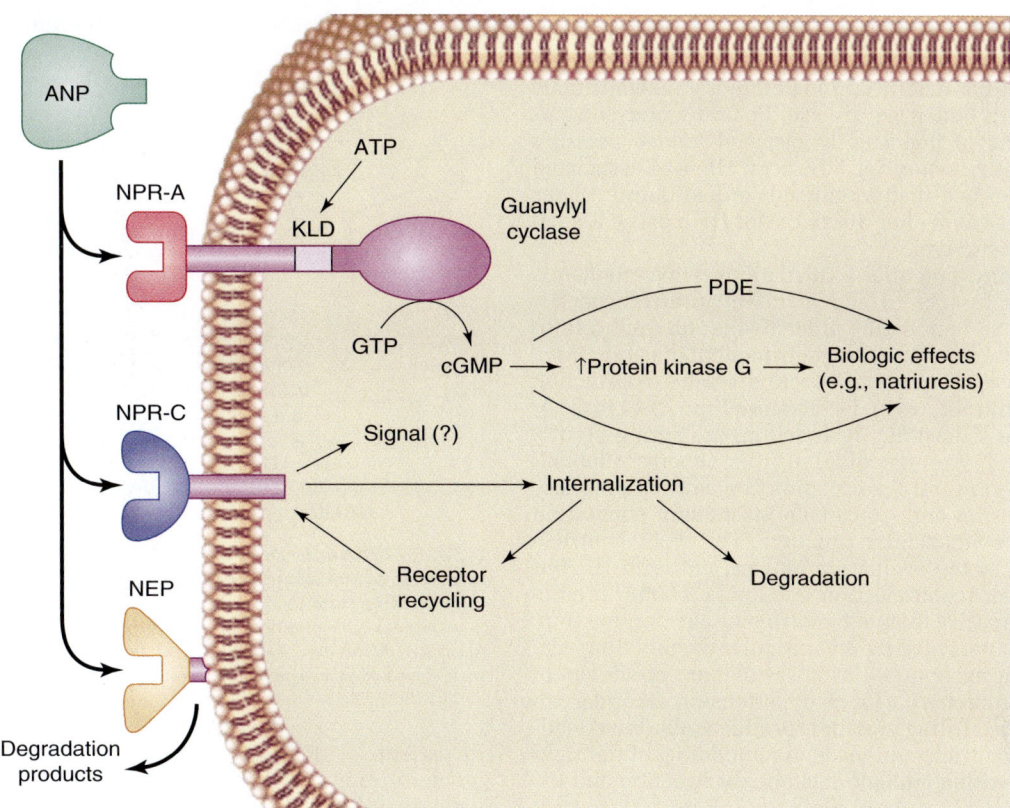

FIGURE 4-13 Natriuretic peptides (atrial natriuretic peptide [ANP] and B-type natriuretic peptide [BNP]) interact with natriuretic peptide receptor A (NPR-A) and natriuretic peptide receptor B (NRP-B), which results in the production of cyclic guanosine monophosphate (cGMP). cGMP can work via multiple pathways, including protein kinase G, phosphodiesterases (PDEs), or directly on amiloride-sensitive sodium channels in the kidney. ANP also interacts with natriuretic peptide receptor C (NPR-C). Neutral endopeptidases (NEPs) in the kidney and vasculature degrade both ANP and BNP. GTP, guanosine triphosphate. *(From Levin ER, Gardner DG, Samson WK. Natriuretic peptides. N Engl J Med. 1998;339:321-328.)*

output, it is more often seen in end-stage disease and may occur for several reasons.[102] Adverse remodeling and ongoing myocardial damage, resulting from either the initiating process or continued neurohormonal stimulation, may impair further the ability of the heart to generate an adequate stroke volume. Remodeling may enlarge the mitral anulus with attendant mitral regurgitation, which may favor ventricular emptying backward into the relatively lower pressure of the left atrium, rather than forward into the aorta.[103] Afterload may remain high and impede forward output further. Atrial fibrillation, especially if uncontrolled, and ventricular arrhythmias may impair ventricular function further.[104,105] Ventricular dyssynchrony as a result of conduction system disease may erode cardiac function further.[106] A cardiac index less than 1.5 L/min/m² has been shown to impair renal perfusion to the degree that kidney function is impaired.[107] Outputs below this level may impair hepatic and cerebral function as well.

As cardiac output declines, blood pressure may decrease as well, which may impair organ perfusion further. At some point, the use of ACEI and beta-blocker therapy becomes problematic because the blood pressure may decrease further when these agents are used. What constitutes an acceptable blood pressure is not always clear, and sometimes the discontinuation of these agents is detrimental.[108] Kittleson and colleagues[109] showed that the discontinuation of an ACEI can be a sentinel event in patients with HF because mortality is 50% in such patients at 1 year. The inability to maintain evidence-based neurohormonal blockade is a sentinel event in HF, signaling a very poor prognosis (Fig. 4-14).

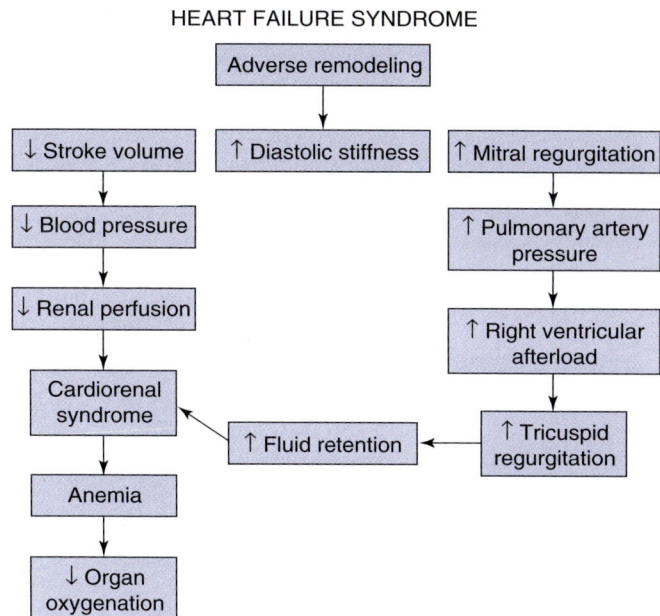

HEART FAILURE SYNDROME

FIGURE 4-14 Heart failure (HF) may progress to stage D via several pathways. Progressive myocardial fibrosis results in progressive dilation and reduced stroke volume. Worsening mitral regurgitation may develop as well, which leads to pulmonary venous hypertension and right ventricular loading. Right ventricular failure plays an important role in exercise limitation and portends a poorer prognosis in advanced HF. High venous filling pressures are associated with reduced renal function (see Figure 4-16).

Many key symptoms associated with HF are related to high filling pressures; the inability to maintain a euvolemic state is associated with end-stage disease. Fonarow and coworkers[110] showed that a persistently elevated wedge pressure after medical optimization for advanced HF was associated with a poorer survival than a reduced cardiac output. Signs of persistent congestion after discharge for HF are also associated with poorer survival.[111]

There are many potential explanations why euvolemia is more difficult to achieve and maintain in advanced HF. Continued adverse remodeling enlarges the left ventricle so that wall stiffness increases to the detriment of diastolic function. Noninvasive indicators of severe diastolic dysfunction in systolic HF (mitral E wave deceleration time <140 msec or irreversible stage 4 diastolic dysfunction) are strong predictors of mortality.[112] Annular dilation from adverse remodeling and associated mitral regurgitation can cause pulmonary venous hypertension and exacerbate pulmonary congestion and impair right ventricular function. The right ventricle is often ignored in the evaluation of a patient with HF, but reduced right ventricular ejection fraction is a better predictor of exercise capacity than left ventricular ejection fraction, and even simple indices of right ventricular dysfunction (e.g., tricuspid annular excursion during systole) are predictors of mortality.[113,114] Pulmonary venous hypertension secondary to increased left-sided filling pressures produces abnormal loading of the right ventricle and leads to remodeling of the right heart structures with attendant diastolic dysfunction and tricuspid regurgitation (Fig. 4-15).[115,116]

Cardiorenal Syndrome

In the past, there was an understandable cardiocentric approach to HF with an emphasis on hemodynamics, cardiac output, and ejection fraction. More recently, there has been a shift of focus to renal function and its role in the development of end-stage HF. Large data sets from randomized trials and registries have shown repeatedly that markers of renal dysfunction are strong predictors of mortality in HF and often overshadow more traditional indicators of cardiac function.[117,118] In the ADHERE (Acute Decompensated Heart Failure National Registry) registry, an admission blood urea nitrogen greater than 42 mg/dL coupled with a systolic blood pressure less than 115 mm Hg was associated with 15% inpatient mortality.[119]

Poor renal function may play an important role in diuretic-resistant fluid retention and can limit the use of RAS blockade to the detriment of the patient, as noted earlier. Reduction of cardiac output with associated renal hypoperfusion is a recognized cause of reduced renal function, but there are other mechanisms as well. High venous pressures are associated with reduced GFR and decreased urine output in animal models.[120,121] More recently, this association has been shown

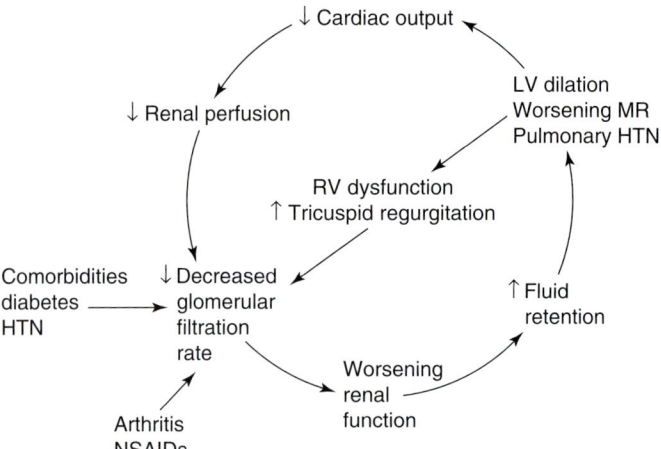

FIGURE 4-15 Prevalence of worsening renal dysfunction is strongly related to increase central venous pressure in patients with severe heart failure (HF). HTN, hypertension; LV, left ventricular; MR, mitral regurgitation; NSAIDs, nonsteroidal anti-inflammatory drugs; RV, right ventricular. *(Redrawn from Mullens W, Abrahams Z, Francis GS, et al. Importance of venous congestion for worsening of renal function in advanced decompensated heart failure. J Am Coll Cardiol. 2009;53:589-596.)*

in patients with acute decompensated HF, and it seems to be more important than cardiac output in predicting which patients will develop renal dysfunction.[122] High venous pressures may be especially important when systemic pressure is low because the resulting reduced transrenal pressure gradient may limit perfusion of the kidney. A negative feedback loop could potentially exist so that reduced sodium excretion caused by the HF syndrome might impair renal function further causing more sodium and fluid retention. Many patients with HF have important comorbidities such as diabetes and hypertension that may produce renal dysfunction that negatively affects cardiac function—the so-called cardiorenal syndrome.[123]

Efforts to improve renal function in HF to normalize volume status and increase survival have largely been disappointing. Early trials of nesiritide and the adenosine blocking drug rolofylline showed favorable results, but questions about increased mortality at 30 days limited the use of nesiritide, and central nervous system toxicity led to the abandonment of the rolofylline.[124,125] Nonetheless, the kidney retains a crucial role in advanced HF, and new strategies are being developed, including "designer BNPs," which specifically improve renal function, and catheter-based sympathectomy of the kidney itself to provide a nonpharmacologic means of blood pressure control (Figs. 4-16 and 4-17).[126,127]

FIGURE 4-16 Worsening renal function is common in advanced heart failure (HF) and is termed the cardiorenal syndrome. The syndrome is complex and is incompletely understood, but several factors play a role, including reduced cardiac output and impaired renal perfusion. High venous pressures may impair renal perfusion and function further. In addition, important comorbidities such as hypertension and diabetes reduce renal function directly, which can cause further fluid retention. Cr, creatinine CVP, central venous pressure.

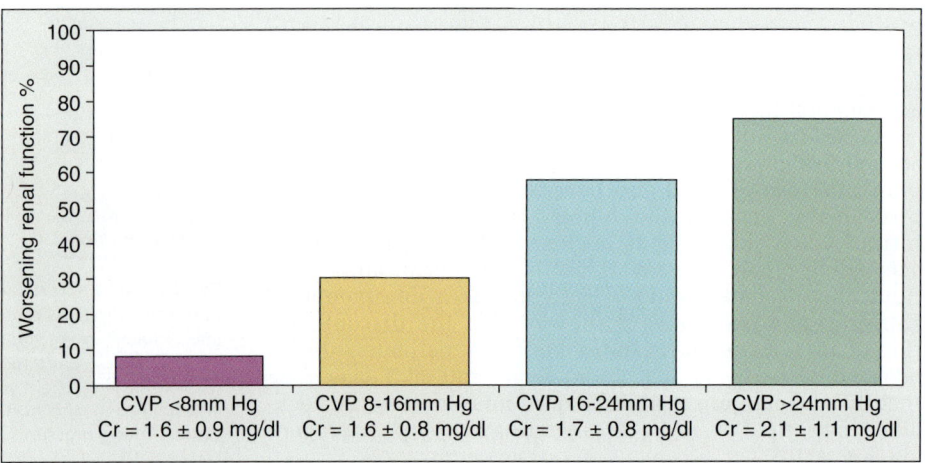

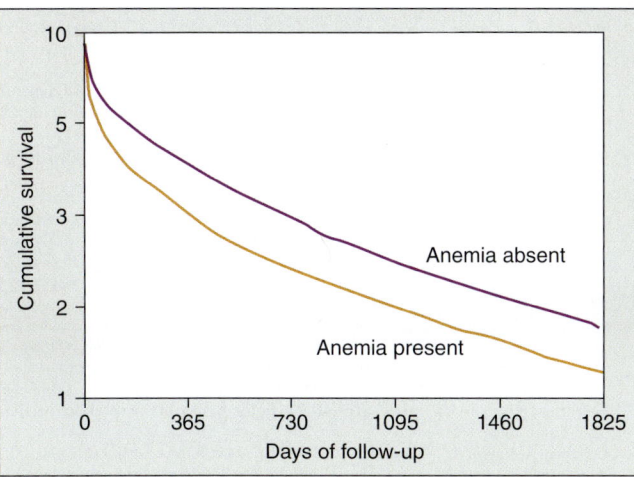

FIGURE 4-17 Effect of anemia on survival in new-onset heart failure (HF) in 12,065 patients with new-onset HF. *(From Ezekowitz JA, McAlister FA, Armstrong PW. Anemia is common in heart failure and is associated with poor outcomes: insights from a cohort of 12,065 patients with new-onset heart failure. Circulation. 2003;107;223-225.*

Sleep Apnea and Heart Failure

Sleep-disordered breathing, including central and obstructive sleep apnea, occurs in a significant minority of patients with CHF and is more frequent in men and with advanced age.[128] Sleep-disordered breathing has profoundly negative hemodynamic and neurohormonal effects in advanced HF, which may lead to further cardiac deterioration. With obstructive sleep apnea, ventricular afterload is increased, while negative intrathoracic pressure may result in right ventricular dilation.[129,130] Repeat episodes of obstruction and arousal increase central sympathetic outflow with the detrimental effects outlined earlier as well as long-term augmentation of systemic blood pressure.[131,132] When controlling for important clinical variables, subjects with central sleep apnea have increased levels of urinary and circulating norepinephrine.[133] The development of sleep-disordered breathing is associated with increased mortality and may be an important exacerbating component of end-stage HF (Fig. 4-18).[134,135]

CONCLUSION

The syndrome of CHF is so distinctive that "dropsy" has been described for more than 2000 years along with speculation as to its cause.[136] Although the tools of hemodynamic investigation, biochemistry, and genetic manipulation have provided a coherent and scientifically testable "explanation" of the pathophysiology of HF, it would be naive to imagine that this complex syndrome has been fully elucidated. The rapid reduction in cost to obtain a complete base pair listing for an individual should provide the opportunity to discover the genetic mechanism responsible for many cases of "idiopathic" HF and provide new means for therapy and prevention. With these new insights, the pathophysiology of HF will expand with each new genetic abnormality detected. Despite the great strides taken in the past few decades, new tools most certainly will render current understanding of HF as quaint.

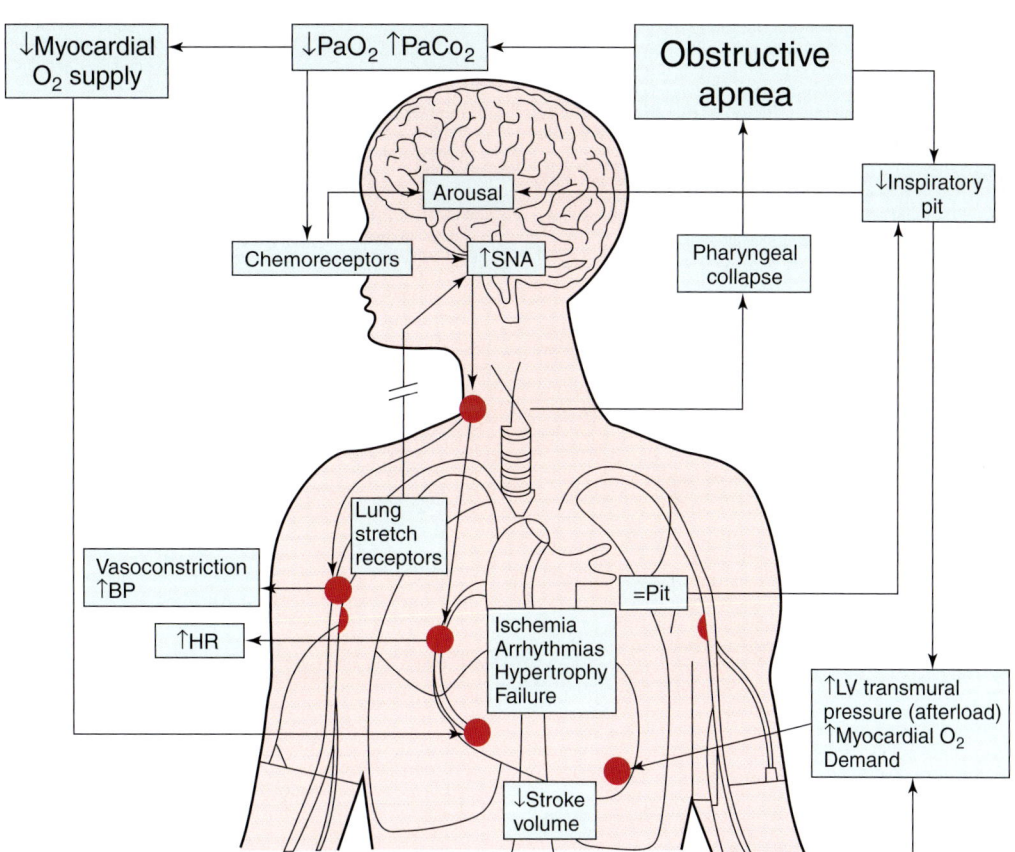

FIGURE 4-18 Effects of obstructive sleep apnea in patients with congestive heart failure (CHF). Obstruction, hypoxia, and arousals increase systemic blood pressure (BP) with stimulation of the sympathetic nervous system. The sympathetic system is also enhanced by the effects of apnea on lung stretch receptors. Increased BP and sympathetic stimulation may increase afterload and impair cardiac performance further. HR, heart rate; SNA, sympathetic nerve activity. *(From Bradley DT, Floras JS. Sleep apnea and heart failure, part I: obstructive sleep apnea. Circulation. 2003;107:1671-1678.)*

REFERENCES

1. Ohno M, Takemura G, Ohno A, et al. "Apoptotic" myocytes in infarct area in rabbit hearts may be oncotic myocytes with DNA fragmentation: analysis by immunogold electron microscopy combined with in situ nick end-labeling. *Circulation.* 1998;98:1422–1430.
2. Koch K, Piek J, de Winter R, et al. Short-term (4 hours) observation after elective coronary angioplasty. *Am J Cardiol.* 1997;80:1591–1594.
3. Koch K, Piek J, Prins M, et al. Triage of patients for short term observation after elective coronary angioplasty. *Heart.* 2000;83:557–563.
4. Gaballa M, Goldman S. Ventricular remodeling in heart failure. *J Card Fail.* 2002;8:S476–S485.
5. Matsumura K, Jeremy R, Schaper J, et al. Progression of myocardial necrosis during reperfusion of ischemic myocardium. *Circulation.* 1998;97:795–804.
6. Lucchesi B. Myocardial ischemia, reperfusion and free radical injury. *Am J Cardiol.* 1990;65:14I–23I.
7. Hahn E, Hartz V, Moon T, et al. The Myocarditis Treatment Trial: design, methods and patients enrollment. *Eur Heart J.* 1995;16(suppl):162–167.
8. Dennert R, Crijns H, Heymans S. Acute viral myocarditis. *Eur Heart J.* 2008; 29:2073–2082.
9. Lee W, Regan T. Alcoholic cardiomyopathy: is it dose-dependent? *Congest Heart Fail.* 2002;8:303–306.
10. Matsumoto S, Hirayama Y, Saitoh H, et al. Noninvasive diagnosis of cardiac sarcoidosis using microvolt T-wave alternans. *Int Heart J.* 2009;50:731–739.
11. Morales A, Painter T, Li R, et al. Rare variant mutations in pregnancy-associated or peripartum cardiomyopathy. *Circulation.* 2010;121:2176–2182.
12. Gentry M, Dias J, Luis A, et al. African-American women have a higher risk for developing peripartum cardiomyopathy. *J Am Coll Cardiol.* 2010;55:654–659.
13. Sliwa K, Fett J, Elkayam U. Peripartum cardiomyopathy. *Lancet.* 2006;368:687–693.
14. Shinbane J, Wood M, Jensen D, et al. Tachycardia-induced cardiomyopathy: A review of animal models and clinical studies. *J Am Coll Cardiol.* 1997;29:709–715.
15. Willis MS, Schisler JC, Portbury AL, et al. Build it up-tear it down: protein quality control in the cardiac sarcomere. *Cardiovasc Res.* 2009;81:439–448.
16. Lionetti V, Bianchi G, Recchia FA, et al. Control of autocrine and paracrine myocardial signals: an emerging therapeutic strategy in heart failure. *Heart Fail Rev.* 2010;15:531–542.
17. Mann DL, Bristow MR. Mechanisms and models in heart failure: the biomechanical model and beyond. *Circulation.* 2005;111:2837–2849.
18. Yang R, Amir J, Liu H, et al. Mechanical strain activates a program of genes functionally involved in paracrine signaling of angiogenesis. *Physiol Genomics.* 2008;36:1–14.
19. Grossman W, Jones D, McLaurin LP. Wall stress and patterns of hypertrophy in the human left ventricle. *J Clin Invest.* 1975;56:56–64.
20. Russell B, Curtis MW, Koshman YE, et al. Mechanical stress-induced sarcomere assembly for cardiac muscle growth in length and width. *J Mol Cell Cardiol.* 2010;48:817–823.
21. Linke WA. Sense and stretchability: The role of titin and titin-associated proteins in myocardial stress-sensing and mechanical dysfunction. *Cardiovasc Res.* 2008;77:637–648.
22. Deschamps AM, Spinale FG. Disruptions and detours in the myocardial matrix highway and heart failure. *Curr Heart Fail Rep.* 2005;2:10–17.
23. Weber KT. Extracellular matrix remodeling in heart failure: a role for de novo angiotensin II generation. *Circulation.* 1997;96:4065–4082.
24. Jugdutt Bodh I. Ventricular remodeling after infarction and the extracellular collagen matrix: when is enough enough? *Circulation.* 2003;108:1395–1403.
25. Borer JS, Truter S, Herrold EM, et al. Responses to volume overload. *Circulation.* 2002;105:1837–1842.
26. Thibault GE. Clinical problem-solving: studying the classics. *N Engl J Med.* 1995;333:648–652.
27. Seward JB, Casaclang-Verzosa G. Infiltrative cardiovascular diseases: cardiomyopathies that look alike. *J Am Coll Cardiol.* 2010;55:1769–1779.
28. Gorlin R. Treatment of congestive heart failure: Where are we going? *Circulation.* 1987;75:IV108–IV111.
29. Levy WC, Mozaffarian D, Linker DT, et al. The Seattle Heart Failure Model: prediction of survival in heart failure. *Circulation.* 2006;113:1424–1433.
30. Levin HR, Oz MC, Chen JM, et al. Reversal of chronic ventricular dilation in patients with end-stage cardiomyopathy by prolonged mechanical unloading. *Circulation.* 1995;91:2717–2720.
31. Miller LW, Pagani FD, Russell SD, et al. Use of a continuous-flow device in patients awaiting heart transplantation. *N Engl J Med.* 2007;357:885–896.
32. Simon MA, Primack BA, Teuteberg J, et al. Left ventricular remodeling and myocardial recovery on mechanical circulatory support. *J Card Fail.* 2010;16:99–105.
33. Saito S, Matsumiya G, Sakaguchi T, et al. Cardiac fibrosis and cellular hypertrophy decrease the degree of reverse remodeling and improvement in cardiac function during left ventricular assist. *J Heart Lung Transplant.* 2010;29:672–679.
34. Merrill AJ, Morrin JL, Brannon ES. Concentration of renin in renal venous blood in patients with chronic heart failure. *Am J Med.* 1946;1:468–472.
35. Davis JO. The control of renin release. *Am J Med.* 1973;55:333–350.
36. Zhang J, Pfaffendorf M, van Zwieten PA. Hemodynamic effects of angiotensin II and the influence of angiotensin receptor antagonists in pithed rabbits. *J Cardiovasc Pharmacol.* 1995;25:724–731.
37. Hall JE, Coleman TG, Guyton AC, et al. Intrarenal role of angiotensin II and (des-Asp) angiotensin II. *Am J Physiol.* 1979;236:F252–F259.
38. Pratt JH. Role of angiotensin II in potassium-mediated stimulation of aldosterone secretion in the dog. *J Clin Invest.* 1982;70:667–672.
39. Ishikawa S, Saito T, Yoshida S. The effect of osmotic pressure and angiotensin II on arginine vasopressin release from guinea pig hypothalamo-neurohypophyseal complex in organ culture. *Endocrinology.* 1980;106:1571–1578.
40. Hirsch AT, Talsness CE, Schunkert H, et al. Tissue-specific activation of angiotensin converting enzyme in experimental heart failure. *Circ Res.* 1991;69:475–482.
41. Burgdorf C, Richardt D, Kurz T, et al. Presynaptic regulation of norepinephrine release in a model of nonfailing hypertrophied myocardium. *J Cardiovasc Pharmacol.* 2003;41:813–816.
42. Sadoshima J, Izumo S. Molecular characterization of angiotensin II-induced hypertrophy of cardiac myocytes and hyperplasia of cardiac fibroblasts: critical role of the AT1 receptor subtype. *Circ Res.* 1993;73:413–423.
43. Weber KT, Brilla CG. Pathological hypertrophy and cardiac interstitium: fibrosis and renin-angiotensin-aldosterone system. *Circulation.* 1991;83:1849–1865.
44. Kim MP, Zhou M, Wahl L. Angiotensin II increases human monocyte matrix metalloproteinase-1 through the AT2 receptor and prostaglandin E2: implications for atherosclerotic plaque rupture. *J Leukoc Biol.* 2005;78:195–201.
45. Cohn JN, Tognoni G, Valsartan Heart Failure Trial Investigators. A randomized trial of the angiotensin-receptor blocker valsartan in chronic heart failure. *N Engl J Med.* 2001;345:1667–1675.
46. McMurray JJ, Ostergren J, Swedberg K, et al. Effects of candesartan in patients with chronic heart failure and reduced left-ventricular systolic function taking angiotensin-converting-enzyme inhibitors: the CHARM-Added trial. *Lancet.* 2003;362:767–771.
47. Leimbach Jr WN, Wallin BG, Victor RG, et al. Direct evidence from intraneural recordings for increased central sympathetic outflow in patients with heart failure. *Circulation.* 1986;73:913–919.
48. Swedberg K, Viquerat C, Rouleau JL, et al. Comparison of myocardial catecholamine balance in chronic congestive heart failure and in angina pectoris without failure. *Am J Cardiol.* 1984;54:783–786.
49. Bristow MR, Ginsburg R, Minobe W, et al. Decreased catecholamine sensitivity and beta-adrenergic-receptor density in failing human hearts. *N Engl J Med.* 1982;307:205–211.
50. Bristow MR, Ginsburg R, Umans V, et al. Beta 1- and beta 2-adrenergic-receptor subpopulations in nonfailing and failing human ventricular myocardium: coupling of both receptor subtypes to muscle contraction and selective beta 1-receptor down-regulation in heart failure. *Circ Res.* 1986;59:297–309.
51. Engelhardt S, Hein L, Wiesmann F, et al. Progressive hypertrophy and heart failure in beta1-adrenergic receptor transgenic mice. *Proc Natl Acad Sci U S A.* 1999;96:7059–7064.
52. Milano CA, Dolber PC, Rockman HA, et al. Myocardial expression of a constitutively active alpha 1B-adrenergic receptor in transgenic mice induces cardiac hypertrophy. *Proc Natl Acad Sci U S A.* 1994;91:10109–10113.
53. Small KM, Wagoner LE, Levin AM, et al. Synergistic polymorphisms of beta1- and alpha2C-adrenergic receptors and the risk of congestive heart failure. *N Engl J Med.* 2002;347:1135–1142.
54. Ichikawa I, Pfeffer JM, Pfeffer MA, et al. Role of angiotensin II in the altered renal function of congestive heart failure. *Circ Res.* 1984;55:669–675.
55. Bell-Reuss E, Trevino DL, Gottschalk CW. Effect of renal sympathetic nerve stimulation on proximal water and sodium reabsorption. *J Clin Invest.* 1976;57:1104–1107.
56. McLeod AA, Brown JE, Kuhn C, et al. Differentiation of hemodynamic, humoral and metabolic responses to beta 1- and beta 2-adrenergic stimulation in man using atenolol and propranolol. *Circulation.* 1983;67:1076–1084.
57. Francis GS, Goldsmith SR, Cohn JN. Relationship of exercise capacity to resting left ventricular performance and basal plasma norepinephrine levels in patients with congestive heart failure. *Am Heart J.* 1982;104(4 Pt 1):725–731.
58. Cohn JN, Levine TB, Olivari MT, et al. Plasma norepinephrine as a guide to prognosis in patients with chronic congestive heart failure. *N Engl J Med.* 1984;311:819–823.
59. Mann DL, Kent RL, Parsons B, et al. Adrenergic effects on the biology of the adult mammalian cardiocyte. *Circulation.* 1992;85:790–804.
60. Communal C, Singh K, Pimentel DR, et al. Norepinephrine stimulates apoptosis in adult rat ventricular myocytes by activation of the beta-adrenergic pathway. *Circulation.* 1998;98:1329–1334.
61. Lijnen PJ, Petrov VV, Fagard RH. Induction of cardiac fibrosis by transforming growth factor-beta(1). *Mol Genet Metab.* 2000;71:418–435.
62. Yanagisawa M, Kurihara H, Kimura S, et al. A novel potent vasoconstrictor peptide produced by vascular endothelial cells. *Nature.* 1988;332:411–415.
63. Agapitov AV, Haynes WG. Role of endothelin in cardiovascular disease. *J Renin Angiotensin Aldosterone Syst.* 2002;3:1–15.
64. Yoshimoto S, Ishizaki Y, Sasaki T, et al. Effect of carbon dioxide and oxygen on endothelin production by cultured porcine cerebral endothelial cells. *Stroke.* 1991;22:378–383.
65. Ishikawa T, Yanagisawa M, Kimura S, et al. Positive inotropic action of novel vasoconstrictor peptide endothelin on guinea pig atria. *Am J Physiol.* 1988;255(4 Pt 2):H970–H973.
66. Ishikawa T, Yanagisawa M, Kimura S, et al. Positive chronotropic effects of endothelin, a novel endothelium-derived vasoconstrictor peptide. *Pflugers Arch.* 1988;413:108–110.
67. Komuro I, Kurihara H, Sugiyama T, et al. Endothelin stimulates c-fos and c-myc expression and proliferation of vascular smooth muscle cells. *FEBS Lett.* 1988;238:249–252.
68. López-Farré A, Montañés I, Millás I, et al. Effect of endothelin on renal function in rats. *Eur J Pharmacol.* 1989;163:187–189.
69. Zeidel ML, Brady HR, Kone BC, et al. Endothelin, a peptide inhibitor of Na(+)-K(+)-ATPase in intact renal tubular epithelial cells. *Am J Physiol.* 1989;257(6 Pt 1): C1101–C1107.
70. Plato CF, Pollock DM, Garvin JL. Endothelin inhibits thick ascending limb chloride flux via ET(B) receptor-mediated NO release. *Am J Physiol Renal Physiol.* 2000;279:F326–F333.
71. Cozza EN, Gomez-Sanchez CE, Foecking MF, et al. Endothelin binding to cultured calf adrenal zona glomerulosa cells and stimulation of aldosterone secretion. *J Clin Invest.* 1989;84:1032–1035.
72. Cunningham ME, Huribal M, Bala RJ, et al. Endothelin-1 and endothelin-4 stimulate monocyte production of cytokines. *Crit Care Med.* 1997;25:958–964.
73. McMurray JJ, Ray SG, Abdullah I, et al. Plasma endothelin in chronic heart failure. *Circulation.* 1992;85:1374–1379.
74. Pacher R, Bergler-Klein J, Globits S, et al. Plasma big endothelin-1 concentrations in congestive heart failure patients with or without systemic hypertension. *Am J Cardiol.* 1993;71:1293–1299.

75. Packer M, McMurray J, Massie BM, et al. Clinical effects of endothelin receptor antagonism with bosentan in patients with severe chronic heart failure: results of a pilot study. *J Card Fail*. 2005;11:12–20.

76. Hedayat M, Mahmoudi M, Rose N, et al. Proinflammatory cytokines in heart failure: double-edged swords. *Heart Fail Rev*. 2010;15:543–562.

77. Katz A. Pathophysiology of heart failure: identifying targets for pharmacotherapy. *Med Clin North Am*. 2003;87:303–316.

78. Siwik D, Pagano P, Colucci W. Oxidative stress regulates collagen synthesis and matrix metalloproteinase activity in cardiac fibroblasts. *Am J Physiol Cell Physiol*. 2001;280:C53–C60.

79. Deardorff R, Spinale F. Cytokines and matrix metalloproteinases as potential biomarkers in chronic heart failure. *Biomark Med*. 2009;3:513–523.

80. Ishibashi Y, Shimada T, Murakami Y, et al. An inhibitor of inducible nitric oxide synthase decreases forearm blood flow in patients with congestive heart failure. *J Am Coll Cardiol*. 2001;38:1470–1476.

81. Katz A. Maladaptive growth in the failing heart: the cardiomyopathy of overload. *Cardiovasc Drugs Ther*. 2002;16:245–249.

82. Boengler K, Hilfiker-Kleiner D, Drexler H, et al. The myocardial JAK/STAT pathway: from protection to failure. *Pharmacol Ther*. 2008;120:172–185.

83. Wagner M, Siddiqui M. Signaling networks regulating cardiac myocyte survival and death. *Curr Opin Investig Drugs*. 2009;10:928–937.

84. Hori M, Nishida K. Oxidative stress and left ventricular remodelling after myocardial infarction. *Cardiovasc Res*. 2009;81:457–464.

85. Kisch B. Electron microscopic investigation of the heart of cattle. 1. The atrium of the heart of cows. *Exp Med Surg*. 1959;17:247–261.

86. Levin ER, Gardner DG, Samson WK. Natriuretic peptides. *N Engl J Med*. 1998;339:321–328.

87. Iwanaga Y, Nishi I, Furuichi S, et al. B-type natriuretic peptide strongly reflects diastolic wall stress in patients with chronic heart failure comparison between systolic and diastolic heart failure. *J Am Coll Cardiol*. 2006;47:742–748.

88. Marcus LS, Hart D, Packer M, et al. Hemodynamic and renal excretory effects of human brain natriuretic peptide infusion in patients with congestive heart failure: a double-blind, placebo-controlled, randomized crossover trial. *Circulation*. 1996;94:3184–3189.

89. Yoshimura M, Yasue H, Morita E, et al. Hemodynamic, renal, and hormonal responses to brain natriuretic peptide infusion in patients with congestive heart failure. *Circulation*. 1991;84:1581–1588.

90. Abraham WT, Lowes BD, Ferguson DA, et al. Systemic hemodynamic, neurohormonal, and renal effects of a steady-state infusion of human brain natriuretic peptide in patients with hemodynamically decompensated heart failure. *J Card Fail*. 1998;4:37–44.

91. Brunner-La Rocca HP, Kaye DM, Woods RL, et al. Effects of intravenous brain natriuretic peptide on regional sympathetic activity in patients with chronic heart failure as compared with healthy control subjects. *J Am Coll Cardiol*. 2001;37:1221–1227.

92. Marin-Grez M, Fleming JT, Steinhausen M. Atrial natriuretic peptide causes preglomerular vasodilatation and post-glomerular vasoconstriction in rat kidney. *Nature*. 1986;324:473–476.

93. La Villa G, Fronzaroli C, Lazzeri C, et al. Cardiovascular and renal effects of low dose brain natriuretic peptide infusion in man. *J Clin Endocrinol Metab*. 1994;78:1166–1171.

94. Jensen KT, Eiskjaer H, Carstens J, et al. Renal effects of brain natriuretic peptide in patients with congestive heart failure. *Clin Sci (Lond)*. 1999;96:5–15.

95. Sackner-Bernstein JD, Skopicki HA, Aaronson KD. Risk of worsening renal function with nesiritide in patients with acutely decompensated heart failure. *Circulation*. 2005;111:1487–1491.

96. Greenberg BH, ed. *Congestive Heart Failure Textbook*. 2nd ed. Philadelphia: Lippincott Williams & Wilkins; 2000.

97. Hawkridge 3rd AM, Heublein DM, Bergen HR, et al. Quantitative mass spectral evidence for the absence of circulating brain natriuretic peptide (BNP-32) in severe human heart failure. *Proc Natl Acad Sci U S A*. 2005;102:17442–17447.

98. Lloyd-Jones D, Adams R, Carnethon M, et al. Heart disease and stroke statistics—2009 update: a report from the American Heart Association Statistics Committee and Stroke Statistics Subcommittee. *Circulation*. 2009;119:e21–e181.

99. Jessup M, Abraham WT, Casey DE, et al. 2009 focused update: ACCF/AHA Guidelines for the Diagnosis and Management of Heart Failure in Adults: a report of the American College of Cardiology Foundation/American Heart Association Task Force on Practice Guidelines: developed in collaboration with the International Society for Heart and Lung Transplantation. *Circulation*. 2009;119:1977–2016.

100. Rose EA, Gelijns AC, Moskowitz AJ, et al. Long-term mechanical left ventricular assistance for end-stage heart failure. *N Engl J Med*. 2001;345:1435–1443.

101. Bain KT, Maxwell TL, Strassels SA, et al. Hospice use among patients with heart failure. *Am Heart J*. 2009;158:118–125.

102. Binanay C, Califf RM, Hasselblad V, et al. Evaluation study of congestive heart failure and pulmonary artery catheterization effectiveness: the ESCAPE trial. *JAMA*. 2005;294:1625–1633.

103. Palardy M, Stevenson LW, Tasissa G, et al. Reduction in mitral regurgitation during therapy guided by measured filling pressures in the ESCAPE trial. *Circ Heart Fail*. 2009;2:181–188.

104. Hsu LF, Jaïs P, Sanders P, et al. Catheter ablation for atrial fibrillation in congestive heart failure. *N Engl J Med*. 2004;351:2373–2383.

105. Bogun F, Crawford T, Reich S, et al. Radiofrequency ablation of frequent, idiopathic premature ventricular complexes: comparison with a control group without intervention. *Heart Rhythm*. 2007;4:863–867.

106. De Nardo D, Antolini M, Pitucco G, et al. Effects of left bundle branch block on left ventricular function in apparently normal subjects: study by equilibrium radionuclide angiocardiography at rest. *Cardiology*. 1988;75:365–371.

107. Ljungman S, Laragh JH, Cody RJ. Role of the kidney in congestive heart failure: relationship of cardiac index to kidney function. *Drugs*. 1990;39(suppl 4):10–21.

108. Schoolwerth AC, Sica DA, Ballermann BJ, et al. Renal considerations in angiotensin converting enzyme inhibitor therapy: a statement for healthcare professionals from the Council on the Kidney in Cardiovascular Disease and the Council for High Blood Pressure Research of the American Heart Association. *Circulation*. 2001;104:1985–1991.

109. Kittleson M, Hurwitz S, Shah MR, et al. Development of circulatory-renal limitations to angiotensin-converting enzyme inhibitors identifies patients with severe heart failure and early mortality. *J Am Coll Cardiol*. 2003;41:2029–2035.

110. Fonarow GC, Stevenson LW, Steimle AE, et al. Persistently high left ventricular filling pressures predict mortality despite angiotensin converting enzyme inhibition in advanced heart failure. *Circulation*. 1994;90(Pt 2):I–488.

111. Gheorghiade M, Gattis WA, O'Connor CM, et al. Effects of tolvaptan, a vasopressin antagonist, in patients hospitalized with worsening heart failure: a randomized controlled trial. *JAMA*. 2004;291:1963–1971.

112. Akkan D, Kjaergaard J, Møller JE, et al. Prognostic importance of a short deceleration time in symptomatic congestive heart failure. *Eur J Heart Fail*. 2008;10:689–695.

113. Di Salvo TG, Mathier M, Semigran MJ, et al. Preserved right ventricular ejection fraction predicts exercise capacity and survival in advanced heart failure. *J Am Coll Cardiol*. 1995;25:1143–1153.

114. Baker BJ, Wilen MM, Boyd CM, et al. Relation of right ventricular ejection fraction to exercise capacity in chronic left ventricular failure. *Am J Cardiol*. 1984;54:596–599.

115. Heywood JT, Grimm J, Hess OM, et al. Right ventricular diastolic function during exercise: effect of ischemia. *J Am Coll Cardiol*. 1990;16:611–622.

116. Heywood JT, Grimm J, Hess OM, et al. Right ventricular systolic function during exercise in patients with coronary artery disease. *Am J Cardiol*. 1991;67:681–686.

117. Hillege HL, Girbes AR, de Kam PJ, et al. Renal function, neurohormonal activation, and survival in patients with chronic heart failure. *Circulation*. 2000;102:203–210.

118. Heywood JT, Fonarow GC, Costanzo MR, et al. High prevalence of renal dysfunction and its impact on outcome in 118,465 patients hospitalized with acute decompensated heart failure: a report from the ADHERE database. *J Card Fail*. 2007;13:422–430.

119. Fonarow GC, Adams Jr J.KF, Abraham WT, et al. Risk stratification for in-hospital mortality in acutely decompensated heart failure: classification and regression tree analysis. *JAMA*. 2005;293:572–580.

120. Firth JD, Raine AE, Ledingham JG. Raised venous pressure: a direct cause of renal sodium retention in oedema? *Lancet*. 1988;1:1033–1035.

121. Doty JM, Saggi BH, Sugerman HJ, et al. Effect of increased renal venous pressure on renal function. *J Trauma*. 1999;47:1000–1003.

122. Mullens W, Abrahams Z, Francis GS, et al. Importance of venous congestion for worsening of renal function in advanced decompensated heart failure. *J Am Coll Cardiol*. 2009;53:589–596.

123. Ronco C, Haapio M, House AA, et al. Cardiorenal syndrome. *J Am Coll Cardiol*. 2008;52:1527–1539.

124. Sackner-Bernstein JD, Kowalski M, Fox M, et al. Short-term risk of death after treatment with nesiritide for decompensated heart failure: a pooled analysis of randomized controlled trials. *JAMA*. 2005;293:1900–1905.

125. Cleland JG, Coletta AP, Yassin A, et al. Clinical trials update from the European Society of Cardiology Meeting 2009: AAA, RELY, PROTECT, ACTIVE-I, European CRT survey, German pre-SCD II registry, and MADIT-CRT. *Eur J Heart Fail*. 2009;11:1214–1219.

126. Lisy O, Huntley BK, McCormick DJ, et al. Design, synthesis and actions of a novel chimeric natriuretic peptide: CD-NP. *J Am Coll Cardiol*. 2008;52:60–68.

127. Krum H, Schlaich M, Whitbourn R, et al. Catheter-based renal sympathetic denervation for resistant hypertension: multicentre safety and proof-of-principle cohort study. *Lancet*. 2009;373:1275–1281.

128. Sin DD, Fitzgerald F, Parker JD, et al. Risk factors for central and obstructive sleep apnea in 450 men and women with congestive heart failure. *Am J Respir Crit Care Med*. 1999;160:1101–1106.

129. Bradley TD, Hall MJ, Ando S, et al. Hemodynamic effects of simulated obstructive apneas in humans with and without heart failure. *Chest*. 2001;119:1827–1835.

130. Brinker JA, Weiss JL, Lappé DL, et al. Leftward septal displacement during right ventricular loading in man. *Circulation*. 1980;61:626–633.

131. Morgan BJ, Denahan T, Ebert TJ. Neurocirculatory consequences of negative intrathoracic pressure vs. asphyxia during voluntary apnea. *J Appl Physiol*. 1993;74:2969–2975.

132. Arabi Y, Morgan BJ, Goodman B, et al. Daytime blood pressure elevation after nocturnal hypoxia. *J Appl Physiol*. 1999;87:689–698.

133. Naughton MT, Benard DC, Liu PP, et al. Effects of nasal CPAP on sympathetic activity in patients with heart failure and central sleep apnea. *Am J Respir Crit Care Med*. 1995;152:473–479.

134. Lanfranchi PA, Braghiroli A, Bosimini E, et al. Prognostic value of nocturnal Cheyne-Stokes respiration in chronic heart failure. *Circulation*. 1999;99:1435–1440.

135. Wang H, Parker JD, Newton GE, et al. Influence of obstructive sleep apnea on mortality in patients with heart failure. *J Am Coll Cardiol*. 2007;49:1625–1631.

136. Katz AM, Katz PB. Disease of the heart in the works of Hippocrates. *Br Heart J*. 1962;24:257–264.

CHAPTER **5**

Risk Factors for Mortality with Heart Failure

Keith D. Aaronson and Donna Mancini

INTRODUCTION

Prognostic indicators for heart failure (HF) include a long list of parameters from every aspect of clinical care, including history, physical examination, laboratory values, hemodynamics, echocardiograms, cardiac procedures, and biomarkers (Table 5-1).[1–5] The number of prognostic variables that have been described constitutes a list that can run more than several pages, and these variables are primarily from univariate analyses. However, the parameters that are readily available and can be easily applied to a patient who pointedly asks his or her physician how much time he or she has left are far fewer. This chapter reviews the most proven univariable and multivariable predictors of survival in HF and compares predictors for acute versus chronic HF, systolic versus diastolic HF, different subpopulations such as transplant candidates versus elderly patients, and mode of death (i.e., HF vs. sudden death). The use of multivariable models to guide prognostication better is examined later in the chapter.

STABLE CHRONIC HEART FAILURE

Although the list of univariable predictors in Table 5-1 is long, there is no perfect prognostic indicator—a variable that in isolation would reliably and easily identify a patient's risk. However, some variables are more powerful than others, and later in this chapter we review peak oxygen consumption (VO_2) extensively. Additional key powerful prognostic indicators include New York Heart Association (NYHA) classification, severely reduced left ventricular ejection fraction (LVEF), chronic hypotension (systolic blood pressure <90 mm Hg), hyponatremia (serum sodium <136 mEq/L), elevated brain natriuretic protein (BNP), troponin, and renal dysfunction. Patients with HF who also have an elevated serum creatinine (>1.5 mg/dL) or reduced glomerular filtration rate (GFR) (<44 mL/min) have significantly increased mortality. However, an ideal biomarker or test—one that has high specificity, has high sensitivity, has high reproducibility, has low cost, is generally available, is easily measured, and has been prospectively tested and validated that can be used across all demographic groups—does not exist (Fig. 5-1).[3] An elevated serum creatinine or a low hemoglobin value as a single marker raises concerns about a patient, but this value alone leaves the physician and patient with no firm trajectory. BNP, troponin, and renal dysfunction are discussed in more detail in subsequent sections.

ACUTE VERSUS CHRONIC HEART FAILURE

Most data on risk prognostication are derived from patients with chronic HF. Acute decompensated HF is a common reason for patients seeking emergency care, and risk stratification in this setting is much less defined. In 2006, 658,000 emergency department visits[6] occurred for acute decompensated HF, with approximately 80% of these patients admitted to the hospital.[7] The in-hospital mortality of these patients averages 3% to 4% with 10% to 12% mortality at 60 to 90 days. Rehospitalization rate and combined mortality and rehospitalization at 60 to 90 days are 30% and 36%.[8–11] Table 5-2 summarizes the OPTIMIZE-HF (Organized Program to Initiate Lifesaving Treatment in Hospitalized Patients with Heart Failure) data on more than 41,000 patients with both systolic HF and HF with preserved ejection fraction hospitalized for acute heart failure in the United States. These data are consistent with the findings of ADHERE (Acute Decompensated Heart Failure National Registry), which reported 4.1% in-hospital mortality in 65,180 patients with similar demographics (mean age 73 to 75 years, 52% women, reduced ejection fraction [<40%] in 51% to 52%, 50% to 57% with coronary heart disease, and 71% to 72% with hypertension). In more than 4000 community-based patients hospitalized in Canada for HF, in-hospital mortality was higher at 8.9%, but 30-day and 1-year mortality were comparable to the U.S. studies at 10.7% and 32.9%.

In the emergency department, physicians are unable to determine which HF patients would respond quickly to treatment and have a low probability of short-term adverse outcomes. The inability to identify low-risk

TABLE 5-1	Univariable Predictors of Survival in Heart Failure
Demographic parameters	Age, etiology, gender, race
Functional parameters	NYHA class, peak VO$_2$, % predicted peak VO$_2$, VE/VCO$_2$ ratio or slope, anaerobic threshold, circulatory power (peak VO$_2$ × systolic blood pressure), cardiac power (cardiac output × mean arterial pressure/451) oxygen kinetics (oxygen debt, recovery time), oxygen uptake efficiency slope, exercise oscillatory breathing pattern, chronotropic incompetence (i.e., failure to achieve 85% of age predicted maximum HR or low chronotropic index HR adjusted to maximal exercise test level), HR recovery, 6-minute walk test
Physical signs	↑ HR, ↓ blood pressure, S$_3$, BMI, mitral regurgitation
Ventricular function	LVEF, ventricular volumes, mitral regurgitation severity, RVEF, tricuspid annular plane systolic excursion
Hemodynamic parameters	RA, PVR, PCW, cardiac output, cardiac index, LVSWI, RVSWI, dP/dt
Laboratory values	Sodium, BUN, creatinine, urinalysis, hemoglobin, hypoalbuminemia, ESR, WBC, urine albumin excretion, insulin resistance, cholesterol
Neurohormones	NE, BNP, N terminal–pro BNP, angiotensin II, aldosterone, endothelin, vasopressin, adrenomedullin, IGF-I, testosterone, dehydroepiandrosterone, pro-ANP, MR-pro-ANP, galectin-3, tumor necrosis factor, C-reactive protein, interleukin-6, soluble CD 14
Biomarkers	Homocysteine, carbohydrate antigen 125, copeptin, troponin I, troponin T, cystatin C, neutrophil gelatinase associated lipocalin, growth differentiation factor 15, ST-2, type 1 collagen telopeptide
Electrocardiogram parameters	↑ QRS duration, ↑ Q-Tc interval, abnormal SAECG, T-wave alternans, ↓ HR variability, history of sudden cardiac death, atrial fibrillation, ventricular tachycardia, nonsustained ventricular tachycardia
Comorbidities	Diabetes, obesity, renal insufficiency, dementia, sleep apnea, mobility disorders
Genetic polymorphisms	Beta-1, beta-2, angiotensin-converting enzymes
Medical therapy	Digoxin, parenteral inotropes, inability to tolerate beta blockers or ACEIs
Recent heart failure hospitalization	

ACEIs, angiotensin-converting enzyme inhibitors; ANP, atrial natriuretic peptide; BMI, body mass index; BNP, brain natriuretic peptide, BUN, blood urea nitrogen; dP/dt, first derivative of pressure measured over time; ESR, erythrocyte sedimentation rate; HR, heart rate; IGF, insulinlike growth factor type I; LVEF, left ventricular ejection fraction; LVSWI, left ventricular stroke work index; NE, norepinephrine; NYHA, New York Heart Association; PCW, pulmonary capillary wedge; PVR, peripheral vascular resistance; RA, right atrium; RVEF, right ventricular ejection fraction; RVSWI, right ventricular stroke work index; SAECG, signal averaged electrocardiogram; VE/VCO$_2$, minute ventilation to CO$_2$ production; VO$_2$, oxygen consumption; WBC, white blood cell count.

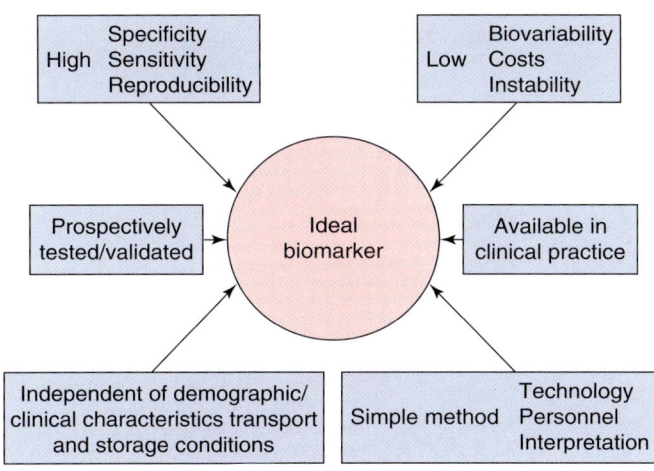

FIGURE 5-1 The ideal biomarker. (From Lainscak M, Anker M, Von Haehling S, et al. Biomarkers for chronic heart failure. Herz 2009;34:589-593.)

HF patients who can be safely discharged coupled with lack of access to quick follow-up care contributes to the high volume of HF admissions. However, large registry databases such as ADHERE[8] and OPTIMIZE-HF[9] have provided insight on patients presenting with acute HF with high and low risk (Table 5-3).

Acute decompensated HF includes a heterogeneous group of patients with a wide range of disease processes. Patients with admission profiles associated with greatest risk include patients with acute myocardial infarction, ischemia as evidenced by electrocardiogram (ECG) changes or elevated troponin T or I,[5] hypotension (systolic blood pressure <115 mm Hg), renal insufficiency (blood urea nitrogen [BUN] >43 mg/dL, creatinine >2.74 mg/dL), increased heart rate, hyponatremia, reduced ejection fraction, increased BNP, older age, and presence of comorbidities such as concomitant pneumonia.[11,12] Patients admitted who require vasoactive drugs have a poor prognosis with increased risk of death.[13] The need for inotropic support in the ADHERE study corresponded to an in-hospital mortality rate of 12% to 13%. Precipitating factors for HF admissions are associated with clinical outcomes independent of other predictive variables; in-hospital mortality ranges from 1.8% to 8% with dietary noncompliance associated with the lowest mortality and worsening renal failure associated with the highest in-hospital mortality (OPTIMIZE).[9]

In contrast, hypertensive patients (systolic blood pressure >160 mm Hg) may appear most acutely ill, but they generally have the best prognosis with a low 60-day mortality.[14] Similarly, patients presenting with acute decompensated HF secondary to medical noncompliance, poorly controlled hypertension, and normal cardiac troponin I levels also have a good prognosis (see Table 5-3). The current data derived on high-risk and low-risk acute HF patients are from hospitalized patients. Much more investigation is needed to determine whether in the future physicians will be able to identify low-risk patients who can be safely sent home from the emergency department. In a Canadian study of almost 51,000 emergency department visits related to HF, of the 16,094 patients who were discharged from the emergency department, 1.3% of these patients died within 7 days, and 4% died within 30 days, raising serious questions about the safety of any emergency department discharge.[15] Later on, we review risk stratification tools and models that have been developed to identify patients with low, intermediate, and high risk so as to triage better resources needed for their care.

Outcomes	Patients With LVSD (n 20,118)	Patients With PSF (EF>40%) (n 21,149)	p Value (LVSD vs.PSF)
TABLE 5-2	Clinical Outcomes from OPTIMIZE-HF Registry for Patients with Heart Failure from Systolic and Preserved Systolic Function		
In-hospital mortality: all patients, % (95% CI)	3.9 (3.6-4.2)	2.9 (2.7-3.1)	.0001
Follow-up cohort	(n=2604)	(n=2294)	
Postdischarge mortality at 60-90 days, % (95% CI)	9.8 (8.2-11.4)	9.5 (7.9-11.0)	.459
Rehospitalization at 60-90 days, % (95% CI)	29.9 (28.1-31.6)	29.2 (28.1-31.6)	.591
Postdischarge mortality/rehospitalization at 60-90 days, % (95% CI)	36.1 (34.3-37.9)	35.3 (33.4-37.3)	.577

CI, confidence interval.

From Fonarow G, Stough W, Abraham W, et al. Characteristics, treatments, and outcomes of patients with preserved systolic heart failure: a report from the OPTIMIZE-HF Registry. J Am Coll Cardiol 2007;50:768-777.

TABLE 5-3	Prognostic Indicators for Acute Decompensated Congestive Heart Failure
Admission Profile Associated with Good Outcome (Low In-Hospital Mortality)	Admission Profile Associated with Poor Outcome
Hypertensive	Elderly
Normal renal function	Blood pressure <100 mm Hg
Serum sodium >136 mEq/L	Creatinine >2.5 mg/dL
Normal troponin	Elevated troponin or ischemic ECG changes
Absence of comorbidity	Pneumonia or significant comorbidity (i.e., dementia, cancer, CVA)
Noncompliance	Good compliance with medications and diet
Diastolic dysfunction	Markedly elevated BNP

BNP, brain natriuretic peptide; CVA, cerebrovascular accident; ECG, electrocardiogram.

HOSPITALIZATIONS

Hospitalizations related to HF continue to increase with 400,000 discharges for HF in 1979 increasing to 1.1 million in 2005.[6] HF is currently the most frequent primary discharge diagnosis, and this number increases to 2 million and 3 million if secondary and tertiary discharge diagnoses listed as HF are also included. Hospitalization for HF is itself a marker for disease progression, increased mortality (Fig. 5-2A), and increased risk of early rehospitalization.[16–19] In the Digitalis Investigation Group Trial, division of patients into patients with at least one HF hospitalization (*n* = 1732) versus no hospitalizations (*n* = 5501) in the 2 years after randomization showed a hazard ratio (HR) of 5.22 for HF mortality in patients with a hospitalization for HF (*P* < .001) (see Fig. 5-2A).[17] Similarly, analysis of the health care usage database during the period 2000-2004 in British Columbia, Canada,[19] showed that in the 14,374 patients admitted with HF, mortality increased with each subsequent hospitalization (Fig. 5-2B). In ambulatory patients with chronic HF, a hospitalization for HF is associated with a marked increase of mortality.

Mortality increases after each hospitalization for HF, and this holds true for systolic and diastolic HF. Examination of data on patients with newly diagnosed chronic HF during the period 1987-2006 identified 1077 patients who experienced

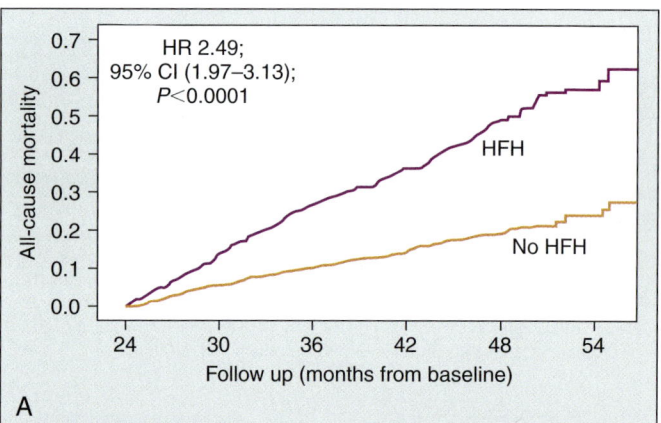

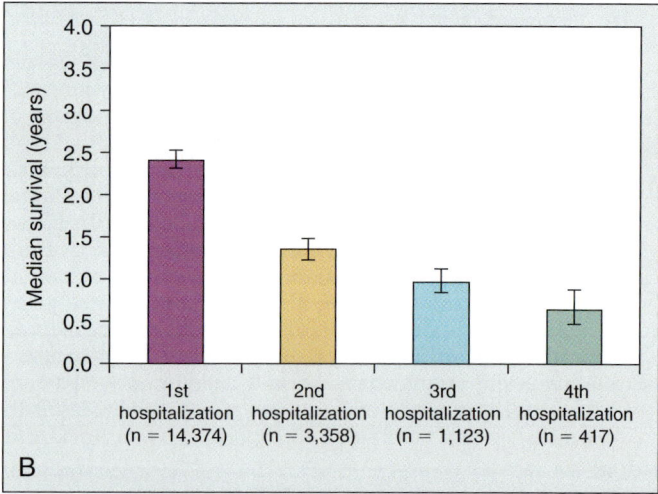

FIGURE 5-2 **A,** Increased mortality in patients with any heart failure hospitalization (HFH). CI, confidence interval; HR, hazard ratio. **B,** Increasing mortality with every subsequent admission. (**A,** From Ahmed A, Allman R, Ponarow G, et al. Incident heart failure hospitalization and subsequent mortality in chronic heart failure: a propensity-matched study. J Card Fail 2008;14:211-218; **B,** from Setoguchi S, Stevenson L, Schneeweiss S. Repeated hospitalizations predict mortality in the community population with heart failure. Am Heart J 2007;154:260-266.)

4.359 hospitalizations over a follow-up of approximately 5 years. Of the patients, 83% were hospitalized at least once, and 67% had multiple admissions. Male gender and comorbid conditions such as diabetes, chronic obstructive pulmonary disease, and renal insufficiency were independent predictors of hospitalization.[20]

Hospital readmission rates are high after the index HF hospitalization and are associated with a substantially increased rate of subsequent hospitalizations. Rehospitalization rates at 1 year are 60% to 69% of patients admitted for any reason, 44% to 50% of patients admitted for a cardiovascular reason, and 14% to 30% of patients admitted for recurrent heart failure. The high rate of rehospitalization of patients admitted for any reason reflects the multiple comorbidities in HF patients. In patients with at least two or more hospitalizations for HF, readmission occurred in 60% at 1 year with 90% of readmissions for cardiovascular reasons and 60% for HF alone.[21,22]

HEART FAILURE WITH PRESERVED SYSTOLIC FUNCTION

The clinical profiles of patients with HF with preserved systolic function versus systolic HF are distinct, with patients with the former condition more frequently female, elderly, hypertensive, and obese, with atrial fibrillation and chronic obstructive pulmonary disease as frequent comorbidities. Survival rates of patients with diastolic dysfunction are reported as either better than or similar to survival rates of patients with systolic dysfunction (Fig. 5-3). There are only a few reports on clinical parameters that predict survival in patients with diastolic HF. As in patients with systolic dysfunction, age, higher NYHA class, higher BNP, expired volume-to-carbon dioxide consumption (VE/VCO_2) ratio, pulmonary pressures, exercise oscillatory breathing, reduced peak VO_2, renal insufficiency, diabetes, anemia, hyponatremia, dementia, and peripheral arterial disease are associated with reduced survival in patients with HF with preserved systolic function. However, male gender and coronary artery disease have not been identified as predictors of reduced survival in diastolic dysfunction.[23–25]

SUDDEN CARDIAC DEATH VERSUS PROGRESSIVE HEART FAILURE

Sudden cardiac death can occur in 50% of patients with HF, but there are a few parameters that specifically identify patients at risk for an arrhythmic death over progressive HF.

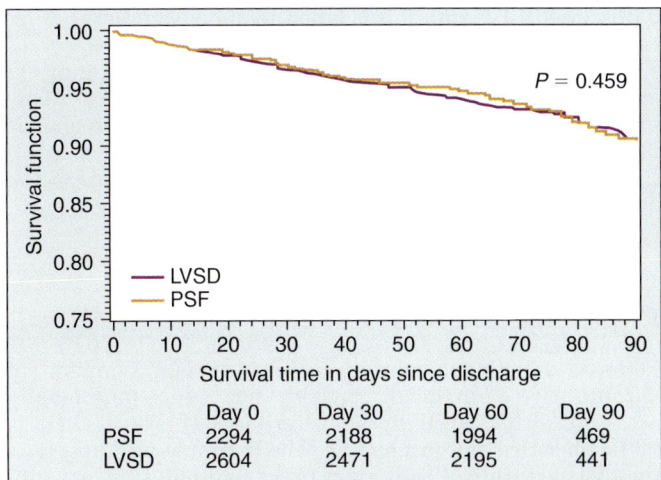

FIGURE 5-3 Survival curves of patients with systolic heart failure and patients with heart failure with preserved ejection fraction. LVSD, left ventricular systolic dysfunction; PSF, preserved systolic failure. *(From Fonarow G, Stough W, Abraham W, et al. Characteristics, treatments, and outcomes of patients with preserved systolic heart failure: a report from the OPTIMIZE-HF Registry. J Am Coll Cardiol 2007;50:768-777.)*

The incidence of sudden cardiac death is higher in patients with mild HF than in patients with advanced disease.[26] Data from MERIT-HF (Metoprolol CR/XL Randomised Intervention Trial in Congestive Heart Failure) showed the change in the distribution of the mode of death as HF advances (Fig. 5-4).[27] In patients with NYHA class II chronic HF, 64% of the deaths were classified as sudden death, and 12% were due to progressive HF, whereas in patients with NYHA class IV chronic HF, 33% died suddenly, and 56% died from progressive HF. Although treatment with angiotensin-converting enzyme inhibitors (ACEIs) and angiotensin II receptor blockers has had a significant impact on HF survival, the impact of these therapies has been through a reduction in HF and not in arrhythmic deaths. In contrast, beta blockers and spironolactone have contributed to a reduction in the incidence of both sudden deaths and progressive HF deaths. Parameters that have been identified as prognostic indicators for sudden cardiac death include presence of severely reduced LVEF; ischemic etiology; prolonged QRS duration; presence of nonsustained ventricular tachycardia; prior episode of sudden cardiac death; history of syncope; elevated BNPs; and, in patients with an ischemic etiology, abnormal T-wave alternans (which is variably predictive in patients with nonischemic etiologies).[28–31] More recently, elevated ST2, an interleukin-1 receptor family member, which has effects on myocardial fibrosis, has been reported to be predictive of sudden cardiac death complementary to BNP.[30]

ELDERLY VERSUS TRANSPLANT REFERRAL POPULATIONS

Despite the growing problem of HF in elderly patients, most of the literature describing prognosis has been derived from younger and middle-aged white male patients being evaluated for advanced HF therapies including clinical trials or cardiac transplantation. The demographic profile of HF in elderly patients is distinct with a greater percentage of female patients, more diastolic dysfunction, and more comorbidities.[32,33] When most elderly patients had limited treatment options, this de-emphasis on elderly patients was more acceptable, but with the advent of the use of left ventricular assist devices as destination therapy, a more exacting approach is needed. A more recent analysis of the elderly population (age 72 ± 6 years [mean $\pm$ SD]) showed that peak VO_2 and the Heart Failure Survival Score (HFSS) were excellent prognostic indicators in an ambulatory elderly population (Fig. 5-5).[34]

In a review of 62,330 elderly patients from a national database of Medicare beneficiaries hospitalized for HF (mean age 80 years, 59% women, 72% with a prior history of HF), 30-day mortality was 9.8%. The best predictors of mortality were presence of dementia, impaired mobility (i.e., inability to walk unaided), elevated serum creatinine, and history of cancer. For this cohort, 5-year mortality was 74.7%.[34] This analysis suggests that the attributable mortality risk from HF in older patients may be age-dependent; among "old-old" HF patients, who are often burdened with many additional comorbidities, HF may be a relatively minor contributor to mortality.

RENAL DYSFUNCTION

Serum creatinine and BUN have frequently been identified as powerful prognostic factors in patients with acute and chronic HF. There is a high prevalence of renal dysfunction in patients admitted with acute decompensated HF. Derivation of GFR using the Modification of Diet in Renal Disease formula for 118,465 patients from the ADHERE database found that only 9% of patients had normal renal function (defined

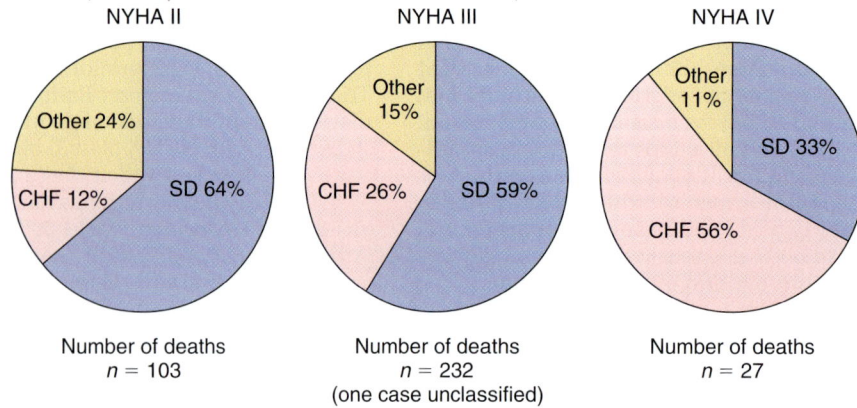

NYHA II — Number of deaths n = 103
NYHA III — Number of deaths n = 232 (one case unclassified)
NYHA IV — Number of deaths n = 27

FIGURE 5-4 Shift in the incidence of sudden death by New York Heart Association (NYHA) class (MERIT-HF). CHF, chronic heart failure; SD, sudden death. *(From Effects of Metoprolol CR/XL in chronic heart failure: Metoprolol CR/XL Randomised Intervention Trial in Congestive Heart Failure [MERIT-HF]. Lancet 1999;353:2001-2007.)*

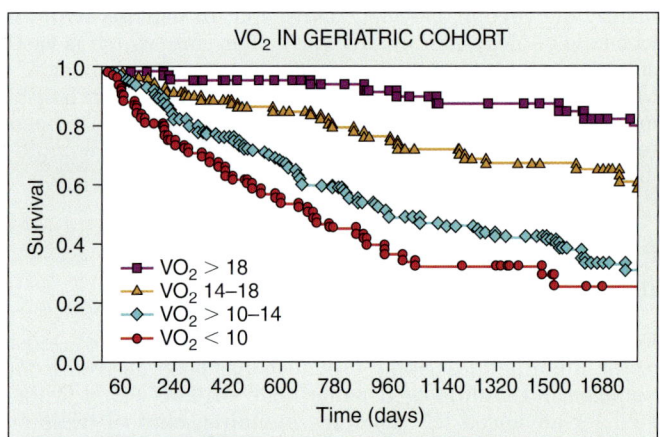

FIGURE 5-5 Prognostic value of peak oxygen consumption (VO₂) in an elderly cohort. *(From Parikh M, Lund L, Goda A, et al. Usefulness of peak exercise oxygen consumption and the Heart Failure Survival Score to predict survival in patients >65 years of age with heart failure. Am J Cardiol 2009;103:998-1002.)*

as GFR >90 mL/min), and 63.5% had moderate to severe renal insufficiency (GFR <60 mL/min).[35] In patients with normal renal function, hospital mortality was 1.9%; this increased to 7.6% in patients with severe renal insufficiency (GFR <30 mL/min). Acute treatment during hospitalization was modified according to renal function with more patients with renal insufficiency receiving inotropic support and nesiritide and fewer patients receiving ACEIs or angiotensin II receptor blockers. It is unclear whether this divergence in therapy affected the mortality rates observed. As discussed later, renal parameters are key variables in the ADHERE risk tool and the EFFECT (Enhanced Feedback for Effective Cardiac Treatment) model for mortality assessment for acute decompensated HF.

Similarly, the development of worsening renal function as evidenced by serum creatinine, GFR, or BUN values during acute hospitalization for HF is associated with poor clinical outcomes. Development of varying degrees of the cardiorenal syndrome and the whole cascade of neurohormonal changes associated with this syndrome likely contributes to the poor clinical outcomes.[36,37]

BIOMARKERS

As discussed earlier, no ideal biomarker has been described yet, but of all the prognostic biomarkers currently identified, BNP comes closest to that ideal parameter.[3] This measurement entails an easily obtainable, rapidly processed, inexpensive blood test that has excellent sensitivity and good specificity for HF. Elevated BNP in a dyspneic patient in the emergency department has assisted in the rapid diagnosis of HF. An elevated BNP probably also provides prognostic information at the time of discharge and provides assistance in the modification of therapies. BNP also has very significant negative predictive accuracy for the diagnosis of HF.[38] Another valuable biomarker in acute and chronic HF is serum troponin both in patients with acute coronary syndrome and in patients with nonischemic acute decompensated HF.[5]

METABOLIC MARKERS

Metabolic markers such as serum cholesterol, uric acid, hemoglobin, and blood glucose all have been variably reported to be predictive of outcome in HF patients.[3] An inverse relationship between serum cholesterol and survival has been described in patients with HF, which is evidenced by a low total cholesterol in HF patients, and reflects malnutrition and cachexia as poor prognostic factors.[39] Insulin resistance is commonly observed in patients with HF and is associated with worse prognosis in HF.[40] Hyperuricemia is another metabolic abnormality associated with an adverse prognosis. Use of the uric acid–lowering agent oxypurinol in 405 patients with class III-IV chronic HF failed to show significant clinical benefit.[41]

Subclinical inflammation is probably the common mechanism that underlies these metabolic abnormalities. Many biomarkers that have been identified as poor prognostic indicators simply reflect the degree of systemic or local inflammation (i.e., C-reactive protein, tumor necrosis factor, and interleukin-6).[3]

OXYGEN CONSUMPTION AS A PROGNOSTIC INDICATOR

Reduced functional capacity is the cardinal symptom of chronic HF. Functional capacity has been traditionally assessed in chronic HF by NYHA criteria. This assessment is both subjective and insensitive. The 6-minute walk test (i.e., the distance walked over a period of 6 minutes) is less subjective than NYHA functional class but still can be heavily influenced by the motivation of the patient or tester or both. Additionally, the 6-minute walk test results cannot estimate how close the patient was to his or her maximal capacity, and this submaximal test approaches maximal effort in patients with severe HF.[42]

Despite these caveats, the 6-minute walk test was first shown to provide prognostic information by the SOLVD (Study of Left Ventricular Dysfunction) investigators, who showed in a substudy of 898 HF patients in their registry that mortality risk was 3.7 times higher in patients with a 6-minute walk distance less than 350m compared with patients who walked more than 450m. Similarly, the risk of HF hospitalization was also 1.4 times higher in patients with reduced walk distance.[43] Subsequent investigators have shown prognostic value with the 6-minute walk test in some cohorts, but others have not. In the context of comparison with other measures of functional capacity such as cardiopulmonary exercise testing, which are reviewed subsequently, the prognostic significance of this test frequently diminishes.[44,45]

Determination of peak oxygen uptake during a maximal symptom limited treadmill or bicycle exercise test is the most objective method to assess maximal functional capacity in patients with chronic HF and has been shown to be the best indicator of prognosis. By identifying the ventilatory threshold, the physician can determine the adequacy of the patient's effort and if not maximal, how close the patient was to achieving his or her maximal effort. Noninvasive cardiopulmonary exercise testing has gained widespread application in functional assessment of patients with congestive HF. It is a useful test to determine the severity of the disease, provide important prognostic information, and assess the efficacy of new drugs and devices.

Peak VO_2 is derived from the Fick principle: Peak VO_2 is the product of peak cardiac output and maximal arteriovenous oxygen difference. Because most sedentary individuals can achieve comparable maximal arteriovenous difference, peak VO_2 provides an indirect assessment of cardiac output reserve, and this largely underlies the effectiveness of peak VO_2 in risk stratification. Several peripheral factors may also affect peak VO_2, such as the metabolic activity of skeletal muscle mass and endothelial function and demographics such as age, gender, and body surface area. Because skeletal muscle mass and its metabolic activity both decrease and endothelial function is progressively impaired as HF severity increases, the prognostic utility of peak VO_2 is enhanced.

The use of peak VO_2 to determine prognosis in patients with HF was first described by Szlachcic and colleagues.[46] In 27 patients, they reported a 77% 1-year mortality rate for patients with VO_2 less than 10mL/kg/min and a 21% mortality rate for patients with VO_2 10 to 18mL/kg/min. In a prospective study of 114 ambulatory patients with chronic HF referred for cardiac transplantation, VO_2 of less than 14mL/kg/min was used as a criterion for acceptance for cardiac transplantation.[47] Patients were divided into three groups based on the results of their cardiopulmonary stress tests: Patients with peak VO_2 less than 14mL/kg/min were accepted as transplant candidates (group 1; $n = 35$); transplant was deferred for patients with peak VO_2 greater than 14mL/kg/min (group 2; $n = 52$); group 3 ($n = 27$) comprised patients with peak VO_2 less than 14mL/kg/min who had a significant comorbidity that precluded transplant (Fig. 5-6). Age, LVEF, and resting hemodynamic parameters were similar in all three groups. In patients with VO_2 greater than 14mL/kg/min, 1-year survival was 94%. Accepted transplant candidates with VO_2 less than 14mL/kg/min had a 1-year survival of 70%; patients with a significant comorbidity and VO_2 less than 14mL/kg/min had a 1-year survival of 47%. Patients accepted for transplant had a falsely elevated survival because all transplants were treated as a censored observation. If urgent transplant was counted as death, the 1-year survival decreased to 48%. This approach permitted the identification of candidates whose transplant could be safely deferred.

Analysis of the ventilatory data obtained during cardiopulmonary testing enables the clinician investigator to determine if a maximal test has been performed and whether an accurate

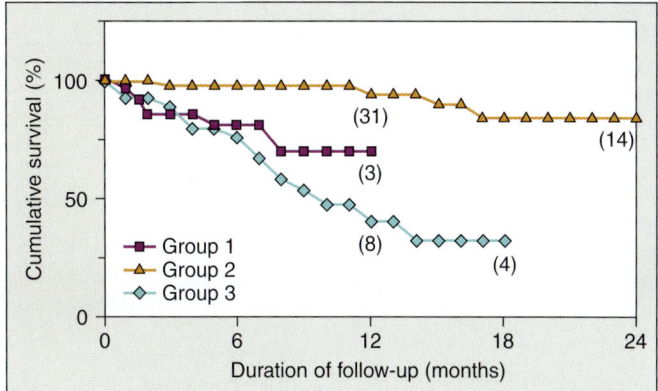

FIGURE 5-6 Survival in patients stratified by peak oxygen consumption (VO_2) and transplant status: peak VO_2 greater than 14 mL/kg/min, transplant deferred (group 1); peak VO_2 less than 14 mL/kg/min, listed for transplant (group 2); peak VO_2 less than 14 mL/kg/min, not listed for transplant because of comorbidities. *(From Mancini DM, Eisen H, Kussmaul W, et al. Value of peak exercise oxygen consumption for optimal timing of cardiac transplantation in ambulatory patients with heart failure. Circulation 1991;83:778-786.)*

peak VO_2 has been measured. Identification of the anaerobic threshold at 50% to 80% of peak VO_2 generally indicates a maximal effort. Peak VO_2 is a continuous variable. Use of statistical methods such as stratum-specific ratios to identify a clear threshold below which the relative risk of death would precipitously increase have yielded a linear relationship of VO_2 with outcome without clear thresholds.[48] Peak exercise VO_2 can be influenced by noncardiac factors such as muscle mass and deconditioning, age, gender, and obesity. Analysis of peak VO_2 normalized by a predicted maximum based on age, obesity, and gender has been performed to determine if better prognostication can be achieved using percent of predicted peak VO_2. Some investigators have suggested the superiority of this approach, whereas others have shown no clear benefit.[49,50] The additional value of adjusting for sex, age, and body composition in any study cohort likely is a function of how these characteristics are distributed across the cohort; in studies of largely middle-aged men of average weight, the methods give similar results, whereas cohorts with greater heterogeneity would likely be better served by reference to sex-specific and age-specific prediction equations with adjustment for weight extremes.[51]

Use of serial measurements of peak VO_2 has also been shown to identify effectively patients in a low-risk category over time.[52] Conversely, a significant decline usually parallels clinical worsening and a worse prognosis; this is particularly important as the therapy for cardiac diseases continue to evolve and improve. Since the initial report of the value of peak VO_2 in guiding transplant candidate selection in 1991, there have been many advances in the treatment of HF. In particular, the use of beta blockade has had a significant impact on long-term survival without significantly improving peak VO_2. Whether VO_2 has retained its predictive power with the advent of beta blockers has been the subject of several reports.[53-55]

Consistent across these reports was the sustained utility of this parameter in predicting survival. Cohorts dichotomized by threshold values of greater than and less than 14 mL/kg/min, or greater than and less than 10 mL/kg/min in patients receiving beta blockers, showed that VO_2 retained its predictive value (Fig. 5-7). The survival for patients receiving beta-blocking agents increased but nevertheless diverged according to peak VO_2. With the improved survival conferred by this therapy, a lower cut point than 14 mL/kg/min for referral or listing for cardiac transplant has generally been accepted, with the American College of Cardiology

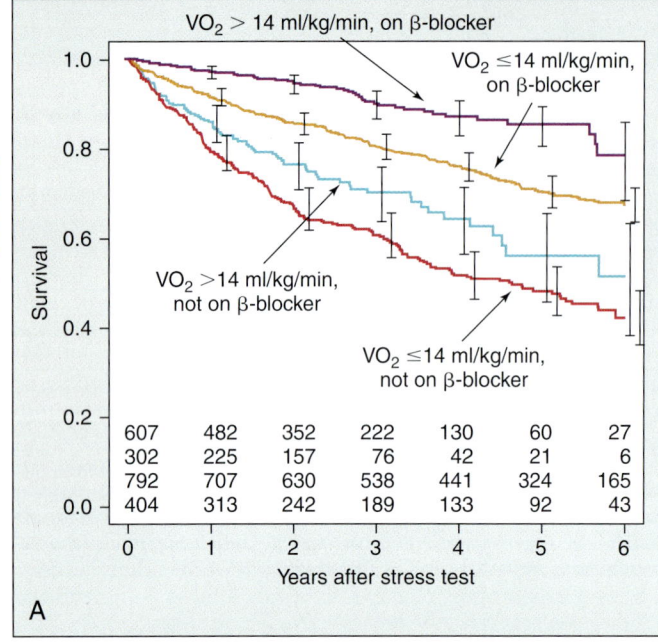

FIGURE 5-7 Survival stratified by peak oxygen consumption (VO_2) (<14 mL/kg/min vs. >14 mL/kg/min) and beta blocker usage. *(From O'Neill J, Young J, Pothier C, et al. Peak oxygen consumption as a predictor of death in patients with heart failure receiving beta blockers. Circulation 2005;111:2313-2318.)*

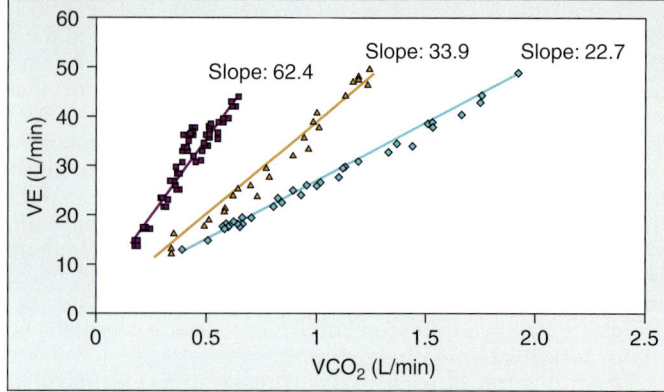

FIGURE 5-8 Examples of expired volume (VE)/carbon dioxide consumption (VCO₂) slope throughout exercise. *(From Arena R, Myers J, Abella J, et al. Development of a ventilatory classification system in patients with heart failure. Circulation 2007;115:2410-2417.)*

Foundation (ACCF)/American Heart Association (AHA) guidelines now selecting a peak VO_2 less than 10 mL/kg/min with achievement of anaerobic threshold as an absolute indication for transplant (in the absence of significant contraindications). A peak VO_2 of 11 to 14 mL/kg/min or 55% of predicted peak VO_2 resulting in major limitation of the patient's daily activities is considered a relative indication for transplant listing.[56]

During cardiopulmonary exercise testing, many variables are collected that also provide prognostic information. Ventilatory response to exercise, most frequently measured by the VE/VCO_2 ratio or slope, has been found by several investigators to be even more predictive of outcome than peak VO_2.[57-59] The abnormal VE/VCO_2 response results from increased ventilation-perfusion mismatching and heightened chemosensitivity and ergoreflex responses. This heightened ventilatory response occurs from the onset of exercise, and in contrast to peak VO_2, the VE/VCO_2 relationship does not require a maximal effort. However, there has been no consensus on how best to derive this parameter. Both VE/VCO_2 ratios and slopes have been reported (i.e., VE/VCO_2 ratio at anaerobic threshold or at peak exercise and VE/VCO_2 slope from onset of exercise to the anaerobic threshold or throughout the total exercise period). The VE/VCO_2 slope derived throughout exercise testing seems to have the greatest prognostic power (Fig. 5-8). A VE/VCO_2 greater than 34 has been the cut point selected in many studies, but similar to peak VO_2, this parameter is a continuous variable with no absolute cut point. Published studies have shown a VE/VCO_2 ratio greater than 30 conferring increased risk with the worst prognosis associated with a VE/VCO_2 ratio greater than 40.[60]

VE/VCO_2 correlates more strongly with pulmonary pressures measured during exercise than does peak VO_2. Both peak VO_2 and VE/VCO_2 are frequently found to have independent prognostic power in studies. The combination of VE/VCO_2 and peak VO_2 may provide the strongest way to determine risk. A patient with a preserved peak VO_2 yet an abnormal VE/VCO_2 remains at greater risk than if the ventilatory response was normal. Similarly, with the converse situation,

in which peak VO_2 is severely reduced but VE/VCO_2 is normal, the patient remains at increased risk despite the normal ventilatory response. Patients with severely reduced VO_2 (<10 mL/kg/min) and large VE/VCO_2 (>40) are in the poorest survival group. Peak VO_2 and VE/VCO_2 slope provide independent and complementary data on prognosis and should be used together to assess risk.[61,62]

Exercise oscillatory breathing is associated with a poor prognosis both in patients with diastolic dysfunction and in patients with systolic dysfunction. There is no uniform definition of this type of breathing; it is a periodic cycling of hyperpnea and hypopnea with appropriate changes in end-tidal oxygen pressure and end-tidal carbon dioxide pressure. This breathing pattern is observed in about 12% to 30% of HF patients during exercise, and most patients with exercise oscillatory breathing have central sleep apnea (Fig. 5-9). A definition for this breathing pattern is not established, but a persistence of periodic breathing for 60% of exercise with amplitude of oscillations greater than 15% over rest has been suggested. The presence of periodic breathing can predict mortality by itself or when combined with the ventilatory slope. In 156 patients with HF, this breathing pattern was strongly correlated with sudden death.[63,64]

Other parameters measured during cardiopulmonary exercise testing that also have been shown to have prognostic power in chronic HF include blood pressure response to exercise (i.e., blunted or failure to increase blood pressure with exercise associated with poor prognosis), heart rate response to exercise (i.e., chronotropic incompetence), ventilatory threshold, circulatory power (peak VO_2 × systolic blood pressure), oxygen kinetics, end-tidal partial pressure of carbon dioxide, and oxygen recovery after exercise.[65-69]

Similar to much HF research, studies of cardiopulmonary exercise have focused largely on systolic HF and have enrolled mainly middle-aged men (reflecting the central role of these studies in the evaluation of heart transplant candidates). However, more recent studies have begun to investigate the prognostic value of peak VO_2 in women, elderly patients, and patients with diastolic HF. In a study by Elimariah and coworkers,[70] peak VO_2 identified women with a worse prognosis, although the overall survival of women was significantly better than their male counterparts (Fig. 5-10). These findings were confirmed by Green and colleagues.[71]

Exercise testing has been used sparingly in elderly populations.[72,73] However, more recently, Parikh and associates[34] showed the prognostic value of peak VO_2 in 396 patients older than 65 years old with HF (see Fig. 5-5).

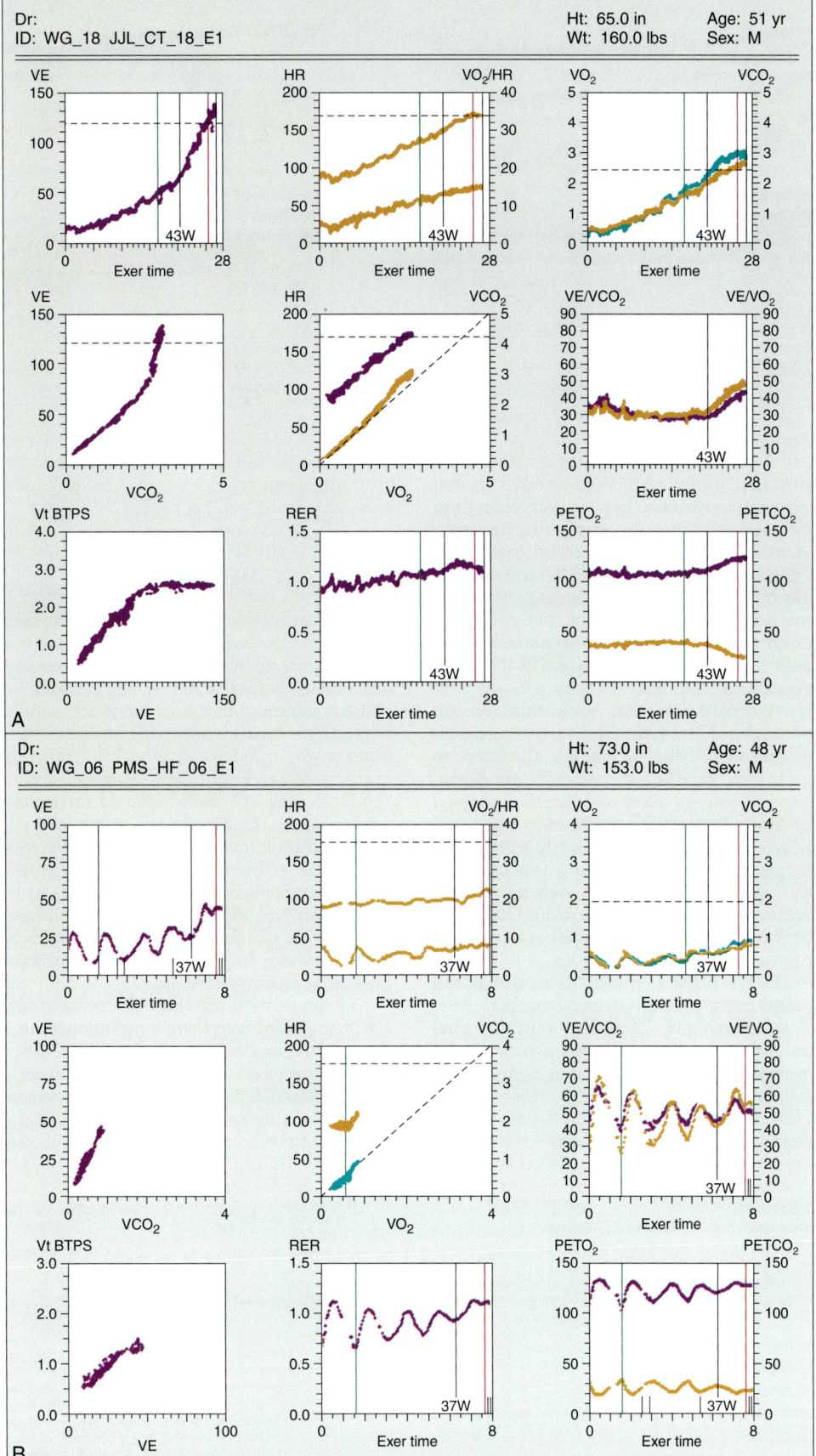

FIGURE 5-9 University of California, Los Angeles (UCLA), montage graphs of a normal subject **(A)** and a heart failure patient **(B)** with oscillatory breathing. VE, minute ventilation; HR, heart rate; VO$_2$, oxygen consumption; VCO$_2$, carbon dioxide production; Vt, tidal volume; BTPS, body temperature and presaturated; RER, respiratory exchange ratio; PETO$_2$, partial pressure of end tidal oxygen; PETCO$_2$, partial pressure of end tidal carbon dioxide.

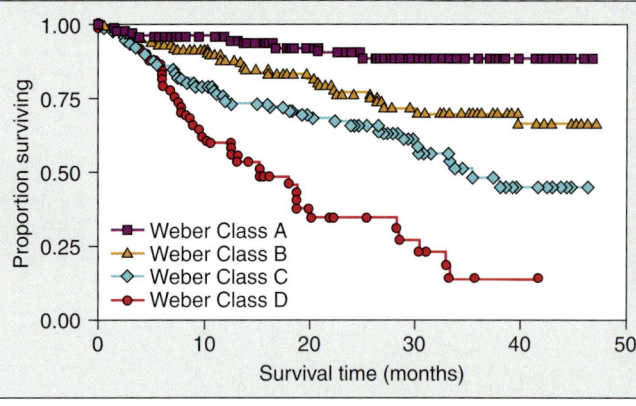
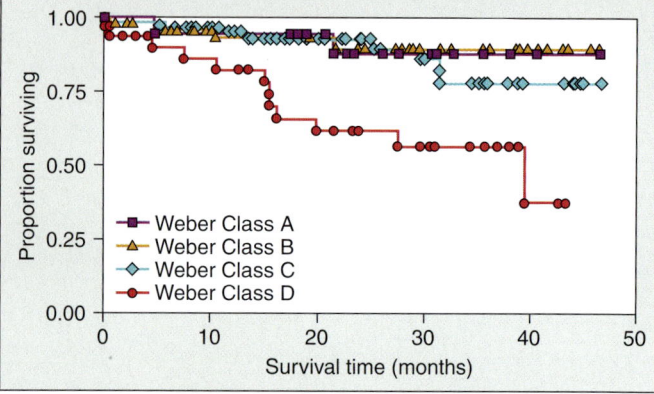

FIGURE 5-10 Kaplan-Meier survival curves by Weber class for men *(left)* and women *(right)*. *(From Elimariah S, Goldberg L, Allen M, et al. Effects of gender on peak oxygen consumption and timing of cardiac transplantation. J Am Coll Cardiol 2006;47:2237-2242.)*

Approximately 40% of patients with HF have HF with preserved systolic function. Use of peak VO_2 to determine outcome in patients with HF with preserved systolic function is controversial[74,75] and much less defined. The cardiopulmonary response of patients with HF with preserved systolic function is essentially indistinguishable from the response of patients with systolic dysfunction.[76]

In a study by Guazzi and colleagues[74] of 50 patients with ejection fractions greater than 50%, both peak VO_2 and VE/VCO_2 slope were univariable predictors of survival, but only the VE/VCO_2 slope was predictive by multivariable analysis. In another study by Guazzi and colleagues[75] in 151 patients with diastolic dysfunction, peak VO_2, VE/VCO_2 slope, and exercise oscillatory breathing all were significant predictors of adverse outcomes with exercise oscillatory breathing being the strongest predictor. Much more study is needed before any conclusions can be drawn about the prognostic value of cardiopulmonary exercise tests in these patients. The number of women studied with exercise testing is significantly smaller than men by a ratio of 1:5-6, but cardiopulmonary exercise testing is likely as valid in both sexes. Data in patients with HF with preserved systolic function and elderly patients are much fewer.

As the therapy of HF has advanced with time so has the technology of metabolic carts. Advances in technology now permit noninvasive measurement of cardiac output using inert gas rebreathing techniques.[76-78] The prognostic value of peak VO_2 has been presumed to be its value as a noninvasive indicator of peak cardiac output response to exercise. Before the availability of newer noninvasive methodologies, several studies suggested that hemodynamically derived variables

from pulmonary artery catheters may enhance risk stratification over peak VO_2 (see Table 5-3).[78]

EXERCISE HEMODYNAMICS

Small to moderate-sized studies have investigated the use of hemodynamic parameters as risk predictors in HF (Table 5-4). The prognostic superiority of hemodynamically derived exercise variables over peak VO_2 was first shown by Griffin and associates,[79] who reported data on 49 HF patients. In this study, left ventricular stroke work index at peak exercise dichotomized at $20 g/m^2$ identified patients with a threefold to fivefold higher mortality compared with the remaining patients. Exercise duration and peak VO_2 were unable to discriminate survivors from nonsurvivors. This study was followed by several studies comparing pulmonary artery catheter measurements with peak VO_2; conclusions varied, but most studies showed the better predictive value of left ventricular stroke work index over peak VO_2.[80-84] This finding is largely in patients with inadequate cardiac output or heart rate responses. The relatively small sample size in this study may explain the lack of equivalent power of cardiopulmonary exercise testing.

Advances in technology in recent years now permit easily obtainable noninvasive measurement of cardiac output at rest and during exercise. In 2001, Williams and colleagues[85] published the first study on the correlation between survival and hemodynamic data obtained by noninvasive measurement of cardiac output using carbon dioxide rebreathing integrated with a standard exercise test. Inert gas rebreathing is a novel, noninvasive method to

TABLE 5-4	Hemodynamic Parameters and Cardiopulmonary Testing				
Study	No.	Method	Hemodynamic	Better than VO_2
Tan[87]	63	Swan-Ganz; TD	Cardiac power output	NA
Griffin[79]	49	Swan-Ganz; TD	SWI	Yes
Roul[80]	50	Swan-Ganz; TD	Peak cardiac power	Yes
Chomsky[82]	185	Swan-Ganz; TD	Cardiac output response	Yes
Mancini[83]	65	Swan-Ganz; TD	Cardiac output response	No
			SWI	Yes
Metra[84]	219	Swan-Ganz; TD	SWI	Yes
Williams[85]	219	CO_2 rebreathing	Peak cardiac power	Yes
Lang[86]	148	Gas rebreathing	Peak cardiac power	Yes

NA, not applicable; SWI, stroke work index; TD, thermodilution.

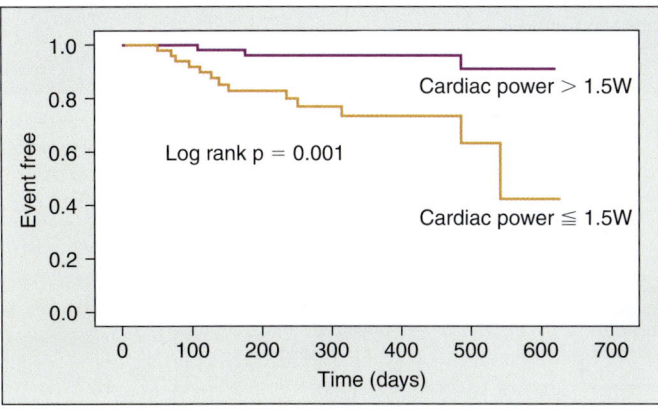

FIGURE 5-11 Survival curves divided by cardiac power. *(From Lang C, Karlin P, Haythe J, et al. Peak cardiac power output measured non-invasively is a powerful predictor of outcome in chronic heart failure. Circ Heart Fail 2009;2:33-38.)*

measure cardiac output during exercise and is reliable, safe, and easily performed in patients with chronic HF.[86]

We applied this technology in 171 consecutive patients with chronic HF during symptom limited bicycle exercise.[86] An accurate measure of peak cardiac output was obtained in 148 patients (85% of patients). Average patient age was 53 ± 14 years, 80% of patients were male, LVEF was $24 \pm 12\%$, and an ischemic etiology was present in 34%. Peak cardiac power was derived from the product of the peak mean arterial blood pressure and cardiac output divided by 451. Peak cardiac power incorporates both flow and pressure-generating ability of the heart and could be viewed as a more comprehensive indicator of cardiac function.[87] Endpoints consisted of death, urgent heart transplant, or left ventricular assist device implantation. Follow-up lasted an average of 1 year. Univariable and multivariable analyses were performed using cardiopulmonary exercise variables (i.e., peak VO_2, peak cardiac output, peak cardiac power, VE/VCO$_2$ slope, and VO_2 at anaerobic threshold). Event-free survival for the entire cohort was 83% with 5 deaths, 4 left ventricular assist device implants, and 16 urgent transplants. In this cohort, peak VO_2 was 12.9 ± 4.5 mL/kg/min, and peak cardiac power was 1.7 ± 0.9 watts. Univariable predictors of adverse outcome were peak VO_2, peak cardiac output, peak cardiac power, VE/VCO$_2$ slope, and VO_2 at anaerobic threshold.

By multivariable analysis, peak cardiac power and peak cardiac output were predictive of outcome with peak cardiac power being the more powerful independent predictor of outcome ($P = .01$) (Fig. 5-11). Additional research is needed to determine if cardiac power is a better prognostic tool than peak VO_2.

MULTIVARIABLE RISK STRATIFICATION FOR INPATIENTS WITH HEART FAILURE

Risk prediction based on a single variable does not make efficient use of routinely obtained clinical measures of known prognostic significance. Multivariable risk models can incorporate a range of prognostic information, often reflecting different pathophysiologic aspects and phenotypic characteristics of the clinical condition, to improve prognostic accuracy. Fonarow and coworkers[12] created a simple bedside tool for risk stratification of individuals hospitalized with acute decompensated HF. Using ADHERE, more than 39 clinical predictors of HF death were evaluated in more than 33,000 patient hospitalizations for acute decompensated HF during the period 2001-2003. Greater than 40% of patients had an ejection fraction of 40% or more, suggesting the diagnosis of HF with preserved ejection fraction. These patients had a mean age of 72.5 years, mean serum sodium of 138 mEq/L,

and mean systolic blood pressure of 143.7 mm Hg. On regression analysis, the best independent predictor of in-hospital mortality was admission BUN level ≥ 43 mg/dL. Other independent predictors included systolic blood pressure less than 115 mm Hg and serum creatinine 2.75 mg/dL or greater.

Figure 5-12 depicts the risk stratification scheme employed in the ADHERE study and the associated mortalities in the derivation cohort at each risk level. Although the overall sample in-hospital mortality was only 4%, the risk stratification model differentiated individuals at very low risk (mortality 2.1%), low-intermediate risk (5.5% and 6.4%), intermediate-high risk (12.4%), and very high risk for in-hospital death (21.9%). When the model was applied to more than 33,000 patient hospitalizations in a validation cohort, the model's predictive ability was maintained with in-hospital mortality rates of 2.3%, 5.7%, 5.6%, 13.2%, and 19.8%.

Rhode and coworkers[88] developed another predictive model for in-hospital HF mortality, termed the HF Revised Score, and compared it with the ADHERE prediction tool applied to 779 consecutive HF admissions in Brazil. Mean population age in the cohort was 67 years, and mean systolic blood pressure, serum sodium, and creatinine were 131 mm Hg, 137 mEq/L, and 1.4 mg/dL, with an in-hospital mortality rate of 10%. Of patients, 53% had an ejection fraction of 40% or more, and 64% had a nonischemic etiology for HF (one of which had Chagas disease). Individuals with severe comorbidities, such as cancer (7%) or acquired immunodeficiency syndrome (AIDS) (1.2%) were not excluded if HF was the primary etiology for admission. Independent predictors of in-hospital death included a history of cancer (odds ratio [OR] 3.6), systolic blood pressure 124 mm Hg or less (OR 3.1), creatinine greater than 1.4 mg/dL (OR 2.1), BUN greater than 37 mg/dL (OR 2.1), serum sodium less than 136 mEq/L (OR 1.8), and age older than 70 years (OR 1.8). Points were assigned for each of the predictors (history of cancer = 1.3 points, systolic blood pressure ≤ 124 mm Hg = 1.1 points, creatinine >1.4 mg/dL = 0.8 points, BUN >37 mg/dL = 0.7 points, sodium <136 mEq/L = 0.6 points, and age >70 years = 0.6 points), and the HF Revised Score was calculated as the sum of the points awarded for the presence of each clinical predictor. Patients were defined as no risk (HF Revised Score 0), low risk (HF Revised Score 0.5 to 1.0), intermediate 1 risk (HF Revised Score 1.0 to 2.0 points), intermediate 2 risk (HF Revised Score 2.0 to 3.0 points), intermediate 3 risk (HF Revised Score 3.0 to 4.0), and high risk (HF Revised Score >4.0 points) with in-hospital mortality rates of 0%, 5%, 7%, 10%, 29%, and 83%.

Evaluating the ADHERE risk stratification score in this sample, the authors found in-hospital mortality rates of 5%, 8%, 12%, 33%, and 58% for patients in very low risk, low-intermediate risk, intermediate-high risk, and very high risk ADHERE strata. Although mortality was higher for each of the ADHERE strata in this study compared with the original ADHERE cohort, patients in this study were burdened by more comorbidities and were potentially exposed to a different structure of health care with disease management decisions that likely varied substantially from that of the original ADHERE cohort.[12,88] As Bayes theorem would predict, the model continued to discriminate between risk groups, but calibration—the accurate prediction of actual, rather than relative, mortality risks—deteriorated in this sicker group of patients. Nonetheless, the utility of the ADHERE risk tool for successfully differentiating high-risk and low-risk patients was validated.

Another predictive model of mortality in acute HF was derived from a retrospective analysis of data obtained from the EFFECT study, which included more than 4000 individuals newly admitted to hospitals in Canada with the primary diagnosis of HF during the period 1997-2001.[89] There were 2624 individuals in the derivation cohort with a mean age of 76 years and a mean serum sodium, creatinine, and systolic blood pressure of 138 mEq/L, 1.45 mg/dL, and 148 mm Hg. More than

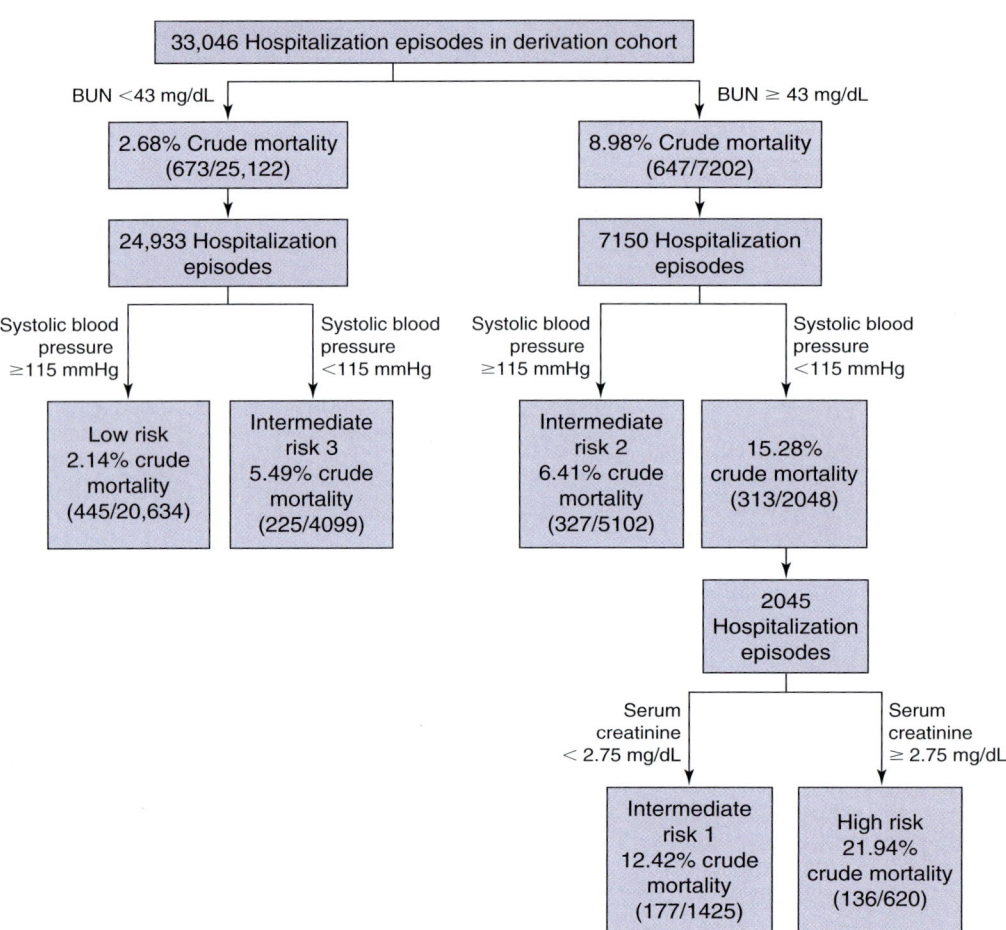

FIGURE 5-12 ADHERE inpatient risk stratification model. Predictors of in-hospital mortality and risk stratification for the derivation cohort. Each node is based on available data from registry patient hospitalizations for each predictive value presented. To convert blood urea nitrogen (BUN) to mmol/L, multiply by 0.357; to convert creatinine to mmol/L, multiply by 88.4.

47% of patients had an ejection fraction of 40% or greater, limiting the generalizability of the EFFECT model to patients undergoing evaluation for transplantation or mechanical circulatory support. In-hospital, 30-day, and 1-year mortality rates were 8.9%, 10.7%, and 32.9%. A multivariable risk score for predicting 30-day and 1-year mortality was derived from independent predictors of mortality and was calculated according to the point allotments depicted in Table 5-5. Risk categories were defined as very low (risk score ≤60), low (risk score 61 to 90), intermediate (risk score 91 to 120), high (risk score 121 to 150), and very high (risk score >150) risk with associated 30-day mortalities of 0.4%, 3.4%, 12.2%, 32.7%, and 59% and associated 1-year mortalities of 7.8%, 12.9%, 32.5%, 59.3%, and 78.8%. The 30-day and 1-year mortality rates were similar in a validation group of 1400 inpatients with HF.

The discriminative ability of the model to predict mortality was slightly higher for patients with systolic dysfunction (receiver operating characteristic curve area 0.81 at 30 days) than for all patients with HF (receiver operating characteristic curve area 0.79 at 30 days). The model incorporates comorbidities that would be contraindicated in transplantation and does not include measures of left ventricular function or functional capacity. These limitations and the inclusion of patients with preserved systolic function in the model derivation sample render this model inapplicable for formal use in patients undergoing evaluation for transplantation or mechanical circulatory support until prospective validation studies for this population are performed. An online version of the EFFECT model can be found at http://www.ccort.ca/CHFriskmodel.asp.

Data from 949 patients hospitalized as part of OPTIME-CHF (Outcomes of a Prospective Trial of Intravenous Milrinone for Exacerbations of Chronic Heart Failure)[90] were used to develop a multivariable model to predict 60-day mortality or combination of rehospitalization and mortality. Independent predictors of 60-day mortality included age, NYHA class (IV vs. I-III), systolic blood pressure, BUN, and serum sodium. The variables that predicted mortality or rehospitalization at 60 days were prior HF hospitalization, systolic blood pressure, BUN, hemoglobin, and history of percutaneous coronary intervention. The multivariable model for mortality was converted into a coefficient-based risk score, which summed the points assigned to each variable. A nomogram was reported that assigned estimated 60-day mortality. The discriminatory power of the model for mortality was good with a c-statistic of 0.77 and excellent calibration. Scores ranged from 124 to 225 with predicted 60-day mortality increasing from 2% to 30%.

In contrast to the ADHERE or EFFECT in-hospital mortality models, these data included only patients with systolic dysfunction (mean ejection fraction of 23% [range 18% to 30%]). The data were also collected in the setting of a randomized clinical trial that used a drug with known long-term adverse effects on survival and excluded patients with severe renal insufficiency, recent ischemia, or unstable arrhythmias. It is unclear how generalizable this model would be to general practice, and it would require validation in a separate cohort. However, these investigators attempted to answer an important question, which is how to identify discharged patients who remain at high risk for early death and rehospitalization.

	TABLE 5-5	**EFFECT Model for Heart Failure In-Hospital Mortality**	
		No. Points	
Variable		**30-day score***	**1-year score†**
Age		+ Age, yr	+ Age, yr
Respiratory rate (minimal value 20, maximum value 45)		+ Rate, breaths/min	+ Rate, breaths/min
Systolic blood pressure, mm Hg			
≥180		−60	−50
160-179		−55	−45
140-159		−50	−40
120-139		−45	−35
100-119		−40	−30
90-99		−35	−25
<90		−30	−20
BUN (maximum value 60 mg/dL)		+ Level, mg/dL	+ Level, mg/dl
Sodium <136 mEq/L		+10	+10
Hemoglobin <10 g/dL		NA	+10
History of comorbidities			
Cerebrovascular disease		+10	+10
Dementia		+20	+15
Chronic obstructive pulmonary disease		+10	+10
Hepatic cirrhosis		+25	+35
Cancer		+15	+15

*Calculated as age + respiratory rate + systolic blood pressure + BUN + sodium + points for individual comorbidities.

†Calculated as age + respiratory rate + systolic blood pressure + BUN + sodium + hemoglobin + points for individual comorbidities.

BUN, blood urea nitrogen; NA, not applicable.

Data from Lee DS, Austin PC, Rouleau JL, et al. Predicting mortality among patients hospitalized for heart failure: derivation and validation of a clinical model. *JAMA* 2003;290:2581-2587.

High-risk patients could be targeted for more aggressive therapy and closer follow-up.

Another more recent study that addressed risk stratification on hospital discharge was developed from the ESCAPE (Evaluation Study of Congestive Heart Failure and Pulmonary Artery Catheterization Effective) trial.[91] The 6-month mortality and mortality or rehospitalization risk for 423 patients whose discharge data were used to form the model were 18.7% and 64%. This patient cohort included congested patients with systolic dysfunction with serum creatinine less than 3.5 mg/dL who had not received inotropic support with milrinone or greater than 3 μg/kg/min of dopamine or dobutamine during the index hospitalization. The best multivariable predictors of mortality were cardiac arrest or need for mechanical ventilation during hospitalization and discharge BNP, BUN, and sodium values. A risk score was developed that included eight variables with a score range of 0 to 13 (Table 5-6). The score was the sum of the parameters. Most patient scores were less than 5. The mortality risk was graded by a nomogram with a 6-month mortality of 5% for patients with a score of 0 to 94% in patients with scores greater than or equal to 8.

TABLE 5-6	**Simplified ESCAPE Discharge Score Model**
Criteria (Based on Discharge Measurements)	**Score if Yes (No = 0)**
Age >70 yr	1
BUN >40 mg/dL	1
BUN >90 mg/dL*	1
6-min walk <300 ft	1
Sodium <130 mEq/L	1
CPR/mechanical ventilation, yes/no	2
Diuretic dose >240 mg at discharge, yes/no	1
No beta blocker at discharge	1
Discharge BNP >500 pg/mmol	1
Discharge BNP >1300 pg/mmol	3
Total of column 2 (score)	

BNP, brain natriuretic peptide; BUN, blood urea nitrogen; CPR, cardiopulmonary resuscitation.

*If BUN >90, both BUN values are coded as 1.

This model was "validated" using a patient cohort from FIRST (Flolan International Randomized Survival Trial); however, BNP and diuretic dose on discharge were not recorded in that dataset. There were other significant differences in the patient populations, such as the use of beta blockers, and this randomized trial was terminated early because of concerns about a strong trend for reduced survival in patients receiving epoprostenol. All of the inpatient models include a much more heterogeneous sample than would be suitable for heart transplantation (including patients with more advanced age, greater comorbidity, or better systolic function), and none of these models have been validated in a heart transplant candidate sample.

MULTIVARIABLE RISK STRATIFICATION FOR OUTPATIENTS WITH HEART FAILURE

The HFSS was the first prospectively validated multivariable risk stratification model to predict survival in patients with HF.[92] The score was derived from a cohort evaluated during the period 1986-1991 and subsequently validated in another cohort during the period 1993-1995. All patients were ambulatory, were younger than 70 years, had LVEF 40% or less, and were able to perform cardiopulmonary exercise testing. Only 10% of the patients were receiving a beta blocker. Independent predictors of mortality included an ischemic etiology for HF (HR 2.0), resting heart rate (HR 1.02), ejection fraction (HR 0.96), QRS duration greater than 120 msec of any cause (HR 1.84), mean resting blood pressure (HR 0.98), peak VO_2 (HR 0.95), and serum sodium (HR 0.95) with the HRs for the continuous variables representing the hazard for a 1-unit increase.

The HFSS is calculated from the following equation: HFSS = $-1 \times$ ([0.0216 × resting heart rate] + [−0.0255 × mean blood pressure] + [−0.0464 × ejection fraction] + [−0.0470 × serum sodium] + [−0.0546 × peak VO_2] + [0.6083 × presence (1) or absence (0) of a QRS >120 msec] + [0.6931 × presence (1) or absence (0) of an ischemic cardiomyopathy]). For patients in the derivation group ($n = 268$) with low-risk (HFSS ≥8.10), medium-risk (HFSS 7.20-8.09), and high-risk (HFSS ≤7.19) scores, 1-year, event-free survivals were 93%, 72%, and 43%. Survival in the validation group ($n = 199$) was similar, with significantly ($P <.001$) better survival in the low-risk versus medium-risk groups and low-risk versus high-risk groups. Patients with high-risk and medium-risk HFSS were considered appropriate for cardiac transplant referral.

The HFSS tool was generated before the widespread use of many therapeutic interventions known to improve HF morbidity and mortality, including beta blockers, aldosterone inhibitors, implantable cardioverter defibrillators, and biventricular pacemakers, raising questions regarding the prognostic utility of the score in the contemporary era of HF care. The impact of beta blocker use and biventricular pacing on two of the seven variables in the model, heart rate and peak VO$_2$, has also been questioned.[93] In response to these concerns, the prognostic accuracy of the HFSS was re-examined in 524 consecutive patients referred for cardiac transplant during the years 1994-2001.[55] Of patients, 80% were receiving an ACEI, 8.4% were receiving an angiotensin II receptor blocker, 32.8% were receiving spironolactone, and 46% were receiving a beta blocker. When the population was dichotomized by the presence or absence of beta blocker therapy, patients receiving beta blocker therapy had higher event-free survival at 2 years compared with patients not receiving beta blocker therapy for each of the HFSS strata. In patients receiving a beta blocker, 1-year and 2-year survivals were 95% and 94% in the low-risk HFSS stratum, 86% and 80% in the medium-risk HFSS stratum, and 83% and 60% in the high-risk stratum. In contrast, 1-year and 2-year survivals for patients not receiving beta blockers were 89% and 85% (low-risk stratum), 82% and 62% (medium-risk stratum), and 47% and 32% (high-risk stratum).

Similarly, Butler and colleagues[94] examined the HFSS in a sample of patients on an improved background of guideline-recommended HF therapies (93% ACEI, 72% beta blocker, 41% spironolactone). In patients with low-risk, medium-risk, and high-risk HFSS, 1-year event-free survival rates were 91%, 71%, and 64%. Because 1-year and 2-year survival in patients with a medium-risk HFSS on beta blocker therapy is comparable in the present era to the survival 1 year after heart transplantation, the authors (and we) believe that patients with HF receiving a beta blocker who have a medium-risk HFSS can have transplant deferred with close monitoring. However, these studies report survival only and do not take into account quality of life and functional impairment.

The Seattle Heart Failure Model (SHFM) was developed more recently by Levy and coworkers[95] to predict 1-year, 2-year, and 3-year survival in patients with HF. The SHFM is simple to use and employs easily obtained variables that do not rely on a patient's ability to complete cardiopulmonary stress testing. Web-based and smartphone SHFM calculators can be found at http://depts.washington.edu/shfm. The model was partially derived from the demographic, laboratory, and clinical data of patients in the PRAISE (Prospective Randomized Amlodipine Survival Evaluation) cohort, which included 1125 patients with an ejection fraction less than 30% and NYHA functional class IIIB and IV symptoms.[96] Mean age was 65 years, mean sodium was 139 mEq/L, and mean systolic blood pressure was 118 mm Hg. HRs for certain HF medications and devices (defibrillators and biventricular pacemakers) were derived from published randomized trials or meta-analyses owing to low baseline rates of use (e.g., 0% were receiving a beta blocker and 0% had an implantable cardioverter-defibrillator) in the PRAISE derivation cohort. Multivariable predictors of survival in the analysis included demographic and clinical factors (age, gender, NYHA class, LVEF, systolic blood pressure); medication use (ACEI, angiotensin II receptor blocker, beta blocker, statin, allopurinol, aldosterone blocker, loop diuretic, metolazone, and hydrochlorothiazide); laboratory values (hemoglobin, percent lymphocytes, uric acid, cholesterol, sodium, QRS duration ≥120 msec); and devices (implantable cardioverter-defibrillator, biventricular pacemaker).

The SHFM model was validated in five independent samples (four from large multicenter clinical trials and one from a university HF clinic). Mean LVEF was less than 36% in all cohorts. In both the derivation and the validation cohorts, predicted survival from the SHFM was similar to actuarial survival at 1 year, 2 years, and 3 years. In addition to predicting survival, the model is useful for showing the expected mortality benefit of adding a medication or device to a patient's HF management. The selected, prescreened, trial populations from which the medication and device HRs were derived and from which the SHFM was validated may not match "typical" outpatients with HF; however, with respect to their relative lack of comorbidities, these patients may be more similar to patients who present for transplant evaluation. The SHFM has subsequently been investigated in a sample of patients presenting to an advanced HF clinic for transplant evaluation.[97] As Bayes theorem would predict for a model developed from cohorts with less advanced HF, discrimination remained excellent, but the SHFM tended to underestimate mortality in patients with the greatest observed mortality.

Contemporary use of implantable mechanical circulatory support is limited to the bridge to transplant and destination therapy indications in patients with very advanced HF. The larger potential of mechanical circulatory support is for its use as permanent therapy in patients with less advanced HF. At the present state of technology development, HF patients with a 1-year expected mortality of approximately 30% have been proposed as an appropriate target for a clinical trial to explore this indication.[98,99] In this context, we evaluated the SHFM in a combined dataset of 9528 patients from three clinical trials (PRAISE, ValHEFT [Valsartan Heart Failure Trial] ACCLAIM [Advanced Chronic Heart Failure Clinical Assessment of Immune Modulation Therapy Heart Failure Trial]) and the University of Washington, identifying 3238 patients (34%) who were older than age 60 years, were NYHA class III or higher, had LVEF 35% or less, and had a serum creatinine value 2.5 mg/dL or less. Within this cohort, the SHFM predicted and observed 1-year survivals were both 18%, and model discrimination was excellent (Fig. 5-13). An SHFM score threshold of 1.5 or greater separated patients into low-risk (61%) and high-risk (39%) groups. The estimated mortality in the low-risk group was 9.6% versus an observed mortality at 1 year of 10.4%. In the 39% of patients with an SHFM score 1.5 or greater, the estimated 1-year mortality was 31% with an observed 1-year mortality of 29% (Levy WC, Mancini DM, Pagani FD, et al; unpublished data).

Direct comparison of the SHFM and HFSS in 715 patients referred to Columbia Presbyterian Medical Center for cardiac transplantation showed comparable risk stratification. For

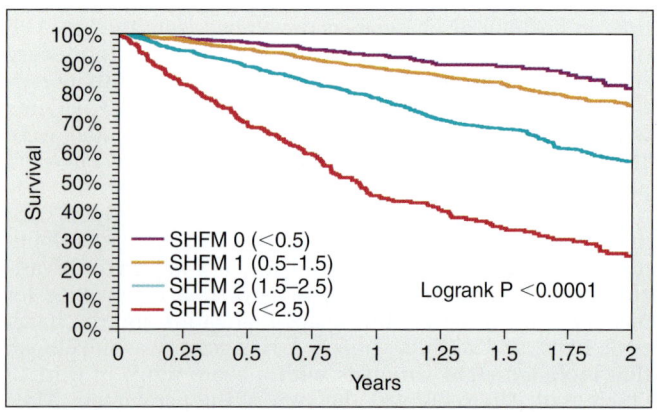

FIGURE 5-13 Observed mortality in 3238 patients with age older than 60 years, New York Heart Association class III or greater, left ventricular ejection fraction 35% or less, and creatinine 2.5 mg/dL or less stratified by Seattle Heart Failure Model (SHFM) score rounded to the nearest integer.

the HFSS, 1-year survivals for low-risk, medium-risk, and high-risk groups were 89%, 72%, and 60% versus 1-year survivals of 93%, 76%, 59%, and 54% for SHFM scores of 0, 1, 2, and 3. Receiver operating curve analysis showed similar 1-year area under the curve analysis of 0.772 versus 0.73 for the HFSS and SHFM.

A major limitation of all of the HF risk tools discussed is the limited data currently available on the utility of repeated risk assessments and the optimal frequency with which to reassess patient risk. At the present time, only one study exists examining the prognostic value of serial HFSS and peak VO$_2$ measurements. Lund and colleagues[53] subjected 227 adults (22% female) to repeat cardiopulmonary testing an average of 1 year after baseline measurement with a subsequent recalculation of the HFSS. Patients whose HFSS or peak VO$_2$ deteriorated from low risk to medium risk or high risk had lower survival rates than patients whose values remained at low risk (P <.01 and P <.001). Patients who started at medium risk or high risk and improved to low risk tended to have higher survival rates than patients who remained medium risk or high risk (P = .06 and P <.16). Patients who improved to low risk based on a repeat HFSS or peak VO$_2$ had a 1-year survival of 72%. However, patients treated with beta blockers who improved to low risk had a 1-year survival comparable to that after transplant (89% for HFSS and 83% for peak VO$_2$).

The optimal timing of HF risk reassessment has not been studied. In our practices, scores are recalculated on a semiannual or annual basis and with any change in clinical status. Patients who are intermediate risk may warrant closer monitoring. It is reasonable to employ more than one scoring system, especially in patients with intermediate risk. Finally, neither the HFSS nor the SHFM has been adequately studied in the assessment of inpatients with decompensated HF, although a limited evaluation of the SHFM is available.[100]

CONCLUSION

Many HF risk stratification tools have been developed, each differing in the type of sample from which they were derived and validated, the variables used for risk stratification, their utility in predicting mortality at varying time points, and in their ease of use (Table 5-7). Risk prediction tools are invaluable for determining HF prognosis. They can be useful in helping clinicians, patients, and families make informed decisions to help guide the implementation of further medical or surgical interventions and in the setting of end-of-life discussions.

Risk prediction tools must be selected carefully, matching the clinical characteristics of the particular patient with that of the sample from which the tool was derived. Validated risk prediction tools should be used whenever possible. No tool can encompass all of the relevant information crucial for informed decision making. These tools should not be used in isolation but rather should be used to enhance clinical decision making. Because HF is a dynamic condition with high morbidity and mortality, HF prognosis should be reassessed frequently with one or more of the tools discussed in this chapter, particularly in patients for whom transplantation or destination therapy with an implantable circulatory support device may be considered.

TABLE 5-7	Comparisons of Current Risk Models for Mortality and Rehospitalization in Patients with Heart Failure					
Model	Development	Derivation Cohort	Systolic vs HFPEF	Acute vs chronic	Model parameters	Endpoints
ADHERE	2001-2003	33,046	Both	Acute admission	BUN >43, systolic BP <115, creatinine >2.75	In-hospital mortality
HF Revised Score		779		Acute admission	History of cancer, systolic BP <124, creatinine >1.4, BUN >37, sodium <136, age >70	In-hospital mortality
EFFECT	1997-2001	2624	Both	Acute admission	Age>70, hemoglobin <10, systolic BP*, respiratory rate 20-45, sodium <136, BUN (maximum 60), comorbid conditions	In-hospital mortality
OPTIME-CHF		949	Systolic	Acute discharge	Age, NYHA class IV vs. I-III, systolic BP*, BUN, sodium, hemoglobin, prior HF hospitalization, PCI during admission	60-day mortality and rehospitalization
ESCAPE	2000-2003	423	Systolic	Acute discharge	BNP >500 and/or >1300, sodium <130, 6-min walk <300 m, cardiac arrest or mechanical ventilation during hospitalization, BUN >40 and/or >90, diuretic dose >240 mg/day	6-mo mortality
HFSS	1986-1991 (derivation); 1993-1995 (validation)	268; 199	Systolic	Chronic	LVEF, presence or absence of QRS >120 msec, presence or absence of CAD, HR, BP, VO$_2$, sodium	Low-risk, medium-risk, and high-risk groups; 1-yr mortality
SHFM	1992-1994 (derivation)	1125; 9942	Systolic	Chronic	Age, gender, NYHA class, weight, LVEF, systolic BP*, presence or absence of CAD, hemoglobin, % lymphocytes, uric acid, sodium, cholesterol, QRS >120, medications and devices, diuretic dose	1-yr, 2-yr, and 3-yr survival

BNP, brain natriuretic peptide; BP, blood pressure; BUN, blood urea nitrogen; CAD, coronary artery disease; HF, heart failure; HR, heart rate; LVEF, left ventricular ejection fraction; NYHA, New York Heart Association; PCI, percutaneous coronary intervention; VO$_2$, oxygen consumption.

*The point value varies over the range of >180 mm Hg and <90 mm Hg; see Table 5-5.

1. Khush K, Tasissa G, Burker J, et al. Effect of pulmonary hypertension on clinical outcomes in advanced heart failure: analysis of the Evaluation Study of Congestive Heart Failure and Pulmonary Artery Catheterization Effectiveness (ESCAPE) database. *Am Heart J.* 2009;157:126–134.
2. Chung Chen W, Tran K, Maisel A. Biomarkers in heart failure. *Heart.* 2010;96:314–320.
3. Lainscak M, Anker M, Von Haehling S, et al. Biomarkers for chronic heart failure. *Herz.* 2009;34:589–593.
4. Parekh N, Maisel A. Utility of B-natriuretic peptide in the evaluation of left ventricular diastolic function and diastolic heart failure. *Curr Opin Cardiol.* 2009;24:155–160.
5. Peacock W, DeMarco T, Fonarow G, et al. Cardiac troponin and outcome in acute heart failure. *N Engl J Med.* 2008;358:2117–2126.
6 Schappert S, Rechtsteiner E. *Ambulatory medical care utilization estimates for 2006.* U.S. Department of Health and Human Services, National Health Statistics Report 2008;8.
7. Peacock W. Using the emergency department clinical decision unit for acute decompensated heart failure. *Cardiol Clin.* 2005;23:569–588.
8. Adams K, Fonarow G, Emerman E, et al. Characteristics and outcomes of patients hospitalized for heart failure in the United States: rationale, design and preliminary observations from the first 100,000 cases in the Acute Decompensated Heart Failure National Registry (ADHERE). *Am Heart J.* 2005;149:209–216.
9. Abraham W, Fonarow G, Albert N, et al. Predictors of in hospital mortality in patients hospitalized for heart failure: insights from the Organized Program to Initiate Life Saving Treatment in Hospitalized Patients with Heart Failure (OPTIMIZE-HF). *J Am Coll Cardiol.* 2008;52:347–356.
10. Smith G, Poses R, McClish D, et al. Prognostic judgements and triage decisions for patients with acute decompensated heart failure. *Chest.* 2002;121:1610–1617.
11. Gheorghiade M, Abraham W, Albert N, et al. Systolic blood pressure at admission, clinical characteristics and outcomes in patients hospitalized with acute heart failure. *JAMA.* 2006;296:2217–2226.
12. Fonarow G, Adams K, Abraham W, et al. Risk stratification for in hospital mortality in acutely decompensated heart failure: classification and regression tree analysis. *JAMA.* 2005;293:572–580.
13. Abraham W, Adams K, Fonarow G, et al. In hospital mortality in patients with acute decompensated heart failure requiring intravenous vasoactive medication: an analysis from the Acute Decompensated Heart failure National Registry (ADHERE). *J Am Coll Cardiol.* 2005;46:57–64.
14. Fonarow G, Stough W, Abraham W, et al. Characteristics, treatments, and outcomes of patients with preserved systolic heart failure: a report from the OPTIMIZE-HF Registry. *J Am Coll Cardiol.* 2007;50:768–777.
15. Lee D, Schull M, Alter D, et al. Early deaths in patients with heart failure discharged from the emergency department: a population based analysis. *Circ Heart Fail.* 2010;3:228–235.
16. O'Connor C, Abraham W, Albert N, et al. Predictors of mortality after discharge in patients hospitalized with heart failure: an analysis from the Organized Program to Initiate Life Saving Treatment in Hospitalized Patients with Heart Failure (OPTIMIZE-HF). *Am Heart J.* 2008;156:662–673.
17. Ahmed A, Allman R, Ponarow G, et al. Incident heart failure hospitalization and subsequent mortality in chronic heart failure: a propensity-matched study. *J Card Fail.* 2008;14:211–218.
18. Setoguchi S, Warner-Stevenson L. Hospitalizations in patients with heart failure: who and why. *J Am Coll Cardiol.* 2009;54:1703–1705.
19. Setoguchi S, Stevenson L, Schneeweiss S. Repeated hospitalizations predict mortality in the community population with heart failure. *Am Heart J.* 2007;154:260–266.
20. Fonarow G. Epidemiology and risk stratification in acute heart failure. *Am Heart J.* 2008;155:200–207.
21. Krumholz H, Wong Y, Paretn E, et al. Quality of care for elderly patients hospitalized with heart failure. *Arch Intern Med.* 1997;157:2242–2247.
22. Gorelik O, Almoznino-Sarafian D, Shteinshnaider M, et al. Clinical variables affecting survival in patients with decompensated diastolic versus systolic heart failure. *Clin Res Cardiol.* 2009;98:224–232.
23. Owan T, Hodge D, Herges R, et al. Trends in prevalence and outcome of heart failure with preserved ejection fraction. *N Engl J Med.* 2006;355:251–259.
24. Acikel S, Akdemir R, Kilic H, et al. Diastolic heart failure in the elderly: the prognostic factors and interventions regarding heart failure with preserved ejection fraction. *Int J Cardiol.* 2009;134:311–313.
25. Perez de Isla L, Canadas V, Contereras L, et al. Diastolic heart failure in the elderly: in hospital mortality and long term outcome after the first episode. *In J Cardiol.* 2009;134:265–270.
26. Goldstein S. The changing epidemiology of sudden death in heart failure. *Curr Heart Fail Rep.* 2004;1:93–97.
27. Effects of Metoprolol CR/XL in chronic heart failure: Metoprolol CR/XL Randomized Intervention Trial in congestive heart Failure (MERIT-HF). *Lancet.* 1999;353:2001–2007.
28. Olshansky B, Poole JE, Johnson G, et al. Syncope predicts the outcome of cardiomyopathy patients. *J Am Coll Cardiol.* 2008;51:1277–1282.
29. Uriarte-Salerno J, De Ferrari G, Klersy C, et al. Prognostic value of T-wave alternans in patients with heart failure due to nonischemic cardiomyopathy: results of the ALPHA Study. *J Am Coll Cardiol.* 2007;50:1896–1904.
30. Berger R, Huelsman M, Strecker K, et al. B-type natriuretic peptide predicts sudden death in patients with chronic heart failure. *Circulation.* 2002;105:2392–2397.
31. Pascual-Figa DA, Odonez-Llanos J, Tornel P, et al. Soluble ST2 for predicting sudden cardiac death in patients with chronic heart failure and left ventricular systolic dysfunction. *J Am Coll Cardiol.* 2009;54:2174–2179.
32. Saczynski J, Darling C, Spencer F, et al. Clinical features, treatment practices, and hospital and long-term outcomes of older patients hospitalized with decompensated heart failure: the Worcester Heart Failure Study. *J Am Geriatr Soc.* 2009;57:1587–1594.
33. Chaudhry SI, Wang Y, Gill TM, et al. Geriatric conditions and subsequent mortality in older patients with heart failure. *J Am Coll Cardiol.* 2010;55:309–316.
34. Parikh M, Lund L, Goda A, et al. Usefulness of peak exercise oxygen consumption and the Heart Failure Survival Score to predict survival in patients >65 years of age with heart failure. *Am J Cardiol.* 2009;103:998–1002.
35. Heywood J, Fonarow G, Costanzo M, et al. High prevalence of renal dysfunction and its impact on outcome in 118,465 patients hospitalized with acute decompensated heart failure: a report from the ADHERE database. *J Cardiac Fail.* 2007;13:422–430.
36. Klein K, Massie B, Leimberger J, et al. Admission or changes in renal function during hospitalization for worsening heart failure predicts postdischarge survival. *Circ Heart Fail.* 2008;1:25–33.
37. Filippatos G, Rossi J, Lloyd-Jones D, et al. Prognostic value of BUN in patients hospitalized with worsening heart failure: insights from the acute and chronic therapeutic impact of a vasopressin antagonist in chronic heart failure (ACTIV in CHF) study. *J Card Fail.* 2007;13:360–364.
38. Maisel A, Mueller M, Adams K, et al. State of the art: using natriuretic peptide levels in clinical practice. *Eur J Heart Fail.* 2008;10:824–839.
39. Rauchhaus M, Clark A, Doehner W, et al. The relationship between cholesterol and survival in patients with chronic heart failure. *J Am Coll Cardiol.* 2003;42:1933–1940.
40. Doehner W, Rauchhaus M, Ponikowski P, et al. Improved insulin sensitivity as an independent risk factor for mortality in patients with stable chronic heart failure. *J Am Coll Cardiol.* 2005;46:1019–1026.
41. Hare J, Mangal B, Brown T, et al. Impact of oxypurinol in patients with symptomatic heart failure: results of the OPT-CHF study. *J Am Coll Cardiol.* 2008;51:2301–2309.
42. Jehn M, Halle M, Schuster T, et al. The 6 min walk test in heart failure: is it a max or sub-maximum test? *Eur J Appl Physiol.* 2009;107:317–323.
43. Bittner V, Weiner D, Yusuf S, et al. SOLVD investigators. Prediction of mortality and morbidity with 6 minute walk test in patients with left ventricular dysfunction. *JAMA.* 1993;270:1702–1707.
44. Roul G, German P, Bareiss P. Does the 6 minute walk test predict the prognosis in patients with NYHA class II and III heart failure? *Am Heart J.* 1998;136:449–457.
45. Rostagno C, Olivo G, Cormeglio M, et al. Prognostic value of 6 minute walk corridor test in patients with mild to moderate heart failure: comparison with other methods of functional evaluation. *Eur J Heart Fail.* 2003;5:247–252.
46. Szlachcic J, Massie B, Kramer B, et al. Correlates and prognostic implication of exercise capacity in chronic congestive heart failure. *Am J Cardiol.* 1985;55:1037–1042.
47. Mancini DM, Eisen H, Kussmaul W, et al. Value of peak exercise oxygen consumption for optimal timing of cardiac transplantation in ambulatory patients with heart failure. *Circulation.* 1991;83:778–786.
48. Aaronson K, Chen T, Mancini D. Demonstration of the continuous nature of peak VO2 for predicting survival in ambulatory patients evaluated for transplant. *J Heart Lung Transplant.* 1996;15:S66.
49. Aaronson K, Mancini D. Is percent predicted VO2 a better selection criterion than peak VO2 for cardiac transplantation? *J Heart Lung Transplant.* 1995;14:981–989.
50. Stelken AM, Younis LT, Jennison SH, et al. Prognostic value of cardiopulmonary exercise testing using percent achieved of predicted peak oxygen uptake for patients with ischemic and dilated cardiomyopathy. *J Am Coll Cardiol.* 1996;27:345–352.
51. Wasserman K, Hansen JE, Sue DY, et al. *Principles of Exercise Testing and Interpretation.* Philadelphia, PA: Lea & Febiger; 1994.
52. Lund L, Aaronson K, Mancini D. Validation of peak VO2 and the heart failure survival score for serial risk stratification in advanced heart failure. *J Am Coll Cardiol.* 2005;95:734–741.
53. Lund L, Aaronson K, Mancini D. Predicting survival in ambulatory patients with severe heart failure on beta blocker therapy. *Am J Cardiol.* 2003;92:1350–1354.
54. Koelling T, Joseph S, Aaronson K. Heart failure survival score continues to predict clinical outcomes in heart failure patients receiving beta blockers. *J Heart Lung Transplant.* 2004;23:1414–1422.
55. O'Neill J, Young J, Pothier C, et al. Peak oxygen consumption as a predictor of death in patients with heart failure receiving beta blockers. *Circulation.* 2005;111:2313–2318.
56. Jessup M, Abraham WT, Casey DE, et al. 2009 focused update: ACCF/AHA Guidelines for the Diagnosis and Management of Heart Failure in Adults: a report of the American College of Cardiology Foundation/American Heart Association Task Force on Practice Guidelines: developed in collaboration with the International Society for Heart and Lung Transplantation. *Circulation.* 2009;119:1977–2016.
57. Osada N, Chaitman BR, Miller LW, et al. Cardiopulmonary exercise testing identifies low risk patients with heart failure and severely impaired exercise considered for heart transplantation. *J Am Coll Cardiol.* 1998;31:577–582.
58. Robbins M, Francis G, Pashkow F, et al. Ventilatory and heart rate responses to exercise: better predictors of mortality then peak oxygen consumption. *Circulation.* 1999;100:2411–2417.
59. Kleber F, Vietzke G, Wernecke K, et al. Impairment of ventilatory efficiency in heart failure: prognostic impact. *Circulation.* 2000;103:967–972.
60. Balady G Arena R, Sietsema K, et al. Clinician's Guide to cardiopulmonary exercise testing in adults: a scientific statement from the American Heart Association. *Circulation.* 2010;122:191–225.
61. Arena R, Myers J, Abella J, et al. Development of a ventilatory classification system in patients with heart failure. *Circulation.* 2007;115:2410–2417.
62. Arena R, Myers J, Guazzi M. The clinical and research application of aerobic capacity and ventilatory efficiency in heart failure: an evidence-based review. *Heart Fail Rev.* 2008;13:245–269.
63. Guazzi M, Arena R, Ascione A, et al. Exercise oscillatory breathing and increased ventilation to carbon dioxide production slope in heart failure: an unfavorable combination with high prognostic value. *Am Heart J.* 2007;153:859–867.
64. Sun X, Hansen J, Beshai J, et al. Oscillatory breathing and exercise gas exchange abnormalities prognosticate nearly mortality and morbidity in heart failure. *J Am Coll Cardiol.* 2010;55:1814–1823.

65. Cohen-Solal A, Laperche T, Morvan D, et al. Prolonged kinetics of recovery of oxygen consumption after maximal graded exercise in patients with chronic heart failure: analysis with gas exchange measurements and NMR spectroscopy. *Circulation.* 1995;91:2924–2932.

66. Gitt A, Wasserman K, Kilkowski C, et al. Exercise anaerobic threshold and ventilatory efficiency identify heart failure patients for high risk of early death. *Circulation.* 2002;106:3079–3084.

67. Nanas S, Anastasiou-Nana M, Dimopoulos S, et al. Early heart rate recovery after exercise predicts mortality in patients with chronic heart failure. *Int J Cardiol.* 2006;110:393–400.

68. Arena R, Guazzi M, Myers J, et al. Prognostic value of heart rate recovery in patients with heart failure. *Am Heart J.* 2006;151:851–813.e7–13.

69. Arena R, Myers J, Abella J, et al. The partial pressure of resting end-tidal carbon dioxide predicts major cardiac events in patients with systolic heart failure. *Am Heart J.* 2008;156:982–988.

70. Elimariah S, Goldberg L, Allen M, et al. Effects of gender on peak oxygen consumption and timing of cardiac transplantation. *J Am Coll Cardiol.* 2006;47:2237–2242.

71. Green P, Lund L, Mancini D. Comparison of peak exercise oxygen consumption and the heart failure survival score for predicting prognosis in women versus men. *Am J Cardiol.* 2007;99:399–403.

72. Davies L, Francis D, Piepoli M, et al. Chronic heart failure in the elderly: value of cardiopulmonary exercise testing in risk stratification. *Heart.* 2000;83:147–151.

73. Brubaker P, Marburger C, Morgan T, et al. Exercise responses of elderly patients with diastolic versus systolic heart failure. *Med Sci Sports Exerc.* 2003;35:1477–1485.

74. Guazzi M, Myers J, Arena R. Cardiopulmonary exercise testing in the clinical and prognostic assessment of diastolic heart failure. *J Am Coll Cardiol.* 2005;46:1883–1889.

75. Guazzi M, Myers J, Peberdy M, et al. Exercise oscillatory breathing in diastolic heart failure: prevalence and prognostic insights. *Eur Heart J.* 2008;29:2751–2759.

76. Farr M, Lang C, Lamanca J, et al. Cardiopulmonary exercise variables in diastolic versus systolic heart failure. *Am J Cardiol.* 2008;102:203–206.

77. Lang C, Karlin P, Haythe J, et al. Ease of noninvasive measurement of cardiac output coupled with peak VO2 determination at rest and during exercise in patients with heart failure. *Am J Cardiol.* 2007;99:404–405.

78. Lang C, Agostoni P, Mancini D. Prognostic significance and measurement of exercise-derived hemodynamic variables in patients with heart failure. *J Card Fail.* 2007;13:672–679.

79. Griffin BP, Shah PK, Ferguson J, et al. Incremental prognostic value of exercise hemodynamic variables in chronic congestive heart failure secondary to coronary artery disease or to dilated cardiomyopathy. *Am J Cardiol.* 1991;67:848–853.

80. Roul G, Moulichon ME, Bareiss P, et al. Prognostic factors of chronic heart failure in NYHA class II or III: value of invasive exercise hemodynamic data. *Eur Heart J.* 1995;16:1387–1398.

81. Wilson JR, Rayos G, Yeoh TK, et al. Dissociation between peak exercise oxygen consumption and hemodynamic dysfunction in potential heart transplant candidates. *J Am Coll Cardiol.* 1995;26:429–435.

82. Chomsky DB, Lang CC, Rayos GH, et al. Hemodynamic exercise testing: a valuable tool in the selection of cardiac transplantation candidates. *Circulation.* 1996;94:3176–3183.

83. Mancini D, Katz SD, Donchez L, et al. Coupling of hemodynamic measurements with oxygen consumption during exercise does not improve risk stratification in patients with heart failure. *Circulation.* 1996;94:2492–2496.

84. Metra M, Faggiano P, D'Aloia A, et al. Use of cardiopulmonary exercise testing with hemodynamic monitoring in the prognostic assessment of ambulatory patients with chronic heart failure. *J Am Coll Cardiol.* 1999;33:943–950.

85. Williams SG, Cooke GA, Wright DJ, et al. Peak exercise cardiac output: a direct indicator of cardiac function strongly predictive of prognosis in chronic heart failure. *Eur Heart J.* 2001;22:1496–1503.

86. Lang C, Karlin P, Haythe J, et al. Peak cardiac power output measured non-invasively is a powerful predictor of outcome in chronic heart failure. *Circ Heart Fail.* 2009;2:33–38.

87. Tan LB. Cardiac pumping capability and prognosis in heart failure. *Lancet.* 1986;ii:1360–1363.

88. Rhode LE, Goldraich L, Polanczyk CA, et al. A simple clinically based predictive rule for heart failure in-hospital mortality. *J Card Fail.* 2006;12:587–593.

89. Lee DS, Austin PC, Rouleau JL, et al. Predicting mortality among patients hospitalized for heart failure: derivation and validation of a clinical model. *JAMA.* 2003;290:2581–2587.

90. Felker G, Leimberger J, Califf R, et al. Risk stratification after hospitalization for decompensated heart failure. *J Card Fail.* 2004;6:460–465.

91. O'Connor CM, Hasselblad V, Mehta RH, et al. Triage after hospitalization with advanced heart failure: the ESCAPE (Evaluation Study of Congestive Heart Failure and Pulmonary Artery Catheterization Effectiveness) risk model and discharge score. *J Am Coll Cardiol.* 2010;55:872–878.

92. Aaronson KD, Schawrtz JS, Chen TM, et al. Development and prospective validation of a clinical index to predict survival in ambulatory patients referred for cardiac transplant evaluation. *Circulation.* 1997;95:2660–2667.

93. Pohwani AL, Murali S, Matheir MM, et al. Impact of β-blocker therapy on functional capacity criteria for heart transplant listing. *J Heart Lung Transplant.* 2003;22:78–86.

94. Butler J, Khadim G, Paul KM, et al. Selection of patients for heart transplantation in the current era of heart failure therapy. *J Am Coll Cardiol.* 2004;43:787–793.

95. Levy WC, Mozaffarian D, Linker DT, et al. The Seattle Heart Failure Model: prediction of survival in heart failure. *Circulation.* 2006;113:1424–1433.

96. Packer M, O'Connor CM, Ghali JK, et al. Effect of amlodipine on morbidity and mortality in severe chronic heart failure. *N Engl J Med.* 1996;335:1107–1114.

97. Kalogeropoulos AP, Georgiopoulou W, Giamouzis G, et al. Utility of the Seattle Heart Failure Model in patients with advanced heart failure. *J Am Coll Cardiol.* 2009;53:324–342.

98. Neaton JD, Normand SL, Gelijns A, et al. Designs for mechanical circulatory support device studies. *J Card Fail.* 2007;13:63–74.

99. *Randomized Evaluation of VAD InterVEntion before Inotropic Therapy.* Available at http://www.clinicaltrial.gov/ct2/show/NCT01369407?term=Left+Ventricular+Assist&rank=20: Accessed July 21, 2011.

100. Levy WC, Mozaffarian D, Linker DT, et al. REMATCH Investigators. Can the Seattle Heart Failure Model be used to risk-stratify heart failure patients for potential left ventricular assist device therapy? *J Heart Lung Transplant.* 2009;28:231–236.

CHAPTER **6**

Candidate Selection for Long-Term Left Ventricular Assist Device Therapy for Advanced Heart Failure

Leslie W. Miller and Stuart D. Russell

INTRODUCTION

There have been variable estimates of the number and percentage of all patients with systolic heart failure (HF) who have advanced or end-stage disease, but this group probably accounts for roughly 5% to 10% of the total population of approximately 3.5 million with estimates ranging from 50,000 to 150,000 (Fig. 6-1).[1–5] Although these patients with the most advanced HF constitute only a small percentage of all patients with systolic HF, they consume more than 60% of health care expenditures for patients with HF.[6,7] This added expense is due to frequent hospitalizations and use of expensive lifesaving devices and therapies such as the biventricular pacemaker and the implantable cardioverter-defibrillator (see Chapter 2).[8] The increasing prevalence and very limited functional capacity and poor quality of life for patients with advanced-stage HF, plus the limited medical options, have provided the stimuli for the development of new and, it is hoped, cost-effective therapies.

LEFT VENTRICULAR ASSIST DEVICES

Cardiac transplantation currently represents the most definitive treatment for end-stage HF with greater than 85% 1-year survival and 70% 5-year survival (Fig. 6-2) and excellent functional capacity.[9] This survival is much better than the 20% survival at 1 year observed with optimal medical therapy in the REMATCH (Randomized Evaluation of Mechanical Assistance for the Treatment of Congestive Heart Failure) trial in patients with end-stage HF who were not considered eligible for heart transplantation.[10] Only 2200 donor hearts are available each year, and these hearts are usually reserved for patients younger than 65 years of age.[9,11,12] Older patients with the highest prevalence of the disease are typically not eligible for this optimal form of therapy. The survival with heart transplantation

is not uniform and decreases with each decade of life of the recipient as shown in Figure 6-2. An increasingly used alternative therapeutic option for patients with refractory HF has been mechanical circulatory support (MCS) with the use of ventricular assist devices (VADs).[13–17] Although the original focus of funding for research in this area was on the total artificial heart, the main success and almost total type of MCS has been with VADs. (See Chapter 1 for a detailed account of this evolution of funding and device development.)

INDICATIONS FOR MECHANICAL CIRCULATORY SUPPORT

The indications for VAD use have evolved over time based on increasing experience and duration of use. VADs originally were used for patients who failed to wean from cardiopulmonary bypass after cardiotomy. The VAD usually employed left-sided support alone with a simple centrifugal pump interposed between a drainage cannula drawing blood from the left atrium and a return cannula to the proximal aorta; this was essentially extracorporeal membrane oxygenation or peripheral cardiopulmonary bypass (see Chapter 8). This type of support was designed for use for only hours to a few days. However, the technology evolved rapidly to development and use of pulsatile volume displacement pumps designed for support for months. This improvement led to the use of VADs in what has become the most common indication for MCS, known as *bridge to transplant* (BTT), in patients who deteriorate and develop refractory HF or shock while on an active heart transplant waiting list (>12,000 patients).[18–24] The success with these devices has remained quite good over the past 2 decades, despite their use in patients with ever-increasing severity of HF and comorbidities, including emergency rescue of patients in cardiogenic shock, such as after acute myocardial infarction[25,26] or cardiac arrest. Historically, 20%

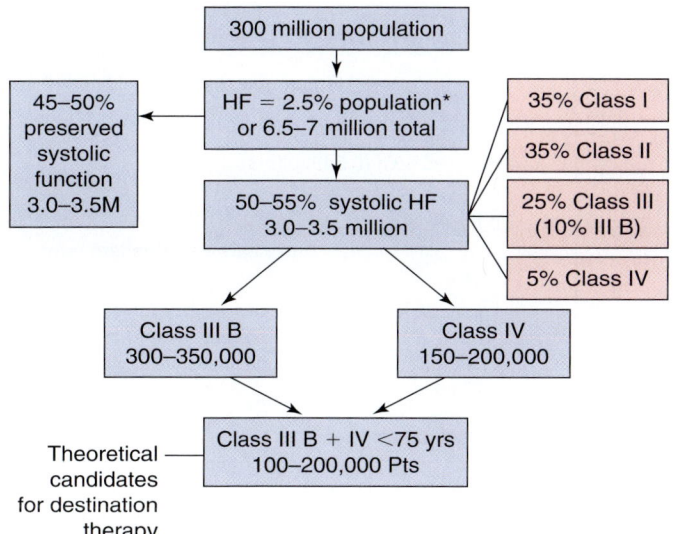

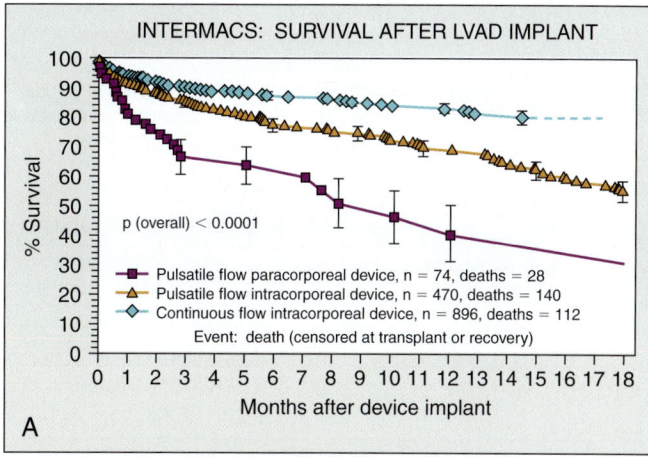

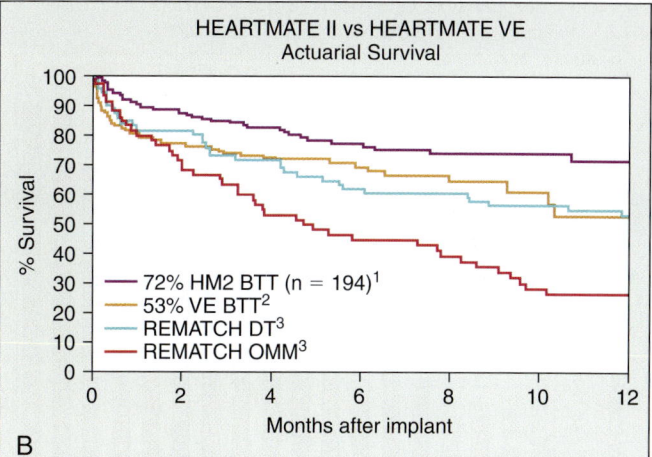

FIGURE 6-1 Projected number of patients with varying types and severity of heart failure (HF) with overall prevalence as estimated by the American Heart Association. Estimated numbers are provided by the author. *(From Writing Group Members, Lloyd-Jones D, Adams RJ, Brown TM, Carnethon M, et al; American Heart Association Statistics Committee and Stroke Statistics Subcommittee. Heart disease and stroke statistics—2010 update: a report from the American Heart Association. Circulation. 2010;121:e46-e215.)*

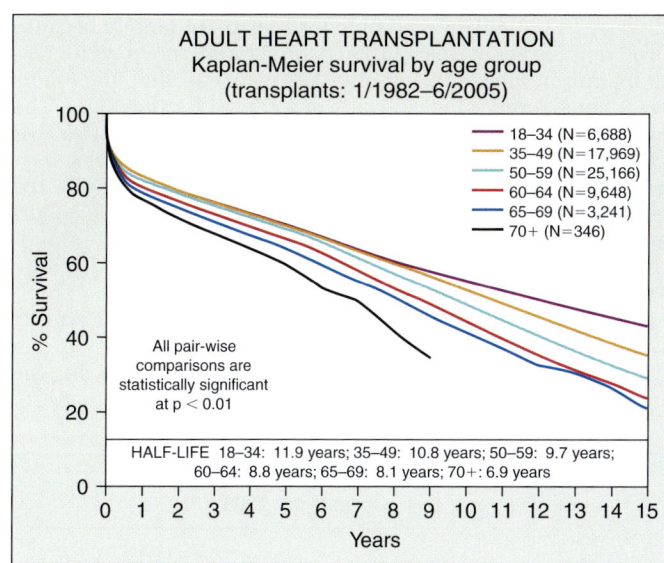

FIGURE 6-2 Kaplan-Meier survival plots show reduced survival with increasing age, from the Registry of the International Society of Heart and Lung Transplantation. *(From Taylor DO, Edwards LB, Aurora P, et al. Registry of the International Society for Heart and Lung Transplantation: twenty-fifth official adult heart transplant report—2008. J Heart Lung Transplant. 2008;27:943-956).*

FIGURE 6-3 A, Kaplan-Meier survival for patients with implantation of a first-generation pulsatile, volume displacement left ventricular assist device (LVAD) (either paracorporeal or intracorporeal) versus a second-generation continuous flow LVAD. **B,** Kaplan-Meier survival curves for patients in the primary cohort and an additional 61 patients enrolled after full enrollment and closure of the Heartmate II bridge to transplant (BTT) trial but before U.S. Food and Drug Administration (FDA) approval compared with a published multicenter trial of the XVE LVAD for BTT versus the outcome of the XVE and optimal medical management (OMM) cohorts in the REMATCH study of destination therapy (DT). *(B, Data from [1]Miller LW, Pagani FD, Russell SD, et al; HeartMate II clinical investigators. Use of a continuous-flow device in patients awaiting heart transplantation. N Engl J Med. 2007;357:885-896; [2]Frazier OH, Rose EA, Kormos RL. J Thorac Cardiovasc Surg. 2001;66:669-674; and [3]Rose EA, Gelijns AC, Moskowitz AJ, et al; Randomized Evaluation of Mechanical Assistance for the Treatment of Congestive Heart Failure [REMATCH] Study Group. Long-term mechanical left ventricular assistance for end-stage heart failure. N Engl J Med. 2001;345:1435-1443.)*

to 30% of patients who had a VAD implanted as a BTT did not survive to transplantation regardless of the device used or year of implantation owing to the severity of HF[24] and the complications associated with the device. More recently, this mortality has been reduced significantly with use of the new generation of continuous flow devices (Fig. 6-3).[13]

Most deaths still occur early after implantation of a VAD, typically before discharge from the index hospitalization. There is an estimated 10% to 15% mortality in patients placed on the heart transplant waiting list who are not supported with MCS.[27] The number of those deaths that could have been averted with use of VADs is unknown, but it is

likely a substantial percentage. The more recent changes in the United Network for Organ Sharing (UNOS) guidelines for organ sharing to prioritize use of donors for primarily status 1A patients (defined as the highest risk for survival of >1 week) has had a significant impact on the use of left ventricular assist devices (LVADs) for BTT (Table 6-1). Patients who are status 1B are now much less likely to get a donor heart, and patients who are status 2 now rarely undergo transplantation. This change toward performing transplantation on only the sickest patients and continual increases in waiting time for a donor have contributed to a rapidly increasing use of LVADs, with current estimates ranging from 40% to 85% of patients having LVADs at the time of heart transplant (Fig. 6-4).

There are few alternative strategies for patients with the most advanced HF. Data from several studies have shown that the outcome with VADs is significantly better than

Table 6-1	Changes in Number of Patients Listed as Status 1A Related to Change in United Network for Organ Sharing (UNOS) Policy To Prioritize Donors for Status 1A		
US Heart Transplants By Status: Change from 2000-2008			
Status	2000	2008	% Change
1A	870	1100	+26
1B	755	714	−5
2	573	188	−67
All	2199	2002	−9

Source: UNOS published data to November 30, 2008 (UNOS/SSTR Database, 2009).

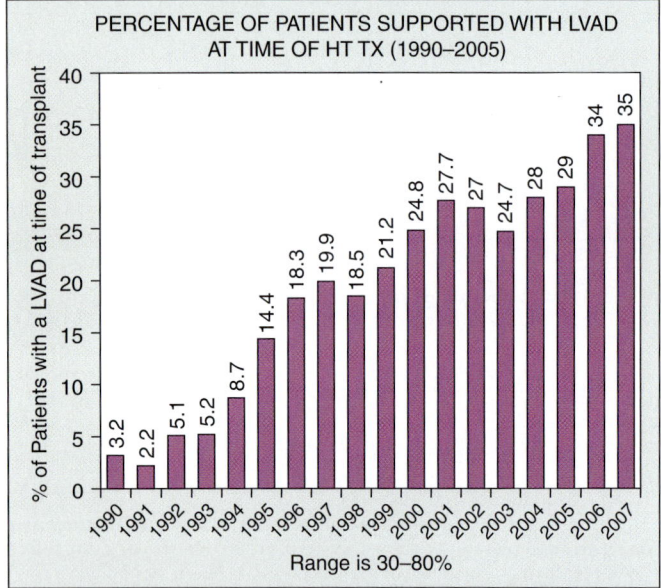

FIGURE 6-4 Increasing percentage of patients who are on left ventricular assist device (LVAD) support at the time of heart transplant (HT TX). *(UNOS data 2008 from UNOS/SSTR Database.)*

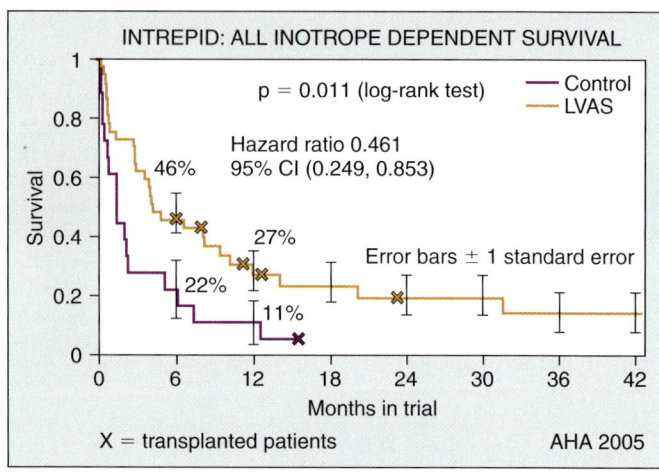

FIGURE 6-5 Kaplan-Meier survival plot for patients enrolled in the INTrEPID trial, which compared Novacor left ventricular assist device (LVAD) with continued inotropic therapy in patients who all were inotrope-dependent at initiation of the trial. LVAS, left ventricular assist system. *(From Rogers JG, Butler J, Lansman SL, et al; INTrEPID investigators. Chronic mechanical circulatory support for inotrope-dependent heart failure patients who are not transplant candidates: results of the INTrEPID trial. J Am Coll Cardiol. 2007;50:741-747.)*

therapy with intravenous inotropes.[28,29] More recently, a cohort of patients followed as a contemporary control group that declined LVAD implantation in the INTREPID (Investigation of Non Transplant-Eligible Patients Who Are Inotrope Dependent) trial had a 20% survival at 1 year (Fig. 6-5).[29] The decision to delay VAD implantation and to support a patient with intravenous inotrope therapy is often based on a shorter expected waiting time for a heart donor; the waiting time varies considerably across the United States according to blood group, body size, and other variables. The success in terms of improved survival, reduced adverse events, and proven device durability reported with several of the new generation of continuous flow LVADs compared with the very low survival reported with use of outpatient inotrope therapy has all but eliminated intravenous inotropes as an alternative to LVADs.[13,15–17]

DESTINATION THERAPY

VADs were not developed for the BTT indication but were designed primarily as an alternative to transplantation, known as *destination therapy* (DT). The development of DT was due largely to the significant increase in prevalence of HF in patients older than age 60 years,[10] the very limited availability of donor hearts, and the age cutoff for transplant of 65 years in most programs.[30]

Two prospective randomized trials[10,16] and one registry[31] have examined the outcome of MCS in DT patients, or patients not eligible for heart transplant. The first was the REMATCH study, which compared the outcome of LVADs versus medical therapy in patients not eligible for transplant largely because of advancing age.[10] Nearly 1000 patients were screened for participation in the study, but only 129 were enrolled; the others were considered either too sick or too well for the study. The entry criteria included New York Heart Association (NYHA) class IV HF, low ejection fraction, and very low peak oxygen consumption (VO$_2$) (target <10 mL/kg/min). Despite the goal of studying stable patients with advanced HF, the cohort enrolled was the sickest HF population ever studied, including 65% who were deemed inotrope-dependent and whose average peak VO$_2$ was 8.5 mL/kg/min. Similar to the experience in BTT, the mortality at 1 month in the LVAD arm[10,32] was high (17%), but it was identical to the mortality of the control group on medical therapy (Fig. 6-6), emphasizing the importance of candidate selection in outcomes with MCS.

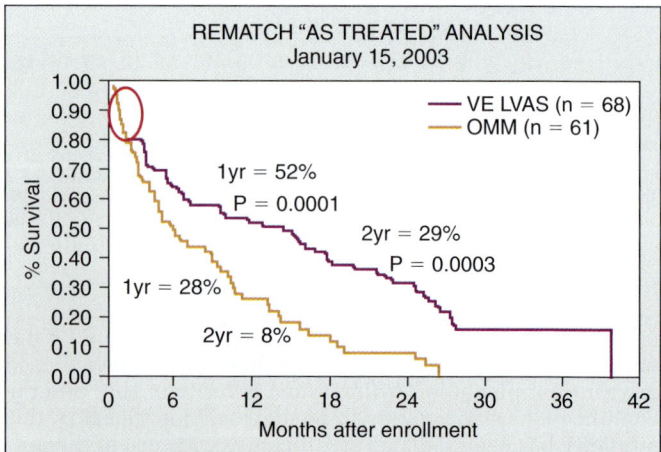

FIGURE 6-6 Kaplan-Meier survival in the REMATCH study comparing XVE left ventricular assist system (LVAS) with optimal medical management (OMM) and showing equal 17% mortality in the first 30 days between the two groups. *(From Rose EA, Gelijns AC, Moskowitz AJ, et al; Randomized Evaluation of Mechanical Assistance for the Treatment of Congestive Heart Failure [REMATCH] Study Group. Long-term mechanical left ventricular assistance for end-stage heart failure. N Engl J Med. 2001;345:1435-1443.)*

Similar to most surgical studies, death was defined at less than 30 days, but many patients had a prolonged postoperative course and died before hospital discharge (65% of all deaths in the first year) from complications that occurred early after surgery.

The trend for most deaths to occur before hospital discharge persisted because 65% of all deaths during the first year after implant occurred before hospital discharge in the subsequent Post-REMATCH. Post-REMATCH was a post-marketing registry study mandated by the U.S. Food and Drug Administration (FDA)[31] that reviewed 250 patients implanted with the HeartMate XVE device (Thoratec Corp, Pleasanton, CA) after the REMATCH study was completed and the XVE device was approved for commercial use (2003-2005) (Fig. 6-7). In the PRM Registry, 66 centers implanted devices; most of the centers were not involved in the REMATCH study and reflected outcomes of broad general use of the device.[31]

More recently, the outcomes with MCS in DT patients were examined in a comparison of the first-generation pulsatile XVE device versus the second-generation continuous flow HeartMate II device.[16] Although there was a significant reduction in the total number and the absolute percentage of patients who died in the first year, the greatest risk of death remained before discharge from the index hospitalization (56%) (Fig. 6-8). The percentage of patients who died before discharge was similar in both devices.

This persisting high percentage of all deaths in the first year occurring before discharge may have been due to the persisting inclusion of patients with the most advanced stage of HF, with 75% of patients receiving intravenous inotropes at the time of enrollment in the study. These data further emphasized candidate selection as the most important determinant of outcomes with MCS, regardless of the indication for use and largely independent of the device used. There are other important targets for improvement that would have a favorable impact on outcomes with LVADs beyond patient selection, including improved durability of the devices[33,34]; better troubleshooting of device dysfunction[35,36]; and adherence to new published clinical management guidelines for patients with continuous flow devices, including such important areas as infection[37,38] and nutrition.[39]

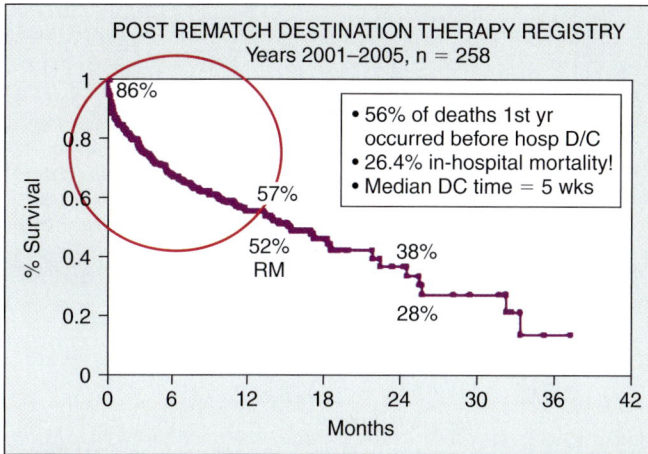

FIGURE 6-7 Kaplan-Meier survival curve for patients enrolled in the U.S. Food and Drug Administration (FDA) mandated postmarketing study for the Heartmate XVE left ventricular assist device (LVAD) shows the high percentage of deaths before hospital discharge (D/C). *(From Lietz K, Long JW, Kfoury AG, et al. Outcomes of left ventricular assist device implantation as destination therapy in the post-REMATCH era: implications for patient selection. Circulation. 2007;116:497-505.)*

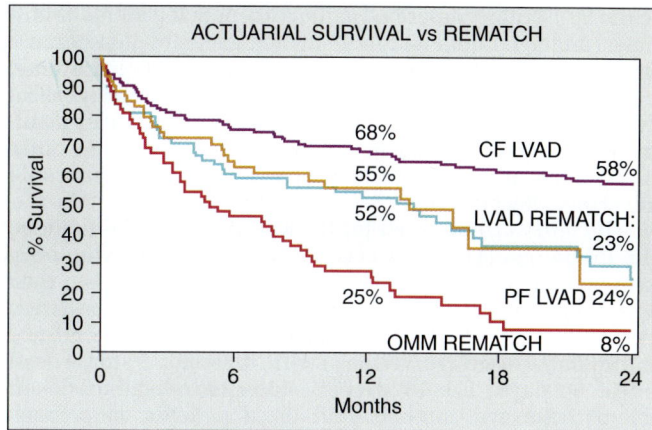

NEJM 2009; 361(23): 2241-51   NEJM 2001; 345(20): 1435-43

FIGURE 6-8 Data from Heartmate II destination therapy (DT) trial comparing Heartmate II with Heartmate XVE left ventricular assist devices (LVADs) and data from the REMATCH study for Heartmate XVE and medically managed patients. CF, continuous flow; PF, pulsatile flow. OMM, optimal medical management. *(Data from Slaughter MS, Rogers JG, Milano CA, et al; HeartMate II investigators. Advanced heart failure treated with continuous-flow left ventricular assist device. N Engl J Med. 2009;361:2241-2251; and Rose EA, Gelijns AC, Moskowitz AJ, et al; Randomized Evaluation of Mechanical Assistance for the Treatment of Congestive Heart Failure [REMATCH] Study Group. Long-term mechanical left ventricular assistance for end-stage heart failure. N Engl J Med. 2001;345:1435-1443.)*

GENERAL CRITERIA FOR CANDIDACY FOR MECHANICAL CIRCULATORY SUPPORT

The assessment of mortality risk with medical therapy alone and potential candidacy for MCS is based primarily on the risk models and factors discussed in detail in Chapter 4, especially recurrent HF hospitalizations. Specific selection criteria for candidacy for cardiac transplantation have been established and endorsed by the International Society for Heart and Lung Transplantation (ISHLT) and the American College of Cardiology, American Heart Association, and Heart Failure Society of America (ACC/AHA/HFSA) and updated by Mehra et al.[30] However, until more recently, there were no approved guidelines for MCS; guidelines have recently been published on overall management of patients with implantation of the new generation of continuous flow VADs and endorsed by the ISHLT. These new guidelines include a section on candidate selection.[40]

The generally accepted criteria for use of MCS as BTT are based on several parameters, including hemodynamics, clinical examination, and laboratory data that show impaired systemic perfusion and end-organ function. General hemodynamic criteria include a cardiac index greater than 2.0 L/min but should be better defined by calculated stroke volume because some patients may have a cardiac index greater than 2.0 L/min but are using tachycardia to compensate for low stroke volume; this represents an advanced phase of decompensation. Other hemodynamic criteria include requirement for adequate intracardiac filling pressures (e.g., right atrial pressure >10 mm Hg, pulmonary capillary wedge pressure >15 mm Hg), to distinguish low cardiac output that might occur with overdiuresis. Additional factors supporting the need for MCS include cool and constricted extremities reflective of poor perfusion, low blood pressure, tachycardia, rales or distended neck veins, laboratory evidence of prerenal azotemia or hepatic dysfunction, prolonged coagulation levels, and reduced urine output in response to diuretics.

The criteria used for patient selection for patients considered not to be transplant candidates, or DT patients, are similar to the BTT criteria described earlier except that patients almost never undergo implantation in an emergent situation because they are typically older and warrant a more detailed evaluation for possible comorbidities that could adversely affect outcomes. Potential candidates should undergo a cardiopulmonary exercise test whenever possible to determine cardiac limitations and a rigorous review for comorbidities that could adversely affect outcomes.[2]

The entry criteria used for the REMATCH study included the following: (1) NYHA class IV or stage D HF symptoms, (2) ejection fraction less than 25%, (3) peak VO_2 less than 12 mL/kg/min, and (4) significant functional limitation despite use of maximally tolerated doses of drugs outlined in the more recent guidelines for HF treatment[2,6] for at least 60 of 90 days. The REMATCH study enrolled the sickest HF patients ever studied, and these patients were much sicker than anticipated. These same criteria were adopted by the Centers for Medicare and Medicaid Services (CMS), however, and remain the criteria used for CMS reimbursement patients not eligible for transplant, or DT patients (Box 6-1).[41,42] Similar guidelines for VO_2[30] and exclusion criteria described earlier apply to this patient population as well. However, the use of percent of predicted VO_2, which is based on nomograms that are adjusted for age, gender, and body surface area, may be more reliable than absolute VO_2 in older candidates because the predicted peak VO_2 decreases with age and body size and is lower in women than men at all ages and sizes (Table 6-2).[43,44]

The target population includes patients who are refractory to all oral HF medications and are being managed with long-term intravenous inotrope therapy, typically as a continuous infusion at the time of VAD implant.[28] This situation is a paradox because long-term outpatient use of intravenous inotropes is not endorsed by national guidelines for HF treatment and typically is reserved for patients with low cardiac output, poor perfusion, end-organ dysfunction, and congestion. In addition, data have consistently shown that use of intravenous inotropes is a very inferior long-term alternative therapy to mechanical support with VADs because it is associated with a 1-year mortality of 80% to 90% (see Fig. 6-5).[45–49] However, the absence of intravenous inotropes at the time of LVAD implantation has been shown to be associated with a significant increase in risk of mortality before index LVAD hospitalization, and INTERMACS (Interagency Registry for Mechanically Assisted Circulatory Support) data show that patients given intravenous inotropes may have the best survival with LVAD use.[17]

The likely explanation for this paradox is that patients who are stable on intravenous inotropes have improved perfusion and end-organ function, especially renal and hepatic function, and are in a lower risk category. Patients who deteriorate on inotrope therapy are at very high risk of death and have poor end-organ function and do worse with LVAD use. Any patient who is deemed to have a sufficient 1- to 2-year survival with a reasonable quality of life to be managed with long-term inotropes should be referred for consideration of possible candidacy for VAD therapy instead.

Body size has historically been a significant limitation to MCS for most women, smaller adults, and adolescents because of the relatively large size of nearly all pulsatile devices because these devices required the patient to have a body surface area greater than 1.5 m^2. However, new continuous flow LVADs are one-fifth the size of the pulsatile devices, and patients with a body surface area of 1.3 m^2 are being studied in trials recently completed or under way in the hope of expanding the use of MCS to this underserved population who were previously excluded due to body size. The percentage of women who have received VAD therapy has increased from 8% with pulsatile devices to nearly 30% in the most recent trials. Although the outcomes for VAD therapy are the same in women as in men, women typically have a longer waiting time for transplant (Fig. 6-9).

BOX 6-1 Centers for Medicare and Medicaid Services Criteria for Eligibility for Coverage for Payment for Use of Left Ventricular Assist Devices as Destination Therapy

MCS for Destination Therapy
CMS Patient Selection Criteria
- Not a transplant candidate
- New York Heart Association class IV heart failure on maximal medical therapy >60-90 days
- Ejection fraction <25%
- Peak oxygen consumption <12 mL/kg/min

Data from Boyle AJ. Risk of bleeding with continuous flow ventricular assist device. *J Heart Lung Transplant* 2009;28:881–887.

TABLE 6-2	Risk Stratification in Heart Failure: Peak Oxygen Consumption (VO_2) Absolute versus % Predicted	
		P Value
% Predicted VO_2		.0005
Peak VO_2		.007
LVEF		.01
Age		.42
PCWP		.42
Etiology		.77

Note: Percent predicted VO_2, which is derived from nomograms factoring age, gender, and body surface area, is compared with commonly used and accepted risk factors for mortality in patients with heart failure.
LVEF, left ventricular ejection fraction; PCWP, pulmonary capillary wedge pressure.
From Stelken A, Younis LT, Jennison SH, et al. Prognostic value of cardiopulmonary exercise testing using percent achieved of predicted peak oxygen uptake for patients with ischemic and dilated cardiomyopathy. *J Am Coll Cardiol.* 1993;27:345-352.

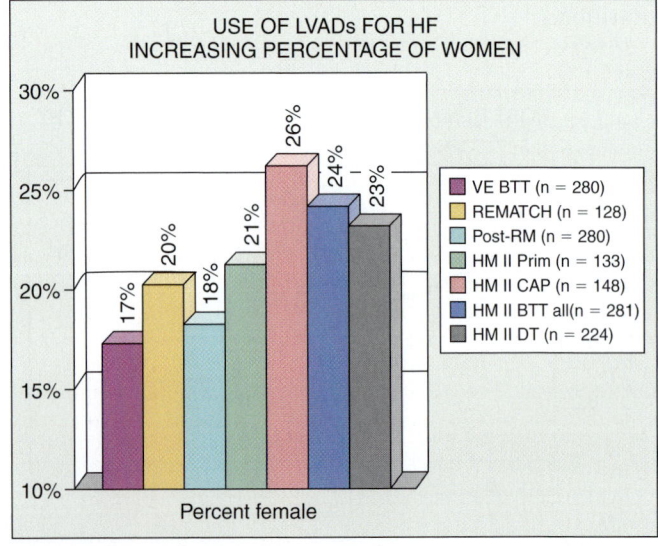

FIGURE 6-9 Increasing percentage of women in left ventricular assist device (LVAD) trials with introduction of continuous flow LVADs. VE BTT, vented electric XVE pump in bridge to transplant (BTT) multicenter study; Post-RM, Thoratec postmarketing registry study of XVE patients with implantation as destination therapy (DT); HM II Prim, original cohort in the HM II BTT trial; HM II CAP, continuous access protocol patients studied after original cohort enrolled and before U.S. Food and Drug Administration (FDA) approval; HM II DT, Heartmate II DT trial (more recently completed).

SPECIFIC RISK FACTORS FOR ADVERSE OUTCOME WITH VENTRICULAR ASSIST DEVICE USE

The leading causes of morbidity and mortality with use of VADs have not changed over the past 30 years and are the same regardless of indication (BTT or DT). These include sepsis, bleeding, renal failure, right HF, multiorgan failure, and stroke.[31,50] Many of these complications can be traced to significant abnormalities in laboratory data, organ function, or clinical status before implantation that constitute significant risk factors for adverse outcome with MCS.

Renal Function

Renal dysfunction has consistently been one of the greatest risks for morbidity and mortality with the use of LVADs.[40] Several measures of renal function have been used to define this risk, including serum creatinine greater than 2.5 mg/dL and blood urea nitrogen greater than 40 mg/dL; alternatively, an estimated glomerular filtration rate less than 0.5 mL/kg/min is used in the new renal formula because serum creatinine can seriously underestimate the severity of renal impairment, especially in women and patients with reduced muscle mass. The assessment of renal function should also include 24-hour urine measurement not only for creatinine clearance but also total protein and standard urinalysis to look for the presence of inflammatory cells or eosinophils suggesting interstitial nephritis secondary to drug allergy or primary interstitial disease. High urine protein excretion detected in a 24-hour urine collection or the presence of cells in the urine may warrant renal biopsy to exclude the presence of a primary renal disease rather than HF, especially if the patient does not have diabetes mellitus. In addition, patients with a high serum creatinine should have an abdominal ultrasound to confirm the presence of two kidneys, to assess the size and cortical thickness of the kidneys as a good index of the chronicity and severity of any renal dysfunction, and to rule out obstruction.

The cut point for exclusion owing to renal function in the REMATCH study[10] was a serum creatinine 3.5 mg/dL or greater, but this has been reduced to 2.5 mg/dL in more recent trials. Future trials are expected to use estimated creatinine clearance rather than serum creatinine. All of these variables are not dichotomous but are continuous variables, with increased risk with progressive abnormality of the variable. Generally, patients who are on long-term dialysis support are considered very high risk candidates for use of LVAD as DT because of long-term increased risk of complications, often related to infection of vascular access. It is often difficult to assess the reversibility of renal dysfunction[51] in patients with HF because it can be secondary to decreased perfusion of the kidney in low cardiac output states typical of advanced HF but may also be due to direct nephrotoxic effect of commonly prescribed drugs such as angiotensin-converting enzyme inhibitors and angiotensin II receptor blockers or nonsteroidal anti-inflammatory drugs. Many centers do not measure creatinine clearance until the patient is on an intravenous drug regimen that is associated with a cardiac index greater than 2.4 L/min for 1 to 2 days.

Although there is a reasonable correlation between cardiac output and renal blood flow, it is not a linear correlation, and many agents, particularly vasodilator drugs (e.g., nitroprusside) and inotropes (e.g., milrinone), may reduce afferent arterial pressure and decrease the perfusion gradient across the glomerulus, leading to failure to improve or worsening serum creatinine despite good cardiac output.[52] Chronic renal dysfunction (e.g., creatinine >3.0 mg/dL), which is associated with a reduction in kidney size and a thinning of the renal cortex, may not be associated with much improvement with the use of mechanical support devices. However, many patients who had LVADs implanted as an alternative to transplantation, or DT, owing to poor renal function subsequently underwent transplantation because of reversal of renal dysfunction with a period of mechanical support.[31] In the HeartMate II BTT trial, many patients with preoperative blood urea nitrogen and creatinine values above normal had improvement after 6 months of support, from 37 mg/dL to 23 mg/dL for blood urea nitrogen and from 1.8 mg/dL to 1.4 mg/dL for creatinine.[53]

Right Ventricular Function: Risk Stratification for Right Ventricular Failure

Right ventricular (RV) failure is one of the most important causes of mortality or morbidity after LVAD therapy for both volume displacement and continuous flow LVADs. RV failure is a major contributing factor to serious adverse events such as bleeding, renal failure, and prolonged hospitalization and often results in many other complications, which can lead to multiorgan failure. Most RV failure occurring after implantation can be anticipated preoperatively, and various therapies that optimize RV function can be used. Optimizing RV function is one of the most important targets for preoperative optimization (see Chapter 7). RV failure is estimated to occur in 20% to 30% of patients undergoing MCS. Patients with a nonischemic etiology often present with significant RV and left ventricular failure and may be at a threefold to fourfold increased risk of needing RV support.[54,55]

RV failure after LVAD is most commonly due to preexisting RV failure, altered RV geometry caused by significantly reduced left ventricular size by the LVAD unloading, and increased venous return resulting from increased left ventricular and LVAD blood flow and output. Left ventricular unloading with a left ventricular assist system (LVAS) should decrease RV afterload by reducing pulmonary artery pressure.[56] However, the LVAD may increase systemic venous return to a myopathic right heart that is unable to accommodate the additional volume. Reduction in left ventricular pressure can cause the interventricular septum to shift leftward, potentially causing disadvantageous geometric changes in the right ventricle that reduce septal contribution to RV stroke volume and exacerbate tricuspid regurgitation (see Chapters 12 and 13).[56]

Two models for prediction of RV failure after LVAD implantation have been reported more recently.[57,58] One model used a weighted scale (Box 6-2) that included measures of bilirubin 2.0 mg/dL or greater, aspartate aminotransferase 80 IU or

---

BOX 6-2 Variables Found to Be Most Associated with Risk of Right Ventricular (RV) Failure after Left Ventricular Assist Device Implantation

RV Failure Risk Score
Points derived from model coefficients:
4 points = presence of vasopressor requirement
3 points = creatinine ≥2.3 mg/dL (or RRT)
2.5 points = bilirubin ≥2.0 mg/dL
2 points = AST ≥80 IU/L
RV failure risk score = vasopressor points + AST points + bilirubin points + creatinine points

AST, aspartate aminotransferase; RRT, renal replacement therapy.

From Matthews JC, Koelling TM, Pagani FD, et al. The right ventricular failure risk score: a pre-operative tool for assessing the risk of right ventricular failure in left ventricular assist device candidates. *J Am Coll Cardiol.* 2008;51:2163-2172.

greater, and creatinine 2.3 mg/dL or greater but importantly identified use of vasopressor support before LVAD implantation as the greatest risk (HF = 4.0) to predict the probability of RV failure and the need for right ventricular assist device (RVAD) support.[57] This model has been shown to predict survival with RVAD support (Fig. 6-10). The other model is based more on hemodynamics, including cardiac index, RV stroke work index, and systolic blood pressure,[58] and severe preoperative RV dysfunction on echocardiogram, serum creatinine, and previous cardiac surgery. In one study, inotropic support for more than 14 days postoperatively was required in 38% of patients with RV stroke work index less than or equal to 600 mm Hg × mL/m² compared with 29% of patients with RV stroke work index 600 to 900 mm Hg × mL/m² and only 3% with RV stroke work index greater than 900 mm Hg × mL/m².[59] RV stroke work index provides a quantitative measure of the ability of the right ventricle to generate pressure and flow. Formulas for calculating RV stroke work index are detailed in the guidelines for continuous flow LVADs.[40]

The largest cohort examined for risk of RV failure after implantation of an LVAD was the analysis of 484 patients in the HeartMate II BTT clinical trial, which identified RV stroke work index less than 300 mm Hg × mL/m², central venous pressure greater than 15 mm Hg, elevated blood urea nitrogen, and elevated white blood cell count as risk factors by univariate analysis and preoperative ventilatory support, central venous pressure-to-pulmonary capillary wedge pressure ratio greater than 0.63, and blood urea nitrogen greater than 39 mg/dL as risk factors by multivariate analysis.[60] There was no difference in the incidence of RV failure in the HeartMate II trial in patients with a nonischemic versus an ischemic etiology for HF. However, several other centers have reported up to a fourfold increased risk of severe RV failure or need for RVAD in patients with a nonischemic etiology who had a pulsatile pump. A high right atrial pressure (>18 mm Hg) leads to poor renal function because of retrograde transmission of this elevated venous pressure to the kidney causing a reduced perfusion gradient in the kidney and resistance to diuretic therapy (see Chapter 7).[61] In addition, these patients often have increased bleeding because of high venous pressure.

The largest series examining risk factors for RV failure after LVAD implantation identified preoperative use of temporary mechanical support, female gender, and nonischemic etiology as the only significant risk factors by multivariate analysis.[54] However, univariate analysis identified several hemodynamic risk factors, including reduced RV stroke work index and low mean and diastolic pulmonary artery pressures but not pulmonary vascular resistance. Other important risk factors include right atrial pressure greater than pulmonary capillary wedge pressure and a significantly enlarged RV end-diastolic volume or dimension.

Other methods to define poor preoperative RV function include measurements made on echocardiogram before implantation including RV dimension or volume and severe tricuspid regurgitation, which can also be associated with early postoperative RV failure. Some surgeons have advocated repair of tricuspid regurgitation at the time of LVAD implantation if the severity is judged to be more than moderate either preoperatively or intraoperatively by echocardiogram. Other surgeons have found this added procedure to increase cardiopulmonary bypass time and not improve outcomes.

Pulmonary hypertension and the risk of severe postoperative RV failure are major concerns in the assessment of patients for heart transplant or BTT. However, the assessment of the risk of postoperative RV failure is of greater importance in the setting of DT because there are currently no good long-term options for outpatient biventricular mechanical support with most current devices typically requiring either a hybrid combination of device types or use of bilateral paracorporeal devices.

EVALUATION OF POTENTIAL CANDIDATES FOR MECHANICAL CIRCULATORY SUPPORT

Hemodynamics

Hemodynamic assessment with use of a Swan-Ganz catheter is an essential part of the evaluation of a potential candidate for MCS. There is no one specific hemodynamic criterion that defines candidacy for MCS, although low cardiac index (e.g., <2.0 L/min) or stroke volume less than 25 mL/beat despite use of vasoactive drugs, especially vasopressors, is a general criterion. Data showing that any individual parameter is an independent predictor of outcome are lacking, although high filling pressure and congestion seem more correlated with poor outcome in patients with HF. Tachycardia may lead to underestimation of the severity of HF if cardiac index alone is examined. It is important to focus more on stroke volume (cardiac output divided by heart rate) than cardiac index, especially in patients with significant tachycardia whose ventricular function is usually much worse than may be suggested by simple measurements of cardiac output alone.

The technique used to measure cardiac output should probably include both Fick and thermodilution methods. The Fick determination may be much less affected by significant tricuspid regurgitation, which may cause a significant amount of the injectant used with the thermodilution method to be ejected back up into the right atrium, which would result in smaller temperature differential and falsely elevate the cardiac output measured. In addition, attention should be given to measurement of mixed venous or pulmonary artery saturation, especially with good measured cardiac output in patients who appear very compromised. Right atrial pressure is the best assessment of RV function regardless of the pulmonary artery pressure. Low cardiac output may lead to deceptively modest elevations of pulmonary artery pressure. Patients with pulmonary artery pressure less than 25 to 30 mm Hg and high poor RV function on echocardiogram or high right atrial pressure are at significant risk

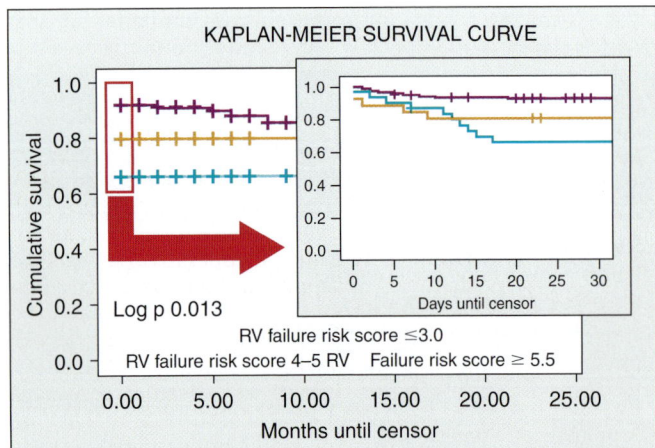

FIGURE 6-10 Use of Michigan right ventricular (RV) failure risk score is associated with prediction of survival after left ventricular assist device (LVAD) surgery. *(From Matthews JC, Koelling TM, Pagani FD, et al. The right ventricular failure risk score a pre-operative tool for assessing the risk of right ventricular failure in left ventricular assist device candidates. J Am Coll Cardiol. 2008;51:2163-2172.)*

of RV failure after LVAD implantation and reduced survival because the low pressure is reflective of very reduced RV function.

Hematologic Evaluation and Coagulation

Thrombocytopenia and anemia (hematocrit <30 mg/dL) are two hematologic parameters associated with poor outcomes with MCS (see Box 6-1). Patients should be thoroughly assessed for the etiology of either problem, and attempts should be made to correct any abnormalities before implantation. Preoperative platelet counts less than 149,000/μL have been shown to be the highest risk factor for death before discharge, with a sevenfold increase in risk of death before hospital discharge. Similarly, any prolongation of the international normalized ratio above normal is associated with a significant increased risk of death, and the international normalized ratio should be normalized in all patients before LVAD implantation. Lietz and colleagues[31] showed that the cause of death before discharge was directly linked to preoperative laboratory abnormalities, and the closest correlation was with abnormal coagulation values and death caused by bleeding. In addition, some centers check protein C, protein S, and anticardiolipin antibodies to identify coagulation abnormalities that may be used to guide postoperative management (see Chapter 7).

Pulmonary Function

Patients with severe obstructive or restrictive pulmonary disease are at increased risk related to LVAD therapy. Significant underlying pulmonary dysfunction or disease often leads to prolonged time in the intensive care unit and mechanical ventilation after implantation of an LVAD, especially the larger pulsatile devices owing to impairment of diaphragm motion. There are no absolute pulmonary function criteria or limits for exclusion of use of an LVAS, but assessment and suggested thresholds are detailed in more recent guidelines.[40]

Severe cardiac dysfunction may preclude accurate assessment of pulmonary function or give falsely low values if significant pulmonary congestion is present at the time of the test.[63] When pulmonary function testing can be performed reliably, and the forced vital capacity, forced expiratory volume at 1 second, and carbon monoxide diffusing capacity all are less than 50% predicted, exclusion from LVAD implantation should be considered. Mechanical ventilation before implantation has been shown to be one of the highest risk factors for poor outcome.[64] The evaluation of a patient with underlying pulmonary disease or demonstrated hypoxemia is detailed in more recent guidelines.[40]

Patients with low oxygen saturations (<92%) on room air also warrant an injection of sonicated saline during echocardiography to rule out a right-to-left shunt from an atrial septal defect or patent foramen ovale. If this test is negative, a spiral computed tomography or nuclear scan is indicated to rule out chronic thromboembolic disease.

One important and often underappreciated cause of hypoxemia, pulmonary hypertension, and RV failure is sleep-disordered breathing with central or secondary sleep apnea. Screening tests for this diagnosis should include measurement of nocturnal oximetry and respiratory function. If these screening tests are suggestive, a formal sleep study should be performed with home oxygen supplementation. The phenotype of a patient with sleep-disordered breathing is not always that described for pickwickian syndrome with morbid obesity. It is estimated that up to 40% of patients with HF have some degree of sleep-disordered breathing. Patients who are proven to have significant obstructive sleep apnea or sleep-disordered breathing should have LVAD surgery delayed for several months if possible to judge response to home therapy and allow possible recovery of RV function and reduction in risk of needing an RVAD.

Evaluation for Gastrointestinal Bleeding

Because all continuous flow LVADs require systemic anticoagulation with warfarin, patients with a history of gastrointestinal bleeding should be carefully screened. Documented current evidence of gastrointestinal blood loss should be assessed before LVAD implantation with both upper and lower endoscopy to define the cause and rule out malignancy.

Hepatic Function

Hepatic dysfunction has long been shown to be associated with poor outcomes after LVAD implantation.[65] It is often associated with abnormal coagulation, which leads to greater need for intraoperative and perioperative blood transfusion, which can result in worsened right heart function and the need for RVAD. The most common laboratory marker of hepatic dysfunction is hyperbilirubinemia, the etiology of which may be multifactorial, including "cardiac congestion," which typically gives a higher bilirubin level than cellular enzyme derangements but may also be due to multiple medications or cholestatic jaundice, infiltrative diseases, or exposure to toxins.

A previous history of significant alcohol use should be reviewed in all potential candidates for VAD therapy, especially patients with abnormal liver function. Previous studies have reported that total bilirubin levels and cellular enzymes greater than three times normal are independent risk factors for adverse outcomes.[66–69] Patients should also be tested for previous infection with hepatitis A, B, C or other viruses. Simple ultrasound visualization of the liver is a good screen for patients with significant hepatomegaly to rule out infiltrative disease, mass, or other pathology that may warrant biopsy. Many centers screen patients with clinical evidence of significant serologic evidence of hepatic dysfunction even in the presence of significant RV failure with hepatic ultrasound or transjugular or transhepatic liver biopsy to rule out cirrhosis. The most common cause of hepatic dysfunction is right HF, which may improve with mechanical support (LVAS or bilateral VAD); cirrhosis is predictive of poor outcome.

As with renal function, there is evidence that hepatic function improves after implantation of a continuous flow LVAD.[53,70–72] In the HeartMate II BTT trial, alanine aminotransferase, aspartate aminotransferase, and total bilirubin values in patients with abnormal baseline parameters improved to normal over 6 months.[53] Several strategies can be used to help improve hepatic function before LVAD implantation, and these are outlined in the recent guidelines[40] and discussed in Chapter 7.

Peripheral Vascular Disease Evaluation

Most LVAD clinical trials exclude patients with significant peripheral vascular disease because these patients often have atherosclerotic disease in multiple other locations in addition to claudication, which may limit postoperative ambulation and recovery. Abdominal ultrasound and measurement of the ankle-brachial index may be warranted to evaluate the degree of disease in susceptible patients being considered for LVAS support, including all patients with diabetes.

The other major form of peripheral vascular disease is carotid stenosis. It is imperative that any patient with an audible carotid bruit or history suggestive of transient ischemic attacks undergo a carotid ultrasound and formal study if significant stenosis is suggested. Generally, patients with a previous stroke who have significant paresis and reduced ambulation or impaired cortical function are not good candidates for LVAD therapy.

Evaluation for Infection

Infection and sepsis have been the leading cause of mortality and morbidity since the beginning of use of VADs for patients with advanced HF. Other risks for infection include the presence of indwelling catheters, which have been in place for several days before the time of surgery; mechanical ventilation; poorly controlled diabetes; renal failure; generalized debilitation; and current infection. Correcting as many of these factors as possible before device implantation can minimize the risk of infection and optimize long-term outcomes. Most patients are hospitalized for days to weeks for evaluation and optimization before implantation of the LVAD, which leads to changes in skin flora and significantly increases the risk of nosocomial infection after LVAD. Patients with active systemic infection should not be considered for LVAS support, and LVAD implantation should be delayed, if clinically feasible, for patients with localized infections that can be effectively treated.

Nutrition

Because of the importance of infection in causing post-LVAD morbidity and mortality, preoperative nutrition is crucial. Malnutrition is quite common in HF patients. Data have shown that 60% of patients in a stable HF clinic had a serum albumin less than 3.2 mg/dL. Serum albumin alone is a crude marker of malnutrition, but a level less than 3.2 mg/dL was associated with a fivefold risk of death before hospital discharge in DT patients receiving a pulsatile XVE pump in the Post-REMATCH study.[31] Almost all the patients who died of infection after LVAD implantation had a preoperative albumin less than 3.2 mg/dL.

The cause of malnutrition in HF patients is multifactorial and includes poor appetite, owing partly to elevated inflammatory cytokines such as tumor necrosis factor,[73] limited exertion, the work of breathing, and nausea and early satiety in patients with significant hepatomegaly. Malnutrition can adversely affect outcomes in surgical patients in many ways,[74] including poor wound healing and increased risk of infection and impaired T-lymphocyte function as manifested by cutaneous skin test anergy. As with non-VAD cardiac surgery data, the risk of operative death, but not infection, was correlated with cachexia and a low body mass index (BMI) (<22).[75,76]

There is an "obesity paradox" with regard to body size in HF because obese patients have a better survival than patients with cachexia. This paradox is also true with cardiac surgery; obesity is not associated with increased mortality risk, although it represents a significant risk of wound and other postoperative infections. Conversely, patients with a BMI less than 22 are at increased risk of death with cardiac surgery and at higher risk of infectious complications because of reduced immunologic response, poor wound healing, and typically impaired motor strength leading to prolonged limitation of ambulation.

Obesity is very common in patients with HF. In the HeartMate II BTT and DT trials, a BMI greater than 40 kg/m² was an exclusion criterion for study purposes. However, a more recent report showed that there were no deleterious effects of obesity on outcome in patients receiving LVAS support.[77] In some cases, LVADs have been used in obese patients as BTT eligibility, with the goal that during LVAS support obese patients will lose sufficient weight to become eligible for transplant. Generally, however, few patients have achieved sufficient weight loss to qualify for transplantation. Providing hemodynamic support with an LVAD as a means for weight loss should be undertaken with a multidisciplinary team approach that includes physicians, nurses, dietitians, exercise physiologists, and, potentially, bariatric surgeons. (See Chapter 7 for a discussion of management of malnutrition before LVAD implantation.)

Neurologic, Psychosocial, and Psychiatric Considerations

Patients with a neurologic or psychiatric disease that compromises their ability to use and care for external system components or to ambulate and exercise are poor candidates for LVAS support. Psychiatric disorders, drug abuse, and other psychosocial issues must be investigated to assess a patient's ability to understand and comply with care instructions. Patients with known recent drug abuse or a history of noncompliance may be unsuitable candidates. Adequate family or caregiver support, housing, and community infrastructure are additional determining factors for potential candidates for LVAS support. Although not an absolute requirement, patients receiving LVAS support should have family or friends nearby to provide supportive care when necessary. Patients must have a reliable means of transportation for follow-up visits and a convenient, reliable telephone service to call for medical help in an emergency.

The guidelines for cardiac transplantation clearly stipulate that all patients seriously considered for this form of advanced therapy should have a formal mental health evaluation by a trained health care professional.[78] This evaluation is as critical to long-term success of VAD therapy as it is for transplant recipients. The evaluation should focus not only on an assessment for significant underlying psychiatric illness but also on some measure of neurocognitive function. Several centers employ a brief training course on the operations and management of the mechanical devices and follow up with a test on these skills within 1 or 2 days of teaching to assess the mental competence and learning capacity of potential candidates, with the recognition that chronic HF may predispose to reversible mental or cognitive dysfunction.

Preoperative screening should also include assessments of medication compliance, compliance with medical recommendations (e.g., weight loss and smoking cessation), and compliance with physician appointments and assessment of any history of chemical dependency. One of the most crucial aspects, which may be even more important in considering a patient for mechanical support as an alternative to transplant, is the availability of a social support network. Support may ideally include a spouse, significant other, or committed family member or friend. Patients usually are not discharged home without the availability of someone who has passed the device education test and would be able to respond to alarms from the device for at least the first several months after hospital discharge should there be a mechanical device failure that results in a significant compromise of hemodynamic status and mental functioning of the patient.

One area that is a potential problem for both heart transplantation and MCS is a patient who is unknown to the program and presents in cardiogenic shock, often from a massive myocardial infarction. Such patients often require intubation and mechanical ventilation or are so compromised that they are virtually unable to participate in any type of preoperative evaluation or discussion regarding the decision to undergo LVAD implantation. This situation represents a significant challenge because some patients may be found later to have an unfavorable past history of chemical dependency or other social situations that may seriously complicate postoperative recovery and management. This potentially serious problem warrants concerted attempts to obtain as much background information as possible on all such patients who present for emergency support and are unable to speak and participate in the decision for an LVAD.

Screening for Malignancy

Many patients who receive an LVAD, especially as an alternative to transplant, are of an age at which malignancy is an increasing risk. Preoperative screening for cancer should be determined by age and gender, as defined by the American Cancer Society,[79] or directed by abnormal findings such as a guaiac-positive stool specimen and anemia. It is not recommended for a patient older than 55 years who has not had a previous colonoscopy to undergo LVAD implantation until appropriate endoscopy can be completed and found to be negative. Patients with a previous malignancy that is associated with significant reduction in expected survival should have a reasonable period of time from the original diagnosis until device implant to maximize the survival with this technology. In contrast, patients with a malignancy that is considered to have a good prognosis may be reasonable candidates for LVAD support.

Use of Composite Scores to Assess Risk for Operative Mortality

Many investigators have examined specific and composite risk factors that are associated with early mortality with use of VADs. Most of the risk factors have been similar or identical over the various time periods examined. Reedy and colleagues[66] used clinical intuition for assignment of relative risk and weighted scale for numerous clinical and laboratory variables to create one of the earliest risk scores. The results of each variable studied were collated into a composite risk score that identified low-risk, medium-risk, and high-risk populations. The low-risk group had nearly a 90% survival to transplant, whereas the high-risk group had only a 30% survival. More recently, the HF survival score, which includes several parameters, was shown retrospectively to be helpful in predicting outcome in patients such as the patients in the REMATCH study with the ability to factor in comorbidities such as use of inotropes or an intra-aortic balloon pump before LVAD implantation.[80]

The largest series examining a composite score of risk factors that correlate with outcomes in patients supported by VADs was reported by Lietz and colleagues[31] and comprised 250 patients who received a HeartMate XVE device between November 2003 and September 2005 after FDA approval of the device for commercial use. The initial analysis showed no improvement in outcomes with subsequent use of the XVE device for DT, but it also showed the very high mortality (70% of all deaths in the first year occurred before hospital discharge; Table 6-3). The analysis was directed at risk factors for these numerous early deaths.

There were 22 centers in the REMATCH study and 66 in the follow-up report by Leitz and colleagues.[31] All patients were in stage D HF and met nearly all the criteria for eligibility in the REMATCH study. The parameters entered into the score all were laboratory or clinical data recorded just before implantation. More than 65 variables were entered into a univariate analysis, and the variables shown to correlate with death before hospital discharge included inability to undergo a cardiopulmonary exercise test (largely owing to dependence on long-term inotrope therapy), right atrial pressure greater than 14 mm Hg, significant renal dysfunction, RV dysfunction, and white blood cell count greater than 12,000/μL. The significant risk factors by multivariate analysis are shown in Table 6-4. A hazard ratio was derived by statistical analysis, and a weighted value was given to each variable in rank order. Most of these risk factors are additive in the estimation of overall risk. The combination of creatinine greater than 1.6 mg/dL and albumin less than 3.3 mg/dL nearly doubled the risk of either factor alone.

The cut point used for each variable was derived by analysis of the range of values for each variable. The patients were divided into quartiles of risk. The laboratory values of each patient were similarly divided by quartiles. The value that defined the highest risk category was used as the cut point for estimating the risk score, and a risk value assigned by hazard ratio was calculated from the data Figure 6-11.

These parameters all were clearly continuous variables, and relative risk exists with degree of abnormality of the laboratory value. A patient with a platelet count of 155,000/μL is not free of risk, but a patient with a platelet count of 85,000/μL is at significant risk. Each patient in the analysis had a composite risk score calculated based on the presence or absence of the abnormal laboratory cut point and grouped into four quartiles defined as follows: 0 to 8, low risk; 9 to 16, medium risk; 17 to 19, high risk; and greater than 19, very high risk. The composite score was shown to have a very tight correlation with risk of death before discharge: 87.5%, 70.5%, 26%, and 13.7% (Fig. 6-12).

The scores were analyzed for prediction of death at 1 year and shown to have very strong positive predictive accuracy. The survival at 2 years after implantation was 87% in the lowest risk group ($n = 41$) and 60% in the next lowest quintile ($n = 53$); in the highest risk group, survival to hospital discharge was 12% and survival at 14 months was zero

Table 6-3	Percentage of Deaths in the First Year That Occur before Hospital Discharge in Left Ventricular Assist Device Trials for Destination Therapy (DT) and Bridge to Transplant (BTT)		
	Year	No. Patients	% Deaths
Pre-Match	1997	20	75
REMATCH	2001	68	62
Post-REMATCH	2005	268	56
HM II BTT	2007	271	59
HM II DT	2009	200	44

TABLE 6-4	Risk Factors Associated with In-Hospital Mortality after Left Ventricular Assist Device Implantation by Multivariate Analysis
Destination Therapy Risk Score – For 90-day in-hospital death	

Patient Variable	Weighted Risk Score
Platelets ≤148 × 10³/μL	7
Albumin ≤3.3 g/dL	5
INR >1.1	4
Vasodilator therapy	4
MPAP ≤25 mm Hg	3
AST >45 U/mL	2
Hematocrit ≤34%	2
BUN >51 U/dL	2
No intravenous inotropes	2

Note: Hazard ratio for each variable is converted to a weighted number. Risk score represents total of all risk factors present in each patient.

AST, aspartate aminotransferase; BUN, blood urea nitrogen; INR, international normalized ratio; MPAP, mean pulmonary arterial pressure.

From Lietz K, Long JW, Kfoury AG, et al. Outcomes of left ventricular assist device implantation as destination therapy in the post-REMATCH era: implications for patient selection. Circulation. 2007;116:497-505.

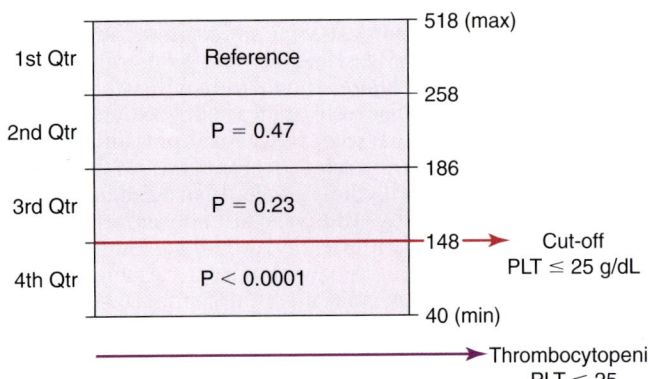

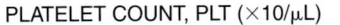

FIGURE 6-11 Derivation of hazard ratio of each risk factor shown to be associated with in-hospital mortality after left ventricular assist device (LVAD) implantation. Data for each parameter are divided into quartiles, and the cut point of the lowest quartile is used as the numerical cut point in the table to derive the risk score. *(From Lietz K, Long JW, Kfoury AG, et al. Outcomes of left ventricular assist device implantation as destination therapy in the post-REMATCH era: implications for patient selection. Circulation. 2007;116:497-505.)*

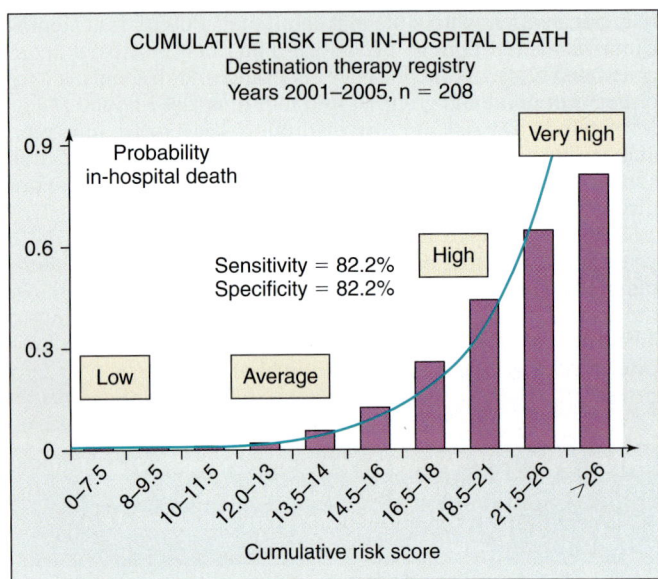

FIGURE 6-12 Cumulative risk of in-hospital death compared with the Lietz-Miller risk score described in Figure 6-13, with scores divided into quartiles of low, medium, high, and very high risk categories. Risk score is highly correlated with in-hospital death. *(From Lietz K, Long JW, Kfoury AG, et al. Outcomes of left ventricular assist device implantation as destination therapy in the post-REMATCH era: implications for patient selection. Circulation. 2007;116:497-505.)*

(Fig. 6-13). These data confirm the ability to use preoperative risk assessment to identify patients with LVAD implantation as DT who are at a high risk for poor outcome. The risk score showed that death before hospital discharge in patients receiving an implant as DT was strongly influenced by preoperative factors, including poor nutritional status, hematologic abnormalities, signs of end-organ and right heart dysfunction, and the lack of inotropic use. An additional strength of the risk score is that it was able to predict the specific cause of death by the high correlation with specific preoperative laboratory abnormalities. Patients who exhibited malnutrition died of infection, patients with coagulopathy died of bleeding, and patients with significant renal dysfunction died of renal or multiorgan failure.

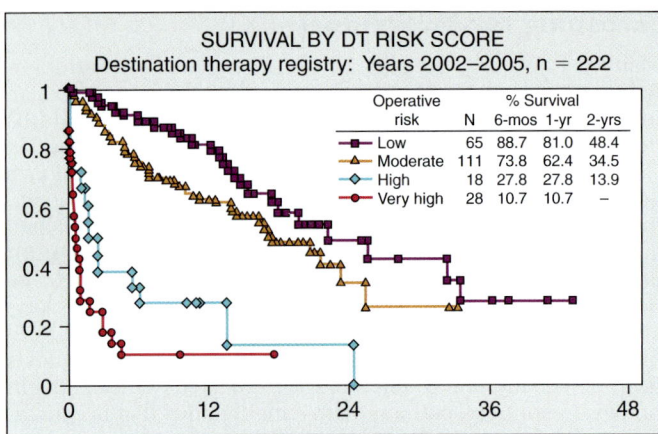

FIGURE 6-13 Survival following hospital discharge after left ventricular assist device (LVAD) implantation by cumulative Lietz-Miller risk score quartiles of low, medium, high, and very high risk categories at months postdischarge. DTRS, destination therapy risk score. *(From Lietz K, Long JW, Kfoury AG, et al. Outcomes of left ventricular assist device implantation as destination therapy in the post-REMATCH era: implications for patient selection. Circulation. 2007;116:497-505.)*

The original derivation of the Lietz risk score was with the use of the pulsatile, volume displacement HeartMate XVE device in exclusively DT patients. However, more recently, Lietz reported use of the risk score in patients with implantation of the new generation of continuous flow devices, primarily implanted for DT, but also included data on a significant number of BTT patients. Although the overall scores were not as high as the scores reported in the original DT cohort, the risk score had significant ability to risk stratify these patients as well. A comparison of the results of the derivation and validation scores is shown in Figure 6-14. This study showed that the Lietz-Miller risk score could be used in any patient undergoing MCS with any device for any indication.

The risk score was not derived as a litmus test to exclude patients in the highest risk category but to describe estimated risk at a given point in time and help guide the timing of LVAD implantation. The authors have suggested that aggressive medical therapy focused on the major risks of postoperative morbidity and mortality—malnutrition, significant RV failure, renal insufficiency, and coagulopathy—could result in reduction in the calculated risk score (Fig. 6-15). A patient with a prohibitive risk score may be an unacceptable candidate at the time of initial evaluation, but with intensive medical therapy and optimization of several parameters such as nutrition, abnormal coagulation values, and right heart function, he or she may become an acceptable risk (see Chapter 7). Patients whose risk score fails to improve after aggressive medical intervention are unlikely to survive the LVAD procedure in most centers. There are no prospective data confirming that this preoperative optimization can reduce the operative risk in a given patient, but this issue is discussed in detail in Chapter 7.

INTERAGENCY REGISTRY FOR MECHANICALLY ASSISTED CIRCULATORY SUPPORT

INTERMACS (Interagency Registry for Mechanically Assisted Circulatory Support) is a collaborative initiative by the National Heart, Lung, and Blood Institute (NHLBI), the FDA, the device industry, and physicians and nurses involved in the care of patients receiving VADs. This registry follows all long-term VADs implanted in the United States, and the submission of data on all patients is a requirement for

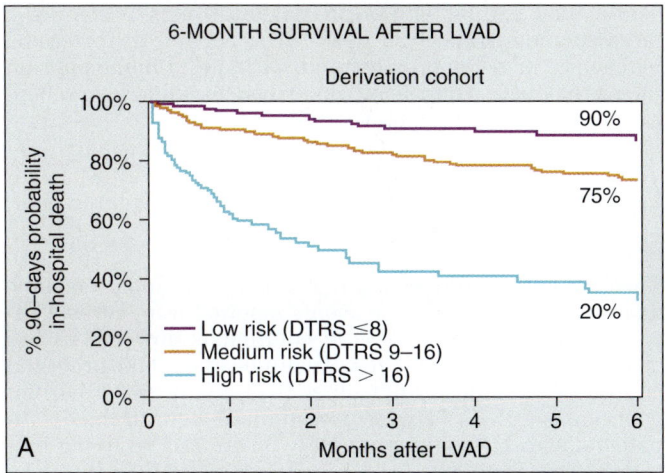

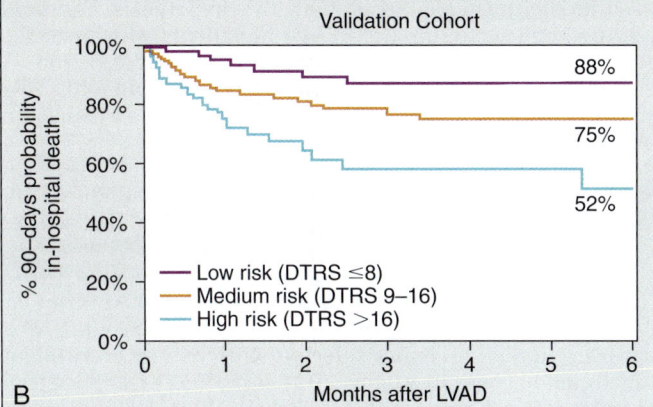

FIGURE 6-14 Survival following hospital discharge after left ventricular assist device (LVAD) implantation by cumulative Lietz-Miller risk score quartiles of low, medium, high, and very high risk categories at months postdischarge. Comparison of original derivation cohort from Thoratec postmarketing registry **(A)** and validation cohort from Columbia University **(B)**. DTRS, destination therapy risk score. *(From Lietz K, Long JW, Kfoury AG, et al. Outcomes of left ventricular assist device implantation as destination therapy in the post-REMATCH era: implications for patient selection. Circulation. 2007;116:497-505.)*

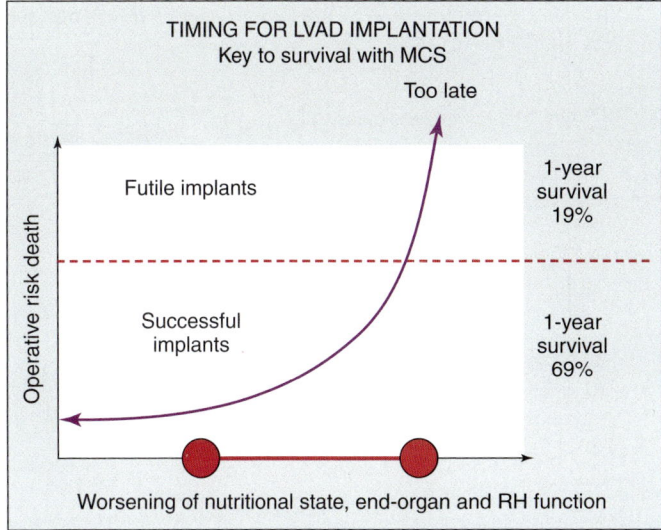

FIGURE 6-15 Use of Lietz-Miller risk score to aid timing of left ventricular assist device (LVAD) implantation. *Bidirectional arrow* indicates potential degree of reversibility of many risk factors that increase the risk of in-hospital mortality. MCS, mechanical circulatory support; RH, right heart. *(From Lietz K, Long JW, Kfoury AG, et al. Outcomes of left ventricular assist device implantation as destination therapy in the post-REMATCH era: implications for patient selection. Circulation. 2007;116:497-505.)*

CMS reimbursement, which has ensured accurate reporting. Although an unfunded mandate for VAD centers, INTERMACS has had nearly 100% data capture, and the analyses already reported have shown the enormous importance of this database, including significant contributions to the understanding of outcomes for patients with VADs as a function of preimplant status or severity of HF and improved risk stratification (see Chapter 24 for details).

The improved risk stratification is due to development of a more descriptive classification than the old, commonly used NYHA classification of HF severity, which is quite subjective. Most patients implanted with VADs since the beginning of INTERMACS in 2005 have been in the two most severe categories of patient status (i.e., in cardiogenic shock or very unstable despite maximal intravenous medical support), and usually the VAD was implanted under emergent conditions.[17,62] INTERMACS has confirmed that survival for profile no. 1, cardiogenic shock, is worse at 6 months (64%) compared with profile no. 2 (74%), profile no. 3 (85%), and profile no. 4 (86%) (Fig. 6-16).[16] Many other important observations have already been reported from INTERMACS, including encouraging changes in patient selection for MCS toward patients with less severe HF at the time of VAD implantation.

These data suggest that patients with cardiogenic shock in particular may be too sick for initial use of permanent LVAD support. Increasing consideration is given for immediate use of univentricular or biventricular support, employing temporary percutaneous or surgically placed systems, to stabilize and optimize the condition of these patients if possible before permanent LVAD implantation (see Chapter 7 for detailed discussions of these devices and their use). These data also support the increasing practice of careful patient selection and implanting an LVAD earlier in the progression of HF. Most patients who are stable on inotrope therapy in INTERMACS category 3 would be appropriate candidates who potentially would have good outcomes from LVAD therapy. The INTERMACS classification of HF severity has been shown to correlate not only with outcome but also worse laboratory abnormalities (Fig. 6-17).

Similarly, more recent data from INTERMACS show that there is a direct correlation of better survival with higher INTERMACS levels and significantly shorter length of hospital stay (Fig. 6-18).[81] This trend toward implanting patients

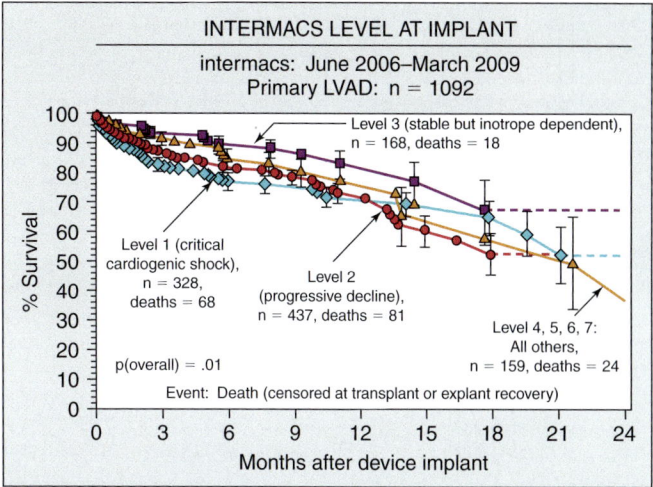

LVAD, left ventricular assist device;

FIGURE 6-16 Inverse correlation of worse survival for patients with most severe heart failure (HF) and clinical status and lowest INTERMACS score. LVAD, left ventricular assist device. *(INTERMACS data 2009, available at http://www.intermacs.org.)*

CH 6

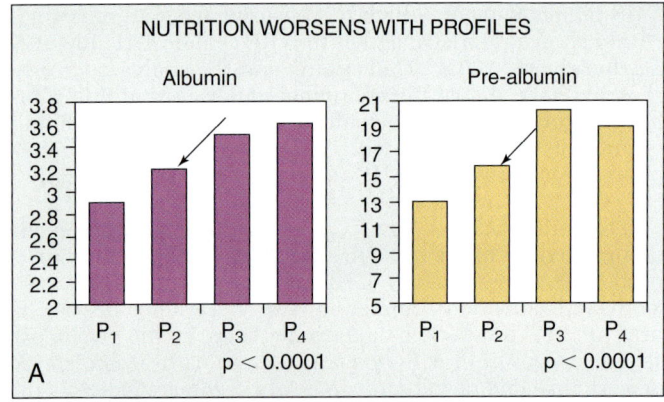

FIGURE 6-17 **A,** Worsening markers of nutrition correlate with more severe heart failure (HF) and lower INTERMACS level. **B,** Worsening markers of hepatic function correlate with more severe HF and lower INTERMACS level. AST, aspartate aminotransferase; INR, international normalized ratio. *(INTERMACS data 2009, available at http://www.intermacs.org.)*

before they exhibit end-organ dysfunction is becoming a more common strategy in most VAD centers. An increasing percentage of patients is being discharged to home after an intense evaluation and stabilization and admitted for a scheduled elective LVAD implant.

PATIENTS WITH LESS SEVERE HEART FAILURE

The enormous improvement in survival, functional capacity, quality of life, and adverse events reported from clinical trials with the new generation of continuous flow LVADs has brought the field to a position of equipoise about the projected equivalent or superior outcomes likely with use of current continuous flow LVADs versus optimized medical therapy in patients who have advanced HF who are not receiving inotropes. This equipoise has created increasing interest in the need for a clinical trial to evaluate this hypothesis. The field cannot continue to implant LVADs in patients who are at the stage of inotrope dependence and end-organ dysfunction. A clinical trial in patients at an earlier stage of HF but with clear criteria of reduced survival is needed to justify an extension into less sick patients (Fig. 6-19) .

In March 2008, the NHLBI convened a meeting of an advisory panel of more than 20 experts in the field of HF that resulted in a consensus recommendation that a trial is warranted to test this hypothesis. A request for applications was extended and subsequently funded for a trial called REVIVE-IT (Randomized Evaluation of Ventricular Assist Device in Patients Not on Inotropic Therapy), which has been funded and sites selected, with patient enrollment scheduled to begin in August 2011. REVIVE-IT is a pilot trial of only 100 patients, with 50 each in the VAD and medical arms. The decision not to conduct a large pivotal trial was based almost entirely on lack of confidence in the current ability to predict mortality reliably in the medical therapy patients because most of the risk models were derived more than 10 years ago and lack important variables shown to be strongly correlated with death with HF, such as recurrent hospitalization for HF or presence of renal dysfunc-

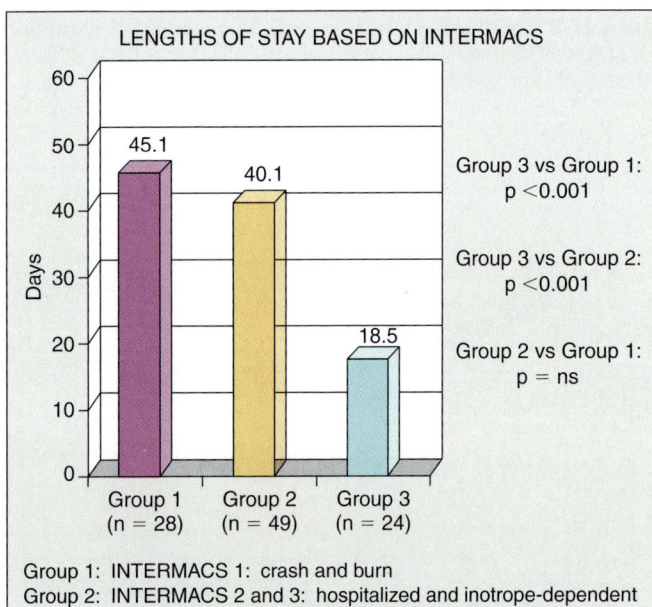

FIGURE 6-18 Correlation of reduced length of stay for patients undergoing left ventricular assist device (LVAD) implantation who are in higher INTERMACS levels and less severe heart failure (HF) at the time of LVAD implantation. *(From Miller LW. LVADs are underutilized. Circulation 2011; 123:1548–1559.)*

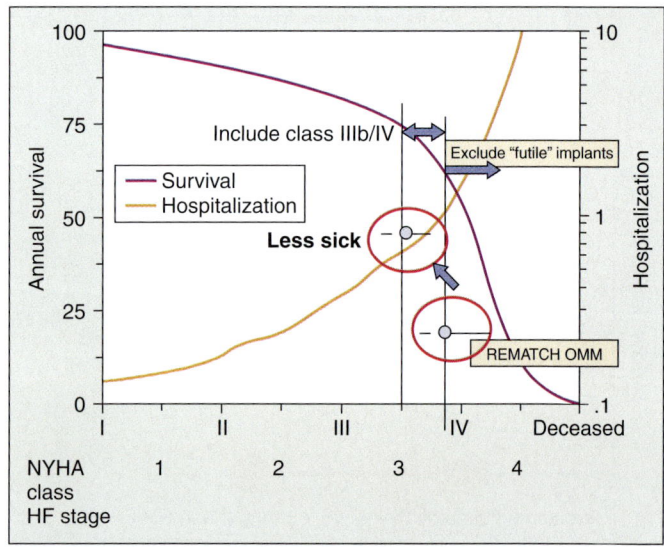

FIGURE 6-19 Correlation of increasing mortality with advancing heart failure (HF). Graph shows patient profile for patients enrolled in the REMATCH study with very advanced end-stage HF versus projected patients to be enrolled in the upcoming National Heart, Lung, and Blood Institute REVIVE-IT trial of patients with less severe heart failure. NYHA, New York Heart Association; OMM, optimal medical management.

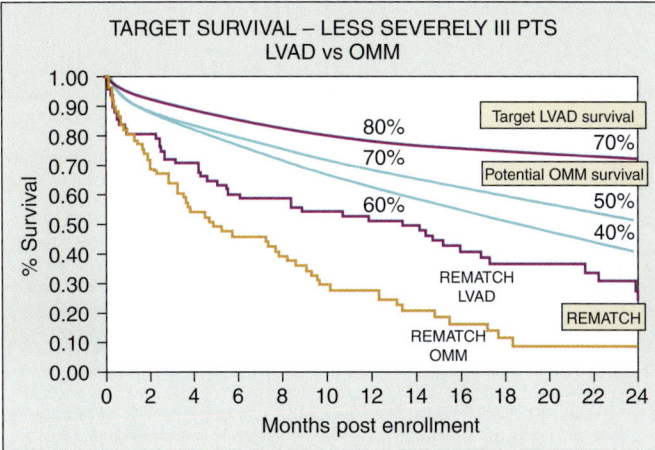

FIGURE 6-20 Sample model of possible projected survival of the two cohorts to be enrolled in the REVIVE-IT trial of medical management versus left ventricular assist device (LVAD) therapy. OMM, optimal medical management.

tion (i.e., cardiorenal syndrome). Renal function has not been shown to be a significant variable when added to the receiver operating characteristic curve of the Seattle model because patients with significant renal insufficiency are not included in most HF trials. The results of the REVIVE-IT trial are likely to lead to refinement in the entry criteria of a subsequent pivotal trial that may lead to a change in indications for VAD use and criteria for CMS and other payer reimbursement. Projections for the projected mortality in the medical therapy group versus the LVAD group are shown in Figure 6-20.

The question of the cost-effectiveness of MCS has been raised and is discussed in detail in Chapter 25. The data from Russo and associates[82] in the medically treated REMATCH patients showed that the cost of care for the last 6 months of life in patients with an 85% mortality and terrible quality of life was nearly $70,000 (Table 6-5). More money is spent on medical care of end-stage HF than any other terminal condition in the Medicare system (Table 6-6). Data such as these and the awareness of the rapidly growing population with HF, a percentage of which are likely to develop advanced HF, have brought the focus on LVADs as a potential cost-effective therapy. The encouraging trends to implant LVADs under elective conditions, in patients who have had risk factor assessment and optimization, should lead to improved success with the therapy in the years ahead.

TABLE 6-6 Comparative Cost of End-of-Life Care for End-Stage Heart Failure (ESHF) with Other Terminal Conditions in the Medicare System*

Pancreatic cancer	$17,000-$49,000
Lung cancer	$26,000
COPD	$34,000
ESHF	$83,000

*Mean costs during the final 6 months of life.
COPD, chronic obstructive pulmonary disease.
From Russo MJ, Gelijns AC, Stevenson LW, et al; REMATCH investigators. The cost of medical management in advanced heart failure during the final two years of life. *J Card Fail.* 2008;14:651-658.

SUMMARY

The use of LVADs is an important treatment option for management of patients with chronic, advanced HF, especially patients who because of either age or comorbidities are not considered candidates for cardiac transplantation. Physicians involved in the selection of candidates for mechanical support need to be familiar with factors that have been shown to have an adverse impact on outcome regardless of the indication. More recent data have suggested that well-selected candidates can have a 2-year survival that may equal or exceed the 2-year survival reported for heart transplantation in a matched age population. Smaller and more durable devices with a single moving part are associated with lower morbidity and mortality and better functional capacity and quality of life with this therapy. Future trials with new devices are needed to confirm these findings in patients with less severe HF and to validate the predictive accuracy and benefit of preoperative risk scoring to guide patient selection and optimize the results of this therapy.

REFERENCES

1. Miller LW, Missov E. The epidemic of heart failure. *Cardiol Clin.* 2001;19:547–555.
2. Hunt SA, American College of Cardiology; American Heart Association Task Force on Practice Guidelines (Writing Committee to Update the 2001 Guidelines for the Evaluation and Management of Heart Failure). ACC/AHA 2005 guideline update for the diagnosis and management of chronic heart failure in the adult: a report of the American College of Cardiology/American Heart Association Task Force on Practice Guidelines (Writing Committee to Update the 2001 Guidelines for the Evaluation and Management of Heart Failure). *J Am Coll Cardiol.* 2005;46:e1–e82.
3. Redfield MM. Heart failure: an epidemic of uncertain proportions. *N Engl J Med.* 2002;347:1142–1144.
4. Lloyd-Jones D, Adams RJ, Brown TM, et al, American Heart Association Statistics Committee and Stroke Statistics Subcommittee. Heart disease and stroke statistics—2010 update: a report from the American Heart Association. *Circulation.* 2010;121:e46–e215.
5. McMurray JV. Systolic heart failure. *N Engl J Med.* 2010;362:228–238.
6. O'Conell JB, Bristow MR. Economic impact of heart failure in the United States: time for a different approach. *J Heart Lung Transplant.* 1994;13:S107–S112.
7. Mackowiak J. Cost of heart failure to the healthcare system. *Am J Manag Care.* 1998;4(6 suppl):S338–S342.
8. Liao L, Anstrom KJ, Gottdiener JS, et al. Long-term costs and resource use in elderly participants with congestive heart failure in the Cardiovascular Health Study. *Am Heart J.* 2007;153:245–252.
9. Christie JD, Edwards LB, Aurora P, et al. The Registry of the International Society for Heart and Lung Transplantation: Twenty-sixth Official Adult Lung and Heart-Lung Transplantation Report—2009. *J Heart Lung Transplant.* 2009;28:1031–1049.
10. Rose EA, Gelijns AC, Moskowitz AJ, et al, Randomized Evaluation of Mechanical Assistance for the Treatment of Congestive Heart Failure (REMATCH) Study Group. Long-term mechanical left ventricular assistance for end-stage heart failure. *N Engl J Med.* 2001;345:1435–1443.
11. Lietz K, Miller LW. Will left ventricular assist device therapy replace heart transplantation in the foreseeable future? *Curr Opin Cardiol.* 2005;20:132–137.
12. Miller LW. Limitations of current medical therapy for the treatment of heart failure. *Rev Cardiovasc Med.* 2003;4:S21–S29.
13. Miller LW, Pagani FD, Russell SD, et al, HeartMate II clinical investigators. Use of a continuous-flow device in patients awaiting heart transplantation. *N Engl J Med.* 2007;357:885–896.
14. Morshuis M, El-Banayosy A, Arusoglu L, et al. European experience of DuraHeart magnetically levitated centrifugal left ventricular assist system. *Eur J Cardiothorac Surg.* 2009;35:1020–1027.

TABLE 6-5 Resource Use and Outcome in Patients with End-Stage Heart Failure in Terms of Inpatient Deaths, Days in the Hospital, and Average

Final 6 Months of Life	All Medicare Enrollees*	Study Population	
% Deaths as inpatients	35.2	53.7	
Average days in the hospital	11.3	41.7	× 3.7
Average days in the ICU	2.4	9.9	× 4.1
Average inpatient costs	$9,400	$68,116	× 7.2

*Source: The Dartmouth Areas of Healthcare 1993.
ICU, intensive care unit.
From Russo MJ, Gelijns AC, Stevenson LW, et al; REMATCH investigators. The cost of medical management in advanced heart failure during the final two years of life. *J Card Fail.* 2008;14:651-658.

15. Pagani F, Miller L, Russell S, et al. Extended mechanical circulatory support with a continuous-flow rotary left ventricular assist device. *J Am Coll Cardiol.* 2009;54:312–321.

16. Slaughter MS, Rogers JG, Milano CA, et al, HeartMate II investigators. Advanced heart failure treated with continuous-flow left ventricular assist device. *N Engl J Med.* 2009;361:2241–2251.

17. Kirklin JK, Naftel DC, Kormos RL, et al. Second INTERMACS annual report: more than 1,000 primary left ventricular assist device implants. *J Heart Lung Transplant.* 2010;29:1–10.

18. Stevenson LW, Shekar P. Ventricular assist devices for durable support. *Circulation.* 2005;112:111–115.

19. Stevenson LW, Rose EA. Left ventricular assist devices: bridges to transplantation, recovery, and destination for whom? *Circulation.* 2003;103:3059–3063.

20. Frazier OH, Delgado RM. Mechanical circulatory support for advanced heart failure: where does it stand in 2003? *Circulation.* 2003;108:3064–3068.

21. Goldstein D, Oz M, Rose E. Implantable left ventricular assist devices. *N Engl J Med.* 1998;339:1522–1533.

22. Morgan JA, John R, Rao V, et al. Bridging to transplant with the Heartmate left ventricular assist device: the Columbia Presbyterian 12-year experience. *J Thorac Cardiovasc Surg.* 2004;127:1309–1316.

23. DiBella I, Pagani FC, Banfi C. Results with the Novacor assist system and evaluation of long-term assistance. *Eur J Cardiothorac Surg.* 2000;18:112–116.

24. Deng MC, Edwards LB, Hertz MI, et al. Mechanical circulatory support device database of the International Society of Heart and Lung Transplantation: third annual report. *J Heart Lung Transplant.* 2005;24:1182–1187.

25. Park SJ, Bank AJ, Miller LW. Left ventricular assist device bridge therapy for acute myocardial infarction. *Ann Thorac Surg.* 2000;69:1146–1151.

26. Dang NC, Topkara VK, Leache MD, et al. Left ventricular assist device implantation after acute anterior wall myocardial infarction and cardiogenic shock: a two center study. *J Thorac Cardiovasc Surg.* 2005;130:693–699.

27. Johnson MR, Meyer KH, Haft J, et al. Heart transplantation in the United States, 1999-2008. *Am J Transplant.* 2010;10(4 Pt 2):1035–1046.

28. Stevenson LW, Miller LW, Desvigne-Nickens P, et al, REMATCH investigators. Left ventricular assist device as destination for patients undergoing intravenous inotropic therapy: a subset analysis from REMATCH (Randomized Evaluation of Mechanical Assistance in Treatment of Chronic Heart Failure). *Circulation.* 2004;110:975–981.

29. Rogers JG, Butler J, Lansman SL, et al, INTrEPID investigators. Chronic mechanical circulatory support for inotrope-dependent heart failure patients who are not transplant candidates: results of the INTrEPID Trial. *J Am Coll Cardiol.* 2007;50:741–747.

30. Mehra MR, Kobashigawa J, Starling R, et al. Listing criteria for heart transplantation: International Society for Heart and Lung Transplantation guidelines for the care of cardiac transplant candidates—2006. *J Heart Lung Transplant.* 2006;25:1024–1042.

31. Lietz K, Long JW, Kfoury AG, et al. Outcomes of left ventricular assist device implantation as destination therapy in the post-REMATCH era: implications for patient selection. *Circulation.* 2007;116:497–505.

32. Park SJ, Tector A, Picconi W, et al. Left ventricular assist devices as permanent heart failure therapy: a new look at survival. *J Thorac Cardiovasc Surg.* 2005;129:9–17.

33. Dowling RD, Park SJ, Pagani FD, et al. HeartMate VE LVAS design enhancements and its impact on device reliability. *Eur J Cardiothorac Surg.* 2004;25:958–963.

34. Pagani FD, Long JW, Dembitsky WP, et al. Improved mechanical reliability of the Heartmate XVE left ventricular assist system. *Ann Thorac Surg.* 2006;82:1413–1418.

35. Birks E, Tansley P, Yacoub M, et al. Incidence and clinical management of life- threatening left ventricular assist device failure. *J Heart Lung Transplant.* 2004;23:964–969.

36. Horton SC, Khodaverdian R, Powers A, et al. Left ventricular assist device malfunction: a systematic approach to diagnosis. *J Am Coll Cardiol.* 2004;43:1574–1583.

37. Holman WL, Park SJ, Long JW, et al. REMATCH investigators. Infection in permanent circulatory support: experience from the REMATCH trial. *J Heart Lung Transplant.* 2004;23:1359–1365.

38. Chinn R, Dembitsky W, Eaton L, et al. Multicenter experience: prevention and management of left ventricular assist device infections. *ASAIO J.* 2005;51:461–470.

39. Holdy K, Dembitsky W, Eaton LL, et al. Nutrition assessment and management of left ventricular assist device patients. *J Heart Lung Transplant.* 2005;24:1690–1696.

40. Slaughter MS, Pagani FD, Rogers JG, et al, HeartMate II Clinical investigators. Clinical management of continuous-flow left ventricular assist devices in advanced heart failure. *J Heart Lung Transplant.* 2010;29(4 suppl):S1–S39.

41. Centers for Medicare and Medicaid Services. Artificial heart and related devices. In: *Medicare National Coverage Determinations Manual, Chapter 1, Part 1, Section 20.9.* 2003. Available at http://www.cms.hhs.gov.manuals/103_cov_determ/ncd103cl-Part 1.pdf.

42. Centers for Medicare and Medicaid Services. Medicare approved LVAD destination therapy facilities. 2005. Available at http://www.cms.hhs.gov/coverage/map/lvadfacilityrev4.asp Accessed 18.04.05.

43. Stelken AM, Younis L, Miller LW, et al. Prognostic value of cardiopulmonary exercise using percent achieved of predicted peak oxygen consumption for patients with ischemic and dilated cardiomyopathy. *J Am Coll Cardiol.* 1996;27:345–352.

44. Arena R, Myers J, Abella J, et al. Determining the preferred percent-predicted equation for peak oxygen consumption in patients with heart failure. *Circ Heart Fail.* 2009;2:113–120.

45. Hershberger RE, Nauman D, Walker TL, et al. Care processes and clinical outcomes of continuous outpatient support with inotropes (COSI) in patients with refractory end stage heart failure. *J Card Fail.* 2003;9:180–187.

46. Stevenson LW. Clinical use of inotropic therapy for heart failure: looking backward or forward? Part II: chronic inotropic therapy. *Circulation.* 2003;108:492–497.

47. Jaski BE, Kim JC, Naftel DC, et al. Cardiac transplant outcome of patients supported on a left ventricular assist device vs intravenous inotropic therapy. *J Heart Lung Transplant.* 2001;20:449–456.

48. Aaronson KD, Eppinger MJ, Dyke DB, et al. Left ventricular assist device therapy improves utilization of donor hearts. *J Am Coll Cardiol.* 2002;39:1247–1254.

49. Gorodeski EZ, Chu EC, Reese JR, et al. Prognosis on chronic dobutamine or milrinone infusions for stage D heart failure. *Circ Heart Fail.* 2009;2:320–324.

50. Holman WL, Kormos RL, Naftel DC, et al. Predictors of death and transplant in patients with a mechanical circulatory support device: a multi-institutional study. *J Heart Lung Transplant.* 2009;28:44–50.

51. Smith GL, Vaccarino V, Watnick SG, et al. Worsening renal function: what is a clinically meaningful change in creatinine during hospitalization with heart failure. *J Card Fail.* 2003;9:13–25.

52. Klein L, Massie BM, Leimberger JD, et al, OPTIME-CHF investigators. Admission or changes in renal function during hospitalization for worsening heart failure predict postdischarge survival: results from the Outcomes of a Prospective Trial of Intravenous Milrinone for Exacerbations of Chronic Heart Failure (OPTIME-CHF). *Circ Heart Fail.* 2008;1:25–33.

53. Russell SD, Rogers JG, Milano CA, et al, HeartMate II Clinical investigators. Renal and hepatic function improve in advanced heart failure patients during continuous-flow support with the HeartMate II left ventricular assist device. *Circulation.* 2009;120:2352–2357.

54. Kavarana MN, Pessin-Minsley MS, Urtecho J, et al. Right ventricular dysfunction and organ failure in left ventricular assist device recipients: a continuing problem. *Ann Thorac Surg.* 2002;73:745–753.

55. Ochiai Y, McCarthy PM, Smedira NG. Predictors of severe right ventricular failure after implantable left ventricular assist device insertion: analysis of 245 patients. *Circulation.* 2002;106:I-198–I-202.

56. Frazier OH, Rose EA, Oz MC, et al. Multicenter clinical evaluation of the HeartMate vented electric left ventricular assist system in patients awaiting heart transplantation. *J Thorac Cardiovasc Surg.* 2001;122:1186–1195.

57. Matthews JC, Koelling TM, Pagani FD, et al. The right ventricular failure risk score: a pre-operative tool for assessing the risk of right ventricular failure in left ventricular assist device candidates. *J Am Coll Cardiol.* 2008;51:2163–2172.

58. Fitzpatrick 3rd JR, Frederick JR, Hsu VM, et al. Risk score derived from pre-operative data analysis predicts the need for biventricular mechanical circulatory support. *J Heart Lung Transplant.* 2008;27:1286–1292.

59. Schenk S, McCarthy PM, Blackstone EH, et al. Duration of inotropic support after left ventricular assist device implantation: risk factors and impact on outcome. *J Thorac Cardiovasc Surg.* 2006;131:447–454.

60. Kormos RL, Teuteberg JJ, Pagani FD, et al, HeartMate II Clinical investigators. Right ventricular failure in patients with the HeartMate II continuous-flow left ventricular assist device: incidence, risk factors, and effect on outcomes. *J Thorac Cardiovasc Surg.* 2010;139:1316–1324.

61. Chen JM, Rose EA. Management of perioperative right-sided circulatory failure. In: Goldstein DJ, Oz M, eds. *Cardiac Assist Devices.* Armonk, NY: Futura Publishing Co; 2000:83–101.

62. Dewald O, Schmitz DO, Reichart B, et al. Platelet activation markers in patients with heart assist devices. *Artif Organs.* 2005;29:292–299.

63. Aaronson KD, Patel H, Pagani FD. Patient selection for left ventricular assist device therapy. *Ann Thorac Surg.* 2003;75:S29–S35.

64. Heilmann C, Geisen U, Beyersdorf F, et al. Acquired von Willebrand syndrome in patients with ventricular assist device or total artificial heart. *Thromb Haemost.* 2010;103:962–967.

65. Reinhartz O, Farrar DJ, Hershon JH, et al. Importance of preoperative liver function as a predictor of survival in patients supported with Thoratec ventricular assist devices as a bridge to transplantation. *J Thorac Cardiovasc Surg.* 1998;116:633–640.

66. Reedy JE, Swartz MT, Miller LW, et al. Bridge to transplantation: importance of patient selection. *J Heart Lung Transplant.* 1990;9:473–480.

67. Farrar DJ. Preoperative predictors of survival in patients with Thoratec ventricular assist devices as a bridge to transplantation. *J Heart Lung Transplant.* 1994;13:93–100.

68. Stevenson LW. Patient selection for mechanical bridging to transplantation. *Ann Thorac Surg.* 1996;61:380–387.

69. Aaronson KD, Patel H, Pagani FD. Patient selection for left ventricular assist device therapy. *Ann Thorac Surg.* 2003;75(6 suppl):S29–S35.

70. Radovancevic B, Vrtovec B, de Kort E, et al. End-organ function in patients on long-term circulatory support with continuous- or pulsatile-flow assist devices. *J Heart Lung Transplant.* 2007;26:815–818.

71. Letsou GV, Myers TJ, Gregoric ID, et al. Continuous axial-flow left ventricular assist device (Jarvik 2000) maintains kidney and liver perfusion for up to 6 months. *Ann Thorac Surg.* 2003;76:1167–1170.

72. Kamdar F, Boyle A, Liao K, et al. Effects of centrifugal, axial, and pulsatile left ventricular assist device support on end-organ function in heart failure patients. *J Heart Lung Transplant.* 2009;28:352–359.

73. Sharma R, Anker SD. Cytokines, apoptosis, and cachexia: The potential for TNF antagonism. *Int J Cardiol.* 2002;85:161–171.

74. Chinn R, Dembitsky W, Eaton L, et al. Multicenter experience: prevention and management of left ventricular assist device infections. *ASAIO J.* 2005;51:461–470.

75. Mano A, Fujita K, Uenomachi K, et al. Body mass index is a useful predictor of prognosis after left ventricular assist system implantation. *J Heart Lung Transplant.* 2009;28:428–433.

76. Holdy K, Dembitsky W, Eaton LL, et al. Nutrition assessment and management of left ventricular assist device patients. *J Heart Lung Transplant.* 2005;24:1690–1696.

77. Coyle LA, Ising MS, Gallagher C, et al. Destination therapy: one-year outcomes in patients with a body mass index greater than 30. *Artif Organs.* 2010;34:93–97.

78. Miller LW. Listing criteria for heart transplantation: results of an American Society of Transplant Physicians-NIH conference. *Transplantation.* 1998;66:947–951.

79. Smith RA, Cokkinides V, Brooks D, et al. Cancer screening in the United States, 2010: a review of current American Cancer Society guidelines and issues in cancer screening. *CA Cancer J Clin.* 2010;60:99–119.

80. Lund L, Aaronson KD, Mancini DM. Validation of peak exercise oxygen consumption and the heart failure survival score for serial risk stratification in advanced heart failure. *Am J Cardiol.* 2005;95:734–741.

81. Boyle AJ, Ascheim DD, Russo MJ, et al. Clinical outcomes for continuous flow left ventricular assist device patients stratified by pre-operative INTERMACS classification. *J Heart Lung Transplant.* 2011;30:402–407.

82. Russo MJ, Gelijns AC, Stevenson LW, et al, REMATCH investigators. The cost of medical management in advanced heart failure during the final two years of life. *J Card Fail.* 2008;14:651–658.

CH 6

Candidate Selection for Long-Term Left Ventricular Assist Device Therapy for Advanced Heart Failure

CHAPTER 7

Preoperative Patient Optimization for Mechanical Circulatory Support

Ranjit John and Andrew Boyle

IS OPTIMIZATION OF PATIENTS AWAITING VENTRICULAR ASSIST DEVICE IMPLANTATION BENEFICIAL?

Cardiac transplantation remains the "gold standard" for treatment of patients with advanced end-stage heart failure (HF), although its widespread application is limited by severe donor shortages. The discrepancy between the limited availability of donor hearts and the ever-increasing number of patients with HF who deteriorate while on the waiting list or are in advanced HF with end-organ dysfunction at the time of listing has led to the increasing use of left ventricular assist devices (LVADs) as a bridge to transplant (BTT).[1–5] The use of mechanical circulatory support (MCS) as BTT has evolved to become the standard of care for these patients in most cardiac transplant programs. Success with LVADs as BTT therapy has led to their successful use as an alternative to a transplant (i.e., as destination therapy [DT]).[6,7] Risk stratification of candidates for MCS has emerged as an important tool in patient selection and outcomes assessment. Outcomes with MCS have gradually improved over time as a result of improvements in device technology, experience gained in intraoperative and perioperative patient management, attention to patient selection, and timing of LVAD implant.

Over the past decade, evidence has accumulated regarding the impact of patient selection on outcomes with MCS.[8–12] Because the major goal of device implantation in both BTT and DT is to be able to discharge patients home in better condition than they were before LVAD surgery, appropriate assessment of the candidate's perioperative risk is of paramount importance. The tremendous impact of patient selection on outcomes after LVAD implantation has been well recognized because implantation in patients with severe functional impairment, right ventricular (RV) failure, malnutrition or cachexia, or infection has resulted in significantly poorer outcomes. Data have shown that the period of greatest risk of dying after LVAD implantation is before hospital discharge, when an average of 70% of deaths occur.[13]

Several risk factors have been identified that have correlated well with outcomes after LVAD placement. Many investigators have examined composite risk scores that are associated with early mortality after ventricular assist device (VAD) implantation. The largest series examining a composite of risk factors that correlate with mortality before hospital discharge in patients supported by VADs was reported by Lietz and colleagues[13] and comprised 250 patients receiving a HeartMate XVE device (Thoratec Corp, Pleasanton, CA) between November 2003 and September 2005 after U.S. Food and Drug Administration (FDA) approval of the device for commercial use. All patients were in stage D HF and met all the criteria for eligibility in the REMATCH (Randomized Evaluation of Mechanical Assistance for the Treatment of Congestive Heart Failure) study. The parameters entered into the score were laboratory or clinical data recorded just before implantation. More than 65 variables were entered into a univariate analysis, and the variables shown to correlate with operative death were entered into a multivariate analysis. There were 11 variables shown to be significant predictors (Table 7-1). The patients were divided into quartiles of risk, and the laboratory values of each patient were similarly divided by quartiles. The risk of survival to hospital discharge between the risk groups ranged from 10% to 82%.

The risk score showed that death before hospital discharge in patients receiving an implant as DT was strongly influenced by worsening nutritional status, hematologic abnormalities, end-organ dysfunction, and right heart dysfunction. These preoperative clinical characteristics identified patients who were at high risk for not surviving to hospital discharge. Preoperative risk factors associated with the highest risk of mortality were severe functional impairment, markers of global cardiac dysfunction, end-organ damage, and malnutrition. The strength of the Lietz risk score is that it also predicted the cause of death in patients who died before discharge. Patients with malnutrition died of infection, patients with coagulopathy died of bleeding, and patients with renal insufficiency died of renal or multiorgan failure (Fig. 7-1). The original derivation and description of the

TABLE 7-1	Predictors of In-Hospital Death*	
Risk Factors	Risk Ratio (CI)	Weight
Platelets ≤148,000	9.7 (3.1-28.4)†	8.5
INR >1.1	4.9 (1.2-19.7)‡	4
Serum CrCl ≤30 mL/min	5.3 (1.1-24.8)‡	4.5
MPAP ≤25 mm Hg	4.7 (1.6-14.0)†	3.5
WBC >12,000/µL	4.1 (1.2-14.0)‡	3
Vasodilatory treatment	3.7 (1.3-10.5)‡	2.5
Albumin ≤3.3 g/dL	3.2 (1.2-8.7)‡	2
BSA ≤1.8 m	5.3 (1.6-17.4)†	4.5
ALT or AST >90 U/L	2.9 (1.0-8.3)‡	2
No beta blockers	2.5 (1.0-6.4)‡	1.5

*Destination therapy registry, 2001-2005, N = 208.
†P < .001.
‡P < .05.
ALT, alanine aminotransferase; AST, aspartate aminotransferase; BSA, body surface area; CI, confidence interval; CrCl, creatinine clearance; INR, international normalized ratio; MPAP, mean pulmonary artery pressure; WBC, white blood cell count.

POST-REMATCH STUDY
RISK FACTORS FOR MORTALITY

Risk factor		Cause of death
Nutrition	→	Infection
Renal dysfunction	→	Renal failure
Coagulopathy	→	Bleeding
RV failure	→	RV/MO failure

Therefore these should be the primary focus of
Optimization Pre-LVAD

FIGURE 7-1 Post-REMATCH study risk factors for mortality. LVAD, left ventricular assist device.

Lietz risk score was with use of the pulsatile, volume displacement HeartMate XVE device in DT patients only, but the risk score has been validated more recently in patients receiving the new generation of continuous flow devices and a significant number of BTT patients. This study suggested that the risk score could be used in any patient undergoing MCS to help not only with patient selection but also timing of implantation to optimize outcomes.

It is arguable whether risk scores are used frequently in many centers on a prospective basis to calculate a risk score on individual patients to aid patient selection (or favor nonselection or a delay in implantation) or whether their major role has been to draw attention to factors in patients who that are at greater risk before LVAD implantation.[14,15] Although objective data on the prospective use of the risk score are not presently unavailable, this paradigm may be shifting to one in which attempts to modify risk factors before LVAD placement is becoming the standard of care. A patient with a prohibitive risk score may be an unacceptable candidate at the time of initial evaluation, but with intensive medical therapy and optimization of several parameters, such as nutrition, abnormal coagulation profile, right heart dysfunction, and infections, the patient may be at lesser risk after LVAD placement (Table 7-2 and Box 7-1). We do not advocate delaying LVAD implantation

TABLE 7-2	Goals before Left Ventricular Assist Device Implantation
Parameter	Desirable Value
Renal	BUN <50 mg/dL Serum creatinine <2.5 mg/dL
Hematologic	INR <1.2 Hemoglobin >10 g/dL Platelets >150,000/µL
Nutritional	Albumin >3 g/dL Prealbumin >15 mg/dL Transferrin >250 mg/dL
Hepatic	Total bilirubin <2.5 mg/dL ALT, AST <2× normal
Hemodynamic	RA pressure <15 mm Hg PCWP <24 mm Hg

ALT, alanine aminotransferase; AST, aspartate aminotransferase; BUN, blood urea nitrogen; INR, international normalized ratio; PCWP, pulmonary capillary wedge pressure; RA, right atrial.

 BOX 7-1 Guidelines for Preoperative Left Ventricular Assist Device Optimization

- May require 24-48 hours preoperative support
- Hemodynamic monitoring
- Drug therapy focusing on right atrial pressure and renal function
- Intra-aortic balloon pump for ischemic or nonischemic etiology
- Normalize coagulation factors
- Intravenous or enteral nutrition, or both
- Consider ultrafiltration

in a patient who is rapidly deteriorating to improve adverse or unfavorable risk profiles. However, as discussed later in this chapter, patients who are at imminent risk of death may be best supported by means other than permanent LVADs, including a wide variety of temporary circulatory support options.

The development of INTERMACS (Interagency Registry for Mechanically Assisted Circulatory Support), a collaborative initiative by the National Heart, Lung, and Blood Institute, the FDA, industry, and health care professionals involved in the care of patients with VADs, has led to a descriptive classification of various clinical subgroups of patients receiving VADs that is far superior to the more subjective New York Heart Association (NYHA) classification used in the past.[16,17] This classification might help in understanding risk factors that affect patient outcomes simply by providing a standardized classification to understand severity of illness among patients.[18] There are six levels of HF severity in the INTERMACS classification that all fit the description of NYHA class IV HF (Table 7-3). Until more recently, most patients undergoing VAD implantation have been in the two most severe categories of patient illness—cardiogenic shock or deteriorating despite inotrope therapy and maximal medical management. These are also the two categories with the poorest survival after permanent VAD placement. These and other data have led to strategies to avoid or at least limit emergency permanent VAD placement in this sometimes futile group in favor of various temporary circulatory support options and to consider permanent VAD support when the risk profile of these patients has improved after a period of temporary MCS.[19]

TABLE 7-3	INTERMACS Patient Profiles and Time Frame for Initiating Mechanical Circulatory Support
Profile No.	Description
1	"Crashing and burning"—critical cardiogenic shock
2	"Progressive decline"—inotrope dependence with continuing deterioration
3	"Stable but inotrope-dependent"—clinical stability on mild to moderate doses of intravenous inotropes (patients stable on temporary circulatory support without inotropes are within this profile)
4	"Recurrent advanced heart failure"—"recurrent" rather than "refractory" decompensation
5	"Exertion intolerant"—comfortable at rest but exercise intolerant
6	"Exertion limited"—able to do some mild activity, but fatigue results within a few minutes or with any significant physical exertion
7	"Advanced NYHA III"—clinically stable with a reasonable level of comfortable activity, despite history of previous decompensation that is not recent

NYHA, New York Heart Association.

STRATEGIES IN PATIENT OPTIMIZATION: IMPORTANT CAUSES OF MORBIDITY AND MORTALITY WITH LEFT VENTRICULAR ASSIST DEVICE USE

Nutrition

Malnutrition as a predictor of outcomes after MCS has gained increased recognition in recent years (Fig. 7-2). A low serum albumin (<3.3 mg/dL) was the most significant risk factor for mortality and was associated with a 6.6-fold increase in mortality in the Lietz-Miller risk score profile.[13] However, albumin is a crude marker of nutrition, and prealbumin is a more sensitive and specific marker of malnutrition. The adverse effects of malnutrition on outcomes after surgical intervention have been well documented (see Fig. 7-2).[20] Significant nutritional deficiency is associated with poor wound healing, increased risk of infection, and impaired T-lymphocyte function and immune response.

Screening for malnutrition in potential patients for LVAD implantation should include serum albumin; prealbumin; total cholesterol, which is often much reduced with malnutrition (<100 mg/dL); absolute lymphocyte count; and possibly transferrin. One additional simple but very sensitive test is skin test anergy; controls need to be used, such as mumps,

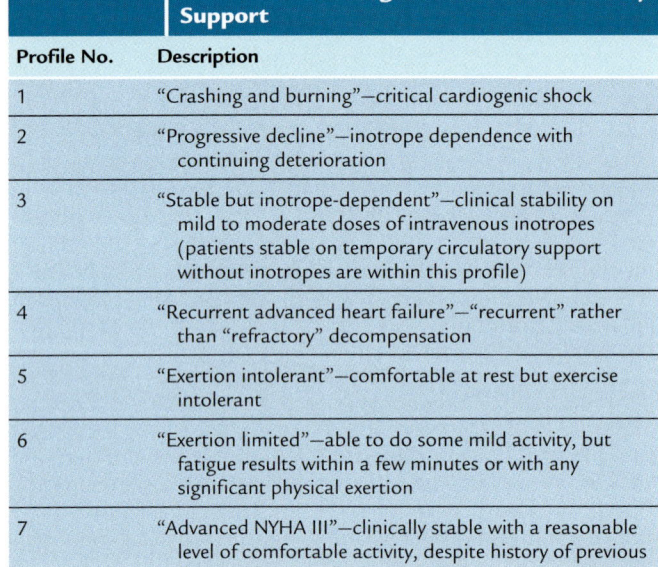

BOX 7-2 Markers of Malnutrition

- Body mass index <20*
- Albumin <3.2 g/dL*
- Prealbumin <15 mg/dL*
- Low total cholesterol <130 mg/dL*
- Low absolute lymph count <100/μL*
- Skin test anergy
- Anthropomorphic measurements

* All continuous variables

to prove anergy versus a negative reaction. Anergy is a definitive sign of impaired T-cell response and vulnerability to infection (Box 7-2).

When a patient is identified as malnourished, efforts can be undertaken to improve the patient's nutritional status. However, the malnourished state did not develop overnight, and it is unlikely to resolve over the short-term, partly owing to atrophy of the intestinal mucosa and frequent development of diarrhea with most oral formulations or supplements (Box 7-3). There is no evidence to support the use of tube feeding or parenteral feeding (i.e., prove that providing nutrients to a patient before LVAD implant has been shown to reduce infection or adverse events) to improve a patient's candidacy for MCS. Rather, a malnourished state is a risk factor for adverse outcomes after MCS that is not easily modified. Without a resolution of the patient's underlying HF, caloric supplementation alone, regardless of the route of administration, may be inadequate to provide for resolution of the malnourished state; this is true even if appropriate caloric supplementation is given. Delaying surgical intervention may worsen the underlying medical condition and increase the patient's surgical risk further.

The state of nutrition for a patient should be used to assess the patient's risk of and candidacy for surgery rather than as a target for preoperative therapeutic intervention. This approach is viewed as controversial because many clinicians believe that proceeding with LVAD placement in a malnourished patient is associated with a significant increase in risk of adverse outcomes, especially given the data from the Lietz-Miller risk score. It is very uncommon for a patient with significant malnutrition to have that risk in isolation; malnourished patients often have abnormal liver function and other risk factors that collectively constitute increased risk. However, a cohort of patients may be LVAD candidates who can be hemodynamically stabilized with measures other than LVAD and undergo aggressive nutritional support for days to weeks before LVAD placement. It remains to be seen if such short-term to intermediate-term nutritional support will improve outcomes in such patients. However, given that infection has remained the number

NUTRITION AND LVAD SURVIVAL
HOW BIG A FACTOR IS IT?

Nutritional correlates →
- Infection
- Immunocompromise
- Wound healing problems
- Organ mass reduction
- Inflammatory response
- Multi-organ failure

FIGURE 7-2 Nutrition and left ventricular assist device (LVAD) survival.

BOX 7-3 Nutritional Considerations before Ventricular Assist Device Implantation

- Nutrition consultation
- Liberalize diet to include oral nutritional supplements; food from home, snacks
- Multivitamin, iron, erythropoietin
- Prealbumin, albumin, and liver function tests 2× weekly
- Pantoprazole (Protonix)
- Nocturnal tube feeds
- Appetite stimulants
- Rule out gastroparesis, mesenteric ischemia, depression, hypothyroidism, gastritis
- Antidepressants

one cause of morbidity and mortality with MCS for the past 20 years, it seems incumbent on the field to use new benchmarks for risks such as nutrition in an attempt to reduce this major problem.

To improve nutrition before LVAD implantation, the suggested goal is a prealbumin level greater than 15 mg/dL; however, it is equally important to maintain adequate nutrition after the procedure (Box 7-4). Studies have shown protein synthesis is reduced by 50% with 24 hours of starvation in normal laboratory animals. Because most patients undergoing LVAD implantation have reduced nutritional status to begin with and then undergo a major surgical procedure and are often without meaningful calorie support for the first 2 to 3 days postoperatively, the risk of infection is not surprising. Figure 7-3 shows an algorithm that can be used to define various levels of malnutrition preoperatively and goals and routes for repletion of relevant metabolic markers.

Patients with cachexia secondary to advanced HF often do not normalize or recover nutritional markers as rapidly as patients with acute illnesses when using only oral nutrition because of impaired intestinal mucosal uptake of calories and nutrients.[21] Patients with prealbumin levels less than 10 mg/dL are at significant risk of infection after LVAD implantation and are the patients who potentially would be most benefited from a period of parenteral nutrition. Typically, there is a reluctance to use parenteral nutrition in candidates for LVAD implantation, including patients with very severe markers of malnutrition who may not tolerate oral or enteral supplements or feedings because of hepatomegaly, diarrhea induced by the high osmotic load of the high-carbohydrate formulas, or relative gastroparesis from low cardiac output. This reluctance is based partly on surgical studies showing

increased risk of systemic infection with parenteral nutrition and the need for central venous catheters for delivery. However, the parenteral route may be the best way to resume intake of nutrients in these patients and should be continued in the early postoperative period until prealbumin levels are greater than 15 mg/dL and the patient is tolerating adequate oral nutrition.

Correction of Abnormal Coagulation Parameters

Bleeding is very common with LVAD implantation and is associated with a fourfold higher requirement for re-exploration (25% to 30%) than any other open heart procedure. This increased incidence of bleeding is due to multiple factors, including hepatic dysfunction from high right-sided cardiac pressures that are reflected back to the liver and cause increased venous bleeding owing to reduced synthesis of coagulation factors in the liver, previous sternotomy, and the frequent use of anticoagulant or antiplatelet medications before LVAD implantation in these patients (Box 7-5).[22,23] Several studies have identified the development of postoperative bleeding and the need for transfusions as a common complication after MCS and as a major risk factor for adverse outcomes. The presence of an elevated preoperative international normalized ratio (INR) may reflect underlying RV failure and the presence of cardiac or other causes of cirrhosis. A prolonged INR, a low platelet count, and the use of anticoagulation or antiplatelet medications contribute to significant perioperative bleeding, which can lead to right ventricular failure, infections, and multiorgan failure. Patients with severe HF often have a nutritional basis for abnormal coagulation secondary to depletion of several specific coagulation factors, such as factor VII. The minimum preoperative screen for coagulation abnormalities should include prothrombin time, partial thromboplastin time, INR, platelet count, platelet aggregation studies, and possibly heparin-induced thrombocytopenia (HIT) assay.

Abnormalities of these tests should result in additional evaluation for their cause. Delay in the institution of MCS is warranted in the presence of gross coagulation abnormalities unless it is an emergency. The use of vitamin K is encouraged in patients with an elevated INR. Platelet inhibitors such as clopidogrel, which are given after placement of intracoronary stents, have an irreversible inhibitory effect on platelet aggregation. Surgery should be delayed a minimum of 5 days, and preferably 7 days, to allow for new platelets to be generated that would be unaffected by clopidogrel. There are few data in LVAD patients to define the best management practice in patients with drug-eluting coronary stents in whom clopidogrel has to be stopped. Abnormalities in coagulation parameters, especially a low platelet count (<149,000/μL) and an elevated INR (>1.1) have been shown

---

BOX 7-4 Preoperative and Postoperative Nutritional Support

- Critical to patient complications and mortality
- Oral diet—limited success
- SBFT enteral feeding—nocturnal vs. continuous
- Peripheral intravenous feeding—limited calories
- TPN—underused
- Risk of infection vs. gain
- Important role of micronutrients—amino acids, arginine, glutamine, zinc, coenzyme Q10
- HF patients do not resume nutritive intake normally

HF, heart failure; SBFT, small bowel feeding tube; TPN, total parenteral nutrition.

PRE-LVAD OPTIMIZATION OF NUTRITION

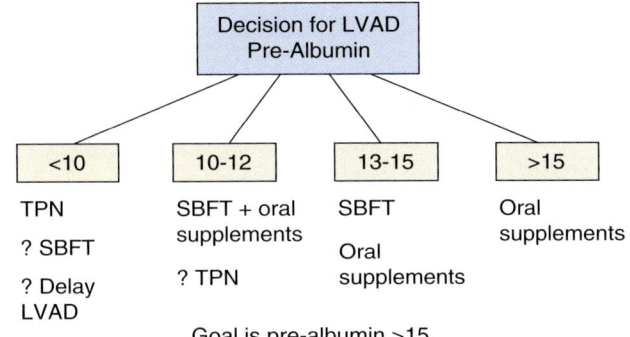

FIGURE 7-3 Optimization of nutrition before left ventricular assist device (LVAD) implantation. SBFT, small bowel feeding tube; TPN, total parenteral nutrition.

BOX 7-5 Coagulation Factors

- Long-term warfarin or multiple antiplatelet drugs
- Prolonged INR
  - Perioperative bleeding
  - RV failure
  - Hemodynamic instability
  - Multiorgan failure
  - Factor VII (nutritional basis)
- Minimal screening
  - PTT/PT, platelet count, platelet aggregation. and HIT

HIT, heparin-induced thrombocytopenia; INR, international normalized ratio; PTT/PT, partial thromboplastin time/prothrombin time; RV, right ventricular.

to be associated with a significant increased risk of death. Strong attempts should be made to normalize these parameters before LVAD placement and, if possible, to defer LVAD placement appropriately.

HIT is a clotting abnormality that warrants consideration for patients undergoing LVAD implantation.[24–26] Although not measured routinely in all patients, HIT should be assessed preoperatively in patients with platelet counts less than 150,000/μL and in patients have who had a recent decrease in platelet count of greater than 20%. Clinical manifestations of HIT include a significant decrease in platelet count (even if the value is within the normal range) or occurrence of any thrombotic event while receiving heparin. Laboratory evaluation should include a coagulation profile and heparin antibody assay. Routine screening of all patients for HIT antibody can be misleading. The serotonin release assay is the most reliable test for establishing the diagnosis of HIT. Alternative anticoagulants to heparin (e.g., argatroban and bivalirudin) have been used anecdotally in patients with HIT undergoing LVAD implantation when significant reductions in platelet counts are noted before LVAD implantation and shown to be associated with the HIT antibody.[27–29] The presence or development of HIT is associated with a high risk of bleeding and thrombosis of both mechanical assist devices and total artificial heart pumps.[27]

Renal Function

Renal dysfunction has consistently been one of the highest risks for morbidity and mortality after LVAD implantation. Heart performance and kidney function are closely interrelated both in health and in disease states. A meta-analysis of studies evaluating the relationship between renal dysfunction and HF revealed that 63% of patients had at least mild renal impairment, and 20% had moderate or severe renal dysfunction. At least one in four patients hospitalized for acute decompensated HF has significant renal dysfunction.[30–34] Measures to evaluate the degree of renal dysfunction include serum creatinine, blood urea nitrogen (BUN), urine output and glomerular filtration rate. New formulas that are available for estimating glomerular filtration rate are more accurate. Serum creatinine may significantly underestimate the degree of renal impairment in women, smaller adults, older patients, and patients with reduced muscle mass. Renal function is often adversely affected in patients with HF as a result of decreased renal perfusion secondary to low cardiac output states and renal venous congestion but may also be affected as a result of direct nephrotoxic effect of medications or concomitant diseases such as diabetes and hypertension.

The pathophysiology of cardiorenal syndrome is multifactorial but is generally related to intrarenal hemodynamics, transrenal perfusion pressure, and systemic neurohormonal factors.[30–34] In the setting of acute decompensated HF in patients being considered for MCS, there is generally inadequate cardiac output and decreased perfusion pressure. In the presence of risk factors such as diabetes and hypertension, there may be a further reduction of glomerular filtration rate. However, a more important contributor is likely the neurohormonal activation mediated by activation of arterial baroreceptors and intrarenal sensors. These reflexes lead to the activation of the renin-angiotensin system, sympathetic nervous system, and arginine-vasopressin system. All of these factors lead to peripheral and intrarenal vasoconstriction, decreasing renal blood flow and glomerular filtration rate further and leading to a decrease in renal function. In addition, high-dose diuretics cause activation of adenosine receptors in the kidney, further increasing renal vasoconstriction. The consequences also lead to renal hypoxia, inflammation, cytokine release, and progressive structural and functional loss.

Transrenal perfusion pressure is calculated as mean arterial pressure minus central venous pressure (CVP). For a patient with volume overload and decompensated HF, the combination of increased pulmonary artery pressure and CVP with low systemic pressure may lead to a severe compromise of the net renal perfusion pressure. Aggressive attempts should be made to reduce the increased CVP in patients awaiting LVAD placement because this can lead to significant improvements in renal blood flow and urine output (Box 7-6). Several risk profile scores have included renal dysfunction and increased CVP as important risk factors for adverse outcomes after LVAD placement.

Patients whose urine output is low (e.g., <1 mL/kg) before LVAD placement along with worsening creatinine and BUN may benefit from attempts to optimize renal function. Initially, high-dose diuretics may be attempted along with close monitoring of hemodynamic parameters with a Swan-Ganz catheter. However, patients who are refractory to these measures may benefit from use of ultrafiltration (see discussion later) and temporary MCS such as intra-aortic balloon pump (IABP) and temporary percutaneous and surgical devices.

Although intravenous loop diuretics are often the first-line therapy in patients with acute decompensated HF, the efficacy of loop diuretics is reduced by repeated exposure as resistance develops. Loop diuretics have been shown to be associated with increased morbidity and mortality attributable to deleterious effects on neurohormonal activation, electrolyte balance, and cardiac and renal function. These agents may even lead to systemic and renal vasoconstriction, leading to further reductions in renal function. In some cases, combination diuretics (loop diuretic preceded by a thiazide diuretic) can produce a more effective diuresis, overcome some diuretic resistance, and increase fractional sodium excretion. The use of the recombinant human B-type natriuretic peptide (nesiritide) has been associated with mixed clinical results in trials in patients with acute decompensated HF.[35] Although it may be useful as an effective vasodilator, it has not been shown to be a superior diuretic or natriuretic agent.

Several clinical trials have confirmed the superiority of ultrafiltration over intravenous loop diuretics.[36,37] Because sodium and its anion are the major determinants of extracellular fluid volume, total body fluid volume can be reduced more by ultrafiltration than by diuretics. Urine produced by loop diuretics is hypotonic compared with plasma, whereas ultrafiltrate is iso-osmotic and isonatremic. The decision to use ultrafiltration over diuretic therapy can sometimes be challenging; however, the natriuretic effect of diuretics can be

---

BOX 7-6 Preoperative Optimization: Renal Dysfunction

Incidence
20%-40% after LVAD implantation

Risk Factors
Renal function before VAD implantation
RA pressure >20 mm Hg
Hypotension
Vasopressor use
Bleeding or transfusion
Nephrotoxins

Etiology
Decreased perfusion, high RA pressure (>20 mm Hg)
Shift from medullary to cortical nephrons

Goal
1 mL/kg/hr urine output

LVAD, left ventricular assist device; RA, right atrial; VAD, ventricular assist device.

measured as a surrogate for diuretic resistance, and patients with continued volume overload combined with diuretic and natriuretic resistance should be considered for ultrafiltration therapy.[38] The goal of ultrafiltration in these circumstances is to reduce an abnormally elevated CVP to improve renal perfusion and renal function before LVAD placement.

If these previously discussed measures do not result in improved renal function, it is prudent to assess if such patients need an IABP to improve renal perfusion. Patients who are anuric (as a result of acute cardiogenic shock) and who are undergoing temporary dialysis can be considered for temporary MCS (either percutaneous or surgical) to improve cardiac output and assess reversibility of renal dysfunction.[39]

Infection

Infection and sepsis have been the leading causes of mortality and morbidity since the beginning of use of VADs for patients with advanced HF.[40,41] Sepsis resulted in 41% of the deaths in the LVAD group of the REMATCH study. Within 3 months after LVAD implantation, the probability of LVAD infection was 28%.[40] It has been well recognized that a reduction in LVAD-related infections is possible with close attention to infection control and prevention guidelines, optimal implantation techniques, and meticulous surgical site care.

Patients undergoing LVAD placement are generally debilitated with varying degrees of malnutrition (see earlier).[42] These patients have many risk factors that increase postoperative infections. Many of these risks are inherent to this patient population and include diabetes mellitus, malnutrition from cardiac cachexia, and azotemia. Additional risks for infection include dental problems, use of indwelling catheters that have been in place for several days before the time of surgery, and mechanical ventilation. Correcting as many of these factors as possible before device implantation can minimize the risk of infection and optimize long-term outcomes. Most patients are hospitalized for days to weeks for evaluation and optimization before LVAD implantation, which leads to changes in skin flora and significantly increases the risk of nosocomial infection after LVAD implantation. Patients with active systemic infection should not be considered for LVAD support, and LVAD implantation should be delayed for patients with localized infections that can be effectively treated, if clinically feasible. Antibiotic therapy may have to be continued for a prolonged period postoperatively in these patients.

Strict attention to correcting or attempting to modify some of the risk factors that contribute to postoperative wound infections should be a primary strategy. The focus in the preimplant period should be on indwelling central lines. Most of these patients may have central lines for prolonged periods, especially for hemodynamic monitoring and adjustment of inotropes or other vasoactive agents. It may be beneficial to remove these lines for at least a short time before surgery. It may also be prudent to send microbial studies of the tips of the lines removed before surgery. If any of these lines show signs of infection, they need to be removed as soon as possible, and the infectious disease service should be consulted to obtain additional information on the type and duration of antibiotic therapy and to decide on whether to delay LVAD implantation. Central lines placed under unknown conditions should be immediately removed in potential candidates for LVAD implantation.

Prophylactic antibiotic regimens are used routinely in patients undergoing LVAD placement. Although the exact antibiotics used vary among medical centers, it is imperative that all regimens include an antibiotic to cover *Staphylococcus* because this is the most common organism implicated in device infections. Also, data suggest that *Staphyloccocus*

aureus nasal carriage is a risk factor for infections in cardiac surgical patients, and it may warrant decolonization in candidates for LVAD implantation if time permits. Close attention to prevention of infections should be continued intraoperatively and in the postoperative period. A detailed discussion of infection prevention is beyond the scope of this chapter, but prevention includes removal of lines and catheters when no longer necessary, aggressive nutritional support, and careful monitoring of the driveline exit site wound.

STRATEGIES TO OPTIMIZE RIGHT VENTRICULAR FUNCTION AND AVOIDANCE OF RIGHT VENTRICULAR FAILURE IN PATIENTS WITH LEFT VENTRICULAR ASSIST DEVICE IMPLANTATION

A major source of morbidity and mortality after MCS relates to RV failure, which leads to multiorgan failure and, in particular, renal and hepatic failure.[43,44] A thorough knowledge of risk factors for RV failure is important because it may help in selecting patients preoperatively who would benefit from biventricular support at the time of LVAD implantation as opposed to isolated LVAD support.[45-51] It has been shown that planned biventricular implantation results in superior outcomes compared with patients receiving LVAD support with delayed institution of right ventricular assist device (RVAD) support.[52,53] More recent studies involving the use of continuous flow pumps have suggested a reduced need for RVAD support; however, mortality for patients requiring RVAD support remains high.[54,55] It was previously suggested that increased mortality in patients requiring biventricular support is related to the direct use of either the additional RVAD or the biventricular VADs.

There is a general hesitancy to use biventricular support because of the significantly worse outcome. However, patients who have an RVAD implanted for significant RV failure days following LVAD implantation do much worse than patients who have an RVAD implanted at the time of the LVAD implant. Historically, there is a wide range of reported use of RVADs or biventricular support in various studies to manage RV failure after LVAD implantation. In the early paracorporeal Thoratec VAD BTT study, 48% of 213 patients received planned biventricular support, and an additional 17% were converted to biventricular support with the later addition of an RVAD.[9] In the HeartMate XVE LVAD BTT study, 11% of 280 patients received an RVAD.[1] More recently in the HeartMate II BTT trial, right HF was defined as the need for RVAD support or inotropic support for at least 14 days after implantation or inotropic support starting after 14 days. The incidence of right HF in the trial was 20%. Of patients, 6% required RVAD support, 7% required extended inotropic support for longer than 14 days, and 7% required use of inotropes after 14 days of support.[51]

Similarly in the HeartMate II DT trial, there was a 4% use of RVADs.[56] Patients with RV failure had increased length of stay and reduced survival compared with patients without RV failure.[51] The incidence of RV failure in patients with the continuous flow HeartMate II is comparable to or better than previous pulsatile devices; but it remains a significant factor for morbidity and mortality. Although improved patient selection algorithms over time have improved outcomes in this regard, the ability to adjust pump speed in real time, as guided by surface echocardiography to define RV and left ventricular size and function, may also have contributed significantly to the ability to manage patients on the new continuous flow pumps and to reduce RVAD use.

Numerous previous studies designed to help predict patients with a high likelihood of developing RV failure after LVAD implantation have identified female gender, nonischemic HF etiology, preoperative need for IABP support, increased right atrial pressure, low pulmonary artery pressure, and decreased RV stroke work index to be predictors of RV failure. Other studies have identified as predictors abnormal biochemical parameters such as elevated bilirubin, creatinine, and aspartate aminotransferase suggestive of preexisting severe multiorgan dysfunction and, importantly, any use of a vasopressor agent (Table 7-4).[45–51] Numerous studies have suggested that patients with an etiology of nonischemic cardiomyopathy are at significantly higher risk for RV failure because both the right ventricle and the left ventricle are involved in the disease process. The complex pathophysiology of RV failure, which could potentially be related to RV myocardial dysfunction, interventricular dependence, and RV afterload, has led to inconsistencies in predicting risk factors for RV dysfunction.[57,58] Most of these studies were done using pulsatile pumps as opposed to the current era, in which predominantly continuous flow pumps are used, which might limit the usefulness and relevance of those studies.

Kormos and associates[51] studied the risk factors for RV failure in a large cohort of almost 500 patients receiving the HeartMate II continuous flow LVAD as part of a multicenter clinical trial. By multivariate analysis, the following variables were predictive of RV failure: a CVP/pulmonary capillary wedge pressure (PCWP) ratio of greater than 0.63, need for preoperative ventilator support, and BUN level greater than 39 mg/dL. Variables that were significant by univariate analysis in addition to the latter included an elevated white blood cell count, increased CVP and decreased RV stroke work index. The value of using the CVP/PCWP as opposed to an elevated CVP alone is that patients with a CVP level that approaches the left-sided filling pressures may be at the highest risk for the development of RV failure after LVAD placement.

Several strategies have evolved over the years of experience with MCS that have aimed to avoid and reduce the incidence of postoperative RV failure (Fig. 7-4). It is imperative that patients who definitely need biventricular support are identified. Despite the numerous risk factors identified in many studies and the development of risk factor profile scores, identifying these patients continues to be a challenging problem. Each potential candidate for LVAD implantation must be carefully evaluated for the risk of developing RV failure after LVAD placement. Also, although the initial biochemical, hemodynamic, and echocardiographic profile of a patient at admission may suggest the need for biventricular support, many of these risk factors may be favorably modified by various strategies that may result in the avoidance of severe RV failure. These strategies include delaying LVAD implantation until the patient's hemodynamics are optimized using therapies such as aggressive diuretic therapy, ultrafiltration, and temporary IABP use.

It is important to proceed with LVAD placement with CVP as low as possible. Generally, the higher the PCWP, the more improvement will be seen with LVAD placement and normalization of left atrial pressure. More recently, the CVP/PCWP ratio has been identified as a significant predictor of RV failure after LVAD implantation.[51] In some patients, temporary biventricular MCS can be used to improve RV function, making the patient a candidate for isolated permanent LVAD support.[39]

In some patients, the development of intraoperative and postoperative bleeding and the subsequent transfusion requirements, especially when given rapidly in large volumes, might predispose to perioperative RV failure.[22]

TABLE 7-4	Literature Review of Risk Factors for Right Ventricular Failure		
Study	No. Patients	Type of VAD	Risk Factors (Multivariable)
Fukamachi et al, 1999[46]*	100	Pulsatile	Younger age Smaller patients Myocarditis Female gender Decreased RVSWI Decreased MPAP
Kavarana et al, 2002[43]*	69	Pulsatile	Decreased RVSWI Increased bilirubin
Ochiai et al, 2002[45]	245	Pulsatile	Pre-LVAD circulatory support Female gender Nonischemic etiology
Dang et al, 2006[47]	108	Pulsatile	Elevated CVP
Patel et al, 2008[49]	77	Pulsatile (55%) Continuous (45%)	Preoperative IABP
Mathews et al, 2008[48]	197	Pulsatile (84%) Continuous (16%)	Vasopressor requirement AST >80 IU/L Bilirubin >2.0 mg/dL Creatinine >2.3 mg/dL
Fitzpatrick et al, 2009†[53]	266	Pulsatile (>90%)	Cardiac index <2.2 L/min/m² RVSWI <0.25 mm Hemoglobin 1/m² Severe preoperative RV dysfunction Creatinine >1.9 mg/dL Prior cardiac surgery Systolic BP <96 mm Hg
Kormos et al, 2010[51]	484	Continuous	CVP/PCWP ratio >0.63 Preoperative ventilator support BUN >39 mg/dL
Drakos et al, 2010	175	Pulsatile (86%) Continuous (14%)	Preoperative IABP Increased PVR Destination therapy

Data from Drakos SG, Janicki L, Horne BD, et al. Risk factors predictive of right ventricular failure after left ventricular assist device implantation. *Am J Cardiol* 2010;105:1030-1035.

*Included only univariate analysis.

†Included patients with planned biventricular support.

AST, aspartate aminotransferase; BP, blood pressure; BUN, blood urea nitrogen; CVP/PCWP, central venous pressure/pulmonary capillary wedge pressure; LVAD, left ventricular assist device; MPAP, mean pulmonary artery pressure; IABP, intra-aortic balloon pump; PVR, pulmonary vascular resistance; RV, right ventricular; RVSWI, right ventricular stroke work index.

Excessive transfusion requirements can also transform a right ventricle that could otherwise tolerate an LVAD in isolation into one with profoundly decreased contractility from which the patient may never recover, particularly if RV MCS is delayed, and high doses of vasopressors and inotropes are used. As discussed earlier, optimization of a patient's coagulation profile in the preoperative period is crucial. Strategies to optimize the coagulation profile include delaying LVAD implantation if a patient has recently received anticoagulant therapy and administration of vitamin K therapy appropriately. Meticulous intraoperative hemostasis is also essential.

OPTIMIZING RIGHT VENTRICULAR FUNCTION

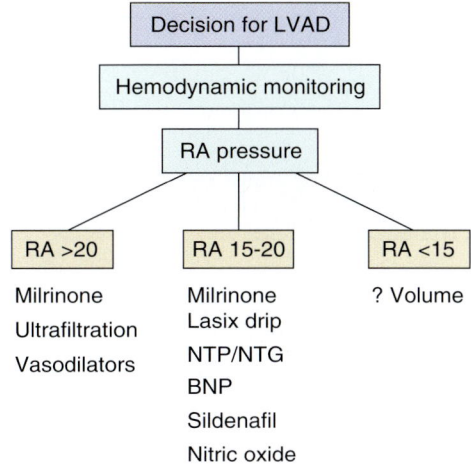

FIGURE 7-4 Optimizing right ventricular (RV) function. LVAD, left ventricular assist device; NTP/NTG, nitroprusside/nitroglycerin; RA, right atrial.

There has been a misconception that the presence of pulmonary hypertension is a risk factor for RV failure after RVAD placement. Patients with severe pulmonary hypertension that is associated with elevated left-sided filling pressures do very well with an LVAD in isolation because as the left ventricle is decompressed, RV function is enhanced further by afterload reduction, and the right ventricle is capable of generating plenty of force.[59] Low pulmonary artery pressure, particularly when associated with high right atrial pressures, suggests a higher risk for RV failure because the poor RV contractile function is unable to generate adequate pulmonary artery pressures. In patients with preoperative pulmonary hypertension undergoing LVAD implantation, aggressive pulmonary vasodilator therapy such as inhaled nitric oxide or inhaled epoprostenol (Flolan) may significantly reduce RV afterload, favorably influencing RV hemodynamics.[60] The use of oral sildenafil postoperatively may also result in a therapeutic benefit and is routinely used at some centers, although data are lacking to recommend this practice.[61]

After HeartMate II implantation, there is a trend toward a reduction in tricuspid regurgitation severity as loading conditions improve.[54] This finding suggests that tricuspid regurgitation severity of moderate grade or less would not need to be corrected by either tricuspid valve repair or replacement at the time of HeartMate II implantation. If severe RV dysfunction does develop in the operating room despite aggressive measures such as adequate inotropic support and use of nitric oxide, immediate use of a temporary RVAD is mandatory. It has been shown that delayed placement of RVAD in such patients is associated with poorer outcomes as opposed to early placement in the operating room.[44] Further details on the management of RV failure are beyond the scope of this chapter.

DELAYING PERMANENT LEFT VENTRICULAR ASSIST DEVICE IMPLANTATION: THE CONCEPT OF BRIDGE TO DECISION

Despite the many advances in the management of patients with acute HF, the outcome for patients with refractory acute cardiogenic shock remains disproportionately poor.[39] Most of these patients are often in hospitals that do not have access to advanced circulatory support technologies or resources to manage these patients optimally. Delay in referral to tertiary centers exacerbates further the poor outcomes in this group of patients. There is a definitive role for wider application of temporary circulatory support in such patients. Questions remain regarding the ideal device, the optimal duration of temporary support, and the ideal timing to bridge these patients to a long-term device.

Acute cardiogenic shock that is refractory to medical treatment with an IABP, multiple inotropes, and pressors continues to be the leading cause of death in patients hospitalized with myocardial infarction with an early mortality rate of greater than 50% despite adequate revascularization. Circulatory support with either mechanical assist devices or extracorporeal membrane oxygenation (ECMO) remains the only means of survival in these very sick patients who often have extreme hemodynamic instability, coagulopathy, and multiorgan dysfunction such as significant renal and liver failure and acidosis. Adding a complex and lengthy operation for placement of a permanent VAD increases the morbidity and mortality associated with this condition further. Outcomes of permanent LVAD implantation in patients with multisystem organ failure (MSOF) with prior cardiac arrest or severe hemodynamic instability are extremely poor. Additionally, transplant candidacy is uncertain with the combination of MSOF, uncertain neurologic status, and uncertain social support (owing to lack of time to perform such an evaluation adequately). There is clearly a role for temporary circulatory support in this population as a bridge to decision.[39] This support must be easy to place, rapidly stabilize the patient's hemodynamics, be transported easily with the patient, and allow time to address the patient's MSOF and neurologic status. Several options for circulatory support are available, including surgically implanted VADs, percutaneous assist devices, and ECMO.[62-65]

Experience with Temporary Mechanical Support as Bridge to Decision

Several centers use the CentriMag ventricular assist system (Levitronix, Waltham, MA) as a bridge to decision device for patients with acute refractory cardiogenic shock secondary to any etiology, including acute myocardial infarction, myocarditis, postcardiotomy, and complications from cardiac catheterization. We have developed an algorithm for treatment of patients with refractory acute cardiogenic shock (Fig. 7-5). This algorithm is being used as a guide for patients who are transferred to our institution in MSOF on multiple inotropes and pressors with IABP. At the time of admission, these patients (bridge to decision patients) typically have contraindications to permanent VAD implantation and uncertain transplant candidacy secondary to uncertain neurologic status, uncertainty of adequate social support (because of the unavailability of adequate time to complete such an evaluation), and unknown reversibility of MSOF. We have found that placement of the device is "user-friendly" because virtually any cannula (including cannulas used for routine cardiopulmonary bypass) can be used.

Generally, the placement of these devices requires the use of a median sternotomy, often with cardiopulmonary bypass. Placement allows for rapid hemodynamic stabilization with restoration of adequate systemic perfusion, which allows end-organ function to recover. The amount of support on the right, left, or both sides can be weaned in various combinations to assess recovery of native cardiac function. This weaning capability permits time to evaluate the patient adequately for recovery, withdrawal of support, need for permanent LVAD, or transplant and allows for recovery of renal, hepatic, and respiratory systems during the support period.

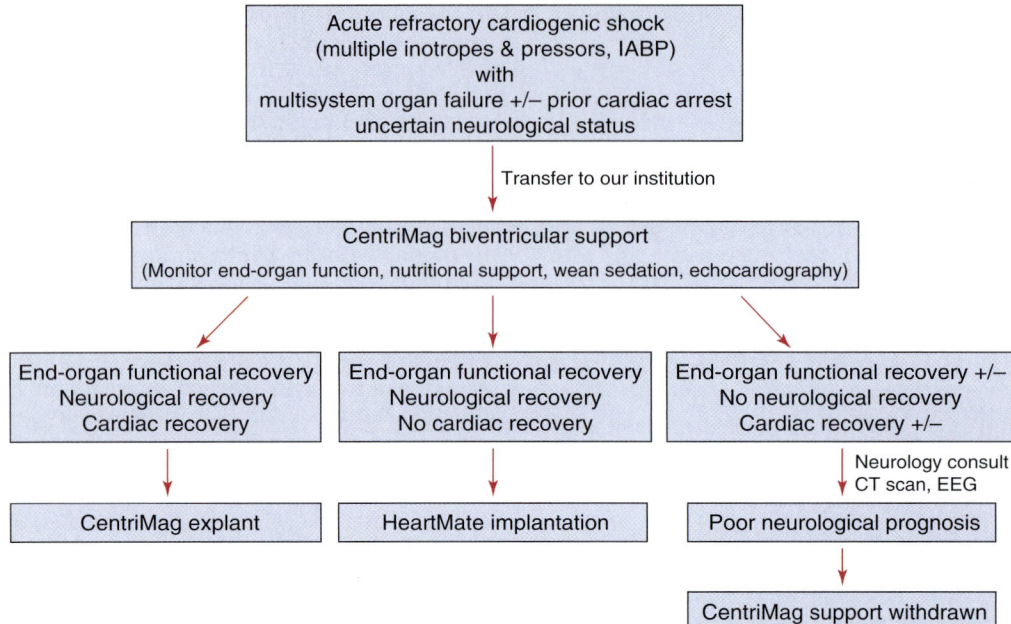

FIGURE 7-5 Algorithm for treatment of patients with refractory acute cardiogenic shock. CT, computed tomography; EEG, electroencephalogram; IABP, intra-aortic balloon pump.

Additional advantages with CentriMag support include the absence of stringent requirements for anticoagulation. Many patients who require urgent MCS are receiving clopidogrel or glycoprotein IIb/IIIa inhibitors; as a result, they have significant postoperative bleeding that is often refractory to correction of coagulopathy. In such patients, anticoagulation with heparin can often be withheld for 48 to 72 hours until all mediastinal bleeding resolves without pump malfunction owing to thrombosis or thromboembolic events. When anticoagulation is withheld, flows greater than 4 L/min reduce the risk of thrombosis even in the absence of anticoagulation.[39]

There are currently many percutaneous options for temporary mechanical support in patients presenting with acute refractory cardiogenic shock.[62–65] These patients historically have been treated with an IABP and inotropic support or ECMO. Although ECMO is suitable for cardiopulmonary support, it does not always unload the ventricles to the degree possible with a VAD, it requires stringent anticoagulation, and it has a high rate of device-related complications. Temporary VADs may be able to provide adequate circulatory support to allow MSOF to recover and neurological status to be assessed adequately. Although questions remain regarding the ideal device, the optimal duration of temporary support, and the timing to bridge to a long-term device, individual patients seem to continue to benefit from LVAD placement.

The cost-benefit ratio of implantable support therapy does not justify its use in all potential recipients. Identification of preoperative variables that accurately predict risk is important for planning and for devising management strategies. A study from Columbia-Presbyterian Hospital identified the following risk factors for increased operative mortality: mechanical ventilation, postcardiotomy shock, previous LVAD support, elevated CVP, and elevated prothrombin time.[66] The presence of all of these factors was associated with nearly 50% postoperative mortality rate. This screening scale did not take into account the patient's neurological status, which we have found to be a risk factor for poor outcomes. Another study from the same group reported a 30-day survival rate of 56% in 46 patients who underwent urgent HeartMate LVAD implantation after being transferred from outside institutions with cardiogenic shock.[67]

Percutaneous temporary VADs represent a relatively new technology that has an obvious appeal in that the devices are easily implanted in the cardiac catheterization laboratory. Eliminating an additional major surgery and possible cardiopulmonary bypass helps to decrease morbidity and mortality for these very sick patients. The Impella 5.0 (Abiomed, Danvers, MA) and the TandemHeart (CardiacAssist, Pittsburgh, PA) both can achieve flows of up to 5.0 L/min, which can provide adequate support in patients with a larger body mass index. The Impella 5.0 requires a femoral cutdown to access the femoral artery, which increases the risk of femoral artery and wound complications after device implantation. The Impella LD is similar in function to the Impella 5.0, but it is inserted surgically via a graft into the aorta. Although this device still functions similar to the percutaneous device, the benefits of the percutaneous approach are lost by the invasive surgical insertion. Percutaneous VAD cannulas can also become dislodged necessitating readjustment, and lower extremity ischemia from femoral vascular occlusion remains a problem. The Impella 2.5 device is currently widely available and easy to implant. Although theoretically adding 2 to 2.5 L of flow might reverse shock in some patients, this amount of support has been inadequate in numerous patients and has not provided much more support than an IABP.[63,64]

Two important questions must be considered in patients with acute cardiogenic shock, MSOF, or a prior cardiac arrest. First, how can patients who would benefit from temporary circulatory support be identified? Any patient with acute cardiogenic shock with contraindications for permanent support can be considered as a candidate for temporary mechanical support (Box 7-7). Second, what modality of temporary circulatory support should be used? Our recommendation is to use whatever temporary device that is available to the team at hand and can best serve the needs of the patient. One must be careful when comparing studies on temporary VADs. Each institution has a different mortality rate associated with the device that they currently employ for patients in acute HF. Comparing survival outcomes between single-center studies does not allow a proper or accurate comparison between different support devices because there are many variations in patient selection and management strategies among the centers. Comparisons

BOX 7-7 Identifying a Bridge to Decision Patient

- Current or ongoing definite contraindications for permanent support
  - Uncertain neurological status (cardiac arrest, prolonged CPR)
  - Major end-organ dysfunction (renal and hepatic dysfunction)
  - Severe hemodynamic instability
  - Major coagulopathy
  - Active, untreated infections
- Relative contraindications for permanent support
  - High-risk social situations
  - Mechanical ventilation

among different therapeutic modalities for acute cardiogenic shock are inherently biased based on the experience and outcomes of a single center. However, temporary MCS is an essential part of the algorithm in the optimization of select candidates for permanent MCS. In such patients, temporary mechanical support may provide an opportunity to improve multiorgan dysfunction and allow for assessment of an unclear neurological status, making this cohort of patients better candidates for permanent support.

SUMMARY

MCS has clearly evolved over the past decade with an increasing emphasis on patient selection in addition to understanding the pathophysiology of various complications such as RV failure and bleeding after LVAD implantation. The development of risk models has allowed investigators to study the impact of various risk factors on outcomes to aid not only patient selection but also timing of implantation.[68] Although objective prospective data on the use of these risk scores are presently unavailable, this paradigm may be shifting to one in which attempts to modify risk factors before LVAD placement is becoming the standard of care. A patient with a prohibitive risk score may be an unacceptable candidate at the time of initial evaluation, but with intensive medical therapy and optimization of several parameters, such as nutrition, abnormal coagulation profile, right heart dysfunction, and infections, it is likely that the patient may be at less risk after LVAD placement (Fig. 7-6).

We do not advocate delaying LVAD implantation in a patient who is rapidly deteriorating to improve adverse or unfavorable risk profiles. However, such patients who are at imminent risk of death may be best supported by means other than permanent LVADs, such as a wide variety of temporary circulatory support options. The field has developed to a point where there may be a need for a prospective trial to assess if modifying risk factors before implantation can improve outcomes.

REFERENCES

1. Frazier OH, Rose EA, Oz MC, et al. Multicenter clinical evaluation of the HeartMate vented electric left ventricular assist system in patients awaiting heart transplantation. *J Thorac Cardiovasc Surg.* 2001;122:1186–1195.
2. Frazier OH, Rose EA, McCarthy P, et al. Improved mortality and rehabilitation of transplant candidates treated with a long-term implantable left ventricular assist system. *Ann Surg.* 1995;222:327–336.
3. John R, Kamdar F, Liao K, et al. Improved survival and decreasing incidence of adverse events using the HeartMate II left ventricular assist device as a bridge-to-transplant. *Ann Thorac Surg.* 2008;86:1227–1235.
4. Miller LW, Pagani FD, Russell SD, et al. Use of a continuous-flow device in patients awaiting heart transplantation. *N Engl J Med.* 2007;357:885–896.
5. Morgan JA, John R, Rao V, et al. Bridging to transplant with the HeartMate left ventricular assist device: the Columbia Presbyterian 12-year experience. *J Thorac Cardiovasc Surg.* 2004;127:1309–1316.
6. Rose EA, Gelijns AC, Moskowitz AJ, et al. Long-term mechanical left ventricular assistance for end-stage heart failure. *N Engl J Med.* 2001;345:1435–1443.
7. Long JW, Kfoury AG, Slaughter MS, et al. Long-term destination therapy with the Heartmate XVE left ventricular assist device: improved outcomes since the REMATCH trial. *Congest Heart Fail.* 2005;11:133–138.
8. Reedy JE, Swartz MT, Miller LW, et al. Bridge to transplantation: importance of patient selection. *J Heart Lung Transplant.* 1990;9:473–480.
9. Farrar DJ. Preoperative predictors of survival in patients with Thoratec ventricular assist devices as a bridge to transplantation. *J Heart Lung Transplant.* 1994;13:93–100.
10. Stevenson LW. Patient selection for mechanical bridging to transplantation. *Ann Thorac Surg.* 1996;61:380–387.
11. Aaronson KD, Patel H, Pagani FD. Patient selection for left ventricular assist device therapy. *Ann Thorac Surg.* 2003;75(6 suppl):S29–S35.
12. Miller LW. Patient selection for the use of ventricular assist devices as a bridge to transplantation. *Ann Thorac Surg.* 2003;75(6 suppl):S66–S71.
13. Lietz KL, Long JW, Kfoury AG, et al. Outcomes of left ventricular assist device implantation as destination therapy in the post-REMATCH era: implications for patient selection. *Circulation.* 2007;116:497–505.
14. Rao V, Oz MC, Flannery MA, et al. Revised screening scale to predict survival after insertion of a left ventricular assist device. *J Thorac Cardiovasc Surg.* 2003;125:855–862.
15. Golstein D, Oz M, Rose E. Implantable left ventricular assist devices. *N Engl J Med.* 1998;339:1522–1533.
16. Holman W, Pae W, Teuteberg J, et al. INTERMACS: interval analysis of registry data. *J Am Coll Surg.* 2009;208:755–762.
17. Stevenson L, Pagani F, Young J, et al. INTERMACS profiles of advanced heart failure: the current picture. *J Heart Lung Transplant.* 2009;28:535–541.
18. Alba A, Rao V, Ivanov J, et al. Usefulness of the INTERMACS scale to predict outcomes after mechanical assist device implantation. *J Heart Lung Transplant.* 2009;28:827–833.
19. Lietz K, Miller LW. Left ventricular assist devices: evolving devices and indications for use. *Curr Opin Cardiol.* 2004;19:613–618.
20. Engelman DJ. Impact of body mass index (BMI) and albumin on morbidity and mortality after cardiovascular surgery. *J Thorac Cardiovasc Surg.* 1999;118:866–873.
21. Filippatos GS, Anker SD, Kremastinos DT. Pathophysiology of peripheral muscle wasting in cardiac cachexia. *Curr Opin Clin Nutr Metab Care.* 2005;8:249–254.
22. Goldstein DJ, Beauford RB. Left ventricular assist devices and bleeding: adding insult to injury. *Ann Thorac Surg.* 2003;75:S42–S47.
23. John R, Lee S. The biological basis of thrombosis and bleeding in patients with ventricular assist devices. *J Cardiovasc Transl Res.* 2009;2:63–70.
24. Warkentin TE, Kelton JG. A 14-year study of heparin-induced thrombocytopenia. *Am J Med.* 1996;101:502–507.
25. Koster A, Sanger S, Hansen R, et al. Prevalence and persistence of heparin/platelet factor 4 antibodies in patients with heparin coated and noncoated ventricular assist devices. *ASAIO J.* 2000;46:319–322.
26. Koster A, Loebe M, Sodian R, et al. Heparin antibodies and thromboembolism in heparin-coated and non-coated ventricular assist devices. *J Thorac Cardiovasc Surg.* 2001;121:331–335.
27. Schenk S, El-Banayosy A, Prohaska W, et al. Heparin-induced thrombocytopenia in patients receiving mechanical circulatory support. *J Thorac Cardiovasc Surg.* 2006;131:1373–1381.e4.
28. Samuels LE, Kohout J, Casanova-Ghosh E, et al. Agratroban as a primary or secondary postoperative anticoagulant in patients implanted with ventricular assist devices. *Ann Thorac Surg.* 2008;85:1651–1655.
29. Schroder JN, Dnaeshmand MA, Villamizar NR, et al. Heparin-induced thrombocytopenia in left ventricular assist device bridge-to-transplant patients. *Ann Thorac Surg.* 2007;84:841–846.
30. Heywood JT. Cardio-renal syndrome: lessons from the ADHERE database and treatment options. *Heart Fail Rev.* 2004;9:195–201.
31. Boerritger G, Burnett JC. Cardio-renal syndrome in decompensated heart failure: prognostic and therapeutic implications. *Curr Heart Fail Rev.* 2004;1:113–120.

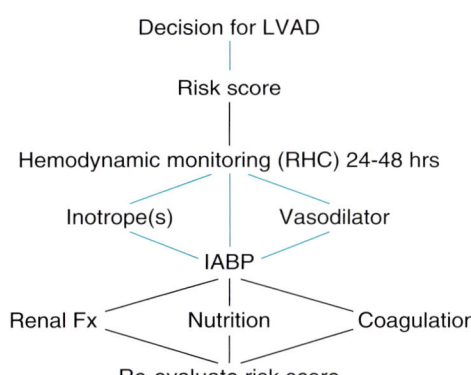

PRE-OP MANAGEMENT VAD CANDIDATES

Decision for LVAD

Risk score

Hemodynamic monitoring (RHC) 24-48 hrs

Inotrope(s)   Vasodilator

IABP

Renal Fx   Nutrition   Coagulation

Re-evaluate risk score

FIGURE 7-6 Preoperative management for candidates for ventricular assist device (VAD) implantation. Fx, function; IABP, intra-aortic balloon pump; LVAD, left ventricular assist device; RHC, right heart catheterization.

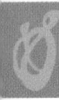

32. Butler J, Forman DE, Abraham WT, et al. Relationship between heart failure treatment and development of worsening renal function among hospitalized patients. *Am Heart J.* 2004;147:331–338.

33. Smith GL, Lichtman JH, Bracken MB, et al. Renal impairment and outcomes in heart failure: systematic review and meta-analysis. *J Am Coll Cardiol.* 2006;47:1987–1996.

34. Liu PP. Cardiorenal syndrome in heart failure: a cardiologist's perspective. *Can J Cardiol.* 2008;24:25B–29B.

35. Aaronson KD, Sackner-Bernstein J. Risk of death associated with nesiritide in patients with acutely decompensated heart failure. *JAMA.* 2006;296:1465–1466.

36. Bart BA, Boyle A, Bank AJ, et al. Ultra filtration versus usual care for hospitalized patients with heart failure: relief for acutely fluid overloaded patients with decompensated heart failure. The RAPID-CHF trial. *J Am Coll Cardiol.* 2005;46:2043–2046.

37. Costanzo MR, Guglin ME, Saltzberg MT, et al. Ultra filtration versus intravenous diuretics for patients hospitalized for acute decompensated heart failure. *J Am Coll Cardiol.* 2007;49:675–683.

38. Ali SS, Olinger CC, Sobotka PA, et al. Loop diuretics can cause clinical natriuretic failure: a prescription for volume expansion. *Congest Heart Fail.* 2009;15:1–4.

39. John R, Liao K, Lietz K, et al. Experience with the Levitronix CentriMag circulatory support system as a bridge to decision in patients with refractory acute cardiogenic shock and multisystem organ failure. *J Thorac Cardiovasc Surg.* 2007;134:351–358.

40. Holman WL, Park SJ, Long JW, et al, REMATCH investigators. Infection in permanent circulatory support: experience from the REMATCH trial. *J Heart Lung Transplant.* 2004;23:1359–1365.

41. Zierer A, Melby SJ, Voeller RK, et al. Late-onset driveline infections: the Achilles' heel of prolonged left ventricular assist device support. *Ann Thorac Surg.* 2007;84:515–521.

42. Chinn R, Dembitsky W, Eaton L, et al. Multicenter experience: prevention and management of left ventricular assist device infections. *ASAIO J.* 2005;51:461–470.

43. Kavarana MN, Pessin-Minsley MS, Urtecho J, et al. Right ventricular dysfunction and organ failure in left ventricular assist device recipients: a continuing problem. *Ann Thorac Surg.* 2002;73:745–750.

44. Morgan JA, John R, Lee BJ, et al. Is severe right ventricular failure in left ventricular assist device recipients a risk factor for unsuccessful bridging to transplant and post-transplant mortality. *Ann Thorac Surg.* 2004;77:859–863.

45. Ochiai Y, McCarthy PM, Smedira NG, et al. Predictors of severe right ventricular failure after implantable left ventricular assist device insertion: analysis of 245 patients. *Circulation.* 2002;106:I–198–I-202.

46. Fukamachi K, McCarthy PM, Smedira NG, et al. Preoperative risk factors for right ventricular failure after implantable left ventricular assist device insertion. *Ann Thorac Surg.* 1999;68:2181–2184.

47. Dang NC, Topkara VK, Mercando M, et al. Right heart failure after left ventricular assist device implantation in patients with chronic congestive heart failure. *J Heart Lung Transplant.* 2006;25:1–6.

48. Mathews JC, Koelling TM, Pagani FD, et al. The right ventricular failure risk score: a preoperative tool for assessing the risk of right ventricular failure in left ventricular assist device candidates. *J Am Coll Cardiol.* 2008;51:2163–2172.

49. Patel ND, Weiss ES, Schaffer J, et al. Right heart dysfunction after left ventricular assist8device implantation: a comparison of the pulsatile HeartMate I and axial-flow HeartMate II devices. *Ann Thorac Surg.* 2008;86:832–840.

50. Furukawa K, Motomura T, Nose Y. Right ventricular failure after left ventricular assist device implantation: the need for an implantable right ventricular assist device. *Artif Organs.* 2005;29:369–377.

51. Kormos RL, Teuteberg JT, Pagani FD, et al. Right ventricular failure in patients with the HeartMate II continuous-flow left ventricular assist device: incidence, risk factors, and effect on outcomes. *J Thorac Cardiovasc Surg.* 2010;139:1316–1324.

52. Tsukui H, Teuteberg JJ, Murali S, et al. Biventricular assist device utilization for patients with morbid congestive heart failure: a justifiable strategy. *Circulation.* 2005;112(9 suppl):I–65–I-72.

53. Fitzpatrick JR, Frederick JR, Hiesinger W, et al. Early planned institution of biventricular mechanical circulatory support results in improved outcomes compared with delayed conversion of a left ventricular assist device to a biventricular assist device. *J Thorac Cardiovasc Surg.* 2009;137:971–977.

54. Lee S, Kamdar F, Madlon-Kay R, et al. Effects of the HeartMate II continuous-flow left ventricular assist device on right ventricular function. *J Heart Lung Transplant.* 2010;29:209–215.

55. Maeder MT, Leet A, Ross A, et al. Changes in right ventricular function during continuous-flow left ventricular assist device support. *J Heart Lung Transplant.* 2009;28:360–366.

56. Slaughter MS, Rogers JG, Milano CA, et al. Advanced heart failure treated with continuous-flow left ventricular assist device. *N Engl J Med*, 2009;361:1–11.

57. Farrar DJ, Compton PG, Hershon JJ, et al. Right ventricular function in an operating room model of mechanical left ventricular assistance and its effects in patients with depressed left ventricular function. *Circulation.* 1985;72:1279–1285.

58. Moon MR, DeAnda A, Castro LJ, et al. Effects of mechanical left ventricular support on right ventricular diastolic function. *J Heart Lung Transplant.* 1997;16:398–407.

59. John R, Liao K, Kamdar F, et al. Effects on pre- and posttransplant pulmonary hemodynamics in patients with continuous-flow left ventricular assist devices. *J Thorac Cardiovasc Surg.* 2010;140:447–452.

60. Argenziano M, Choudhri AF, Moazami N, et al. Randomized, double-blind trial of inhaled nitric oxide in LVAD recipients with pulmonary hypertension. *Ann Thorac Surg.* 1998;65:340–345.

61. Klodell CT, Morey TE, Lobato EB, et al. Effect of sildenafil on pulmonary artery pressure, systemic pressure, and nitric oxide utilization in patients with left ventricular assist devices. *Ann Thorac Surg.* 2007;83:68–71.

62. De Robertis F, Rogers P, Amrani M, et al. Bridge to decision using the Levitronix CentriMag short-term ventricular assist device. *J Heart Lung Transplant.* 2008;27:474–478.

63. Seyfarth M, Sibbing D, Bauer I, et al. A randomized clinical trial to evaluate the safety and efficacy of a percutaneous left ventricular assist device versus intra-aortic balloon pumping for treatment of cardiogenic shock caused by myocardial infarction. *J Am Coll Cardiol.* 2008;52:1584–1588.

64. Siegenthaler MP, Brehm K, Strecker T, et al. The Impella Recover microaxial left ventricular assist device reduces mortality for postcardiotomy failure: a three-center experience. *J Thorac Cardiovasc Surg.* 2004;127:812–822.

65. Doll N, Kiaii B, Borger M, et al. Five-year results of 219 consecutive patients treated with extracorporeal membrane oxygenation for refractory postoperative cardiogenic shock. *Ann Thorac Surg.* 2004;77:151–157.

66. Oz MC, Goldstein DJ, Pepino P, et al. Screening scale predicts patients successfully receiving long-term implantable left ventricular assist devices. *Circulation.* 1995;92(suppl II):169–173.

67. Kherani AR, Cheema FH, Oz MC, et al. Implantation of a left ventricular assist device and the hub-and-spoke system in treating acute cardiogenic shock: who survives? *J Thorac Cardiovasc Surg.* 2003;126:1634–1635.

68. Levy W, Mozaffarian D, Linker D, et al. The Seattle Heart Failure Model. *Circulation.* 2006;113:1424–1433.

CHAPTER **8**

Current Types of Devices for Mechanical Circulatory Support

Igor Gregoric and Christian A. Bermudez

DEVELOPMENT OF MECHANICAL CIRCULATORY SUPPORT SYSTEMS

Methods for providing mechanical circulatory support (MCS) have varied greatly over the past 60 years. The evolution of MCS technology has been gradual because the biologic barriers to progress have remained constant and difficult.[1] Clinicians and engineers have collaborated for many years to develop an arsenal of devices rather than a single ideal system that could support all patients. The numerous MCS systems that have been developed range from very small catheter-mounted devices to fully implantable total cardiac replacement systems. This variety of device types is necessary to support the vast and complex population of patients with heart failure (HF). Although considerable progress has been made in recent years with medical technology and medical care, the future of HF treatment remains complex and dynamic. MCS is increasingly a key component of HF management.

Various types of blood pumps have evolved with the continuing search for smaller, biocompatible, and durable devices. Figure 8-1 provides a concise timeline of MCS technology development. The modern era of MCS began in the early 1950s when cardiopulmonary bypass (CPB) was first used to support patients during open heart operations for the repair of congenital heart defects.[2,3] As the field of cardiac surgery proliferated throughout the 1960s, a need for MCS beyond the operating room became apparent. Patients with cardiogenic shock needed temporary circulatory support to avoid other organ failure and to allow time for recovery of myocardial function. Counterpulsation with the intra-aortic balloon pump (IABP) was introduced in 1968 as a means to augment cardiac function by improving cardiac output and decreasing myocardial work.[4] Since that time, the IABP has effectively supported large numbers of patients with HF and remains the most commonly used MCS device. During this early era, it was also realized that some form of long-term circulatory support was necessary to treat the expanding population of patients with HF. Cardiac replacement with heart transplantation or a total artificial heart (TAH) and temporary support with a left ventricular assist device (LVAD) were attempted in a few cases during the 1960s,[5–7] but the dismal results led to a moratorium on these treatments, and researchers continued developing MCS technologies.

Throughout the 1970s, researchers continued work on developing artificial heart technology with the goal of providing near-total circulatory support with an implantable device for durations of many years.[8] Because heart transplantation was ineffective therapy owing to immunologic barriers and relatively primitive availability of immunosuppressant agents, scientists believed that MCS systems must replace cardiac function and closely mimic the function of the natural heart. Early devices were large and bulky but could provide 10 L/min of cardiac output with a stroke volume and pump rate in the normal physiologic range. Early in the 1980s, heart transplantation was renewed with the development of effective immunosuppressive therapy, and MCS technology had undergone more than a decade of research and development. Under the direction of and with funding support from the National Heart, Lung and Blood Institute, pulsatile blood pumps for use as a TAH or ventricular assist device (VAD) were developed. As the limitations of heart transplantation were realized, and a suitable population for testing these devices was needed, clinical trials for bridge to transplant (BTT) and bridge to recovery (BTR) with LVADs were initiated. Most of these systems were based on pulsatile designs. At the same time, the TAH was implanted in a few patients as destination therapy (DT) and for BTT with mixed and controversial results.[9,10]

Axial flow blood pumps were first introduced in the late 1980s with a catheter-mounted device that was inserted either percutaneously via the femoral artery or directly through an open chest to the left ventricle and across the aortic valve.[11] Clinical studies showed that continuous blood flow generated by a miniature pump was feasible and that there may be a broader application of this type of pump.[12] The early concerns of excessive hemolysis from these small devices were eventually dispelled as clinical results indicated that this type of pump was safe. In the 1990s, implantable axial flow devices were developed owing to the need for smaller and more reliable devices

Roller Pumps	Pulsatile Pumps Counterpulsation	Centrifugal Flow		Axial Flow			Maglev Centrifugal Flow
1950	1960	1970	1980	1990	2000	2010	
CPB 1951	LVAD 1963	TAH 1969	ECMO 1972	Implantable Pulsatile Devices 1982–1986	Implantable Axial Flow LVADs 1998–2000	Percutaneous LVADs	

FIGURE 8-1 Timeline showing the evolution of the various types of blood pumps used for mechanical circulatory support (MCS). CPB, cardiopulmonary bypass; ECMO, extracorporeal membrane oxygenation; LVAD, left ventricular assist device; TAH, total artificial heart.

for long-term support. Having a single moving component and durable bearings, these devices have been proven to provide long-term support with a very low incidence of pump failure. The smaller size of these devices and their improved durability have contributed to a reduction in life-threatening complications and enhanced survival.[13,14] More recent LVAD designs have centrifugal flow pumps that use magnetic or hydrodynamic bearings or both to eliminate friction and wear of the rotating impeller. This type of pump design is used in short-term and long-term MCS systems. With miniaturization of the centrifugal and axial flow blood pumps and improved catheter designs, LVADs that are inserted percutaneously are now being used for first-line support of patients with cardiogenic shock.

Heart transplantation has been considered the best treatment option for patients with end-stage HF. However, the shortage of donor organs has encouraged the continued development of MCS systems for long-term use. The persistent high mortality rate of cardiogenic shock requires that MCS devices be inserted rapidly and with minimal invasiveness. In the last 6 decades, MCS with VADs and artificial hearts has matured substantially, with outcomes now similar to that of heart transplantation.

BRIDGE TO DECISION WITH TEMPORARY VENTRICULAR ASSIST DEVICES

Bridge to decision with temporary VADs is an evolving paradigm in the management of patients who present in acute refractory cardiogenic shock (Fig. 8-2). The etiologies of cardiogenic shock are most commonly acute myocardial infarction (MI), failure to wean from CPB (postcardiotomy), acute decompensation of chronic HF, acute myocarditis, peri-

partum cardiomyopathy, and other cardiac disorders such as valvular disorders and congenital defects. Despite maximal medical therapy with multiple inotropes, vasoactive medications, and IABP support, the mortality rate remains high for these patients.[15] Patients who are marginally stabilized with medical therapy and IABP may be candidates for revascularization or other surgical treatment. In these cases, the interventional or surgical procedure can be performed with MCS on standby. For patients who experience cardiac arrest or are hemodynamically unstable, the only means of survival is with temporary MCS for BTR, BTT, and bridge to bridge with a long-term implantable device or for stabilization until corrective surgery can be performed. The primary goal of circulatory assist with a temporary VAD is to restore adequate hemodynamics rapidly to avoid the development of multisystem organ failure (MSOF). Patients with MSOF secondary to cardiogenic shock or cardiac arrest have very poor outcomes with long-term implantable LVADs[16]; these devices also require extensive surgery for implantation, and the cost is sizable.

Temporary MCS for patients with cardiogenic shock for bridge to decision can be applied with devices that use a percutaneous insertion or cannulation (Table 8-1) or devices that require surgery (Table 8-2). Each approach has different advantages and disadvantages, and it has not been determined if there is a survival benefit of either approach over the other. Early implementation of circulatory assist after the onset of cardiogenic shock is an important factor in avoiding MSOF. The availability of the specialized technology and personnel needed for the different approaches may determine which type of device is used at individual institutions. The percutaneous technique avoids surgery and its associated complications, but support is limited to LVAD only,

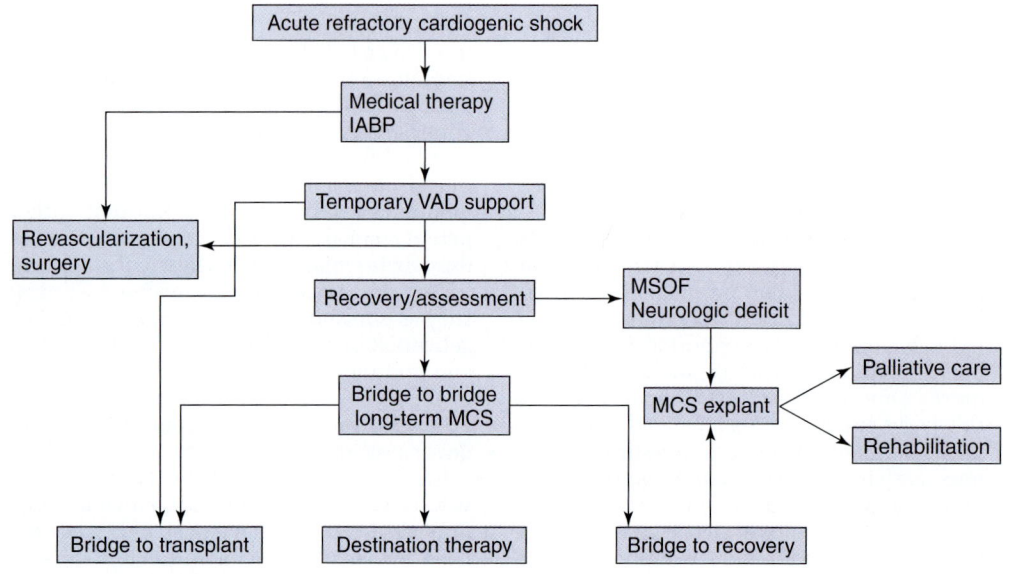

FIGURE 8-2 Algorithm for bridge to decision with temporary ventricular assist devices. IABP, intra-aortic balloon pump; MCS, mechanical circulatory support; MSOF, multisystem organ failure; VAD, ventricular assist device.

TABLE 8-1	Temporary Mechanical Circulatory Support Systems with Percutaneous Cannulation			
Device Name	Manufacturer	Type of Pump	Type of Support	Pump Position
IABP	Maquet Cardiovascular, Fairfield, NJ; Teleflex Medical, Research Triangle Park, NC	Aortic balloon	Counterpulsation	Intra-aortic
ECMO	Various components from different manufacturers	Centrifugal continuous flow	Venoarterial and venovenous	Extracorporeal; peripheral cannulation
Impella Recover	ABIOMED, Inc, Danvers, MA	Axial flow	LVAD	Transvalvular; LV to ascending aorta
TandemHeart	Cardiac Assist, Inc, Pittsburgh, PA	Centrifugal flow	LVAD	Extracorporeal; atrial transseptal cannulation

ECMO, extracorporeal membrane oxygenation; IABP, intra-aortic balloon pump; LV, left ventricle; LVAD, left ventricular assist device.

TABLE 8-2	Temporary Mechanical Circulatory Support Systems That Require Surgical Implantation		
Device Name	Manufacturer	Type of Pump	Type of Support
CentriMag	Levitronix, LLC, Waltham, MA	Centrifugal flow with magnetically levitated impeller	Biventricular or univentricular
BVS 5000 and AB 5000	ABIOMED, Inc, Danvers, MA	Pneumatic pulsatile sac-type	Biventricular or univentricular

and the amount of blood flow is less than that of surgically placed devices. The devices implanted surgically can provide biventricular support of 5 to 10 L/min, which is substantially greater than the percutaneous devices. It has not been determined if the higher flow rate of the surgical devices is advantageous. Percutaneous extracorporeal membrane oxygenation (ECMO) may be a preferred method of support for patients with severe hypoxemia secondary to fulminant pulmonary edema that may occur in cardiogenic shock.[17,18] Because all MCS devices require anticoagulation therapy during support, bleeding complications are more significant for surgically implanted devices.

Assessing the potential for myocardial recovery begins with the initiation of temporary VAD support and continues throughout the support time. Renal, hepatic, pulmonary, and neurologic dysfunctions are frequently assessed to determine severity and reversibility. During MCS, many patients with MSOF show improvements, which enable other treatment options, such as bridge to bridge with a long-term device or even heart transplant if a donor organ becomes available.[19–21] Patients with MSOF and severe irreversible neurologic deficit should not undergo implantation with a long-term device, and discontinuing VAD support should be considered. Assessment of neurologic function is vital before the conversion from a short-term device to a long-term implantable device to avoid use of a costly device in patients with a low probability of surviving. Recovery and device explant is considered only when renal, hepatic, pulmonary, and neurologic functions are adequate, and the patient successfully undergoes VAD weaning. Palliative care with device removal may be necessary for patients without hope for substantial recovery of neurologic function. Ideally, mechanical ventilation, dialysis, and inotropic support have been discontinued or are in the final stages of weaning before VAD support is discontinued.

Patients receiving temporary VAD support who have recovery of end-organ function and good neurologic function but have poor cardiac function should be considered for an implantable long-term LVAD as BTT or DT. A few patients may undergo BTT during support with a short-term device.[22] Patients may not be approved candidates at the time of implantation of the short-term device or at the time of conversion to a long-term device, but as their condition continues to improve, their candidacy may change. Patients being supported by a long-term device for BTT or DT may

also experience sufficient myocardial recovery and become candidates for device removal. Myocardial recovery should be assessed throughout support, especially in patients with nonischemic HF.

TEMPORARY SUPPORT DEVICES

Percutaneous Insertion

Temporary MCS devices that are applied by percutaneous cannulation techniques are intended for rapid support of the left ventricle (see Table 8-1). The potential advantage of this approach to MCS is that circulatory assistance can be provided within a short time after the onset of cardiogenic shock. The disadvantage of these devices is that the maximum flow rate that can be achieved is 2.5 to 5 L/min, which may be insufficient for large patients and patients with cardiac arrest or trivial cardiac function. Cannulation is accomplished via peripheral vessels, which renders the patient nonambulatory during the support time. These devices are used most often for durations of 1 week or less.

Intra-aortic Balloon Pump

Circulatory support with the IABP has been the mainstay of treatment of acute HF for more than 40 years. Since the first use of the IABP for support of patients with cardiogenic shock in 1968,[23] this device has been the most widely used MCS system; more than 42,000 implants are performed in the United States annually.[24] The IABP initially required surgical insertion because of its large size; however, the introduction of a percutaneous version of the IABP catheter in the early 1980s allowed widespread use. Further improvements, including prefolded balloons and smaller device sizes, have made the IABP one of the preferred systems for the management of left ventricular dysfunction by cardiologists and cardiothoracic surgeons.

The IABP consists of a polyethylene balloon mounted on a double-lumen catheter. The external lumen allows the flux of gas needed for inflation with helium, which has a low density and rapid diffusion coefficient, or carbon dioxide, which has a high solubility in blood and reduces the potential consequences of gas embolization. The central lumen provides access to the guidewire used for percutaneous placement.

The IABP catheter is usually inserted into the descending thoracic aorta via the femoral artery and is attached to an external control console (Fig. 8-3). After placement in the proximal descending aorta, the balloon is connected to a drive console that includes a pressurized gas reservoir and a monitor for electrocardiogram (ECG) and pressure wave recording and allows adjustments in inflation-deflation timing, ideally coordinating inflation with the onset of diastole and deflation just before the onset of systole. This coordination is accomplished using the patient's ECG signal, arterial waveform, or an intrinsic pump rate. The principal effects of the IABP are to increase myocardial oxygen supply and decrease myocardial oxygen demand (left ventricular wall tension) associated with the improvement in diastolic coronary blood flow and the observed reduction in left ventricular afterload. Secondary effects are improvement in cardiac output and ejection fraction and decreases in heart rate and pulmonary capillary wedge pressure.[25,26]

The indications for IABP use have evolved throughout the years. Originally developed to be used for cardiogenic shock complicating an acute MI, the IABP has been applied to diverse unstable cardiac conditions, including unstable angina refractory to medical therapy, mechanical complications of acute MI, postcardiotomy failure, ischemia-related ventricular arrhythmias, HF refractory to medical therapy, and support for high-risk percutaneous coronary intervention and surgical coronary revascularization.[27] Contraindications to IABP use include severe aortic regurgitation, aortic dissection, significant peripheral vascular disease, and contraindications to heparinization. Different complications have been described; vascular, embolic, and hemorrhagic complications are the most clinically relevant. Limb ischemia ranged from 2% to 5% in some series, and careful assessment and heparinization should be considered if prolonged support is required.[28]

Despite wider indications for IABP use, cardiogenic shock after an acute MI continues to be one of the most frequent indications. Different trials have studied the effects of IABP in ST segment elevation MI and shown better outcomes when IABP was added to thrombolytic therapy versus thrombolytic therapy alone.[29] These results may not be applicable to patients undergoing primary percutaneous interventions, however.[30] To date, no randomized prospective trial has examined the role of IABP in patients with post–acute

MI cardiogenic shock undergoing pharmacologic or mechanical reperfusion.[31] A more recent meta-analysis suggests insufficient evidence endorsing the current recommendations for the use of IABP therapy in the setting of ST segment elevation MI complicated by cardiogenic shock.[32]

Another common use of the IABP is as adjunct therapy in patients undergoing high-risk cardiac surgery or presenting with postoperative left ventricular dysfunction. Of patients undergoing cardiac surgery, 10% to 15% receive an IABP either preoperatively to reduce risk or postoperatively in case of difficulty weaning from CPB. The use of the IABP preoperatively in patients undergoing high-risk coronary artery bypass grafting with the use of CPB may have a beneficial effect on mortality and morbidity.[33] Despite the absence of definitive scientific evidence showing the impact of the IABP on the clinical outcomes of patients presenting with advanced HF, the IABP continues to play a role in the management of these patients. IABP support can be initiated rapidly by percutaneous techniques and is used to stabilize patients before a more permanent therapeutic option is offered.

Extracorporeal Membrane Oxygenation

ECMO is a well-established mechanism to provide short-term circulatory support for patients presenting with cardiogenic shock. Initially used in the early 1970s in patients with advanced respiratory failure, ECMO use was rapidly expanded to pediatric and adult patients with acute cardiogenic shock refractory to medical therapy.[34,35] It has since been successfully used as BTR,[36] BTT,[37] or bridge to bridge[38] to a more permanent LVAD in patients with various etiologies of overt cardiac failure, including acute MI, end-stage dilated cardiomyopathy, acute myocarditis, inability to wean from bypass after cardiac surgery, or cardiac arrest.[39,40]

ECMO support combines the use of a centrifugal or roller pump and a membrane oxygenator and has the ability to provide rapid and complete respiratory and hemodynamic support in advanced clinical decompensation with up to 6 L/min of nonpulsatile flow (Fig. 8-4). The ability of the system to resolve organ injury and provide complete cardiopulmonary support has several advantages over some other percutaneous and surgically implanted temporary devices. ECMO support can be implanted centrally (open surgical technique) via sternotomy with a cannula placed in the right atrium for venous drainage and in the aorta for oxygenated blood return; this is the most frequent approach used for ECMO implantation after an unsuccessful weaning from CPB (postcardiotomy failure). The peripheral cannulation strategy is more frequently used in acute hemodynamic collapse or cardiac arrest. Peripheral cannulation is performed percutaneously using the Seldinger technique (femoral vein and femoral artery) with cannulas ranging from 17-Fr to 21-Fr for arterial cannulation and 25-Fr to 29-Fr for venous cannulation, depending on the size of the patient and other characteristics. Occasionally, an 8-mm Dacron graft is anastomosed to the femoral artery for cannula placement to minimize the risk of ischemic complications of the lower extremity,[41] but this graft can be impractical in emergent situations and is associated with significant bleeding in the presence of coagulopathy.

The ability to provide cardiac and respiratory support and improve oxygenation is an added benefit of ECMO over other temporary support systems, especially in cases of severe hypoxemia and pulmonary edema, which is frequent in these critically ill patients. The ease of implantation, transport capabilities, and lower component costs are unique features that make ECMO a first-line alternative for emergent resuscitation after a cardiac arrest.[42] The relatively high incidence of complications from ECMO, including bleeding, infections, and embolic and vascular events, limits the duration of support to less than 7 days in most cases and is considered the Achilles heel of the system.[43] Several technologic

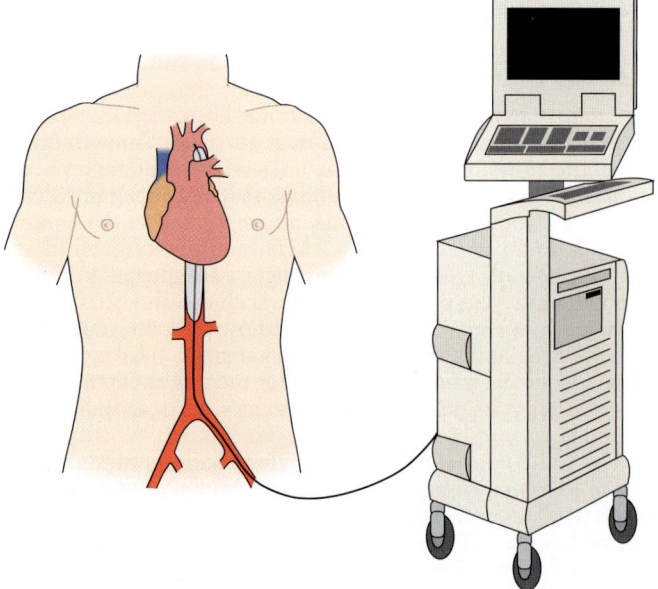

FIGURE 8-3 Intra-aortic balloon pump (IABP) and drive console.

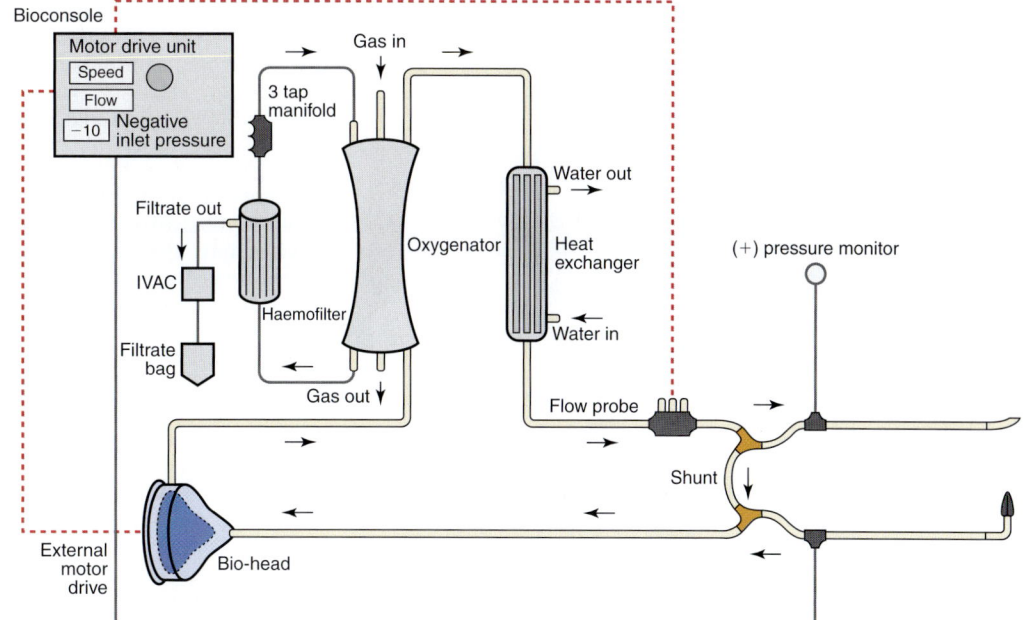

FIGURE 8-4 Schematic illustration of extracorporeal membrane oxygenation (ECMO) circuit. IVAC, intravenous accurate control.

improvements, including the use of magnetically levitated centrifugal pumps and more biocompatible low-gradient oxygenators, have reinvigorated the use of ECMO as a rapidly available percutaneous support to perform the first stabilization in acutely decompensated patients, allowing transfer to tertiary institutions or simply time to resuscitate and design an individualized treatment strategy. The most commonly used ECMO systems are depicted in Figure 8-5.

An important consideration is the inability of the percutaneous support to unload the left ventricle in the presence of severe cardiac dysfunction, which may limit the chances of later myocardial recovery. The central cannulation strategy may facilitate ventricular unloading, especially when ventricular contraction is absent or limited, in which case the peripheral approach may have limited use. Despite the increasing experience gained with the use of ECMO over the last 20 years and the availability of more biocompatible systems, the success of ECMO for the management of cardiogenic shock has been modest with hospital survival rates of 15% to 50%, depending on the institutional experience.[44] The initiation of support under active cardiopulmonary resuscitation and the rapid institution of renal and hepatic failure are associated with considerable risk for mortality in the intensive care unit. Institutions specialized in the management of these patients have noted that the involvement of a multidisciplinary team in the management of patients is beneficial and considerably improves results.[45]

Impella Recover

The Impella Recover (ABIOMED Inc, Danvers, MA) is used for temporary hemodynamic support in patients with acute HF. This device uses a small axial flow blood pump that is positioned in the ascending aorta with its cannula placed across the aortic valve and the tip within the left ventricular cavity. There are two versions of this device, the 2.5 and the 5.0, which are designations indicating the maximum blood flow rate of each device. The 2.5 version is percutaneously inserted via a peripheral artery with fluoroscopic guidance. The 5.0 device can be inserted through a femoral artery cutdown but is most often inserted directly through the ascending aorta and may be used either as an alternative to CPB or for postcardiotomy failure.

The Impella 2.5 is a small 12-Fr axial flow pump that aspirates up to 2.5 L/min of blood from the left ventricle into the ascending aorta (Fig. 8-6). The device is inserted percutaneously from a femoral artery through a 13-Fr sheath and is mounted on a 9-Fr pigtail catheter (Fig. 8-7). With fluoroscopic guidance, a guidewire is first passed retrograde through the aorta and into the left ventricle, and the pump is passed over the wire until the J-tipped portion is within the left ventricular cavity. A dual pressure sensor located on the cannula near the rotor provides a display of the aortic and ventricular pressures when the device is in proper position. The catheter is connected to an external console that monitors and controls the function of the device. The pump seal is continuously purged with a solution of glucose and heparin

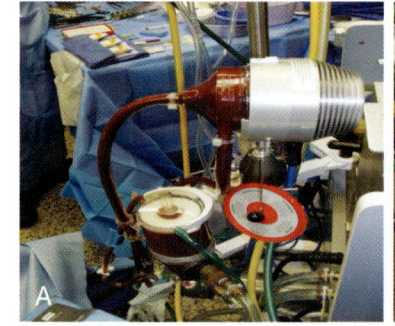
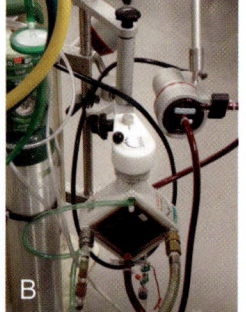
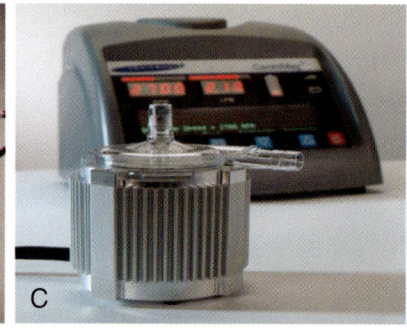

FIGURE 8-5 Most frequently used extracorporeal membrane oxygenation (ECMO) pumps. A, Biomedicus (Medtronic). B, Rotaflow (Maquet). C, CentriMag (Levitronix).

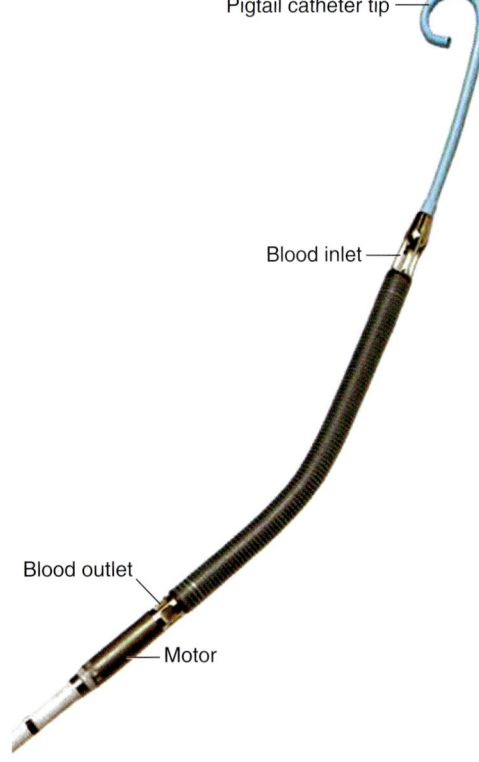

Pigtail catheter tip

Blood inlet

Blood outlet

Motor

FIGURE 8-6 Impella Recover 2.5 blood pump and cannula.

to prevent blood from entering the motor and clot formation at the seal. The console is portable and battery operated for patient transport, but patients are not ambulatory because of the presence of the catheter in the femoral artery.

The Impella 2.5 has been used for rapid short-term support of patients with acute HF and in high-risk patients undergoing percutaneous coronary intervention (PCI). Contraindications for the use of the Impella 2.5 are severe peripheral vascular disease, presence of a mechanical aortic valve, and a severely calcified aortic valve. Patients with a cardiac index less than $2.0 \, L/min/m^2$, arterial blood pressure less than 90 mm Hg, and pulmonary capillary wedge pressure or left atrial pressure greater than 18 mm Hg and who have a potentially reversible etiology may benefit from support with this device. The Impella 2.5 has successfully supported patients with postcardiotomy low cardiac output,[46–49] post-MI cardiogenic shock,[50–54] acute myocarditis,[55,56] and severe allograft rejection.[57,58] This device may also be useful to stabilize patients with acute decompensated chronic HF who are then bridged to transplant or to implantation of a long-term device.[53]

Randomized controlled trials comparing the Impella 2.5 with the IABP in patients with cardiogenic shock showed that patients treated with the Impella device had better hemodynamics; however, these differences are not significant, and 30-day mortality is not improved.[59,60] These preliminary findings are limited by the small sample size in the studies ($n = 25$ and $n = 41$), and the superiority of Impella support over the IABP remains undecided. Studies evaluating the Impella 2.5 during high-risk PCI have shown that this device is safe and provides adequate hemodynamic support.[61] However, in a subsequent randomized trial comparing support of the Impella 2.5 and the IABP during PCI, the authors concluded that proven superiority of Impella support would require a very large trial. Although the Impella 2.5 consistently produces higher cardiac output and left ventricular unloading than the IABP, the IABP generates better coronary perfusion.

TandemHeart

The TandemHeart percutaneous LVAD (CardiacAssist, Inc, Pittsburgh, PA) provides support by pumping blood from the left atrium to the femoral artery (Fig. 8-8). Blood flow is provided by a centrifugal flow pump that has hydrodynamic bearings. The pump's impeller rotates at speeds of 3000 to 7000 rpm and can generate flow up to 4 L/min. The unique feature of this device is the requirement for placement of the inflow cannula transseptally into the left atrium. The 21-Fr polyurethane inflow cannula has a large end hole and multiple side

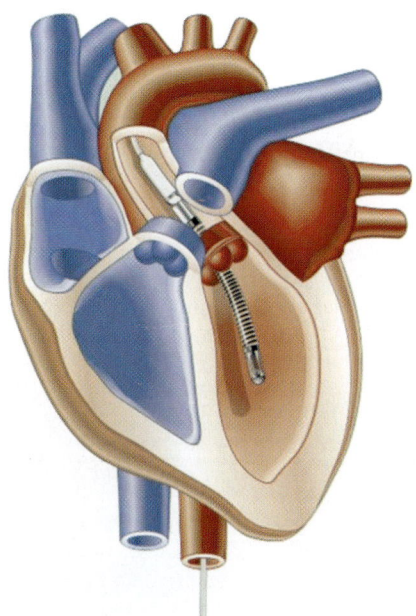

FIGURE 8-7 Position of the Impella 2.5 pump and cannula. The pump and blood exit point are in the ascending aorta, and the cannula is across the aortic valve with its tip in the left ventricle.

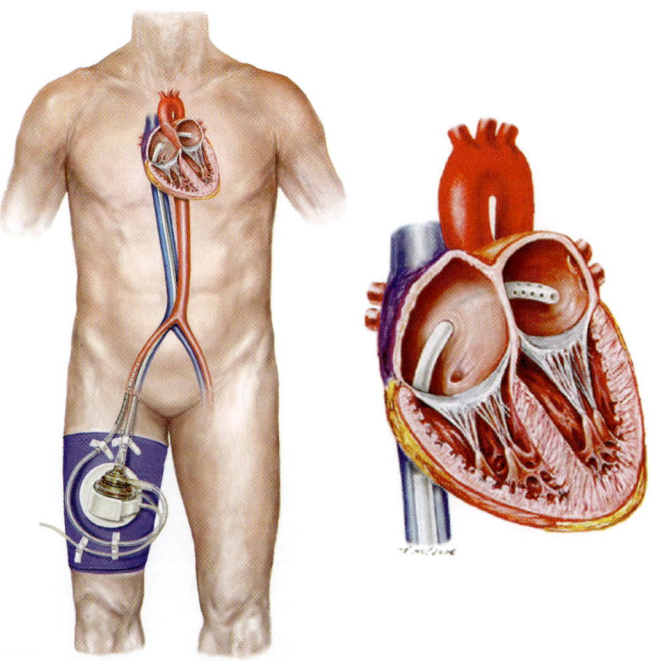

FIGURE 8-8 *Left*, TandemHeart percutaneous left ventricular assist device (LVAD) blood pump resides on a patient's thigh with the inflow cannula inserted through the femoral vein and the outflow cannula in the contralateral femoral artery. *Right*, Transseptal cannula position.

holes to maintain patency. Cannulation for device implementation is usually performed in the cardiac catheterization laboratory with fluoroscopic guidance. A septal puncture is first performed with a Brockenbrough needle passed through a Mullins sheath in the right atrium. A 0.035-inch pigtail guidewire is inserted into the left atrium, and a two-stage (14-Fr and 21-Fr) dilator is used to dilate the opening in the atrial septum. The inflow cannula is passed over the wire into the left atrium. Outflow is provided through a 15-Fr or 17-Fr cannula that is placed in the contralateral femoral artery. The pump resides on the patient's leg near the arterial return cannula. A bedside console provides monitoring and control functions, and it supplies a continuous flow of a heparinized solution to the bearing of the pump. With optimal facilities, equipment, and personnel, support with the TandemHeart can be accomplished within 1 hour of initial presentation.[62]

The TandemHeart has been used mainly for temporary support in patients with cardiogenic shock[21,53,63–65] and for brief support during high-risk PCI.[66–68] When compared with the IABP in patients with cardiogenic shock, TandemHeart support resulted in significantly higher cardiac index and mean arterial pressure and a significantly greater decrease in pulmonary capillary wedge pressure; however, the difference in 30-day mortality was not significant.[69] The TandemHeart has also been used for support during cardiac surgery and for postcardiotomy failure.[70–72] Patients with cardiogenic shock who are successfully stabilized with TandemHeart support have multiple potential therapeutic options. Corrective valvular surgery or surgical revascularization may be sufficient to allow patients to recover myocardial function and to be discharged from the hospital. Patients who do not recover myocardial function to allow device explant may undergo heart transplantation or bridge to an implantable LVAD for BTT.[21,22,73] Successful support until resolution of acute fulminant myocarditis has also been reported.[74,75]

Contraindications to TandemHeart support include isolated right ventricular failure and ventricular septal defect because of the potential for significant right-to-left shunting and severe peripheral vascular disease.[76] Potential serious device-related complications are persistent patent foramen ovale, limb ischemia, and thromboembolism. In addition, there is a potential for dislodgment of the inflow cannula into the right atrium, which would result in right-to-left shunting and a loss of support. Patients are usually sedated to avoid accidental cannula dislodgment. Although these complications have been observed, the incidence is low, and there is a positive risk-benefit for use with this device.

Surgical Insertion

Support of patients with postcardiotomy cardiogenic shock is best accomplished by implantation of a temporary VAD system that is capable of univentricular or biventricular support (see Table 8-2). For patients who fail to wean from CPB, conversion to another VAD system is sometimes possible with the existing cannulas. Continued VAD support may be required for many days to a few weeks until there is sufficient myocardial recovery allowing device removal, or in the absence of recovery, a long-term VAD or heart transplant may be required. Most patients with postcardiotomy failure are adequately supported with a biventricular VAD, but some may require pulmonary support with ECMO. Cannulation for ECMO may be accomplished percutaneously or surgically and is discussed in the section on percutaneously inserted devices.

CentriMag Ventricular Assist System

The CentriMag (Levitronix LLC, Waltham, MA) is a centrifugal flow blood pump that uses a magnetically levitated (Maglev) impeller for contact-free rotation (Fig. 8-9).

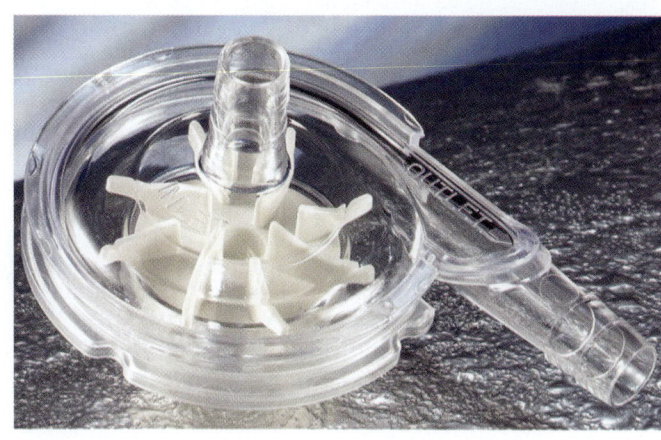

FIGURE 8-9 CentriMag blood pump.

The magnetic levitation of the impeller eliminates wear of moving components and any heat generation from friction. The VAD system consists of a pump, electromagnetic motor, ultrasonic flow probe, and drive console. Standard ⅜-inch tubing and user selected cannulas are used with the pump. Cannulation for biventricular support is usually accomplished with inflow cannulas placed in the left and right atria and outflow cannulas placed in the ascending aorta and main pulmonary artery (Fig. 8-10). The pump has a priming volume of 31 mL and can generate blood flow up to 10 L/min at a maximum rotational speed of 5500 rpm. An ultrasonic flow probe attached to the tubing provides a continuous display of the pump flow rate. The console can be placed at the bedside on a wheeled cart or in the patient's bed during transport.

The Maglev pump is designed to provide high blood flow rates but with low shear stress on blood components. The small artificial surface area of this pump, the absence of device-generated heat, and the high blood flow rate minimize thrombogenicity and may allow for moderate levels of anticoagulation during support. Hemolysis has been minimal in most patients supported.

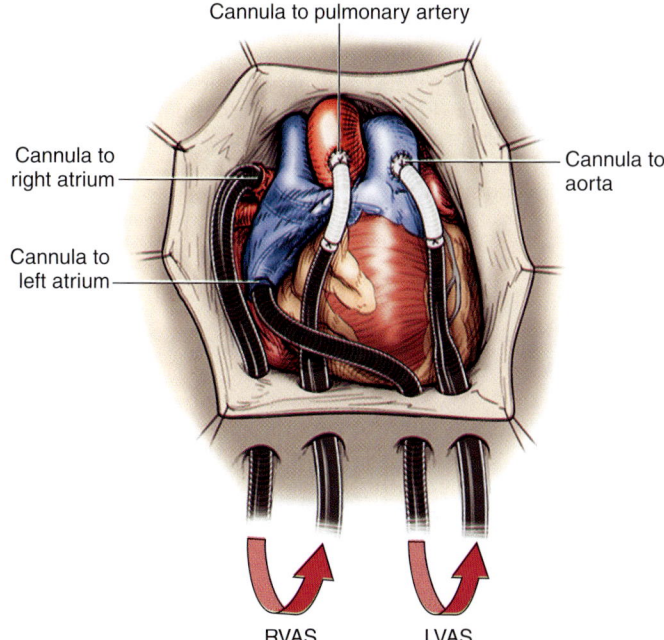

FIGURE 8-10 Typical cannulation sites for biventricular support with CentriMag. LVAS, left ventricular assist system; RVAS, right ventricular assist system.

The CentriMag is a versatile VAD system that can be used in various clinical scenarios. This system can provide univentricular or biventricular support, by surgical or percutaneous approaches, and it can be used as the pump in ECMO circuits. Reported uses include support in postcardiotomy failure, post-transplant rejection, congenital heart disease, right ventricular failure after LVAD implant, cardiogenic shock after acute MI, and acute myocarditis.[77-83] The versatility of cannulation, the flow range of 0 to 10 L/min, and the extracorporeal placement allow for this device to be used in patients of various sizes including small children.[84] Because of the clinical versatility and relatively low cost of the CentriMag, the use of this device as a bridge to decision is increasing in frequency.[9,80,84-86]

ABIOMED BVS 5000 and AB 5000

The ABIOMED biventricular system (ABIOMED Inc) is a temporary support system available in two versions, the BVS 5000 and the AB 5000. Both devices are pneumatically powered pumps that contain trileaflet valves that are integral with a flexible polyurethane blood sac. The BVS 5000 was developed as a short-term (<2 weeks) support system with the initial intention of assisting patients with acute HF and was the first cardiac assist device approved by the U.S. Food and Drug Administration (FDA) for postcardiotomy support in 1992.

The BVS 5000 is a cylindrical polycarbonate device that contains atrial and ventricular chambers (Fig. 8-11). The device is placed at the bedside on an intravenous catheter pole. This short-term, external pulsatile assist device is capable of providing left, right, or biventricular support as required and can provide 5 L/min of flow. The upper chamber (atrium) fills by gravity, and a lower chamber (ventricle) propels the blood out of the pump. Each chamber contains a 100-mL polyurethane bladder with the ventricular pump collapsing under compressed air, ejecting blood to the patient. Inflow cannulas (32-Fr to 42-Fr) are placed in the right atrium, left atrium, or left ventricle, and outflow cannulas are connected through a 10- to 12-mm Dacron graft to the pulmonary artery or aorta depending on the type of support required. The cannula design, graft sizes, and implantation techniques have been adapted in case removal of the device is considered after myocardial recovery.

Different institutional reports have shown the efficacy of the BVS 5000 as a short-term support device for many indications, including postcardiotomy failure, allograft dysfunction after heart transplantation, and as a bridge to heart transplant.[87-89] In ABIOMED's World Registry report, more than 60% of BVS 5000 implantations were performed for postcardiotomy failure, mean duration of support was 5 days, longest duration of support was 90 days, and 52% of patients required biventricular support. Survival with postcardiotomy support ranged from 30% to 60% with improved outcomes in cases of left ventricular versus biventricular support.[90]

The AB 5000 pump differs in size from the BVS 5000, does not have an atrial chamber, and resides paracorporeally on the anterior surface of the abdomen (Fig. 8-12). In addition, filling of the AB 5000 pump is vacuum-assisted. Supported patients are not ambulatory with the BVS version, but the console allows mobilization with the AB 5000 pump. When used in postcardiotomy failure, the available information suggests improved performance of the AB 5000 if longer support is required.[91] The AB 5000 allows right ventricular, left ventricular, or biventricular support. The pump, connected to cannulas placed in the heart, fills with blood by gravitational force and by vacuum assistance from the drive console. The cannulas and drive console are the same as used for the BVS 5000. The AB 5000 can provide flow rates of 6 L/min.

The general criteria for implantation of the ABIOMED VAD are based on persistent cardiogenic shock parameters despite maximal medical efforts to restore hemodynamic stability including the use of an IABP. Specific criteria have been described by investigators and are based on low cardiac output in the setting of multiple high-dose inotropic drugs[92] or surrogates of low cardiac output in the presence of an IABP.[93] The rationale behind these "formulas" is based on the hospital mortality of 80% to 100% if shock parameters cannot be reversed despite an IABP and inotropic drugs. It is imperative to identify patients in acute shock states rapidly and to institute VAD support quickly because the relationship between survival and time to VAD implantation is inversely proportional.[94]

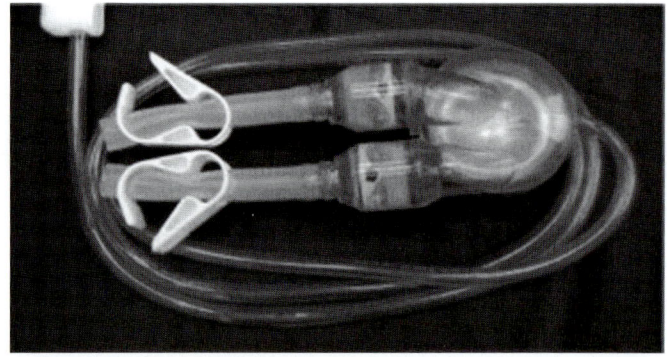

FIGURE 8-12 ABIOMED AB 5000 blood pump.

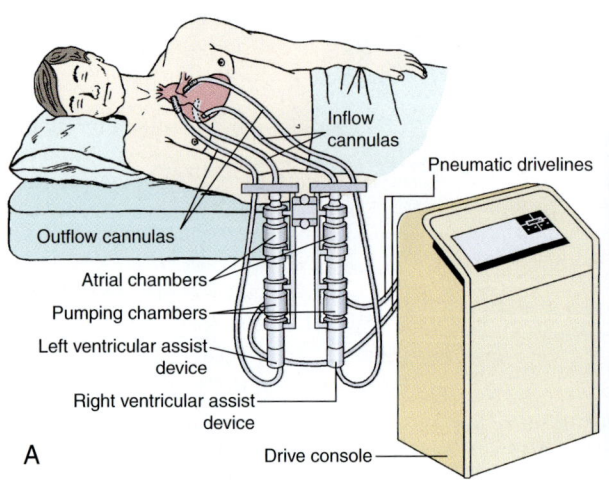

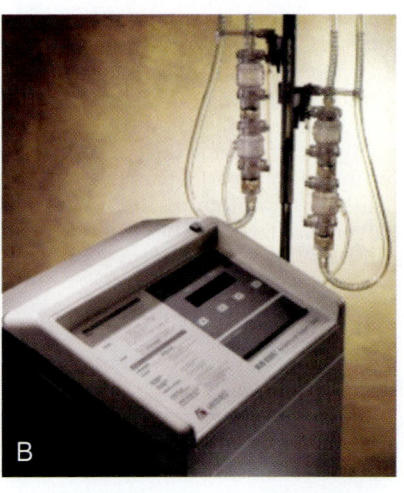

Inflow cannulas

Pneumatic drivelines

Outflow cannulas

Atrial chambers

Pumping chambers

Left ventricular assist device

Right ventricular assist device

Drive console

A

B

FIGURE 8-11 A and **B,** ABIOMED BVS 5000 blood pumps positioned at the bedside **(A)** and the drive console **(B)**.

The timing of VAD insertion for acute cardiogenic shock is crucial. At the present time, it is advisable to use a post-cardiotomy VAD within 1 hour from the first failed attempt to wean from CPB. During this critical hour, an IABP and inotropic drugs can be instituted and their success (or failure) assessed. The timing of insertion in the medical setting is less well defined, but the principles are the same. Delaying VAD insertion results in MSOF and other systemic problems; in addition, univentricular failure can deteriorate into biventricular failure, and biventricular support may become necessary. Although it is acceptable to place biventricular assist devices in patients with profound shock states, surgical or otherwise, it is also appropriate to start with an LVAD and determine if right-sided mechanical support is necessary. In most cases, the usual culprit for acute cardiac failure is the left ventricle. Beginning with an LVAD is a reasonable approach followed by the addition of a right ventricular assist device (RVAD) as needed.

Cannulation Techniques and Strategies

The BVS 5000 and the AB 5000 use the same inflow and outflow cannulas. The inflow cannula choices are 32-Fr and 42-Fr, and the outflow cannula is a "one size fits all" 10-mm Hemashield (Maquet, GmbH & Co Kg, Rastatt, Germany) graft bonded to the cannula; it does not require coagulation beforehand. The important decisions that need to be made regarding cannulation depend on the best and most suitable locations for establishing inflow and outflow and chamber size. LVAD inflow cannulation generally can be accomplished from either the left atrium or the left ventricle. The outflow graft is generally anastomosed to the anterolateral aspect of the ascending aorta. Similarly, RVAD implantation uses the same inflow and outflow cannulas except that the structures are right-sided (i.e., right atrium, right ventricle, pulmonary artery). Alternative cannulation sites have been described and include any sites in which inflow and outflow can be established.[95] Peripheral cannulation can be used in special circumstances.[96]

An advantage of ABIOMED cannulas is that they can be placed with or without CPB and use techniques familiar to any cardiac surgeon. The left atrial cannula is placed through two purse-string sutures and secured with rubber tourniquets. In the past, the left ventricular cannula was similarly placed and secured via the left ventricular apex. More recently, an inflow "sleeve" is available for better fixation to the left ventricle. The sleeve is secured to the left ventricular apex through which the cannula is placed and secured.[97] On explantation, the cannula is removed, and the sleeve is stapled or tied flush to its base.

In terms of inserting the cannula in the atrium or the ventricle, no tissue removal is necessary; this feature makes off-pump insertion simple and safe. In terms of a preferred LVAD cannulation strategy, two things need to be considered: (1) whether or not CPB is needed to restore and maintain hemodynamic stability while the VAD is being placed, and (2) whether to establish left atrial or left ventricular inflow for an LVAD. The need for CPB is answered by the hemodynamic state of the patient and whether or not the goal of placing the VAD can be accomplished in the shock state with or without CPB support. Both surgical and anesthetic considerations need to be taken into account during an off-pump implantation,[98] and rapid conversion to a CPB-assisted implantation should always be available.

With regard to left atrial or left ventricular cannulation, experienced VAD surgeons would argue that the left ventricular location is superior for two main reasons: (1) Left ventricular drainage is optimal from the ventricle directly compared with the left atrium, and (2) stagnation of blood in the left ventricle is more likely with left atrial cannulation increasing the risk of systemic thromboembolization and

stroke, particularly with left ventricular recovery or weaning that allows the left ventricle to begin ejecting. However, cannulation via the left atrium has advantages: (1) It can be accessed directly between the pulmonary veins or indirectly via the pulmonary vein itself or the left atrial appendage (if large enough) using the smaller (32-Fr) cannula; (2) minimal manipulation of the heart is needed, particularly if the dome of the left atrium is accessed[99]; and (3) a freshly infarcted left ventricle can be avoided eliminating the concern of an left ventricular cannula disrupting this friable area. In one unique situation of a postinfarction ventricular septal defect, a cannulation strategy was chosen in which a biventricular VAD was placed with biatrial inflow to avoid the infarcted ventricle altogether. The ventricular septal defect was deliberately not addressed, and the circulation was effectively rerouted around the septal hole. Nearly 2 months of support was accomplished, and successful BTT was achieved.[100]

Despite the similarities in cannulation between the BVS 5000 and the AB 5000, one important distinction between the two units is how the blood pumps are attached to the cannulas. In the BVS 5000, the cannulas are secured to the blood pump by pushing the tubing onto the hub and applying plastic bands to tighten the connection. In the case of the AB 5000, the cannula is also pushed onto the hub of the blood pump but secured with restraints that are screwed overtop.

Considerations for Biventricular Support

One feature of the ABIOMED BVS 5000 and AB 5000 is biventricular capability. Although univentricular support is appealing from many perspectives, biventricular support is sometimes necessary. Addition of an RVAD to an LVAD is not without complications, however, including (1) technical aspects of crowding the mediastinum with extra cannulas that may prevent sternal closure, (2) additional bleeding sites associated with inflow and outflow attachments to the right heart, and (3) balancing left and right flows. The advantage of adding an RVAD is total control of the circulation; this is particularly valuable in the setting of profound circulatory collapse or ventricular dysrhythmia.[101,102] The indication for additional RVAD support in the acute setting is also simple: inadequate hemodynamic parameters in the presence of an LVAD alone. Such conditions may arise if there is direct right ventricular dysfunction, such as right ventricular infarct or ischemia, or secondary conditions affecting the right ventricle, such as massive pulmonary embolism or right ventricular failure secondary to left ventricular failure. Occasionally (10% to 20%), a right ventricle may fail after LVAD implantation—specifically when inflow is established from the left ventricle proper—because of distortion of the ventricular septum resulting in geometric disfigurement of the right ventricle and subsequent dysfunction.[103] Although originally described in association with implantable LVADs in patients with chronic HF, this phenomenon has been observed with short-term devices as well. Regardless of the cause, management of the right ventricle in the setting of an LVAD is similar to management without an LVAD.

The usual considerations for right ventricular protection and enhancement of function include the following:

1. Ensure adequate coronary circulation to the right ventricle—repair stenotic graft or occluded right coronary artery vessels if warranted.
2. Allow any inadvertent air embolization within the right coronary artery territory to dissipate—vent the aortic root to remove air as the LVAD is ejecting and wait for the ST segment elevation associated with air emboli to the right coronary artery to normalize.
3. Avoid fluid (crystalloid or colloid products) overload—control bleeding.
4. Treat reversible pulmonary hypertension—use inhalational or intravenous agents that can augment right ventricular

performance and reduce pulmonary artery pressure with agents such as milrinone, epoprostenol, and nitric oxide.

5. Consider leaving the sternum open to avoid myocardial compression, affording enough "play" for the heart to beat without the extra compression caused by sternal approximation.

The RVAD (if added to an LVAD) may be necessary only for a short duration, and removal may be an option while leaving the LVAD in place.

LONG-TERM MECHANICAL CIRCULATORY SUPPORT

Pulsatile Devices

Implantable pulsatile VADs are used for BTT or BTR and DT (Table 8-3). These devices were developed during the 1970s and 1980s when the common design concepts of blood pumps for long-term use mimicked the function of the natural heart. The stroke volume, pump rate, and total blood flow were in the normal physiologic range. This design requirement resulted in large LVADs and TAHs that could be implanted only in large patients. Because of the size of these devices, the number of patients with HF that could be supported by implantable devices was limited, and extracorporeal devices were developed to broaden their application. Large implantable devices required extensive surgery for implantation, and the extracorporeal devices required multiple percutaneous cannulas, which led to persistent complications of bleeding and infection. Thromboembolism resulting from the large blood-contacting surface area has also limited the effectiveness of these devices. Despite these unrelenting problems, numerous patients have been successfully supported for extended durations, and these devices remain in use today for selected patients.

HeartMate XVE Left Ventricular Assist Device

The HeartMate XVE LVAD (Thoratec Corp, Pleasanton, CA) is an electrically powered pusher-plate device that is implanted in the left upper quadrant of the abdomen and pumps blood from the left ventricle to the ascending aorta (Fig. 8-13). The blood pump housing is made from a titanium alloy, and a flexing polyurethane diaphragm separates the internal blood and motor chambers. Porcine valves located in the inlet and outlet conduits direct blood flow through the pump and prevent regurgitant flow. A 19-mm textured titanium inflow cannula is inserted into the left ventricle and is secured in place by a Silastic and Dacron apical cuff. Outflow from the pump is via a 20-mm Dacron graft that is sewn to the ascending aorta. The XVE LVAD has a stroke volume of 83 mL and pumps at 50 to 120 strokes per minute. A constant pump rate can be set in the fixed rate mode, or the auto rate mode can be selected with the rate adjusted according to the filling volume. This portable system is powered by batteries and is controlled by a microprocessor controller, both worn by the patient dur-

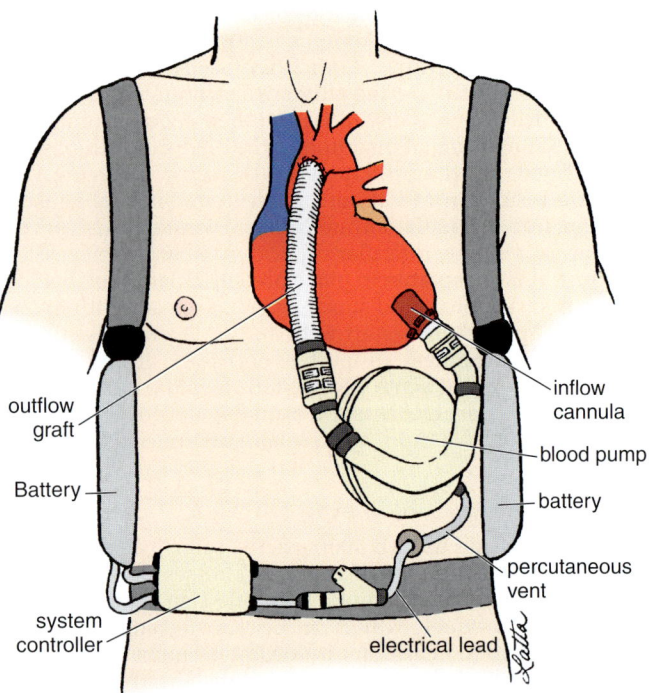

FIGURE 8-13 HeartMate XVE left ventricular assist device (LVAD).

ing ambulatory operation. Audible and visual indicators provide information regarding proper operation of the implanted pump. Backup actuation is provided pneumatically with a portable hand pump or by a pneumatic drive console.

The HeartMate XVE LVAD is implanted via a sternotomy and requires the development of a preperitoneal pocket or intra-abdominal pocket. The advantages of a preperitoneal pocket include isolation of the pump from abdominal contents; easier reoperation for explant or replacement; and less posterior compression on the stomach, which could lead to early satiety. Disadvantages of this technique include the time required to create the pocket and potential for prolonged pocket drainage with more bleeding and increased risk of infection. An alternative method is to place the pump into an abdominal pocket. Advantages of this technique are no pocket dissection with less chance for postoperative hematoma, the ability to use an omental wrap of housing, and a percutaneous lead resulting in the potential for less infection. The disadvantages are potential for visceral contact or erosion, a more complex re-exposure at replacement or at transplantation, and visceral compression and early satiety. Some surgeons create a pocket using Gore-Tex mesh to prevent erosion into the viscera and to facilitate explantation. The pump itself can be placed in the pocket before instituting CPB; however, the anastomosis of the outflow graft and implantation of the left ventricular apical cannulation connector are usually

TABLE 8-3	Pulsatile Mechanical Circulatory Support Systems for Long-Term Support			
Device Name	**Manufacturer**	**Type of Pump**	**Type of Support**	**Pump Position**
HeartMate XVE LVAD	Thoratec Corp, Pleasanton, CA	Electric pulsatile pusher-plate	LVAD	Preperitoneal or intraperitoneal pocket
Thoratec PVAD	Thoratec Corp, Pleasanton, CA	Pneumatic pulsatile sac-type	Biventricular or univentricular	Paracorporeal
Thoratec IVAD	Thoratec Corp, Pleasanton, CA	Pneumatic pulsatile sac-type	Biventricular or univentricular	Preperitoneal pocket
CardioWest TAH	SynCardia Systems, Inc, Tucson, AZ	Pneumatic pulsatile sac-type	Biventricular	Intrapericardial

IVAD, intracorporeal ventricular assist device; LVAD, left ventricular assist device; PVAD, paracorporeal ventricular assist device; TAH, total artificial heart.

done on cardiopulmonary bypass. Both the outflow graft and the inflow valved conduit required preoperative coagulation to prevent bleeding.

A unique feature of the XVE LVAD is its textured blood-contacting surfaces, which attract circulating blood cells that adhere to the surface and create a nonthrombogenic cellular lining.[104] The titanium surfaces are textured by the sintering of titanium microspheres, and the diaphragm is textured by the extrusion of polyurethane fibrils. The pseudoneointimal lining that forms on the surfaces consists of various cell types and a collagen-fibrin matrix that is uniform throughout the pump. This nonthrombogenic surface eliminates the need for continuous anticoagulation therapy during support. Although this surface is thromboresistant, it is immunologically active, which may lead to defects in immunity and increases the potential for infection.[1,105,106]

The XVE LVAD was the first implantable device approved for both BTT and DT and has been used extensively worldwide.[107,108] The landmark REMATCH (Randomized Evaluation of Mechanical Assistance for the Treatment of Congestive Heart Failure) trial showed a significant survival and quality-of-life benefit of support with the XVE LVAD over continued medical therapy.[108] The REMATCH trial and subsequent use of the XVE LVAD for DT resulted in lengthening support times, which revealed that the life of this device was limited by wear and failure of the valves and motor. Modifications of the valve conduits and the control software provided some improvement, but the durability of the system has been limited to approximately 18 months. Although the present preferences are to use the newer axial and centrifugal flow LVADs, the XVE LVAD is used for patients who cannot tolerate continuous anticoagulation therapy.

Thoratec VAD

The Thoratec VAD (Thoratec Corp) is a pneumatically powered sac-type device that is available in paracorporeal and intracorporeal versions. Both devices may be used for univentricular or biventricular support. The external pneumatic drive console and portable pneumatic driver allow ambulatory outpatient support. Thoratec VADs are used for BTR and BTT. Thoratec VADs have been considered a mainstay of ventricular support since approval as BTT in 1995 and approval for postcardiotomy failure in 1998, with more than 3000 patients receiving implants worldwide.[109,110] The Thoratec VAD is the only long-term device other than the TAH that can be used for biventricular support and, in particular, still retain the ability to be weaned in the presence of myocardial recovery. The risk of biventricular failure is especially high in specific instances, such as low pulmonary artery pressure in the presence of poor right ventricular function, in the setting of cardiogenic shock with end-organ failure where the risk of postoperative bleeding is high, giant cell myocarditis, in patients in whom retransplantation is considered, in the presence of postcardiotomy failure after interventricular septal rupture, in the presence of severe pulmonary edema despite maximal medical therapy, and in patients with ischemic cardiomyopathy where surgery threatens the right ventricular viability.

The Thoratec VAD has a 65-mL stroke volume polyurethane blood pumping chamber and two mechanical valves. With the use of a console or a portable pneumatic driver, the Thoratec VAD produces a clinical beat range of 40 to 110 beats/min and a flow rate of 1.3 to 7.2 L/min. The paracorporeal ventricular assist device (PVAD) (Fig. 8-14) is positioned paracorporeally on the anterior abdominal wall and is suitable for use in smaller patients (body surface area >0.73 m²). This device requires surgical implantation; the most frequently used cannulation configuration for left ventricular support is the left ventricular apex, with a 12- to 15-mm inflow cannula and a 14- to 18-mm Dacron outflow graft anastomosed to the ascending aorta. Right ventricular support has most frequently drained the right atrium with an 11-mm inflow cannula, and a 14- to 18-mm graft is anastomosed to the pulmonary artery. Although left atrial cannulation can be used, making it easy to insert and remove with minimal dissection or myocardial damage, it is used only for the right atrium. Direct left ventricular cannulation provides higher VAD flows with a lower risk of thromboembolism especially after acute MI and allows for better decompression of the left ventricle, which may reduce infarct size, improving chances of recovery.

The PVAD requires CPB for insertion after a brief period of pump preparation. Pump preparation involves flushing the pump itself with 250 mL of 5% albumin with 100 U of heparin to passivate the biomer surface of the blood pump sac over a period of 15 minutes. There are several cannula configurations for the VAD for both inflow and outflow. Most typically, the straight ventricular inflow cannula is used for the left ventricle, and the atrial beveled tip is used for the right atrium.

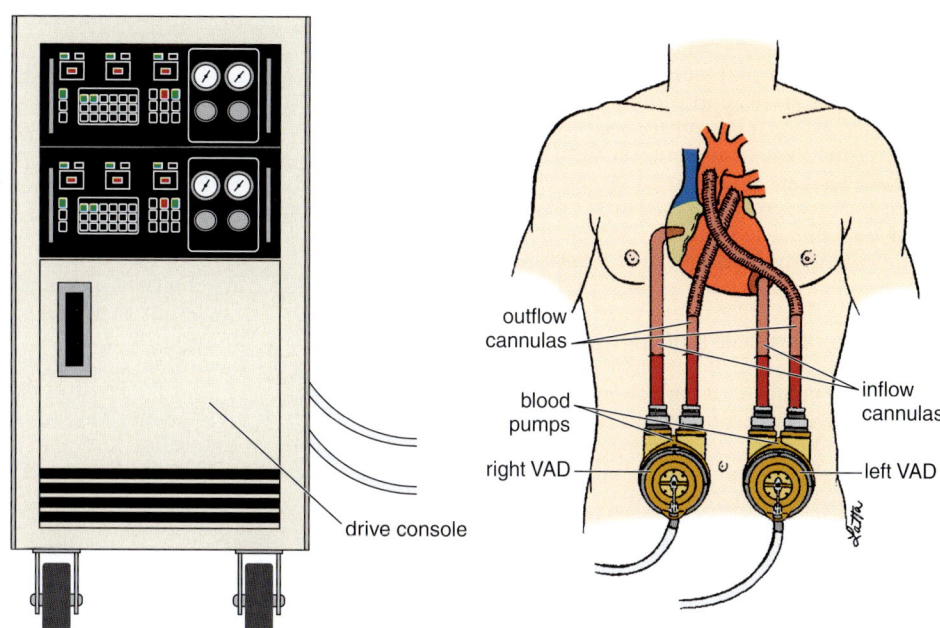

FIGURE 8-14 Thoratec paracorporeal ventricular assist device (PVAD). VAD, ventricular assist device.

The outflow grafts are coated to avoid the need for coagulation before the procedure. For most patients, the 14-mm size is adequate for both pulmonary artery and aortic outflow. Many surgeons prefer to use the 18-mm graft for the aorta, however, because it provides a lower outflow resistance; for patients with a body surface area that is greater than $2.0\,m^2$, the larger graft is also used for the pulmonary artery.

A tunnel is made for the left ventricular apical inflow conduit, which travels through the pericardium at its apex and subsequently under the left costal margin to exit two finger breadths below the ribs. The conduit is sewn into the apex after making a 1-cm core with 12 pledgeted sutures, and the cannula is passed through the tunnel. A de-airing cannula is attached to drain the left ventricle, and the aortic outflow, which has been measured, is then sewn end-to-side to the ascending aorta. The outflow cannula can be tunneled unless the patient requires an RVAD as well. In this case, the right atrial inflow cannula is brought through a subcostal tunnel into the mediastinum, and a premeasured length of the outflow graft is sewn to the pulmonary artery end-to-side.

The placement of the cannulas and grafts is optimized in the mediastinum to make re-entry for transplantation easier; this is accomplished by placing the aortic graft to the right lateral side of the mediastinum next to the right atrium and placing the pulmonary artery graft to the right over the right ventricle. The atrial drainage cannula is placed in the right atrial appendage with its tip directed toward the inferior vena cava–pericardial juncture, but the cannula itself is placed over the aortic graft to protect it at resternotomy. The outflow grafts are covered with a second layer of remaining trimmed graft. The right and left pumps are de-aired and connected to their respective inflow and outflow cannulas with collet nuts. The air line and Hall switch line are connected. Most surgeons wean from CPB and start the pumps at a fixed rate of 40 beats/min, gradually increasing to 60 beats/min and adding chamber vacuum to enhance pump filling. At this point, the pump is switched to a volume mode. The device heart rate is totally dependent on the rate of filling of the pump.

The PVAD allows the intermediate-term to long-term support that is needed if recovery of the patient and myocardial recovery are expected before heart transplantation. Support for more than 3 years has been possible with the PVAD in selected patients. The capability of long-term support with acceptable results and of biventricular support makes the PVAD one of the pumps of choice in patients presenting acutely or with marginal right ventricular function in whom relatively long support is expected. The rates of survival using the PVAD as BTT or bridge to myocardial recovery are comparable to other implantable pulsatile devices, especially with left ventricular support alone, with similar rates of embolic and hemorrhagic complications.[110]

An important consideration with the use of the PVAD is the potential of skin entry site infection requiring frequent and skilled nursing management. Despite acceptable survival with the use of the PVAD for left ventricular support, the results with the use of the PVAD for biventricular support have been more variable, reflecting institutional patient selection because the PVAD has been frequently used in patients with more advanced HF and biventricular dysfunction.[111] Worldwide, clinical experience with the PVAD as BTT shows that more than 50% of the patients had biventricular support, whereas right ventricular support alone was used in only 3% of the patients. The average support was 51.8 days, and patients transplanted or weaned from the device after cardiac recovery had adequate long-term survival.[112]

The Thoratec intracorporeal ventricular assist device (IVAD) (Fig. 8-15) is designed to provide the same features as the PVAD and to improve results in cases of long-term support by minimizing the risk of the infectious complications associated with the paracorporeal design of the PVAD. The

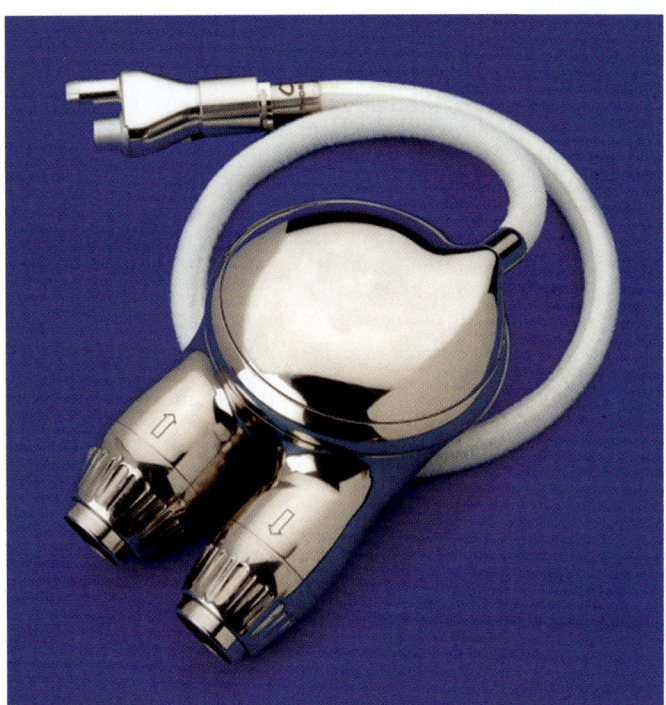

FIGURE 8-15 Thoratec intracorporeal ventricular assist device (IVAD).

pumping chamber, mechanical valves, and stroke volumes are similar. The differences include titanium housing; reduced weight; and the presence of a more narrow, 9-mm percutaneous lead. The pump can be placed in an intraperitoneal or preperitoneal position and is actuated pneumatically by the dual-drive console for in-hospital use or a portable pneumatic driver for home use. A prospective, multicenter clinical trial of 39 patients supported device approval in 2004 and showed successful outcomes as BTT and as postcardiotomy BTR, similar to other pulsatile devices.[113,114]

The Thoratec PVAD and IVAD require an external pneumatic driver, which has become portable enough to allow for patient discharge. This device weighs only 9.8 kg (with batteries and carrying case) and can provide LVAD, RVAD, and biventricular VAD support in fixed and auto modes of operation. There is a mobility cart to facilitate patient ambulation, and the console is approved to allow patients to go home and travel by air.

Total Artificial Heart

The TAH is designed to replace the cardiac structures completely and to provide long-term support as BTT.[115] It has been considered as an alternative to the LVAD in patients with massive myocardial damage, such as patients with post-MI ventricular septal defects, intractable arrhythmias, and valvular or ischemic disease with extensive myocardial damage, in whom biventricular support is required. Various types of TAHs have been designed with variable success in completing approval for human device exemption. The SynCardia CardioWest C70 TAH (SynCardia Systems, Inc., Tucson, AZ) is approved in the United States for support. With an extensive developmental history since the 1960s, the first successful application of a TAH as BTT was performed in 1985.[116]

The SynCardia TAH (Fig. 8-16) is a biventricular, pneumatic pulsatile pump that replaces the native ventricle and all four valves. The ventricles consist of a rigid spherical outer housing that supports a blood-contacting diaphragm, two intermediate diaphragms, and an air diaphragm, all made of segmented polyurethane. Two Medtronic Hall (Medtronic, Minneapolis, MN) 25-mm and 27-mm mechanical valves

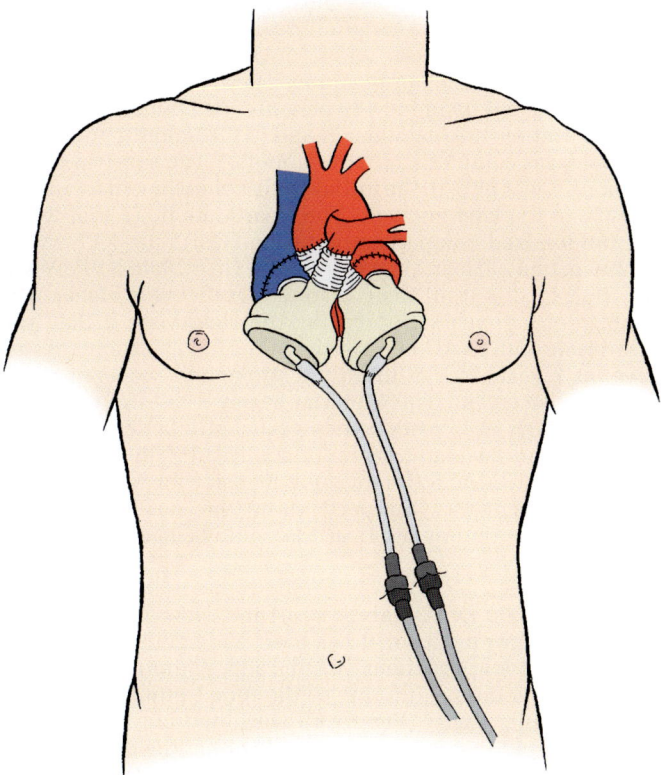

FIGURE 8-16 CardioWest total artificial heart (TAH).

separate the areas of each ventricle. The complete displacement of the diaphragm generates a displacement of 70 mL per beat for a total cardiac output of 7 to 8 L/min. The pumps are placed in orthotopic position after suturing polyurethane inflow connectors to the left and right atrial cuffs of the recipient. Dacron outflow conduits are snapped to the mounts of the TAH ventricles after completion of the anastomoses to the great vessels. A driveline, passed percutaneously, connects to the external console that contains the pneumatic drivers. Changes to the console and a newly designed mobile and fully portable pneumatic driver allow patients to ambulate and potentially to be discharged from the hospital.

Because of the size of the device and because it is fully implanted in the pericardial cavity, careful considerations are necessary before implantation to avoid size mismatch and compression of left superior pulmonary vein or inferior vena cava when fitting the device in small patients. Selection criteria include a left ventricular end-diastolic diameter greater than 70 mm, cardiothoracic ratio greater than 0.5, computed tomography scan volume greater than 1500 mL, and anteroposterior chest diameter (from sternum to spine) greater than 10 cm. The adverse events seen in TAH support are the same adverse events frequently seen for any type of mechanical support. Infection is the most common complication, probably associated with the device size and the advanced state of the patient's disease. Other events, including bleeding and neurologic complications, are similar to events seen with other VADs. The accumulated experience of the centers using this TAH and the lessons learned regarding patient selection and complication management have made support using this TAH a valid alternative to BTT in patients who have irreversible biventricular failure and are at imminent risk of dying. The pivotal U.S. multicenter investigational trial involving this device showed adequate survival to transplant of patients supported with the TAH and acceptable midterm outcomes (5 years) after transplant compared with patients supported with an LVAD.[117]

Continuous Flow Left Ventricular Assist Devices

More recently, implantable LVADs with continuous flow blood pumps have been developed and are used for BTT and DT (Table 8-4). These axial and centrifugal flow LVADs are smaller and more durable compared with the pulsatile devices. Reports of studies with large numbers of patients have indicated that these new devices can provide safe long-term support with fewer adverse events than the pulsatile devices.[118,119] Most of the continuous flow devices are undergoing clinical trials, and more information on the use of these devices is forthcoming.

HeartMate II

The HeartMate II (Thoratec Corp) is an implantable axial flow LVAD that is intended for long-term support for BTT and DT in patients with chronic HF. When implanted, the pump resides in a preperitoneal pocket below the left hemidiaphragm, with the inflow cannula in the left ventricle and the outflow graft anastomosed to the ascending aorta. A percutaneous driveline from the pump exits the right upper quadrant of the abdomen. A microprocessor-based controller, worn by

TABLE 8-4	Continuous Flow Mechanical Circulatory Support Systems for Long-Term Support				
Device Name	**Manufacturer**	**Type of Pump**	**Type of Support**	**Pump Position**	
HeartMate II	Thoratec Corp, Pleasanton, CA	Axial flow with blood-immersed bearings	LVAD	Preperitoneal pocket	
Jarvik 2000	Jarvik Heart, Inc, New York, NY	Axial flow with blood-immersed bearings	LVAD	LV	
Synergy	CiruLite, Inc, Saddle Brook, NJ	Axial flow with blood-immersed bearings	LVAD	Chest wall pocket	
INCOR	Berlin Heart, Berlin, Germany	Axial flow with blood-immersed bearings	LVAD	Preperitoneal pocket	
DuraHeart	Terumo Cardiovascular, Ann Arbor, MI	Centrifugal flow; magnetic and hydrodynamic bearings	LVAD	Preperitoneal pocket	
HVAD	HeartWare, Inc, Framingham, MA	Centrifugal flow; magnetic and hydrodynamic bearings	LVAD	Intrapericardial	
Levacor	WorldHeart, Inc, Salt Lake City, UT	Centrifugal flow; magnetic bearings	LVAD	Preperitoneal pocket	

LV, left ventricle; LVAD, left ventricular assist device.

the patient, monitors and controls the pump's function. The device can provide 10 L/min of cardiac output support with a speed operating range of 6000 to 15,000 rpm. The usual operating speed range is 8000 to 10,000 rpm. Power is provided by AC and DC power sources, with wearable batteries for ambulatory operation. A system monitor is used to make changes in pump speed, collect data on device function, and display pump parameters in the acute care setting.

The HeartMate II left ventricular assist system (LVAS) components include the HeartMate II LVAD, system controller, power base unit, system monitor, rechargeable batteries, and battery clips (Fig. 8-17). The HeartMate II LVAD axial flow rotary pump contains a magnet that is rotated by the electromotive force generated by the motor. Rotation of the rotor provides the driving force to propel the blood from the left ventricle through the pump out to the natural circulation. Pump output depends on the rotational speed of the rotor and the pressure difference between the inlet and outlet of the pump making this device, similar to other axial flow pumps, very sensitive to changes in afterload. The primary operating mode of the HeartMate II LVAD is fixed speed control. In fixed speed mode, the device operates at a constant speed, which may be varied via commands from the system monitor under the control of a qualified individual. In fixed speed mode, the set speed can be reduced below the normal range to allow (1) evaluation of the patient under reduced levels of augmented flow or (2) slow start of the pump at implant to reduce risk of air embolism. The patient does not have access to change the fixed speed set-point. The internal pump surfaces (rotor, thin-walled duct, inlet stator, and outlet stator) have a smooth polished titanium surface. The inflow conduit and outflow graft have a textured titanium microsphere surface similar to the textured, blood-contacting surface on the HeartMate XVE system. Although these surfaces are designed to help resist the development of thrombi, anticoagulation is required in all patients.

This device has been the most widely used implantable LVAD in recent years. Large clinical trials for BTT and DT have shown that the use of this device is safe and effective when used for these applications. The BTT clinical trial for the HeartMate II included 489 patients with published results for the initial 133 patients,[119] and an 18-month follow-up analysis was completed in 281 patients.[13] The survival rate at 12 months was 68% in the initial study cohort, and it increased to 73% in the later analysis. The HeartMate II DT trial was a 2:1 randomized comparison with the HeartMate XVE LVAD in 200 patients (HeartMate II, n = 134; HeartMate XVE LVAD, n = 66). In this trial, there were a significantly higher percentage of patients supported by the HeartMate II than the HeartMate XVE LVAD who reached the study endpoint of survival at 2 years free of disabling stroke and reoperation for pump replacement. The actuarial survival rates of 68% at 1 year and 58% at 2 years were significantly better than 55% at 1 year and 24% at 2 years for the HeartMate XVE LVAD. Data in INTERMACS (Interagency Registry for Mechanically Assisted Circulatory Support) show the survival rate for patients supported by the HeartMate II to be near 90%.

Jarvik 2000

The Jarvik 2000 LVAD (Jarvik Heart Inc, New York, NY) is a small axial flow device that has been undergoing clinical trials for BTT for approximately a decade. A unique feature of this device is the positioning of the blood pump within the left ventricular cavity (Fig. 8-18). Outflow from the pump is through a graft that is anastomosed to either the ascending or the descending aorta. A percutaneous driveline that exits the skin in the right upper quadrant of the abdomen provides the means for power and control to the blood pump. An analog controller provides a display of alarm conditions and allows for adjustment of the pump speed from 8000 to 12,000 rpm in increments of 1000. Patients are allowed to make speed changes as their requirement for support changes. There is no method for monitoring the pump flow with this device. The Jarvik LVAD is powered only by DC battery power; AC power sources are needed to recharge batteries. Portable lithium ion batteries are available for ambulatory operation and larger lead-acid batteries are available for nonambulatory use.

Although the clinical trials with this device have not been completed, numerous reports indicate that outcomes have been largely positive.[120–122] Patients have been successfully

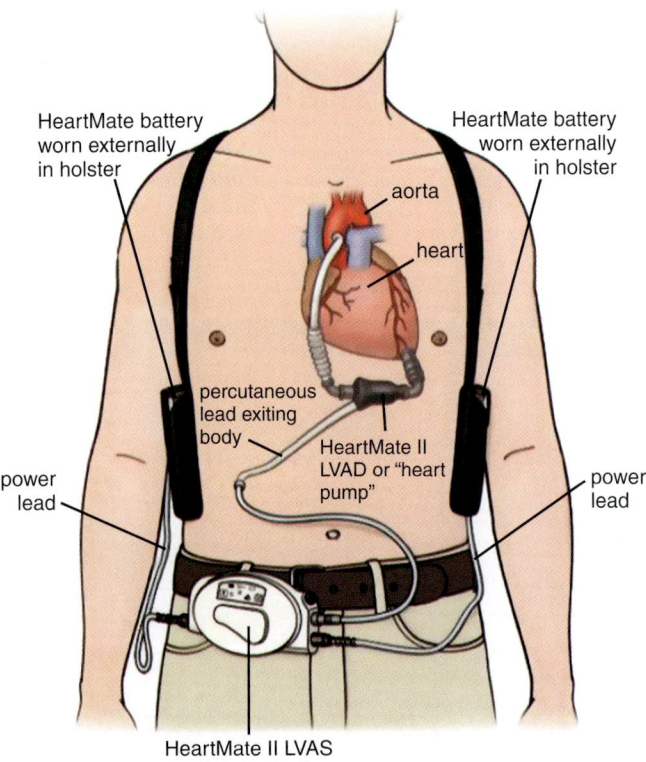

FIGURE 8-17 HeartMate II left ventricular assist system (LVAS). LVAD, left ventricular assist device.

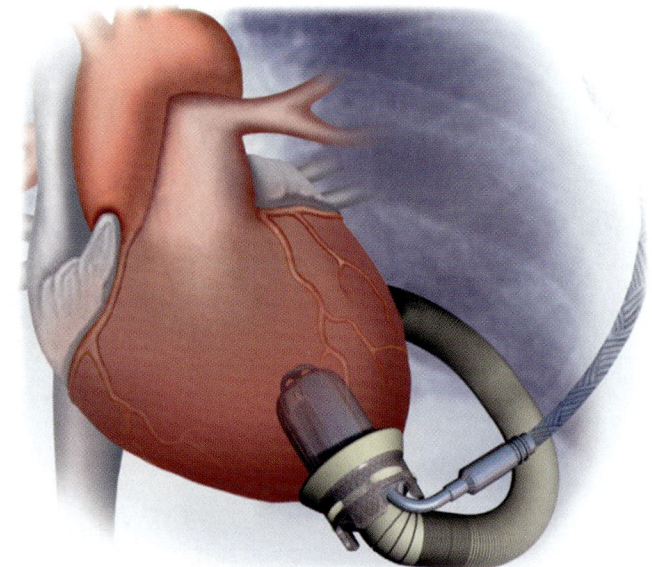

FIGURE 8-18 Implanted Jarvik 2000 left ventricular assist device (LVAD).

supported by this device for durations greater than 7 years with no device failures, and the mean survival time for patients supported for DT is 402 days.[123] A unique skull-pedestal power cable connector appears to allow for long-term use with a low incidence of driveline infections. An early report described an observed high incidence of gastrointestinal bleeding in patients supported by this device,[124] and this observation was later made in patients supported by the HeartMate II.[125] Detailed analysis of patients supported by axial flow devices indicates that the gastrointestinal bleeding is related to acquired von Willebrand disease.[126–128] This form of von Willebrand disease is shear-induced and may be a characteristic of continuous flow devices.

HVAD

The HeartWare Ventricular Assist Device (HVAD) (HeartWare, Inc, Framingham, MA) is a centrifugal flow pump that is implanted in the pericardial space at the apex or diaphragmatic surface of the left ventricle (Fig. 8-19). The HeartWare system is intended for use as BTT in patients with end-stage HF. It is designed for in-hospital and out-of-hospital use. A short integrated inflow cannula and the small size of the pump allow for the pericardial positioning and avoidance of a pump pocket.

The HeartWare system consists of the following major components: HVAD pump, HeartWare controller with rechargeable batteries, and HeartWare monitor. The HeartWare blood pump (HVAD pump) incorporates an integrated inflow cannula, a 10-mm gel-impregnated polyester outflow graft with strain relief, a percutaneous driveline, and an apical sewing ring. Strain relief is used in conjunction with the outflow graft to prevent kinking. The driveline is wrapped with woven polyester fabric to encourage tissue ingrowth at the skin exit site.

The HVAD pump has a displaced volume of 50 mL and weighs 140 g. The pump has one moving part, an impeller that can generate 10 L/min of flow and has a pump speed operating range of 1800 to 4000 rpm. The impeller has integrated motor magnets and uses a passive, noncontacting suspension system for rotation of the impeller.[129] A hermetically sealed electric motor within the pump housing generates electromagnetic fields to move the impeller with dual motor stators. The frictionless movement of the impeller eliminates heat generation and wear of the components. A short integrated inflow cannula is inserted into the left ventricle, and the outflow graft connects the HVAD pump to the ascending aorta through an end-to-side anastomosis. A sewing ring secures the pump to the left ventricle.

An external microprocessor-based system controller, which is connected to the pump by a percutaneous driveline, controls and monitors the implanted device. Suction detection and alternating speed modes are automatically regulated by the controller, but their use is determined by the operator. A light-emitting diode display on the controller provides information on pump-operating parameters and alarm conditions. A system monitor is used to make changes in operating parameters and for collection of data regarding pump function. The device can be operated with AC or DC power sources. Lithium-ion batteries are used during ambulatory operation, and an automobile DC adapter allows for extended travel time.

The HVAD is a new LVAD that is undergoing international clinical trials for BTT and DT. This device has been used for BTR and for long-term biventricular support.[130,131] Initial clinical reports have indicated that long-term support with this device has been safe and effective with a 1-year survival rate of 86% in BTT patients.[132] The potential clinical advantage of this device is a reduction in bleeding and infection complications owing to its small size and placement in the pericardial space. Avoidance of an abdominal pump pocket minimizes surgery and eliminates complications associated with abdominally placed LVADs. At the time of this writing in 2011, the results of clinical trials are pending, and assessment of the potential benefits is inconclusive.

DuraHeart

The Terumo DuraHeart LVAS (Terumo Heart, Inc, Ann Arbor, MI) includes a centrifugal flow pump with magnetic and hydrodynamic bearings for frictionless impeller rotation (Fig. 8-20).[133] The DuraHeart magnetically levitated centrifugal LVAS is designed for long-term circulatory support in patients with late-stage HF and is initially used as MCS as BTT in patients who are at risk of death from end-stage left

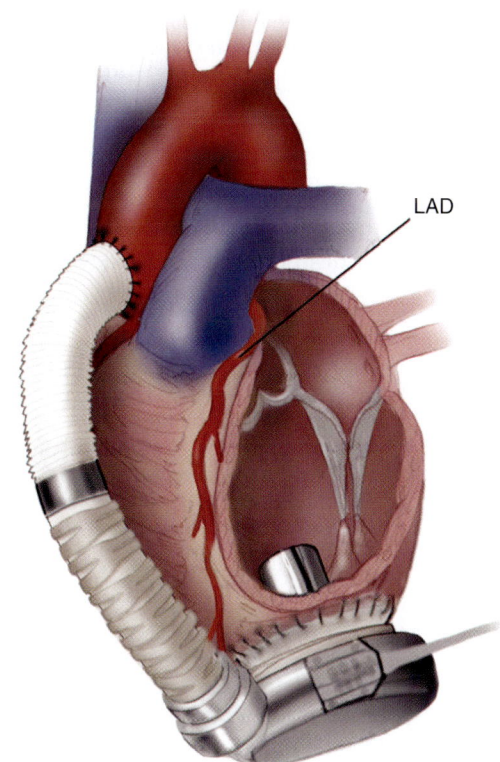

FIGURE 8-19 Implanted HeartWare HVAD. LAD, left anterior descending (artery).

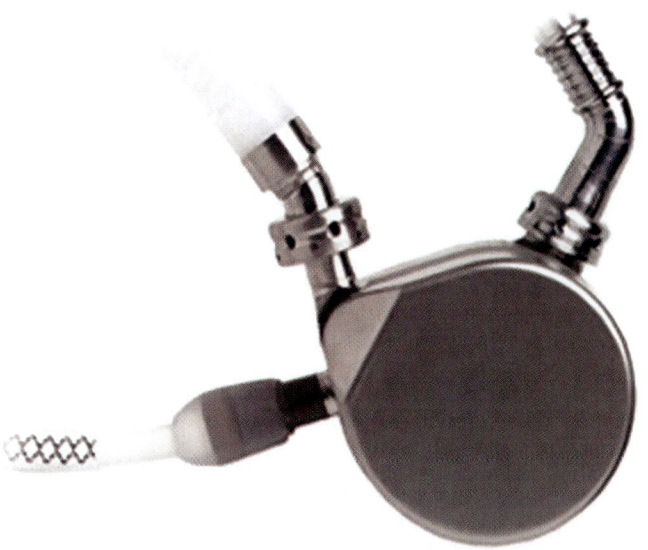

FIGURE 8-20 Terumo DuraHeart left ventricular assist device (LVAD).

ventricular failure. The DuraHeart LVAS is suitable for use inside and outside of the hospital.

Made of titanium, the DuraHeart centrifugal pump employs magnetic levitation to achieve friction-free blood propulsion. Through electromagnets and position sensors, the impeller is rigidly suspended within the blood chamber, leaving a 500-μm gap between the impeller and the device housing. Secondary blood flow around the impeller assists washout to eliminate areas of stasis that may lead to thrombus formation. The DuraHeart pump is 73 mm in diameter and 46.2 mm thick and weighs approximately 540 g. The impeller rotational speed range is 1200 to 2400 rpm, which generates continuous blood flow of 2.0 to 9.0 L/min. The internal surface of the pump is coated with covalently bonded heparin. The pump is positioned in a subdiaphragmatic abdominal pocket with a titanium inflow conduit in the left ventricle and an outflow graft anastomosed to the ascending aorta. The inflow cannula is available in various lengths to accommodate patients of different sizes. The outflow conduit measures 350 mm long and has a 14-mm outer diameter and a 12-mm inner diameter. It incorporates a 12-mm Vascutek Gelweave graft (Terumo Cardiovascular Systems, Ann Arbor, MI), a polyethylene reinforcement sleeve, and a titanium connector. During system implantation, the graft is anastomosed to the aorta and secured to the outflow port of the pump using the DuraHeart wrench. A percutaneous lead is attached to an external controller that controls and monitors the pump, and it stores data on multiple operating parameters. The controller can be connected to the patient's bedside monitor for a continuous display of pump function parameters. A pair of batteries provides 4 to 5 hours of continuous ambulatory operation.

Initial clinical studies with the DuraHeart LVAS for BTT and DT have shown that this device provides adequate hemodynamic support with a low incidence of thromboembolism and hemolysis. Results of the European clinical experiences as of July 31, 2009, showed survival at 18 months to be 73%. Stroke-free survival at 1 year and 2 years in the trial (33 patients) was 94% for the last 22 patients after implementing a less intensive anticoagulation and antiplatelet regimen.[133-135] The DuraHeart LVAS is the only device of its kind that combines a centrifugal pump with magnetic impeller levitation and is designed for long-term durability. There have been no reported pump failures. The low operating speed range seems to minimize blood trauma from shear stress, the power requirements are low, and device wear has not occurred. The heparin-coated surface also seems to result in a low thromboembolic rate; however, patients are routinely anticoagulated with heparin or warfarin (Coumadin) and aspirin. The target international normalized ratio is 2 to 3. More complete results from ongoing clinical trials are pending.

INCOR

The INCOR LVAD (Berlin Heart AG, Berlin, Germany) is an implantable pump that is intended for long-term support for BTT or DT (Fig. 8-21). The unique design feature of this axial flow pump is the contact-free impeller, which differs from other axial flow pumps that use blood-immersed bearings. The pump has a displacement volume of 82 mL and weighs 200 g. Active and passive magnetic force is used to suspend and rotate the impeller along the axis of the cylindrical pump housing. The operational impeller speed range is 5000 to 10,000 rpm. The pump is positioned below the left hemidiaphragm in a pump pocket with the inflow in the left ventricle, and the outflow is attached to the ascending aorta. The blood-contacting surfaces are heparin-coated to reduce thrombogenicity. A percutaneous driveline connects to an external controller that monitors and controls the function of the implanted pump. The device can be powered by AC and DC sources, with small batteries for portable operation. A laptop computer interfaced with the controller may be used to set operating parameters.

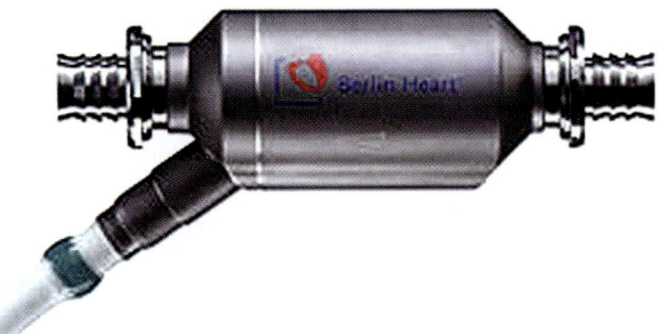

FIGURE 8-21 Berlin INCOR left ventricular assist device (LVAD).

The INCOR device was developed for long-term support and has been used for DT, BTT, and BTR.[136-138] This device has been used mainly in Europe and has not been tested in controlled trials. Clinical results indicate that hemodynamic support, incidence of adverse events, and outcomes are similar to other axial flow and pulsatile LVADs.[138-140]

Synergy Micropump

The Synergy micropump (CircuLite, Inc, Saddle Brook, NJ) is a very small LVAD that can provide 3 L/min of blood flow from the left atrium to the subclavian artery. The concept of support with this device is to provide partial cardiac output support for patients who have chronic HF but do not require complete left ventricular support. Candidates for this device are in New York Heart Association class IIIb or IV HF and are INTERMACS category of 2 or greater. The pump is approximately the size of a AA battery, has an outer diameter of 14 mm, and weighs 25 g. The pump is implanted subcutaneously in a pocket about the size of a typical pacemaker pocket. The Synergy micropump generates axial, centrifugal, and orthogonal flow paths with a single-stage impeller that is powered by an integrated brushless microelectric motor (Fig. 8-22). A rechargeable dual battery pack system and controller provide control and power to the implanted device. The batteries weigh 3.3 lb and power the system for approximately 16 to 18 hours. The controller provides information on the battery status and alerts the patient to any problems. The micropump is connected to the power system via a percutaneous lead that exits the body in the abdominal area.

A feasibility study was conducted in 17 patients who were supported for a mean duration of 81 days (range 6 to 213 days).[141] In this initial study group, three patients died, nine patients underwent transplant, four patients had support ongoing, and one patient required conversion to a biventricular VAD. Of the 17 patients, 13 were discharged from the hospital while supported by the Synergy micropump. Assessment of postoperative hemodynamic parameters showed a significant improvement ($P < .001$) in the cardiac index. The only device-related adverse events that were noted were pump pocket hematoma in three cases. The preliminary studies are encouraging, and larger controlled trials are ongoing.

Levacor

The Levacor VAD (Worldheart Corp, Salt Lake City, UT) is the most recent MCS device to be introduced clinically (Fig. 8-23). The centrifugal flow pump is positioned in an abdominal pocket and pumps blood from the left ventricle to the ascending aorta. The titanium pump contains a magnetically levitated impeller that rotates with friction. The outer surface of the inflow cannula is covered with titanium microspheres to create a textured surface to allow cellular

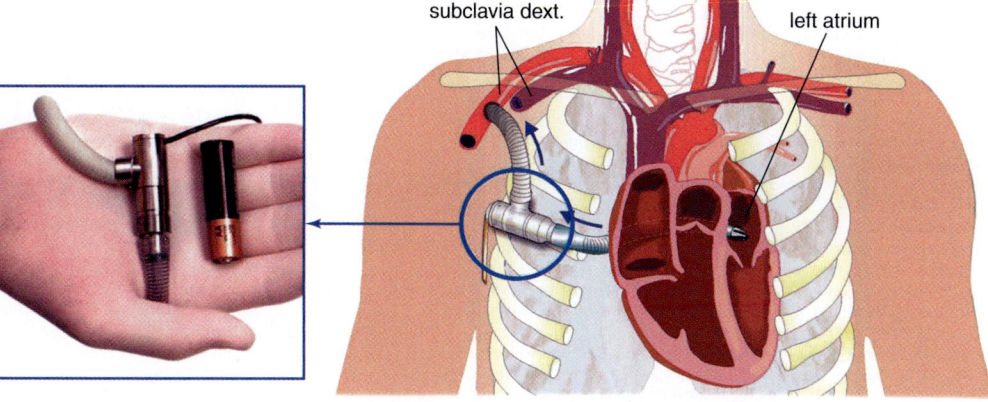

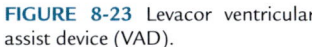

FIGURE 8-22 CircuLite Synergy left ventricular assist device (LVAD).

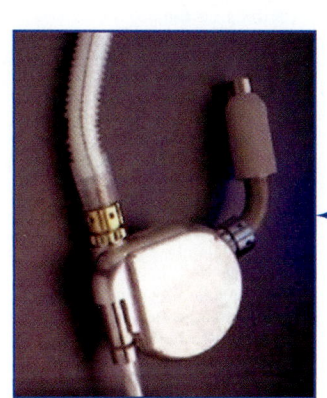

FIGURE 8-23 Levacor ventricular assist device (VAD).

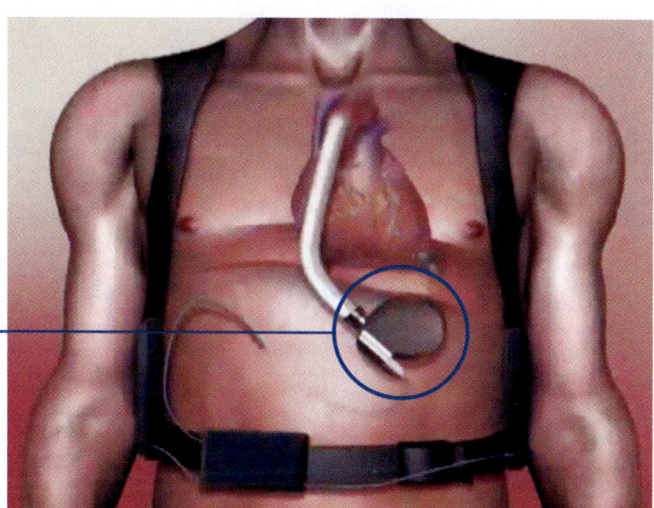

adhesion and to promote fixation within the left ventricle. A percutaneous lead connects to the external controller that provides the power and control to the implanted pump. A switch on the controller allows the patient to choose one of three preset speed settings. An automatic control mode is used to prevent suction in the left ventricle and may be used later to respond to changes in patient cardiac output needs. The device can be powered by AC or DC power sources and is designed for ambulatory operation. The initial clinical trials with the Levacor VAD are ongoing, but little has been published on the results to date. Anecdotal experience has been positive.[142,143]

SUMMARY

Various devices are available for short-term and long-term MCS that can be used to support a wide range of patients with severe HF. Continued research and development with MCS technology should allow for safer and longer use in the future. In the absence of an ideal MCS that may be used for all HF cases, hybrid use and bridge to bridge with different devices seem to provide some patients with the best opportunity for long-term survival. As clinical experience progresses and as more devices become available, more patients with HF are expected to be treated with MCS. Increased availability in regions where the incidence of HF deaths is high is essential to revealing the potential impact of MCS on the growing population of patients with HF.

REFERENCES

1. Holman WL, Teitel ER, Itescu S. Biologic barriers to mechanical circulatory support. In: Frazier OH, Kirklin JK, eds. *Ishlt Monograph Series*. New York: Elsevier; 2006:9–32.
2. Dennis C, Gorayeb EJ, Iticovici HN, et al. The artificial heart-lung apparatus, experimental creation and repair of interventricular septal defects. *Surg Forum*. 1956;6:185–189.
3. Gibbon Jr JH. Application of a mechanical heart and lung apparatus to cardiac surgery. *Minn Med*. 1954;37:171–185.
4. Kantrowitz A, Tjonneland S, Krakauer J, et al. Clinical experience with cardiac assistance by means of intraaortic phase-shift balloon pumping. *Trans Am Soc Artif Intern Organs*. 1968;14:344–348.
5. Liotta D, Hall CW, Henly WS, et al. Prolonged assisted circulation during and after cardiac or aortic surgery: prolonged partial left ventricular bypass by means of intracorporeal circulation. *Am J Cardiol*. 1963;12:399–405.
6. DeBakey ME. Left ventricular bypass pump for cardiac assistance: clinical experience. *Am J Cardiol*. 1971;27:3–11.
7. Cooley DA, Liotta D, Hallman GL, et al. Orthotopic cardiac prosthesis for two-staged cardiac replacement. *Am J Cardiol*. 1969;24:723–730.
8. Szycher M, Clay W, Gernes D, et al. Thermedics' approach to ventricular support systems. *J Biomater Appl*. 1986;1:39–105.
9. Gunby P. Utah group to implant "Jarvik 7" heart soon. *JAMA*. 1982;248:1944–1946.
10. Copeland JG, Smith RG, Icenogle TB, et al. Early experience with the total artificial heart as a bridge to cardiac transplantation. *Surg Clin North Am*. 1988;68:621–634.
11. Frazier OH, Nakatani T, Duncan JM, et al. Clinical experience with the hemopump. *ASAIO Trans*. 1989;35:604–606.
12. Wieblalck AC, Wouters PF, Waldenberger FR, et al. Left ventricular assist with an axial flow pump (hemopump): clinical application. *Ann Thorac Surg*. 1993;55:1141–1146.
13. Pagani FD, Miller LW, Russell SD, et al. HeartMate III: extended mechanical circulatory support with a continuous-flow rotary left ventricular assist device. *J Am Coll Cardiol*. 2009;54:312–321.
14. Kormos RL, Teuteberg JJ, Pagani FD, et al. Right ventricular failure in patients with the HeartMate II continuous flow left ventricular assist device: incidence, risk factors, and impact on outcomes. *J Thorac Cardiovasc Surg*. 2010;139:1316–1324.
15. Aggarwal S, Slaughter MS. Acute myocardial infarction complicated by cardiogenic shock: role of mechanical circulatory support. *Expert Rev Cardiovasc Ther*. 2008;6:1223–1235.

16. Kirklin JK, Naftel DC, Kormos RL, et al. Second INTERMACS annual report: more than 1,000 primary left ventricular assist device implants. *J Heart Lung Transplant.* 2010;29:1–10.
17. Saeed D, Kizner L, Arusoglu L, et al. Prolonged transcutaneous cardiopulmonary support for postcardiotomy cardiogenic shock. *ASAIO J.* 2007;53:e1–e3.
18. Hoefer D, Ruttmann E, Poelzl G, et al. Outcome evaluation of the bridge-to-bridge concept in patients with cardiogenic shock. *Ann Thorac Surg.* 2006;82:28–33.
19. John R, Liao K, Lietz K, et al. Experience with the Levitronix Centrimag circulatory support system as a bridge to decision in patients with refractory acute cardiogenic shock and multisystem organ failure. *J Thorac Cardiovasc Surg.* 2007;134:351–358.
20. Gregoric ID, Jacob LP, La Francesca S, et al. The TandemHeart as a bridge to a long-term axial-flow left ventricular assist device (bridge to bridge). *Tex Heart Inst J.* 2008;35:125–129.
21. Bruckner BA, Jacob LP, Gregoric ID, et al. Clinical experience with the TandemHeart percutaneous ventricular assist device as a bridge to cardiac transplantation. *Tex Heart Inst J.* 2008;35:447–450.
22. Reverdin S, Gregoric ID, Kar B, et al. Bridge to transplantation with the TandemHeart: bending the indications in a chronic aortic dissection patient with postcardiotomy shock. *Tex Heart Inst J.* 2008;35:340–341.
23. Kantrowitz A, Tjonneland S, Freed PS, et al. Initial clinical experience with intraaortic balloon pumping in cardiogenic shock. *JAMA.* 1968;203:113–118.
24. *National Hospital Discharge Survey: 2002 annual summary with detailed diagnosis and procedural data.* National Center for Health Statistics; 2002.
25. Sarnoff SJ, Braunwald E, Welch Jr GH, et al. Hemodynamic determinants of oxygen consumption of the heart with special reference to the tension-time index. *Am J Physiol.* 1958;192:148–156.
26. Gutterman DD, Cowley Jr AW. Relating cardiac performance with oxygen consumption: historical observations continue to spawn scientific discovery. *Am J Physiol Heart Circ Physiol.* 2006;291:H2555–H2556.
27. Cohen M, Urban P, Christenson JT, et al. Intra-aortic balloon counterpulsation in US and non-US centres: results of the benchmark registry. *Eur Heart J.* 2003;24:1763–1770.
28. Ferguson 3rd JJ, Cohen M, Freedman Jr RJ, et al. The current practice of intra-aortic balloon counterpulsation: results from the benchmark registry. *J Am Coll Cardiol.* 2001;38:1456–1462.
29. Sanborn TA, Sleeper LA, Bates ER, et al. Impact of thrombolysis, intra-aortic balloon pump counterpulsation, and their combination in cardiogenic shock complicating acute myocardial infarction: a report from the shock trial registry. Should we emergently revascularize occluded coronaries for cardiogenic shock? *J Am Coll Cardiol.* 2000;36:1123–1129.
30. Barron HV, Every NR, Parsons LS, et al. The use of intra-aortic balloon counterpulsation in patients with cardiogenic shock complicating acute myocardial infarction: data from the National Registry of Myocardial Infarction 2. *Am Heart J.* 2001;141:933–939.
31. Trost JC, Hillis LD. Intra-aortic balloon counterpulsation. *Am J Cardiol.* 2006; 97:1391–1398.
32. Sjauw KD, Engstrom AE, Vis MM, et al. A systematic review and meta-analysis of intra-aortic balloon pump therapy in ST-elevation myocardial infarction: should we change the guidelines? *Eur Heart J.* 2009;30:459–468.
33. Christenson JT, Cohen M, Ferguson 3rd JJ, et al. Trends in intraaortic balloon counterpulsation complications and outcomes in cardiac surgery. *Ann Thorac Surg.* 2002;74:1086–1090.
34. Hill JD, Rodvien R, Snider MT, et al. Clinical extracorporeal membrane oxygenation for acute respiratory insufficiency. *Trans Am Soc Artif Intern Organs.* 1978;24:753–763.
35. Pennington DG, Merjavy JP, Codd JE, et al. Extracorporeal membrane oxygenation for patients with cardiogenic shock. *Circulation.* 1984;70:I130–I137.
36. Chen JS, Ko WJ, Yu HY, et al. Analysis of the outcome for patients experiencing myocardial infarction and cardiopulmonary resuscitation refractory to conventional therapies necessitating extracorporeal life support rescue. *Crit Care Med.* 2006;34:950–957.
37. Pagani FD, Aaronson KD, Dyke DB, et al. Assessment of an extracorporeal life support to LVAD bridge to heart transplant strategy. *Ann Thorac Surg.* 2000;70:1977–1984.
38. Pagani FD, Aaronson KD, Swaniker F, et al. The use of extracorporeal life support in adult patients with primary cardiac failure as a bridge to implantable left ventricular assist device. *Ann Thorac Surg.* 2001;71:S77–S81.
39. Rastan AJ, Dege A, Mohr M, et al. Early and late outcomes of 517 consecutive adult patients treated with extracorporeal membrane oxygenation for refractory postcardiotomy cardiogenic shock. *J Thorac Cardiovasc Surg.* 2010;139:302–311.
40. Cardarelli MG, Young AJ, Griffith B. Use of extracorporeal membrane oxygenation for adults in cardiac arrest (E-CPR): a meta-analysis of observational studies. *ASAIO J.* 2009;55:581–586.
41. Smith C, Bellomo R, Raman JS, et al. An extracorporeal membrane oxygenation-based approach to cardiogenic shock in an older population. *Ann Thorac Surg.* 2001;71:1421–1427.
42. Haft JW, Pagani FD, Romano MA, et al. Short- and long-term survival of patients transferred to a tertiary care center on temporary extracorporeal circulatory support. *Ann Thorac Surg.* 2009;88:711–717.
43. Wu MY, Lin PJ, Tsai FC, et al. Postcardiotomy extracorporeal life support in adults: the optimal duration of bridging to recovery. *ASAIO J.* 2009;55:608–613.
44. Smedira NG, Moazami N, Golding CM, et al. Clinical experience with 202 adults receiving extracorporeal membrane oxygenation for cardiac failure: survival at five years. *J Thorac Cardiovasc Surg.* 2001;122:92–102.
45. Combes A, Leprince P, Luyt CE, et al. Outcomes and long-term quality-of-life of patients supported by extracorporeal membrane oxygenation for refractory cardiogenic shock. *Crit Care Med.* 2008;36:1404–1411.
46. Granfeldt H, Hellgren L, Dellgren G, et al. Experience with the Impella recovery axial-flow system for acute heart failure at three cardiothoracic centers in Sweden. *Scand Cardiovasc J.* 2009;43:233–239.
47. Lauten A, Franke U, Strauch JT, et al. Postcardiotomy failure after Ross operation: implantation of intravascular flow pump through pulmonary autograft. *Thorac Cardiovasc Surg.* 2007;55:399–400.
48. Siegenthaler MP, Brehm K, Strecker T, et al. The Impella recover microaxial left ventricular assist device reduces mortality for postcardiotomy failure: a three-center experience. *J Thorac Cardiovasc Surg.* 2004;127:812–822.
49. Jurmann MJ, Siniawski H, Erb M, et al. Initial experience with miniature axial flow ventricular assist devices for postcardiotomy heart failure. *Ann Thorac Surg.* 2004;77:1642–1647.
50. Patane F, Centofanti P, Zingarelli E, et al. Potential role of the Impella recover left ventricular assist device in the management of postinfarct ventricular septal defect. *J Thorac Cardiovasc Surg.* 2009;137:1288–1289.
51. Gupta A, Allaqaband S, Bajwa T. Combined use of Impella device and intra-aortic balloon pump to improve survival in a patient in profound cardiogenic shock post cardiac arrest. *Cathet Cardiovasc Interv.* 2009;74:975–976.
52. Cheng JM, den Uil CA, Hoeks SE, et al. Percutaneous left ventricular assist devices vs. intra-aortic balloon pump counterpulsation for treatment of cardiogenic shock: a meta-analysis of controlled trials. *Eur Heart J.* 2009;30:2102–2108.
53. Windecker S. Percutaneous left ventricular assist devices for treatment of patients with cardiogenic shock. *Curr Opin Crit Care.* 2007;13:521–527.
54. Meyns B, Stolinski J, Leunens V, et al. Left ventricular support by catheter-mounted axial flow pump reduces infarct size. *J Am Coll Cardiol.* 2003;41:1087–1095.
55. Garatti A, Colombo T, Russo C, et al. Different applications for left ventricular mechanical support with the Impella Recover 100 microaxial blood pump. *J Heart Lung Transplant.* 2005;24:481–485.
56. Colombo T, Garatti A, Bruschi G, et al. First successful bridge to recovery with the Impella Recover 100 left ventricular assist device for fulminant acute myocarditis. *Ital Heart J.* 2003;4:642–645.
57. Rajagopal V, Steahr G, Wilmer CI, et al. A novel percutaneous mechanical biventricular bridge to recovery in severe cardiac allograft rejection. *J Heart Lung Transplant.* 2010;29:93–95.
58. Beyer AT, Hui PY, Hauesslein E. The Impella 2.5 l for percutaneous mechanical circulatory support in severe humeral allograft rejection. *J Invasive Cardiol.* 2010;22:E37–E39.
59. Thiele H, Sick P, Boudriot E, et al. Randomized comparison of intra-aortic balloon support with a percutaneous left ventricular assist device in patients with revascularized acute myocardial infarction complicated by cardiogenic shock. *Eur Heart J.* 2005;26:1276–1283.
60. Seyfarth M, Sibbing D, Bauer I, et al. A randomized clinical trial to evaluate the safety and efficacy of a percutaneous left ventricular assist device versus intra-aortic balloon pumping for treatment of cardiogenic shock caused by myocardial infarction. *J Am Coll Cardiol.* 2008;52:1584–1588.
61. Dixon SR, Henriques JP, Mauri L, et al. A prospective feasibility trial investigating the use of the Impella 2.5 system in patients undergoing high-risk percutaneous coronary intervention (the PROTECT I trial): initial U.S. experience. *JACC Cardiovasc Interv.* 2009;2:91–96.
62. Kar B, Adkins LE, Civitello AB, et al. Clinical experience with the TandemHeart percutaneous ventricular assist device. *Tex Heart Inst J.* 2006;33:111–115.
63. Gregoric ID, Loyalka P, Radovancevic R, et al. TandemHeart as a rescue therapy for patients with critical aortic valve stenosis. *Ann Thorac Surg.* 2009;88:1822–1826.
64. Solomon H, Lim DS, Ragosta M. Percutaneous ventricular assist device to rescue a patient with profound shock from a thrombosed prosthetic mitral valve. *J Invasive Cardiol.* 2008;20:E320–E323.
65. Burkhoff D, O'Neill W, Brunckhorst C, et al. Feasibility study of the use of the TandemHeart percutaneous ventricular assist device for treatment of cardiogenic shock. *Catheter Cardiovasc Interv.* 2006;68:211–217.
66. Aragon J, Lee MS, Kar S, et al. Percutaneous left ventricular assist device: "TandemHeart" for high-risk coronary intervention. *Catheter Cardiovasc Interv.* 2005;65:346–352.
67. Kar B, Forrester M, Gemmato C, et al. Use of the TandemHeart percutaneous ventricular assist device to support patients undergoing high-risk percutaneous coronary intervention. *J Invasive Cardiol.* 2006;18:93–96.
68. Vranckx P, Schultz CJ, Valgimigli M, et al. Assisted circulation using the TandemHeart during very high-risk PCI of the unprotected left main coronary artery in patients declined for CABG. *Catheter Cardiovasc Interv.* 2009;74:302–310.
69. Burkhoff D, Cohen H, Brunckhorst C, et al. TandemHeart investigators group. A randomized multicenter clinical study to evaluate the safety and efficacy of the TandemHeart percutaneous ventricular assist device versus conventional therapy with intraaortic balloon pumping for treatment of cardiogenic shock. *Am Heart J.* 2006;152:e461–e468.
70. Gregoric ID, Bruckner BA, Jacob L, et al. Techniques and complications of TandemHeart ventricular assist device insertion during cardiac procedures. *ASAIO J.* 2009;55:251–254.
71. Pitsis AA, Visouli AN, Burkhoff D, et al. Feasibility study of a temporary percutaneous left ventricular assist device in cardiac surgery. *Ann Thorac Surg.* 2007;84:1993–1999.
72. Cohn WE, Morris CD, Reverdin S, et al. Intraoperative TandemHeart implantation as an adjunct to high-risk valve surgery. *Tex Heart Inst J.* 2007;34:457–458.
73. Brinkman WT, Rosenthal JE, Eichhorn E, et al. Role of a percutaneous ventricular assist device in decision making for a cardiac transplant program. *Ann Thorac Surg.* 2009;88:1462–1466.
74. Khalife WI, Kar B. The TandemHeart PVAD in the treatment of acute fulminant myocarditis. *Tex Heart Inst J.* 2007;34:209–213.
75. Chandra D, Kar B, Idelchik G, et al. Usefulness of percutaneous left ventricular assist device as a bridge to recovery from myocarditis. *Am J Cardiol.* 2007;99:1755–1756.
76. Lee MS, Makkar RR. Percutaneous left ventricular support devices. *Cardiol Clin.* 2006;24:265–275.
77. Loforte A, Montalto A, Lilla Della Monica P, et al. Simultaneous temporary CentriMag right ventricular assist device placement in HeartMate II left ventricular assist system recipients at high risk of right ventricular failure. *Interact Cardiovasc Thorac Surg.* 2010;10:847–850.
78. Jaroszewski DE, Marranca MC, Pierce CN, et al. Successive circulatory support stages: a triple bridge to recovery from fulminant myocarditis. *J Heart Lung Transplant.* 2009;28:984–986.

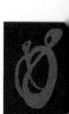

79. Bhama JK, Kormos RL, Toyoda Y, et al. Clinical experience using the Levitronix Centrimag system for temporary right ventricular mechanical circulatory support. *J Heart Lung Transplant*. 2009;28:971–976.

80. Shuhaiber JH, Jenkins D, Berman M, et al. The Papworth experience with the Levitronix Centrimag ventricular assist device. *J Heart Lung Transplant*. 2008;27:158–164.

81. Khan NU, Al-Aloul M, Shah R, et al. Early experience with the Levitronix Centrimag device for extra-corporeal membrane oxygenation following lung transplantation. *Eur J Cardiothorac Surg*. 2008;34:1262–1264.

82. Favaloro RR, Bertolotti A, Diez M, et al. Adequate systemic perfusion maintained by a Centrimag during acute heart failure. *Tex Heart Inst J*. 2008;35:334–339.

83. Santise G, Petrou M, Pepper JR, et al. Levitronix as a short-term salvage treatment for primary graft failure after heart transplantation. *J Heart Lung Transplant*. 2006;25:495–498.

84. Kouretas PC, Kaza AK, Burch PT, et al. Experience with the Levitronix Centrimag in the pediatric population as a bridge to decision and recovery. *Artif Organs*. 2009;33:1002–1004.

85. Haj-Yahia S, Birks EJ, Amrani M, et al. Bridging patients after salvage from bridge to decision directly to transplant by means of prolonged support with the Centrimag short-term centrifugal pump. *J Thorac Cardiovasc Surg*. 2009;138:227–230.

86. De Robertis F, Rogers P, Amrani M, et al. Bridge to decision using the Levitronix Centrimag short-term ventricular assist device. *J Heart Lung Transplant*. 2008;27:474–478.

87. Morgan JA, Stewart AS, Lee BJ, et al. Role of the Abiomed BVS 5000 device for short-term support and bridge to transplantation. *ASAIO J*. 2004;50:360–363.

88. Samuels LE, Holmes EC, Thomas MP, et al. Management of acute cardiac failure with mechanical assist: experience with the Abiomed BVS 5000. *Ann Thorac Surg*. 2001;71:S67–S72.

89. Petrofski JA, Patel VS, Russell SD, et al. BVS5000 support after cardiac transplantation. *J Thorac Cardiovasc Surg*. 2003;126:442–447.

90. Jett GK. Abiomed BVS 5000: experience and potential advantages. *Ann Thorac Surg*. 1996;61:301–304.

91. Anderson M, Smedira N, Samuels L, et al. Use of the AB5000 ventricular assist device in cardiogenic shock after acute myocardial infarction. *Ann Thorac Surg*. 2010;90:706–712.

92. Samuels LE, Kaufman MS, Morris RJ, et al. Pharmacologic criteria for ventricular assist device insertion: experience with the Abiomed BVS 5000 system. *J Cardiac Surg*. 1999;14:288–293.

93. Hausmann H, Potapov EV, Koster A, et al. Predictors of survival one hour after implantation of an intra-aortic balloon pump in cardiac surgery. *J Card Surg*. 2001;16:72–77.

94. Samuels LE, Darze ES. Management of acute cardiogenic shock. *Cardiol Clin*. 2003;21:43–49.

95. Samuels LE, Thomas MP, Morris RJ, et al. Alternative sites for Abiomed BVS5000 left ventricular assist device implantation. *J Congest Heart Fail Circ Support*. 1999;1:85–89.

96. Anderson MB, Plate JM, Krause TJ, et al. Peripheral arterial cannulation for Abiomed BVS 5000 left ventricular assist device support. *J Heart Lung Transplant*. 2005;24:1445.

97. Akhter SA, Raman J, Jeevanandam V. Technique for left ventricular apical cannulation for short-term mechanical circulatory support. *Ann Thorac Surg*. 2010;89:994–995.

98. Leyvi G, Taylor DG, Hong S, et al. Intraoperative off-bypass management of the Abiomed AB5000 ventricle. *J Cardiothorac Vasc Anesth*. 2005;19:76–78.

99. Jett GK. Atrial cannulation for left ventricular assistance: superiority of the dome approach. *Ann Thorac Surg*. 1996;61:1014–1015.

100. Samuels LE, Entwistle 3rd JC, Holmes EC, et al. Mechanical support of the unrepaired post-infarction VSD with the Abiomed BVS 5000. *J Thorac Cardiovasc Surg*. 2003;126:2100–2101.

101. Tsukui H, Teuteberg JJ, Murali S, et al. Biventricular assist device utilization for patients with morbid congestive heart failure: A justifiable strategy. *Circulation*. 2005;112:165–172.

102. Zhang L, Kapetanakis EI, Cooke RH, et al. Bi-ventricular circulatory support with the Abiomed AB5000 in a patient with idiopathic refractory ventricular fibrillation. *Ann Thorac Surg*. 2007;83:298–300.

103. Kormos RL, Gasior T, Antaki J, et al. Evaluation of right ventricular function during clinical left ventricular assistance. *ASAIO Trans*. 1989;35:554–560.

104. Rose EA, Levin HR, Oz MC, et al. Artificial circulatory support with textured interior surfaces: a counterintuitive approach to minimizing thromboembolism. *Circulation*. 1994;90:II87–II91.

105. John R, Lietz K, Burke E, et al. Intravenous immunoglobulin reduces anti-HLA alloreactivity and shortens waiting time to cardiac transplantation in highly sensitized left ventricular assist device recipients. *Circulation*. 1999;100:II229–II235.

106. Ankersmit HJ, Edwards NM, Schuster M, et al. Quantitative changes in T-cell populations after left ventricular assist device implantation: relationship to T-cell apoptosis and soluble CD95. *Circulation*. 1999;100:II211–II215.

107. Frazier OH, Rose EA, Oz MC, et al. Multicenter clinical evaluation of the HeartMate vented electric left ventricular assist system in patients awaiting heart transplantation. *J Thorac Cardiovasc Surg*. 2001;122:1186–1195.

108. Rose EA, Gelijns AC, Moskowitz AJ, et al. Long-term mechanical left ventricular assistance for end-stage heart failure. *N Engl J Med*. 2001;345:1435–1443.

109. El-Banayosy A, Korfer R, Arusoglu L, et al. Bridging to cardiac transplantation with the Thoratec ventricular assist device. *Thorac Cardiovasc Surg*. 1999;47(suppl 2):307–310.

110. Farrar DJ. The Thoratec ventricular assist device: a paracorporeal pump for treating acute and chronic heart failure. *Semin Thorac Cardiovasc Surg*. 2000;12:243–250.

111. Fitzpatrick 3rd JR, Frederick JR, Hiesinger W, et al. Early planned institution of biventricular mechanical circulatory support results in improved outcomes compared with delayed conversion of a left ventricular assist device to a biventricular assist device. *J Thorac Cardiovasc Surg*. 2009;137:971–977.

112. Farrar DJ, Holman WR, McBride LR, et al. Long-term follow-up of Thoratec ventricular assist device bridge-to-recovery patients successfully removed from support after recovery of ventricular function. *J Heart Lung Transplant*. 2002;21:516–521.

113. Slaughter MS, Tsui SS, El-Banayosy A, et al. Results of a multicenter clinical trial with the Thoratec implantable ventricular assist device. *J Thorac Cardiovasc Surg*. 2007;133:1573–1580.

114. Samuels LE, Holmes EC, Hagan K, et al. The Thoratec implantable ventricular assist device (IVAD): initial clinical experience. *Heart Surg Forum*. 2006;9:E690–E692.

115. Copeland JG, Dowling R, Tsau PH. Total artificial hearts. In: Kirklin JK, Frazier OH, eds. *Ishlt Monograph Series*. New York: Elsevier; 2006:105–125.

116. Copeland JG, Levinson MM, Smith R, et al. The total artificial heart as a bridge to transplantation: a report of two cases. *JAMA*. 1986;256:2991–2995.

117. Copeland JG, Smith RG, Arabia FA, et al. Cardiac replacement with a total artificial heart as a bridge to transplantation. *N Engl J Med*. 2004;351:859–867.

118. Slaughter MS, Rogers JG, Milano CA, et al. Advanced heart failure treated with continuous-flow left ventricular assist device. *N Engl J Med*. 2009;361:2241–2251.

119. Miller LW, Pagani FD, Russell SD, et al. Use of a continuous-flow device in patients awaiting heart transplantation. *N Engl J Med*. 2007;357:885–896.

120. Feller ED, Sorensen EN, Haddad M, et al. Clinical outcomes are similar in pulsatile and nonpulsatile left ventricular assist device recipients. *Ann Thorac Surg*. 2007;83:1082–1088.

121. Siegenthaler MP, Frazier OH, Beyersdorf F, et al. Mechanical reliability of the Jarvik 2000 heart. *Ann Thorac Surg*. 2006;81:1752–1758.

122. Frazier OH, Myers TJ, Westaby S, et al. Clinical experience with an implantable, intracardiac, continuous flow circulatory support device: physiologic implications and their relationship to patient selection. *Ann Thorac Surg*. 2004;77:133–142.

123. Westaby S, Siegenthaler M, Beyersdorf F, et al. Destination therapy with a rotary blood pump and novel power delivery. *Eur J Cardiothorac Surg*. 2010;37:350–356.

124. Letsou GV, Shah N, Gregoric ID, et al. Gastrointestinal bleeding from arteriovenous malformations in patients supported by the Jarvik 2000 axial-flow left ventricular assist device. *J Heart Lung Transplant*. 2005;24:105–109.

125. Stern DR, Kazam J, Edwards P, et al. Increased incidence of gastrointestinal bleeding following implantation of the HeartMate II LVAD. *J Card Surg*. 2010;25:352–356.

126. Malehsa D, Meyer AL, Bara C, et al. Acquired von Willebrand syndrome after exchange of the HeartMate XVE to the HeartMate II ventricular assist device. *Eur J Cardiothorac Surg*. 2009;35:1091–1093.

127. Geisen U, Heilmann C, Beyersdorf F, et al. Non-surgical bleeding in patients with ventricular assist devices could be explained by acquired von Willebrand disease. *Eur J Cardiothorac Surg*. 2008;33:679–684.

128. Yoshida K, Tobe S, Kawata M, et al. Acquired and reversible von Willebrand disease with high shear stress aortic valve stenosis. *Ann Thorac Surg*. 2006;81:490–494.

129. Larose JA, Tamez D, Ashenuga M, et al. Design concepts and principle of operation of the Heartware ventricular assist system. *ASAIO J*. 2010;56:285–289.

130. Wood C, Maiorana A, Larbalestier R, et al. First successful bridge to myocardial recovery with a Heartware HVAD. *J Heart Lung Transplant*. 2008;27:695–697.

131. Hetzer R, Krabatsch T, Stepanenko A, et al. Long-term biventricular support with the Heartware implantable continuous flow pump. *J Heart Lung Transplant*. 2010;29:822–824.

132. Wieselthaler GM, O'Driscoll G, Jansz P, et al. Initial clinical experience with a novel left ventricular assist device with a magnetically levitated rotor in a multi-institutional trial. *J Heart Lung Transplant*. 2010;29:1218–1225.

133. Griffith K, Jenkins E, Pagani FD. First American experience with the Terumo DuraHeart left ventricular assist system. *Perfusion*. 2009;24:83–89.

134. Yoshitake I, El-Banayosy A, Yoda M, et al. First clinical application of the DuraHeart centrifugal ventricular assist device for a Japanese patient. *Artif Organs*. 2009;33:763–766.

135. Morshuis M, El-Banayosy A, Arusoglu L, et al. European experience of DuraHeart magnetically levitated centrifugal left ventricular assist system. *Eur J Cardiothorac Surg*. 2009;35:1020–1027.

136. Komoda T, Komoda S, Dandel M, et al. Explantation of Incor left ventricular assist device after myocardial recovery. *J Card Surg*. 2008;23:642–647.

137. Garatti A, Bruschi G, Colombo T, et al. Clinical outcome and bridge to transplant rate of left ventricular assist device recipient patients: comparison between continuous-flow and pulsatile-flow devices. *Eur J Cardiothorac Surg*. 2008;34:275–280.

138. Galantier J, Moreira LF, Benicio A, et al. Hemodynamic performance and inflammatory response during the use of VAD-Incor as a bridge to transplant. *Arq Bras Cardiol*. 2008;91:327–334.

139. Schmid C, Jurmann M, Birnbaum D, et al. Influence of inflow cannula length in axial-flow pumps on neurologic adverse event rate: results from a multi-center analysis. *J Heart Lung Transplant*. 2008;27:253–260.

140. Schmid C, Tjan TD, Etz C, et al. First clinical experience with the Incor left ventricular assist device. *J Heart Lung Transplant*. 2005;24:1188–1194.

141. Meyns B, Klotz S, Simon A, et al. Proof of concept: hemodynamic response to long-term partial ventricular support with the synergy pocket micro-pump. *J Am Coll Cardiol*. 2009;54:79–86.

142. Pitsis AA, Visouli AN, Ninios V, et al. Elective bridging to recovery after repair: the surgical approach to ventricular reverse remodeling. *Artif Organs*. 2008;32:730–735.

143. Pitsis AA, Visouli AN, Vassilikos V, et al. First human implantation of a new rotary blood pump: design of the clinical feasibility study. *Hellenic J Cardiol*. 2006;47:368–376.

CHAPTER 9

Special Clinical Settings for Mechanical Circulatory Support

Shahab A. Akhter and Valluvan Jeevanandam

POSTCARDIOTOMY FAILURE

Despite the increasingly complex and high-risk patient population undergoing cardiac surgery, the overall incidence of postcardiotomy heart failure (HF) remains relatively low with the need for mechanical circulatory support (MCS) estimated to be 0.2% to 0.6%.[1] Potential etiologies include inadequate myocardial protection; myocardial ischemia as a result of graft failure, nonrevascularization, air or particulate embolism; native or prosthetic valvular dysfunction; metabolic abnormality; aortic dissection; and preoperative risk factors including severe ventricular dysfunction and emergent operation. More recent studies have shown that early institution of short-term MCS after unsuccessful weaning from cardiopulmonary bypass (CPB) is associated with improved chances of myocardial recovery and patient survival.[2] Escalation of inotropic support is associated with much poorer outcomes compared with a strategy of myocardial unloading using temporary circulatory support (Fig. 9-1).

The definition of postcardiotomy shock includes cardiac index less than 1.8 to 2.0 L/min/m[2], mean arterial blood pressure less than 65 mm Hg, pulmonary arterial wedge pressure greater than 20 mm Hg, venous oxygen saturation less than 50%, ongoing metabolic acidosis, and end-organ hypoperfusion. A single-center study of more than 3000 patients who underwent cardiac surgery showed the rapid increase in postcardiotomy mortality based on the number and doses of inotropic agents used to separate from CPB. Mortality doubled from 2% to 4% with the use of one low-dose inotrope and increased to 8% with one moderate-dose inotrope.[3] Mortality increased to 20% with one high-dose inotrope, 42% with two high-dose inotropes, and 80% with three high-dose inotropic agents. Biologic mechanisms for these poor outcomes include increased myocardial oxygen consumption and cardiac myocyte apoptosis.[4]

Counterpulsation

Following the inability to wean from CPB with the addition of one moderate-dose to high-dose inotropic agent, early placement of an intra-aortic balloon pump (IABP) is typically performed in the absence of significant contraindications such as severe peripheral vascular disease. Counterpulsation increases coronary arterial flow, reduces afterload and myocardial oxygen consumption, and experimentally reduces infarct size early after infarction.[5] Timing of IABP insertion has been shown to affect hospital mortality: Preoperative insertion is associated with a mortality rate of 18.8% to 19.6%; intraoperative insertion, 27.6% to 32.3%; and postoperative insertion, 39% to 40.5%.[6] Given the overall ease of IABP insertion, excellent physiologic augmentation of coronary blood flow, and left ventricular unloading, this form of therapy is considered as the first line of mechanical support rather than continuing to escalate inotropic agents. Some studies also suggest that preoperative prophylactic IABP insertion in high-risk patients (left ventricular ejection fraction <30%, unstable angina, severe left main stenosis, redo coronary artery bypass grafting) can improve cardiac index, reduce length of intensive care unit stay, and decrease mortality.[7,8] However, there are no controlled studies to prove the benefit of this strategy.

Mechanical Circulatory Support

Postcardiotomy ventricular failure that is refractory to inotropic or IABP support requires use of MCS, which can provide a greater degree of cardiac output (Fig. 9-2). An ideal device should support adequate flow, maximize hemodynamics, and unload the ventricle. Current temporary assist devices all have the capability of biventricular support, provided that the lungs can support oxygenation and ventilation. In cases of acute lung injury in conjunction with circulatory failure, extracorporeal membrane oxygenation (ECMO) is the only device currently approved that can support an in-line oxygenator.

To date, the most common postcardiotomy support system after an IABP has been the ABIOMED BVS 5000 blood pump (ABIOMED, Inc, Danvers, MA), which was approved by the U.S. Food and Drug Administration (FDA) in 1992 (Fig. 9-3). This system delivers pulsatile flow and can

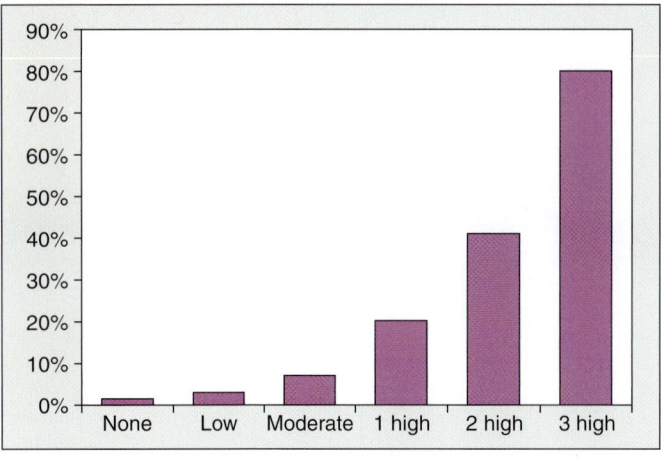

FIGURE 9-1 Postcardiotomy inotrope mortality score. *(Adapted from Samuels LE, Kaufman MS, Thomas MP, et al. Pharmacological criteria for ventricular assist device insertion following postcardiotomy shock: experience with the Abiomed BVS system. J Card Surg. 1999;14:288-293.)*

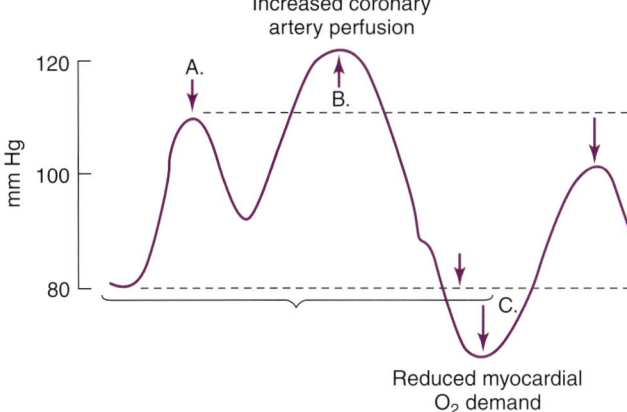

FIGURE 9-2 Hemodynamic effects of the intra-aortic balloon pump (IABP) on aortic pressure. After native left ventricular ejection produces the pulse *(A)*, inflation of the balloon increases aortic diastolic pressure *(B)* and coronary artery perfusion. At end diastole, deflation of the balloon decreases aortic end-diastolic pressure *(C)* below that of an unassisted beat and reduces afterload and myocardial oxygen demand.

be used for univentricular or biventricular support. It has been used in Europe and the United States for the primary purpose of postcardiotomy ventricular failure. The system is a simple, user-friendly, extracorporeal pulsatile pump; it is available in more than 550 centers in the United States, with most being used in nontransplant centers.

The pump is configured as a dual-chamber device containing an atrial chamber that fills passively by gravity and a ventricular chamber that pneumatically pumps the blood to the outflow cannula. The two chambers and the outflow tract are divided by trileaflet polyurethane valves, which allows for unidirectional blood flow. The rate of pumping and the duration of pump systole and diastole are adjusted by the pump microprocessor that operates asynchronously to the native heart rate. The pump makes adjustments to account for changes in preload and afterload and delivers a constant stroke volume of approximately 80 mL. The maximum output is approximately 5 to 6 L/min. The device has not shown any significant hemolysis, and the pulsatile flow may have some degree of physiologic benefit. As opposed to ECMO, patients can be extubated and have limited mobility.

Many centers that previously utilized the BVS 5000 blood pumps have transitioned to the ABIOMED AB5000 system as these ventricles can provide long-term support if the patient cannot be weaned. Patients can also be discharged home with uni- or bi-ventricular AB5000 support. Cannula selection and placement are very straightforward for the ABIOMED BVS or AB5000 systems (Fig. 9-4). For left ventricular assist device (LVAD) support, left atrial cannulation can be achieved via the interatrial groove, the dome of the left atrium, or the left atrial appendage. Alternatively, the left ventricular apex can be directly cannulated and offers the advantage of excellent ventricular decompression, which may improve ventricular recovery.[9] Our group has described a simple and reliable method for left ventricular apical cannulation for short-term LVAD support.[10] Left-sided outflow is to the ascending aorta (Fig. 9-5). For right-sided support, inflow is from the right atrial appendage, the right atrial free wall, or the body of the right ventricle. Right ventricular assist device (RVAD) outflow is to the main pulmonary artery. It is technically much easier to use cardiopulmonary bypass for placement of these cannulas; however, off-pump insertion is possible and may be preferable in certain clinical scenarios, particularly for isolated right-sided support.

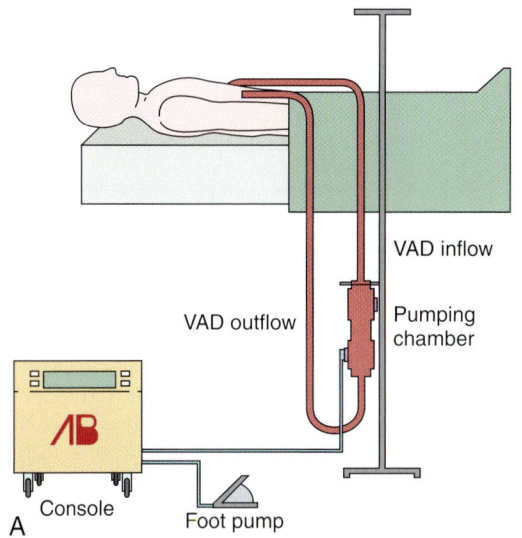

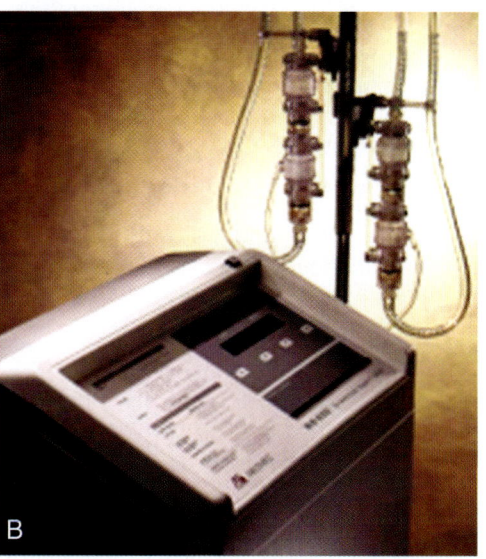

FIGURE 9-3 ABIOMED BVS 5000 system (ABIOMED, Inc). **A,** Illustration shows gravity drainage for inflow to the dual-chamber blood pump. Pulsatile outflow is generated pneumatically by the console in asynchronous fashion relative to the native cardiac rhythm. **B,** Console and blood pumps. VAD, ventricular assist device.

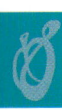

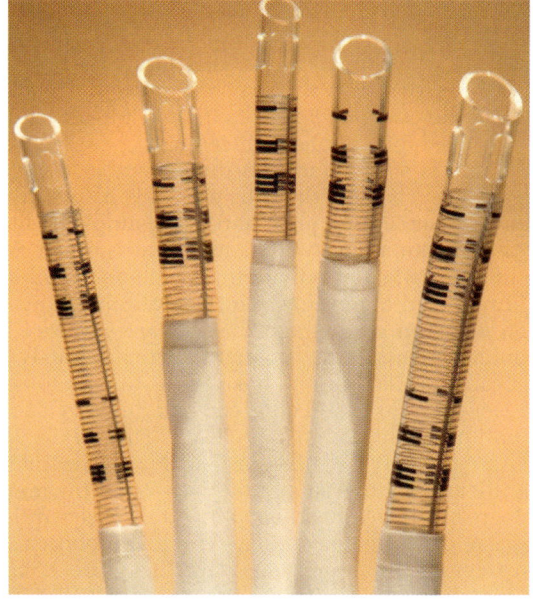

FIGURE 9-4 ABIOMED inflow and outflow cannulas. Outflow cannulas have either a 12-mm or 14-mm Dacron graft at the end allowing anastomosis to either the aorta or the pulmonary artery.

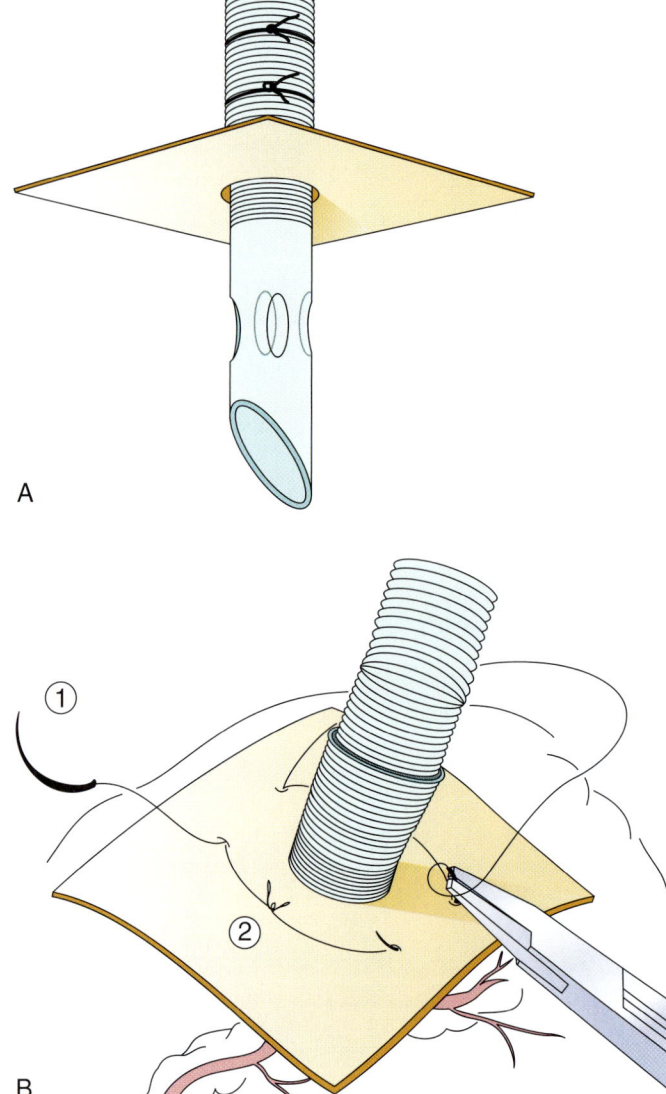

A

B

FIGURE 9-5 **A,** Technique for left ventricular apical cannulation for short-term ventricular assist device (VAD) support. Before placement of the cannula, an anastomosis is created between a 12-mm Hemashield (MAQUET Cardiovascular, Wayne, NJ) graft and a 4 × 4 cm square of soft Teflon felt with a 12-mm circle excised from the center. The Hemashield graft length is cut to 5 cm, and the left ventricular apical cannula is passed through the graft with the inflow holes approximately 4 cm proximal to the felt square. The cannula is secured to the graft with two heavy silk ties placed outside the graft. **B,** Completion of left ventricular apical cannulation. The cannula is passed into the left ventricle until the Teflon felt square is in apposition with the epicardium. The Teflon square is sewn to the left ventricular apex using 2-0 polypropylene (Prolene) sutures on MH (Ethicon, Inc., Somerville, NJ) needles in a horizontal mattress technique very close to the Hemashield graft and in a circumferential manner.

There has been a recent transition to greater use of centrifugal flow pumps to support patients with acute cardiogenic shock of any etiology. This includes the Levitronix CentriMag (Levitronix LLC, Waltham, MA) ventricular assist system, which can provide up to 10 L/min of flow (Fig. 9-6). This device has been used in nearly 4000 patients worldwide for indications ranging from postcardiotomy cardiogenic shock to primary graft failure after heart transplantation. It is also frequently used as the pump for an ECMO circuit. The device is driven with a bearingless motor that enables the spinning component within the pump to be magnetically levitated and rotated without contact or wear. This allows for a greatly reduced incidence of hemolysis and thrombus formation. The devices are relatively easy to implant as they require cannulation techniques routinely used in cardiac surgery. Postoperative management is also simplified by an intuitive user interface and relatively low anticoagulation requirements. The CentriMag pumps are currently FDA approved in the United States for left- or right-sided support of 6 hours' duration and 30 days in Europe; however, these devices have been used very successfully with low complication rates for extended periods.

Extracorporeal Membrane Oxygenation

Some centers have used ECMO as the device of choice for postcardiotomy failure after inotropic and IABP support (Fig. 9-7). Central (right atrium and ascending aorta) or peripheral (femoral) cannulation can be performed, and this serves as biventricular and pulmonary support; this can provide 6 L/min of flow. The primary components of an ECMO circuit include a hollow-fiber membrane oxygenator, a centrifugal pump, a heat exchanger, and tubing for the system. The experience in adults with ECMO for postcardiotomy cardiogenic shock is limited because of nearly universal bleeding problems associated with the chest wound in combination with heparin anticoagulation for the ECMO circuit.[11]

Another potential shortcoming of ECMO in this setting is that the left ventricle is not unloaded even though left ventricular preload is reduced.[12] If the left ventricle is poorly contracting, the marked increase in afterload provided by ECMO offsets any change in left ventricular end-diastolic volume resulting from bypassing the heart. The heart remains dilated because the left ventricle cannot eject sufficient volume against the increased afterload. ECMO may theoretically increase left ventricular wall stress and myocardial oxygen consumption, unless an IABP or other means is used to unload the left ventricle mechanically and reduce wall stress. A separate drainage cannula inserted into the left atrium can also provide left-sided decompression in the postcardiotomy setting.

Investigators at the Cleveland Clinic reported on 107 adult patients who were supported with ECMO after cardiac surgery and observed the following complications: infections in 48%, renal failure requiring dialysis in 39%, neurologic events

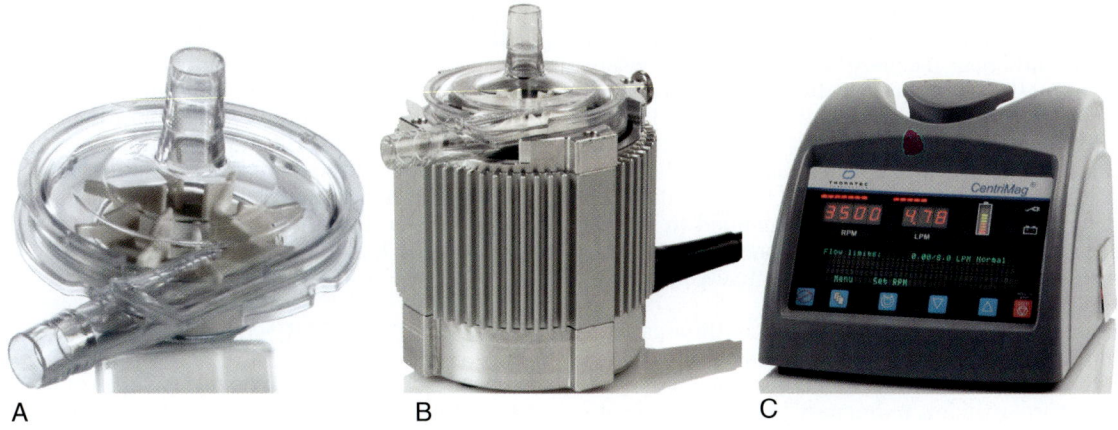

FIGURE 9-6 The Levitronix CentriMag is the first disposable, extracorporeal, short-term magnetically levitated blood pump. The components are a polycarbonate pump **(A)**, which sits in the motor **(B)** and is driven by a console **(C)**. *(Courtesy Thoratec Corp., Pleasanton, CA.)*

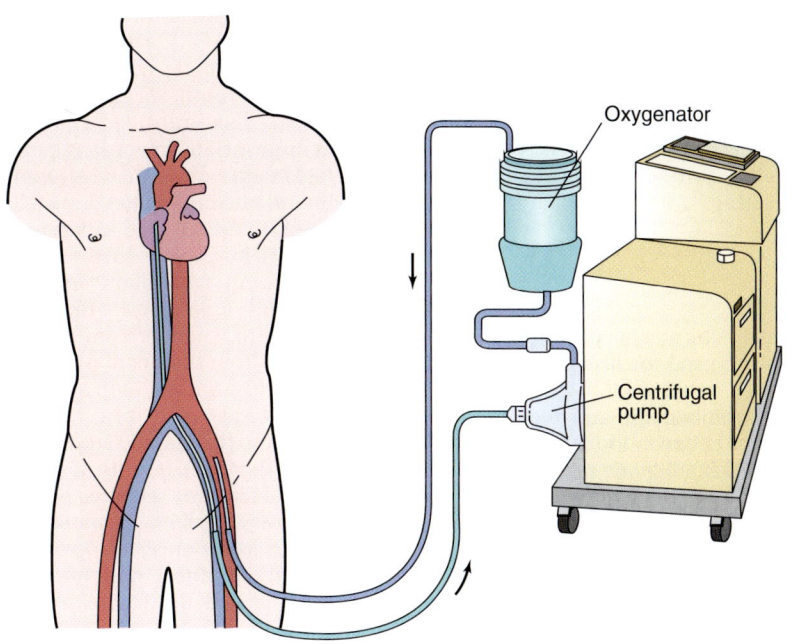

FIGURE 9-7 Percutaneous extracorporeal membrane oxygenation (ECMO) circuit. Right atrial blood is drained via a catheter inserted into the femoral vein and advanced into the right atrium. Oxygenated blood is delivered retrograde via the femoral artery. A smaller cannula can also be placed for distal femoral artery perfusion (not shown).

in 29%, pump thrombus in 5%, and limb complications in 27%.[13] The infections were not related to the ECMO system or cannulation sites. The median number of transfused units of packed red blood cells was 18. In this study, 18 of 107 (17%)

TABLE 9-1	Representative Clinical Trials Evaluating Extracorporeal Membrane Oxygenation for Treatment of Postcardiotomy Cardiogenic Shock			
Reference	No. Patients	Duration of Support (hr)	No. Weaned from Device (%)	No. Survived to Hospital Discharge (%)
Magovern	21	9-92	16 (76)	11 (52)
Wang	18	7-456	10 (55)	6 (33)
Muehrcke	23	0.5-144	9 (39)	7 (30)
Magovern	55	8-137	36 (65)	20 (36)

patients supported by ECMO were bridged to transplant, and 42 (39%) were weaned with intent for survival. ECMO support was withdrawn from 47 (44%) patients. This yielded an overall survival to discharge of 35%. Magovern and colleagues[14] reported improved results in 14 patients supported by a heparin-coated ECMO circuit after operations for myocardial revascularization. Of 14 patients with revascularization, 11 (79%) survived, but none of 3 patients with mitral valve surgery and none of 4 patients who underwent elective circulatory arrest survived. Overall, 52% of the whole group survived, but two patients had strokes during the perfusion period (Table 9-1).

PATIENT MANAGEMENT AND WEANING FROM SUPPORT

The ultimate goal of ventricular assist device (VAD) support for postcardiotomy failure is to maintain optimal perfusion of all end organs, to allow time for myocardial recovery, and to prevent deterioration of organ function. Ideally, pump flow would achieve a mixed venous saturation greater than 70%.

A weaning trial is usually attempted after 48 to 72 hours of support. It is crucial not to rush weaning and to allow time for myocardial and end-organ recovery. The principle of weaning is common to all devices because they have the capability to allow for reduction of flow, enabling more work to be performed by the native ventricle. Flow is gradually reduced in increments of 0.5 to 1 L/min. Adequate anticoagulation is important during these low-flow periods to prevent pump thrombosis, and it is generally not recommended to reduce flow to less than 2.0 L/min for a prolonged period. Heparin is titrated during this period to maintain an activated coagulation time of greater than 300 seconds.

With optimal pharmacologic support and continuous evaluation of ventricular function with transesophageal echocardiography, flows are reduced while monitoring systemic blood pressure, cardiac index, pulmonary pressures, and ventricular dimensions. Maintenance of cardiac index and low pulmonary pressures with preserved left ventricular function by echocardiography suggests weaning is likely. A failed attempt at weaning requires resumption of full flow support. Absence of ventricular recovery after several wean attempts is a poor prognostic sign, particularly after 1 week of support. Patients who are transplant candidates should undergo a full evaluation and subsequently be staged to a long-term VAD as a bridge to cardiac transplantation. Early conversion to long-term ventricular support is beneficial and improves the low survival that is associated with cardiogenic shock, particularly in the postcardiotomy setting.[15,16]

COMPLICATIONS

Complications tend to increase with greater duration of support. Generally, these devices are used for less than 2 weeks, but longer durations have been reported.[17,18] Currently, all short-term assist devices are thrombogenic and require anticoagulation. The delicate balance between too much anticoagulation resulting in bleeding and inadequate anticoagulation leading to thromboembolism is a major determinant of morbidity. Early in the postoperative period, bleeding is a significant problem, occurring at suture lines and cannulation sites or often consisting of a diffuse coagulopathy that becomes difficult to localize. The high incidence of coagulopathy and bleeding is due partially to the hemostatic disarray associated with the operation, the low-flow physiologic state that necessitates pump placement, and the need for anticoagulation early in the course of support.

Current recommendations are to begin anticoagulation with heparin when mediastinal bleeding is less than 100 mL/hr. Intraoperative and early postoperative coagulopathy can be corrected until this goal is achieved before initiating heparin. The target activated coagulation time is 180 to 200 seconds during full flow conditions. The level of anticoagulation should be increased during weaning of these devices. The use of heparin-coated circuits has failed to reduce the coagulopathy and bleeding associated with ECMO effectively. Peripheral ECMO cannulation is associated with less bleeding, however, than transthoracic approaches in the postcardiotomy setting. Similarly, with the ABIOMED BVS devices, the incidence of significant bleeding has been reported to be 40%.[19]

The incidence of thromboembolism remains a constant threat despite the development of heparin-coated systems. Thrombin deposition in centrifugal pumps with increasing duration of support is a well-known phenomenon. In a study of 202 adult patients supported with ECMO, pump head thrombus was present in 5%, and neurologic complications occurred in 29%.[20] Both factors were found to have a profound negative impact on survival and the ability to be weaned from support. Similarly, the incidence of thromboembolic events has been reported to be 13% for the ABIOMED device, but this may be an underestimate of the actual number of thromboembolic episodes. One additional risk for thrombosis is the development of heparin-induced thrombocytopenia. This risk is increased when there is a significant decrease in platelet count or an absolute value of less than 75,000/μL. The development of heparin-induced thrombocytopenia is typically secondary to re-exposure to intravenous heparin, and if this condition is present, alternative strategies for anticoagulation are warranted until platelet counts normalize or VAD support is no longer required.

SUMMARY OF RESULTS

No data indicate that one device is superior over others with regard to weaning from support and survival in the setting of postcardiotomy cardiogenic shock. Published reports suggest that weaning can be accomplished in approximately 45% to 60% of patients; however, overall survival is less than 30%, and only 50% of weaned patients are discharged alive from the hospital.[21,22] Long-term follow-up results are unavailable. In all series, sepsis, multisystem organ failure, and neurologic complications are prominent causes of death. The overall survival rate in reported series over the last decade has improved significantly at transplant centers where appropriate transplant candidates are bridged to transplantation after a period of support.

Minami and colleagues[23] reported on 68 patients supported by the ABIOMED BVS 5000 with the primary indication of postcardiotomy failure; 32 patients were weaned, and 13 underwent transplant for an overall survival of 47%. Guyton and associates[24] reported 55% of postcardiotomy patients were weaned from support (n = 31), and 29% were discharged from the hospital. In another report of 500 patients treated with the BVS 5000 system, including 265 (53%) who could not be weaned from cardiopulmonary bypass, 27% of patients were discharged from the hospital.[19] More recent data using this device in a wide range of clinical situations, including postcardiotomy failure, have reported successful weaning in 83% with 45% of patients being discharged to home. Körfer and associates[25] also reported 50% hospital discharge in 50 postcardiotomy patients supported with the ABIOMED system. The ABIOMED worldwide registry experience shows that earlier transfer of these patients to a transplant center after device implantation results in improved overall survival.

Results with the Levitronix CentriMag ventricular assist device in the postcardiotomy setting have also been very favorable, but relatively small numbers have been reported. A report from the Papworth group[26] in the United Kingdom showed a 42% survival when this device was implanted for postcardiotomy shock (n = 7 patients). De Robertis and colleagues[27] reported an identical survival rate (42%) for a group of 12 postcardiotomy patients who required either RVAD, LVAD, or bi-VAD support for a duration of 1 to 27 days.

TIMING OF MECHANICAL CIRCULATORY SUPPORT FOR END-STAGE HEART FAILURE

Continued improvement in LVAD technology and clinical outcomes has made this option available to more patients with advanced HF. The current generation of continuous flow devices has significantly decreased the incidence of perioperative and long-term complications including bleeding, adverse neurologic events, infection, right HF, arrhythmias, and rate of hospital readmission relative to the previous generation of pulsatile, volume displacement pumps.[28] In addition, the durability of these continuous flow devices is far superior to the pulsatile devices with patients having been supported for 5 years without any device-related issues.

The timing of LVAD implantation is crucial to both short-term and long-term outcomes. Most patients being referred for MCS continue to be hospitalized for decompensated HF and are being supported with inotropes or an IABP or both. Postoperative survival and rate of discharge to home is far superior for patients who are not in critical cardiogenic shock at the time of implant.[29] For patients who are transplant candidates, the timing of LVAD implantation should be based on the balance of the clinical status and factors that may prolong the time on the waiting list. These factors include an elevated panel reactive antibody level, greater weight, and O blood type. Another important factor in the timing of LVAD implantation is the inability to tolerate short-term inotropic support, typically as a result of stimulating ventricular arrhythmias. Long-term inotropic support is associated with a 1-year survival of less than 10%,[30] and patients who are inotrope-dependent should be considered for earlier LVAD implantation if the waiting time for transplant is prolonged. In addition, patients who need a combined heart-kidney or other abdominal organ transplant have longer wait times because of the limitation of typically needing a local donor. Patients with these characteristics that prolong wait list time should be considered for earlier referral for MCS before decompensation occurs and they become critically ill.

Each of the following clinical factors has a significant negative impact on 1-year survival and should be taken into consideration for patients who are being evaluated for transplant or are already listed with regard to referral for MCS: worsening renal function with creatinine greater than 1.8 mg/dL; inability to tolerate angiotensin-converting enzyme inhibitors, angiotensin II receptor blockers, or beta blockers; diuretic dose greater than 1.5 mg/kg/day; recurrent admission for HF; no clinical improvement with cardiac resynchronization therapy (CRT); inability to walk one block without dyspnea; and dyspnea at rest.[31] Another indication for earlier consideration of MCS is irreversible elevated pulmonary vascular resistance, which is a contraindication to heart transplant, generally greater than 4 Wood units. Pulmonary hypertension has been shown to have a favorable response to unloading with LVAD implantation allowing subsequent transplantation without the high risk of right ventricular failure.[32]

More recent data for patients with HeartMate II (Thoratec Corp, Pleasanton, CA) devices shows the relationship between clinical status at the time of implantation and short-term and long-term outcomes.[33] Patients were stratified into three groups based on INTERMACS (Interagency Registry for Mechanically Assisted Circulatory Support) score (Table 9-2): group 1 (INTERMACS 1), group 2 (INTERMACS 2 and 3),

and group 3 (INTERMACS 4-7). Survival to discharge was 70.4% for group 1 (n = 28), 93.5% for group 2 (n = 49), and 95.8% for group 3 (n = 24). Length of stay also correlated with INTERMACS score: group 1, 44 days; group 2, 41 days; and group 3, 17 days. One-year survival was greatest for patients in group 3 at 95.8% versus 73% for patients in groups 1 and 2. Longer-term survival at 18 months was also significantly improved for group 3 (95.8%) versus group 1 (50.2%) and group 2 (72.7%). In addition, a more recent study of 468 patients who underwent HeartMate II LVAD implantation at 36 centers as bridge to transplant showed equivalent 30-day and 1-year survival compared with conventional cardiac transplantation (97% and 87%).[34] Post-transplant survival was not found to be influenced by duration of LVAD support. The authors concluded that the improved durability and reduced short-term and long-term morbidity associated with the HeartMate II LVAD has reduced the need for urgent cardiac transplantation, which may have adversely influenced post-transplant survival in the pulsatile LVAD era.

There is a more recent trend to consider implantation of most LVADs on an elective, scheduled basis. Patients are typically evaluated and accepted for LVAD therapy for bridge to transplant or destination therapy (DT). Most patients can tolerate 2 to 3 days off of inotropic agents so that they can be discharged from the hospital, return home, and be admitted electively on the day of surgery. This practice reduces the risk of nosocomial infection and other comorbidities. This trend is increasing; a recent poll indicated that 85% of programs reported using this strategy with increasing practice because of good associated results.

LEFT VENTRICULAR ASSIST DEVICE VERSUS BIVENTRICULAR ASSIST DEVICE OR TOTAL ARTIFICIAL HEART

The incidence of right HF requiring RVAD implantation at the time of LVAD implantation has decreased with the transition to continuous flow devices. The reasons for this decrease are unclear but may be related to less volume loading of the right heart by this new generation of pumps and possibly the ability to adjust pump speed to avoid overdistention of the right ventricle with echocardiographic guidance. Only 4% of patients in the HeartMate II bridge to transplant trial required RVAD support; however, 13% required extended inotropic support.[35] Patients who require RVAD support at the time of LVAD implantation have significantly worse survival than patients with adequate right heart function.[36] In addition, planned biventricular support has much better outcomes than LVAD implantation followed by RVAD implantation.[37]

It is imperative to be able to identify patients who are at high risk for right ventricular failure and plan for bi-VAD or total artificial heart support. The University of Michigan group has developed a right ventricular failure risk score (RVFRS) as a preoperative tool for assessing the risk of right ventricular failure in candidates for LVAD implantation (Fig. 9-8).[38] Right ventricular failure was defined as the need for RVAD implantation, inotropic support for more than 14 days, or hospital discharge on an inotrope. Of 197 LVAD implants, 68 (35%) were complicated by postoperative right ventricular failure. These LVAD implants were primarily pulsatile devices; only 15% were continuous flow pumps. A vasopressor requirement (4 points), aspartate aminotransferase 80 U/L or greater (2 points), bilirubin 2.0 mg/dL or greater (2.5 points), and creatinine 2.3 mg/dL or greater (3 points) were independent predictors of right ventricular failure. The odds ratios for right ventricular failure for patients with an RVFRS 3.0 or less, 4.0 to 5.0, and 5.5 or greater were 0.49 (95% confidence interval 0.37 to 0.64), 2.8 (95% confidence interval 1.4 to 5.9), and 7.6

TABLE 9-2	INTERMACS Profiles for Patient Selection
Profile	**Description**
1	Critical cardiogenic shock
2	Progressive decline on inotropic support
3	Stable but inotrope-dependent
4	Resting symptoms home on oral therapy
5	Exertion intolerant
6	Exertion limited
7	Advanced NYHA class III symptoms

NYHA, New York Heart Association.
From Kirklin JK, Naftel DC, Stevenson LW, et al. INTERMACS database for durable devices for circulatory support: first annual report. *J Heart Lung Transplant.* 2008;27:1065-1072.

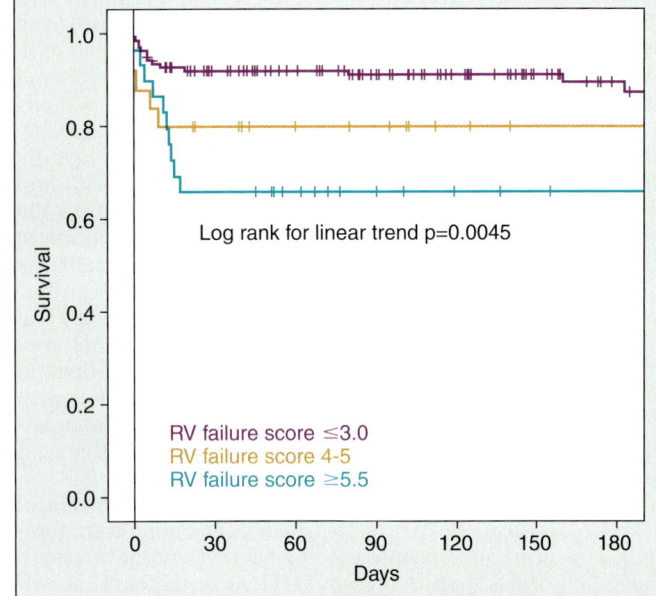

FIGURE 9-8 Kaplan-Meier survival curve for each right ventricular (RV) failure risk score range. The 180-day survival curves after left ventricular assist device (LVAD) implantation for each scoring range are displayed. *(From Matthews JC, Koelling TM, Pagani FD, et al. The right ventricular failure risk score: a pre-operative toll for assessing the risk of right ventricular failure in left ventricular assist device candidates. J Am Coll Cardiol. 2008;51:2163-2172.)*

In our experience at the University of Chicago Medical Center with more than 80 continuous flow LVAD implantations, the ratio of mean pulmonary artery pressure to right atrial pressure has been very predictive of the degree of right ventricular dysfunction and potential need for an RVAD. When this ratio was 2 or greater, none of the patients required RVAD support; however, this ratio was less than 2 for patients who did require an RVAD at the time of HeartMate II LVAD implantation ($n = 5$). We have observed that higher pulmonary artery pressures are associated with better right ventricular function.

The typical hemodynamic scenario during weaning from cardiopulmonary bypass with severe right ventricular dysfunction is poor LVAD flow, elevated right atrial pressure, and low pulmonary artery and systemic blood pressures. Transesophageal echocardiography shows poor right ventricular function and dilation with bowing of the interventricular septum to the left. Inotropic support should be initiated before weaning from bypass, and inhaled nitric oxide can be used as an adjunctive therapy in the setting of right ventricular dysfunction. If two high-dose inotropes are required to achieve adequate hemodynamics, consideration should be given to short-term RVAD support. In the absence of any technical issues with the LVAD, high-dose vasoconstrictor support in the presence of poor LVAD flow and low venous oxygen saturation is a very high-risk situation, which should be avoided by early placement of a temporary RVAD. At our center, we have primarily used the Levitronix CentriMag device as an RVAD because of its ease of use and cost-effectiveness. Weaning of the RVAD can be done at the bedside, and the device usually can be removed within 3 to 5 days of implantation using low- to moderate-dose inotropic support.

For transplant candidates with severe biventricular dysfunction and very high risk scores for right ventricular failure after LVAD implantation, the Thoratec paracorporeal and intracorporeal VADs (Fig. 9-9), SynCardia total artificial heart (SynCardia, Tuscon, AZ) (Fig. 9-10), and ABIOMED AB 5000 (Fig. 9-11) are the current options for long-term biventricular support as bridge to transplant. The ABIOMED and Thoratec devices are approved by the FDA for discharge to home. Long-term biventricular support should be strongly considered in patients in need of bridge to transplant with the combination of severe right ventricular dysfunction by echocardiography, high right atrial pressure, and low pulmonary artery pressure and in patients with ischemic cardiomyopathy with a history of right ventricular infarction.

(95% confidence interval 3.4 to 17.1), and 180-day survival was 90 ± 3%, 80 ± 8%, and 66 ± 9% for each group.

Fitzpatrick and colleagues[39] identified risk factors for requiring RVAD implantation at the time of LVAD implantation based on 266 patients who underwent LVAD placement at the University of Pennsylvania during the period 1995-2007 (Table 9-3). Of these patients, 99 (37%) required RVAD support. The most significant predictors for RVAD support at the time of LVAD implantation were cardiac index 2.2 L/min/m² or less, right ventricular stroke work index 0.25 mm Hg • L/m² or less, severe preoperative right ventricular dysfunction, creatinine 1.9 mg/dL or greater, previous cardiac surgery, and systolic blood pressure 96 mm Hg or less. Each of these criteria that are met is assigned a score of 1 or 0 if it is not met, and a risk score is derived from the following equation: 18 • (cardiac index) + 18 • (right ventricular stroke work index) + 17 (creatinine) + 16 • (previous cardiac surgery) + 16 • (right ventricular dysfunction) + 13 • (systolic blood pressure). The maximum possible score is 98, and a score of 50 or greater is predictive of the need for biventricular VAD support with a sensitivity of 83% and specificity of 80%.

DESTINATION THERAPY

It is estimated that 250,000 patients in the United States are in the terminal phase of systolic HF and have severe symptoms that are refractory to maximal medical therapy.[40] Heart transplantation is the best long-term solution for these patients,

TABLE 9-3	Results of Multivariate Logistic Regression		
Variable	**Odds Ratio**	**95% Confidence Interval**	**P Value**
Cardiac index ≤2.2 L/min/m²	5.7	1.3-24.4	.0192
RVSWI ≤0.25 mm Hg • L/m²	5.1	2.1-12.2	.0002
Severe pre-VAD RV dysfunction	5.0	2.0-12.5	.0006
Creatinine ≥1.9 mg/dL	4.8	1.9-12.0	.0010
Previous cardiac surgery	4.5	1.7-11.8	.0023
SBP ≤96 mm Hg	2.9	1.2-6.9	.0162

RV, right ventricular; RVSWI, right ventricular stroke work index; SBP, systolic blood pressure; VAD, ventricular assist device.
From Fitzpatrick 3rd JR, Frederick JR, Hsu VM, et al. Results of multi-variable logistic regression (Penn bi-VAD study). *J Heart Lung Transplant.* 2008;27:1286-1292.

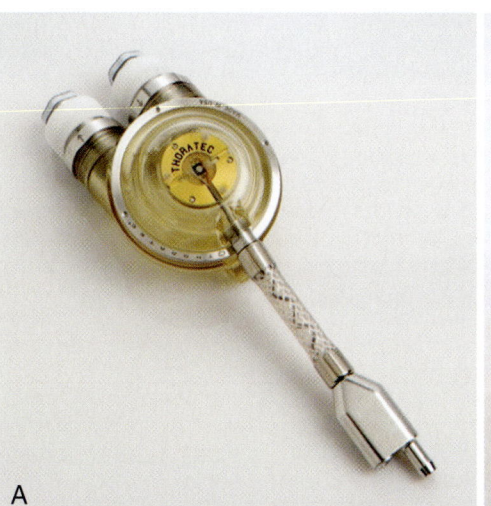
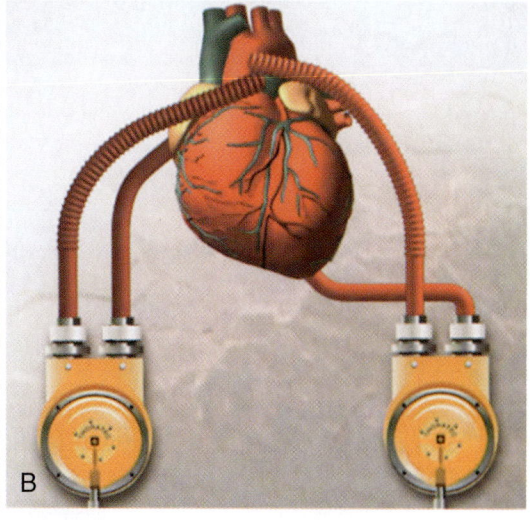

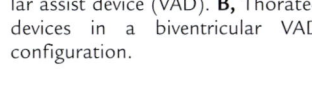

FIGURE 9-9 **A,** Thoratec ventricular assist device (VAD). **B,** Thoratec devices in a biventricular VAD configuration.

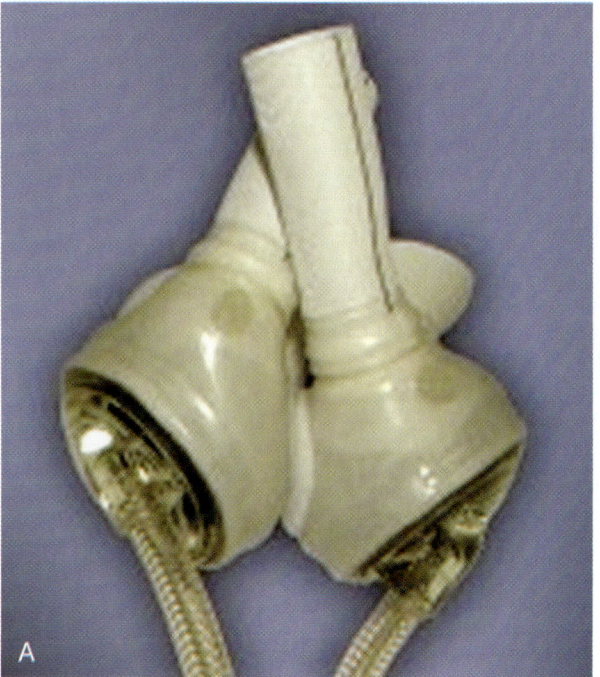
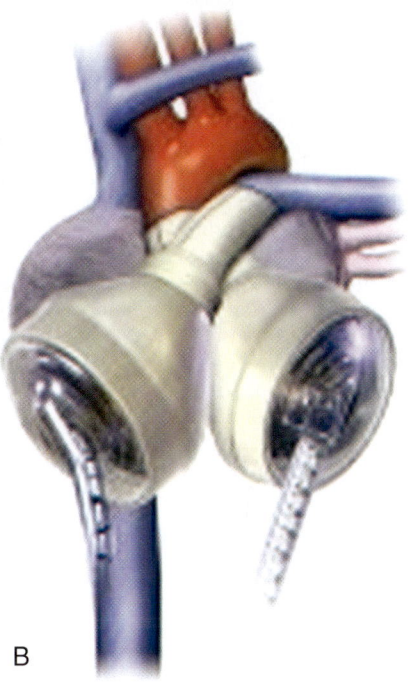

FIGURE 9-10 **A,** SynCardia total artificial heart. **B,** SynCardia total artificial heart illustrating atrial anastomoses.

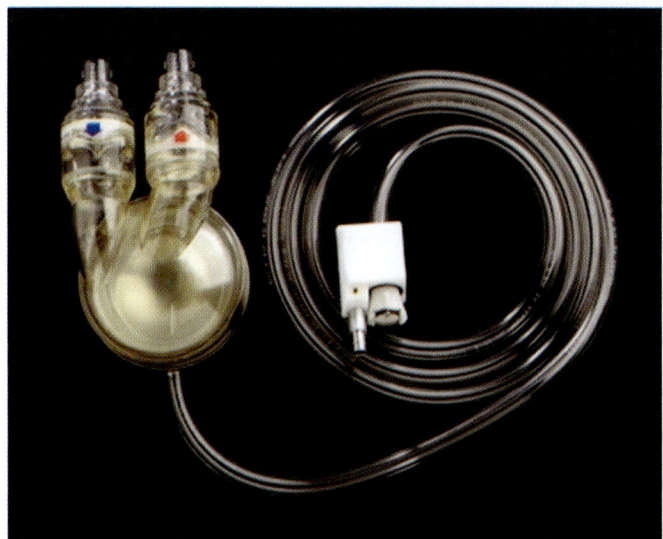

FIGURE 9-11 ABIOMED AB 5000 ventricle for long-term univentricular or biventricular support.

but it is available to only a very small fraction of these patients because of the extremely limited number of donor organs available. Also, many patients are not suitable candidates for transplantation because of other comorbidities. Long-term MCS with a pulsatile LVAD was shown to be superior at 1 year and 2 years to optimal medical therapy in the landmark REMATCH (Randomized Evaluation of Mechanical Assistance for the Treatment of Congestive Heart Failure) trial on patients ineligible for cardiac transplant, which was published in 2001.[41] This was the first trial to evaluate the LVAD as DT and it showed a marked improvement in functional capacity and quality of life (Table 9-4). The enthusiasm for DT was tempered by the 2-year survival rate of only 23% versus 8% with medical therapy and a high postoperative mortality. The results of the HeartMate II DT trial showed significantly better survival rates, device durability, and lower incidence of device-related complications.[42] In the HeartMate II trial, 1-year and 2-year survivals were 68% and 58%, which is far superior compared with the pulsatile device used in the REMATCH trial.

Candidate selection and timing of LVAD implantation are crucial for achieving excellent outcomes in DT. The most common indication for DT LVAD implantation versus listing for

TABLE 9-4	Multivariable Analysis of Risk Factors for 90-Day In-Hospital Mortality after Left Ventricular Assist Device Implantation as Destination Therapy (N = 222)			
Patient Characteristics	Odds Ratio (CI)	P Value		Weighted Risk Score
Platelet count ≤148 × 10³/μL	7.7 (3.0-19.4)	< .001		7
Serum albumin ≤3.3 g/dL	5.7 (1.7-13.1)	< .001		5
INR >1.1	5.4 (1.4-21.8)	.01		4
Vasodilator therapy	5.2 (1.9-14.0)	.008		4
Mean PAP ≤25 mm Hg	4.1 (1.5-11.2)	.009		3
AST >45 U/L	2.6 (1.0-6.9)	.002		2
Hematocrit ≤34%	3.0 (1.1-7.6)	.02		2
BUN >51 mg/dL	2.9 (1.1-8.0)	.03		2
No intravenous inotropes	2.9 (1.1-7.7)	.03		2

AST, aspartate aminotransferase; BUN, blood urea nitrogen; CI, confidence interval; INR, international normalized ratio; PAP, pulmonary artery pressure.
From Lietz K, Long JW, Kfoury AG, et al. Outcomes of left ventricular assist device implantation as destination therapy in the post-REMATCH era: implications for patient selection. Circulation. 2007;116:497-505.

heart transplantation is age. Other comorbidities that may be a contraindication to listing for transplantation include significant end-organ dysfunction, treated malignancy within the past 5 years, severe pulmonary hypertension (pulmonary vascular resistance >5 Wood units), peripheral vascular disease, obesity (body mass index >35), substance abuse, and psychosocial factors. Patients with any of these issues who are refractory to optimal medical therapy should be considered for LVAD implantation as DT. Renal failure and pulmonary dysfunction may be relative contraindications for DT; however, the experience with continuous flow devices and long-term dialysis is very limited, and long-term results have not been published to date.

Lietz and coauthors[43] developed a risk score for in-hospital mortality after pulsatile LVAD implantation for DT by studying 309 patients who underwent implantation in the post-REMATCH period 2002-2005 at 66 hospitals (Fig. 9-12) Overall survival on LVAD support was 86.1% at 30 days, 56.0% at 1 year, and 30.9% at 2 years. The following predictors of 90-day in-hospital mortality after LVAD implantation were identified by multivariable analysis: platelet count 148,000/μL or less, serum albumin 3.3 g/dL or less, international normalized ratio greater than 1.1, vasodilator therapy at time of implantation, mean pulmonary artery pressure 25.3 mm Hg or less, aspartate aminotransferase greater than 45 U/L, hematocrit 34% or less, blood urea nitrogen greater than 51 mg/dL, and lack of intravenous inotropic support. Each risk factor was weighted, and the operative risk score was calculated with results shown in Table 9-5. The risk factors and scoring are likely to be

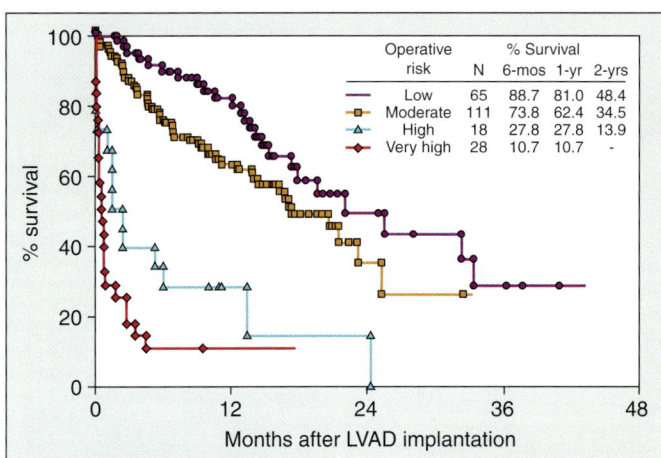

FIGURE 9-12 Survival after left ventricular assist device (LVAD) implantation as destination therapy (DT) by the candidate's operative risk. (From Lietz K, Long JW, Kfoury AG, et al. Outcomes of left ventricular assist device implantation as destination therapy in the post-REMATCH era: implications for patient selection. Circulation. 2007;116:497-505.)

different in the current era of continuous flow LVADs but are very useful to estimate the risk of operative mortality.

The ideal scenario is to perform LVAD implantation for DT as an elective procedure with patients being admitted to the hospital on the day of scheduled surgery. Patients who are

TABLE 9-5	Operative Risk Categories with Corresponding Cumulative Risk Score for 90-Day In-Hospital Mortality after Left Ventricular Assist Device Implantation as Destination Therapy and Survival to Hospital Discharge and 1-Year Survival Depicted by Operative Risk Categories*							
			In-Hospital Mortality within 90 Days			% Survival		
Operative Risk Categories	Risk Score	No.	No. Observed	No. Predicted	% Probability (CI)	To Discharge	90 Days	1 Year
Low	0-8	65	2	1.6	2 (1.1-5.4)	87.5	93.7	81.2
Medium	9-16	111	12	13.7	12 (8.0-18.5)	70.5	86.5	62.4
High	17-19	28	10	7.9	44 (32.8-55.9)	26	38.9	27.8
Very high	>19	18	22	22.8	81 (66.0-90.9)	13.7	17.9	10.7

* Analysis limited to 208 patients with available measures of pulmonary artery pressure and serum albumin level.
From Lietz K, Long JW, Kfoury AG, et al. Outcomes of left ventricular assist device implantation as destination therapy in the post-REMATCH era: implications for patient selection. Circulation. 2007;116:497-505.

classified as INTERMACS 4 to 7 are at the lowest risk for perioperative complications, including right ventricular failure, multisystem organ failure, and sepsis. Right ventricular failure is a much more problematic issue in patients receiving DT compared with bridge to transplant. Only 4% of the patients required RVAD support in the HeartMate II DT trial, and 20% were managed with extended use of inotropes.[42] Right HF was the cause of death in 5% of patients who underwent HeartMate II device implantation. These data underscore the significance of patient selection, optimization, timing of surgery, and meticulous surgical technique to minimize right ventricular–related morbidity and mortality.

REFERENCES

1. Torchiana DF, Hirsch G, Buckley MJ, et al. Intra-aortic balloon pumping for cardiac support: trends in practice and outcome, 1968 to 1995. *J Thorac Cardiovasc Surg.* 1997;113:758–769.
2. Potapov EV, Loforte A, Weng Y, et al. Experience with over 1000 implanted ventricular assist devices. *J Card Surg.* 2008;23:185–194.
3. Samuels LE, Kaufman MS, Thomas MP, et al. Pharmacological criteria for ventricular assist device insertion following postcardiotomy shock: experience with the Abiomed BVS system. *J Card Surg.* 1999;14(4):288–293.
4. Dunser MW, Hasibeder WR. Sympathetic overstimulation during critical illness: adverse effects of adrenergic stress. *J Intensive Care Med.* 2009;24:293–316.
5. Maroko PR, Bernstein EF, Libby P, et al. Effects of intraaortic balloon counterpulsation on the severity of myocardial ischemic injury following acute coronary occlusion. *Circulation.* 1972;45:1150–1159.
6. Creswell LL, Moulton MJ, Cox JL, et al. Revascularization after acute myocardial infarction. *Ann Thorac Surg.* 1995;60:19–26.
7. Christenson JT, Badel P, Simonet F, et al. Preoperative intra-aortic balloon pump enhances cardiac performance and improves the outcome of redo CABG. *Ann Thorac Surg.* 1997;64:1237–1244.
8. Christenson JT, Schmuziger M, Simonet F. Effective surgical management of high-risk coronary patients using preoperative intra-aortic balloon counterpulsation therapy. *Cardiovasc Surg.* 2001;9:383–390.
9. Lohmann BP, Swartz RC, Pendelton DJ, et al. Left ventricular versus left atrial cannulation for the Thoratec ventricular assist device. *ASAIO J.* 1995;41:M17–M22.
10. Akhter SA, Raman J, Jeevanandam V. Technique for left ventricular apical cannulation for short-term mechanical circulatory support. *Ann Thorac Surg.* 2010;89:994–995.
11. Pennington DG, Merjavy JP, Codd JE, et al. Extracorporeal membrane oxygenation for patients with cardiogenic shock. *Circulation.* 1984;70:I–130–I-137.
12. Pagani FD, Lynch W, Swaniker F, et al. Extracorporeal life support to left ventricular assist device bridge to heart transplant: a strategy to optimize survival and resource utilization. *Circulation.* 1999;100:II–206–II-210.
13. Smedira NG, Blackstone EH. Postcardiotomy mechanical support: risk factors and outcomes. *Ann Thorac Surg.* 2001;71:S60–S66.
14. Magovern GJ, Magovern JA, Benckart DH, et al. Extracorporeal membrane oxygenation versus the biopump: preliminary results in patients with postcardiotomy cardiogenic shock. *Ann Thorac Surg.* 1994;57:1462–1468.
15. DeRose JJ, Umana JP, Argenziano M, et al. Improved results for postcardiotomy cardiogenic shock with the use of implantable left ventricular assist devices. *Ann Thorac Surg.* 1997;64:1757–1762.
16. Samuels LE, Holmes EC, Garwood P, et al. Initial experience with the ABIOMED AB5000 ventricular assist device system. *Ann Thorac Surg.* 2005;80:309–312.
17. Couper GS, Dekkers RJ, Adams DH. The logistics and cost-effectiveness of circulatory support: advantages of the ABIOMED BVS 5000. *Ann Thorac Surg.* 1999;68:646–649.
18. Morgan JA, Stewart AS, Lee BJ, et al. Role of the Abiomed BVS 5000 device for short-term support and bridge to transplantation. *ASAIO J.* 2004;50:360–363.
19. Jett GK. ABIOMED BVS 5000: Experience and potential advantages. *Ann Thorac Surg.* 1996;61:301–304.
20. Smedira NG, Moazami N, Golding CM, et al. Clinical experience with 202 adults receiving extracorporeal membrane oxygenation for cardiac failure: survival at five years. *J Thorac Cardiovasc Surg.* 2001;122:92–102.
21. Paul S, Leacche M, Unic D, et al. Determinants of outcomes for postcardiotomy VAD placement: an 11-year, two-institution study. *J Card Surg.* 2006;21:234–237.
22. Mehta SM, Aufiero TX, Pae Jr WE, et al. Results of mechanical ventricular assistance for the treatment of postcardiotomy cardiogenic shock. *ASAIO J.* 1996;42:211–1208.
23. Minami K, Posival H, el-Bynayosy A, et al. Mechanical ventricular support using pulsatile Abiomed BVS 5000 and centrifugal Biomedicus-pump in postcardiotomy shock. *Int J Artif Organs.* 1994;17:492–498.
24. Guyton RA, Schonberger J, Everts P, et al. Postcardiotomy shock clinical evaluation of the BVS 5000 biventricular support system. *Ann Thorac Surg.* 1993;56:346–356.
25. Körfer R, El-Banayosy A, Arusogul L, et al. Temporary pulsatile ventricular assist devices and biventricular assist devices. *Ann Thorac Surg.* 1999;68:678–683.
26. Shuhaiber JH, Jenkins D, Berman M, et al. The Papworth experience with the Levitronix CentriMag ventricular assist device. *J Heart Lung Transplant.* 2008;27(2):158–164.
27. De Robertis F, Birks EJ, Rogers P, et al. Clinical performance with the Levitronix CentriMag short-term ventricular assist device. *J Heart Lung Transplant.* 2006;25(2):181–186.
28. Miller LW, Pagani FD, Russell SD, et al. Use of a continuous-flow device in patients awaiting heart transplantation. *N Engl J Med.* 2007;357:885–896.
29. Kirklin JK, Naftel DC, Kormos RL, et al. Second INTERMACS annual report: more than 1,000 primary left ventricular assist device implants. *J Heart Lung Transplant.* 2010;29:1–10.
30. Hershberger RE, Nauman D, Walker TL, et al. Care processes and clinical outcomes of continuous outpatient support with inotropes (COSI) in patients with refractory end stage heart failure. *J Card Failure.* 2003;9:180–187.
31. Russell SD, Miller LW, Pagani FD. Advanced heart failure: a call to action. *Congest Heart Fail.* 2008;14:316–321.
32. Torre-Amione G, Southard RE, Loebe MM, et al. Reversal of secondary pulmonary hypertension by axial and pulsatile mechanical circulatory support. *J Heart Lung Transplant.* 2010;29:195–200.
33. Boyle AJ. Ascheim DD, Russo MJ, et al: Clinical outcomes for continuous-flow left ventricular assist device patients stratified by pre-operative INTERMACS classification. *J Heart Lung Transplant.* 2011;30(4):402–407.
34. John R, Pagani FD, Naka Y, et al. Post-cardiac transplant survival after support with a continuous-flow left ventricular assist device: impact of duration of left ventricular assist device support and other variables. *J Thorac Cardiovasc Surg.* 2010;140:174–181.
35. Miller LW, Pagani FD, Russell SD, et al. Use of a continuous-flow device in patients awaiting heart transplantation. *N Engl J Med.* 2007;357:885–896.
36. Dang NC, Topkara VK, Mercando M, et al. Right heart failure after left ventricular assist device implantation in patients with chronic congestive heart failure. *J Heart Lung Transplant.* 2006;25:1–6.
37. Fitzpatrick 3rd JR, Frederick JR, Hiesinger W, et al. Early planned institution of biventricular mechanical circulatory support results in improved outcomes compared with delayed conversion of a left ventricular assist device to a biventricular assist device. *J Thorac Cardiovasc Surg.* 2009;137:971–977.
38. Matthews JC, Koelling TM, Pagani FD, et al. The right ventricular failure risk score: a pre-operative toll for assessing the risk of right ventricular failure in left ventricular assist device candidates. *J Am Coll Cardiol.* 2008;51:2163–2172.
39. Fitzpatrick 3rd JR, Frederick JR, Hsu VM, et al. Risk score derived from pre-operative data analysis predicts the need for biventricular mechanical circulatory support. *J Heart Lung Transplant.* 2008;27:1286–1292.
40. *Heart Disease and Stroke Statistics: 2008 Update.* American Heart Association; 2008.
41. Rose EA, Gelijns AC, Moskowitz AJ, et al. Long-term mechanical left ventricular assistance for end-stage heart failure. *N Engl J Med.* 2001;345:1435–1443.
42. Slaughter MS, Rogers JG, Milano CA, et al. Advanced heart failure treated with continuous-flow left ventricular assist device. *N Engl J Med.* 2009;361:2241–2251.
43. Lietz K, Long JW, Kfoury AG, et al. Outcomes of left ventricular assist device implantation as destination therapy in the post-REMATCH era: implications for patient selection. *Circulation.* 2007;116:497–505.

Perioperative Anesthetic Management for Ventricular Assist Device Implantation

Theresa Gelzinis

The anesthetic management of patients undergoing placement of a ventricular assist device (VAD) is complex and requires knowledge of the indication for the device, the extent of preoperative end-organ damage, the presence of concurrent comorbidities, and the type and physiology of the device to be implanted. This chapter reviews the perioperative management of these patients from the preoperative assessment to transport to the intensive care unit (ICU).

PATIENT SELECTION

The three indications for placement of a VAD include bridge to recovery, bridge to transplantation, and destination therapy. In 80% of these patients, the indication is bridge to transplantation.[1] Patients who receive a device as a bridge to recovery require short-term support; this group includes patients who have had a myocardial infarction, patients after cardiotomy, and patients requiring a bridge to further corrective surgery because they have developed heart failure while awaiting their definitive procedure. Patients who receive a VAD as destination therapy are generally not candidates for cardiac transplantation, although there is a subgroup of patients whose condition stabilizes after VAD placement, qualifying them later for cardiac transplantation.

Patient selection depends on the patient's hemodynamic status and on the presence and degree of end-organ dysfunction. Patients who may benefit from a VAD include patients who require long-term inotropic therapy, who develop intolerance to angiotensin-converting enzyme inhibitor therapy as manifested by progressive cardiac and renal dysfunction, who have a peak oxygen consumption of $12\,mL/kg^{-1}/min^{-1}$ or less, or who cannot be restored to New York Heart Association (NYHA) class III despite maximal medical therapy.[2] The hemodynamic parameters that define cardiogenic shock, developed by Norman and colleagues,[3] apply to patients receiving maximal pharmacologic therapy, preload optimization, and intra-aortic balloon pump (IABP) support (Box 10-1).

Multiple scoring systems have been developed in an effort to risk stratify patients receiving left ventricular assist devices (LVADs), including the Acute Physiology and Chronic Health Evaluation II (APACHE II) score and the Seattle Heart Failure Model (SHFM), originally validated in critically ill patients and then applied to patients receiving LVADs, and the Columbia, Leitz-Miller, and INTERMACS (Interagency Registry for Mechanically Assisted Circulatory Support) scores, generated and validated from patients receiving LVADs to assess the risk of mortality after device implantation.[4] The Leitz-Miller scale measures the extent of preoperative renal, hepatic, and pulmonary dysfunction and assesses the need for inotropic or vasodilator support and is commonly used to identify high-risk patients and to predict 1-year survival after LVAD insertion.[5] The INTERMACS scale uses similar variables to determine the appropriate time for LVAD insertion.[6] Finally, Schaffer and colleagues[4] showed that in patients receiving continuous flow VADs, the SHFM[7]—which uses clinical characteristics, including age, weight, and gender; the extent and etiology of heart failure; laboratory data, including hemoglobin, total cholesterol, and uric acid levels; ECG findings, including a prolonged QRS; and the presence of a biventricular pacemaker, automatic implantable cardioverter-defibrillator (AICD), or both—was able to stratify patients into high risk and low risk of mortality after VAD implantation.

PREOPERATIVE EVALUATION

The preoperative assessment should be comprehensive, focusing on the cardiac history, the presence and degree of end-organ dysfunction, and any concurrent diseases (Box 10-2).

Cardiac Assessment

The cardiac assessment includes the etiology and extent of heart failure; the ventricles affected; a history of previous cardiac interventions, including intracoronary stent placement, coronary or intracardiac procedures,

BOX 10-1 Hemodynamic Criteria for Cardiogenic Shock

Cardiac index <2.0 L/m²/min
Stroke volume <25 mL/beat
Systemic vascular resistance >2100 dyne•s•cm⁻⁵
Left atrial pressure >20 mm Hg
Urine output <20 mL/hr

BOX 10-2 Preoperative Assessment

Cardiac
Etiology
NYHA class
Previous interventions
  Stents
  Coronary or valve surgery
  Correction of congenital heart disease
Prior sternotomy
Right ventricular function
  Pulmonary hypertension
  Peripheral venous congestion
Arrhythmias
Pacer, AICD, IABP

Pulmonary
Pulmonary hypertension
Pulmonary edema
Intrinsic pulmonary disease
  Chronic obstructive pulmonary disease
  Restrictive lung disease
  Pneumonia
  Pleural effusion

Renal
BUN and creatinine
Acute vs. chronic renal insufficiency
Dialysis

Hepatic
AST, ALT, and bilirubin
Albumin
INR and prothrombin time

Vascular
Cerebrovascular disease
Hypertension
Peripheral vascular disease

Endocrine and Metabolic
Diabetes mellitus
Cachexia

ALT, alanine aminotransferase; AST, aspartate aminotransferase; AICD, automatic implantable cardioverter-defibrillator; BUN, blood urea nitrogen; IABP, intra-aortic balloon pump; INR, international normalized ratio; NYHA, New York Heart Association.

or previous sternotomy; the presence of malignant arrhythmias, pulmonary hypertension, or central or peripheral venous congestion; and the presence of pre-existing mechanical support devices such as a pacemaker, AICD, or IABP. Although sinus rhythm is the preferred rhythm, patients may often present with atrial arrhythmias, such as atrial fibrillation or flutter. For optimal right ventricular function and VAD filling, both atrial and ventricular arrhythmias should be treated whenever possible.[8] In some patients, normalized hemodynamic values produced by VAD support may ablate the arrhythmogenic

activity. Patients with malignant or refractory tachyarrhythmia may be candidates for biventricular support.

For patients with coronary artery disease who are receiving an LVAD, it is important to diagnose and treat right ventricular ischemia to prevent the need for a right ventricular assist device (RVAD). Treatment of right ventricular ischemia includes optimal medical management, coronary artery stent placement, or coronary artery bypass grafting during LVAD implantation. If coronary stents are to be placed, a bare metal stent is advisable, and the patient should receive at least 4 to 6 weeks of dual antiplatelet therapy with aspirin and clopidogrel to prevent stent thrombosis.

If the etiology of ventricular failure is congenital heart disease, any lesions that produce right-to-left shunting need to be corrected to prevent postimplantation hypoxia. For patients undergoing LVAD placement, the most important assessment is preimplantation right ventricular function. Primary right ventricular failure (RVF) has been defined as right atrial pressure greater than 20 mm Hg on maximal inotropic support or right atrial pressure greater than pulmonary capillary wedge pressure.

Primary RVAD insertion is much less common than LVAD insertion because the right ventricle recovers more readily than the left ventricle. RVF after LVAD implantation occurs in 15% to 20% of patients and is a major cause of morbidity and mortality. RVF after implantation is associated with prolonged cardiopulmonary bypass (CPB) time, nonsurgical coagulopathy requiring multiple transfusions and surgical re-explorations, increased incidence of end-organ dysfunction including an increased incidence of dialysis, increased ICU length of stay, and decreased survival to cardiac transplantation.[9] Patients with significant preoperative right ventricular dysfunction who receive a planned biventricular VAD had superior outcomes compared with patients who received an LVAD followed by an RVAD.[10]

Many studies have attempted to predict patients who will require postimplantation right ventricular support. The problems with these studies are that most are retrospective, they have different definitions of postimplantation RVF, and they include patients receiving both pulsatile and continuous flow VADs. The risk factors for postimplantation RVF can be divided into demographic, clinical, hemodynamic, echocardiographic, and biochemical factors (Box 10-3). Demographic risk factors include younger age, female sex, and small body surface area.[2,9,11–13] Clinical risk factors include nonischemic cardiomyopathy that may involve the right ventricle, reoperation, preoperative mechanical ventilation or circulatory support, vasopressor requirements,[2,12] preoperative pulmonary edema, and noninfectious fever (an indication of inflammation).[14]

Hemodynamic risk factors include a low mean arterial pressure; low mean pulmonary artery pressure, an indication of poor right ventricular contractility in the presence of elevated pulmonary vascular resistance[11]; central venous pressure greater than 15 mm Hg or greater than left atrial pressure; decreased right ventricular stroke work index; and pulmonary vascular resistance greater than 3.8 Wood units. Echocardiographic risk factors include severe right ventricular dysfunction, right ventricular dilation with increased end-systolic and end-diastolic volumes, severe tricuspid regurgitation, moderate to severe pulmonic regurgitation, and low estimated pulmonary artery systolic pressure. Biochemical risk factors include elevated blood urea nitrogen and creatinine; elevated hepatic enzymes including total bilirubin, aspartate aminotransferase, and alanine aminotransferase; elevated white blood cell count; decreased platelet count; elevated international normalized ratio (INR); elevated glucose levels; and elevated markers of inflammation, including C-reactive protein, procalcitonin, neopterin, N-terminal prohormone brain natriuretic peptide, and endothelin-1.[15]

BOX 10-3 Predictors of Postimplantation Right Ventricular Failure

Demographic
Younger age
Female sex
Small body surface area

Clinical
Nonischemic cardiomyopathy
Reoperation
Preoperative mechanical ventilation
Preoperative circulatory support
Vasopressor requirement
Preoperative pulmonary edema
Noninfectious fever

Hemodynamic
Low MAP
CVP >15 mm Hg
RAP > LAP
RVSWI >300 mm Hg × mL/m²
Low mean and diastolic PAP
PVR >3.8 Wood units
Transpulmonary gradient >15 mm Hg
PAP – RAP <4 mm Hg
CVP/PCWP ratio >0.63

Echocardiographic
Severe tricuspid regurgitation
Moderate to severe pulmonic regurgitation
Estimated low pulmonary artery systolic pressure
Right ventricular dilation with increased EDV and ESV
    RVEDV >200 mL
    RVESV >177 mL
Severe right ventricular systolic dysfunction with FAC <20%
Right ventricle S/L <0.6

Biochemical
Elevated creatinine
    Renal replacement
Elevated BUN
Elevated AST, ALT, and total bilirubin
Elevated glucose
Complete blood count
    Decreased platelet count
    Increased white blood cell count
    Decreased hematocrit
Elevated INR
Elevated markers of inflammation
    C-reactive protein
    Procalcitonin
    Neopterin
    NT-proBNP
    Endothelin-1

ALT, alanine aminotransferase; AST, aspartate aminotransferase; BUN, blood urea nitrogen; CVP, central venous pressure; EDV, end-diastolic volume; ESV, end-systolic volume; FAC, fractional area change; INR, international normalized ratio; LAP, left atrial pressure; MAP, mean arterial pressure; NT-proBNP, N-terminal prohormone brain natriuretic peptide; PAP, pulmonary artery pressure; PCWP, pulmonary capillary wedge pressure; PVR, pulmonary vascular resistance; RAP, right atrial pressure; RVEDV, right ventricular end-diastolic volume; RVESV, right ventricular end-systolic volume; RVSWI, right ventricular stroke work index; S/L, short axis to long axis ratio.

In an attempt to predict the incidence of postimplantation RVF, Matthews and coworkers[12] developed the right ventricular failure risk score (RVFRS) (Box 10-4). Performing a retrospective analysis of LVAD recipients, they found that the strongest predictors of postimplantation RVF included a preoperative vasopressor requirement, elevated aspartate

BOX 10-4 Right Ventricular Failure Risk Score

Vasopressor requirement: 4 points
AST ≥80 U/L: 2 points
Bilirubin ≥2.0 mg/dL: 2.5 points
Creatinine ≥2.3: 3 points

AST, aspartate aminotransferase.

aminotransferase and bilirubin, and elevated creatinine or renal replacement therapy. Each predictor was assigned a numerical value, and patients with an RVFRS 5.5 or greater had a 15-fold increase in postimplantation RVF compared with patients with an RVFRS 3 or less.

Kormos and associates[16] used the central venous pressure-to-pulmonary capillary wedge pressure (CVP/PCWP) ratio to distinguish RVF caused by increased left-sided filling pressures and pulmonary hypertension from RVF caused by a progressive myocardial disease. Patients with RVF secondary to elevated filling pressures have a low CVP/PCWP ratio, whereas patients with intrinsic myocardial disease have an elevated CVP/PCWP ratio. In the study by Kormos and associates,[16] patients with CVP/PCWP ratios 0.63 or less were less likely to develop postimplantation RVF.

Pulmonary Assessment

The pulmonary examination should quantify the presence of chronic obstructive pulmonary disease, pulmonary edema, and pulmonary hypertension. Mechanical ventilation is one of the most important predictors of morbidity and mortality after VAD insertion, and all acute processes, such as pneumonia, should be treated before VAD insertion. Chronic lung disease may lead to irreversible pulmonary hypertension. Aaronson and colleagues[17] suggested guidelines for successful VAD placement that include pulmonary vascular resistance less than 3 Wood units, forced expiratory volume in 1 second 50% or greater predicted, forced vital capacity ≥50% or greater predicted, and carbon dioxide diffusing capacity 50% or greater.

Renal Assessment

Renal insufficiency is a significant risk factor for poor outcome after VAD implantation. Increased risk occurs with blood urea nitrogen greater than 40 mg/dL,[18] creatinine greater than 3.0 mg/dL, long-term dialysis, and urine output of 20 to 30 mL/hr for 6 to 8 hours after VAD implantation.[19] If there is renal insufficiency, it should be determined whether the cause is organic or it is due to decreased cardiac output. Although renal dysfunction resulting from inadequate cardiac output is often reversible, it is also a risk factor for poor outcome after VAD implantation.

Hepatic Assessment

Preoperative hepatic dysfunction is another risk factor for adverse outcome after VAD implantation, especially postimplantation RVF requiring biventricular support. It is important to determine whether the etiology of the hepatic dysfunction is primary or secondary, either due to decreased cardiac output or due to hepatic congestion caused by right ventricular dysfunction.

The hepatic artery and portal vein are the two main vessels that perfuse the liver. Of the two, the portal vein contributes most of the total blood flow. The portal vein and hepatic artery ultimately merge and drain into the hepatic vein, which has a pressure that closely correlates to the central venous pressure. The pressure difference between the portal and hepatic veins is approximately 5 to 10 mm Hg, and any increase in central venous pressure that is due to right ventricular dysfunction would increase hepatic vein pressure, decrease the portal to hepatic vein pressure gradient, and impair portal vein flow to the liver. The decreased portal vein flow reduces intrahepatic oxygen delivery, leading to hepatocyte hypoxia and centrilobar damage. Hepatocyte hypoxia also impairs hepatocyte secretion of bile into the canaliculi, and as a result, bilirubin is excreted into the systemic circulation.[20] Hepatic congestion also decreases the production of coagulation factors, contributing to post-CPB coagulopathy.

The incidence of adverse outcomes increases with an INR greater than 1.5, alanine aminotransferase and aspartate aminotransferase levels three times normal, and a total bilirubin greater than 5 mg/dL. An elevated total bilirubin greater than 5 mg/dL has been shown to be the most predictive hepatic marker associated with mortality.[2] Patients with significant hepatic impairment may benefit from a planned biventricular VAD. Hepatic dysfunction may or may not improve after LVAD implantation. Hepatic function improves if the decrease in pulmonary artery pressure and right ventricular afterload improves right ventricular function. Some patients may continue to have deteriorating hepatic function secondary to increased activation of proinflammatory cytokines.[21]

Vascular Assessment

The presence of hypertension and its sequelae can adversely affect VAD implantation and function. Severe systemic hypertension produces systolic and diastolic dysfunction that impedes LVAD ejection and should be controlled before VAD implantation. The presence of severe peripheral vascular disease may lead to difficulty in obtaining arterial access both for monitoring and for aortic cannula placement. Patients with severe carotid disease may be difficult to manage because they require a higher mean arterial pressure to maintain cerebral perfusion pressure, which may impede VAD emptying. Severe neurologic deficits are a contraindication to VAD placement.

Endocrine and Metabolic Assessment

A body surface area greater than 1.5 m^2 is required to accommodate abdominal implantation of the larger pulsatile VADs. Smaller patients may experience intra-abdominal crowding, leading to chronic abdominal discomfort, poor appetite, and nutritional impairment. Cachexia and other markers of poor nutrition, such as low serum albumin, prealbumin, and total protein, are strong independent predictors of mortality. Prior abdominal surgeries can produce adhesions that may preclude proper VAD placement and may increase the risk of bleeding, infection, or recurrent abdominal complications.[2] Many of these patients have diabetes mellitus, which should be controlled before VAD placement to prevent complications from hyperglycemia.

Medications

Medications commonly administered to patients are listed in Box 10-5. Medications that have been known to affect anesthetic management include anticoagulants, which contribute to post-CPB coagulopathy; milrinone, associated with a decreased risk of postimplantation RVF; amiodarone, associated with an increased risk of postimplantation RVF[11]; and diuretics, which can lead to electrolyte disturbances, including hypokalemia and hypomagnesemia, and intraoperative arrhythmias.

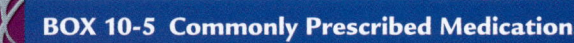

> **BOX 10-5 Commonly Prescribed Medications**
>
> Inotropic agents
>   Dobutamine, milrinone, digoxin
> Antihypertensive agents
>   Beta blockers, angiotensin-converting enzyme inhibitors, angiotensin II receptor blockers, direct vasodilators, diuretics
> Antiarrhythmic agents
>   Amiodarone
> Antianginal agents
> Antilipid agents
> Hypoglycemic agents
> Anticoagulants
>   Antiplatelet agents
>   Warfarin
>   Heparin and low-molecular-weight heparin

Laboratory Studies

Preoperative laboratory studies include electrolytes, especially in patients receiving diuretics or with chronic renal insufficiency; blood urea nitrogen and creatinine to diagnose chronic renal insufficiency; baseline hematocrit and platelet counts; baseline glucose level; liver function tests to diagnose underlying hepatic insufficiency; and coagulation studies, such as a functional platelet count, prothrombin time, partial thromboplastin time, INR, and fibrinogen. Cardiac studies include an electrocardiogram (ECG) to detect the presence of arrhythmias; echocardiogram to determine right ventricular function and to detect the presence of valvular disease; right-sided cardiac catheterization to determine pulmonary vascular resistance and the response to vasodilators, the transpulmonary gradient, and ventricular filling pressures[1]; and left-sided cardiac catheterization to determine left ventricular filling pressures and the patency of pre-existing grafts. Posteroanterior and lateral chest x-rays can be obtained to identify the presence of pleural effusions; pulmonary edema; or, in patients who have had a previous sternotomy, the retrosternal space. It is advisable to review a noncontrast computed tomography (CT) scan to help delineate ascending aortic size and degree of calcification and amount of pleural effusion and proximity of cardiac structures to the sternum. For patients with a history of peripheral vascular disease, CT scan should extend into the abdomen to assess the degree of calcification of abdominal vasculature including the renal and mesenteric vessels.

INDUCTION AND MONITORING

The anesthetic management of patients with severe cardiomyopathy is associated with increased morbidity and mortality, and the induction of these patients is one of the most critical aspects of anesthetic management. Before induction, the patient's AICD should be turned off, and external defibrillator pads should be applied, particularly in patients with a previous sternotomy. In addition to standard monitors, intra-arterial access via an IABP or an arterial catheter is mandatory to monitor beat-to-beat blood pressure during induction. A Swan-Ganz catheter is crucial not only to understand better the levels of preoperative support required after induction of anesthesia but also for making determinations regarding post-LVAD right heart function. A simple thermodilution catheter is adequate for pulsatile devices where the cardiac output determination is more reliable. In the case of the rotary blood pumps in which the algorithms for flow or cardiac output are more derived, a continuous cardiac output Swan-Ganz catheter is mandatory to obtain a reliable output measurement.

This catheter becomes very important in situations in which one needs to know the total cardiac output, which may be a combination of the VAD and the native cardiac function. Strict aseptic technique should be used during the insertion of invasive monitors to prevent infection.

The goal of induction is to produce hypnosis and analgesia while maintaining cardiac output. If the patient presents with inotropic support, it should be continued throughout the pre-CPB period. Induction agents such as etomidate, midazolam, and fentanyl provide stable hemodynamics. In these patients, the circulation time for intravenous anesthetics is prolonged, whereas the circulation time for inhalational agents is decreased. To prevent hypotension and decreased cardiac output owing to the loss of sympathetic tone during induction, inotropic support, such as low-dose dobutamine, milrinone, and epinephrine, may be initiated before or during induction. Large doses of vasopressor agents to treat hypotension can increase left ventricular afterload and can lead to pulseless electrical activity and cardiac arrest.

Except for the Jarvik 2000 VAD, which can be placed through a thoracotomy, most VADs are implanted through a median sternotomy. After intubation, large bore central and peripheral access should be obtained, especially if the patient has undergone a prior sternotomy or presents with a preoperative coagulopathy. A pulmonary artery catheter with mixed venous saturation capabilities is useful to measure pulmonary artery pressure; calculate the CVP/PCWP ratio; and measure mixed venous saturation, which may be the first indicator of poor perfusion owing to decreased cardiac output. After induction and institution of mechanical ventilation, baseline laboratory studies are obtained, and any abnormalities are corrected. These studies include arterial blood gases, potassium, hematocrit, glucose, a functional platelet test, activated clotting time (ACT), and thromboelastogram (TEG). Commonly seen abnormalities include hypokalemia, hyperglycemia, and anemia, which may be unmasked during induction.

The TEG is a valuable tool in assessing the presence of perioperative coagulopathy. The TEG evaluates clot initiation, formation, and stability using whole blood[22] and provides a graphic representation of the rate of fibrin polymerization and the overall strength of the clot. Within 30 minutes, the TEG can provide a measure of platelet function, coagulation proteases and inhibitors, and the fibrinolytic system. The time from the beginning of the test to the initial clot formation is known as the R time. A prolonged R time indicates reduced clotting factor activity and is treated with fresh frozen plasma. The clot formation time, or k time, measures time from the beginning of clot formation (R time) until the amplitude of the TEG reaches a specific level of clot strength of 20 mm and represents the dynamics of clot formation. The k time is affected by the activity of intrinsic clotting factors, fibrinogen, and platelets,[23] but the most common cause of a prolonged k time is fibrinogen deficiency, which is corrected with cryoprecipitate.[24] The alpha angle is the angle formed from the slope between the R and k values, and it measures the speed of fibrin buildup and cross-linking. It represents the rate at which a clot is formed. A decreased alpha angle also denotes a fibrinogen deficiency. The maximum amplitude represents clot strength and is dependent on platelet quantity and function and its interaction with fibrin. Decreases in maximum amplitude are treated with platelets. The LY30 is the clot lysis 30 minutes after the maximum amplitude and is a measure of clot stability. LY30 of greater than 7.5% denotes increased fibrinolysis and requires administration of antifibrinolytic agents such as tranexamic acid or aminocaproic acid.[24] A schematic of normal and abnormal TEGs is shown in Figure 10-1. In the absence of any anticoagulants, an abnormal TEG, especially with a prolonged R time, may be indicative of underlying hepatic disease owing to right ventricular dysfunction, and a biventricular VAD should be considered.

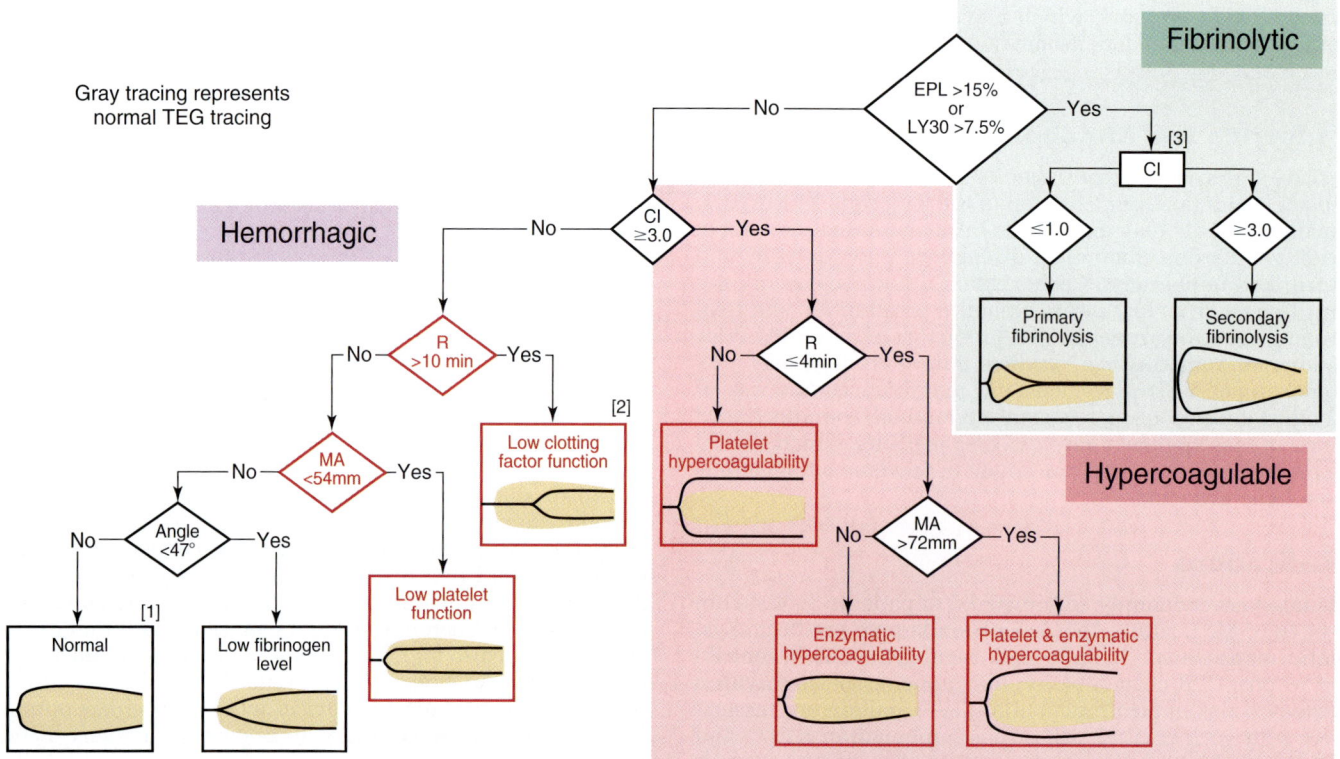

FIGURE 10-1 Thromboelastogram (TEG) analysis algorithm showing normal, hemorrhagic, and fibrinolytic states. *(From Haemonetics Inc., Braintree, MA.)*

The anesthetic goals of the pre-CPB period are to maintain cardiac output using inotropic support if necessary; to restrict fluid volume to avoid excessive central venous pressure and right ventricular end-diastolic pressure; and to correct any electrolyte abnormalities, anemia, and pre-CPB coagulopathy. If the INR is elevated or the R time is prolonged, fresh frozen plasma should be infused to minimize pre-CPB bleeding and to prevent post-CPB coagulopathy. To prevent postoperative infections, serum glucose levels are maintained between 100 mg/dL and 150 mg/dL using insulin infusions. If the patient has had a previous sternotomy, blood should be available in the operating room before incision. In cases where the patient is a candidate for heart transplantation, it is important to use a white blood cell filter or use white blood cell–poor packed red blood cell components to prevent subsequent HLA antibody sensitization.

TRANSESOPHAGEAL ECHOCARDIOGRAPHY

Before the patient is placed on CPB, a comprehensive transesophageal echocardiography (TEE) examination is performed to evaluate right ventricular function and to detect any intracardiac or aortic abnormalities that may impede proper VAD implantation and function. These abnormalities include a patent foramen ovale (PFO); aortic, mitral, and tricuspid valve abnormalities; the presence of intracardiac thrombi; and severe aortic atherosclerosis.

During proper LVAD function, left atrial pressure may decrease below right atrial pressure, producing right-to-left shunting, leading to hypoxemia or paradoxical embolism through a PFO. The interatrial septum should be interrogated using color flow Doppler and agitated saline contrast. A Valsalva maneuver can be performed to optimize right-to-left shunting. Conditions when a Valsalva maneuver may not detect a PFO include patients with elevated left atrial pressure that markedly exceeds right atrial pressure and patients with biventricular dysfunction in whom both the right atrial pressure and the left atrial pressure are elevated, decreasing the interatrial pressure gradient.[25] A Valsalva maneuver must be performed carefully because it may produce hemodynamic instability. A ventricular septal defect can also produce profound right-to-left shunting, and the interventricular septum should be interrogated in patients suspected to have a ventricular septal defect.

The detection of aortic valve insufficiency is a critical element of the TEE examination. The initiation of LVAD therapy decreases left ventricular diastolic pressure, increasing the transvalvular gradient and the degree of aortic regurgitation. Aortic regurgitation distends the left ventricle, producing hemodynamically compromising volume overload and inadequate forward flow. The degree of aortic insufficiency can be exacerbated when the position of the aortic outflow cannula is too close to the aortic valve, producing valvular distortion and turbulence.[2] The degree of aortic insufficiency before CPB may be underestimated in patients with heart failure because of a decreased transvalvular gradient secondary to increased left ventricular end-diastolic pressure and low aortic diastolic pressure.[26] Patients with moderate to severe aortic insufficiency require surgical treatment. If the LVAD is a continuous flow device or is placed as a bridge to recovery, a bioprosthetic valve may be placed. If the LVAD is pulsatile or is placed as a bridge to transplantation or for destination therapy, the valve may be oversewn to prevent regurgitation and peripheral embolism. Many surgeons have also performed aortic valve repair for central aortic insufficiency with rotary blood pumps.

The presence of aortic stenosis does not affect pulsatile devices because they do not depend on systolic blood flow through the aortic valve to generate cardiac output. With continuous flow devices, intermittent aortic valve opening may contribute to the cardiac output, and the aortic valve may need to be replaced. Because the aortic valve may not open or may open sporadically, mechanical aortic valves may develop thrombi on the aortic side of the prosthesis, leading to systemic embolization, and may require replacement with a bioprosthetic valve or need to be oversewn with a patch.[25]

Mitral stenosis produces low cardiac output by impeding LVAD filling and by exacerbating pulmonary hypertension and right ventricular dysfunction. Significant mitral stenosis requires correction at the time of LVAD implantation. Mitral regurgitation does not affect LVAD function. When LVAD therapy is initiated, the left ventricle reduces in size resulting in improved mitral leaflet coaptation and decreased mitral regurgitation. Significant postimplantation mitral regurgitation may be a sign of inadequate left ventricular decompression.

Other echocardiographic findings that affect LVAD implantation and function include significant tricuspid regurgitation, which decreases LVAD filling and should be treated with an annuloplasty ring; intracardiac thrombi, especially in the left atrium and left ventricle, which may lead to systemic embolization; and aortic atherosclerotic disease, especially at the aortic cannulation site. If severe atherosclerotic disease is present, epiaortic scanning may be useful in determining a cannulation site.

Evaluation of the right ventricle is one of the most important components of the TEE examination because the left and right ventricles are in series, and if the right ventricle is impaired, LVAD filling becomes impaired. The examination should include the evaluation of the right ventricular free wall and septal function, the presence of right ventricular dilation, the presence and degree of tricuspid regurgitation, the measurement of the right ventricle and right ventricular outflow tract fractional area change, and the tricuspid annular plane systolic excursion (TAPSE).[27,28]

Catena and Milazzo[28] devised a scale of echocardiographic and hemodynamic predictors of postimplantation RVF. Grade I right ventricular dysfunction is characterized by 2+ to 3+ tricuspid regurgitation, a right ventricular right atrial pressure difference decrease from 30 to 50 mm Hg, right ventricular fractional area change (FAC) from 30% to 35%, right ventricular outflow tract FAC from 20% to 40%, TAPSE between 10 mm and 15 mm, and pulmonary artery acceleration time of less than 90 seconds. Grade I right ventricular dysfunction primarily is due to a significant increase in pulmonary artery pressure caused by elevated left atrial and pulmonary venous pressures. Patients with grade I right ventricular dysfunction rarely require RVAD support because the decrease in right ventricular afterload is sufficient to improve right ventricular function. Grade II right ventricular dysfunction is characterized by severe right ventricular hypokinesis, right ventricular FAC 25% or less, right ventricular outflow tract fractional shortening (FS) ≥20% or less, and TAPSE 10 mm or less. These patients have intrinsic right ventricular dysfunction and many develop RVF when device therapy is initiated. These patients usually require maximal inotropic and pulmonary vasodilator support to obtain a gradual improvement in right ventricular function. Grade III right ventricular dysfunction is characterized by severe right ventricular hypokinesis or akinesis with right ventricular dilation and end-diastolic dimension greater than 85 mm, end-diastolic volume greater than 200 mL, and end-systolic volume greater than 177 mL. These patients are best treated with a planned biventricular VAD.[28]

When right ventricular dilation is present, Potapov and colleagues[29] showed that the right ventricular short axis-to-long axis ratio can be used to predict postimplantation RVF. A ratio less than 0.6 has been shown to predict right ventricular dysfunction after LVAD placement.

CARDIOPULMONARY BYPASS MANAGEMENT

Many patients have been exposed to heparin and have acquired antithrombin III deficiency. Antithrombin III deficiency can be treated with the administration of fresh frozen plasma or recombinant antithrombin III. The advantage of recombinant antithrombin III is that it is a nonhuman product and can prevent sensitization to blood products, especially in patients who are transplant candidates. An antifibrinolytic agent—either the lysine analog tranexamic acid or aminocaproic acid—is also administered to aid in postoperative coagulation. After the adequacy of heparinization is determined by ACT, the patient is placed on CPB. The ascending aorta and right atrial appendage are the usual cannulation sites. Once the patient is placed on CPB, the aortic valve should be reinterrogated for the presence of aortic insufficiency, which may be unmasked when the transvalvular gradients are closer to the values after VAD insertion.[26]

The management of these patients on CPB differs slightly from management of patients undergoing other cardiac procedures. Anesthetic management includes maintaining normoglycemia, normal electrolyte levels, urine output, and mean arterial pressure and treating preoperative coagulopathy. The neurohormonal stress of CPB producing insulin resistance and pre-existing diabetes mellitus predispose patients to hyperglycemia, which may increase the incidence of postoperative infections. Hyperglycemia is treated with an insulin infusion, with the goal of maintaining the glucose level less than 150 mg/dL. Electrolyte disturbances are common because of preoperative renal dysfunction, diuretic use, and intraoperative insulin infusions. Hypokalemia and hypomagnesemia are treated before weaning from bypass to prevent postoperative atrial and ventricular arrhythmias.

To optimize right ventricular function after CPB, the patient is weaned from bypass in a hypovolemic state, with a low central venous pressure. To obtain this state, fluid has to be removed from the patient and bypass circuit; this can be accomplished by the administration of diuretics, especially if the patient has previously been receiving diuretics, and by ultrafiltration by the perfusionist. In patients who are at risk for postoperative bleeding, such as patients on preoperative warfarin therapy or with hepatic dysfunction, the bypass pump may be primed with fresh frozen plasma to decrease the severity of postoperative coagulopathy.

The last goal is to maintain mean arterial pressure to provide adequate cerebral and end-organ perfusion. Hypotension on CPB leading to the development of postoperative vasoplegia is more common in these patients than in patients undergoing routine cardiac procedures. Vasoplegic syndrome is defined as a low systemic vascular resistance state with a high cardiac output and low filling pressures that are refractory to catecholamine support and is associated with a high postoperative mortality.[30] Risk factors for the development of perioperative vasoplegia include the prolonged use of medications, such as angiotensin-converting enzyme inhibitors, beta blockers, calcium channel blockers, amiodarone, and heparin; patient factors, such as left ventricular ejection fraction less than 35%, symptoms of congestive heart failure, and diabetes mellitus; and intraoperative factors, such as low mean arterial pressure and the use of preoperative vasoconstrictors, the length of CPB, normothermic bypass, and higher preoperative and postoperative hematocrit.[31]

The exact etiology is unknown, but proposed mechanisms include the development of systemic inflammatory response syndrome with the release of proinflammatory vasodilatory mediators such as interleukin (IL)-1, IL-6, IL-8, tumor necrosis factor, and atrial natriuretic peptide[32,33]; a deficiency or depletion of vasopressin on bypass[34]; endothelial injury[35]; or extensive complement activation.[36] The release of inflammatory cytokines may lead to guanylate cyclase and cyclic guanosine monophosphate (cGMP) production, leading to vascular smooth muscle relaxation. The treatment of hypotension on CPB may require the use of alpha agents, such as phenylephrine and norepinephrine or vasopressin.[37] If phenylephrine is unsuccessful in treating hypotension on CPB, vasopressin should be the next therapeutic agent of choice because it increases systemic vascular resistance with minimal increases in pulmonary vascular resistance.[38] In patients in whom the mean arterial pressure is resistant to catecholamine or vasopressin, methylene blue, a guanyl cyclase inhibitor, has been advocated as a second-line therapy to counteract cGMP-mediated vasodilation.[33]

Because VAD insertion does not require the use of cardioplegia, inotropic support with milrinone, dobutamine, or epinephrine is initiated near the end of the CPB run to support the unassisted ventricle. The phosphodiesterase inhibitor milrinone provides both inotropy and pulmonary artery vasodilation. Levosimendan, a calcium sensitizer with inodilator properties, has been shown to improve right ventricular function in patients with biventricular failure; however, this agent is unavailable in the United States.[39,40] In patients with preoperative pulmonary hypertension or who develop post-CPB pulmonary hypertension, inhaled agents, such as nitric oxide, epoprostenol, milrinone, or nitroglycerin, or intravenous agents, such as nitroglycerin or sodium nitroprusside, may be used to decrease pulmonary artery pressure and improve right ventricular function and LVAD filling. In patients receiving biventricular support, small doses of milrinone may be useful to decrease pulmonary artery pressure and to assist VAD filling.

After the cannulas are inserted, the heart and device need to be deaired. Common sites for the accumulation of air include the cannulas, the pulmonary veins, the left ventricular apex, left atrium and appendage, and right coronary sinus of Valsalva.[41,42] Air in the right coronary sinus and artery can produce right ventricular ischemia and RVF after CPB. Once deairing has been accomplished, the patient is weaned from CPB, and the device is started. With pulsatile devices, such as the Thoratec VAD (Thoratec Corp, Pleasanton, CA), the device is started in the asynchronous or fixed mode with a slow fixed rate, low ejection pressure, and moderate vacuum. After the suture lines are inspected for leaks, the ejection pressure and vacuum are adjusted until complete pump filling and emptying is achieved.

With continuous flow devices, such as the HeartMate II (Thoratec Corp., Pleasanton, CA) and CentriMag, the device is started at the lowest speed. When the device is completely deaired and the left ventricle is full, the speed is gradually increased. If the LVAD speed is increased before the left ventricle is full, air can be entrained.

After separating from CPB and once hemodynamically stable, a post-CPB TEE examination is performed. The interatrial septum should be reinterrogated to diagnose a PFO that may have been masked by increased left atrial pressures. For patients undergoing LVAD implantation, the examination should detect the presence or absence of aortic valve opening and should assess the degree of mitral regurgitation, right ventricular function, extent of left ventricular decompression, and cannula placement (Figs. 10-2 and 10-3).

Pulsatile LVADs that provide full support prevent systolic opening of the aortic valve because of the increased aortic to left ventricular pressure gradient produced by the negative pressure generated by the left ventricular inflow cannula and ejection through the aortic cannula. Continuous flow LVADs may provide full or partial support, and the degree of support

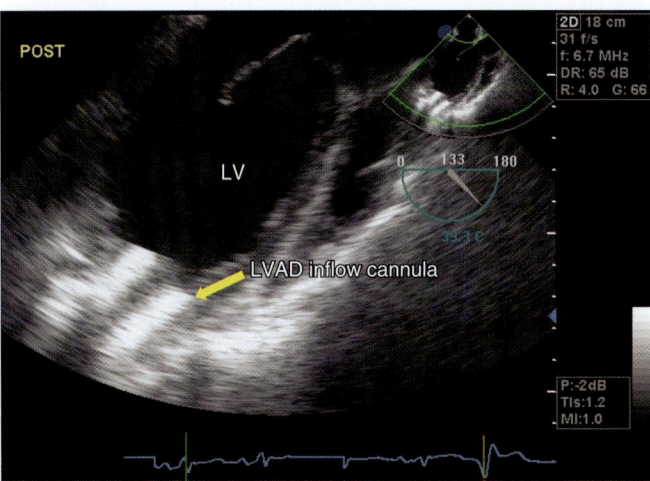

FIGURE 10-2 Transesophageal echocardiography (TEE) midesophageal long axis view of left ventricular assist device (LVAD) cannula. LV, left ventricle.

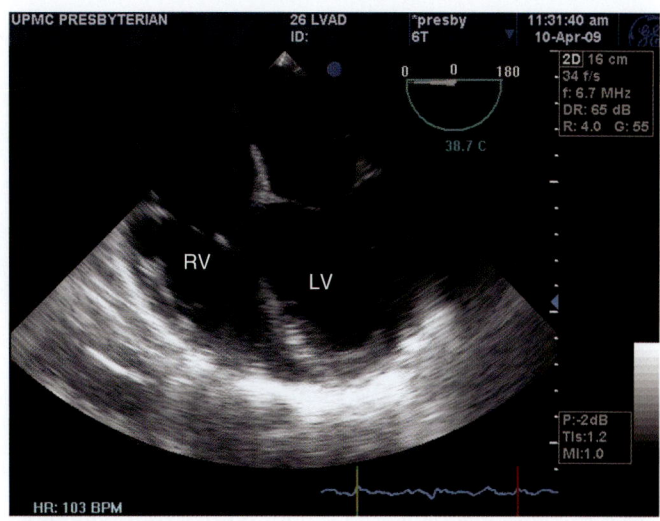

FIGURE 10-4 Transesophageal echocardiography (TEE) four chamber view of decompressed left ventricle (LV) with normal right ventricle (RV).

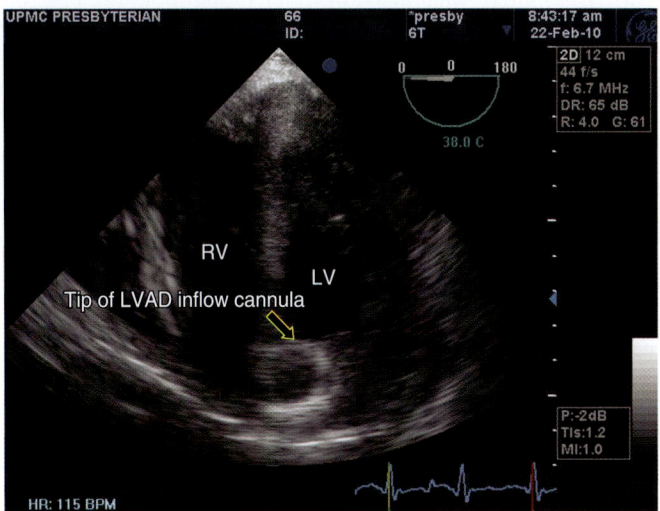

FIGURE 10-3 Transesophageal echocardiography (TEE) transgastric short axis view of left ventricular assist device (LVAD) cannula. LV, left ventricle; RV, right ventricle.

flow devices, such as the HeartMate II and CentriMag, show a pulsatile pattern synchronous with the ECG superimposed on a continuous flow pattern throughout the device cycle with peak filling velocities of 1 to 2 m/sec.[44] The outflow cannula for most devices is located at the right anterolateral aspect of the ascending aorta. An exception is the Jarvik 2000, where the outflow cannula is in the lower one-third of the descending thoracic aorta.

In patients receiving an RVAD or biventricular VAD, placement of the inflow and outflow cannulas should be evaluated by TEE. The inflow cannula is usually placed in the right atrium, and the tip of the cannula should be seen in the middle of the chamber, away from the tricuspid valve and septal wall (Fig. 10-5). The outflow cannula can be sutured to the main or right pulmonary artery or can be inserted into the main pulmonary artery from the right ventricle. The tip of the outflow cannula should be seen 1.5 to 2 cm beyond the pulmonic valve.[45] As with LVAD cannulas, RVAD cannulas should be interrogated using color flow, pulsed wave, and continuous wave Doppler, and RVAD flows should be similar to LVAD flows.

is associated with intermittent opening of the aortic valve. The higher the degree of support, the less frequent the aortic valve opening.[43]

Echocardiographic signs of normal LVAD function include a neutral interventricular septum, a decompressed left ventricle, decreased mitral regurgitation compared with the pre-CPB examination, adequate right ventricular contractility, and minimal tricuspid regurgitation (Fig. 10-4). The inflow cannula, most commonly placed in the left ventricular apex, should be aligned with the left ventricular outflow tract and not abutting any ventricular wall. The inflow cannula can be evaluated with color, pulsed wave, and continuous wave Doppler. A normal color flow Doppler pattern should consist of laminar, unidirectional flow. Abnormally elevated velocities and turbulent flow suggest cannula obstruction.

Pulsed wave Doppler can be used to calculate device stroke volume and output for both inflow and outflow cannulas, and continuous wave Doppler can quantify the amount of flow from the atrium to the VAD. Using pulsed wave Doppler, pulsatile devices show a pattern of pulsatile flow with normal flows of approximately 2.3 m/sec, corresponding with an inflow cannula diameter of 16 mm. Continuous

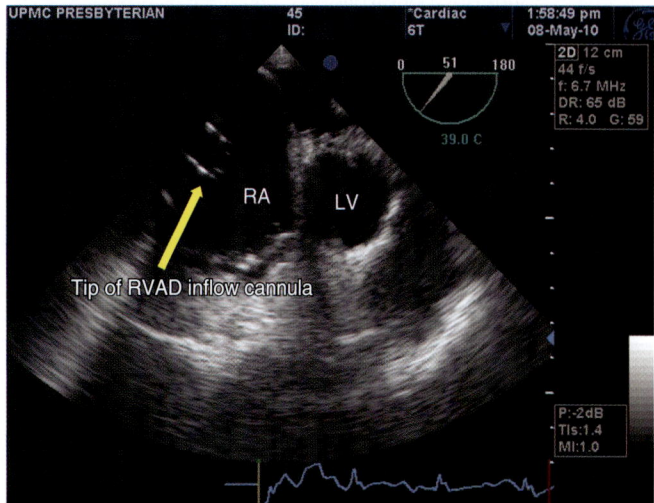

FIGURE 10-5 Transesophageal echocardiography (TEE) four chamber view of right ventricular assist device (RVAD) cannula. LV, left ventricle; RA, right atrium.

MANAGEMENT AFTER CARDIOPULMONARY BYPASS

After the patient is weaned from CPB with an LVAD or RVAD, the goals of anesthetic management are to maintain optimal preload, to allow the pump to fill; to maintain systemic vascular resistance to maintain coronary perfusion pressure of the unassisted ventricle; to prevent systemic hypertension, which would impede LVAD emptying; to prevent pulmonary hypertension, which would impede LVAD filling or RVAD emptying; and to maintain contractility in the unassisted ventricle.

PULSATILE DEVICES

Pneumatic pulsatile devices, such as the Thoratec VAD, have five major settings: mode of operation, device rate, drive pressure, vacuum, and duration of systole. The most important is the mode of operation. There are three different modes: the asynchronous mode, where the device rate is fixed and not in synch with the patient's ECG; the volume mode, another asynchronous mode where the rate and cardiac output depend on VAD filling; and the external asynchronous mode, where the VAD is synchronized to the patient's ECG and is a weaning mode. The device is initially set in the asynchronous mode, and as the patient recovers, the device is switched to the volume mode with a backup rate, which allows increases in cardiac output during normal activity and exercise. The other variables that need to be set include the duration of pump systole, used to permit diastolic filling; the drive pressure, the internal device pressure required to allow blood ejection; and the vacuum, which assists in device filling. Patients with systemic hypertension require a higher driving pressure to allow the device to empty.[46]

Continuous Flow Devices

Continuous flow devices can be divided into axial and centrifugal pumps. Axial flow pumps, such as the HeartMate II, Jarvik 2000, and Impella, produce high flows at low pressures by spinning an impeller, whereas continuous flow devices, such as the CentriMag, produce higher pressures at lower flows using rotating discs of blades or concentric cones.[47,48] Advantages of the axial flow pumps are that they are smaller, are more comfortable, and require less power than centrifugal pumps.[48] The most important setting is the rpm, which is initially set low and then gradually increased until a normal cardiac index is obtained.

Physiology of Ventricular Assist Devices

When a VAD is implanted, depending on the extent of residual native ventricular function, there may be two competing parallel ventricles. They compete for the same left atrial preload, and both are dependent on the systemic or pulmonary vascular resistance. In most cases, the native ventricle acts as a passive conduit to VAD filling.

With pulsatile VADs, the device rate and cardiac output depend on preload and pump filling. In the volume mode, hypovolemia manifests as device bradycardia, whereas hypervolemia manifests as device tachycardia.[46] In contrast, continuous flow pumps can be coupled to the native ventricle and either can replace the entire cardiac output or can augment any residual ventricular function. When augmenting the left ventricle, the aortic valve opens, creating pulsatility. Increasing the rpm setting increases the contribution from the pump.

Biventricular Support

With biventricular support, the native heart does not participate in maintaining cardiac output; therefore the anesthetic management consists of ensuring adequate device preload through fluid administration and by preventing vasodilation, which can decrease device blood return, and to prevent increases in both pulmonary and systemic vascular resistance, which may impede device ejection. With a normally functioning biventricular device, there is always a greater LVAD output than RVAD output because of increased LVAD preload, owing to blood from the bronchial circulation that enters the left atrium through the pulmonary veins. If there is elevated pulmonary hypertension, or if it is difficult for the LVAD to fill, small doses of a pulmonary vasodilator, such as inhaled prostacyclin or nitric oxide, or an inotropic agent, such as milrinone, may be required to augment LVAD filling.

DIFFERENTIAL DIAGNOSIS OF DEVICE MALFUNCTION

The differential diagnosis of device malfunction can be divided into inadequate filling and impaired device ejection.

Inadequate Ventricular Assist Device Filling

The most common causes of inadequate device filling are hypovolemia, tamponade, and RVF. Hypovolemia is common after VAD implantation and can be caused by the intraoperative administration of diuretics, hemofiltration during CPB, and post-CPB coagulopathy. Because VADs are preload-dependent, hypovolemia manifests as a decrease in both mean arterial pressure and cardiac output. TEE may reveal a leftward shift of the interventricular septum and tricuspid regurgitation, which may impair VAD filling further. A serious consequence of severe hypovolemia is the development of air emboli. In patients with pulsatile LVADs, severe hypovolemia can lead to decreased left-sided pressures with collapse of the left ventricular chamber. The LVAD attempts to fill against this collapsed chamber, generating up to 5 mm Hg of subatmospheric pressure. This negative pressure may allow air to enter through surgical sites, such as venting needle holes, grafts, and suture lines, creating a systemic air embolism that may produce RVF secondary to right ventricular ischemia or neurologic complications. Severe hypovolemia is also dangerous in patients with continuous flow RVADs. Because most of these devices create suction, they can entrain air from both surgical sites and from right atrial cannulas or catheters.[49,50]

RVF after LVAD implantation is common and is a major cause of morbidity and mortality. The mechanism for RVF is alteration in right ventricular geometry secondary to either underlying right ventricular dysfunction or LVAD activation. This mechanism can be explained by understanding normal and abnormal right ventricular physiology. Normally, the right ventricle is composed of an interventricular septum, a dual layer of muscle fibers oriented in an oblique formation, and the right ventricular free wall, composed of muscle fibers oriented transversely.[51] The oblique orientation of the muscle fibers allows the septum to twist during contraction, whereas the transverse orientation allows the right ventricular free wall to constrict the right ventricle circumferentially. The septal wall is also responsible for ventricular interdependence because the twisting motion of the septum produces up to 40% of left ventricular output. In the right ventricle, most normal contraction depends on the septum; this has been proven experimentally and clinically when the right ventricular free wall was destroyed or infarcted without significant hemodynamic consequences.[52]

When left ventricular systolic or diastolic dysfunction occurs, septal architecture is disrupted. With systolic dysfunction, as the affected ventricle dilates, the oblique fibers become more transverse, impairing septal twist and shortening, leading to impaired ventricular contraction.[53,54] Left ventricular diastolic dysfunction can increase left-sided filling pressures, leading to bowing and stretching of the septum toward the right ventricle, impairing right ventricular function further. Right ventricular function becomes predominantly dependent on the transverse fibers in the right ventricular free wall. Right ventricular function becomes further impaired with the development of elevated pulmonary artery pressures. Besides RVF secondary to left ventricular failure, RVF secondary to coronary artery disease, myocarditis, or pulmonary hypertension may also be present.

Initiation of LVAD therapy can also affect right ventricular function. Acute unloading of the left ventricle produces a septal shift that alters right ventricular size and shape, leading to decreased systolic function and increased diastolic compliance.[16] LVAD therapy also shifts volume from the central to the peripheral compartment, decreasing pulmonary artery pressure and right ventricular afterload but increasing right ventricular preload. The decreased contractility and increased right ventricular preload can precipitate overt RVF in patients with pre-existing right ventricular dysfunction. Intraoperative factors that can precipitate postimplantation RVF include hypervolemia; right ventricular ischemia or stunning, owing to air in the right coronary artery or untreated coronary artery disease; and increased pulmonary vascular resistance produced by CPB-induced release of thromboxane A_2 and complement, hypoxia, and massive transfusion, which increases the production of the pulmonary vasoconstrictors IL-1β, IL-6, IL-10, and tumor necrosis factor-α.[20,44,55] RVF is poorly tolerated, leading to decreased LVAD filling, systemic hypoperfusion, and end-organ dysfunction, and may require temporary or permanent RVAD placement. Besides RVF, other conditions that impede LVAD filling include tricuspid regurgitation and atrial arrhythmias.

RVF occurring after implantation can be diagnosed with TEE, which reveals right ventricular dilation and hypokinesis and a flattened interventricular septum that bulges into the left ventricle, both resulting in tricuspid regurgitation. RVF may be associated with a low pulmonary artery pressure, which is reflective of poor right ventricular output rather than decreased right ventricular pressure (Figs. 10-6 and 10-7).

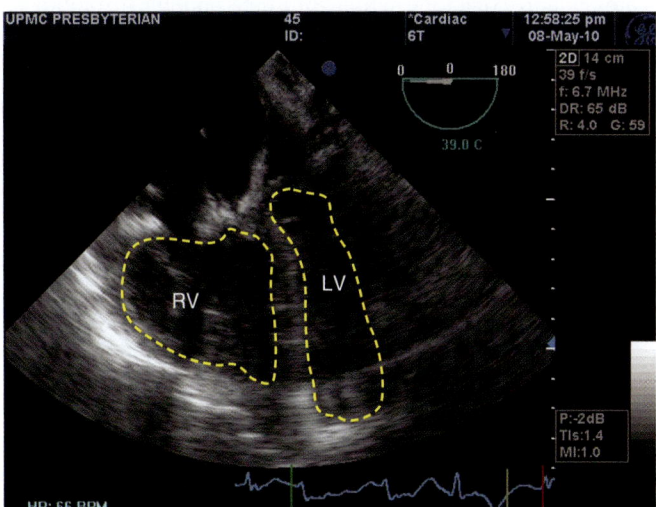

FIGURE 10-6 Transesophageal echocardiography (TEE) midesophageal four chamber view of right ventricular failure (RVF) with left ventricular collapse. LV, left ventricle; RV, right ventricle.

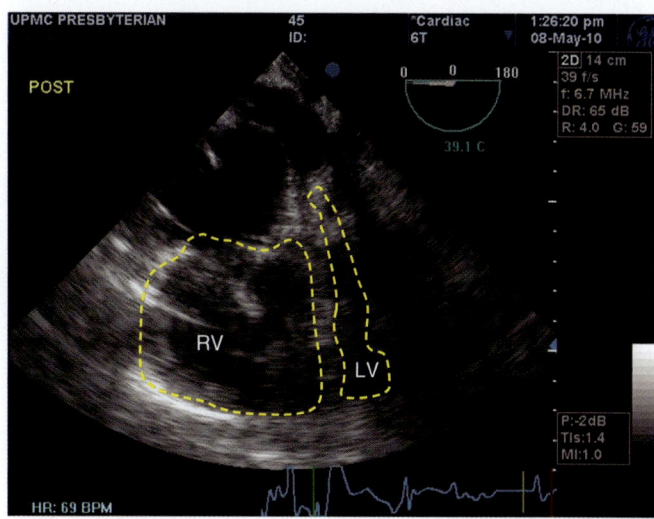

FIGURE 10-7 Transesophageal echocardiography (TEE) midesophageal four chamber view of increased right atrial pressure, right ventricular dilation, and left ventricular collapse. LV, left ventricle; RV, right ventricle.

Strategies to optimize perioperative right ventricular function after implantation include avoiding excessive right ventricular preload when separating from CPB; minimizing perioperative bleeding and administering blood products; augmenting right ventricular function with inotropic agents such as milrinone, epinephrine, and dobutamine; and decreasing right ventricular afterload with inhaled agents, such as prostacyclin, milrinone, nitroglycerin, or nitric oxide. The use of intravenous pulmonary vasodilators, such as nitroglycerin, is limited by systemic hypotension and by the inhibition of hypoxic pulmonary vasoconstriction, leading to decreased alveolar oxygenation.[56]

Impaired Device Ejection

The most common causes of impaired device ejection include excessive systemic or pulmonary vascular resistance, device or native valve regurgitation, cannula obstruction, incompetent device, or the return of native ventricular function. A rare cause of impaired device ejection is primary pump failure.

TEE is useful in diagnosing impaired device ejection. Spontaneous echo contrast in the left atrium or left ventricle and left ventricular dilation are signs of impaired device function or cannula obstruction.[57] Besides RVF, a leftward shift of the septum may be due to excessive decompression caused by high pump speeds.

Cannula obstruction can also be diagnosed using echocardiography. Inflow cannula obstruction is defined as interrupted flow into the cannula during VAD diastole.[58] Causes include hypovolemia, intracardiac thrombus, cannula misalignment, and compression of the interventricular septum. In patients with right atrial cannulas, obstruction may be produced by the anterior leaflet of the tricuspid valve, by the tricuspid subvalvular apparatus, or by an interatrial septum aneurysm. Inflow cannula obstruction can be diagnosed using color flow Doppler, which reveals turbulent flow, and by pulsed or continuous wave Doppler, which reveals turbulent flow with velocities greater than 2.3 m/sec. Outflow cannula obstruction results in accelerated Doppler velocities more proximally compared with distal flows along the cannula and can be diagnosed as turbulent flow with elevated velocities using color flow, pulsed wave, and continuous wave Doppler.[44] A sign of possible cannula obstruction in patients with a biventricular VAD is an RVAD output greater than LVAD output.

Another cause of impaired ejection is native or device valve regurgitation. Valvular regurgitation manifests clinically as fluid overload, inappropriate tachycardia in patients with pulsatile devices, and device malfunction. Normal pulsed wave Doppler flow appears unidirectional and laminar.[27] Using color flow Doppler, inflow valve regurgitation appears as turbulent flow during LVAD ejection, whereas pulsed wave Doppler reveals flow reversal in the inflow cannula during ejection. Other findings include a dilated left ventricle with frequent aortic valve opening, reduced outflow graft velocity time integral and peak velocity, and a differential between the Doppler-derived cardiac output calculated at the pulmonic valve and the device output.[27,58] Outflow graft regurgitation, also associated with device tachycardia with pulsatile devices, is seen as retrograde flow during device diastole using color flow Doppler and a differential between the VAD output and the forward cardiac output.[58,59]

For pulsatile devices, left ventricular recovery may interfere with LVAD function. Normally, the left ventricle acts as a passive conduit for VAD filling. When the left ventricle begins to recover, it can be in phase or out of phase with the device.[60] The left ventricle and LVAD are in phase when left ventricular systole occurs during LVAD diastole, resulting in maximal device filling and decreased filling pressures. When left ventricular systole occurs during device systole, the two are out of phase, competing for the same left ventricular preload, leading to decreased LVAD filling and increased filling pressures.

COAGULATION

After the patient is weaned from CPB and is hemodynamically stable, protamine is administered, and in patients with no perioperative risk factors, this is usually sufficient to reverse heparinization. Post-CPB coagulopathy is the most common complication after VAD insertion; its incidence is 11% to 48%.[44] Preoperative risk factors include prior sternotomy, emergent procedures, hepatic or renal dysfunction, hereditary coagulopathies, and use of anticoagulants or antiplatelet agents. Intraoperative risk factors include the presence of surgical bleeding, length of CPB, hypothermia, and inadequate or excessive protamine administration. Excessive protamine acts as an anticoagulant and can decrease platelet adhesion.[61]

The diagnosis of post-CPB coagulopathy is both a clinical and a laboratory diagnosis. Clinically, coagulopathy is diagnosed when there is no evidence of a surgical source, there is an absence of clot formation, and there is diffuse bleeding from suture lines and puncture sites. The initial laboratory tests that are performed are ACT, functional platelet assay, and TEG.

ACT is the simplest and fastest of the assays, but a major disadvantage is that it is not specific for heparin; elevated ACT can be due to inadequate heparin reversal, thrombocytopenia, or the presence of platelet inhibitors.[62] The Hepcon HMS system has the ability to calculate the concentration of heparin required to achieve a desired ACT, to measure the heparin concentration in the blood at the termination of CPB, and can confirm the complete reversal of heparin after protamine administration, which may lead to decreased blood product administration.

A functional platelet assay provides a measure of the degree of platelet reactivity after CPB. With these tests, whole blood is added to an analyzer along with platelet activators. Depending on the analyzer, the degree of platelet reactivity is determined by the time it takes for a clot to form, as with the PFA-100 (Siemens, New York) and VerifyNow (Accumetrics, San Diego) analyzers, or the ratio between activated and non-activated platelet count, as with the Platelet Works (Helena Laboratories, Beaumont, TX) analyzer. The TEG can also assist in diagnosing platelet deficiency or dysfunction, which appears as a decreased maximum amplitude.[62] To obtain a quantitative platelet count, a complete blood count is required. The TEG is useful in diagnosing deficiencies in coagulation factors or inadequate heparin reversal, hypofibrinogenemia, and the presence of fibrinolysis, which would confirm the diagnosis of coagulopathy; a coagulation profile including a platelet count, prothrombin time, partial thromboplastin time, INR, and fibrinogen may be obtained.

The treatment of coagulopathy should be tailored to the cause. The surgical site should be inspected for bleeding. If there is no evidence of surgical bleeding, patients with a low platelet count, a reduced maximum amplitude, or an abnormal platelet function assay should be treated with platelets. Platelets and desmopressin should also be considered in patients with pre-existing renal dysfunction. Fresh frozen plasma and cryoprecipitate should be reserved for patients with evidence of a prolonged R time or increased angle or k time. Increased LY30 should be treated with an antifibrinolytic, such as aminocaproic acid or tranexamic acid. When multiple blood products are required, care must be taken to prevent anemia, hypocalcemia, and right ventricular distention. Inotropic agents, pulmonary vasodilators, and diuretics may be required to support the right ventricle. Any blood products that are administered must be screened for viral contamination and leukocyte reduced.

Besides an increased incidence of RVF, the consequences of massive transfusion include sensitization to blood products, an increased incidence of transfusion-related acute lung injury, and an induced immunosuppressant state that may increase the incidence of infection.[63–65] Besides desmopressin, pharmacologic treatments include topical procoagulants administered into the surgical field and activated factor VII (factor VIIa). At the present time, factor VIIa is approved only for the prevention and treatment of bleeding in patients with hemophilia A or hemophilia B with inhibitors, in patients with acquired hemophilia, and in patients with congenital factor VII deficiency; the recommended dose in these situations is 90 µg/kg. There has been increasing off-label use of this drug to treat uncontrolled hemorrhage during cardiac, trauma, general, and orthopedic procedures.

Factor VIIa acts by both tissue factor–dependent and tissue factor–independent mechanisms. Damage to the subendothelial surface exposes tissue factor, which forms a complex with circulating factor VIIa. The resulting tissue factor–factor VIIa complex activates factor IX and factor X, leading to the generation of a small quantity of thrombin. This thrombin activates platelets and cofactors, which produce enough thrombin to cleave fibrinogen to produce a clot. If tissue factor is unavailable, factor VIIa can generate thrombin by binding to factor X located on the platelet surface.[66] The optimal dose of factor VIIa to treat post-CPB coagulopathy is unknown because the administration of large doses is associated with thrombotic complications, including stroke, deep vein thrombosis, pulmonary embolus, ventricular thrombus, myocardial infarction, and death.[67] The increased incidence of thromboembolic events is due to the expression of tissue factor present on coronary artery plaques and the initiation of coagulation produced by CPB.[68]

Although there is no suggested dose of factor VIIa, multiple prospective and retrospective studies have shown a reduced incidence of thrombotic side effects with doses of 40 µg/kg or less, and 10 to 20 µg/kg may be effective.[67] Before factor VIIa is considered, it is important to ensure that adequate blood products and platelets are infused to provide the substrate for factor VIIa to be effective.

If the coagulopathy persists after chest closure, the patient may return to the operating room with cardiac tamponade. Signs of tamponade include hypotension, tachycardia, increased right trial and pulmonary artery pressures, decreased

VAD output, and oliguria, with a widened mediastinum on the chest x-ray. These symptoms are similar to symptoms with RVF, and the easiest method to differentiate between the two is TEE. Echocardiography findings consistent with cardiac tamponade include a localized or generalized pericardial effusion with right atrial systolic or right ventricular diastolic collapse, reciprocal respiratory changes in left ventricle and left ventricular volume, inferior vena cava dilation, and respiratory flow variation of transmitral and transtricuspid inflow velocities.[69,70] The treatment of cardiac tamponade consists of surgical exploration of the mediastinum, with removal of the clot and the administration of blood products to treat any residual coagulopathy.

After the patient has been stabilized and the bleeding is under control, the chest is closed. After chest closure, the interatrial septum should be interrogated once more for a PFO, which could be unmasked because chest closure increases right atrial pressure, and chest tube suction decreases left atrial pressure by generating negative intrathoracic pressures, leading to increased right-to-left shunting.[71] After the incision is closed, the patient is transferred to the ICU.

ANESTHESIA FOR PATIENTS WITH VENTRICULAR ASSIST DEVICES UNDERGOING NONCARDIAC SURGERY

Besides the typical preoperative assessment, the preoperative assessment of a patient with a VAD undergoing noncardiac surgery should include the type of device, the coagulation requirements for that device, the function of the unsupported ventricle, any end-organ dysfunction, and the surgical procedure. Before the patient arrives to the operating room, an engineer who understands the device console, the power source, and battery life should be available for transport. For elective procedures, devices that require anticoagulation with warfarin require conversion to heparin. With emergent procedures, fresh frozen plasma is required to reverse the anticoagulation. If the patient has an AICD, it should be turned off, and defibrillator pads should be applied to the patient.

In the operating room, the choice of monitoring depends on the type of device, the surgical procedure, and the function of the unassisted ventricle. Otherwise healthy patients with pulsatile devices undergoing simple procedures require only American Society of Anesthesiologists standard monitors. In patients with continuous flow devices, it may be difficult to obtain an oxygen saturation or noninvasive blood pressure, necessitating invasive blood pressure monitoring. Invasive blood pressure monitoring and possibly central venous pressure monitoring are reserved for patients with impaired right ventricular function or who are undergoing extensive surgical procedures, with expected blood loss. All invasive monitors must be placed with strict aseptic technique to avoid infection. TEE is helpful to assess right ventricular function, hypovolemia, septal shift, and cannula placement.

The goals of induction and anesthetic management are to maintain preload, maintain contractility and rhythm of the unassisted ventricle, and maintain afterload. In patients with right ventricular dysfunction, inotropic drugs and pulmonary vasodilators may be helpful to prevent overt RVF. Because of the abdominal placement of the pump, these patients should be considered to have a full stomach and at risk for aspiration.

After the patient is intubated, it is important to control hypoxia and hypercarbia, especially in laparoscopic or thoracoscopic procedures, and to avoid acidosis to prevent increased pulmonary pressures and RVF. Excessive amounts of positive end-expiratory pressure can also affect right ventricular function. The cautery pad should be placed away from the device, to prevent electrical current from traveling through the pump. If excessive interference occurs with monopolar cautery, bipolar cautery should be considered.[72]

With a pulsatile device, the device cardiac output and heart rate should be monitored. Inappropriate bradycardia could signify hypovolemia. Hypovolemia with continuous flow devices manifests as decreased cardiac output. Decreased systemic vascular resistance should be treated to avoid decreases in cardiac output and coronary perfusion pressure to the unassisted ventricle and can be treated with small doses of phenylephrine or vasopressin, and decreased right ventricular function can be treated with inotropic agents and pulmonary vasodilators. Any blood products administered must be filtered and screened. At the end of the procedure, it is important to prevent emergence hypertension, which may impede VAD emptying, and hypoxia or hypercarbia, which can exacerbate right ventricular dysfunction.

REFERENCES

1. Lietz K, Miller L. Patient selection for left-ventricular assist devices. *Curr Opin Cardiol.* 2009;24:246–250.
2. Wilson S, Mudge G, Stewart G, et al. Evaluation for a ventricular assist device: selecting the appropriate candidate. *Circulation.* 2009;119:2225–2232.
3. Norman J, Cooley D, Iago S. Prognostic indices for survival during postcardiotomy intra-aortic balloon pump support in 728 patients. *J Thorac Cardiovasc Surg.* 1977; 74:709–720.
4. Schaffer J, Allen J, Weiss E, et al. Evaluation of risk indices in continuous-flow left ventricular assist device patients. *Ann Thorac Surg.* 2009;88:1889–1896.
5. Alba A, Rao V, Ivanov J, et al. Usefulness of the INTERMACS scale to predict outcomes after mechanical assist device implantation. *J Heart Lung Transplant.* 2009;28:827–833.
6. Lietz K, Long J, Kfoury A. Outcomes of left ventricular assist device implantation as destination therapy in the post REMATCH era: implications for patient selection. *Circulation.* 2007;116:497–505.
7. Levy W, Mozaffarian D, Linker D, et al. The Seattle Heart Failure Model: prediction of survival in heart failure. *Circulation.* 2006;113:1424–1433.
8. Mielniczuk L, Mussivand T, Davies R, et al. Patient selection for left ventricular assist devices. *Artif Organs.* 2004;28:152–157.
9. Dang N, Topkara V, Mercando M, et al. Right heart failure after left ventricular assist device implantation in patients with chronic congestive heart failure. *J Heart Lung Transplant.* 2006;25:1–6.
10. Fitzpatrick J, Hiesinger W, Hsu V, et al. Early planned institution of biventricular mechanical circulatory support results in improved outcomes compared to delayed conversion of a left ventricular assist device to a biventricular assist device. *J Thorac Cardiovasc Surg.* 2009;137:971–977.
11. Fukamachi K, McCarthy P, Smedira N, et al. Preoperative risk factors for right ventricular failure after implantable left ventricular assist device insertion. *Ann Thorac Surg.* 1999;68:2181–2184.
12. Matthews J, Koelling T, Pagani F, et al. The right ventricular failure risk score. *J Am Coll Cardiol.* 2008;51:2163–2172.
13. Ochiani Y, McCarthy P, Smedira N, et al. Predictors of severe right ventricular failure after implantable left ventricular assist device insertion: analysis of 245 patients. *Circulation.* 2002;106:I-198–I-202.
14. Kormos R, Gasior T, Kawai A, et al. Transplant candidate's clinical status rather than right ventricular function defines need for univentricular versus biventricular support. *J Thorac Cardiovasc Surg.* 1996;111:773–778.
15. Hennig F, Potapov E, Hetzer R, et al. Prediction of right ventricular function after implantation of left ventricular assist device. *J Card Fail.* 2005;11:S140.
16. Kormos KL, Teuteberg JJ, Pagani FD, et al. Right ventricular failure in patients with the HeartMate II continuous-flow left ventricular assist device: incidence, risk factors, and effect on outcomes. *J Thorac Cardiovasc Surg.* 2010;139:1316–1324.
17. Aaronson K, Patel H, Pagani F, et al. Patient selection for left ventricular assist device therapy. *Ann Thorac Surg.* 2003;75:S29–S35.
18. Farrar D. Preoperative predictors of survival in patients with Thoratec ventricular assist devices as a bridge to heart transplantation. Thoratec ventricular assist device principle investigators. *J Heart Lung Transplant.* 1994;13:93–100.
19. Oz M, Rose E, Levin H. Selection criteria for placement of left ventricular assist devices. *Am Heart J.* 1995;129:173–177.
20. Furukawa K, Motomura T, Nose Y. Right ventricular failure after left ventricular assist device implantation: the need for an implantable right ventricular assist device. *Artif Organs.* 2005;29:369–377.
21. Masai T, Sawa Y, Ohtake S, et al. Hepatic dysfunction after left ventricular mechanical assist in patients with end-stage heart failure: role of inflammatory response and hepatic microcirculation. *Ann Thorac Surg.* 2002;73:549–555.
22. Luddington R. Thromboelastography/thromboelastometry. *Clin Lab Haematol.* 2005; 27:81–90.
23. Klein S, Slaughter T, Vail P, et al. Thromboelastography as a perioperative measure of anticoagulation resulting from low molecular weight heparin: a comparison with anti-Xa concentrations. *Anesth Analg.* 2000;91:1091–1095.
24. Narani K. Thromboelastography in the perioperative period. *Indian J Anaesth.* 2005; 49:89–95.

25. Hagen P, Scholz D, Edwards W. Incidence and size of patent foramen ovale during the first 10 decades of life: an autopsy study of 965 normal hearts. *Mayo Clin Proc.* 1984;59:17–20.

26. Rao V, Slater J, Edwards N, et al. Surgical management of valvular disease in patients requiring left ventricular assist device support. *Ann Thorac Surg.* 2001;71:1448–1453.

27. Scalia G, McCarthy P, Savage R, et al. Clinical utility of echocardiography in the management of implantable ventricular assist devices. *J Am Soc Echocardiogr.* 2000;13:754–763.

28. Catena E, Milazzo F. Echocardiography and cardiac assist devices. *Minerva Cardioangiol.* 2007;55:247–265.

29. Potapov E, Stepanecnko A, Dandel M, et al. Tricuspid incompetence and geometry of the right ventricle as predictors of right ventricular function after implantation of a left ventricular assist device. *J Heart Lung Transplant.* 2008;27:1275–1281.

30. Byrne J, Leacche M, Paul S, et al. Risk factors and outcomes for "vasoplegic syndrome" following cardiac transplantation. *Eur J Cardiothorac Surg.* 2004;25:327–332.

31. Levin M, Lin H, Castillo J, et al. Early-on cardiopulmonary bypass hypotension and other factors associated with vasoplegic syndrome. *Circulation.* 2009;120:1664–1671.

32. Wan S, Marchant A, DeSmet J, et al. Human cytokine responses to cardiac transplantation and coronary artery bypass grafting. *J Thorac Cardiovasc Surg.* 1996;111:469–477.

33. Shanmugam G. Vasoplegic syndrome—the role of methylene blue. *Eur J Cardiothorac Surg.* 2005;28:705–710.

34. Argenziano M, Chen J, Choudhri A, et al. Management of vasodilatory shock after cardiac surgery: identification of predisposing factors and use of a novel pressor agent. *J Thorac Cardiovasc Surg.* 1998;116:973–980.

35. Boyle E, Pohlman T, Johnson M, et al. Endothelial cell injury in cardiovascular surgery: the systemic inflammatory response. *Ann Thorac Surg.* 1997;63:277–284.

36. Kirklin J. Prospects for understanding and eliminating the deleterious effects of cardiopulmonary bypass. *Ann Thorac Surg.* 1991;51:529–531.

37. Argenziano M, Choudhri A, Oz M, et al. A prospective randomized trial of arginine vasopressin in the treatment of vasodilatory shock after left ventricular assist device placement. *Circulation.* 1997;96:II-286–II-290.

38. Jeon Y, Ryu J, Lim Y, et al. Comparative hemodynamic effects of vasopressin and norepinephrine after milrinone-induced hypotension in off-pump coronary artery bypass surgical patients. *Eur J Cardiothorac Surg.* 2006;29:952–956.

39. Poelzl G, Zwick R, Grander W, et al. Safety and effectiveness of levosimendan in patients with predominant right heart failure. *Herz.* 2008;33:368–373.

40. Yilmaz M, Yontar C, Erdem A, et al. Comparative effects of levosimendan and dobutamine on right ventricular function in patients with biventricular heart failure. *Heart Vessels.* 2009;24:16–21.

41. Orihashi K, Matsuura Y, Hamanaka Y, et al. Retained intracardiac air in open heart operations examined by transesophageal echocardiography. *Ann Thorac Surg.* 1993;55:1467–1471.

42. Tingleff J, Joyce P, Pettersson G. Intraoperative echocardiographic study of air embolism during cardiac operations. *Ann Thorac Surg.* 1995;60:673–677.

43. Stainback R, Croitoru M, Hernandez A, et al. Echocardiographic evaluation of the Jarvik 2000 axial-flow LVAD. *Texas Heart Inst J.* 2005;32:263–270.

44. Chumnanvej S, Wood M, MacGillivray T, et al. Perioperative echocardiographic examination for ventricular assist device implantation. *Anesth Analg.* 2007;105:583–601.

45. Minami K, Bonkohara Y, Arugoglu L, et al. New technique for the outflow cannulation of right ventricular assist device. *Ann Thorac Surg.* 1999;68:1092–1093.

46. Mudge G. The management of mechanical hearts. *Trans Am Clin Climatol Assoc.* 2005;116:283–291.

47. Bolno P, Kresh J. Physiologic and hemodynamic basis of ventricular assist devices. *Cardiol Clin.* 2003;21:15–27.

48. Song X, Throckmorton A, Untariou A, et al. Axial flow pumps. *ASAIO J.* 2003;49:355–364.

49. Leyvi G, Rhew E, Crooke G, et al. Transient right ventricular failure and transient weakness: a TEE diagnosis. *J Cardiothorac Vasc Anesth.* 2005;19:406–408.

50. Pollock S, Dent J, Kaul S, et al. Diagnosis of ventricular assist device malfunction by transesophageal echocardiography. *Am Heart J.* 1992;124:793–794.

51. Saleh S, Liakopoulos O, Buckberg G. The septal motor of biventricular function. *Eur J Cardiothorac Surg.* 2006;295:S126–S138.

52. Agata Y, Hiraishi S, Misawa H, et al. Two-dimensional echocardiographic determinants of interventricular septal configurations in right or left ventricular overload. *Am Heart J.* 1985;110:819–825.

53. Shapiro E, Rademakers P. Importance of oblique fiber orientation for left ventricular wall deformation. *Technol Health Care.* 1997;5:21–28.

54. Chouraqui P, Rabinowitz B, Livschitz S, et al. Effects of antegrade/retrograde cardioplegia on postoperative septal wall motion in patients undergoing open heart surgery. *Cardiology.* 1997;88:526–529.

55. Kavarana M, Pessin-Minsley M, Urtecho J, et al. Right ventricular dysfunction and organ failure in left ventricular assist device recipients: a continuing problem. *Ann Thorac Surg.* 2002;73:745–750.

56. Rademacher P, Santak B, Becker H. Prostaglandin E1 and nitroglycerin reduce pulmonary capillary pressure but worsen ventilation-perfusion distributions in patients with adult respiratory distress syndrome. *Anesthesiology.* 1989;70:601–606.

57. Peterson G, Brickner M, Reimold S. Transesophageal echocardiography: clinical indications and applications. *Circulation.* 2003;107:2398–2402.

58. Horton S, Khodaverdian R, Chatelain P, et al. Left ventricular assist device malfunction: an approach to diagnosis by echocardiography. *J Am Coll Cardiol.* 2005;45:1435–1440.

59. Amir O, Kar B, Delgado R, et al. Images in cardiovascular medicine: high left ventricular assist device flows resulting from combined native aortic valve and outflow valve regurgitation. *Circulation.* 2005;111:E34.

60. Maybaum S, Williams M, Barbone A, et al. Assessment of synchrony relationships between the native left ventricle and the HeartMate left ventricular assist device. *J Heart Lung Transplant.* 2002;21:509–515.

61. Mochizuli T, Olson P, Szlam F, et al. Protamine reversal of heparin affects platelet aggregation and activated clotting time after cardiopulmonary bypass. *Anesth Analg.* 1998;8:781–785.

62 Enrizuez L, Shore-Lesserson L. Point-of-care coagulation testing and transfusion algorithms. *Br J Anaesth.* 103:I-14–I-22.

63. Speis B. Blood transfusion: the silent epidemic. *Ann Thorac Surg.* 2001;72(suppl):1832–1837.

64. Murphy P, Connery C, Hicks G, et al. Homologous blood transfusion as a risk factor for infection as a risk factor for postoperative infection after coronary artery bypass graft operations. *J Thorac Cardiovasc Surg.* 1992;104:1092–1099.

65. Goldstein D, Seldomridge J, Chen J, et al. Use of aprotinin in LVAD recipients reduces blood loss, blood use, and perioperative mortality. *Ann Thorac Surg.* 1995;59:1063–1068.

66. Hardy J, Belisle S, Van der Linden P. Efficacy and safety of activated recombinant factor VII in cardiac surgical patients. *Curr Opin Anaesthesiol.* 2009;22:95–99.

67. Bruckner B, DiBardino D, Ning Q, et al. High incidence of thromboembolic events in left ventricular assist device patients treated with recombinant activated factor VII. *J Heart Lung Transplant.* 2009;28:785–790.

68. Mayer S, Brun N, Begtrup K, et al. Recombinant activated factor VII for acute intracerebral hemorrhage. *N Engl J Med.* 2005;352:777–785.

69. Fowler N. Cardiac tamponade: a clinical or an echocardiographic diagnosis? *Circulation.* 1993;87:1738–1741.

70. Kuvin J, Harati N, Pandian N, et al. Postoperative cardiac tamponade in the modern surgical era. *Ann Thorac Surg.* 2002;74:1148–1153.

71. Peters J, Fraser C, Stuart R, et al. Negative intrathoracic pressure decreases independently left ventricular filling and emptying. *Am J Physiol.* 1989;257:H120–H131.

72. Riha H, Netuka I, Kotulak T, et al. Anesthesia management of a patient with a ventricular assist device for noncardiac surgery. *Semin Cardiothorac Vasc Anesth.* 2010;14:29–31.

Surgical Methods for Mechanical Circulatory Support

Mark S. Slaughter

Mechanical circulatory support (MCS) systems for treating severe heart failure have evolved rapidly over the past decade as considerable progress has been made in improving blood pump reliability, with a significant reduction in size of devices and patient morbidity and mortality. Various ventricular assist devices (VADs) are now available to support the diverse patient population (from neonates to elderly adults) with indications for device support. Systems range from small, percutaneously inserted catheter pumps to total heart replacement systems, which require an invasive surgical procedure and a highly trained surgical team for implantation. The duration of VAD support can range from a few days to many years depending on the etiology of a patient's condition.

The surgical methods required for implanting MCS devices depend mainly on the VAD system being implanted. Short-term VADs are typically extracorporeal pumps connected to externalized cannulas or catheter-delivered intravascular pumps. Long-term left ventricular assist devices (LVADs) are implantable devices that require extensive thoracic surgery for implantation. Regardless of the type of LVAD, postoperative bleeding is the main adverse event affecting morbidity and mortality in patients supported by these devices.[1–5] Coagulopathy secondary to multiple organ dysfunction, depletion of clotting factors during surgery, required anticoagulant therapy, and the extensive surgery for device implantation all contribute to bleeding complications.[6] Meticulous surgical technique is necessary not only to avoid bleeding complications but also to optimize circulatory support by the device. Surgical measures for optimizing hemostasis include minimizing cardiopulmonary bypass (CPB) time, minimizing dissection, maintaining normothermia, and reinforcing sutures in friable tissues. In addition, careful management of the coagulation system with blood products, anticoagulant reversal agents, and use of procoagulants is imperative.

LEFT VENTRICULAR CANNULATION METHODS

Left ventricular cannulation is required for implanting long-term LVADs but is optional for implanting some short-term devices.

The left ventricular apex is the preferred cannulation site for two reasons: (1) more complete unloading of the ventricle can be achieved, and (2) thrombosis caused by stasis in the ventricle may be avoided. During cannulation of the apex, CPB should be used to avoid air entry into the pump and arterial circulation; this also allows maximal inspection of the left ventricular cavity for potential thrombi. The cannula should be inserted on the anterolateral aspect of the apex 2 to 3 cm from the left anterior descending coronary artery and should be directed toward the central portion of the left ventricle to avoid its obstruction by the septum or the lateral ventricular wall (Fig. 11-1). The cannula position should be verified by transesophageal echocardiography, and adjustments should be made before device support is initiated. The possibility that a patient might have a patent foramen ovale needs to be considered; if a patent foramen ovale exists, it must be closed to prevent right-to-left shunting during LVAD support.

Although apical left ventricular cannulation is preferred for LVAD support, the presence of a left ventricular aneurysm or ischemic friable tissue at the apex may preclude use of this site. In such cases, the left atrium can be cannulated. The left atrium may also be used for cannulation when the support time is expected to be short.

Numerous left ventricular inflow cannula types exist for the Thoratec paracorporeal VAD (Thoratec Corp, Pleasanton, CA) (Table 11-1)[7] and the Thoratec intracorporeal VAD (Table 11-2).[8] The cannulas are chosen based on the type and site of cannulation and whether support is univentricular or biventricular (Fig. 11-2). Each of the Thoratec inflow cannulas incorporates a felt cuff into the exterior cannula wall; the cuff is used to secure the cannula in place. Multiple pledgeted sutures are placed around the apex so that the diameter is approximately 3 to 4 cm (Fig. 11-3). An opening in the left ventricle inside the suture line is created with a scalpel and scissors or by using a 12-mm diameter circular knife. After inspecting the left ventricular opening for thrombi, the cannula is inserted through the opening into the ventricle. The sutures are passed through the cuff and tied to secure the cannula in position. After the

Inferior oblique view | Lateral view

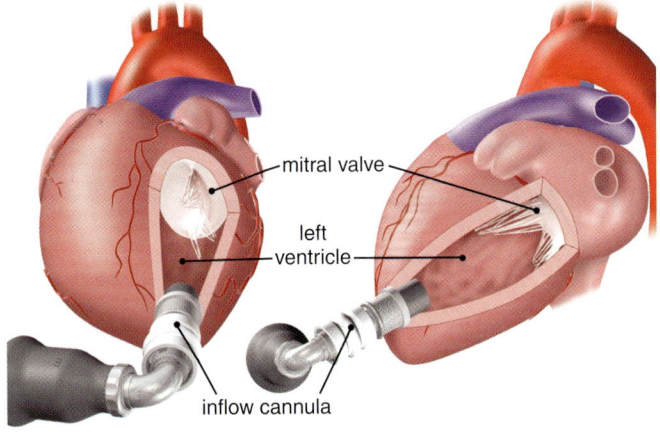

mitral valve

left
ventricle

inflow cannula

FIGURE 11-1 Proper placement of an inflow cannula within the left ventricle.

Table 11-2	Cannulas Available for the Thoratec Intracorporeal Ventricular Assist Device			
Cannula Type	Length	Cannula Internal Diameter	Cannula Tip Internal Diameter	Cannula Shape
Ventricular inflow	Short (blunt tip): 8 cm Short (beveled): 9 cm Long: 13 cm	16 mm	13 mm	Curved
Atrial inflow	Short: 17 cm Long: 22 cm	11-16 mm tapered	11 mm	90-degree bend
Arterial outflow	Short: 8 cm Short curved: 8 cm Long: 11 cm	16 mm	14 mm	Short: Straight and curved Long: Curved
Sealed arterial outflow	Short: 8 cm Long: 11 cm	16 mm	14 mm	Short: Straight Long: Curved

cannula is secured, it is brought straight out through a sub-costal incision in the abdominal wall and connected to the pump. The proper positions of the inflow and outflow cannula exit sites are important to avoid kinking of the cannulas after they are connected to the blood pump. Thoratec cannulas have velour coverings to allow tissue ingrowth at the exit site.

Cannulation locations for univentricular and biventricular support with the ABIOMED BVS/AB 5000 (ABIOMED, Inc, Danvers, MA) are similar to the locations used for the Thoratec VAD.[9,10] ABIOMED inflow cannulas are wire-reinforced, 40 cm long, and available in many sizes (Table 11-3). The cannulas are available in malleable or right-angle and blunt-tip or open-tip versions. Cannulation of the left ventricle is accomplished by first placing two purse-string sutures with tourniquets at the apex of the left ventricle (Fig. 11-4). A stab incision is made in the apex, and the cannula is inserted and secured by tightening the

tourniquets. This method for cannula insertion and removal can be performed without CPB, but the left ventricle must be full to avoid air entry.

Left ventricular cannulation is performed in the same location for most long-term, implanted LVADs, but the sewing cuffs and coring devices used for cannulation differ. Design characteristics that affect surgical implantation of long-term implantable LVADs are summarized in Table 11-4. The HeartMate XVE and HeartMate II LVADs (Thoratec Corp) use the same inflow cannulas, and because both pumps are positioned in the same subdiaphragmatic location, inflow cannulation methods are identical.

TABLE 11-1	Cannulas Available for the Thoratec Paracorporeal Ventricular Assist Device
Arterial outflow cannula	Short, straight, 15-cm straight tube and 30-cm graft (14-mm ID) Short, curved, 15-cm curved tube and 30-cm graft (14-mm ID) Long, straight, 18-cm straight tube and 30-cm graft (14-mm ID) Long, curved, 18-cm curved tube and 30-cm graft (14-mm ID) Long straight, 18-mm graft; 18-cm long straight tube; and 30-cm long graft (18-mm ID) Extra-long, straight, 18-mm graft; 20-cm straight tube; and 30-cm graft (18-mm ID)
Sealed arterial outflow cannula	Short, straight, 15-cm straight tube and 30-cm graft (14-mm ID) Short, curved, 15-cm curved tube and 30-cm graft (14-mm ID) Long, straight, 18-cm straight tube and 30-cm graft (14-mm ID) Long, curved, 18-cm curved tube and 30-cm graft (14-mm ID) Long, straight, 18-mm graft; 18-cm straight tube; and 30-cm graft (18-mm ID) Extra-long, straight, 18-mm, 20-cm straight tube and 30-cm long graft (18-mm ID)
Atrial inflow cannula (caged tip)	Short, 25-cm tube with right-angle bend and 10-cm velour cuff Long, 30-cm tube with right-angle bend and 10-cm velour cuff Long tube, with extra-long velour cuff; 30-cm tube with right-angle bend and 13-cm velour cuff
Beveled-tip atrial inflow cannula	Short, 25-cm tube with right-angle bend and 11-cm velour cuff Long, 30-cm tube with right-angle bend and 11-cm velour cuff
Ventricular inflow cannula	Two side holes; 20-cm straight tube; and 5-cm, 16-mm OD smooth tip (beveled, with two side holes) Extra-long, with two side holes; 25-cm straight tube; and 5-cm, 16-mm OD smooth tip (beveled, with two side holes) Blunt tip, 27-cm straight tube and 2.5-cm, 16-mm OD velour-covered tip (blunt, no side holes) Extra-long, blunt tip, 29-cm straight tube and 2.5-cm, 16-mm OD velour-covered tip (blunt, no side holes) Short, curved, 16-cm curved tube and 3-cm, 16-mm OD velour-covered tip (beveled, no side holes) Long, curved, 21-cm curved tube and 3-cm, 16-mm OD velour-covered tip (beveled, no side holes) Long, large tip, 28-cm straight tube and 4-cm, 19-mm OD smooth tip (beveled, no side holes)

ID, internal diameter; OD, outer diameter.

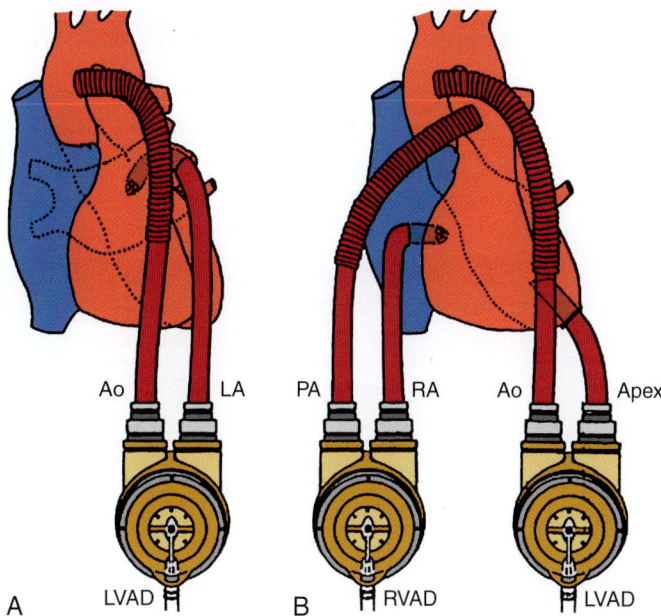

TABLE 11-3	Cannulas Available for the ABIOMED BVS/AB 5000	
Support	**Location**	**Size**
Left inflow	Left atrium, interatrial groove	32-Fr, 42-Fr
Left inflow	Right superior pulmonary vein	32-Fr
Left inflow	Left ventricular apex	32-Fr, 42-Fr
Left outflow	Ascending aorta	10 mm, 14 mm
Right inflow	Right atrial mid-wall	32-Fr, 42-Fr
Right outflow	Pulmonary artery	10 mm, 14 mm

FIGURE 11-2 Cannulation options for univentricular and biventricular assist. **A,** Left ventricular assist with the inflow cannulation site through the left atrial appendage and the outflow graft anastomosed to the ascending aorta. **B,** Biventricular ventricular assist device (VAD) with the right ventricular assist device inflow cannula in the right atrium and the outflow graft anastomosed to the main pulmonary artery. The left ventricular assist device (LVAD) inflow is at the left ventricular apex, and the outflow graft is anastomosed to the ascending aorta.

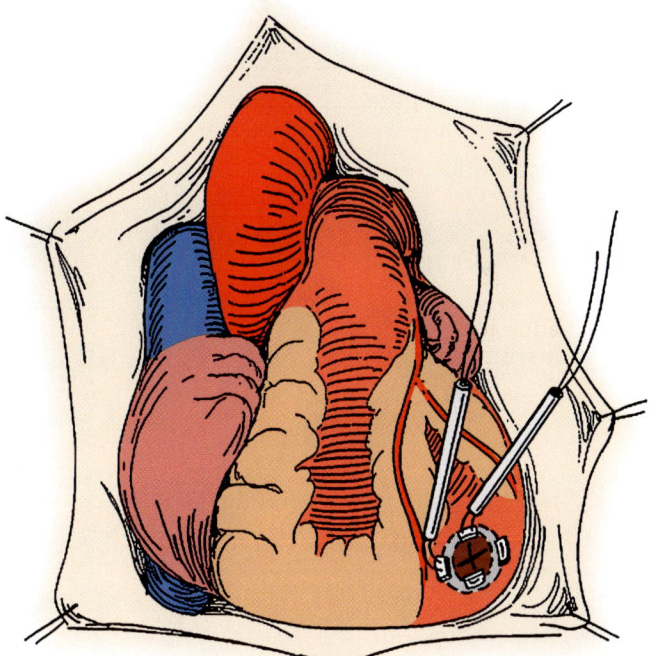

FIGURE 11-4 Preparation for left ventricular cannulation for the ABIOMED BVS/AB 5000. Two pledgeted, purse-string sutures are placed on the apex, and a cruciate incision is made. Tourniquets on each suture are used to secure the cannula after it is inserted. (*From DiCorte CJ, Van Meter CH Jr. Operative Techniques in Thoracic and Cardiovascular Surgery: A Comparative Atlas 1999;4:301-317.*)

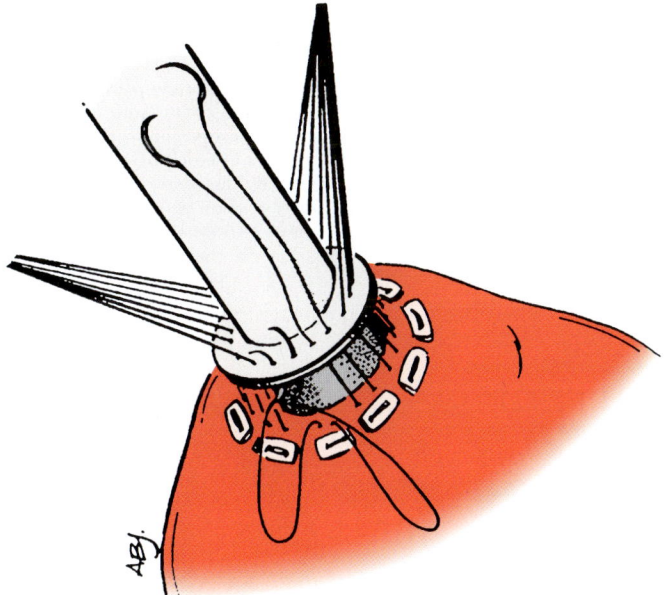

FIGURE 11-3 Insertion of Thoratec paracorporeal and intracorporeal ventricular assist device (VAD) cannulas. The cannulas are inserted into the left ventricle through a cored opening and then secured with 12 pledgeted sutures passed through the myocardium and the felt cuff on the cannula.

With CPB support, a circular knife is placed on the anterolateral epicardial surface approximately 2 to 3 cm from the left anterior descending coronary artery and rotated with inward pressure until a full-thickness core is made in the myocardium (Fig. 11-5A). The myocardial core is removed, and the opening is inspected for thrombi. Full-thickness sutures are placed in the myocardium around the opening and are passed through the felt portion of the sewing cuff (Fig. 11-5B). The sewing cuff is secured to the apical opening by tying down

the sutures (Fig. 11-5C). Because the sewing cuff is made of pliable Silastic and Dacron, a rigid, plastic centering device is placed within the sewing cuff to maintain the circular shape. The sutures around the cuff may be reinforced by placement of a felt strip. The inflow cannula is inserted and secured by tying down the circumferential ligatures around the outer surface of the sewing cuff and cannula.

Placement of the HVAD (HeartWare, Inc, Framingham, MA) differs from placement of the HeartMate VADs. The HVAD sewing cuff is configured differently, the inflow cannula is integrated with the pump, and the coring knife has an obturator tip.[11] The sewing cuff is attached to the anterolateral left ventricular apex, approximately 2 to 3 cm from the left anterior descending coronary artery with 12 pledgeted sutures that are placed through a partial thickness of the myocardium (Fig. 11-6). After CPB is begun, a full-thickness cruciform incision is made within the sewing ring (Fig. 11-7). The obturator tip of the coring device is inserted into the ventricle; with a rotating motion of the circular knife portion, the

Device	Weight and Displacement Volume	Pump Location	Inflow Cannula Diameter	Outflow Graft Diameter
HeartMate XVE	1250 gm; 450 mL	Intraperitoneal or extraperitoneal	19 mm	20 mm
HeartMate II	390 gm; 63 mL	Intraperitoneal or extraperitoneal	20 mm	16 mm
Thoratec PVAD	419 gm; 318 mL	Paracorporeal	16 mm	14 mm or 18 mm
Thoratec IVAD	339 gm; 252 mL	Extraperitoneal	11 or 13 mm	14 mm
ABIOMED BVS	NA	Bedside	32-Fr or 42-Fr	10 mm or 14 mm
ABIOMED AB	NA	Paracorporeal	32-Fr or 42-Fr	10 mm or 14 mm
CentriMag	31-mL priming volume	Bedside	Various	Various
HeartWare HVAD	145 gm; 50 mL	Intrapericardial	21 mm	10 mm
Jarvik 2000	90 gm; 25 mL	Intraventricular	NA	16 mm
DuraHeart	540 gm; 196 mL	Preperitoneal	12 mm	12 mm

TABLE 11-4   Characteristics of Commonly Used Long-Term Left Ventricular Assist Systems

IVAD, intracorporeal ventricular assist device; NA, not applicable; PVAD, paracorporeal ventricular assist device.

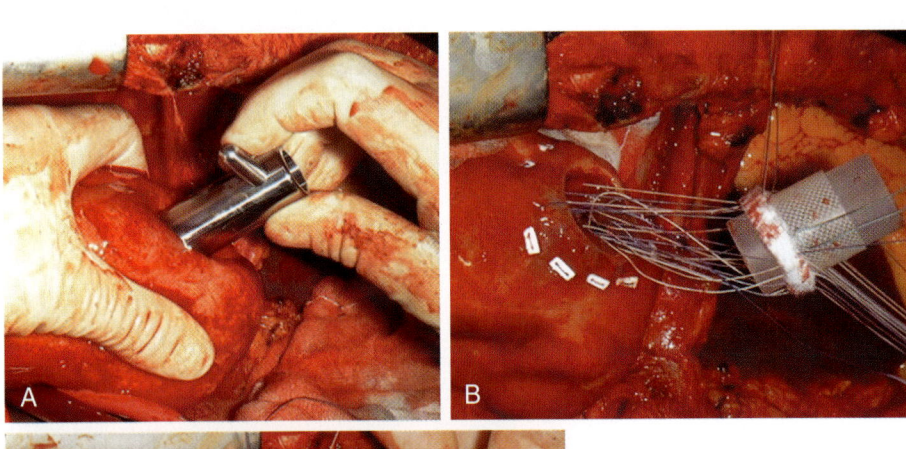

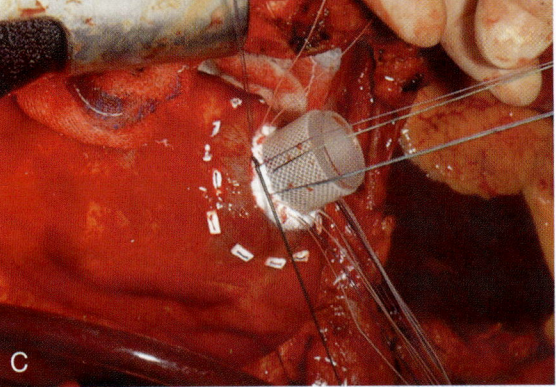

FIGURE 11-5 **A,** Insertion of the HeartMate inflow cannulas. The HeartMate coring knife is used to create the opening in the left ventricle for insertion of the inflow cannula. **B,** The sewing cuff is attached to the ventricle with 12 pledgeted sutures. **C,** Sutures are tied to secure the cuff to the heart.

opening is made into the left ventricle. The pump and the inflow cannula are inserted into the left ventricular opening and secured by tightening the titanium ring within the sewing ring (Fig. 11-8). The advantage of this system is that it reduces CPB time by attaching the sewing ring before making the incision in the left ventricular apex.

Implantation of the Jarvik 2000 device differs from implantation of the HeartMate and HeartWare VADs because there is no inflow cannula, and the entire pump is placed within the left ventricle. Sewing cuff placement and apical coring are nearly identical to the previous descriptions except that the cuff is beveled to direct the pump toward the mitral valve. CPB support is used to make the opening in the left ventricle. First, a cruciate incision is made in the ventricle.

The obturator tip of the circular knife is passed through the cuff, and the cutting edge is brought down to the myocardium. With a rotating motion, the ventricular apex is cored. After the core is removed and the opening inspected for obstruction, the pump is inserted and secured in place by two cotton tapes tied around the cuff and pump (Fig. 11-9).

VENTRICULAR ASSIST DEVICE OUTFLOW

With the exception of percutaneously placed VADs and the CentriMag device (Levitronix, Waltham, MA), each VAD system uses a specific outflow graft and arterial cannula. The diameters

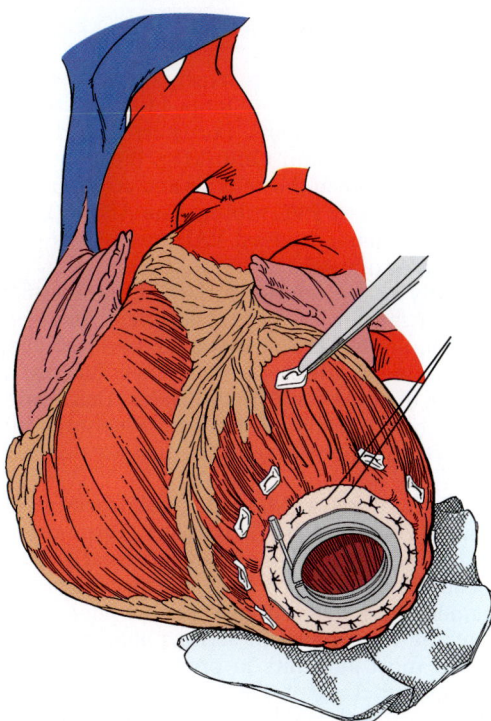

FIGURE 11-6 HVAD sewing cuff sewn to the left ventricular apex.

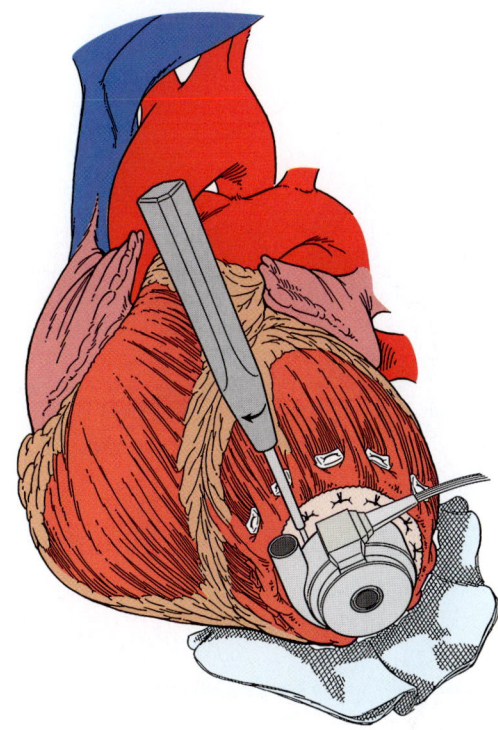

FIGURE 11-8 Tightening a titanium ring within the sewing cuff of the HVAD inflow cannula to secure the pump in position.

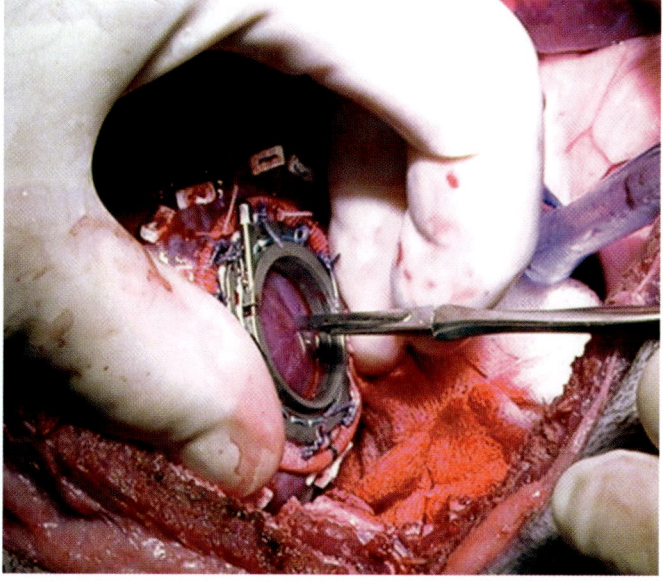

FIGURE 11-7 Full-thickness cruciate incision made within the sewing ring to accommodate insertion of the obturator of the coring knife.

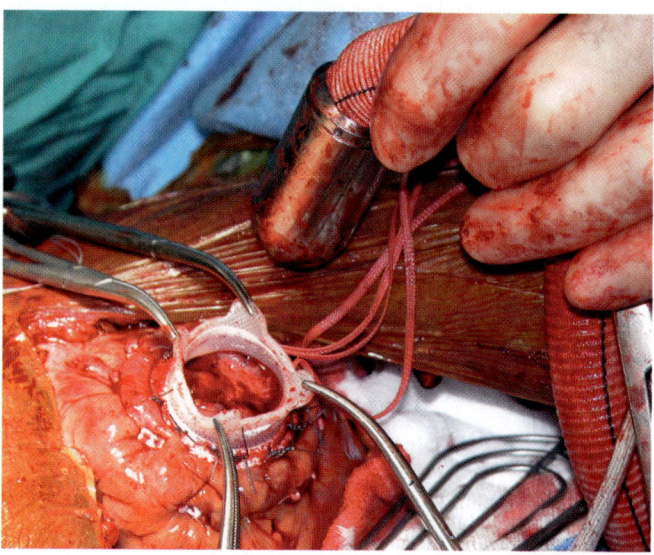

FIGURE 11-9 Insertion of Jarvik 2000 device. With the sewing cuff in place, an opening is made into the left ventricle, and the Jarvik 2000 device is inserted.

of these grafts range from 10 to 20 mm. Some are porous, and others are collagen-coated to reduce porosity. To minimize bleeding, noncoated porous grafts require preclotting with the patient's blood or other materials, such as albumin or a surgical adhesive (e.g., BioGlue, Cryolife, Kennesaw, GA). Tables 11-1 to 11-4 list the sizes of outflow grafts for the various VAD systems. Each VAD system manufacturer has specific, required procedures for preparing the graft before implantation.

Before the outflow graft is anastomosed, it should be trimmed to a proper length, and its tip should be beveled for the direction of the cannula; both of these procedures are necessary to avoid kinking. Grafts that are too long or too short may cause excessive tension on the anastomosis after they are attached to the pump.[12] Grafts that are too short often lie just below the sternum, creating the risk of being cut during a resternotomy. Because the graft stretches after it is pressurized with blood, it should be stretched manually when estimating the proper length. The aortic graft should be beveled at approximately 30 degrees; the pulmonary artery graft bevel should be greater.

The outflow graft is anastomosed to the ascending aorta for LVAD support and to the main pulmonary artery for right ventricular assist device support (Fig. 11-10). The anterolateral portion of the ascending aorta is the preferred location for the LVAD outflow, but location may vary depending on the presence of coronary artery grafts. With a partial occlusion

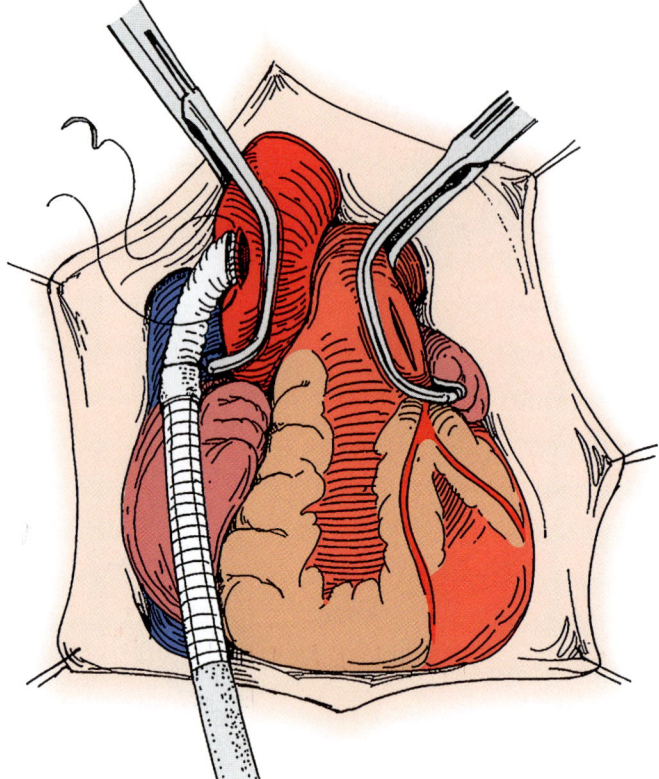

FIGURE 11-10 Ventricular assist device (VAD) outflow anastomosis to the ascending aorta and main pulmonary artery. (From DiCorte CJ, Van Meter CH Jr. Operative Techniques in Thoracic and Cardiovascular Surgery: A Comparative Atlas 1999;4:301-317.)

clamp on the target vessel, a longitudinal aortotomy the length of the graft diameter is made, and the graft is anastomosed with a polypropylene suture. The integrity of the anastomosis is carefully inspected by releasing the partial occlusion clamp, allowing blood to fill the graft and expel air. After the graft fills with blood, a cross clamp is placed. If necessary, the anastomotic site can be reinforced by placing pledgeted, buttressed sutures or a felt strip around the site (Fig. 11-11).

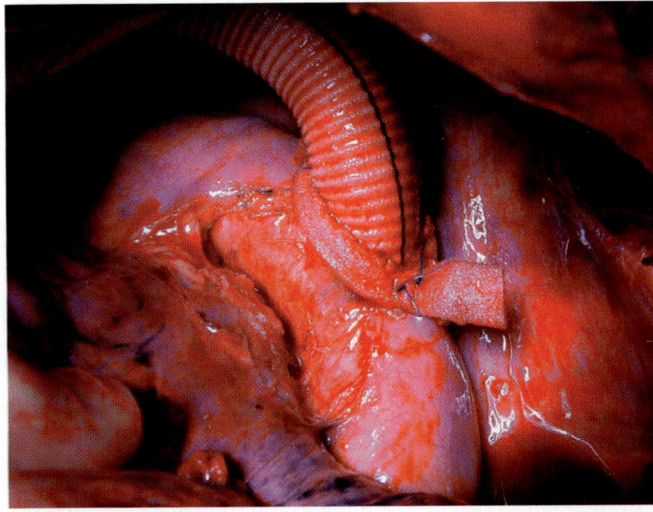

FIGURE 11-11 Aortic outflow graft anastomosis shown reinforced with a felt strip.

BLOOD PUMP PLACEMENT

The placement of blood pumps largely depends on the intended duration of VAD support. Table 11-4 lists the locations for the different VAD systems. For short-term devices, such as the ABIOMED BVS and CentriMag, the pumps are positioned near the patient at the bedside and are connected to the implanted cannulas by PVC tubing. The ABIOMED AB 5000 and the Thoratec paracorporeal VAD pumps are suitable for support durations of weeks to months because they are placed paracorporeally on the anterior surface of the abdomen. Long-term devices used for bridge to transplant and destination therapy are implanted in the abdomen, pericardial space, or left ventricle. Two short-term VAD systems that are uniquely positioned are the Impella (ABIOMED, Inc, Danvers, MA) and the TandemHeart (CardiacAssist, Inc, Pittsburgh, PA). The implantation techniques for these devices are described separately later.

The pumps for the HeartMate XVE and HeartMate II LVADs, the Thoratec IVAD, and the DuraHeart (Terumo Heart, Inc, Ann Arbor, MI) are normally placed subcostally in a preperitoneal pocket (Fig. 11-12).[12–15] Both intraperitoneal placement and placement in a preperitoneal pocket have been controversial, but the occurrence of serious abdominal complications has led most surgeons to prefer placing the pump in a preperitoneal pocket.[16–19] The pocket is created above the posterior rectus sheath and transversalis fascia and below the rectus abdominis and internal oblique muscles. Alternatively, the pump may be placed intraperitoneally in the left upper quadrant of the abdomen. Preperitoneal placement may be preferable for patients who have undergone previous abdominal surgery or for patients with a short torso. Preperitoneal placement also avoids the potential for the bowel to adhere to the device. Potential disadvantages of the preperitoneal position include the risk of pocket hematoma, pocket and exit site infection, wound dehiscence, and erosion of the skin overlying the pump. Intraperitoneal placement may be preferable for thin patients and for patients with automatic implantable cardioverter-defibrillators. The risks of the intraperitoneal

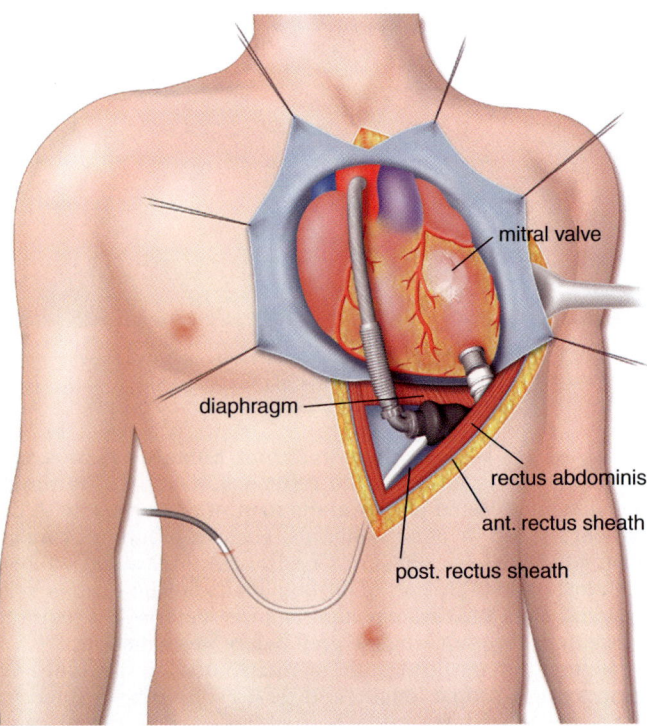

FIGURE 11-12 HeartMate II left ventricular assist device (LVAD) pump positioned in a preperitoneal pocket.

position include diaphragmatic hernia, wound dehiscence, bowel adhesions and obstruction, and erosion of surrounding tissues.[20,21]

Because the Jarvik 2000 blood pump is small, it can be placed within the left ventricle (Fig. 11-13). It can be implanted via sternotomy with the outflow graft placed to the ascending aorta, or it can be implanted through a left thoracotomy with the outflow graft anastomosed to the descending thoracic aorta.[22] The intraventricular position has two potential advantages: (1) abdominal surgery is avoided, and (2) the pericardial space is not occupied by the device. The outflow for the Jarvik 2000 was designed for the descending thoracic aorta, which allows for implantation through a left thoracotomy. However, outflow to the descending aorta may result in stagnant blood flow at the root of the aorta with a subsequent high risk of life-threatening thrombosis.[23,24]

The HVAD is a small pump with an integrated inflow cannula that is implanted via a sternotomy with CPB support.[11] The HVAD is positioned at the apex or at the diaphragmatic surface of the left ventricle within the intrapericardial space, and the outflow graft is anastomosed to the ascending aorta (Fig. 11-14).[25] A low-profile sewing cuff with a titanium C-clamp is necessary to secure the device in this position. Because the abdomen does not have to be entered to place this device, abdominal complications known to be associated with abdominally implanted devices are avoided.

The Impella 5.0 device is a unique, catheter-mounted LVAD that may be implanted through a femoral artery cutdown or directly into the aorta when the chest is open.[26] The "5.0" designation for this model indicates the maximal blood flow rate that can be achieved. The device has two designs: One is for femoral artery insertion, and the other is for direct insertion in the ascending aorta. For peripheral insertion, fluoroscopy is required to deliver the 21-Fr pump and cannula via a 3- to 5-cm cut-down on the femoral artery, retrograde through the aorta and into the left ventricle (Fig. 11-15). Distal and proximal vessel loops are placed to control bleeding during insertion. A 0.025-inch guidewire

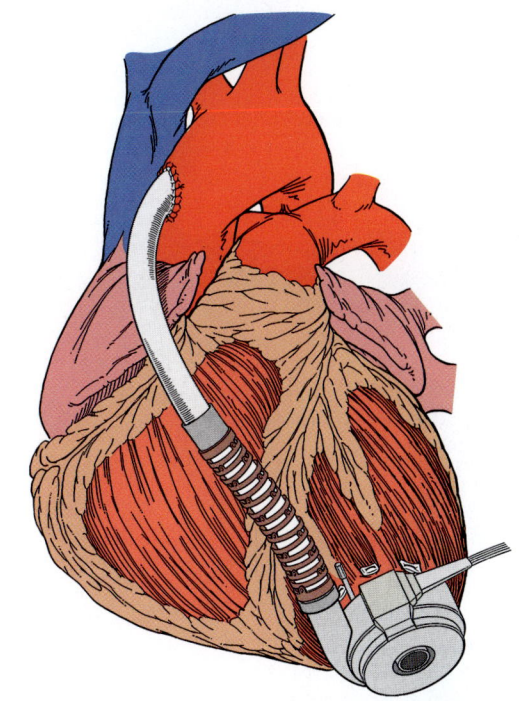

FIGURE 11-14 HeartWare HVAD pump shown positioned at the apex of the left ventricle in the pericardial space.

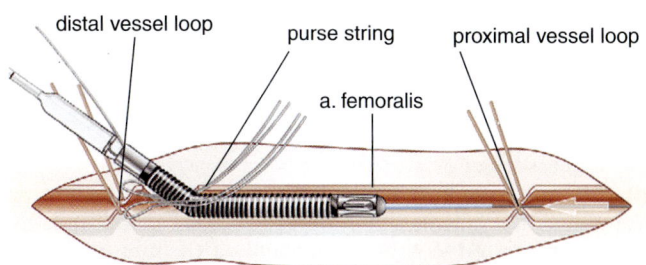

FIGURE 11-15 Impella 5.0 device, inserted through a femoral artery cut-down. Ties are placed to control bleeding from the site.

is inserted first with its tip in the left ventricle. The proximal end of the guidewire is passed through the pigtail catheter tip. The pump is inserted into the femoral artery and directed across the aortic arch and aortic valve. An introducer is passed into the femoral artery and secured with the vessel ties, which normally allow distal blood flow and hemostasis of the insertion site. A pressure waveform from a pressure sensor in the cannula is used to verify proper positioning of the device.

For patients who have undergone sternotomy for other cardiac procedures, the direct aortic insertion technique can be used to insert the Impella 5.0 LVAD if there is a sufficient area in the ascending aorta to accommodate the device.[27-29] For the direct insertion technique, a 10-mm Dacron graft is anastomosed end-to-side to the ascending aorta. The catheter and two silicone plugs are inserted into the graft, and ties are placed around the plugs to achieve hemostasis. The pump is advanced across the aortic valve, and the position is verified by the pressure waveform (Fig. 11-16). Contraindications to use of the Impella 5.0 include the presence of a mechanical aortic valve, aortic valve stenosis, moderate-to-severe aortic insufficiency, and peripheral vascular disease severe enough to prevent insertion of the pump. When the device is removed, the femoral or aortic artery is closed in the standard manner.

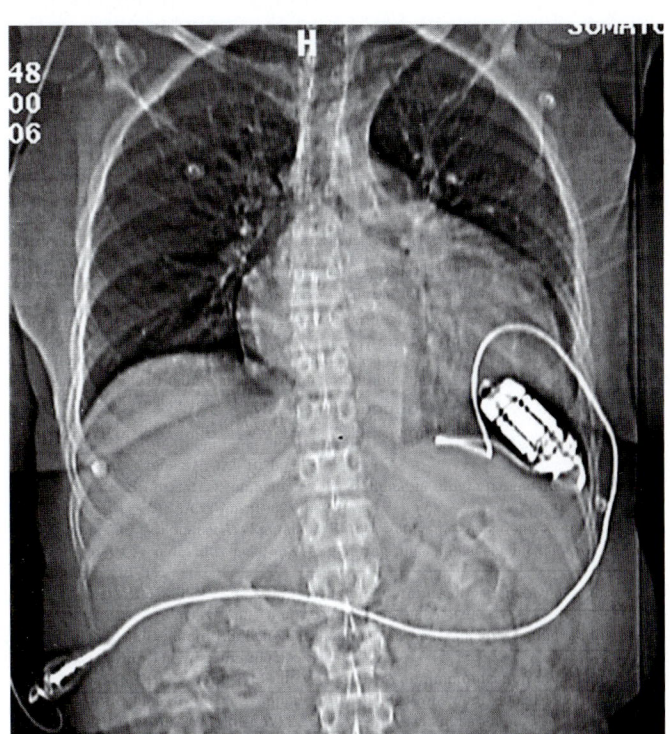

FIGURE 11-13 Chest x-ray shows Jarvik 2000 blood pump in the left ventricle.

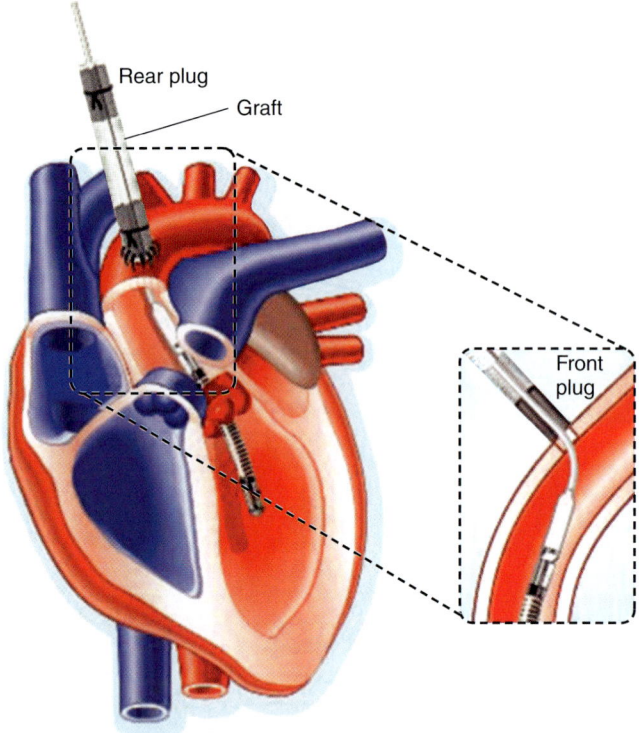

Rear plug

Graft

Front plug

FIGURE 11-16 Impella 5.0 device, directly inserted into the ascending aorta. A graft is sewn to the aorta, and the pump or cannula is inserted with two silicone plugs that are used for hemostasis.

EXTERNALIZING THE PERCUTANEOUS DRIVELINE

All implantable VADs require a percutaneous driveline for communication between the implanted blood pump and the external power and control components. Driveline infections are the most frequent device-related adverse events associated with implantable VADs.[30,31] To minimize infection, drivelines have been developed with a polyester velour covering that allows for subcutaneous tissue ingrowth. Making the driveline tunnel as long as possible and carefully choosing the exit site to minimize movement and trauma can also decrease the incidence of driveline infection. To increase its length, the tunnel can be made in a U-shape, or a loop of driveline can be created near the pump connection before the tunnel (Fig. 11-17).[6] It is important to avoid sharp bends in the driveline because this can cause stress points that may weaken and fracture the driveline. An exit site that is just below the right costal margin along the midclavicular line is suitable for most patients. However, individual anatomic variations in patients should be considered, and the site should be altered to optimize stabilization and care of the exit site. The exit site diameter should be as similar as possible to the diameter of the driveline to minimize exposure of the subcutaneous tissue and to avoid excessive tension on the skin. The exit site should be closed with suture and removed when the skin is well healed. Postoperative stabilization of the driveline exit site is crucial in preventing infection.

DEAIRING AND WEANING FROM CARDIOPULMONARY BYPASS

Deairing of the VAD system and the transition from CPB to VAD support are critical steps for avoiding a catastrophic air embolism. With an open thorax and vacuum to assist in VAD filling, the risk of air entry into the device and the arterial circulation is high. The transition to device support should proceed slowly. The surgeon, anesthesiologist, perfusionist, and VAD operator all must pay meticulous attention to procedures for avoiding air entry into the system. Combined CPB and LVAD support should never exceed 100% of the total cardiac output. After the LVAD is implanted, native heart function should be supported with blood volume, inotropic medications, and cardioversion, as necessary. The amount of CPB should be gradually decreased, and LVAD support should be begun at a minimal support level. Blood volume in the heart must be kept optimized—neither excessively full nor empty. Some centers monitor left atrial pressure to assess left ventricular volume, but this also adds to the risk of air entry by having another point of entry in the left side of the heart.

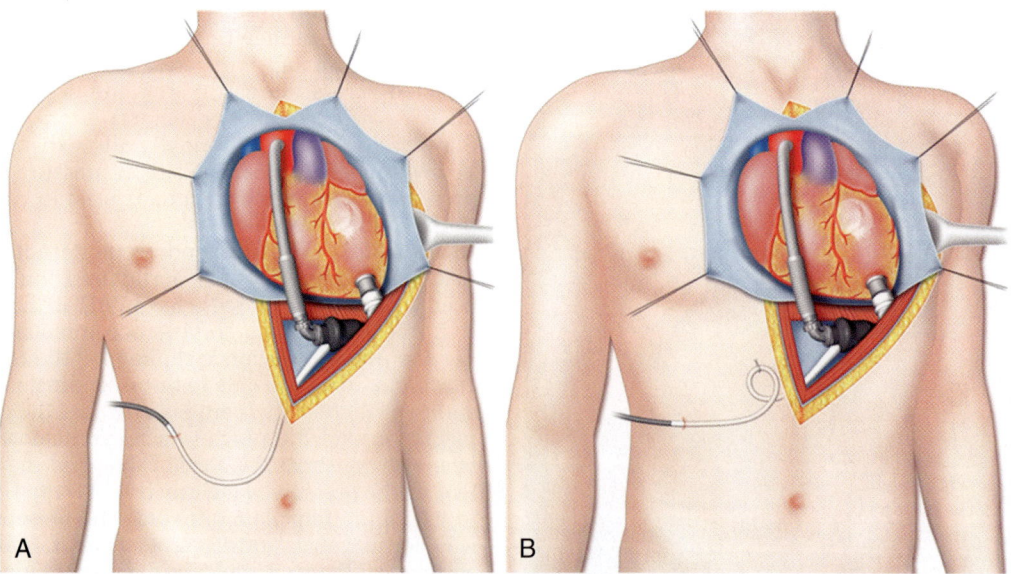

A B

FIGURE 11-17 Two tunneling techniques used for the driveline of the HeartMate II left ventricular assist system to maximize exposure of the velour covering to the subcutaneous tissue. **A,** U-shaped tunnel. **B,** Loop of the driveline with the exit site just subcostal in the midclavicular line.

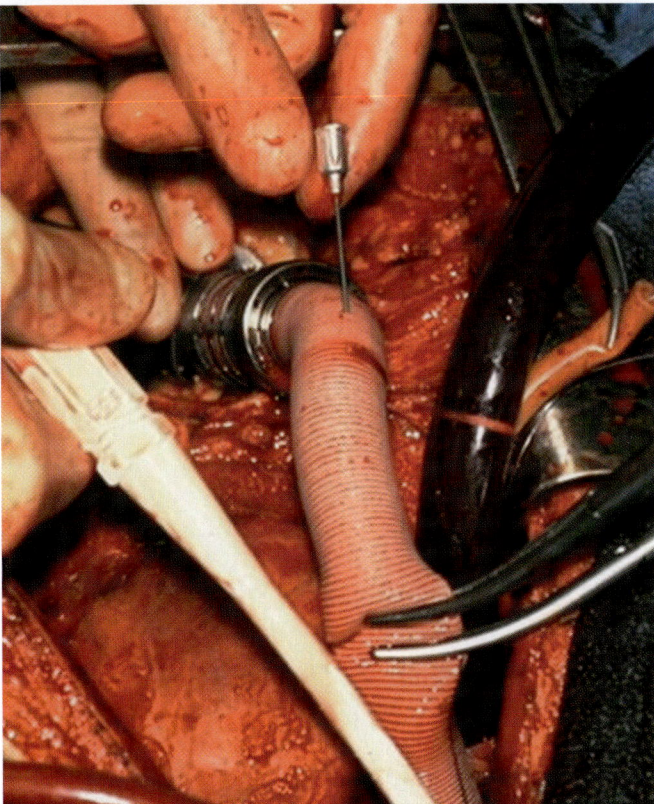

FIGURE 11-18 Deairation of the pump and outflow graft. A needle is placed at the highest point in the graft to allow air to escape while the pump is turned on at a minimal setting.

To avoid air entry into the blood pump during connection of the cannula, the pump and cannula should be filled with saline or blood to allow air to escape. After both inflow and outflow cannulas are in place, the primed blood pump is connected. The cross-clamp on the aorta should be gradually released to allow backflow of blood to occur. Alternatively, saline can be poured continuously over the connector as the connection is gradually made. In most cases, after the cannulas are connected to the blood pump, a cross-clamp is left in place on the outflow graft, and a needle is placed in the graft at its highest point to allow any entrapped air to exit the device (Fig. 11-18). The pump is gently rotated and tapped to dislodge any air in the device. When possible, the device is slowly actuated manually. When it cannot be actuated manually, the pump should be set at a minimal speed.

During the deairation process, it is very important to allow the left ventricle to have sufficient blood volume to cause antegrade flow through the pump and heart. When all air is removed from the graft and pump, CPB support is reduced to a minimal level (1 to 2 L/min). Transesophageal echocardiography is used during this transition to assess for air in the left ventricle, aorta, and outflow graft.[32] When LVAD flows are stable, bleeding is minimal, and native cardiac function is adequate, the CPB cannulas are removed. Some VAD systems have specific auxiliary equipment to aid in the deairation process; this equipment should be used according to manufacturers' recommendations.

PERCUTANEOUS LEFT VENTRICULAR ASSIST DEVICES

The Impella 2.5 and TandemHeart are LVADs intended for short-term support for cardiogenic shock or for support of patients undergoing high-risk coronary interventions.[33–35]

Patients must be nonambulatory and confined to bed during support. Because fluoroscopic guidance is needed for insertion, these devices are most often placed in the cardiac catheterization laboratory. Surgical insertion is uncommon.

The Impella 2.5 device is a catheter-mounted axial flow LVAD that is intended to provide support for up to 5 days. It is used to support patients who have cardiogenic shock or who are undergoing high-risk percutaneous coronary interventions.[36] The device is inserted via a femoral artery and passed retrograde through the aorta and across the aortic valve with the tip of the cannula in the left ventricle (Fig. 11-19). When the pump is operating, blood is withdrawn from the left ventricle through the cannula and pumped into the ascending aorta. A 0.035-inch guidewire, a 6-Fr to 8-Fr dilator, and a 13-Fr introducer are used to insert the pump. The 12-Fr pump and cannula are inserted over the guidewire under fluoroscopic guidance. If there is excessive bleeding after the device is removed, the femoral artery may require surgical closure.

The TandemHeart device is an extracorporeal centrifugal flow LVAD that pumps blood from the left atrium to the femoral artery (Fig. 11-20).[37] With the aid of fluoroscopy, cannulation is accomplished by first performing a standard atrial transseptal puncture. A 0.035-inch pigtail guidewire is inserted into the left atrium, and a two-stage (14-Fr and 21-Fr) dilator is used to enlarge the transseptal puncture. The 21-Fr transseptal inflow cannula with a large end hole and 14 side holes is inserted into the left atrium and connected to the inflow of the pump. A 15-Fr or 17-Fr cannula connected to the outflow of the pump is next placed in a femoral artery. In cases where the femoral artery is small, bilateral femoral arterial cannulation with a 12-Fr or 14-Fr cannula may be performed. When the patient's cardiac function improves enough to allow device removal, the cannulas are removed

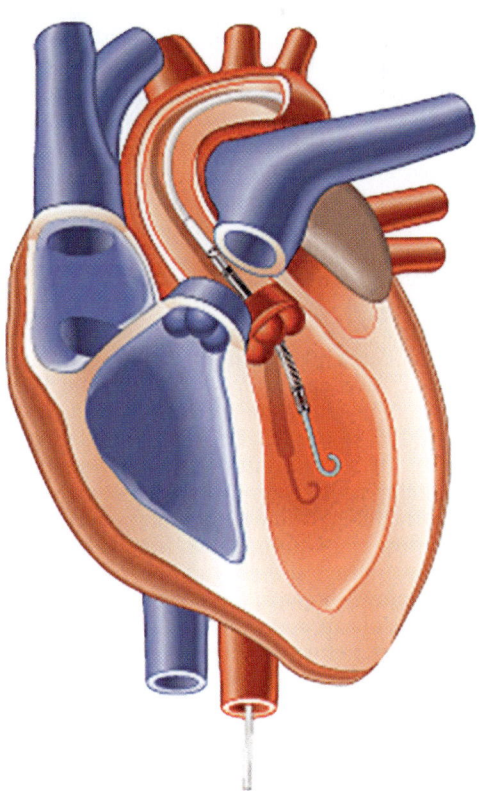

FIGURE 11-19 Position of the Impella 2.5 device after percutaneous insertion from the femoral artery. The cannula tip is in the left ventricle, and the pump is in the ascending aorta.

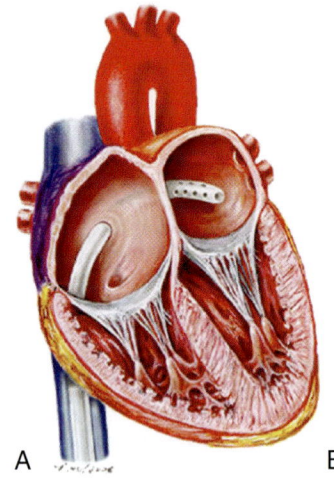

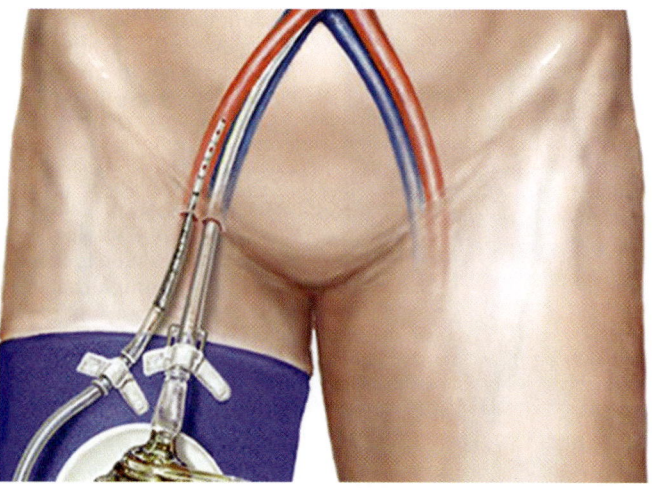

FIGURE 11-20 **A** and **B,** Tandem-Heart device insertion. TandemHeart cannulas are inserted percutaneously via the femoral vein and artery **(B)**. The inflow cannula tip is positioned across the atrial septum in the left atrium **(A)**.

A   B

at the bedside. Manual compression at the puncture site is usually sufficient to stop bleeding. A small septal defect with an insignificant right-to-left shunt normally resolves within weeks.

EXTRACORPOREAL MEMBRANE OXYGENATION

Extracorporeal membrane oxygenation (ECMO) was originally used primarily to support pediatric and adult patients with severe respiratory failure. Since its first use in 1965,[38] the frequency of ECMO use has varied greatly because of its complexity, high rate of complications, and poor outcomes.[39,40] With improved biomaterials and techniques for cannulation, along with advances in medical care, ECMO support has gained in popularity and is being applied more frequently for multiple indications. ECMO is indicated when severe cardiopulmonary failure is refractory to medical therapy and rapid circulatory or respiratory assistance is needed to sustain the patient. Venoarterial ECMO is used for cardiopulmonary support; venovenous ECMO is used only for respiratory support. Cardiac arrest, postcardiotomy and post–myocardial infarction cardiogenic shock, and primary severe respiratory failure are clinical scenarios wherein ECMO may be beneficial.

The basic ECMO circuit consists of arterial and venous cannulas, hollow-fiber oxygenator, a centrifugal flow pump, an oxygen blender, and a heat exchanger (Fig. 11-21). The system configuration varies among institutions, but the most common pumps used are the CentriMag and the BioPump (Medtronic, Eden Prairie, MN). The CentriMag pump offers the advantage of a frictionless and bearingless impeller, which eliminates heat generation and its thrombotic potential. In addition, heparin-coated tubing, cannulas, connectors, oxygenators, and pumps are often used to minimize thrombosis and reduce the requirement for anticoagulation therapy. Continuous heparin anticoagulation is necessary to prevent thrombosis in static blood flow areas, such as the left atrium and left ventricle. For patients undergoing ECMO, activated clotting time is maintained in the range of 180 to 220 seconds.

Numerous cannulation techniques can be used for ECMO, depending on the clinical condition of the patient. For patients who cannot be weaned from CPB, the existing right atrial and aortic cannulas can be used, changing the ECMO circuit to a portable system. The cannulation sites are reinforced with purse-string sutures and tourniquets with buttons; the

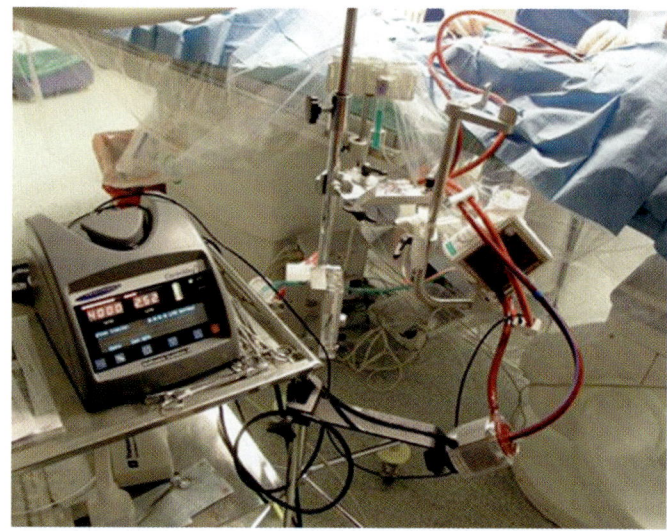

FIGURE 11-21 Typical extracorporeal membrane oxygenation (ECMO) system at the bedside includes a CentriMag console and pump, an oxygenator, a gas source, and a monitor.

cannulas are externalized through stab incisions in the chest wall. The sternum is not wired shut, but the skin is closed. In this situation, some surgeons may prefer to change the cannulation sites to the femoral artery and vein to allow the chest to be completely closed and to allow for eventual decannulation at the bedside. Because large cannulas are required, however, peripheral cannulation in patients with peripheral vascular disease may be impossible.

ECMO can be rapidly executed with percutaneous peripheral venoarterial or venovenous cannulation. A surgical cutdown is not required, and fewer bleeding complications at the insertion site occur with the percutaneous approach. With standard percutaneous procedures, the venous inflow cannula is placed through the femoral vein to the level of the right atrium, and the arterial return cannula is inserted into the femoral artery or alternatively into the femoral vein. Venovenous ECMO has been used with the venous outflow from the right atrium and the return flow to the femoral artery, but higher flow rates and oxygenation can be achieved with reversed flow direction. Because venoarterial ECMO with femoral arterial return increases left ventricular afterload, an intraaortic balloon pump and vasodilator medications may be needed to augment blood flow. For venoarterial ECMO with femoral cannulation, the largest cannulas that the vessels can accommodate should be used (i.e., 18-Fr to 28-Fr for the venous inflow and 16-Fr to 20-Fr for the arterial outflow). A long, two-stage cannula is optimal because it can be inserted to the level of the right atrium. To minimize leg ischemia, arterial cannulation may be performed above and below the cannulation site with a 20-Fr cannula directed toward the aorta and a 10-Fr cannula directed downstream toward the leg.

ECMO is normally used to support patients for durations of 2 to 3 days, but it has been used in rare cases to support patients for weeks. The duration of ECMO support is directly related to the incidence of serious complications, such as bleeding, infection, renal failure, and thromboembolism.[41] Oxygenator failure and pump thrombosis rates also increase with time.

CENTRIMAG VENTRICULAR ASSIST SYSTEM

The CentriMag ventricular assist system (VAS) does not have specific cannula requirements, which allows for versatile use of this device.[42–44] The CentriMag VAS has been used for CPB, ECMO, and postcardiotomy biventricular assist. Cannulation is normally accomplished with standard CPB cannulas and techniques. The versatility of the cannulation options with the CentriMag VAS allows this device to be applied in a wide range of patients. Figure 11-22 shows a typical setup cannulation for biventricular support with the CentriMag VAS. A malleable, wire-reinforced inflow cannula and a large, low-resistance outflow cannula are preferred. For postcardiotomy failure, the existing CPB cannulas can be used. For left VAS support, a 32-Fr inflow cannula is inserted into the left atrium at the level of the junction between the superior and inferior pulmonary veins or directly into the left ventricle. A 22-Fr

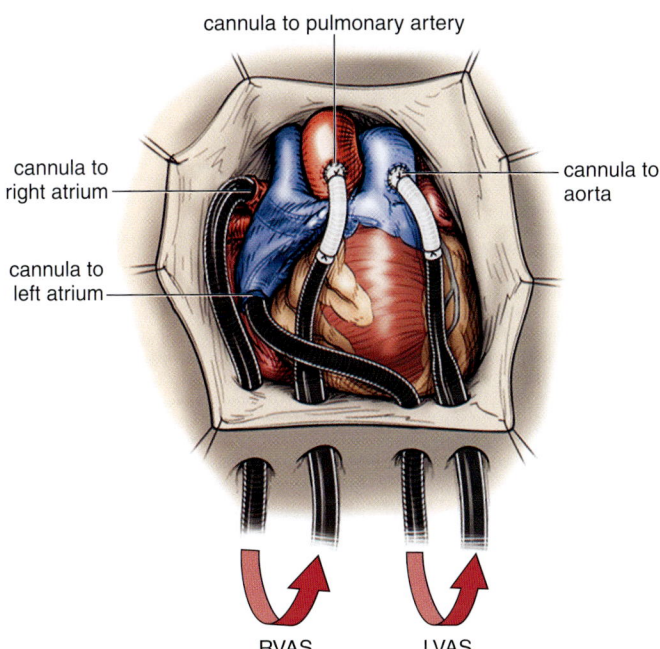

cannula to pulmonary artery

cannula to right atrium

cannula to aorta

cannula to left atrium

RVAS LVAS

FIGURE 11-22 Cannulation for biventricular support with the CentriMag device. The left ventricular assist device (LVAD) inflow cannula is located in the left atrium through the right superior pulmonary vein, and the outflow is at the ascending aorta. The right ventricular assist device inflow cannula is placed through the atrial appendage into the right atrium, and the outflow is at the main pulmonary artery. LVAS, left ventricular assist system; RVAS, right ventricular assist system.

outflow cannula is inserted preferably into the ascending aorta, but when this site is unavailable, the cannula can be inserted via the femoral artery. For right ventricular support, the CPB inflow cannula is used, and the pulmonary artery is cannulated.

After cannulation and the circuit are completed, CPB flow should be decreased to a minimal level (approximately 1 to 2 L/min) to allow for filling of the ventricles. When the VAS is on and functioning properly, CPB is terminated. Pump speed is gradually increased to achieve the desired level of cardiac output and to verify that suction has not occurred. When left atrial pressure is monitored, it should be maintained in the range of 10 to 15 mm Hg. As the flow is increased, the operator should monitor the pump flow rate, the patient's blood pressure, and the circuit for signs of suction. The VAS flow rate and the patient's total cardiac output, central venous pressure, pulmonary capillary wedge pressure, and arterial blood pressure should be monitored frequently because hemodynamic conditions can change rapidly during surgery. Similar to most of the temporary pumps, the speed of the CentriMag pump can be adjusted to allow evaluation of right ventricle or left ventricle recovery over hours to days, rather than a snapshot look at the need for continuing support.

OFF-PUMP VENTRICULAR ASSIST DEVICE IMPLANTATION

The use of CPB is standard during a VAD implantation if the left ventricle is entered or when cardiac manipulation results in compromised cardiac function. However, the effects of CPB may worsen pre-existing, end-organ dysfunction and contribute to abnormal coagulation postoperatively. Implantation of a VAD without the use of CPB (off-pump) may be advantageous for patients with end-organ dysfunction and for patients who have had prior cardiac surgery. There are numerous anecdotal reports of VAD implantation without CPB support, but this technique requires careful planning and should be performed only by surgeons with extensive VAD implant experience.

The greatest risk of a serious problem during off-pump VAD implantation occurs during placement of the left ventricular inflow cannula. After the apex has been cored, air entry into the left ventricle and the arterial circulation is likely. It is important that volume and pressure in the left side of the heart are sufficient to prevent air entry and that the inflow cannula is rapidly inserted into the ventricle. Preferably, the inflow cannula should be inserted at the start of systole to reduce air entry into the left ventricle during diastole. Whenever the left ventricle is open, the patient should be in the Trendelenburg position. Deairation of the system can be accomplished by allowing antegrade blood flow through the device with the outflow temporarily opened. Cardiac stabilization devices may be useful for inserting the cannula into the left ventricle.

The standard technique for HeartMate LVAD implantation is to core the apex and then place full-thickness sutures through the myocardium and the sewing cuff, which exposes the open left ventricle for several minutes. In one off-pump technique for implanting the HeartMate XVE,[45] the coring knife was used to score the epicardial surface where sutures would be placed. The sewing cuff was sewn in place, and a suture was placed in the center of the area to be cored and brought out through the center of the coring knife. The coring knife was used to complete and remove the full-thickness core. The inflow cannula was quickly inserted into the opening and secured. The outflow graft was anastomosed to the aorta and connected to the outflow of the pump. After standard deairing procedures, the pump was started. A potential problem with this technique is inadvertent cutting of the sutures securing the cuff in place during the coring.

The Jarvik 2000 LVAD has been implanted without CPB support in many patients via a left thoracotomy or a subcostal approach.[46,47] In two small series, there was minimal bleeding, and patients recovered more quickly than patients who underwent CPB during implantation of other devices.[48] Because the Jarvik device is small, it can be rapidly inserted into the left ventricle after coring is completed. In addition, use of the obturator coring knife helps to protect the sutures in the sewing cuff when the coring device is passed through the myocardium.

Apical left ventricular cannulation for off-pump implantation of the Thoratec LVAD is accomplished by placing sutures through the myocardium and the felt ring on the cannula, after which a full-thickness stab incision is made through the center of the sutures. The cannula tip is inserted into the left ventricle,[49] and the sutures are tied down to secure the cannula in place.

CONCLUSION

The type of VAD system being implanted determines the surgical methods required for implantation. Regardless of the type of VAD, meticulous surgical technique is required to avoid complications, especially postoperative bleeding, and to optimize device function. This chapter has highlighted the surgical methods that have been determined to be key factors that contribute to the success of short-term and long-term mechanical circulatory support.

REFERENCES

1. Velik-Salchner C, Hoermann C, Hoefer D, et al. Thromboembolic complications during weaning from right ventricular assist device support. *Anesth Analg.* 2009;109:354–357.
2. Stulak JM, Dearani JA, Burkhart HM, et al. ECMO cannulation controversies and complications. *Semin Cardiothorac Vasc Anesth.* 2009;13:176–182.
3. Gregoric ID, Bruckner BA, Jacob L, et al. Techniques and complications of TandemHeart ventricular assist device insertion during cardiac operations. *ASAIO J.* 2009;55:251–254.
4. Lahpor J, Khaghani A, Hetzer R, et al. European results with a continuous-flow ventricular assist device for advanced heart-failure patients. *Eur J Cardiothorac Surg.* 2010;37:357–361.
5. John R, Kamdar F, Liao K, et al. Improved survival and decreasing incidence of adverse events with the HeartMate II left ventricular assist device as bridge-to-transplant therapy. *Ann Thorac Surg.* 2008;86:1227–1234.
6. Slaughter MS, Pagani FD, Rogers JG, et al. Clinical management of continuous-flow left ventricular assist devices in advanced heart failure. *J Heart Lung Transplant.* 2010;29:S1–S39.
7. Thoratec Ventricular Assist Device (VAD) System Instructions for Use. Thoratec, Pleasanton, CA, 2009.
8. Thoratec Implantable Ventricular Assist Device (IVAD) Instructions for Use. Thoratec, Pleasanton, CA, 2008.
9. ABIOMED AB5000 Circulatory Support System AB5000 Ventricle Instructions for Use. Abiomed, Danvers, MA, 2003.
10. ABIOMED BVS5000 Bi-ventricular Support System Operator's Manual. Abiomed, Danvers, MA, 2002.
11. Heartware Ventricular Assist System HVAD Pump Surgical Implant Procedure. HeartWare, Miami Lakes, FL, 2009.
12. Radovancevic B, Frazier OH, Duncan JM. Implantation technique for the HeartMate left ventricular assist device. *J Card Surg.* 1992;7:203–207.
13. Komoda T, Weng Y, Nojiri C, et al. Implantation technique for the DuraHeart left ventricular assist system. *J Artif Organs.* 2007;10:124–127.
14. Slaughter MS, Tsui SS, El-Banayosy A, et al. Results of a multicenter clinical trial with the Thoratec implantable ventricular assist device. *J Thorac Cardiovasc Surg.* 2007;133:1573–1580.
15. Frazier OH, Gemmato C, Myers TJ, et al. Initial clinical experience with the HeartMate II axial-flow left ventricular assist device. *Tex Heart Inst J.* 2007;34:275–281.
16. Capek P, Kadipasaoglu KA, Radovancevic B, et al. Human intraperitoneal response to a left ventricular assist device with a Ti-6Ai-4V alloy surface. *ASAIO J.* 1992;38:M543–M549.
17. el-Amir NG, Gardocki M, Levin HR, et al. Gastrointestinal consequences of left ventricular assist device placement. *ASAIO J.* 1996;42:150–153.
18. Icenogle T, Sandler D, Puhlman M, et al. Intraperitoneal pocket for left ventricular assist device placement. *J Heart Lung Transplant.* 2003;22:818–821.
19. Wasler A, Springer WE, Radovancevic B, et al. A comparison between intraperitoneal and extraperitoneal left ventricular assist system placement. *ASAIO J.* 1996;42:M573–M576.
20. Costantini TW, Taylor JH, Beilman GJ. Abdominal complications of ventricular assist device placement. *Surg Infect (Larchmt).* 2005;6:409–418.
21. Bhama JK, Rayappa S, Zaldonis D, et al. Impact of abdominal complications on outcome after mechanical circulatory support. *Ann Thorac Surg.* 2010;89:522–528.
22. Westaby S, Frazier OH, Pigott DW, et al. Implant technique for the Jarvik 2000 heart. *Ann Thorac Surg.* 2002;73:1337–1340.
23. Delgado 3rd R, Frazier OH, Myers TJ, et al. Direct thrombolytic therapy for intraventricular thrombosis in patients with the Jarvik 2000 left ventricular assist device. *J Heart Lung Transplant.* 2005;24:231–233.
24. Kar B, Delgado 3rd RM, Frazier OH, et al. The effect of LVAD aortic outflow-graft placement on hemodynamics and flow: implantation technique and computer flow modeling. *Tex Heart Inst J.* 2005;32:294–298.
25. Tuzun E, Roberts K, Cohn WE, et al. In vivo evaluation of the HeartWare centrifugal ventricular assist device. *Tex Heart Inst J.* 2007;34:406–411.
26. Impella 5.0 and Impella LD Instructions for Use. Abiomed, Danvers, MA, 2009.
27. LaRocca GM, Shimbo D, Rodriguez CJ, et al. The Impella Recover LP 5.0 left ventricular assist device: a bridge to coronary artery bypass grafting and cardiac transplantation. *J Am Soc Echocardiogr.* 2006;19:468 e465–468 e467.
28. Rossiter-Thornton M, Arun V, Forrest AP, et al. Left ventricular support with the Impella LP 5.0 for cardiogenic shock following cardiac surgery. *Heart Lung Circ.* 2008;17:243–245.
29. Samoukovic G, Rosu C, Giannetti N, et al. The Impella LP 5.0 as a bridge to long-term circulatory support. *Interact Cardiovasc Thorac Surg.* 2009;8:682–683.
30. Holman WL, Park SJ, Long JW, et al. Infection in permanent circulatory support: experience from the REMATCH trial. *J Heart Lung Transplant.* 2004;23:1359–1365.
31. Zierer A, Melby SJ, Voeller RK, et al. Late-onset driveline infections: the Achilles' heel of prolonged left ventricular assist device support. *Ann Thorac Surg.* 2007;84:515–520.
32. Simon P, Owen AN, Moritz A, et al. Transesophageal echocardiographic evaluation in mechanically assisted circulation. *Eur J Cardiothorac Surg.* 1991;5:492–497.
33. Jolly N. Role of Impella 2.5 heart pump in stabilizing diastolic aortic pressure to avert acute hemodynamic collapse during coronary interventions. *J Invasive Cardiol.* 2009;21:E134–E136.
34. Harjai KJ, O'Neill WW. Hemodynamic support using the Impella 2.5 catheter system during high-risk percutaneous coronary intervention in a patient with severe aortic stenosis. *J Interv Cardiol.* 2010;23:66–69.
35. Kar B, Adkins LE, Civitello AB, et al. Clinical experience with the TandemHeart percutaneous ventricular assist device. *Tex Heart Inst J.* 2006;33:111–115.
36. Vecchio S, Chechi T, Giuliani G, et al. Use of Impella Recover 2.5 left ventricular assist device in patients with cardiogenic shock or undergoing high-risk percutaneous coronary intervention procedures: experience of a high-volume center. *Minerva Cardioangiol.* 2008;56:391–399.
37. Pretorius M, Hughes AK, Stahlman MB, et al. Placement of the TandemHeart percutaneous left ventricular assist device. *Anesth Analg.* 2006;103:1412–1413.
38. Spencer FC, Eiseman B, Trinkle JK, et al. Assisted circulation for cardiac failure following intracardiac surgery with cardiopulmonary bypass. *J Thorac Cardiovasc Surg.* 1965;49:56–73.
39. Zwischenberger JB, Cox Jr CS. ECMO in the management of cardiac failure. *ASAIO J.* 1992;38:751–753.
40. Magovern Jr GJ, Magovern JA, Benckart DH, et al. Extracorporeal membrane oxygenation: preliminary results in patients with postcardiotomy cardiogenic shock. *Ann Thorac Surg.* 1994;57:1462–1468.
41. Smedira NG, Blackstone EH. Postcardiotomy mechanical support: risk factors and outcomes. *Ann Thorac Surg.* 2001;71:S60–S66.
42. CentriMag Blood Pump Instructions for Use. 2006.
43. Bhama JK, Kormos RL, Toyoda Y, et al. Clinical experience using the Levitronix CentriMag system for temporary right ventricular mechanical circulatory support. *J Heart Lung Transplant.* 2009;28:971–976.
44. De Robertis F, Birks EJ, Rogers P, et al. Clinical performance with the Levitronix CentriMag short-term ventricular assist device. *J Heart Lung Transplant.* 2006;25:181–186.
45. Piacentino 3rd V, Jones J, Fisher CA, et al. Off-pump technique for insertion of a HeartMate vented electric left ventricular assist device. *J Thorac Cardiovasc Surg.* 2004;127:262–264.
46. Anyanwu AC, Fischer GW, Plotkina I, et al. Off-pump implant of the Jarvik 2000 ventricular assist device through median sternotomy. *Ann Thorac Surg.* 2007;84:1405–1407.
47. Frazier OH, Gregoric ID, Cohn WE. Initial experience with non-thoracic, extraperitoneal, off-pump insertion of the Jarvik 2000 heart in patients with previous median sternotomy. *J Heart Lung Transplant.* 2006;25:499–503.
48. Selzman CH, Sheridan BC. Off-pump insertion of continuous flow left ventricular assist devices. *J Card Surg.* 2007;22:320–322.
49. Collart F, Feier H, Metras D, et al. A safe, alternative technique for off-pump left ventricular assist device implantation in high-risk reoperative cases. *Interact Cardiovasc Thorac Surg.* 2004;3:286–288.

CHAPTER **12**

Intraoperative Management Issues in Mechanical Circulatory Support

Walter Dembitsky and Yoshifumi Naka

There are many technical considerations that confront a surgeon during implantation of ventricular assist devices (VADs). This chapter focuses on intraoperative strategies used to optimize the outcome for patients receiving left ventricular assist devices (LVADs). The overriding principle is to correct the specific physiologic abnormalities in the patient and his or her native heart and then supplement the effort by addressing other specific coexisting problems and conditions. The issues outlined here represent a collation of many current successful strategies, but it is recognized that recommendations for management are certain to change as the field of mechanical circulatory support (MCS) continues to evolve. Primary issues include native valve dysfunction, the presence of prosthetic valves, arrhythmias, apical thrombus and myocardial infarction, and a patent foramen ovale (PFO). The process for weaning patients from cardiopulmonary bypass (CPB) to LVAD support is outlined with special attention to preservation of right ventricular function including the use of temporary right ventricular assist device (RVAD) support. Finally, prevention and treatment of intraoperative bleeding and the use of prosthetic materials to facilitate chest closure at the end of the VAD implantation procedure are summarized.

VALVULAR INCOMPETENCE AND REPAIR

The intraoperative management of native valvular incompetence during LVAD insertion is an ongoing topic for discussion. The management of left-sided mitral and aortic valvular insufficiency may directly affect the integrity of the left ventricular–LVAD pumping complex. If the left-sided system is functioning properly, the entire circulatory system depends on the pumping capacity of the right side. Correction of tricuspid insufficiency reinforces the integrity of the right ventricular pumping complex, which comprises the right ventricle and the pulmonary vascular resistance.

Both the expected duration of LVAD support and patient characteristics influence the decision to repair insufficient native valves. For short-term support (i.e., periods <3 months), native aortic valvular insufficiencies in relatively healthy LVAD recipients are more likely to be well tolerated and less likely to progress and manifest with a late liability. Severely debilitated patients are least likely to tolerate native valvular malfunctions after LVAD insertion. Potential transplant patients who live in areas with short average waiting times for a donor heart and clinical patient characteristics favoring early transplantation, such as small body size, may have only a short wait; however, brevity is not assured because patients can develop conditions during LVAD support that prolong support time.

Patients with very acute heart failure, especially young patients with proven or a high likelihood for myocarditis and a high likelihood of recovery of ventricular function, require special consideration. In cases where myocardial recovery is anticipated, a competent mitral and tricuspid valve and a nonstenotic aortic valve make assessment of a recovered ventricle during VAD support much more reliable. Because the duration of support can never be certain, it seems reasonable to err on the side of being more aggressive about correcting tricuspid and aortic valvular insufficiencies, especially if correction can be accomplished without significant mortality and morbidity.[1]

During and after LVAD insertion, both the right and the left native valves are subjected to new demands that can influence their performance acutely and chronically. Functional demands imposed on the native left-sided valves change not only with VAD insertion but also with the type of LVAD implanted. Volume displacement pumps provide pulsatile flow, which is independent of the native left ventricular pulsatile flow. When the pulses are countersynchronous, the left ventricle can serve to fill the LVAD as a sequential pump, without aortic valve opening and with decreased mitral valve pressure demands commensurate with the reduced pressure generated by the unloaded native left ventricle. During the systolic synchronous relationship, any mitral insufficiency can be reflected by episodic elevations of left atrial pressure with potentially deleterious effects on pulmonary vascular resistance in pulmonary function and possible filling of the left ventricular reservoir. If the native ventricle remains nonfunctional, the effects of mitral regurgitation are minimal.

Tricuspid Valve Incompetence

The new demands imposed on the tricuspid valve are superimposed on the demands the valve has already carried over the time that the heart has progressively failed. Usually the right ventricular pressure requirements are reduced because the left atrial pressure component of the total pulmonary vascular resistance is lowered with LVAD support. Occasionally in patients with high intrinsic pulmonary vascular resistance, the increased flow produced by the left ventricular–LVAD complex can increase the pulmonary artery pressure.

The cause of tricuspid valvular insufficiency in LVAD recipients is multifactorial. Advancing age, chronic atrial fibrillation, and pulmonary hypertension with chronic right heart pressure and volume overload all can dilate the tricuspid anulus. In patients with a compliant interventricular septum, increased venous return to the right heart after LVAD insertion can be accompanied by a septal shift to the left. The resulting increased right ventricular volume can exacerbate existing tricuspid regurgitation by increasing the amount of leaflet tethering or distraction of the septal leaflet. Secondary tricuspid regurgitation in LVAD recipients is often due to the adverse effects of the transvalvular lead components of automatic implantable cardioverter-defibrillators and pacemakers (Fig. 12-1). The degree and incidence of tricuspid regurgitation increase with the number and size of the transvalvular leads.[2] These leads can develop clots within days, inflammation within weeks, and sclerosis within 1 year. Sclerosis has been reported 17 days after insertion. Usually the posterior leaflet is affected. Perforation can occur, as can entanglement of the subvalvular apparatus. Diagnosis preoperatively is difficult because of echocardiographic shadowing produced by the lead.

Secondary tricuspid regurgitation may abate over time if the left ventricular–LVAD complex is functioning properly and is accompanied by a high degree of reduction in pulmonary hypertension and pulmonary insufficiency. In patients with chronic pulmonary hypertension from chronic thrombotic obstruction of the pulmonary arteries, even severe tricuspid regurgitation abated after right ventricular pressures were reduced following pulmonary thromboendarterectomy. However, these patients do not have myopathic ventricles. The corresponding tendency to repair the tricuspid valve using annuloplasty techniques has also been reduced over time in these patients, and this remains a controversial issue. Some data suggest that leaving greater than moderate tricuspid regurgitation is associated with worsening right ventricular function and tricuspid regurgitation over time and need for reoperation for correction.[3]

Other investigators have found that unless there is severe right ventricular failure, the additional time required to repair the tricuspid valve was offset by longer cardiopulmonary bypass (CPB) time and no improvement in outcome.[4] Although patients with tricuspid insufficiency may do well initially, it is likely they will not do as well as patients with a competent tricuspid valve. This statement seems especially true for patients who are not expected to recover right ventricular function or tricuspid valve function, or both. Patients with restrictive cardiomyopathies, severe dilated cardiomyopathy, and ischemic cardiomyopathy with right ventricular infarction and persistent arrhythmias that can produce tricuspid regurgitation and iatrogenic valvular destruction usually do not recover tricuspid function and require correction. Patients without LVADs undergoing mitral and aortic valve surgery have better exercise tolerance and survive longer if their tricuspid valves are competent.

Tricuspid annuloplasty can be effective in decreasing tricuspid regurgitation resulting from a dilated anulus. However, if leaflet tethering is severe, annuloplasty is usually inadequate or unsuccessful.[5] In our experience, in instances where annuloplasty is impossible, tricuspid valve replacement using a bioprosthesis inserted over the pacemaker leads without excision of the tricuspid apparatus has produced excellent long-term results.[6] The disadvantage of having a bioprosthesis in the right heart is the increased possibility of incurring a prosthetic valve infection. Because the hemodynamic function of the right heart after LVAD implantation is largely physiologic, transvalvular flow patterns and reduced pressures are likely to favor longer durability of bioprostheses in the tricuspid position. In general cardiac surgical patients, bioprostheses in the tricuspid position outlast bioprostheses in the mitral position.

Mitral Valve Abnormalities

With continuous flow pumps, the mitral valve may remain open throughout the entire natural cardiac cycle. This open mitral valve is especially noticeable in the early postoperative period when native left ventricular function is most compromised. As the left ventricle recovers, attenuated pulsatile flow becomes the norm. The reduced pressure reduces the work demands on the mitral valve. It is unknown if these abnormal pressure and flow patterns affect the native mitral valve function, but reports of failed mitral valve mechanical prostheses and bioprostheses[7] in patients with LVADs are likely due to these altered hemodynamics. Successful LVAD support in patients with both mechanical prostheses and bioprostheses has also been reported.[8]

Bridge to transplant support has also been successful in a patient with a nonfunctional left ventricle and no mitral valve in place; however, loss of the mitral valve may cause more collapse of the ventricular chamber and potentially compromise left ventricular filling. Management of mechanical mitral valve prostheses is controversial. There is a theoretical liability to mechanical prostheses, which depends on intermittent pulsatile flows to wash areas of stasis and minimize thrombogenicity. In recipients of long-term LVAD support, the long-term bleeding consequences imposed by LVADs sometimes may necessitate the cessation of anticoagulation and antiaggregation medications. Stopping these medications has an unknown but worrisome effect on implanted mechanical valves. LVAD recipients with mechanical mitral prosthetic valves have been successfully supported for 689 days.[9]

Severe secondary mitral regurgitation caused by chordal tethering is diminished during LVAD support because left ventricular volumes are reduced and the intrapapillary muscle distance is lessened by the functioning LVAD. Annular dilation and contraction may recover as left ventricular function recovers. If mitral regurgitation is 2+ or greater, an

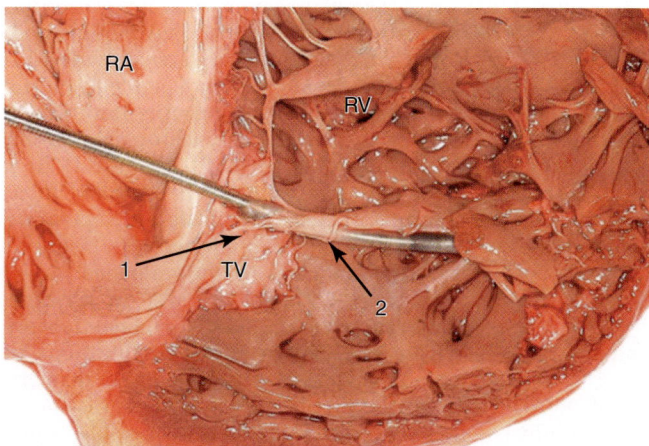

FIGURE 12-1 Transvalvular pacing wires with associated destruction of the tricuspid septal leaflet and the subvalvular mechanism. RA, right atrium; RV, right ventricle; TV, tricuspid valve.

annuloplasty ring can be placed in the unarrested heart and provides a secure remedy at a low risk. In rare cases in which a structural valve leaflet abnormality exists, the abnormality is corrected where indicated by using standard techniques, including chordal replacement, edge-to-edge repair, and annuloplasty. In patients with hypertrophic cardiomyopathy and mitral regurgitation, excision of the mitral valve and concomitant excision of all the papillary muscles that can be accessed through the mitral anulus and through the apex of the heart eliminate intraventricular obstructions to the LVAD inflow cannula. The valve is replaced with a bioprosthesis. The higher profile nature is of no consequence in patients during LVAD performance because very little flow exits the native left ventricular outflow tract during support.

Aortic Valve Abnormalities

The new functional demands on the native aortic valve during LVAD support are not physiologic. Where the left ventricle gains during LVAD support, the aortic valve seems to lose. During pulsatile pumping using displacement pumps, the aortic valve is obliged to hold a continuous barrage of pulsed systolic pressure in addition to its normal diastolic pressure load. Because flows from LVADs are usually directed to the ascending aorta, the aortic root remains well washed; this is especially true with pulsatile VADs. Aortic root flow conditions favoring stasis and recirculation have been observed with continuous flow VADs and are more severe as the distance of aortic inflow cannula from the aortic valve is increased.[10]

Thrombus has been observed in the noncoronary cusp and in the left coronary sinus in patients with previous coronary artery bypass grafting and in patients with aortic root closure, presumably owing to the static flow conditions. This thrombotic liability can result in systemic embolization.

Reduced systolic opening times for the aortic valve have been proposed as a mechanism for aortic valve deterioration in elderly patients.[11] During systole, the diastolic transmural aortic valve gradient is eliminated and may provide the necessary interval for aortic valve leaflets to replenish themselves. Systolic opening times decrease with advancing age and may render the aortic valve stromal cells incapable of properly maintaining leaflet integrity. In vitro studies have shown the increase in leaflet stress during LVAD support. Radial stress was greater than circumferential stress in a model using a continuous flow pump in an LVAD support configuration. These factors may help to explain the increasing incidence of native aortic valve insufficiency in LVAD recipients (20% to 25% at 2 years[12]; 15% at 1 year in patients with HeartMate II [Thoratec Corp, Pleasanton, CA] devices[13]).

AORTIC INSUFFICIENCY

Aortic insufficiency can lead to failure of the left ventricle to reduce in size and lead to progressive congestive heart failure in patients with VADs. The clinical importance of aortic insufficiency depends on many factors, including native left ventricular function and the degree of native mitral valve insufficiency. As aortic insufficiency progresses, more blood recirculates centrally through the left ventricular–LVAD complex and causes systemic hypoperfusion and progressive left ventricular volume loading. Patients with progressive or significant aortic insufficiency have signs of low systemic flow and high LVAD flows with increased pulmonary capillary wedge pressure and pulmonary congestion. The severity of this condition can be confirmed by measuring right heart output (Fick, thermal dilution) and finding that it is less than the left ventricular–LVAD output, which is reflected mostly by the flows calculated by the LVAD performance interpretation displayed on the VAD console. Intraoperative echocardiography

can confirm the correct positioning of the apical cannula. The echocardiogram shows a small right ventricle, dilated left ventricle, and atrial septal shifts to the right. High pulmonary artery pressure and high pulmonary capillary wedge pressure in this setting confirm the presence of intolerable failure owing to aortic insufficiency.

No absolute rules exist to guide treatment of aortic insufficiency seen in the operating room. The amount of aortic insufficiency is determined after CPB is instituted. The high left ventricular end-diastolic pressure in LVAD recipients clouds the echocardiographic diagnosis of aortic insufficiency because the transvalvular gradient is low. Initiating CPB increases the gradient as the left ventricular end-diastolic pressure decreases, and aortic insufficiency becomes more evident on transesophageal echocardiography. Direct examination of the aortic valve leak is also possible by viewing it through the apical cannulation site or through the mitral anulus, if mitral valve repair is performed without cross clamping. A competent aortic valve with good leaflet coaptation may remain competent over time. Thickened leaflets may also be more durable.

Because late repair may become necessary and to date requires reoperation, early valve closure is warranted in patients with existing aortic insufficiency, especially in recipients of long-term LVAD support who have thin leaflets. An effective technique has been described by Adamson[14] (Fig. 12-2). In patients with sclerotic valves where progression is unlikely, simple suture closure of insufficient leaflets may suffice, but central coaptation sutures in otherwise normal valves do not prevent progression of aortic insufficiency and its sequelae.[15]

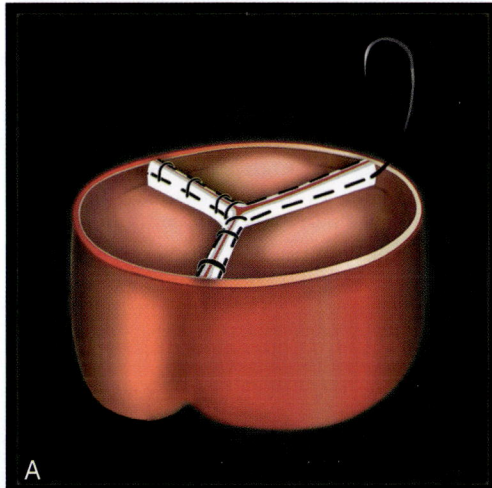

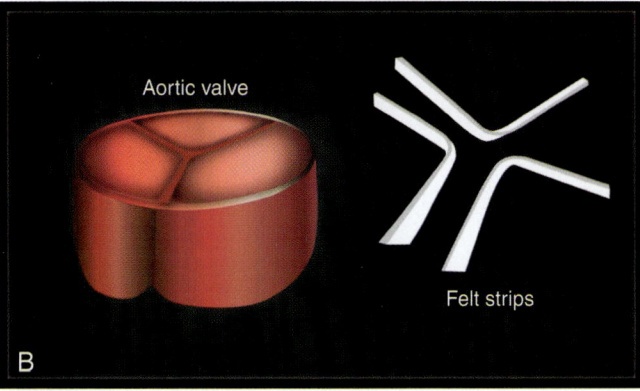

FIGURE 12-2 A, Adamson technique for closure of the aortic valve using 4-0 polypropylene (Prolene) sutures and felt strips. **B,** Adamson technique for closure of the aortic valve using 4-0 Prolene sutures and felt strips.

Prosthetic aortic valve replacement also corrects insufficiency. However, protracted low intermittent transvalvular flows cause both mechanical valves and bioprosthetic valves to thrombose. Permanent closure of these prostheses is probably best because it seems to minimize systemic embolization of valve thrombus during intermittent opening. Patients with existing mechanical aortic prostheses are at extra risk for thromboembolism. Various techniques have been suggested to reduce that liability, including sutures to retard the valve leaflets, patch closure over the valve, replacement of the valve with a bioprosthesis, and replacement of the valve using a patch in the aortic root.

Chronic left ventricular outflow tract closure has been reported and has produced no adverse long-term consequences to date.[14] The incidence of thromboembolism does not seem to be increased but has not been eliminated. Survival seems to be at least as good as in patients without outflow tract closure, and hemodynamics are excellent. Patients with left ventricular outflow tract who recover ventricular function and are able to be weaned from the devices require aortic valve replacement.

PATENT FORAMEN OVALE

An LVAD may create a pressure gradient from the right to the left atrium, which exaggerates right-to-left shunting through a PFO resulting in profound oxygen desaturation. Careful direct inspection can be made to ensure that a PFO is not present. If direct inspection is not made, a transesophageal echocardiography (TEE) Doppler examination can confirm the presence of a physiologically significant PFO, but the atrial septum must be shifted to the left either by increasing LVAD flows or, if tested before LVAD insertion, by compressing the pulmonary artery (Fig. 12-3). Profound hypoxia results from a persistent PFO as the LVAD reduces the left atrial pressure and the right atrial pressure increases. The incidence of PFO is 20% to 30% depending on whether it is defined by physiologic testing with a left shifted septum or by direct inspection. All PFOs should be surgically closed before leaving the operating room, although they have been successfully closed postoperatively using percutaneous technology.[16]

Pal and associates[17] reviewed the influence of associated procedures performed at the time of LVAD implantation. Almost 30% of the patients had closure of the foramen ovale or repair of the tricuspid or aortic valves. Almost half of the patients had a valvular procedure; the most common

valve repaired was the tricuspid valve followed much less frequently by the aortic valve. Overall 30-day mortality was 5.8% for the group receiving the HeartMate II LVAD alone and 11.3% for the group undergoing an associated procedure. Subgroup analysis showed that simultaneous PFO closure was not associated with an increased 30-day mortality rate, but concurrent valvular procedures increased the risk to 8.5%. Patients who underwent an aortic valve procedure had a 30-day mortality rate of 25%, which was higher than the mortality for isolated concurrent mitral (0%) or tricuspid repair (3.3%). Survival at 180 days was 87% for patients receiving the HeartMate II LVAD alone and 80% for the group undergoing an associated procedure. Aortic valve procedures generally require cardioplegic arrest, which may have had a negative impact on right ventricular function, explaining some of the reduced outcomes. In addition, patients who undergo mechanical replacement have abnormal washing of the prosthesis, which may predispose to thrombus formation and embolic complications.

VENTRICULAR ARRHYTHMIAS

Recipients with ventricular severe arrhythmias may require biventricular support, but arrhythmias may improve or are better tolerated after LVAD insertion. Standard ventricular arrhythmia ablation techniques are used to eliminate or attenuate these rhythms. Preoperative mapping, if possible, can serve as a guide to intraoperative ablation. It may also be prudent to connect the apical cannulation site to any proximate scar using cryoablation. This procedure eliminates the formation of an isthmus of myocardium between the scar and the apical cannulation site, which can sustain a postoperative short circuit ventricular tachycardia. During VAD insertion, the left atrial appendage is usually oversewn especially in patients who have atrial fibrillation.

BIVENTRICULAR VENTRICULAR ASSIST DEVICE VERSUS LEFT VENTRICULAR ASSIST DEVICE FOR RIGHT HEART FAILURE

Management of right ventricular failure during LVAD implantation is a major clinical problem with LVAD use. Postoperative right ventricular failure remains a challenge, but its severity and duration are still controversial. Right ventricular failure is defined by the need for the use of an RVAD or use of inotropes beyond 14 days. The use of RVADs was less in more recent trials comparing HeartMate I and HeartMate II devices than it was in the original REMATCH (Randomized Evaluation of Mechanical Assistance for the Treatment of Congestive Heart Failure) trial comparing HeartMate I with optimal medical therapy in 2001.[18]

Right Heart Physiology

The functions of the right ventricle are to maintain a low systemic venous pressure, provide flow to the lungs, and fill the left ventricle adequately. In contrast to the systemic circulation, the low pressure, low resistance, high compliance characteristics of the pulmonary vascular bed with a gradient of 5 mm Hg normally allow almost continuous flow. The right ventricle is anatomically adapted for generating sustained low pressure perfusion. It is predominantly a volume pump, and in contrast to the left ventricle, it is much less capable of tolerating sustained acute afterload increases. The right ventricle comprises two functionally and anatomically different cavities. The sinus generates the systolic pressure, which is

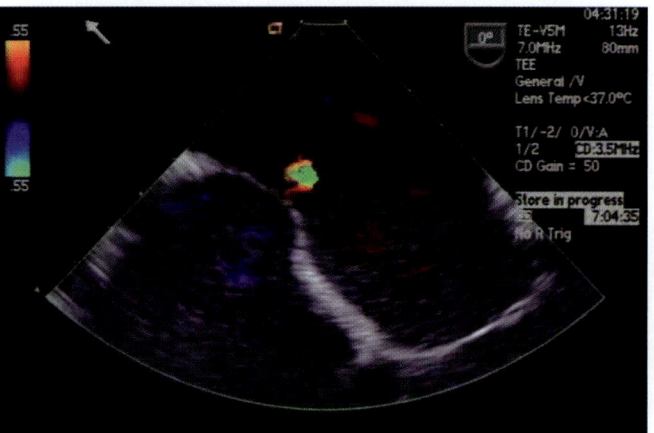

FIGURE 12-3 Confirmation of the physiologic significance of right-to-left shunt through a patent foramen ovale (PFO) using transesophageal echocardiography (TEE) to image the interatrial septum being shifted to the left by compressing the pulmonary artery before the institution of cardiopulmonary bypass (CPB).

attenuated by the cone. Initial systolic pressure is generated in the sinus by the sequential contraction of the papillary muscle, the right ventricular free wall, and the left ventricle. The pressurized blood is transferred to the more compliant conus region, beneath the pulmonary valve, where peak pressure is reduced and prolonged. Experimentally, a pulmonary arterial pulse pressure around 20 mm Hg permits optimal gas exchange. Histologic damage is seen with pressures greater than 20 mm Hg, and interstitial edema forms without pulsatility.[19]

The characteristics of the pulmonary vascular bed permit prolonged right ventricular ejection. The ability of the normal pulmonary vascular bed to accept higher flows is evident in pneumonectomy patients whose pulmonary arterial pressure remains normal. Acute elevations of right ventricular afterload alter these ejection characteristics, and the right ventricular pressure volume loop is no longer triangular but resembles that of the left ventricular pressure volume loop. The right ventricle dilates to maintain stroke volume, albeit with a reduced ejection fraction. The loss of the peristaltic contraction produces an accelerated increase in pulmonary artery pressures and flows. Prolonged isovolumic contraction and ejection time increase myocardial oxygen consumption and the associated demand for increased coronary blood flow. Normally, right ventricular coronary blood flow is equally distributed between diastole and systole. During periods of increased pulmonary artery pressure, the flow becomes similar to the left ventricular coronary blood flow and is almost exclusively diastolic.

Right Ventricular and Left Ventricular Interaction

Ventricular interdependence is influenced by the noncompliant periventricular tissues, usually the pericardium. Numerous studies have defined the beat-to-beat nature of ventricular interdependence and shown that 20% to 70% of right ventricular function is derived from the left ventricle. Contractile septal function independent of systolic deformity appears to be an important determinant of systolic right ventricular function. In addition, changes in septal position alter right ventricular preload by changing right ventricular volume.[20] Reduced systemic blood pressure during periods of acute increases in pulmonary artery pressure produces subendocardial right ventricular ischemia, especially when the right ventricular myocardial tissue perfusion gradient is compromised further by an increased right ventricular end-diastolic pressure and flow restricting coronary arterial occlusive disease.

Influence of Left Ventricular Assist Device Support on Right Ventricular Performance

The interactions between the two ventricles are altered by the use of LVADs. During LVAD support, global right ventricular performance can be impaired by excessive reduction of left ventricular volume and chamber size in patients with a compliant septum resulting in a shift of the interventricular septum to the left and into the left ventricle. This shift distorts the geometry of the right ventricle and reduces its pumping ability. Myocardial efficiency and power output can often be maintained through a decrease in pulmonary artery pressure and an increase in right ventricular filling pressure.[21,22]

Isolated right ventricular free wall ischemia during LVAD support appears to be an insufficient indication for RVAD support[21] compared with isolated right ventricular ischemia caused by right coronary occlusion often found in patients with ischemic cardiomyopathy.[23] In contrast, septal ischemia caused by left anterior artery occlusive disease is more

important and can result in significant degradation of right ventricular function during LVAD support.[24]

Any diminution of right ventricular contractile performance during LVAD support is largely nullified by the reduction in afterload created by reducing the left atrial pressure contribution to elevated pulmonary artery pressure. Reduction of left ventricular end-diastolic pressure is reflected back to the pulmonary circulation resulting in a reduced pulmonary artery pressure, reducing right ventricular afterload and enhancing right ventricular function. Increased systemic blood pressure enhances right coronary blood flow. Increasing the speed of a rotary pump LVAD increases its output, which increases systemic blood flow and secondarily increases venous return to the right ventricle causing distention, which can increase tricuspid regurgitation.

Three experimental observations that separate mild from severe right ventricular depression during LVAD support are (1) underlying right ventricular dysfunction appears to be necessary; (2) degree of right ventricular afterload reduction, especially pulmonary artery pressure, is important; and, (3) regional ischemia from coronary artery occlusive disease (especially septal) is especially important.[20] These experimental conditions all have been observed clinically and have been published.[18,25]

Clinical Experience with Right Ventricular Failure during Left Ventricular Assist Device Support

Overt significant right ventricular dysfunction requiring prolonged use of inotropic drugs, pacing, pulmonary artery dilators, and RVAD support to enhance LVAD flow during initial LVAD implantation remains a clinical problem and is associated with a high mortality (Fig. 12-4). Pulmonary hypertension reflects chronic elevation of left atrial pressure and usually secondary pulmonary artery hypertension. In contrast to high pulmonary artery pressures during heart transplantation, high pulmonary artery pressures during LVAD implantation usually indicate that the right ventricle is well compensated and will perform well. Conversely, high central venous pressure (CVP) and low pulmonary artery pressure in patients with low output left ventricular failure are indicative of a failing right ventricle that is incapable of generating a high pulmonary artery pressure. Right atrial pressure may be the best marker of right ventricular function. One measurement of right ventricular function that has been shown to correlate with right ventricular failure is the right ventricular stroke work index. A decreased right ventricular stroke work index indicates a diminished capacity of the right ventricular complex to perform and helps define patients who might need RVAD support during LVAD implantation.

Intraoperative right ventricular function can be optimized in some patients by preoperative reduction of CVP using pharmacologic or mechanical methods including ultrafiltration (see Chapter 7). Preoperative oral or intravenous pulmonary vasodilation can be beneficial and can augment the effects of nitrous oxide, which may be used intraoperatively. An intra-aortic balloon pump inserted preoperatively may also have a salutary effect on right ventricular function by reducing left atrial and pulmonary artery pressures, increasing mean aortic pressure, and augmenting diastolic coronary artery perfusion pressure.

High preoperative pulmonary artery pressures (and increased right ventricular stroke work index) are not a predictor of RVAD support. The total pulmonary vascular resistance after LVAD implantation is reduced because both the left ventricular end-diastolic pressure and the pulmonary vascular resistance are minimized. The reduced right ventricular afterload permits the preimplantation hypertensive

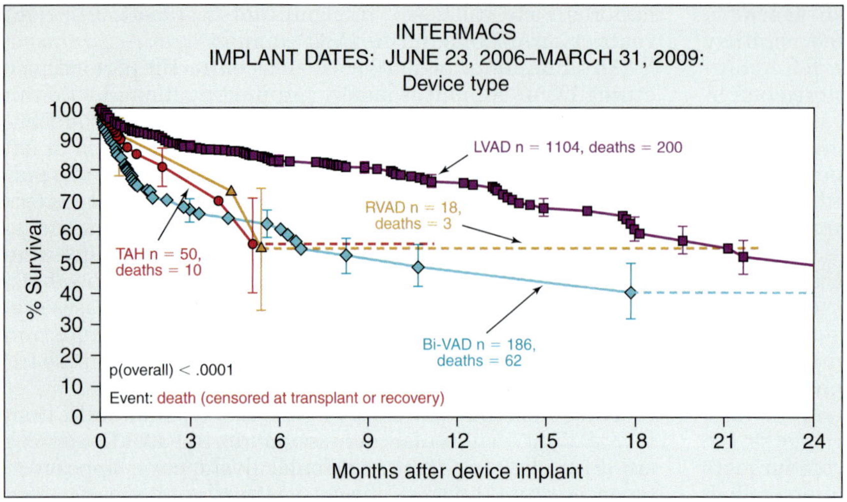

FIGURE 12-4 INTERMACS (Interagency Registry for Mechanically Assisted Circulatory Support) registry data illustrating the adverse survival influence of right ventricular failure. BiVAD, biventricular ventricular assist device; LVAD, left ventricular assist device; RVAD, right ventricular assist device; TAH, total artificial heart.

right ventricle to function well, similar to the immediate improvement seen in right ventricular function after lung transplantation for pulmonary hypertension or after pulmonary thromboendarterectomy in patients with chronic pulmonary hypertension. Right ventricular exercise hemodynamic studies in patients with long-term support by implantable LVADs have indicated that maximal exercise capacity is primarily limited by the performance of the left ventricular–LVAD complex and not the right ventricle, which has been shown to have improved pumping capacity.[26] Histologic and chemical structural changes show reverse remodeling in the right ventricles of patients supported by LVADs.[27] Reduction of right ventricular pressure reduces the duration of the monophasic right ventricular action potentials and lessens the chances of generating right ventricular arrhythmias.[28] Some authors believe that patients who develop post-LVAD right ventricular failure can be identified preoperatively with the use of two right ventricular risk scores, which are detailed in Chapters 6 and 7.

WEANING FROM CARDIOPULMONARY BYPASS AND IMPLANTATION OF RIGHT VENTRICULAR ASSIST DEVICES

Hemodynamic Management of Weaning from Cardiopulmonary Bypass

When the implantation of the LVAD is completed, pharmacologic cardiac support is initiated, and the patient is weaned from CPB. The device is actuated shortly afterward. This sequence allows the left ventricle to be filled and to serve as a safe reservoir to supply the implanted LVAD. During the critical weaning interval, assiduous attention must be directed toward maintaining left ventricular filling volume. If the ventricle is emptied, a suction event can occur in rotary blood pumps. Suction events can create transient ventricular arrhythmias or, at worse, cause gas (carbon dioxide [CO_2], it is hoped) to be aspirated around the apical cannula and pumped into the ascending aorta and then into the right coronary and cerebral circulation. In cases in which the aortic valve is closed, the LVAD is actuated, and its flow is increased as CPB is weaned.

With continuous flow pumps, the revolutions per minute (rpms) are slowly increased as the left ventricle progressively receives more flow from the lungs. The interventricular and interatrial septa are monitored by TEE and are maintained in a neutral position. Correct position of the apical cannula can

be confirmed by increasing the pump rpms and observing a reduction of left ventricular volume. The appropriate shape of the left ventricle in TEE short axis view is a round shape; a flattened or convex septum ("D"-shaped left ventricle) indicates excessive suction by the LVAD. In patients with a compliant septum, dynamic interventricular interaction through the ventricular septum can significantly change after LVAD initiation and compromise right ventricular function especially with continuous flow devices. If the left ventricle is overly aspirated, temporarily decreasing pump speed usually restores the shape of the left ventricle and the hemodynamics.

Right ventricular failure occurs in 20% to 40% of LVAD recipients, and it is related to worse outcomes.[29,30] Optimizing right ventricular function is the key in hemodynamic management in weaning from CPB after LVAD implantation because without device-related mechanical problems, device output depends on the output from the right ventricle, whose function is rarely normal in patients undergoing LVAD placement and is impaired even further during LVAD implantation. Right ventricular function is monitored with direct visualization by the surgeon and more importantly with TEE. During transition from CPB to LVAD support, right ventricular function is optimized by adjusting heart rate, contractility, preload, and afterload.

Proactive and aggressive treatment of subtle signs of right ventricular dysfunction can prevent deterioration of hemodynamics and enable a smooth transition. The fragile nature of the right ventricular myocardium with its dependence on left ventricular function and the influence of right ventricular afterload on right ventricular performance can collectively create right circulatory failure over a short time. Progressive pulmonary circulatory failure proceeds to systemic circulatory failure. A firm treatment plan eliminates this undesirable positive feedback mechanism. During LVAD implantation with CPB, pulmonary vascular resistance is minimized. Patients with chronic vasoactive pulmonary hypertension can be treated pharmacologically with pulmonary vasodilators, including nitric oxide, milrinone, dobutamine, prostacyclin, isoproterenol, iloprost, and sildenafil.

On weaning from CPB, ventilation is adjusted to reduce the end-tidal CO_2 to 24 mm Hg, and oxygen saturation is kept high using appropriate inspired oxygen concentrations. Systemic acidosis should be corrected to optimize the pulmonary vascular response to drugs. Pulmonary effusions should also be evacuated, and endobronchial obstructions are removed endoscopically if necessary. Proper position of the left ventricular or left atrial cannula providing flow to the LVAD can be determined by use of TEE or hand-held echo probes placed on the left ventricle. Left ventricular chamber size is adjusted so that the septum is midline. Excessive suction can cause the apical cannula to impinge on the ventricular septum or free wall and generate ventricular arrhythmias.

Extreme care is taken to avoid air embolization to the right coronary artery. To minimize the impact of coronary gas embolization, the operative field is flooded with CO_2 during the entire implantation procedure. The heavy CO_2 displaces lighter atmospheric gases in the pericardium, and if it is aspirated, it is quickly absorbed from the blood and does not cause significant ischemic myocardial injury. Any occlusive disease in the coronaries supplying myocardium contributing to right ventricular function is bypassed using saphenous vein grafts. The special function of the right ventricle warrants revascularization of the acute marginal branches and posterior descending and left anterior descending arteries to ensure that the free wall and important septal component of the right ventricular pump are well perfused.

As stated earlier, tricuspid valve insufficiency may initially appear to be minimal, but increasing right atrial return from a functioning left ventricular–LVAD complex and associated septal shift may dramatically increase tricuspid regurgitation in some patients. Patients with more than moderate regurgitation should have it corrected with a tricuspid annuloplasty ring or insertion of a bioprosthetic valve. Elevating the right ventricular heart rate by pacing the right atrium to 100 to 110 beats/min minimizes the right ventricular diastolic filling time and enhances right ventricular contractility owing to the treppe effect. Optimal direct right ventricular pacing is probably best initiated in the sinus and not the conus region of the right ventricle. Both interventions reduce tricuspid regurgitation.

Factors Influencing Weaning from Cardiopulmonary Bypass

The following parameters are the key factors in hemodynamic management (Table 12-1): preload (CVP), afterload and pulmonary vascular resistance, contractility of the right ventricle, interventricular interaction, heart rate, rhythm, and coronary perfusion and systemic vascular resistance. Preload is monitored with the CVP. Overdistention of the

right ventricle must be avoided. A CVP greater than 15 mm Hg is a sign of right ventricular dysfunction. Increased stress of the thin right ventricular wall can lead to worsening tricuspid regurgitation and decreased organ perfusion. Afterload is estimated based on the preoperative calculation of pulmonary vascular resistance. Pulmonary vascular resistance is frequently elevated after LVAD implantation. If the lung resistance is high and the cardiac output is low, the pulmonary artery pressures are low. Patients with good right ventricular function can generate a high pressure even with a low cardiac output. Patients with poor right ventricular function and a low cardiac output have low pulmonary artery pressures.

Inotropic therapy with either milrinone (0.25 to 0.5 µg/kg/min) or dobutamine (3 to 5 µg/kg/min) is always administered to support contraction of the right ventricle and provide pulmonary vasodilation. These two drugs may be combined with isoproterenol. All three drugs have a synergistic pulmonary vasodilatory effect when combined with nitric oxide. Inhaled nitric oxide with low tidal volumes is usually begun during CPB. Epinephrine is added for further assistance without delay if subtle signs of right ventricular dysfunction appear. If the patient requires escalation of inotropic or vasopressor support, an RVAD should be promptly inserted. Heart rate and rhythm are controlled with pacing or administration of antiarrhythmic agents, or both. Maintenance of coronary perfusion is achieved by maintaining systemic vascular resistance and adequate perfusion pressure (mean systemic blood pressure approximately 80 mm Hg). Arginine vasopressin has been shown to be effective in treating vasodilatory hypotension in these patients.[31] Excessive afterload can impair pump flow, particularly with continuous flow devices.

Usually the decision to proceed to RVAD support is made in the operating room. Occasionally, the decision to proceed directly to a biventricular VAD or total artificial heart can be made preoperatively. Patients with signs of systemic hypoperfusion presenting with multisystem organ failure may be best managed with biventricular support, which provides the highest cardiac outputs with the lowest venous pressures and the least requirement for adrenergic drugs. When the retained natural heart is a persistent liability, full biventricular support is best. Acute cardiac homograft failure, severe uncontrollable ventricular arrhythmias, extensive ischemic damage including some cases with infarct ventricular septal defects,

CH 12

Intraoperative Management Issues in Mechanical Circulatory Support

TABLE 12-1	Hemodynamic Parameters				
Contractility					
Systemic vasoconstrictors to keep mean BP 80 mm Hg	Avoid overdistention	Prevent subendocardial ischemia	CABG as needed	Inotropic agents: dobutamine, milrinone, isoproterenol, epinephrine	
Afterload Reduction					
LVEDP <10 mm Hg	Pulmonary arterial vasodilators (NO, isoproterenol, dobutamine, milrinone, sildenafil)	Normalize pH, Pa_{O_2}			
Preload					
Keep CVP less than preoperatively; <15 mm Hg better					
Heart Rate					
Atrial pace, RV pace near apex at 100 beats/min	Treat atrial fibrillation and ventricular tachycardia				
Correct Native Heart Abnormalities					
2+ or greater TR, probably 2+ or >MR, CABG 1+ or > AI	Treat VSD	Preserve or replace CABG grafts			

AI, aortic insufficiency; BP, blood pressure; CABG, coronary artery bypass grafting; CVP, central venous pressure; LVEDP, left ventricular end-diastolic pressure; MR, mitral regurgitation; NO, nitric oxide; Pa_{O_2}, partial arterial oxygen tension; RV, right ventricular; TR, tricuspid regurgitation; VSD, ventricular septal defect.

extensive myocarditis with systemic inflammation, and intraventricular clots especially if bilateral all represent clinical situations where retention of native heart may persist as a liability. Most of these clinical conditions have impaired right ventricular pumping capacity combined with elevated pulmonary vascular resistance. If pulmonary vascular resistance is kept low, univentricular support is almost always successful.

After weaning the LVAD recipient from CPB, low pulmonary capillary wedge pressure, low pulmonary artery pressure, and high LVAD output all confirm that the left heart is decompressed and the right ventricular pumping complex is performing well. Transient periods of systemic hypotension and low flow associated with elevations in right ventricular filling pressures lead to progressive right ventricular failure and reduced LVAD filling and resultant circulatory collapse and pulmonary vasoconstriction with worsening right ventricular function. If intrapulmonary shunting is present, the reduced cardiac output and the resultant lowered systemic venous oxygen saturation create systemic hypoxia that can also incite pulmonary vasoconstriction. The increasingly challenged right ventricle progressively fails as oxygen demand increases, coronary blood flow decreases, and the tricuspid valve begins to leak. When this scenario is evident, temporary right heart bypass is used to allow the right ventricle to recover. Other authors have successfully used right heart and lung bypass.

Temporary Right Heart Support with the Cardiopulmonary Bypass Circuit

In patients with low cardiac output with low left atrial pressure or pulmonary capillary wedge pressure and increased CVP in whom the above-described management strategy fails, temporary support can be achieved using the CPB circuit. A cannula is placed in the pulmonary artery through a simple purse-string suture. Using a "Y" connector, the arterial flow from the bypass circuit can be redirected from the aorta into the pulmonary artery (Fig. 12-5).[32] This redirection of flow allows the right ventricle to remain decompressed, gradually elevating the systemic pressure and enhancing the important right ventricular transmyocardial blood flow. Increased cardiac output elevates the systemic venous oxygen saturation, and the arterial oxygen desaturation associated with intrapulmonary shunting is minimized. Systemic acidosis is more easily adjusted. During this period of temporary right heart support, the oxygenator gas flow is reduced, and the gas exchange function of the natural lung can be assessed. The pulmonary vascular resistance is pharmacologically reduced. Gradually, the temporary pump flow is reduced from the initial flows of 4 to 5 L, and the CVP is allowed to increase to 10 to 15 mm Hg. If the native right ventricle cannot assume the burden of pulmonary flow necessary to fill the LVAD within 0.5 to 1 hour, a short-term device is implanted, heparin is reversed, hemostasis is obtained, and the chest is closed.

Pump Selection for Right Heart Support

Published reports of reduced survival for RVAD recipients have incorrectly discouraged the appropriate application of RVADs. Underuse of RVADs may impair patient recovery in the early perioperative period by allowing right ventricular pressure and CVP to remain high and LVAD outputs to be low. The resultant low mean arterial pressure and high systemic venous pressure reduce the tissue perfusion gradient below the desired minimum of 40 mm Hg. This condition and the independent adverse effect of increased CVP compromise right ventricular, hepatic, renal, gastrointestinal, and cerebral recovery and may directly lead to worsening function. Before selecting a pump to support the failing right circulation, the duration of support needed must be estimated. Most patients require only short periods of support. If more than 1 or 2 hours but less than 2 weeks of assistance is needed, widely available short-term pumps may be used. Percutaneously placed continuous flow paracorporeal rotary pumps are well suited for brief use.

If more than 2 weeks of support is anticipated, long-term support devices are inserted. To date, long-term support devices have usually been paracorporeal pulsatile pumps, although successful biventricular support using implantable centrifugal pumps has been reported more recently and is very likely to become more common.

INTRAOPERATIVE BLEEDING ASSOCIATED WITH LEFT VENTRICULAR ASSIST DEVICES

Intraoperative and perioperative bleeding associated with general cardiac surgery is usually easily managed. At the present time, however, the bleeding associated with LVAD insertion is on average three to four times that of routine cardiac surgery. Excessive bleeding increases mortality and morbidity secondary to right heart failure, renal failure, respiratory failure, and multiple organ failure. The hemostatic system is a dynamic balance between thrombotic and thrombolytic influences; when one falters, the other prevails and produces the clinical problem of either thrombosis or bleeding. Often both forces are coincidentally activated creating an uneasy truce without hemorrhagic or thrombotic clinical consequences. Bleeding causes are multifocal, so attempts to manage bleeding should be guided by a studied approach.

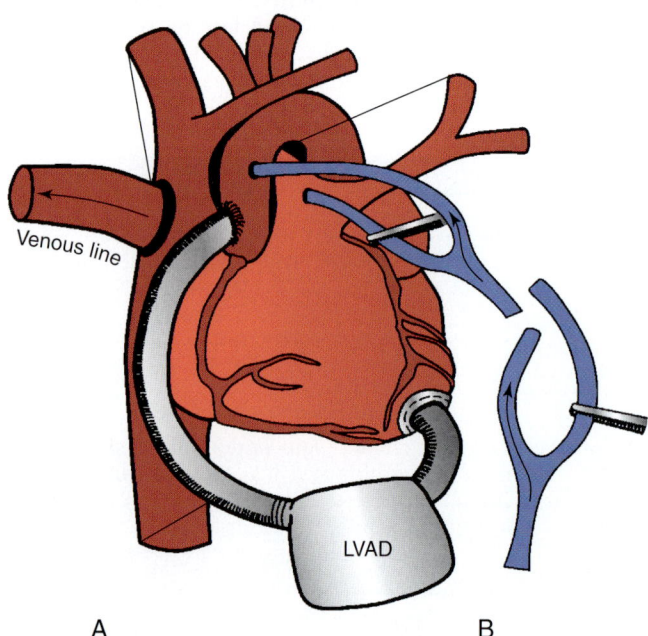

Venous line

A   B

LVAD

FIGURE 12-5 A and **B,** Using standard cardiopulmonary bypass (CPB) **(A)** as a temporary right heart bypass **(B)** by diverting the arterial flow from venoarterial bypass to the pulmonary artery using a "Y" connector and a tubing clamp. LVAD, left ventricular assist device.

Preoperative Definition of Bleeding Risk

An important component of the initial assessment of patients requiring LVAD insertion is to define the patient's likelihood of bleeding. Inherited bleeding problems, such

CH 12

as hemophilia or von Willebrand defects, are uncommon and often obvious from the history. These conditions can usually be managed by the appropriate administration of the deficit factors. An acquired pathology is the most common culprit contributing to intraoperative bleeding diathesis. Acquired pathologies are usually multiple and are more recalcitrant to therapy. Accurately defining these pathologies preoperatively and correcting them when possible help minimize intraoperative blood loss. Because patients receiving LVADs usually have chronic stage D heart failure, they present with low cardiac output and mean blood pressures and high pulmonary artery pressure and CVP. Patients are often malnourished and have varying degrees of renal and hepatic dysfunction and active systemic inflammation, all of which predispose them to excessive intraoperative bleeding.

The high metabolic rate and complex vascular supply of the liver make it particularly vulnerable to circulatory disturbances. Potential LVAD recipients with liver dysfunction should undergo a careful history and physical examination to exclude findings or risk factors for primary liver disease. This evaluation should include asking specifically about prior blood transfusions, tattoos, illicit drug use, sexual promiscuity, a family history of jaundice or liver disease, a history of jaundice or fever following anesthesia, alcohol use, and a complete review of current medications. The severity and characteristics of hepatic injury depend on the blood vessels that are involved and the degree to which injury is related to passive congestion or diminished perfusion.[33] Passive visceral congestion often coexists with reduced cardiac output and lowered blood pressure, making their relative contributions to hepatic injury interdependent. Because most of the proteins needed for proper functioning of the coagulation system are produced in the liver, hepatic dysfunction can affect intraoperative bleeding.

Worsening preoperative coagulopathy correlates with the severity of hepatic dysfunction and usually represents significant hepatic dysfunction because the liver can typically maintain normal synthetic function with 50% reduction of functional mass. In addition to deficiency of coagulant proteins, patients with hepatic failure may develop varying degrees of disseminated intravascular coagulation, fibrinolysis, vitamin K deficiency, dysfibrinogenemia, and thrombocytopenia, all of which may contribute to intraoperative bleeding. The prothrombin time is mildly abnormal in many patients. When the international normalized ratio (INR) is significantly elevated in the absence of anticoagulant medication, it may be due in part to impaired hepatic synthesis of coagulation factors II, V, VII, IX, and X. Because the prothrombin time may not correct completely with administration of vitamin K, other coagulation defects (e.g., disseminated intravascular coagulation) may also contribute.[34]

Mild hyperbilirubinemia totaling less than 3 mg/dL is often present. Other liver biochemical tests are usually only mildly increased. All of these tests can be strikingly elevated with severe acute right heart. Serum albumin levels are decreased in 30% to 50% of patients with liver dysfunction but are rarely less than 2.5 g/dL. Hypoalbuminemia is most likely caused by inflammation, malnutrition, and protein-losing gastroenteropathy. Normal hepatic function tests at rest may belie the ability of the liver to respond to the stress of surgery. Patients with severe liver failure can also have thrombocytopenia mainly caused by portal hypertension with attendant congestive splenomegaly. An enlarged spleen secondary to increased portal pressure from right heart failure can result in temporary sequestration of up to 90% of the circulating platelet mass.[35] Decreased thrombopoietin levels may also contribute to thrombocytopenia. Other considerations include drug effects and heparin-induced thrombocytopenia.

Chronic congestive heart failure can create cirrhosis. The cirrhotic liver may be enlarged, normal in size, or small. When palpable, the cirrhotic liver has a firm and nodular consistency. If cirrhosis is suspected, a biopsy is usually warranted and can confirm the diagnosis in 80% to 100% of cases. Patients with cirrhosis commonly have many hematologic abnormalities, including disorders of coagulation and varying degrees of cytopenia.[36]

Thrombocytopenia is the most common first hematologic abnormality, whereas leukopenia and anemia develop later in the disease course.[37] Compared with other surgical procedures, cardiac surgery is associated with increased mortality in patients with cirrhosis.[38] Patients with advanced cirrhosis are not good candidates for LVAD insertion.

The effect of heart failure on renal function is well described, and the suppressive influence of renal dysfunction on the bone marrow and platelet function is known. Uremia associated with heart failure influences hemostasis mainly by creating platelet dysfunction including intrinsic defects and abnormal platelet-endothelial interactions.[39] Contributing factors are intrinsic to platelets and external. Intrinsic platelet factors include abnormal expression of glycoproteins, altered adenosine diphosphate and serotonin release from platelet alpha granules, faulty arachidonic acid and depressed prostaglandin metabolism, decreased platelet thromboxane A_2 generation, and abnormal platelet cytoskeletal assembly. Extrinsic factors include the action of uremic toxins, anemia, increased nitric oxide production, von Willebrand factor abnormalities, decreased platelet production, and abnormal interactions between the platelet and the endothelium of the vessel wall. Correction of anemia with blood transfusions or erythropoietin often improves platelet function in uremic patients.

Vascular pathology associated with increased sheer stress can create bleeding abnormalities at surgery, probably by causing degradation of the large multimers of von Willebrand factor. Patients with coarctation, aortic valve stenosis, hypertrophic cardiomyopathy, peripheral vascular disease, and pre-existing LVADs all are susceptible to having this abnormality. The normal large multimers of von Willebrand factor are universally absent in patients with axial flow pumps. They were absent preoperatively in 20% of a small series of recipients of the HeartMate II LVAD.[40]

Direct measurement of large von Willebrand factor multimers is costly and time-consuming. The platelet function assay serves as a simple surrogate test for the deficit, but the test is also affected by heparin and anemia. Serum von Willebrand factor antigen levels may be normal because the test measures total von Willebrand factor antigen load and is not specific for the very large multimers. In patients with aortic stenosis, the defect has been seen to be corrected within hours of replacement of the aortic valves using bioprostheses. The degree of correction was found to be proportionate to the residual valve gradient.

Congestive heart failure is associated with alterations in a host of autocrine and paracrine signaling systems, many of which are involved in mediating inflammation, including nitric oxide, inflammatory cytokines, chemokines, and cyclooxygenase. The physiologic and clinical significance of these changes is complex and less well understood. The generalized inflammatory response to end-stage heart failure affects the interdependent clotting cascade and can be partially defined by measuring C-reactive protein, albumin, platelet count, and fibrinogen levels.[41]

Iatrogenic coagulopathies are common in patients with terminal heart failure. Patients are often anticoagulated with warfarin (Coumadin) to prevent thromboembolism from atria, ventricles, or prosthetic valve thrombus or dysfunction. The effects of antiaggregation medications including clopidogrel (Plavix) and aspirin are measured using platelet function tests.

To reduce intraoperative bleeding and its attendant morbidity, coagulopathic drugs are discontinued, and the hemodynamics are optimized. The hemodynamic strategy is directed toward normalizing visceral organ responsiveness by reducing visceral organ congestion while maintaining cardiac output and blood pressure. Congestive hepatopathy and its clinical features including jaundice and ascites may respond dramatically to diuretics to reduce CVP. In addition, blood pressure, cardiac output, and venous pressure are optimized using appropriate inotropes and vasodilators in conjunction with fluid removal techniques including diuretics, hemofiltration, peripheral ultrafiltration, and therapeutic paracentesis. Care should be taken to avoid excessive diuresis, which could impair hepatic perfusion by reducing cardiac output and lowering blood pressure.[42] Lietz and Miller[43] showed that a minimally elevated INR was associated with a fourfold increase in the risk of death before hospital discharge.

Intramuscular or oral vitamin K helps to correct abnormal prothrombin times. Intraoperative bleeding has been reduced in general surgical patients with isolated hepatic failure by using preoperative plasmapheresis and preoperatively administering fresh frozen plasma. LVAD recipients may not tolerate the infused fresh frozen plasma volume. Plasmapheresis has had limited success in LVAD recipients. CPB can exacerbate underlying hepatic coagulopathy by inducing platelet dysfunction, fibrinolysis, and hypocalcemia.[44]

Warfarin should be discontinued 4 to 5 days before surgery, and LVAD insertion is planned when the INR normalizes. Heparin is used when necessary when chronic atrial fibrillation or mechanical valve prostheses are present. Antiplatelet drugs such as clopidogrel should be discontinued 4 to 5 days before surgery when 90% of the effect is thought to be gone. Lack of effect can be estimated by using the P2 Y12 accumetrics test. Patients receiving clopidogrel for recently placed stents are at risk for stent thrombosis and should receive heparin before surgery. Given the compromised condition of most VAD recipients, the known hemorrhagic consequences of the operative intervention may be magnified and reflected by increased intraoperative bleeding. Recipients with previous sternotomy and recipients subjected to the increased trauma of more extensive dissections are at increased risk of bleeding.

The large surface area of intravascular devices, with varying degrees of sheer stress, also influences the coagulopathy of recipient patients. The effect of foreign surfaces on coagulation and lytic interaction is precipitated by the protein race for the surface that occurs when foreign surfaces are inserted into the bloodstream. Indiscriminant attachment of proteins can favor fibrinogen, which precipitates an intravascular coagulopathy. Pacifying the surfaces has been proposed as a means of directing this race and its winners. Certain proteins, including albumin, can passively coat surfaces, and this has been used successfully to minimize initiating this cascade. CPB generates its own universe of coagulopathy; insertion of VADs without CPB may be associated with less bleeding (Sun B, personal communication, Ohio State University). Less bleeding has been observed in off-pump coronary artery bypass grafting versus coronary artery bypass grafting with bypass. The liability of not using CPB for VAD insertion is the relative uncertainty of the presence of clots and the intra–left ventricular anatomy and its potential influence on apical cannula position. Often CPB must be used to insert VADs because ancillary procedures to correct other abnormalities in the host heart are necessary.

Normally, CPB requires heparin even in patients with known heparin allergies. Where heparin cannot be used safely, such as documented heparin-induced thrombocytopenia and thrombocytopenia less than 100,000/mm³, bivalirudin can be used instead.[45]

Technical Intraoperative Factors Influencing Bleeding

The anatomic domain required for LVAD implantation is determined by its size. Larger pulsatile VADs are placed below the diaphragm, either preperitoneal or intraperitoneal. Smaller axial flow pumps to date require less dissection but still require division of the diaphragm. Even smaller centrifugal pumps can be entirely contained within the supradiaphragmatic area, often entirely within the pericardium. Left ventricular apical cannulation is now standard for pump access. Late embolic sequelae are less, and flows are generally higher than the flows afforded by left atrial access. Left ventricular mural thrombi occur in one-third of cases of Q wave acute myocardial infarction, 50% of cases of left ventricular aneurysm, and 18% of cases of hearts with dilated cardiomyopathy.[46] Cardioplegic arrest may be required for adequate visualization of the left ventricular cavity to allow total removal of left ventricular thrombus to prevent subsequent systemic embolization or pump aspiration and resultant impaired function, hemolysis, and possible need for replacement.

Minimizing bleeding from apical cannulation sites requires special attention to detail. A good technique is to use a circumferential polytef (Teflon) felt bolster to attach the cannula to the apical ventriculotomy with horizontal mattress sutures. Extra bleeding between the myocardium and the cannula is controlled using large circumferential cerclage sutures. When inserting the cannula into a friable, infarcted ventricle, it is important to achieve hemostasis without overzealous suture tensions, which can fracture the weakened muscle. A large felt cone extended over the surface of the heart and attached to normal myocardium can rectify this problem. In cases where extensive ventricular apical infarction is present, the effective apical cannulation sites can be reconstructed by sandwiching the myocardium between two felt patches in the affected areas. Because left ventricular pressures during VAD support are greatly reduced, apical bleeding is usually controllable.

Treatment of Bleeding Disorders Associated with Left Ventricular Assist Device Insertion

At the present time, no defined proven strategy exists to treat every bleeding diathesis with LVAD insertion. The general condition of patients with terminal heart failure, large foreign surface areas, medications, and more recently the high sheer stress associated with intravascular rotary pumps all combine to create a clinical nonsurgical bleeding puzzle that has been difficult to decipher. The observed syndrome is dynamic. After initial pump insertion, a period of relative hemostasis is followed by a period of increased nonsurgical bleeding. Measurement of specific clotting factors and assays during this period have shown varying degrees of fibrinolysis (F1.2, D-dimers) and coagulation (thrombomodulant) and platelet activation and destruction. There is also degradation of the ligands necessary to bond platelets to the necessary active sites. Large von Willebrand factor multimers have been shown to be reduced rapidly. The absence of this essential platelet ligand is manifested by a bleeding diathesis that persists despite high platelet counts. Diagnostic strategies in the operating room are crudely directed toward using dynamic tests such as the thromboelastogram and the platelet function assay and platelet counts, fibrinogen levels, and INR to guide administration of blood products.

Correction of anemia with blood transfusions often improves platelet function. When the hematocrit is greater than 30%, the red blood cells primarily occupy the center of the vessel, and platelets are displaced peripherally toward the endothelial surface where they are able to be active. Nitric oxide is often used intraoperatively to reduce pulmonary artery pressure. Experimental observations suggest that the effect of nitric oxide on platelets may enhance intraoperative bleeding[47]; however, clinical documentation does not currently exist.

Platelet dysfunction can be treated with desmopressin acetate (DDAVP); which appears to act by increasing the release of large von Willebrand factor multimers from endothelial storage sites. Avoiding a prolonged postbypass period and hypothermia may optimize hepatic function and facilitate achieving the appropriate balance between the thrombotic and lytic systems. Use of factor VII has been associated with excess thrombus formation but may be advantageous in lower doses.[48]

Aminocaproic acid has been shown to reduce intraoperative bleeding in patients undergoing general cardiac surgery. It is probably beneficial in LVAD patients, but studies are lacking. Aprotinin has been shown to reduce intraoperative bleeding in LVAD patients; however, a small increase in renal failure was seen with its use, and the drug is no longer available in the United States.

The aortic return conduit is most often anastomosed to the ascending aorta; this is the favored position because it creates less prothrombotic static aortic root flow. Grafts are becoming less pervious to blood. Some grafts are prepared with sealants such as heated albumin solutions or organic or synthetic surgical glues. Synthetic sealants may be advantageous.[49] The aortic anastomosis is created by excising a portion of the aorta to accommodate the enlarging influence of the graft diameter, and this may reduce the potential for the aorta to dissect by minimizing abnormal aortic wall stresses.

Covering the Ventricular Assist Device with Antifibrotic Acellular Matrix Material

Sternal re-entry after VAD implantation is frequently needed, most commonly for subsequent heart transplantation, and it is challenging because there is usually development of dense adhesion around the heart and the device. Adhesions extend the time for dissection of the recipient heart with possibly prolonging ischemic time of the donor heart and increase the risk of post-transplant bleeding.[50] Various materials have been tried to reduce the adhesion after cardiac surgery. The most commonly used material may be an expanded polytetrafluoroethylene membrane. This pericardial substitute has been reported to be safe and effective in reducing the risk of sternal re-entry for various types of cardiac reoperations, including operations after VAD implantation.[51] More recently with advances in tissue engineering, elements of the extracellular matrix (ECM) have gained increasing attention as crucial elements in maintaining the characteristics of three-dimensional cardiac cell aggregates.[52] ECM is composed primarily of collagen and is found in all humans and animals. Previously regarded as merely a scaffold for developing tissue, ECM plays an important role in providing essential signals to influence major intracellular pathways such as proliferation, differentiation, and cell metabolism. The ECM has been studied and used in regenerative medicine to replace and reconstruct native tissue including heart and pericardium. The synthetic ECM technology became applicable more recently to reconstruct a pericardium through a commercially available product, CorMatrix (CorMatrix Cardiovascular, Inc).

CorMatrix is made from sterilized and decellularized porcine small intestinal submucosa leaving the complex ECM intact. When used to reconstruct a pericardium, it allows cells to infiltrate the ECM to remodel and form a new pericardial layer. This product has gained attention and increasingly has been used in clinical practice. It has been used for pericardial reconstruction after VAD implantation with satisfactory antifibrotic properties at subsequent VAD explantation and heart transplantation (Naka Y, personal communication, Columbia University). The edge of the CoreMatrix is placed in contact with the edge of opened pericardium with 4-0 polypropylene running suture to cover the entire heart and inflow and outflow conduit. A drain is placed underneath the membrane, and the device is left uncovered in place in the preperitoneal space.

LEFT VENTRICULAR ASSIST DEVICE USE WITH COMPLICATIONS OF ACUTE MYOCARDIAL INFARCTION

Unusual circumstances may exist in the setting of an acute myocardial infarction and add to the complexity of LVAD implantation, especially in cases where long-term devices are used in anticipation of the need for long-term support. One immediate factor is that the size of the heart in these cases is smaller, and the ventricular chamber dimensions are much smaller than with chronic heart failure. This factor dictates that precise positioning of the LVAD is crucial to avoid encroachment of the inflow cannula tip by the septal or left ventricular lateral wall.

The first challenge was discussed previously in relation to the determination of the extent of right ventricular involvement and the degree of impairment of its function. In many cases of left main or left anterior descending artery infarction, it is common to see areas of the right ventricle affected by the extent of septal infarction or edema. For that reason, the surgeon must be prepared to use at least temporary right ventricular support. In cases of right coronary occlusion and infarction, an RVAD alone may suffice. However, the presence of heart block secondary to septal infarction is often a critical problem that can result in severe overpumping of blood to the left ventricle in the setting of bradycardia. In this situation when pacing is not used, severe and acute pulmonary edema may occur with an RVAD pumping at full capacity, while the left ventricle beats at a rate of only 40 beats/min. It is absolutely essential to place reliable pacing wires on the ventricle and overpace the left ventricle at a rate of at least 100 beats/min so that the left ventricle can accommodate the blood being pumped by the RVAD. Should the RVAD become needed on a long-term basis, a permanent pacer should always be placed, and the backup rate should be immediately set to at least 100 beats/min to prevent pulmonary edema.

An acute myocardial infarction may also be associated with acute inflammatory changes and hemorrhagic deterioration of the endocardial walls. In these cases, the surgeon should anticipate the presence of fragile and abundant thrombus within the left ventricular chamber, especially near the apex. This thrombus needs to be meticulously cleaned before inserting the inflow cannula of the LVAD. Often the walls of the left ventricle are edematous and fragile owing to the infarction, and care has to be taken in placing the apical sutures for the inflow cannula so as not to tear the muscle. Many surgeons use strips of felt to buttress the tissue and strengthen the sutures. The reality is that ventricular rupture is rarely, if ever, seen with an LVAD because the chamber pressures are so effectively reduced that the wall tension is low.

An infrequent scenario for LVAD use is in the case of ventricular septal rupture. The most important action in these cases is to achieve complete repair of the ventricular septal defect to prevent severe desaturation from shunting of right ventricular blood into the LVAD. Very little information exists in the literature regarding this situation,[53] but limited reports show successful achievement of transplantation after bridging in this scenario. Associated right ventricular failure is common in this condition, and the use of a biventricular VAD may be warranted.

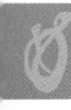

1. Adamson RM, Dembitsky WP, Baradarian S, et al. Aortic valve closure associated with HeartMate LVAD support: technical considerations and long-term results. *J Heart Lung Transplant*. 2011;30:576–582.

2. Lin G, Nishimura RA, Connolly HM, et al. Severe symptomatic tricuspid valve regurgitation due to permanent pacemaker or implantable cardioverter-defibrillator leads. *J Am Coll Cardiol*. 2005;45:1672–1675.

3. Kwak JJ, Kim YJ, Kim MK, et al. Development of tricuspid regurgitation late after left-sided valve surgery: a single-center experience with long-term echocardiographic examination. *Am Heart J*. 2008;155:732–737.

4. Saeed D, Shalli S, Kidambi T, et al. Tricuspid valve repair at the time of left ventricular assist device implantation: is it warranted? *J Heart Lung Transplant* 2011;30:530–535.

5. McCarthy PM, Bhudia SK, Rajeswaran J, et al. Tricuspid valve repair: durability and risk factors for failure. *J Thorac Cardiovasc Surg*. 2004;127:674–685.

6. Adamson R, Dembitsky W, Baradarian S, et al. *Tricuspid valve replacement coincident with HeartMate II LVAD insertion*. ASAIO presentation, Baltimore, 2010.

7. Barbone A, Rao V, Oz MC, et al. LVAD support in patients with bioprosthetic valves. *J Thorac Surg*. 2002;74:232–234.

8. Krishan K, Pinney S, Anyanwu AC. Successful fuse of continuous flow ventricular assist device in a patient with mechanical mitral and aortic valve prosthesis without replacement or exclusion of valves. *Interact Cardiovasc Thorac Surg*. 2010;10:325–327.

9. Greegoric I, Loyalka P, Salem A. HeartMate II LVAD support in patients with mechanical mitral valves (abstract). *ASAIO J*. 2010;56:111.

10. May-Newman K, Hillen B, Dembitsky W. Effect of left ventricular assist device outflow conduit anastomosis location on flow patterns in the native aorta. *ASAIO J*. 2006;52:132–139.

11. Schoen FJ. Evolving concepts of cardiac valve dynamics: the continuum of development, functional structure, pathobiology, and tissue engineering. *Circulation*. 2008;118:1864–1880.

12. Matthews JC, Aaronson KD, Jain R, et al. Aortic insufficiency—trends over time in LVAD support patient. *J Heart Lung Transplant*. 2009;28:S306.

13. Pak SW, Uriel N, Takayama H, et al. Prevalence of de novo aortic insufficiency during long-term support with left ventricular assist devices. *J Heart Lung Transplant*. 2010;29:1172–1176.

14. Adamson RM, Dembitsky WP, Baradarian S, et al. Aortic valve closure associated with HeartMate LVAD support: technical considerations and long-term results. *J Heart Lung Transplant*. 2011;30:576–582.

15. Park SJ, Liao KK, Segurola R, et al. Management of aortic insufficiency in patients with left ventricular assist devices: a simple coaptation stitch method (Park's stitch). *J Thorac Cardiovasc Surg*. 2004;127:264–266.

16. Kapur NK, Conte JV, Resar JR. Percutaneous closure of patient foramen ovale for refractory hypoxemia after HeartMate II left ventricular assist device placement. *J Invasive Cardiol*. 2007;19:E268–E270.

17. Pal JD, Klodell CT, John R, et al. Low operative mortality with implantation of a continuous-flow left ventricular assist device and impact of concurrent cardiac procedures. *Circulation*. 2009;120(suppl 1):S215–S219.

18. Slaughter MS, Pagani FD, Rogers JG, et al. Clinical management of continuous-flow left ventricular assist devices in advanced heart failure. *J Heart Lung Transplant*. 2010;29(suppl 4):S1–S39.

19. Eda K. Optimal pulse pressure of pulmonary circulation under biventricular assist after cardiogenic shock. *Ann Thorac Cardiovasc Surg*. 1999;5:365–369.

20. Klima UP, Lee MY, Guerrero JL, et al. Determinants of maximal right ventricular function: role of septal shift. *J Thorac Cardiovasc Surg*. 2002;123:72–80.

21. Moon MR, Castro LJ, DeAnda A, et al. Right ventricular dynamics during left ventricular assistance in closed-chest dogs. *Ann Thorac Surg*. 1993;56:54–66.

22. Santamore WP, Gray Jr LA. Left ventricular contributions to right ventricular systolic function during LVAD support. *Ann Thorac Surg*. 1996;61:350–356.

23. Farrar DJ, Chow E, Compton PG, et al. Effects of acute right ventricular ischemia on ventricular interactions during prosthetic left ventricular support. *J Thorac Cardiovasc Surg*. 1991;102:588–595.

24. Daly RC, Chandrasekaran K, Cavarocchi NC, et al. Ischemia of the interventricular septum: a mechanism of right ventricular failure during mechanical left ventricular assist. *J Thorac Cardiovasc Surg*. 1992;103:1186–1191.

25. Drakos SG, Janicki L, Horne BD, et al. Risk factors predictive of right ventricular failure after left ventricular assist device implantation. *Am J Cardiol*. 2010;105:1030–1035.

26. Jaski BE, Branch KR, Adamson R, et al. Exercise hemodynamics during long-term implantation of a left ventricular assist device in patients awaiting heart transplantation. *J Am Coll Cardiol*. 1993;22:1574–1580.

27. Kucuker SA, Stetson SJ, Becker KA, et al. Evidence of improved right ventricular structure after LVAD support in patients with end-stage cardiomyopathy. *J Heart Lung Transplant*. 2004;23:28–35.

28. Chen PS, Moser KM, Dembitsky WP, et al. Epicardial activation and repolarization patterns in patients with right ventricular hypertrophy. *Circulation*. 1991;83:104–118.

29. Van Meter Jr CH. Right heart failure: best treated by avoidance. *Ann Thorac Surg*. 2001;71(suppl 3):S220–S222.

30. Patel ND, Weiss ES, Schaffer J, et al. Right heart dysfunction after left ventricular assist device implantation: a comparison of the pulsatile HeartMate I and axial-flow HeartMate II devices. *Ann Thorac Surg*. 2008;86:832–840.

31. Argenziano M, Choudhri AF, Oz MC, et al. A prospective randomized trial of arginine vasopressin in the treatment of vasodilatory shock after left ventricular assist device placement. *Circulation*. 1997;96(9 suppl):II–286–II–290.

32. Loebe M, Potapov E, Sodian R, et al. A safe and simple method of preserving right ventricular function during implantation of a left ventricular assist device. *J Thorac Cardiovasc Surg*. 2001;122:1043.

33. Giallourakis CC, Rosenberg PM, Friedman LS. The liver in heart failure. *Clin Liver Dis*. 2002;6:947.

34. Jafri SM. Hypercoagulability in heart failure. *Semin Thromb Hemost*. 1997;23:543.

35. Pratt D, Kaplan M. Evaluation of the liver: laboratory tests. In: Schiff E, Sorrell M, Maddrey W, eds. *Schiff's Diseases of the Liver*. 8th ed. Philadelphia: Lippincott Williams & Wilkins; 1999:205.

36. Matthews JC, Pagani FD, Haft JW, et al. Model for end-stage liver disease score predicts left ventricular assist device operative transfusion requirements, morbidity, and mortality. *Circulation*. 2010;121:214–220.

37. Qamar AA, Grace ND, Groszmann RJ, et al. Incidence, prevalence, and clinical significance of abnormal hematologic indices in compensated cirrhosis. *Clin Gastroenterol Hepatol*. 2009;7:689.

38. Suman A, Barnes DS, Zein NN, et al. Predicting outcome after cardiac surgery in patients with cirrhosis: a comparison of Child-Pugh and MELD scores. *Clin Gastroenterol Hepatol*. 2004;2:719.

39. Weigert AL, Schafer AI. Uremic bleeding: pathogenesis and therapy. *Am J Med Sci*. 1998;316:94.

40. Crow S, Milano C, Joyce L, et al. Comparative analysis of von Willebrand factor profiles in pulsatile and continuous left ventricular assist device recipients. *ASAIO J*. 2010;56:441–445.

41. Levi M, van der Poll T. Inflammation and coagulation. *Crit Care Med*. 2010;38(suppl 2):S26–S34.

42. Kisloff B, Schaffer G. Fulminant hepatic failure secondary to congestive heart failure. *Am J Dig Dis*. 1976;21:895.

43. Lietz K, Miller LW. Patient selection for left ventricular assist devices. *Curr Opin Cardiol*. 2009;24:246–251.

44. Pollard RJ, Sidi A, Gibby GL. Aortic stenosis with end-stage liver disease: prioritizing surgical and anesthetic therapies. *J Clin Anesth*. 1998;10:253.

45. Mann MJ, Tseng E, Ratcliffe M, et al. Use of bivalirudin, a direct thrombin inhibitor, and its reversal with modified ultrafiltration during heart transplantation in a patient with heparin-induced thrombocytopenia. *J Heart Lung Transplant*. 2005;24:222–225.

46. Cregler LL. Antithrombotic therapy in left ventricular thrombosis and systemic embolism. *Am Heart J*. 1992;123(4 Pt 2):1110–1114.

47. Roberts W, Michno A, Aburima A, et al. Nitric oxide inhibits von Willebrand factor-mediated platelet adhesion and spreading through regulation of integrin alpha(IIb)beta(3) and myosin light chain. *J Thromb Haemost*. 2009;7:2106–2115.

48. Bruckner BA, DiBardino DJ, Ning Q, et al. High incidence of thromboembolic events in left ventricular assist device patients treated with recombinant activated factor VII. *J Heart Lung Transplant*. 2009;28:785–790.

49. Elefteriades JA. How I do it: utilization of high-pressure sealants in aortic reconstruction. *J Cardiothorac Surg*. 2009;4:27.

50. Oz MC, Levin HR, Rose EA. Technique for removal of left ventricular assist devices. *Ann Thorac Surg*. 1994;58:257–258.

51. Leprince P, Rahmati M, Bonnet N, et al. Expanded polytetrafluoroethylene membranes to wrap surfaces of circulatory support devices in patients undergoing bridge to heart transplantation. *Eur J Cardiothorac Surg*. 2001;19:302–306.

52. Akhyari P, Kamiya H, Haverich A, et al. Myocardial tissue engineering: the extracellular matrix. *Eur J Cardiothorac Surg*. 2008;34:229–241.

53. Faber C, McCarthy PM, Smedira NG, et al. Left ventricular assist device for patients with postinfarction ventricular septal defect. *J Thorac Cardiovasc Surg*. 2002;124:400–401.

Adverse Events and Complications of Mechanical Circulatory Support

Robert L. Kormos and William L. Holman

Ventricular assist devices (VADs) provide effective treatment for end-stage heart failure, used as a bridge to transplantation,[1-3] bridge to recovery,[4-9] or destination therapy.[10-14] With VAD support, patients have enhanced cardiac function, which is associated with pretransplant and posttransplant survival rates equal to patients without the need for VAD support and significant improvements in their quality of life and functional status.[1-3,15-23] Continued advances in VAD technology and increasing clinical experience with VADs have resulted in improved patient outcomes over time.[14,24-28] Nevertheless, VAD support is still associated with serious complications or adverse events, which, although reduced in frequency, can limit treatment efficacy and safety.

Although the risk of developing adverse events is clinically well recognized, the frequency and timing of important adverse events are variably characterized in the literature. Historically, most studies reported simple, overall percentages of patients who experienced the most common adverse events, including bleeding, infection, neurologic events such as stroke, and device malfunction.[2,20,29-31] These studies did not adjust for duration of VAD support or consider whether rates varied over time during the period of support. Other studies adjusted for duration of support but provided little evidence of how adverse event incidence rates change over time.[1,10,12,14,22,32,33] The few reports that have rigorously examined the timing of adverse event onset focused on only one or two of the most prominent types of adverse events rather than considering the full spectrum of these events.[1,34-38] Adverse events occur at rates that can be influenced by preoperative status of end-organ function; patient age; urgency of VAD implant; and the type of VAD, in particular, whether a biventricular VAD or single left ventricular assist device (LVAD) is used. It has also been a consistent finding that in every decade since the 1980s there has been a significant reduction in the overall incidence of adverse events that parallels not only the advances in technology but also the experience of the surgical team and timing of implant strategies adopted by the center.

The incidence of adverse events may be characterized by the timing of occurrence: events occurring within the first 60 days and events occurring after 60 days, most commonly after discharge from the hospital. Adverse events occurring early after implantation are related primarily to the preoperative condition of the patient and often reflect the risks associated with preoperative morbidity or laboratory abnormalities or the fact that major cardiovascular surgery is being performed in a patient with decompensated congestive heart failure, whereas the more chronically occurring events result from device design issues or management strategies.

Most importantly, the results from historical studies are difficult to compare because of the lack of standard definitions for specific adverse events. To ensure the potential generalizability of findings, clinical investigators, the device industry, and the U.S. Food and Drug Administration (FDA) have employed the standardized definitions of adverse events from INTERMACS (Interagency Registry for Mechanically Assisted Circulatory Support) (see Appendix 13-1). INTERMACS was established in 2005 as a joint effort of the National Heart, Lung and Blood Institute; the FDA; the Centers for Medicare and Medicaid Services; and the mechanical circulatory support (MCS) device community, which includes industry representatives, cardiac surgeons, cardiologists, nurse coordinators, and scientists.[39]

The first attempt at standardized definitions came with the advent of the Mechanical Circulatory Support Registry that was started by the International Society for Heart and Lung Transplantation.[40] Another source for definitions came from within the device industry because several VAD manufacturers had developed adverse event definitions for their device trials conducted as a condition for premarket approval. Although similar, these definitions were characterized by minor differences often designed to favor a particular device. The FDA approved these definitions based on the ability of a given manufacturer to argue their relevance and completeness for detecting all important events. Specific adverse events have arbitrary definitions, such as bleeding episodes or the number of units transfused to define a bleeding adverse event. Taking these inconsistencies into account, the Adverse Event Subcommittee for INTERMACS began a series of meetings with the MCS device industry, the FDA, and clinicians to standardize iteratively a set of adverse event definitions that could be used across the spectrum of MCS devices. Standard definitions for common device-related adverse events were established, which should simplify future clinical trials, provide standardization for future premarket device approval studies and postmarket surveillance studies, and facilitate the establishment of benchmarks for best site practices with current devices.[41] In addition, one goal of standardization of adverse events is to be able to perform direct side-by-side comparisons of devices and incidence of specific complications (e.g., stroke).

CLINICAL ADVERSE EVENTS IN THE ACUTE POSTIMPLANTATION PERIOD

Genovese and colleagues[42] reported the cumulative incidence rates for the occurrence of the 14 major categories of adverse event and the cumulative incidence of the specific types of adverse events included within the 14 categories. The estimates of the probability of occurrence of each adverse event during the 60-day period after VAD implant, controlling for the competing risks of death, transplant, or recovery or wean, are shown in Table 13-1. Table 13-1 shows that most patients have at least one adverse event in the first 60 days after implantation, with a cumulative incidence rate of 89% by that time point. The most common types of events are bleeding and infection (incidence rates >40%), followed by arrhythmias, tamponade, neurologic events, respiratory events, and reoperations (rates 22% to 33%). Other events are less common.

The cumulative incidence for the onset of any adverse event and for the competing risks of death, transplant, and recovery or wean in the sample are shown in Figure 13-1. Figure 13-1 shows a high incidence of adverse events immediately after VAD implantation, with a leveling off after approximately 30 days. The rate of death and transplant show a steady increase during this early period.

The cumulative incidence for the major categories of adverse events is shown in Figure 13-2; the categories are cardiac/vascular, other organ systems, and other types of adverse events. Many adverse events, such as arrhythmias, tamponade, right ventricular failure, renal and hepatic events, and bleeding, show a high frequency of initial onset early after VAD implantation, and then few, if any, new events occur during the remainder of the first 60 days. In contrast, adverse events such as neurologic events, infection, reoperations, and device malfunction show onsets that are more gradual; events within these categories continued to occur throughout the 60-day period.

The specific rates for each adverse event and their incremental risks are different for each type of early adverse event at 10, 20, and 30 days, as is shown in Table 13-2. Patients have a 24.1% chance of having an arrhythmia by 5 days after VAD implantation. Between 5 days and 10 days, the incremental risk is 4.6% yielding a total, cumulative incidence of arrhythmias at 10 days of 28.7%. Figures 13-1, 13-2 and Table 13-3 show that the greatest incidence of many adverse events occurs in the first 5 to 10 days after VAD implantation, with progressively smaller incremental risk thereafter. In addition, incremental risks of neurologic events and device malfunction steadily continue to increase during the entire period.

The most frequent individual adverse events after VAD implantation are bleeding (in particular, mediastinal or pocket bleeds), major infections, and arrhythmias requiring defibrillation or cardioversion intervention. Beyond cumulative incidence rates, one sees different patterns of timing of

TABLE 13-1	Patient Risk of Clinically Significant Adverse Events during the First 60 Days after Ventricular Assist Device Implantation: Cumulative Incidence at End of Time Period		
		Actuarial Event Rate	
Event Type	No. Patients with Event	Cumulative Incidence*	95% Confidence Interval
Any adverse event	192	88.9	83.9, 92.4
Cardiac/Vascular			
Arrhythmia, any	78	36.1	29.5, 42.5
Ventricular	40	18.5	13.7, 24.0
Atrial	46	21.3	16.1, 27.0
Tamponade	59	27.3	21.6, 33.2
RV failure	25	11.6	7.8, 16.2
Thromboembolism (non-CNS)	18	8.3	5.1, 12.5
Hemolysis	6	2.9	1.1, 5.6
Other Organ Systems			
Respiratory, any	54	25.0	19.4, 30.9
Tracheostomy	30	13.9	9.7, 18.8
Reintubation	27	12.5	8.5, 17.3
Neurologic	50	23.2	17.8, 29.0
Infarct or hemorrhagic CVA	31	14.4	10.1, 19.4
TIA	24	11.2	7.4, 15.8
Renal	33	15.3	10.8, 20.4
Hepatic	20	9.2	5.9, 13.6
Gastrointestinal	1	0.5	0.0, 2.4
Other			
Bleeding, any	105	48.6	42.0, 55.1
Coagulopathy	38	17.6	12.9, 23.0
Mediastinum or pocket	59	27.3	21.6, 33.4
Thorax	20	9.2	5.9, 13.6
Gastrointestinal	13	6.0	3.4, 9.7
Infection, any	92	42.6	35.9, 49.1
Driveline	35	16.2	11.6, 21.4
Bloodstream	40	18.5	13.7, 24.0
Pulmonary	43	19.9	14.9, 25.5
Mediastinum or pocket	13	6.0	3.4, 9.7
Reoperation, any	71	32.9	26.7, 39.2
Bleeding	51	23.6	18.1, 29.4
Infection	12	5.6	3.0, 9.2
Wound dehiscence	7	3.2	1.4, 6.2
Wound débridement	15	6.9	4.1, 10.8
Device malfunction	20	9.2	5.9, 13.6

*Adjusted for the competing hazards of transplant, death, or recovery/wean.
CNS, central nervous system; CVA, cerebrovascular accident; RV, right ventricular; TIA, transient ischemic attack.

onset of adverse events, with some (i.e., arrhythmias, tamponade, bleeding, renal events, hepatic events) occurring frequently in the first several days after VAD implantation. The rates of onset then slow dramatically so that few, if any, new events occur beyond 2 weeks after implantation. In contrast, adverse events such as neurologic events, infection, reoperations, and device malfunction have patterns of more gradual onset; events within these categories continued to occur throughout the 60-day period. These findings are consistent with other reports that these types of adverse events are of ongoing, long-term concern for VAD recipients[35,37,38] and represent challenges for extended-term use of these devices, particularly as destination therapy.

A review of larger cohorts from INTERMACS[43] shows that the most common major adverse events occurring within the first year of implant (measured in events per 100 patient-months)

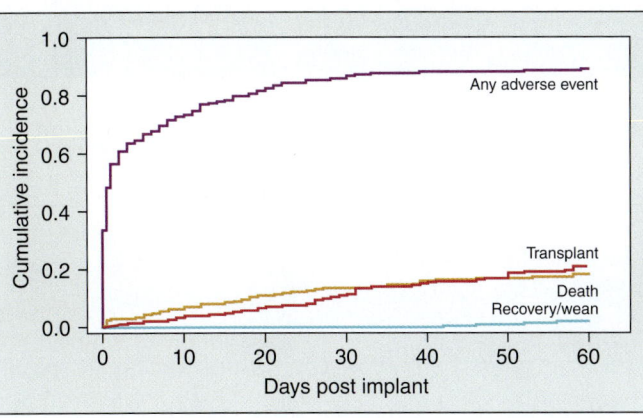

FIGURE 13-1 Cumulative incidence of any adverse event during the first 60 days after ventricular assist device (VAD) implant, controlling for competing risks of transplant, death, and recovery/wean.

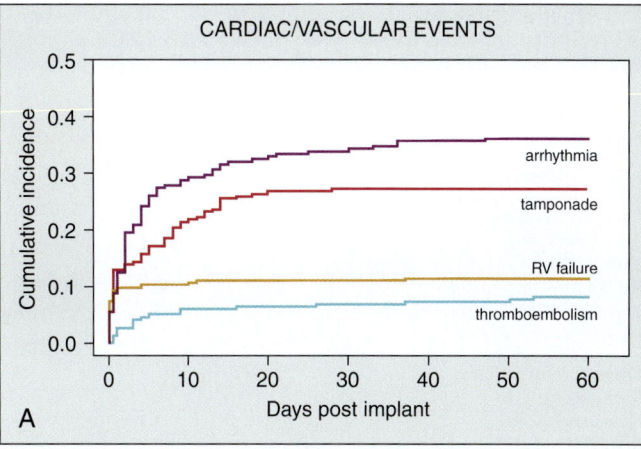

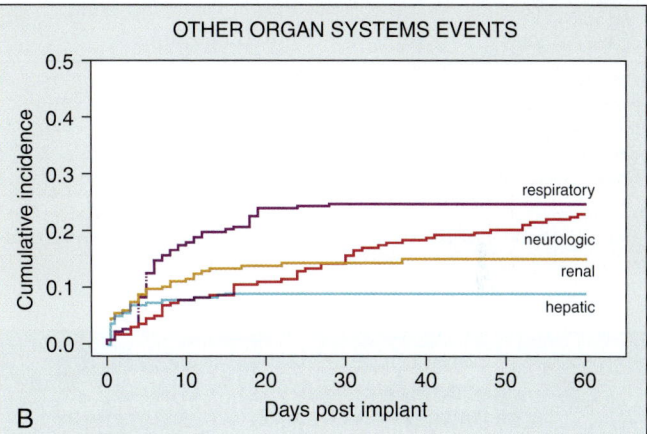

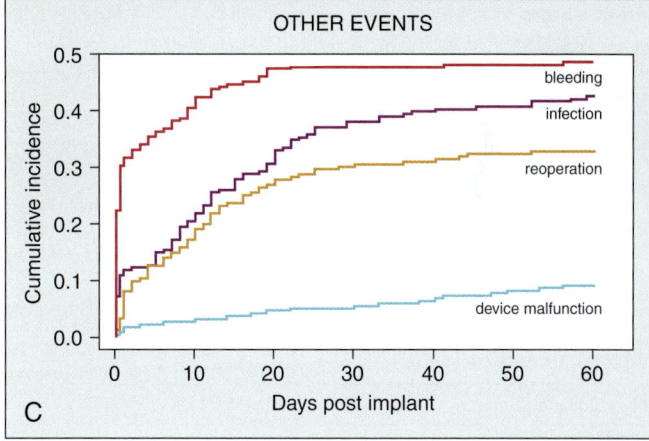

FIGURE 13-2 Cumulative incidence of major categories of adverse events during the first 60 days after ventricular assist device (VAD) implant. **A,** Cardiovascular and vascular events. **B,** Other organ system events. **C,** Other events.

include infection (17.46), bleeding (16.52), and cardiac arrhythmias (7.68) (see Table 13-3). Other events seen less frequently in decreasing order include respiratory failure (4.50), neurologic dysfunction (2.87), renal dysfunction (2.48), and hypertension (2.31). These data also show that for primary LVAD recipients the rates of adverse events are significantly less for patients receiving newer second-generation rotary blood pumps as opposed to the first-generation pulsatile systems (Table 13-4). Rates for infection, hepatic dysfunction, and neurologic dysfunction are more than twice as high with the pulsatile pumps compared with rotary pumps, whereas hypertension occurs at a rate six times higher in patients with a pulsatile pump.

Perioperative respiratory failure requiring reintubation or tracheostomy is associated with a significant decrease in late survival. Respiratory failure occurs in one-fourth of patients and carries a high risk of mortality with only 35% surviving at 1 year (compared with 65% of patients without respiratory failure). These respiratory adverse events may be associated with episodes of decreased tissue oxygenation, increased right ventricular afterload, risks of prolonged mechanical ventilation, and decreased mobility that contributes to deconditioning, all of which are likely to have an impact on survival.

Several early adverse events have an influence on subsequent survival at 1 year while on the VAD as shown in Table 13-5.[44] The adverse events that correlate most with mortality are renal and respiratory complications, bleeding, and the need for reoperations while on the VAD. Of these, renal adverse events are the most influential on survival by multivariable analyses, whereas neurologic events and the occurrence of right ventricular failure do not exert an effect on long-term morality.

Bleeding is one of the most common adverse events after VAD implantation,[42,45–47] and the associated transfusions have been shown to increase risk of infection, allosensitization, and acute lung injury.[48,49] Early nonfatal bleeding has a substantial impact on late-term mortality as well. Although patients with major bleeding events are often successfully managed with transfusions or reoperations or both, their 1-year survival rate of 48% is significantly poorer than the 71% survival rate in patients without bleeding events. Bleeding events may require multiple transfusions and lead to acute lung injury, which may compromise right ventricular function, increase the risk of end-organ ischemia, and require reoperations to ensure hemostasis.

Reoperations also confer an increased risk of mortality and include procedures for bleeding events and severe infections requiring débridement or flaps or both, and their association with decreased late survival may represent the impact of severe bleeding events and infections. Wound dehiscence

may be indicative of significant, chronic infections that are associated with malnutrition because a prealbumin less than 15 mg/dL at 2 weeks after VAD implantation is highly correlated with death pre-discharge, a prolonged inflammatory response, deconditioning, and risk of sepsis, all which have long-term consequences on patient outcomes.[50,51]

Acute renal failure that occurs early in VAD support is associated with a significantly decreased survival rate at 1 year. Chronic heart failure may result in renal dysfunction via persistently elevated filling pressures, marginal cardiac output, and an adverse neurohormonal milieu.[52,53] Equally common is primary underlying renal disease secondary to

TABLE 13-2 Patient Risk of Clinically Significant Adverse Events at Specific Time Points during the First 60 Days after Ventricular Assist Device Implantation

Event Type	Actuarial Event Rate (Cumulative Incidence) at 5 Days	Increment to Incidence by*			
		10 Days	20 Days	30 Days	60 Days
Any adverse event	64.4	8.3	8.8	4.1	3.3
Cardiac/Vascular					
Arrhythmia, any	24.1	4.6	3.7	1.4	2.3
Tamponade	15.7	5.6	5.1	0.4	0.5
RV failure	10.2	0.0	0.9	0.0	0.5
Thromboembolism (non-CNS)	5.6	0.4	0.5	0.4	1.4
Hemolysis	1.4	0.5	0.0	0.5	0.5
Other Organ Systems					
Respiratory	8.8	8.8	6.5	0.9	0.0
Neurologic	3.7	4.2	3.2	3.3	8.8
Renal	8.3	2.8	2.8	0.4	1.0
Hepatic	6.9	1.0	1.3	0.0	0.0
Gastrointestinal	0.0	0.0	0.0	0.5	0.0
Other					
Bleeding	35.2	5.1	6.9	0.5	0.9
Infection	12.5	7.9	10.2	7.4	4.6
Reoperation	12.5	4.6	9.7	3.4	2.8
Device malfunction	2.3	0.5	1.8	0.5	4.1

*Each incremental value indicates the increased risk accrued since the previous period. The increase in risk of any adverse event by 10 days was 8.3 beyond the risk of 64.4 (i.e., cumulative incidence) at 5 days. The increase by 20 days was 8.8 over the total risk (cumulative incidence) at 10 days.
CNS, central nervous RV, right ventricular.

TABLE 13-3 Adverse Events Rates (Events/100 Patient-Months) in First 12 Months after Implantation for 1092 Primary Left Ventricular Assist Devices*

Adverse Event	Events	Rate
Device malfunction	113	1.98
Bleeding	944	16.52
Cardiac/vascular		
Right heart failure	108	1.89
MI	4	0.07
Cardiac arrhythmia	439	7.68
Pericardial drainage	86	1.50
Hypertension†	132	2.31
Arterial non-CNS thrombosis	20	0.35
Venous thrombotic event	83	1.45
Hemolysis	31	0.54
Infection	998	17.46
Neurologic dysfunction	164	2.87
Renal dysfunction	142	2.48
Hepatic dysfunction	52	0.91
Respiratory failure	257	4.50
Wound dehiscence	27	0.47
Psychiatric episode	112	1.96
Total burden	3712	64.96

*INTERMACS (Interagency Registry for Mechanically Assisted Circulatory Support), June 2006–March 2009. Unadjudicated data.
†With current reporting, identification of hypertension with continuous flow pumps is unreliable.
CNS, central nervous system; MI, myocardial infarction.

diabetes, hypertension, or other causes. Ventricular support restores end-organ perfusion, improves the neurohormonal milieu, and allows for more effective volume removal, all of which have potentially salutary effects on renal function.[54–57] However, a small proportion of patients still develop renal failure while on VAD support. The development of renal failure after VAD implantation is particularly ominous because previous reports have shown a 6-month mortality of 71% in such patients.[58–60] The prognosis for late-term survival is poor among patients who develop renal failure and survive the first 60 days. Only 50% of such patients are alive at 6 months, and 30% are alive at 12 months.

The overriding impact of early renal events warrants further investigation into the mechanisms behind the development of acute renal failure after implantation to identify clinical targets to modify in daily practice. Previous reports have suggested that the development of renal failure may be associated with a high-risk presentation,[61] where the insult to the renal system from prolonged periods of cardiogenic shock and typical use of high-dose or multiple vasopressors cannot be ameliorated by VAD support. Although significant right ventricular failure after LVAD implantation is one of the primary causes of early post-LVAD renal dysfunction, others have suggested that renal failure after VAD support is the result of pre-existing diffuse intrarenal vascular changes owing to primary disease vasculopathy,[61] which limits renal reserve and contributes to increased mortality.

Further examination of the INTERMACS data (Table 13-6) confirms that major adverse events occur most commonly within the first 3 months after implantation. Within the first 3 months after device implantation, the most common adverse events were bleeding and infection. These two events occurred more frequently in the biventricular VAD group likely reflecting the consequences of patients being more critically ill and requiring a more extensive procedure. In particular, bleeding is seen three times more frequently primarily because of the associated coagulopathy that often accompanies pre-existing right ventricular failure. Many patients have been receiving one or multiple antiplatelet medications and warfarin, which increase the risk of bleeding, as does reoperation. High venous pressure also increases the risk of bleeding. Even in the LVAD group, bleeding and infectious events occur with the highest frequency reflecting the critically ill nature of VAD recipients. Most pulsatile VADs were implanted in very critically ill patients as shown by the fact that 80% of patients were in INTERMACS profile 1 or 2.

TABLE 13-4 Adverse Event Rates (Events/100 Patient-Months) in the First 12 Months after Implantation of Primary Left Ventricular Assist Devices for 954 Bridge to Transplant and Bridge to Candidacy Patients*

Adverse Event	Pulsatile (n = 406)		Continuous (n = 548)		Pulsatile/Continuous	
	Events	Rate	Events	Rate	Ratio	P Value
Device malfunction	45	2.95	17	0.82	3.60	< .0001
Bleeding	369	24.22	360	17.41	1.39	< .0001
Cardiac/vascular						
Right heart failure	48	3.15	46	2.23	1.41	.05
MI	2	0.13	2	0.10	1.30	.37
Cardiac arrhythmia	154	10.11	218	10.54	0.96	.65
Pericardial drainage	44	2.89	30	1.45	1.99	.003
Hypertension†	75	4.92	17	0.82	6.00	< .0001
Arterial non-CNS thrombosis	7	0.46	6	0.29	1.59	.21
Venous thrombotic event	38	2.49	32	1.55	1.61	.03
Hemolysis	11	0.72	12	0.58	1.24	.29
Infection	431	28.29	244	11.80	2.40	< .0001
Neurologic dysfunction	66	4.33	40	1.93	2.24	< .0001
Renal dysfunction	63	4.14	45	2.18	1.90	.0007
Hepatic dysfunction	24	1.58	14	0.68	2.32	.009
Respiratory failure	121	7.94	89	4.31	1.84	< .0001
Wound dehiscence	8	0.53	9	0.44	1.20	.34
Psychiatric episode	43	2.82	38	1.84	1.53	.03
Total burden	1549	101.69	1219	58.96	1.72	< .0001

*INTERMACS (Interagency Registry for Mechanically Assisted Circulatory Support), June 2006–March 2009.
†With current reporting, identification of hypertension with continuous flow pumps is unreliable.
CNS, central nervous system; MI, myocardial infarction.

TABLE 13-5 Actuarial Survival at 12 Months (by Kaplan-Meier) Stratified by the Presence or Absence of Early Nonfatal Adverse Events (AEs)

Adverse Event	Percentage Surviving on Device		Test of Significance*
	≥1 AEs	No AE	
Renal	32.0%	65.1%	$\chi^2 = 15.464$ $P < .001$
Respiratory	35.3%	68.7%	$\chi^2 = 8.623$ $P = .003$
Bleeding	48.3%	70.9%	$\chi^2 = 4.945$ $P = .026$
Reoperation	47.9%	67.7%	$\chi^2 = 4.343$ $P = .037$
Right ventricular failure	43.0%	66.7%	$\chi^2 = 3.714$ $P = .054$
Infection	53.9%	65.2%	$\chi^2 = 2.717$ $P = .099$
Neurologic event	57.3%	60.6%	$\chi^2 = 1.026$ $P = .311$
Tamponade	58.0%	61.2%	$\chi^2 = .001$ $P = .980$
Cardiovascular dysfunction	57.7%	62.1%	$\chi^2 = .000$ $P = .984$

*Statistical test: log-rank analysis.

The need for biventricular VAD use because of severe right ventricular failure is associated with several complications that occur more commonly than with the use of an LVAD alone. These complications include respiratory failure, hypertension, neurologic dysfunction, cardiac arrhythmias, and respiratory failure, which typically occur early after biventricular VAD implantation. After the first 3 months of support, the characteristics of the adverse events change. In LVAD recipients, the rates of most adverse events decrease substantially except for infection, which continues to be a persistent problem. In patients receiving a biventricular VAD, bleeding still continued to occur at a rate that was three times higher than in the LVAD group. Late infection rates were not any different from the late infection rates in the LVAD group.

SPECIFIC TYPES OF ADVERSE EVENTS

Bleeding

Bleeding is the most common adverse event associated with MCS. The preoperative optimization of the coagulation status that is necessary for reducing the risk of postoperative bleeding is outlined in Chapter 10, and the complex interaction between anticoagulation, bleeding, and thromboembolism is well delineated in Chapter 19. Preoperatively, impaired nutritional status and acute decompensation associated with cardiogenic shock leading to hepatic and renal dysfunction (with associated uremic platelet dysfunction) and severe right ventricular failure and high central venous pressure are the primary risk factors that influence the incidence of postoperative and intraoperative bleeding. In addition, the use of preoperative anticoagulation, especially platelet inhibitors used with acute coronary interventions, exacerbates the intraoperative and postoperative problems. It has been shown that an increased international normalized ratio (INR) is associated with high risk of bleeding and pre-discharge death and needs to be normalized in all patients before LVAD implantation.

The complexity and number of previous cardiac surgeries aggravate bleeding. In addition to the need for increased blood product transfusions, bleeding significantly increases LVAD operative morbidity. Bleeding is associated with a

TABLE 13-6	Major Adverse Events Occurring in Left Ventricular Assist Device (LVAD) and Biventricular Ventricular Assist Device (VAD) Recipients

	Events per 100 Patient-Months	
Adverse Event	≤3 Months	>3 Months
LVAD		
Device malfunction	2.6	3.3
Bleeding	29.1	5.5
Cardiac/vascular		
Right heart failure	4.0	0.3
MI	0.2	0
Cardiac arrhythmia	13.7	0.7
Pericardial drainage	3.4	0.1
Hypertension	6.1	1.4
Arterial emboli	0.7	0.1
Venous thrombus	3.5	0.3
Hemolysis	0.5	0.5
Infection	31.0	11.1
Neurologic event	6.7	1.4
Renal dysfunction	6.1	0.4
Hepatic dysfunction	2.1	0.4
Respiratory failure	11	1.0
Wound dehiscence	1.2	0.1
Psychiatric episode	3.7	0.7
Biventricular VAD		
Device malfunction	5.6	2.5
Bleeding	102.0	18.4
Cardiac/vascular		
Right heart failure	2.3	0
MI	0	0
Cardiac arrhythmia	10.3	2.0
Pericardial drainage	10.3	0
Hypertension	4.2	0.6
Arterial emboli	1.4	1.3
Venous thrombus	1.4	0
Hemolysis	5.6	1.9
Infection	47.6	10.8
Neurologic event	10.7	3.2
Renal dysfunction	11.7	1.3
Hepatic dysfunction	9.8	1.3
Respiratory failure	11	1.0
Wound dehiscence	0	0
Psychiatric episode	5.6	1.2

MI, myocardial infarction.

threefold increased risk of reoperation compared with other cardiac surgery, with greater than 30% of patients requiring reoperation for bleeding. Massive blood transfusions can trigger cytokine storms that may provoke respiratory insufficiency and reactive pulmonary vascular hypertension with resultant right ventricular failure.[62] Blood transfusions are also associated with increased risk for nosocomial infections and allosensitization.[63] The meticulous intraoperative hemostasis management of patients is crucial to the avoidance of bleeding, and judicious application of blood products as outlined in Chapter 10 is mandatory. Surgical sites need to be carefully checked before sternal closure. Potential non-LVAD surgical bleeding sites include cardiopulmonary bypass cannulation sites, the sternal edges, the pleural fat pads, and, in reoperative cases, the adhesions between the epicardium and pericardium and exposed lung surface. The aortic outflow anastomosis and left ventricular apical cannulation sites are sites to be wary of; however, the most troublesome area is often the muscle edges of the diaphragm that result from dissection for the pump pocket.

Many surgeons have used several adjuvant compounds to reduce suture line bleeding. One such agent, CoSeal, is a biocompatible polyethylene glycol polymer that rapidly cross-links with proteins in tissue to adhere immediately to the area of application.[64] Another agent, TISSEEL, is a fibrin sealant that is vapor-heated and solvent detergent–treated. It is a two-component fibrin sealant made from pooled human plasma. When combined, the two components, sealer protein (human) and thrombin (human), mimic the final stage of the blood coagulation cascade. This agent is also often used to reduce bleeding in reoperative surgery. In cases of heavier suture line bleeding, FLOSEAL,[65] a hemostatic matrix that is a proprietary combination of cross-linked gelatin granules and topical human thrombin, can be used.

In cases of reoperative surgery, the bleeding is often made worse by the fact that petechial hemorrhage from lysed adhesions usually stops when the ventricle and pericardium are approximated. In the case of an LVAD, the left ventricle is often decompressed significantly from the preoperative dimension, creating a large pericardial space, and the pericardium does not tamponade the bleeding resulting in continuous hemorrhage. As devices become more compact, patient selection practices turn toward less ill patients, and the surgical procedures become shorter, the amount of postoperative bleeding has been seen to decrease. Postoperative bleeding is common, but through more judicious use of anticoagulation with the advent of better pump design, bleeding requiring reoperation with significant transfusion has been found to be reduced from previous levels with use of first-generation LVADs. Cardiac tamponade, the most common secondary complication of bleeding, can result in dramatically reduced right ventricular function and poor LVAD filling. Several surgeons elect to leave the sternum opened for 24 hours after LVAD implantation to reduce the risk of cardiac tamponade and to avoid the need for reoperation because of bleeding.

A more recent study from the University of Michigan found a strong correlation between the preoperative Model for End-Stage Liver Disease (MELD) score, which is a weighted sum of serum creatinine, bilirubin, and INR and risk of bleeding and death after LVAD implantation.[66] The authors found that for each 10 total perioperative blood product exposures, the odds of perioperative death were increased by 5% with equivalent 8% increases in the odds of developing postoperative right ventricular and renal failure. They also found a 70% increase in the odds of developing a postoperative device infection for each 5-unit increase in MELD score. The MELD score showed independent risk prediction for operative bleeding and death as a continuous variable as opposed to identifying a dichotomous cut point. These data are important inasmuch as none of the patients in their series had cirrhosis, a population in which the MELD score was originally validated.

Late bleeding in LVAD recipients has been seen more frequently with the advent of rotary LVADs owing to the requirement for oral warfarin therapy and typically manifests as chronic gastrointestinal bleeding. One of the first reports of this problem[67] compared multiple rotary pumps with pulsatile systems and found that after 30 days the rate of gastrointestinal bleeding was 46.5 events/100 patient-years for nonpulsatile devices versus 4.7 events/100 patient-years for pulsatile devices. Approximately 96% of patients with pulsatile pumps were free of bleeding at 2 years, whereas only 66% of patients with rotary pumps were free from gastrointestinal bleeding. The most common finding on gastrointestinal endoscopy is angiodysplasia—often multiple and typically in the stomach or early portions of the small bowel. This pattern was believed to be associated with a low pulse pressure in rotary pump patients similar to patients with aortic stenosis.

Patients with aortic stenosis[68] who develop angiodysplasia and gastrointestinal bleeding have been shown to have a decrease in high-molecular-weight multimers of von Willebrand factor (vWF). Nonpulsatile flow has been proposed to increase the development of gastrointestinal angiodysplasia through a pathophysiology similar to that seen with the narrow pulse pressure that occurs in aortic stenosis, and recipients of nonpulsatile devices may see a chronic increase in intraluminal pressure that dilates mucosal veins, leading to development of arteriovenous malformation and significant reduction in vWF multimers, which makes the patient vulnerable to bleeding with anticoagulation.[69] In another study, investigators measured vWF in patients who had gastrointestinal bleeding and showed that all 18 patients who had documented gastrointestinal bleeding while on a rotary pump had near-total depletion of levels of vWF at the time of the bleed. The investigators also found that the preoperative levels of vWF were almost totally depleted in a similar number of patients with rotary VADs at the time of heart transplantation.[70] The need for blood transfusion after transplantation was twice as high in the patients with rotary pumps compared with patients who underwent heart transplantation after having been on a pulsatile LVAD. This finding has led many clinicians to make adjustments in pump flow to enhance pulsatility and to reduce the level of anticoagulation. Many anecdotal reports describe cessation of oral anticoagulation for months after significant gastrointestinal bleeding without apparent thrombus formation in the LVAD.

However, both of these maneuvers are highly controversial, and the risk of thrombosis in patients insufficiently anticoagulated has yet to be carefully reported.

It is also unclear whether patients require an antithrombotic or antiplatelet agent or both. It remains to be seen whether other rotary pumps of centrifugal design will have the same findings as pumps of axial type in which the current problem has been seen. A review of INTERMACS data reveals that the incidence of bleeding is high early after implantation and most predominant in pulsatile VADs, in particular, biventricular VADs (Fig. 13-3). The time to the first bleeding event is shorter and cumulative events are higher in biventricular VADs. Although adverse event rates have been decreased by more than half in rotary devices compared with pulsatile devices, bleeding rates, which are lower in the first 30 days after implantation, are not reduced late after implantation. Approximately 62% of patients required at least 2 to 3 U of red blood cells, 21% required 4 to 7 U, and 14% required 8 U or more. Of bleeding episodes, 31% occurred in patients on no anticoagulation and presumably immediately after surgery, 24% occurred in patients on heparin alone, 16% occurred in patients on warfarin (Coumadin) alone, and 18% occurred in patients on aspirin alone. Also, women and patients 60 years old or older seemed more likely to experience bleeding.

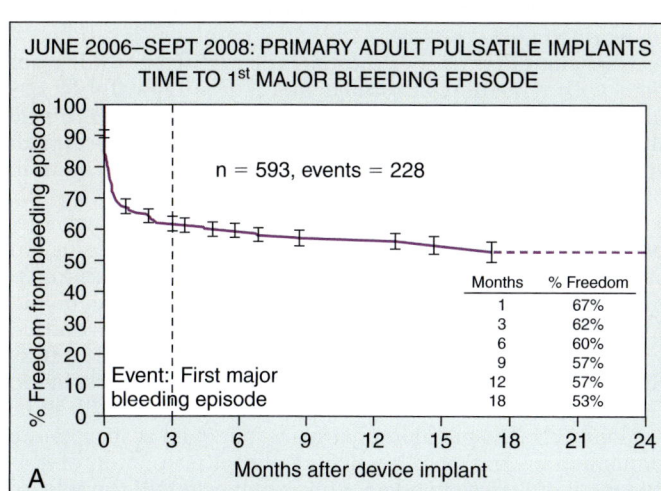

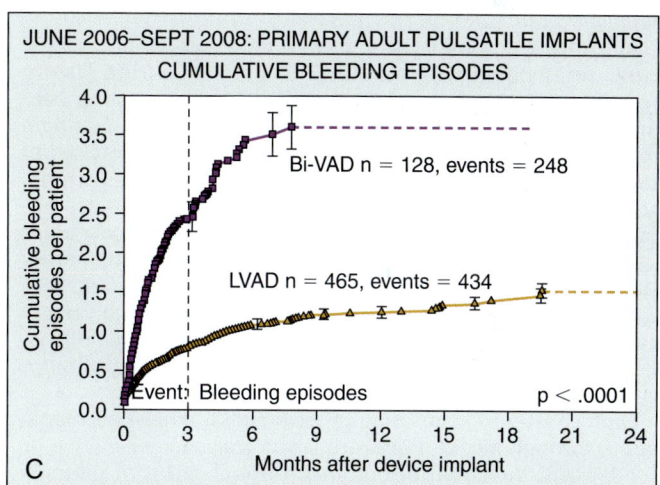

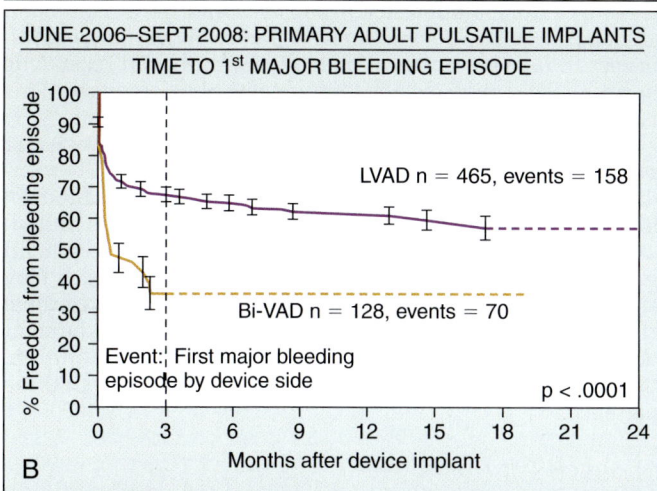

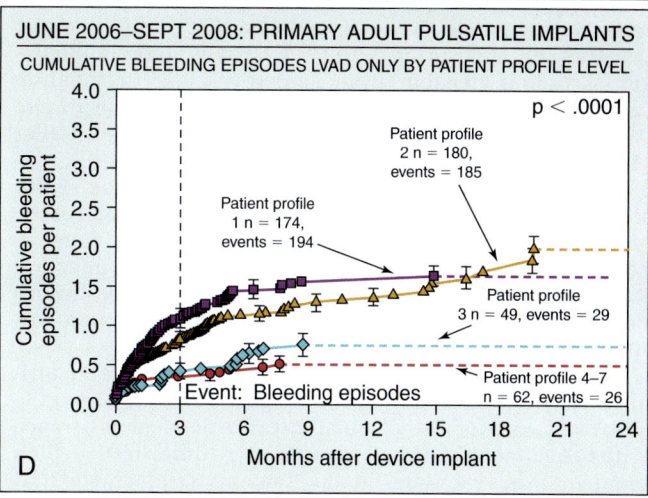

FIGURE 13-3 A, Actuarial freedom from major bleeding episode for pulsatile ventricular assist devices (VADs). **B,** Actuarial freedom from major bleeding episode for pulsatile VADs grouped by left ventricular assist devices (LVADs) versus bilateral ventricular assist devices (BiVADs). **C,** Cumulative incidence of major bleeding episodes for pulsatile VADs grouped by LVADs versus BiVADs. **D,** Cumulative incidence of major bleeding episodes for pulsatile LVADs grouped according to INTERMACS patient profile.

Neurologic complications in LVAD recipients can be the most devastating and frustrating of all adverse events; they are a leading cause of morbidity, mortality, increased hospital stay, and cost.[71] The causes of cerebrovascular events are multifactorial, but embolic episodes play a substantial role. These are usually attributed to (1) low flow states or areas of flow stagnation within the device, (2) thrombogenic surfaces, (3) hypercoagulable states, (4) ineffective or overzealous anticoagulation therapy, or (5) thrombus within the left atrioventricular cavities.

The device design has a lot to do with the incidence of neurologic events. In the INCOR device (Berlin Heart GmbH, Berlin), a small change in the inlet cannula length had a large effect on the incidence of neurologic events.[72] Patients with a long inflow cannula had a better survival rate than patients with a short inflow cannula (63.4% vs. 52.9%). The thromboembolic adverse event rate was also significantly lower. Only 3 (3.8%) of 78 patients with a long inflow cannula had a thromboembolic adverse event (thromboembolic events per patient-year) compared with 32 (23.2%) patients with a short inflow cannula (thromboembolic events per patient-year). The Novacor device (World Heart, Salt Lake City, UT) eventually failed to reach market potential because of the high rate (>35%) of neurologic events.[73] Similarly, the trial of the LionHeart device (Arrow International, Inc., Reading, PA),[74] the first totally implantable LVAD, failed because of a neurologic event rate of greater than 55%.

Multiple comorbidities or factors may lead to neurologic events in a patient with an LVAD. In patients with a history of peripheral vascular and cerebrovascular disease and ischemic cardiomyopathy, the stage is set for events at a later date when blood flow conditions and post-LVAD hypertension may work together to increase the risk of stroke. Similarly, the preoperative state of multiorgan failure leading to postoperative bleeding restricts the implementation of anticoagulant therapy. The effects of right ventricular failure on preventing optimal filling of the left ventricle and the LVAD also can predispose to thrombus formation. As noted earlier, the further limitations on anticoagulation driven by the presence of gastrointestinal bleeding may also predispose to pump thrombosis and thromboembolic complications.

One constant factor that is associated with neurologic events throughout the literature is the presence of device or bloodstream infection. In one institutional series of patients receiving multiple different devices,[75] cerebrovascular accidents were seen in 25% of patients. Of cerebrovascular accidents, 66% occurred within 4 months after implantation. Actuarial freedom from cerebrovascular accident at 6 months was 75%, 64%, 63%, and 33% with the HeartMate XVE (Thoratec Corp, Pleasanton, CA), Thoratec biventricular VAD (Thoratec Corp), Thoratec LVAD (Thoratec Corp), and Novacor device. Of all events, 42% occurred in patients with infections. The mean white blood cell count at the time of the cerebrovascular accident was greater than the normal range in patients with infection (12,900/mm³) and without infection (9500/mm³). The mean maximum amplitude of the thromboelastogram in the presence of infection (63.6 mm) was higher than in the absence of infection (60.7 mm).

To put the issues of neurologic events into more historical perspective, one needs only to look at the results from the REMATCH (Randomized Evaluation of Mechanical Assistance for the Treatment of Congestive Heart Failure) trial, which heralded the advent of destination therapy. Although the trial was deemed a success because of the survival of LVAD recipients over patients randomly assigned to medical therapy, 44% of the patients in the LVAD arm had a neurologic event compared with 7% of the patients in the medical arm. Stroke occurred in 16% of the patients in the LVAD arm compared

with 3% of patients in the medical arm.[76] Most (65%) of these events were transient, and 40% were related to the metabolic state of the patient. In more recent data from INTERMACS, the incidence of neurologic events in pulsatile devices still approaches 17%. Approximately 43% of the events were deemed embolic, 27% were hemorrhagic, and 26% were encephalopathic. Although there was no difference between LVADs and biventricular VADs with respect to the actuarial freedom from events, the patients receiving biventricular VADs had significantly more cumulative events at 1 year.

Data from the HeartMate II bridge to transplant and destination therapy trials[77,78] placed the incidence of stroke at 19% and 17%. In these series, the hemorrhagic and ischemic stroke rates were 2% and 6% for the bridge to transplant patients and 11% and 8% for the destination therapy patients reflecting the longer period of support. It is possible that overaggressive anticoagulation protocols in the early stages of use of the HeartMate II device combined with overconfident restricted anticoagulant use by some clinicians have predisposed to neurologic event rates not that different from rates seen with the HeartMate XVE. This possibility is borne out in a study that emphasized the benefits of careful control of anticoagulation[79] where the ischemic stroke rate was 2.4% and the hemorrhagic stroke rate was 1.2% in more than 300 patients in whom the INR was maintained between 1.5 and 2.5. However, as in patients undergoing standard open heart surgery using cardiopulmonary bypass, changes may occur in executive cognitive function if tested for even in the absence of overt stroke.[80]

The mortality with hemorrhagic stroke is much higher than with embolic causes, and this is due typically to significant hypertension. It has become clear only more recently that the blood pressure measured by a routine arm blood pressure cuff measures mean arterial pressure rather than systolic blood pressure.

Finally, a rare but recognized side effect of increasing cerebral perfusion with LVAD use is cerebral hyperperfusion syndrome.[81] Cerebral hyperperfusion is a life-threatening syndrome that can occur in patients with chronically hypoperfused cerebral vasculature whose normal cerebral circulation was re-established. Complications with excessive LVAD flow include severe brain edema and hemorrhage.[82] Cerebral blood flow in LVAD candidates is probably markedly impaired as evidenced by the mental impairment that often is seen before implantation. It is possible that an abrupt restoration of normal cardiac output after device implantation could overwhelm cerebral autoregulation leading to the findings of confusion and encephalopathy sometimes seen after LVAD implantation in cases where a normal computed tomography (CT) scan fails to find an organic cause for the mental status changes. This pathophysiology is largely presumptive, however.

Neurologic events occur in a complex setting of pre-existent pathology that is prone to neurologic dysfunction. The conditions of implantation are aggravating to such pathology; implantation is often performed in the setting of acute inflammation and multiorgan failure, which leads to peripheral vasodilation and the need for vasoconstrictor agents that may affect cerebral perfusion. Postoperative bleeding and variable anticoagulation management contribute to an environment that predisposes patients to neurologic events. In addition, the varied effects of pump design contribute to stroke in these patients.

Device Failure

One of the most important aspects of design of MCS devices is reliability. Engineers who develop MCS devices have a different view of device reliability than INTERMACS or the FDA because the engineers are attempting to predict device failure rather than report it accurately.

An engineering definition for device failure is "the non-performance or inability of a component or system to perform its intended function for a specified time under specified environmental conditions."[83] Failure rates are defined as the number of failures that occur during the accumulated operating time of the device. For MCS devices, failures include hardware and software failures. Hardware failure may occur secondary to degradation of components or unrecognized defects in fabrication. Defects in fabrication that result in failure are minimized by specifying appropriately low tolerance limits for variation in components, excellent quality control in the assembly process, and adequate prepackaging testing of the assembled MCS device. Such prepackaging testing may include a wet-test. During a wet-test, the MCS device is run in sterile fluid (e.g., saline) for a specified period. If the performance falls outside of specified limits, the device is discarded. The wet-test also provides a period of "burn in" that is useful for identifying a substandard component. Such early failure is more typical of the controller than the pump itself. Failure of a substandard component can lead to an unanticipated early failure of the MCS device.

Software failures usually equate with controller failure. Software deficiencies have been identified in several devices during premarket testing or postmarket surveillance. Software failures often can be resolved by installing a new version of the software on existing hardware.

Failures resulting from user error or deficiencies in the human-device interface are extremely important in MCS. Human factors are defined as "the application of the scientific knowledge of human capabilities and limitations to the design of systems and equipment to produce products with the most efficient, safe, effective, and reliable operation."[84] Engineers are assigned to develop the human-device interface during initial MCS device design. Before initiating human trials, the engineers subject their design to a formal hazard and operability study to identify the consequences of MCS device misuse. The human-device interface takes into account numerous factors, including the need to change energy sources (e.g., battery power to power base unit and vice versa), appropriate recognition and response to various alarm conditions, and environmental factors (e.g., exposure to water, extreme heat, or repetitive bending of the driveline). The human-device interface should minimize the chance of a catastrophic mistake by the patient or the caregivers. The alarm conditions must be relatively simple so that persons with limited hearing, cognitive ability, or reading capability can easily understand the condition and respond appropriately to the alarm.

Examples of Device Failure

Pulsatile pumps were the first MCS devices to enter clinical trials. Various causes of device failure have been identified, which are unique to specific design types and specific devices. The Novacor LVAD was the only MCS device during the pulsatile pump era to be fully validated on mock circulatory loop testing. The dual pusher plate mechanism for this pump led to a relatively gentle increase in pressure during the early part of pump systole. The dual pusher plate mechanism and biologic valves in this pump tolerated numerous cycles before failure. The driveline of the Novacor was robust and had relatively few failures. However, the design of the inflow graft led to numerous embolic strokes. Ultimately, redesign of the inflow cannula successfully diminished the frequency of this problem.

The HeartMate vented electric LVAD (later known as HeartMate XVE and HeartMate I LVAD) went through several design iterations. The HeartMate XVE and HeartMate I LVADs were used for the REMATCH trial of permanent MCS device use in patients who were not candidates for transplantation. This trial showed the failure modes and the expected life of the device.

One of the early causes of device failure identified was inflow graft failure. The valves in the HeartMate XVE are porcine valves that are sutured directly to the Dacron inflow and outflow conduits. Bending of the inflow conduit at implantation could slightly distort the geometry of the leaflets leading to suboptimal coaptation. More importantly, the pusher plate is driven by a DC electric motor that is capable of rapidly generating a high dP/dt (i.e., rate of pressure increase) during pump systole. After the inflow valve failure problem was recognized, modification of the inflow conduit and the controller software was developed. The software change mitigated the force of pumping by rapid interruption of the power signal during the first few milliseconds of systole. Other software modifications were installed to ensure nearly complete filling of the pump sac, which optimizes contact between the pusher plate and the cam followers of the electric motor before systole is initiated. As a result of these modifications, the dP/dt of the pump was decreased, and inflow graft failure became less common during the useful life of the pump.

The increase in durability of the HeartMate XVE inflow valves exposed a second cause of device failure that was related to failure of bearings in the central cam and cam followers. The forces on the bearings in the HeartMate XVE electric motor are substantial, and severe bearing wear is common within 18 to 24 months. As a result, the power demands of the pump increase leading to intermittent high-voltage alarms. These alarms serve as a warning of impending device failure. Specifically, the central cam or cam followers eventually freeze in place, and the pump stops. Pump stoppage is not catastrophic for two reasons. First, the inflow and outflow valves ensure that there is no retrograde movement of blood from the aorta to the left ventricle. Second, the pusher plate can be driven by air pressure using a pneumatic drive console or by using a hand pump. The hand pump is employed in emergency situations until the patient reaches a hospital or other place where a pneumatic drive console is available. Most patients at the University of Alabama-Birmingham tolerated pneumatic driving of a failed HeartMate XVE or HeartMate I LVAD without significant problems. The propensity for thrombus formation may be higher in the pneumatically driven mode; these patients are given systemic anticoagulation with heparin or warfarin. In our experience, thromboembolic events during pneumatic actuation of the HeartMate XVE or HeartMate I LVAD are rare.

Examples of human-device interface failures are instances where the patient or the caregiver mistakenly disconnects all power from the pump while changing batteries or while changing from battery power to a power base unit. Removing all power from a rotary pump can be catastrophic because these pumps have no valves, and retrograde flow occurs immediately after cessation of forward pumping. The capacity for retrograde flow depends on the pressure differential between the aorta and the left ventricle and is not quantified for the various rotary pumps currently available. Based on anecdotal reports, some patients seem to tolerate retrograde flow from a stopped rotor quite well, whereas other patients develop acute heart failure and cardiogenic shock within minutes. If the patient is alone at this time, an acute decrease in blood pressure can cause syncope that is followed by death. The number of deaths that occurred in elderly patients suggests that the mistake was not recognized and successfully resolved by the patient before he or she lost consciousness. The need for a caregiver within hearing range of the device alarms is increased for patients with limited cognitive abilities.

Prediction and Management of Device Failure

Important device failure refers to events that lead to serious adverse events or death if the failure condition is not promptly recognized and resolved. These events primarily include pump stoppage. Some pulsatile pumps driven by electric motors have the possibility for pneumatic actuation as a backup in the event of complete device failure. Experience with electrically driven pulsatile LVADs is sufficiently extensive that failure modes have been identified, and methods for detecting abnormal device performance and predicting imminent device failure have been developed. The aforementioned intermittent yellow alarms for increased voltage use by the electric motor of the HeartMate I is one such example.

Rotary pumps are early enough in their development that failure modes have not been fully identified. However, the potential for rapid decompensation and death owing to pump stoppage applies to essentially all rotary devices. An ingenious protocol for dealing with such pump failures that occur at a distance from the implant hospital has been devised by the group at Integress Health Care in Oklahoma.[85] The solution of this group is to send patients with failure of a rotary pump directly to the interventional catheterization laboratory at the local hospital whether or not there are signs of decompensation. The interventional cardiologist is asked to occlude the outflow graft of the device by retrograde cannulation of the graft with an appropriately sized balloon catheter. With the catheter in place, the pump has a high chance of developing thrombus, but retrograde flow is eliminated. If the patient tolerates this intervention, the device exchange can be deferred to allow for patient transport and preparation of the operating room.

Early experience with rotary pumps suggests that they are likely to have markedly superior durability compared with pulsatile devices. However, repetitive strain secondary to bending of the driveline can cause wire fractures and interruption of power to the motor. One solution to this problem and the problem of driveline infection is to anchor the driveline to a pedestal on the skull (see Fig. 13-11 on p. 177).[86] Other solutions include patient education and design modification to increase the strength of the driveline itself. The ultimate elimination of drivelines would eliminate driveline failure and infections related to percutaneous drivelines. However, the demands for implanted components are high from the standpoint of durability and resistance to fluid ingress. These requirements substantially increase the cost of a fully implanted MCS device. Experience with the LionHeart LVAD showed that it is feasible to design and implant a controller, a battery for temporary support, and other necessary components (e.g., a compliance chamber for a pulsatile device).[87,88] The use of a transcutaneous energy transmission system is a challenging but essential step toward an MCS device that has minimal impact on the patient's daily life.

Infection

Infection of MCS devices was recognized early in the development of these devices as the highest cause of morbidity and mortality with threat to patient survival and quality of life. During the 1990s, individual center experiences and multicenter trials confirmed that infection was a relatively common adverse event and mode of death[89,90] with a prevalence ranging from 20% to 70% of implants.[89] By 2000, investigators recognized the importance of reporting the incidence rather than the prevalence of infection because of the steadily increasing duration of MCS as a bridge to cardiac transplantation, the advent of permanent device implantation in patients who were not candidates for cardiac transplantation (i.e., destination therapy), and the need to identify time points during implantation with the greatest risk for infection (e.g., the first 30 days after implantation).

Gordon and colleagues[91] documented time-related adverse events associated with the time from LVAD implantation to the first diagnosis of bloodstream infection and the duration of infection-free survival (Fig. 13-4). This analysis showed

that blood-borne infections most commonly manifested within the first 30 days after implantation but could manifest later. Subsequently, a post-hoc analysis of the REMATCH trial examined infection complications in patients receiving pulsatile LVADs as destination therapy (HeartMate I).[92] The importance of sepsis syndrome as a mode of death was confirmed, and a comparison of the LVAD group with the medically treated control group verified the importance of infection to MCS device therapy. The frequency of sepsis and septic death as an early adverse event within 30 to 60 days of implantation was depicted using a hazard function of instantaneous risk after VAD implant (Fig. 13-5), and the negative influence of sepsis to survival for MCS device recipients was documented (Fig. 13-6).

INTERMACS defined infection adverse events for durable MCS devices.[93] Analysis of INTERMACS infection data has shown the following risk factors for cumulative number of infection adverse events: greater severity of preimplantation illness (i.e., INTERMACS level I), use of biventricular support, patient age, and higher blood urea nitrogen at implantation.[94]

Most recently, analysis of INTERMACS data confirmed that rotary MCS devices have a significantly lower incidence of infection adverse events than pulsatile devices, as measured 6 months after implantation.[95] Prior single-institution

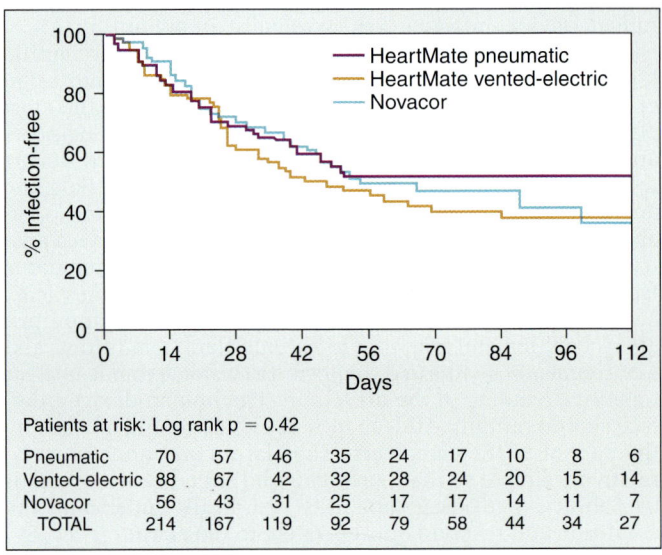

FIGURE 13-4 Actuarial freedom from bloodstream infection for common first-generation pulsatile left ventricular assist devices (LVADs).

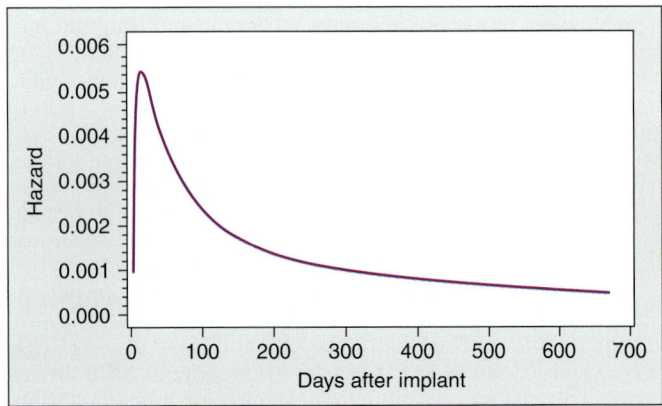

FIGURE 13-5 Instantaneous risk (hazard function) for sepsis and septic death after ventricular assist device (VAD) implantation.

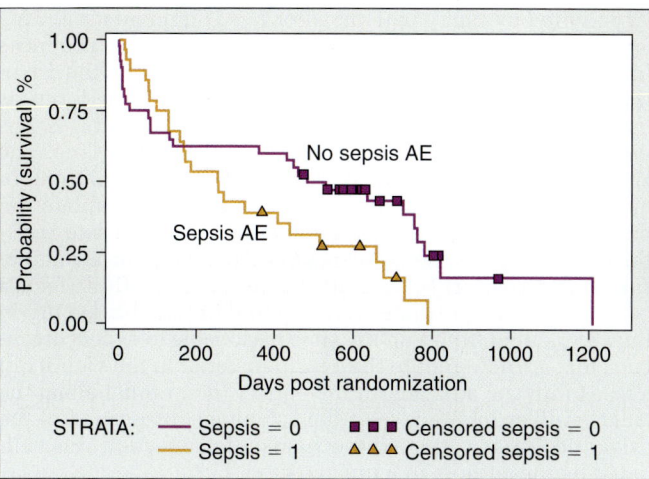

FIGURE 13-6 Influence of ventricular assist device (VAD) sepsis on actuarial survival after VAD implantation. AE, adverse event.

nonrandomized studies suggested that this was the case.[96,97] The lower infection rates may relate to the smaller size of rotary pumps because a major contributor to pulsatile pump infection is the infection in the pump pocket. The smaller rotary pumps offer less surface area for colonization and typically collect less fluid and clot around the pump at the time of implant compared with pulsatile pumps. The space between the inflow and outflow cannulas of the pulsatile HeartMate I LVAD provides room for fluid and clot collections, which then become a nidus for infection. Modification of the implant technique for pulsatile MCS devices to place them intraperitoneally appears to decrease pocket infection[98,99]; however, the technique is cumbersome compared with placing a small rotary pump that requires a small pocket or no pocket at all. This section is focused on device-related infections (i.e., percutaneous driveline, pump pocket, and internal pump components) but includes other aspects of infection (e.g., sepsis) that often involve the MCS device.

Microbiology of Device Infection

A brief consideration of the microbiology of device infection is important to understand how these infections occur, how to prevent them, how to manage them, and how to develop rationally new therapies to prevent or eradicate infections. The concepts of inoculation of pump surfaces, microbial adhesion, colony proliferation, and biofilm formation are fundamental to this understanding.[100]

Preoperative cleansing of the patient's skin with antimicrobial substances (e.g., disinfectants such as chlorhexidine) and detergents in conjunction with clipping of body hair rather than shaving decreases the microbial burden at the cutaneous incision site. However, viable bacteria remain in the epidermis and deep in hair follicles that can inoculate the wound at the time of implant. There is evidence that pathogenic bacteria (e.g., methicillin-resistant *Staphylococcus aureus* [MRSA]) from sites such as the nose or perineum are additional risk factors for postimplantation infection. Some centers use rapid screening for nasal or perineal MRSA based on polymerase chain reaction assays to identify patients colonized with MRSA, and there are reports of lower sternal infection rates after application of topical antimicrobials to eradicate MRSA.[101]

Despite all of these measures, some inoculation of bacteria into the surgical wound and onto the exterior surface of the implanted pump components is inevitable. The battle between prophylactic antimicrobial drugs, native host defenses, and microbes (bacteria and fungi) then begins. Bacteria that find a safe haven, such as retained clot in a pump pocket, may survive prophylactic antibiotics. As they multiply, some organisms

contact and adhere to the surface of implanted MCS device components. The individual microbes that initially colonize the surface are able to detect the presence of other microbes in the immediate vicinity through a process termed *quorum sensing*.[102] Quorum sensing is the mechanism for triggering alterations in microbial gene expression that result in biofilm formation. The colony encases itself in a slime layer or biofilm, defined as "a structured community of bacterial cells enclosed in a self-produced polymeric matrix."[103] The biofilm stabilizes the microbial colony on the prosthetic surface and markedly increases the resistance of the individual organisms to antimicrobial drugs or host immune attack (Fig. 13-7).[102,104] At this point, the patient begins to manifest signs of infection (e.g., fever and leukocytosis) that can progress to sepsis syndrome.

Bacteria and fungi that exist in biofilms have several characteristics that make their eradication challenging (Fig. 13-8).[102] First, some members of the colony may switch on genes for substances that cleave or otherwise inactivate antimicrobial drugs. Second, organisms that live in relatively nutrient-poor and oxygen-poor regions of the biofilm slow their metabolism and develop higher tolerance to antimicrobial drugs that depend on actively metabolizing cells for their microbicidal activity. A third mechanism for survival has been described that represents an extreme form of slowed metabolism. This is the "persister state," whereby an individual organism becomes essentially metabolically inert and is highly tolerant to environmental stresses including antimicrobial drugs.[105,106] The state of persistence seems to be a spontaneously occurring phenotype that is present in a small percentage of organisms within a biofilm and that can be responsible for resurgence of a colony after eradication of the actively metabolizing organisms.

Based on the ingenious and robust properties of microbes for attaching to prosthetic surfaces, thriving on the surface, and surviving efforts at eradication, it is not surprising that device-related infection has emerged as a major challenge to the survival and quality of life for recipients of MCS devices. Prevention of infection is based on minimizing the inoculation of the wound and pump surfaces at the time of surgery and meticulous care of the percutaneous driveline exit site. Management of established device infection is based on removal of the biofilm by any means possible and extended therapy with antimicrobial drugs, disinfectants, or host

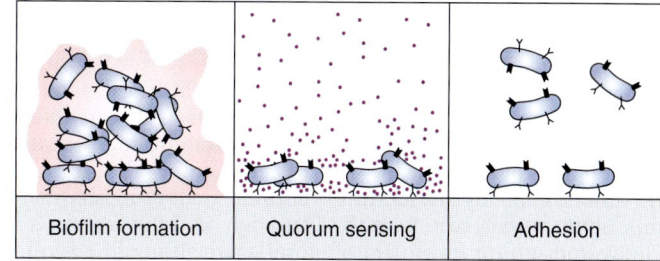

FIGURE 13-7 Relationship of biomaterial biofilm to bacterial adhesion.

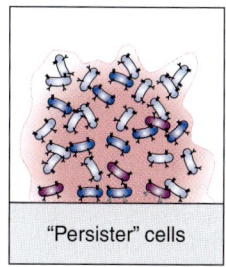

FIGURE 13-8 Depiction of "persister" state of infected biofilm layer.

defenses (e.g., omental coverage of infected pump pocket) to suppress or eradicate any resurgence of infection.

Management of Device-Related Infections

Percutaneous Driveline Infections. Prevention of driveline infection begins with careful intraoperative management. It is important to minimize movement to and fro across the percutaneous exit site that can rub bacteria off the skin edge and into the fabric that is ultimately left in a subcutaneous position. Some groups routinely soak the driveline fabric in antimicrobial solutions.[107] The group at the University of Alabama-Birmingham uses a plastic sheath from a pulmonary artery catheter insertion kit to cover the driveline, and the driveline is soaked in a solution of vancomycin and gentamicin. As a final step in the implantation procedure, the plastic sheath is pulled out of the driveline tunnel, and the driveline is stabilized by skin stitches and an external appliance (Horizontal Drain/Tube Attachment Device; Hollister, Inc, Libertyville, IL). Consistent stabilization of the driveline and focus on reinforcement to the patient to minimize or avoid any pulling or twisting of the driveline is essential to preventing late infections of the percutaneous driveline site. The optimal management for the percutaneous site has not yet been defined but probably involves periodic cleaning to remove shed epithelial cells and kill microbes followed by a dry dressing to minimize contamination.

The optimal driveline design to prevent infection is controversial. Points to be considered are the following. There is general agreement that the percutaneous driveline should be covered in a fabric that encourages ingrowth by fibroblasts to create a stable and infection-resistant collagen bond to the fabric. However, the exact fabric material, the diameter and flexibility of the driveline, and whether or not the fabric crosses the dermis are debated. A fabric that has adequate durability against degradation and physical stresses (e.g., pulling, repetitive flexion, and torque) is required. The driveline should be supple so that bending forces are not transmitted to the healed edge of the skin-driveline junction, but there must be resistance to overbending that jeopardizes the integrity of the electrical wires within the driveline. Smaller driveline circumference minimizes the area at risk for infection, but after a certain point the circumferential length of healed tissue has insufficient strength to resist pulling or torque.

The question of whether to bring the fabric (velour) across the skin or leave it a few millimeters below the dermal layer has been studied for many years.[108] Most of this research focused on the design of catheters for long-term peritoneal dialysis (e.g., Tenckhoff and related catheters)[109] or for intravenous access. Designs for peritoneal dialysis catheters typically employ a fibrous cuff at the level of the fascia to discourage leakage of the dialysate and a second fibrous cuff in the subcutaneous tissue 10 to 15 mm below the dermis. In humans, an epithelial-lined sinus forms from the dermis down to the fibrous cuff. The edge of the fibrous cuff is covered with a small rim of granulation tissue.[110] Makers of the C-Pulse counterpulsation MCS device have chosen this approach for their pneumatic percutaneous driveline (Sunshine Heart, Inc, Tustin, CA), whereas makers of other implanted and paracorporeal MCS devices have chosen to have the velour-covered percutaneous driveline or cannulas cross the dermal junction. There have not been any trials that compare MCS device driveline design in humans, and long-term animal models are unlikely to provide useful information to answer this question.

If initial driveline healing is adequate, infection can still occur. Cumulative driveline infection rates approach 100% in some studies.[110] The mechanism for late infection is probably a tear in the dermal-fabric healing because of abrupt pulling or twisting. This problem is a testimony to, and a consequence of, the marked increase in mobility and activity reported by many patients after LVAD implantation. This opening can allow a nidus of infection to begin that produces further loosening of the collagen that has grown into the driveline velour. Exuberant and moist granulation tissue forms as the infection progresses. This moist tissue encourages further bacterial growth and tunneling along the driveline. The group at Columbia University[111] published an elegant microbiologic study that examined one mechanism to explain the propensity for *Staphylococcus epidermidis* to cause late driveline infections. These investigators isolated a surface adhesion molecule (SdrF) of *S. epidermidis* that has affinity for the collagen and the polyester velour found in fully healed drivelines explanted from humans. It is reasonable to expect organisms that are adherent to tissue and material in the vicinity of a tear to invade a breach in the barrier then tunnel along the collagen-fiber interface over the subcutaneous portion of the driveline. This postulated mechanism for infection was validated by the authors in a murine model.[112]

The management of a driveline infection should begin with a call from the patient whenever injury occurs to the percutaneous insertion site. The advent of cameras in many cell phones allows the patient or caregiver to take a picture of the driveline and upload it directly to the implant center coordinator or physician to visualize the state of the driveline. Topical disinfectants such as chlorhexidine can be added to the regimen for driveline care if they are not already part of it. If there is erythema or an obvious tear at the junction of the dermis and fabric, antibiotics that cover *Staphylococcus* may be added. If the infection has progressed to the point where moist granulation tissue has formed at the percutaneous insertion site, cauterization with silver nitrate would make it regress. If the infection begins to tunnel along the driveline, débridement of the infected tissue should be considered. Some groups have used vacuum-assisted healing devices (Vacuum Assisted Closure; Kinetic Concepts, Inc, San Antonio, TX) to accelerate the healing of the resulting wound,[113,114] but our group has been disappointed by the high recurrence rate of tunnel infection. The approach at the University of Alabama-Birmingham is to débride the infected tunnel widely (Fig. 13-9) and treat it with strong disinfectants (e.g., full-strength hydrogen peroxide). Disinfectants slow the healing process, but in some cases a collagen bond forms again between the granulation tissue and the velour (Fig. 13-10). Wound cultures are used to guide antimicrobial therapy and are prescribed in consultation with infectious disease experts.

Pump Pocket Infections. The tissue (pocket) surrounding an intracorporeal MCS device may become infected. Larger

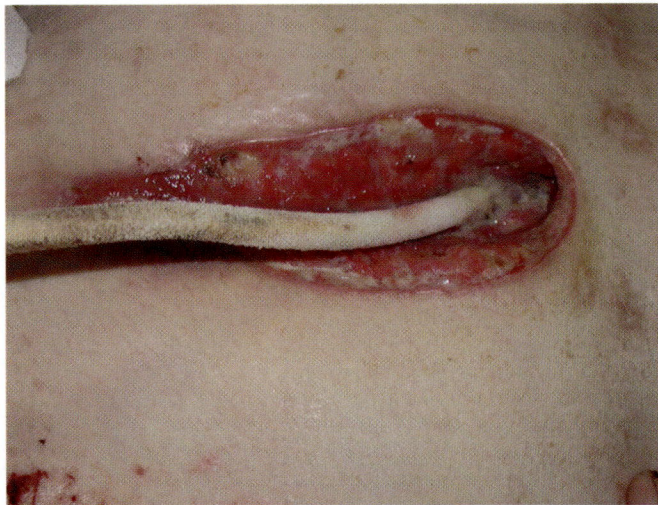

FIGURE 13-9 Infected left ventricular assist device (LVAD) driveline that has undergone surgical débridement.

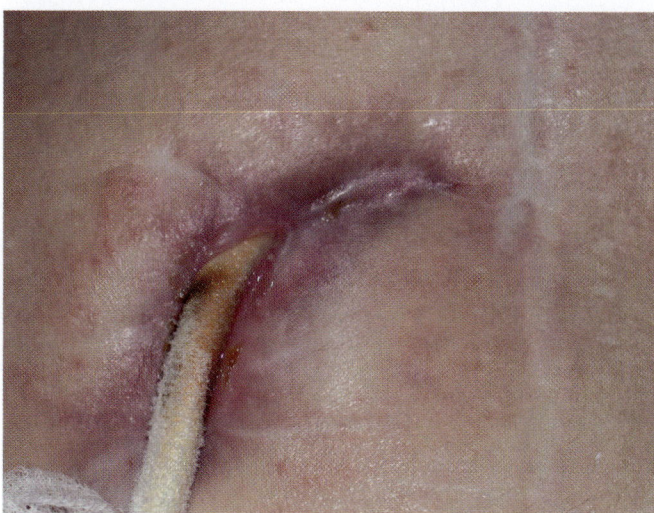

FIGURE 13-10 Chronic driveline infection bonded with granulation tissue.

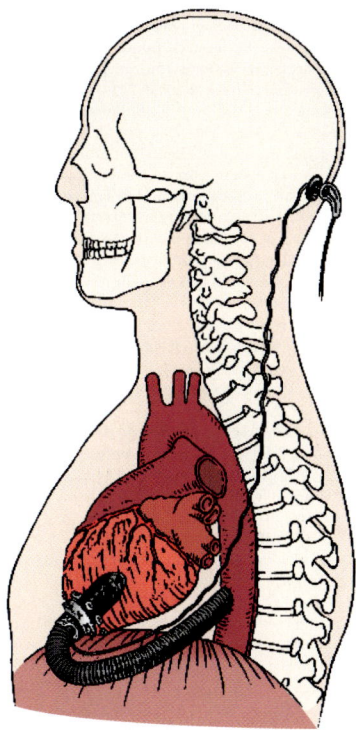

FIGURE 13-11 Skull pedestal configuration for driveline: Jarvik Flowmaker LVAD.

pumps with a configuration that creates a potential space for retention of blood clot or other fluids are prone to this problem. An example is the HeartMate I LVAD that creates a space between the inflow and outflow conduits.

Patients with infected pump pockets may present with sepsis syndrome, fevers without other symptoms, or minimal signs and symptoms (e.g., low-grade fever and mild leukocytosis). Infection of the pocket should be suspected when the patient has positive blood cultures (often *Staphylococcus* species) and mild to severe pain over the device. The diagnosis can be confirmed by either CT scan or ultrasound evidence of fluid around the implanted pump. Patients with other reasons for positive blood cultures, such as long-term indwelling intravenous lines, pose a diagnostic challenge because an ultrasound scan of the pump pocket may show fluid that is uninfected and

occupying the potential space around the device. Our practice has been to eliminate other sources for bacteremia and then explore the pump pocket for culture and treatment. We have not used needle aspiration of the pocket because of the possibility of false-negative or false-positive diagnoses and the potential for infecting an otherwise sterile space. Some centers have used radiolabeled leukocyte scans to assist with this diagnosis, although the results can be confusing because of noninfectious regional inflammation and other artifacts.

The incidence of pump pocket infection can be diminished by alterations in surgical technique, such as placing a pulsatile pump in the peritoneal space together with a polytetrafluoroethylene sheet (W.L. Gore & Associates, Flagstaff, AZ) to protect the abdominal viscera from adhesions or bowel herniation.[17,18] Rotary pumps are generally smaller than pulsatile devices and need only a small or no preperitoneal pocket. The incidence of pump pocket infection has been lower with rotary pumps, but this complication still occurs.

Management of an infected pump pocket begins with the initial drainage. Cultures for bacteria and fungi are obtained, and the tissue and pump surfaces are thoroughly cleaned. We use a dilute solution of povidone-iodine soap (Betadine; Purdue Pharma L.P., Stamford, CT) consisting of 5 to 10 mL of Betadine soap per liter of sterile saline and a pulsating irrigation device (Pulsavac Irrigation System; Zimmer, Inc, Warsaw, IN). The irrigation device cleanses and débrides the pocket, and the detergent action of the soap disrupts biofilms. After irrigation, beads of bone cement are fabricated with heat stabile antibiotic powder and left in the wound.[115,116] These beads elute antibiotics at cidal levels for about 6 to 8 weeks after placement, depending on the size of the beads and the number that are placed.

Initially, the regional concentration of antibiotics is extremely high, and absorption of the antibiotics into the body is detectable in peripheral blood samples. The levels are typically well below toxic levels; however, if the patient is receiving the same antibiotic intravenously (e.g., vancomycin), the treating physician may wish to obtain one or two serum levels to ensure safety. Many patients require more than one round of therapy with pump pocket irrigation and antibiotic beads. With multiple rounds of therapy, patients can live as outpatients with their infection, and in some instances the infection appears to be eradicated. Appropriate systemic antibiotics are given long-term and stopped only with careful monitoring (e.g., temperature, leukocyte count, and surveillance blood cultures).

Wound dehiscence over an implanted pump may occur, although this is much less common with smaller rotary pumps. When wound dehiscence occurs, the assistance of a plastic surgeon is invaluable in planning surgical reconstruction.[116–119] Rotational myocutaneous flaps and omental coverage have been used successfully even in grossly infected wounds with large areas of exposed pump. In cases where the tissue lying over the pump is attenuated or weak, we reinforce the inner layer with a sheet of acellular dermal matrix (e.g., Alloderm; LifeCell Corporation, Branchburg, NJ).

Infections of Blood Contacting Pump Components (Pump Endocarditis). Pump endocarditis is rare compared with other infection adverse events. Infection with or without vegetations can occur in inflow cannulas, outflow cannulas, valves, and pumping sacs. Rotary pumps do not have valves or pumping sacs, which limits the possibilities for pump endocarditis.

Differentiating bloodstream infection from pump endocarditis is challenging. Taking blood cultures from the left ventricle and outflow graft and nuclear tagged leukocyte scans[120] can help, but the diagnosis may ultimately be by exclusion. The options for treating pump endocarditis are limited and entail substantial risk. If the infection is low grade, device removal with transplantation is an option.[121] Other options include replacing an infected component of the pump[120] or device replacement.[122]

Various types or duration of arrhythmias may occur in patients using the INTERMACS definition, which classifies cardiac arrhythmias as one of two types: (1) sustained ventricular arrhythmia requiring defibrillation or cardioversion or (2) sustained supraventricular arrhythmia requiring drug treatment or cardioversion. Arrhythmias are an important consideration for patients with LVADs but are less important for patients with biventricular VADs. Arrhythmias are of no consequence for patients with a total artificial heart.

Patients with LVADs depend on delivery of blood from the right-sided circulation for effective LVAD pumping, and the symptoms, especially sustained ventricular tachycardia, are directly related to the function of the right ventricle. Contraction of the native left ventricle aids in filling of the VAD. This situation is analogous to atrial filling of the native left ventricle.

Supraventricular arrhythmias that lead to atrioventricular dyssynchrony can affect right ventricular output. Control of supraventricular arrhythmias using standard medical therapy optimizes LVAD function. In patients with chronic atrial fibrillation and slow ventricular response, ensuring an adequate ventricular rate with the use of temporary pacing wires may be beneficial in the immediate postoperative period.

Sustained ventricular tachycardia usually results in diminished LVAD output, whereas ventricular fibrillation diminishes LVAD flow further. LVAD flow during ventricular fibrillation varies from patient to patient. In some cases, the residual flow is sufficient for the patient to maintain consciousness and ambulation. During the era of pulsatile LVAD therapy, the ability of an LVAD to support patients with ventricular fibrillation for minutes to days was documented by the group at Columbia University.[123] This same group documented the effects of VAD therapy on nonischemic ventricular arrhythmias.[124] Generally, patients with ischemic ventricular arrhythmias improve with LVAD therapy alone. If a patient has a history of medically refractory arrhythmias and biventricular support is feasible, this is a preferred mode of therapy over single ventricle support. If it is available, the total artificial heart is the best solution for the management of refractory ventricular arrhythmias.

When patients with an LVAD have sustained ventricular arrhythmias and as a consequence experience a decrease in flow, they can be treated with cardioversion or defibrillation. The patient should be adequately sedated before receiving external electrical shocks if flow remains adequate for consciousness. MCS devices are designed to withstand internal and external electrical shocks for cardioversion and defibrillation. However, the instructions for use should be consulted before employing external shocks. Detaching the driveline from the controller or other measures may be required. Implantable cardioverter-defibrillators (ICDs) use sufficiently low energy levels that their potential for affecting pump components is substantially less. The ICD should be checked after VAD implantation to ensure that the pacing and sensing thresholds have not changed and that the device is functioning properly.

In some instances, the radiofrequency energy emitted by the implanted pump (e.g., HeartMate II) interferes with radiofrequency signals sent transcutaneously to the ICD. In such cases, the power to the pump must be temporarily interrupted to allow communication with the ICD. This interruption is usually well tolerated by the patient but not always. The patient should be comfortable and in a supine position if interruption of pump power is necessary. If the patient develops syncope or presyncope, power is immediately restored

to the pump. The most recent versions of ICDs have successfully resolved this problem with radiofrequency interference by using another frequency.

REFERENCES

1. Miller LW, Pagani FD, Russell SD, et al. Use of a continuous-flow device in patients awaiting heart transplantation. *N Engl J Med.* 2007;357:885–896.
2. Frazier OH, Rose EA, Oz MC, et al. Multicenter clinical evaluation of the HeartMate vented electric left ventricular assist system in patients awaiting heart transplantation. *J Thorac Cardiovasc Surg.* 2001;122:1186–1195.
3. Frazier OH, Rose EA, Macmanus Q, et al. Multicenter clinical evaluation of the HeartMate 1000 IP left ventricular assist device. *Ann Thorac Surg.* 1992;53:1080–1090.
4. Ueno T, Bergin P, Richardson M, et al. Bridge to recovery with a left ventricular assist device for fulminant acute myocarditis. *Ann Thorac Surg.* 2000;69:284–286.
5. Simon MA, Kormos RL, Murali S, et al. Myocardial recovery using ventricular assist devices: prevalence, clinical characteristics, and outcomes. *Circulation.* 2005;112(suppl 9):I–32–I-36.
6. Farrar DJ, Holman WR, McBride LR, et al. Long-term follow-up of Thoratec ventricular assist device bridge-to-recovery patients successfully removed from support after recovery of ventricular function. *J Heart Lung Transplant.* 2002;21(5):516–521.
7. Chen JM, Spanier TB, Gonzalez JJ, et al. Improved survival in patients with acute myocarditis using external pulsatile mechanical ventricular assistance. *J Heart Lung Transplant.* 1999;18:351–357.
8. Westaby S, Katsumata T, Pigott D, et al. Mechanical bridge to recovery in fulminant myocarditis. *Ann Thorac Surg.* 2000;70:278–282.
9. Frazier OH, Myers TJ. Left ventricular assist system as a bridge to myocardial recovery. *Ann Thorac Surg.* 1999;68:734–741.
10. Rose EA, Gelijns AC, Moskowitz AJ, et al. Long-term mechanical left ventricular assistance for end-stage heart failure. *N Engl J Med.* 2001;345:1435–1443.
11. Rogers JG, Butler J, Lansman SL, et al. Chronic mechanical circulatory support for inotrope-dependent heart failure patients who are not transplant candidates: results of the INTrEPID Trial. *J Am Coll Cardiol.* 2007;50:741–747.
12. Richenbacher WE, Naka Y, Raines EP, et al. Surgical management of patients in the REMATCH trial. *Ann Thorac Surg.* 2003;75(suppl 6):S86–S92.
13. Stevenson LW, Miller LW, Desvigne-Nickens P, et al. Left ventricular assist device as destination for patients undergoing intravenous inotropic therapy: a subset analysis from REMATCH (Randomized Evaluation of Mechanical Assistance in Treatment of Chronic Heart Failure). *Circulation.* 2004;110:975–981.
14. Park SJ, Tector A, Piccioni W, et al. Left ventricular assist devices as destination therapy: a new look at survival. *J Thorac Cardiovasc Surg.* 2005;129:9–17.
15. Burnett CM, Duncan JM, Frazier OH, et al. Improved multiorgan function after prolonged univentricular support. *Ann Thorac Surg.* 1993;55:65–71.
16. Frazier OH, Macris MP, Myers TJ, et al. Improved survival after extended bridge to cardiac transplantation. *Ann Thorac Surg.* 1994;57:1416–1422.
17. DeRose Jr JJ, Umana JP, Argenziano M, et al. Implantable left ventricular assist devices provide an excellent outpatient bridge to transplantation and recovery. *J Am Coll Cardiol.* 1997;30:1773–1777.
18. Morrone TM, Buck LA, Catanese KA, et al. Early progressive mobilization of patients with left ventricular assist devices is safe and optimizes recovery before heart transplantation. *J Heart Lung Transplant.* 1996;15:423–429.
19. Dew MA, Kormos RL, Roth LH, et al. Life quality in the era of bridging to cardiac transplantation: bridge patients in an outpatient setting. *ASAIO J.* 1993;39(2):145–152.
20. Frazier OH, Rose EA, McCarthy P, et al. Improved mortality and rehabilitation of transplant candidates treated with a long-term implantable left ventricular assist system. *Ann Surg.* 1995;222:327–336.
21. Aaronson KD, Eppinger MJ, Dyke DB, et al. Left ventricular assist device therapy improves utilization of donor hearts. *J Am Coll Cardiol.* 2002;39:1247–1254.
22. Esmore D, Kaye D, Spratt P, et al. A prospective, multicenter trial of the VentrAssist left ventricular assist device for bridge to transplant: safety and efficacy. *J Heart Lung Transplant.* 2008;27:579–588.
23. Frazier OH, Benedict CR, Radovancevic B, et al. Improved left ventricular function after chronic left ventricular unloading. *Ann Thorac Surg.* 1996;62:675–681.
24. Portner PM, Jansen PG, Oyer PE, et al. Improved outcomes with an implantable left ventricular assist system: a multicenter study. *Ann Thorac Surg.* 2001;71:205–209.
25. Strauch JT, Spielvogel D, Haldenwang PL, et al. Recent improvements in outcome with the Novacor left ventricular assist device. *J Heart Lung Transplant.* 2003;22:674–680.
26. Long JW, Kfoury AG, Slaughter MS, et al. Long-term destination therapy with the HeartMate XVE left ventricular assist device: improved outcomes since the REMATCH study. *Congest Heart Fail.* 2005;11:133–138.
27. Lietz K, Long JW, Kfoury AG, et al. Outcomes of left ventricular assist device implantation as destination therapy in the post-REMATCH era: implications for patient selection. *Circulation.* 2007;116:497–505.
28. Long JW, Healy AH, Rasmusson BY, et al. Improving outcomes with long-term "destination" therapy using left ventricular assist devices. *J Thorac Cardiovasc Surg.* 2008;135:1353–1360.
29. Thomas CE, Jichici D, Petrucci R, et al. Neurologic complications of the Novacor left ventricular assist device. *Ann Thorac Surg.* 2001;72:1311–1315.
30. Morgan JA, John R, Rao V, et al. Bridging to transplant with the HeartMate left ventricular assist device: the Columbia Presbyterian 12-year experience. *J Thorac Cardiovasc Surg.* 2004;127:1309–1316.
31. Haj-Yahia S, Birks EJ, Rogers P, et al. Midterm experience with the Jarvik 2000 axial flow left ventricular assist device. *J Thorac Cardiovasc Surg.* 2007;134:199–203.

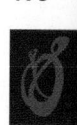

32. Sharples LD, Cafferty F, Demitis N, et al. Evaluation of the clinical effectiveness of the Ventricular Assist Device Program in the United Kingdom (EVAD UK). *J Heart Lung Transplant.* 2007;26:9–15.
33. Deng MC, Edwards LB, Hertz MI, et al. Mechanical circulatory support device database of the International Society for Heart and Lung Transplantation: third annual report—2005. *J Heart Lung Transplant.* 2005;24:1182–1187.
34. Gordon SM, Schmitt SK, Jacobs M, et al. Nosocomial bloodstream infections in patients with implantable left ventricular assist devices. *Ann Thorac Surg.* 2001;72:725–730.
35. Birks EJ, Tansley PD, Yacoub MH, et al. Incidence and clinical management of life-threatening left ventricular assist device failure. *J Heart Lung Transplant.* 2004;23:964–969.
36. Holman WL, Rayburn BK, McGiffin DC, et al. Infection in ventricular assist devices: prevention and treatment. *Ann Thorac Surg.* 2003;75(suppl 6):S48–S57.
37. Navia JL, McCarthy PM, Hoercher KJ, et al. Do left ventricular assist device (LVAD) bridge-to-transplantation outcomes predict the results of permanent LVAD implantation? [erratum in *Ann Thorac Surg.* 2004;77(1):383]. *Ann Thorac Surg.* 2002;74:2051–2062.
38. Tsukui H, Abla A, Teuteberg JJ, et al. Cerebrovascular accidents in patients with a ventricular assist device. *J Thorac Cardiovasc Surg.* 2007;134:114–123.
39. Holman WL, Kormos RL, Naftel DC, et al. Predictors of death and transplant in patients with a mechanical circulatory support device: a multi-institutional study. *J Heart Lung Transplant.* 2009;28:44–50.
40. Deng MC, Edwards LB, Hertz MI, et al. Mechanical Circulatory Support Device Database of the International Society for Heart and Lung Transplantation—first annual report, 2003. *J Heart Lung Transplant.* 2003;22:653–662.
41. INTERMACS. *Adverse Event Definitions.* Available at http://www.uab.edu/ctsresearch/intermacs/manuals.htm. Accessed Sept 10, 2010.
42. Genovese EA, Dew MA, Teuteberg JJ, et al. Incidence and patterns of adverse event onset during the first 60 days after ventricular assist device implantation. *Ann Thorac Surg.* 2009;88:1162–1170.
43. Kirklin JK, Naftel DC, Kormos RL, et al. Second INTERMACS annual report: more than 1,000 primary left ventricular assist device implants. *J Heart Lung Transplant.* 2010;29:1–10.
44. Genovese EA, Dew MA, Teuteberg JJ, et al. Early adverse events as predictors of late mortality during mechanical circulatory support. *J Heart Lung Transplant.* 2010;29:981–988.
45. Miller LW, Pagani FD, Russell SD, et al. Use of a continuous-flow device in patients awaiting heart transplantation. *N Engl J Med.* 2007;357:885–896.
46. Holman WL, Pae WE, Teutenberg JJ, et al. INTERMACS: interval analysis of registry data. *J Am Coll Surg.* 2009;208:755–761.
47. Pagani FD, Miller LW, Russell SD, et al. Extended mechanical circulatory support with a continuous-flow rotary left ventricular assist device. *J Am Coll Cardiol.* 2009;54:312–321.
48. McKenna Jr DH, Eastlund T, Segall M, et al. HLA alloimmunization in patients requiring ventricular assist device support. *J Heart Lung Transplant.* 2002;21:1218–1224.
49. Sihler KC, Napolitano LM. Complications of massive transfusion. *Chest.* 2010;137:209–220.
50. Schulman AR, Martens TP, Russo MJ, et al. Effect of left ventricular assist device infection on post-transplant outcomes. *J Heart Lung Transplant.* 2009;28:237–242.
51. Asadollahi K, Beeching NJ, Gill GV. Leukocytosis as a predictor for non-infective mortality and morbidity. *QJM.* 2010;103:285–292.
52. Forman DE, Butler J, Wang Y, et al. Incidence, predictors at admission, and impact of worsening renal function among patients hospitalized with heart failure. *J Am Coll Cardiol.* 2004;43:61–67.
53. Hillege HL, Girbes AR, de Kam PJ, et al. Renal function, neurohormonal activation, and survival in patients with chronic heart failure. *Circulation.* 2000;102:203–210.
54. Russell SD, Rogers JG, Milano CA, et al. Renal and hepatic function improve in advanced heart failure patients during continuous-flow support with the HeartMate II left ventricular assist device. *Circulation.* 2009;120:2352–2357.
55. Sandner SE, Zimpfer D, Zrunek P, et al. Renal function after implantation of continuous versus pulsatile flow left ventricular assist devices. *J Heart Lung Transplant.* 2008;27:469–473.
56. Radovancevic B, Vrtovec B, de Kort E, et al. End-organ function in patients on long-term circulatory support with continuous- or pulsatile-flow assist devices. *J Heart Lung Transplant.* 2007;26:815–818.
57. James KB, McCarthy PM, Jaalouk S, et al. Plasma volume and its regulatory factors in congestive heart failure after implantation of long-term left ventricular assist devices. *Circulation.* 1996;93(8):1515–1519.
58. Sandner SE, Zimpfer D, Zrunek P, Rajek A, Schima H, Dunkler D, et al. Renal function and outcome after continuous flow left ventricular assist device implantation. *Ann Thorac Surg.* 2009;87:1072–1078.
59. Kanter KR, Swartz MT, Pennington DG, et al. Renal failure in patients with ventricular assist devices. *ASAIO Trans.* 1987;33:426–428.
60. Kaltenmaier B, Pommer W, Kaufmann F, et al. Outcome of patients with ventricular assist devices and acute renal failure requiring renal replacement therapy. *ASAIO J.* 2000;46:330–333.
61. Gaudino M, Luciani N, Giungi S, et al. Different profiles of patients who require dialysis after cardiac surgery. *Ann Thorac Surg.* 2005;79:825–829.
62. Goldstein DJ, Beauford RB. Left ventricular assist devices and bleeding: adding insult to injury. *Ann Thorac Surg.* 2003;75:S42–S47.
63. McKenna Jr DH, Eastlund T, Segall M, et al. HLA alloimmunization in patients requiring ventricular assist device support. *J Heart Lung Transplant.* 2002;21:1218–1224.
64. Wallace DG, Cruise GM, Rhee WM, et al. A tissue sealant based on reactive multifunctional polyethylene glycol. *J Biomed Mater Res.* 2001;58:545–555.
65. Oz MC, Cosgrove III DM, Badduke BR, et al. Controlled clinical trial of a novel hemostatic agent in cardiac surgery. *Ann Thorac Surg.* 2000;69:1376–1382.
66. Matthews JC, Pagani FD, Haft JW, et al. Model for End-Stage Liver Disease score predicts left ventricular assist device operative transfusion requirements, morbidity, and mortality. *Circulation.* 2010;121:214–220.
67. Crow S, John R, Boyle A, et al. Gastrointestinal bleeding rates in recipients of nonpulsatile and pulsatile left ventricular assist devices. *J Thorac Cardiovasc Surg.* 2009;137:208–215.
68. Warkentin TE, Moore JC, Morgan DG. Aortic stenosis and bleeding gastrointestinal angiodysplasia: is acquired von Willebrand's disease the link? *Lancet.* 1992;340:35–37.
69. Letsou GV, Shah N, Gregoric ID, et al. Gastrointestinal bleeding from arteriovenous malformations in patients supported by the Jarvik 2000 axial-flow left ventricular assist device. *J Heart Lung Transplant.* 2005;24:105–109.
70. Uriel N, Pak SW, Jorde UP, et al. Acquired von Willebrand syndrome after continuous-flow mechanical device support contributes to a high prevalence of bleeding during long-term support and at the time of heart transplantation. *J Am Coll Cardiol.* 2010;56:1207–1213.
71. Lazar RM, Shapiro PA, Jaski BE, et al. Neurological events during long-term mechanical circulatory support for heart failure: the Randomized Evaluation of Mechanical Assistance for the Treatment of Congestive Heart Failure (REMATCH) experience. *Circulation.* 2004;109:2423–2427.
72. Schmid C, Jurmann M, Birnbaum D, et al. Influence of inflow cannula length in axial-flow pumps on neurologic adverse event rate: results from a multi-center analysis. *J Heart Lung Transplant.* 2008;27:253–260.
73. Thomas CE, Jichici D, Petrucci R, et al. Neurologic complications of the Novacor left ventricular assist device. *Ann Thorac Surg.* 2001;72:1311–1315.
74. Pae WE, Connell JM, Boehmer JP, et al. Neurologic events with a totally implantable left ventricular assist device: European LionHeart Clinical Utility Baseline Study (CUBS). *J Heart Lung Transplant.* 2007;26:1–8.
75. Tsukui H, Abla A, Teuteberg JJ, et al. Cerebrovascular accidents in patients with a ventricular assist device. *J Thorac Cardiovasc Surg.* 2007;134:114–123.
76. Lazar RM, Shapiro PA, Jaski BE, et al. Neurological events during long-term mechanical circulatory support for heart failure: the Randomized Evaluation of Mechanical Assistance for the Treatment of Congestive Heart Failure (REMATCH) experience. *Circulation.* 2004;109:2423–2427.
77. Miller LW, Pagani FD, Russell SD, et al. Use of a continuous-flow device in patients awaiting heart transplantation. *N Engl J Med.* 2007;357:885–896.
78. Slaughter MS, Rogers JG, Milano CA, et al. Advanced heart failure treated with continuous-flow left ventricular assist device. *N Engl J Med.* 2009;361:2241–2251.
79. Boyle AJ, Russell SD, Teuteberg JJ, et al. Low thromboembolism and pump thrombosis with the HeartMate II left ventricular assist device: analysis of outpatient anti-coagulation. *J Heart Lung Transplant.* 2009;28:881–887.
80. Komoda T, Drews T, Sakuraba S, et al. Executive cognitive dysfunction without stroke after long-term mechanical circulatory support. *ASAIO J.* 2005;51:764–768.
81. Lietz K, Brown K, Ali SS, et al. The role of cerebral hyperperfusion in postoperative neurologic dysfunction after left ventricular assist device implantation for end-stage heart failure. *J Thorac Cardiovasc Surg.* 2009;137:1012–1019.
82. Boyle AJ, Park SJ, Colvin-Adams MM, et al. Cerebral hyperperfusion syndrome following LVAD implantation (abstract). *J Heart Lung Transplant.* 2003;22(suppl):S203.
83. Fries RC. The concept of failure. In: *Reliable Design of Medical Devices.* New York: Marcel Dekker; 1997:11–21.
84. Fries RC. Human factors. In: *Reliable Design of Medical Devices.* New York: Marcel Dekker; 1997:313–355.
85. Chrysant GS, Hostmanshof DA, Snyder TA, et al. Successful percutaneous management of acute left ventricular assist device stoppage. *ASAIO J.* 2010;56:483–485.
86. Haj-Yahia S, Birks EJ, Rogers P, et al. Midterm experience with the Jarvik 2000 axial flow left ventricular assist device. *J Thorac Cardiovasc Surg.* 2007;134:199–203.
87. el-Banayosy A, Arusolglu L, Kizner L, et al. Preliminary experience with the LionHeart left ventricular assist device in patients with end-stage heart failure. *Ann Thorac Surg.* 2003;75:1469–1475.
88. Pae WE, Connell JM, Adelowo A, et al. Does total implantability reduce infection with the use of a left ventricular assist device? The LionHeart experience in Europe. *J Heart Lung Transplant.* 2007;26:219–229.
89. Holman WL, Rayburn BK, McGiffin DC, et al. Infection in ventricular assist devices: prevention and treatment. *Ann Thorac Surg.* 2003;75(suppl):S48–S57.
90. Simon D, Fischer S, Grossman A, et al. Left ventricular assist device-related infection: treatment and outcome. *Clin Infect Dis.* 2005;40:1108–1115.
91. Gordon SM, Schmitt SK, Jacobs M, et al. Nosocomial bloodstream infections in patients with implantable left ventricular assist devices. *Ann Thorac Surg.* 2001;72:725–730.
92. Holman WL, Park SJ, Long JW, et al. Infection in permanent circulatory support: experience from the REMATCH trial. *J Heart Lung Transplant.* 2004;23:1359–1365.
93. INTERMACS. *Manual of Operations.* Available at http://www.uab.edu/ctsresearch/intermacs/manuals.htm. Accessed Sept 10, 2010.
94. Holman WL, Kirklin JK, Naftel DC, et al. Infection after implantation of pulsatile mechanical circulatory support devices. *J Thorac Cardiovasc Surg.* 2010;139:1632–1636.
95. Milano CA, Naftel DC, Padera RF, et al. Infection during mechanical circulatory support: can we really expect a better outlook with continuous flow technology (abstract). *J Heart Lung Transplant.* 2010;29:S52.
96. Siegenthaler MP, Martin J, Pernice K, et al. The Jarvik 2000 is associated with less infections than the HeartMate left ventricular assist device. *Eur J Cardiothorac Surg.* 2003;23:748–755.
97. Schulman AR, Martens TP, Christos PJ, et al. Comparisons of infection complications between continuous flow and pulsatile flow left ventricular assist devices. *J Thorac Cardiovasc Surg.* 2007;133:841–842.

98. Icenogle T, Sandler D, Puhlman M, et al. Intraperitoneal pocket for left ventricular assist device placement. *J Heart Lung Transplant.* 2003;22:818–821.

99. Holman WL, Pamboukian SV, Bellot SC, et al. Use of an intraperitoneal ventricular assist device with a polytetrafluoroethylene barrier decreases infection. *J Heart Lung Transplant.* 2008;27:268–271.

100. Holman WL. Microbiology of infection in mechanical circulatory support. *Int J Artif Organs.* 2007;30:764–770.

101. Cimochowski GE, Harostock MD, Brown R, et al. Intranasal mupirocin reduces sternal wound infection after open heart surgery in diabetics and nondiabetics. *Ann Thorac Surg.* 2001;71:1572–1578.

102. Fux CA, Costerton JW, Stewart PS, et al. Survival strategies of infectious biofilms. *Trends Microbiol.* 2005;13:34–40.

103. Rani SA, Pitts B, Stewart PS. Rapid diffusion of fluorescent tracers into Staphylococcus epidermidis biofilms visualized by time lapse microscopy. *Antimicrob Agents Chemother.* 2005;49:728–732.

104. Hall-Stoodley L, Costerton JW, Stoodley P. Bacterial biofilms: from the natural environment to infectious diseases. *Nature.* 2004;2:95–108.

105. Kussell E, Kishony R, Balaban NQ, et al. Bacterial persistence: a model of survival in changing environments. *Genetics.* 2005;169:1807–1814.

106. Balaban NQ, Merrin J, Chait R, et al. Bacterial persistence as a phenotypic switch. *Science.* 2004;305:1622–1625.

107. Hernandez MD, Mansouri MD, Aslam S, et al. Efficacy of combination of N-acetylcysteine, gentamicin, and amphotericin B for prevention of microbial colonization of ventricular assist devices. *Infect Control Hosp Epidemiol.* 2009;30:190–192.

108. Poirier VL. *Percutaneous drivelines: developmental history.* 2010 Personal communication.

109. Twardowski ZJ. History and development of the access for peritoneal dialysis. *Contrib Nephrol.* 2004;142:387–401.

110. Twardowski ZJ, Dobbie JW, Moore HL, et al. Morphology of peritoneal dialysis catheter tunnel: macroscopy and light microscopy. *Perit Dial Int.* 1991;11:237–251.

111. Zierer A, Melby SJ, Voeller RK, et al. Late-onset driveline infections: the Achilles' heel of prolonged left ventricular assist device support. *Ann Thorac Surg.* 2007;84:515–520.

112. Arrecubieta C, Toba FA, von Bayern MP, et al. SdrF, a Staphylococcus epidermidis surface protein, contributes to the initiation of ventricular assist device driveline-related infections. *PLoS Pathog.* 2009;5:1–13.

113. Yuh DD, Albaugh M, Ullrich S, et al. Treatment of ventricular assist device driveline infection with vacuum-assisted closure system. *Ann Thorac Surg.* 2005;80:1493–1495.

114. Baradarian S, Stahovich M, Krause S, et al. Case series: clinical management of persistent mechanical assist device driveline drainage using vacuum-assisted closure therapy. *ASAIO J.* 2006;52:354–356.

115. McKellar SH, Allred BD, Marks JD, et al. LVAD pocket infection controlled with antibiotic-impregnated polymethylmethacrylate beads. *Ann Thorac Surg.* 1999;67:554–555.

116. Holman WL, Fix RJ, Foley BA, et al. Management of wound and left ventricular assist device pocket infection. *Ann Thorac Surg.* 1999;68:1080–1082.

117. Buck DW, McCarthy PM, McGee Jr E, et al. Exposed left ventricular assist device salvage using the components separation technique. *Plast Reconstr Surg.* 2008;122:225e–227e.

118. Piper HM, Siegmund B, Ladilov YV, et al. Calcium and sodium control in hypoxic-reoxygenated cardiomyocytes. *Basic Res Cardiol.* 1993;88:471–482.

119. Sajjadian A, Valerio IL, Acurturk O, et al. Omental transposition flap for salvage of ventricular assist devices. *Plast Reconstr Surg.* 2006;118:919–926.

120. de Jonge KC, Laube HR, Dohmen PM, et al. Diagnosis and management of left ventricular assist device valve-endocarditis: LVAD valve replacement. *Ann Thorac Surg.* 2000;70:1404–1405.

121. Poston RS, Husain S, Sorce D, et al. LVAD bloodstream infections: therapeutic rationale for transplantation after LVAD infection. *J Heart Lung Transplant.* 2003;22:914–921.

122. Nurozler F, Argenziano M, Oz MC, et al. Fungal left ventricular assist device endocarditis. *Ann Thorac Surg.* 2001;71:614–618.

123. Oz MC, Rose EA, Slater J, et al. Malignant ventricular arrhythmias are well tolerated in patients receiving long-term left ventricular assist devices. *J Am Coll Cardiol.* 1994;24:1688–1691.

124. Ziv O, Dizon J, Thosani A, et al. Effects of left ventricular assist device therapy on ventricular arrhythmias. *J Am Coll Cardiol.* 2005;45:1428–1434.

APPENDIX

INTERMACS (Interagency Registry for Mechanically Assisted Circulatory Support) Definitions of Clinically Significant Acute Adverse Events after Ventricular Assist Device Implantation

Event Type	Definition
Cardiac/Vascular	
Arrhythmia (ventricular or atrial)	Any documented ventricular or atrial arrhythmia that results in a clinical compromise (e.g., diminished VAD outflow, oliguria, presyncope or syncope) that requires hospitalization or occurs during the hospital stay *Ventricular arrhythmia:* Sustained ventricular arrhythmia requiring defibrillation or cardioversion *Atrial arrhythmia:* Sustained supraventricular arrhythmia requiring drug treatment or cardioversion
Right heart failure	Symptoms and signs of persistent right ventricular dysfunction (central venous pressure >18 mm Hg with cardiac index <2.0 L/min/m² in the absence of elevated left atrial or pulmonary capillary wedge pressure [>18 mm Hg], tamponade, ventricular arrhythmias, or pneumothorax) requiring RVAD implantation or inotropic therapy, ≥14 days after LVAD implantation
Hypertension	New-onset blood pressure elevation ≥140 mm Hg systolic or 90 mm Hg diastolic (pulsatile pump) or 110 mm Hg mean pressure (rotary pump)
Thromboembolism (arterial or venous)	*Arterial thromboembolism:* Acute systemic arterial perfusion deficit in any noncerebrovascular organ system confirmed by clinical and laboratory findings, operative or autopsy *Venous thromboembolism:* Evidence of deep vein thrombosis or other venous thrombotic event
Hemolysis	Plasma free hemoglobin >40 mg/dL in association with clinical signs of hemolysis (e.g., anemia, low hematocrit, hyperbilirubinemia) occurring within the first 72 hours after implantation. Hemolysis related to documented non–device-related causes (e.g., transfusion or drug) is excluded from this definition

Continued

Event Type	Definition
MI	Two categories of MI: *Perioperative MI:* Clinical suspicion of MI together with CK-MB or troponin >10 times the local hospital upper limits of normal, found within 7 days after VAD implant together with ECG findings consistent with acute MI. This definition uses the higher suggested limit for serum markers because of apical coring at the time of VAD placement and does not use wall motion changes because the apical sewing ring inherently creates new wall motion abnormalities *Nonperioperative MI:* The presence at >7 days after implantation of two of the following three criteria: (1) Chest pain that is characteristic of myocardial ischemia (2) ECG with a pattern or changes consistent with MI (3) Troponin or CK (measured by standard clinical pathology or laboratory medicine methods) greater than the normal range for the local hospital with positive MB fraction (≥3% total CK). This should be accompanied by a new regional left ventricular or right ventricular wall motion abnormality on a myocardial imaging study

Other Organ Systems

Event Type	Definition
Respiratory (tracheostomy or reintubation)	Impairment of respiratory function requiring reintubation, tracheostomy, or (for patients >5 years old) the inability to discontinue ventilator support within 6 days (144 hours) after VAD implantation. This excludes intubation for reoperation or temporary intubation for diagnostic or therapeutic procedures
Neurologic (infarct or hemorrhagic CVA or TIA)	Any new, temporary or permanent, focal or global neurologic deficit ascertained by standard neurologic examination (administered by a neurologist or other qualified physician and documented with appropriate diagnostic tests and consultation note). The examining physician distinguishes between TIA, which is fully reversible within 24 hours (and without evidence of infarction), and stroke, which lasts >24 hours (or <24 hours if there is evidence of infarction). The NIH Stroke Scale (for patients >5 years old) must be readministered at 30 days and 60 days after the event to document the presence and severity of neurologic deficits. Each neurologic event must be subcategorized as: (1) TIA (acute event that resolves completely within 24 hours with no evidence of infarction) (2) Ischemic or hemorrhagic CVA (event that persists >24 hours or <24 hours and associated with infarction on an imaging study) In addition, for patients <6 months old, any of the following: (3) New abnormality on head ultrasound (4) EEG positive for seizure activity with or without clinical seizure
Renal	Acute renal dysfunction (abnormal kidney function requiring dialysis in patients who did not require this procedure before implantation or increase in serum creatinine >3 times normal baseline or >5 mg/dL) and chronic renal dysfunction (increase in serum creatinine of ≥2 mg/dL above baseline or requirement of hemodialysis for at least 90 days)
Hepatic	Increase in any two hepatic laboratory values (total bilirubin, AST, or ALT) to a level >3 times the upper limit of normal 14 days after implantation (or if hepatic dysfunction is the primary cause of death)
Gastrointestinal	Cholecystitis, Crohn disease, diverticulitis, esophagitis, gastroesophageal reflux disease, hiatal hernia, ischemic bowel requiring surgical exploration, pancreatitis with abnormal amylase or lipase requiring nasogastric suction therapy, polyps, or ulcer
Bleeding (coagulopathy, mediastinum or pocket, thorax, gastrointestinal)	Episode of internal or external bleeding in the mediastinum, pocket, thorax, or gastrointestinal system that results in death or the need for reoperation or hospitalization or necessitates transfusions of red blood cells (≥4 U packed red blood cells within any 24-hour period in the first 7 days after implantation or ≥2 U packed red blood cells within any 24-hour period after 7 days after implantation)
Infection (driveline, bloodstream, pulmonary, mediastinum, or pocket)	Driveline, bloodstream, or pulmonary infection accompanied by pain, fever, drainage, or leukocytosis that is treated by antimicrobial agents (nonprophylactic) *Driveline infection:* Positive culture from the skin or tissue or both surrounding the driveline or from the tissue surrounding the external housing of a pump, with the need for treatment, when there is clinical evidence of infection (pain, fever, drainage, leukocytosis). A positive culture from the infected site or organ should be present unless strong clinical evidence indicates the need for treatment despite negative cultures. The general categories of infection are: *Localized nondevice infection:* Infection localized to any organ system or region (e.g., mediastinitis) without evidence of systemic involvement (see sepsis definition), ascertained by standard clinical methods and either associated with evidence of bacterial, viral, fungal, or protozoal infection or requiring empirical treatment *Percutaneous site or pocket infection:* Positive culture from the skin or tissue surrounding the driveline or from the tissue surrounding the external housing of a pump implanted within the body, coupled with the need to treat with antimicrobial therapy, when there is clinical evidence of infection, such as pain, fever, drainage, or leukocytosis *Internal pump component, inflow or outflow tract infection:* Infection of blood-contacting surfaces of LVAD documented by positive site culture. There should be a separate data field for paracorporeal pump that describes infection at the percutaneous cannula site (e.g., Thoratec PVAD) *Sepsis:* Evidence of systemic involvement by infection, manifested by positive blood cultures or hypotension or both
Reoperation (bleeding, infection, wound dehiscence, wound débridement)	Return operation secondary to bleeding, infection, or disruption of the apposed surfaces of a surgical incision requiring surgical repair
Pericardial fluid collection	Accumulation of fluid or clot in the pericardial space that requires surgical intervention or percutaneous catheter drainage This event is subdivided into events with clinical signs of tamponade (e.g., increased central venous pressure and decreased cardiac or VAD output) and events without signs of tamponade

Continued

Event Type	Definition
Device malfunction	Device malfunction denotes a failure of one or more of the components of the MCS device system, which either directly causes or could potentially induce a state of inadequate circulatory support (low cardiac output state) or death. The manufacturer must confirm device failure. A failure that was iatrogenic or recipient-induced would be classified as an iatrogenic/recipient-induced failure Device failure should be classified according to which components fail: (1) Pump failure (blood-contacting components of pump and any motor or other pump-actuating mechanism that is housed with the blood-contacting components). In the special situation of pump thrombosis, thrombus is documented to be present within the device or its conduits that results in or could potentially induce circulatory failure (2) Nonpump failure (e.g., external pneumatic drive unit, electric power supply unit, batteries, controller, interconnect cable, compliance chamber)
Psychiatric episode	Disturbance in thinking, emotion, or behavior that causes substantial impairment in functioning or marked subjective distress requiring intervention. Intervention is the addition of new psychiatric medication, hospitalization, or referral to a mental health professional for treatment. Suicide is included in this definition

ALT, alanine aminotransferase; AST, aspartate aminotransferase; CK-MB, creatine kinase muscle-band; CVA, cerebrovascular accident; ECG, electrocardiogram; EEG, electroencephalogram; LVAD, left ventricular assist device; MCS, mechanical circulatory support; MI, myocardial infarction; NIH, National Institutes of Health; PVAD, paracorporeal ventricular assist device; RVAD, right ventricular assist device; TIA, transient ischemic attack; VAD, ventricular assist device.

CHAPTER **14**

Predischarge and Outpatient Management

Jeffrey Teuteberg and Kathleen L. Lockard

ECHOCARDIOGRAPHY

Echocardiography is an indispensable tool in all patients undergoing cardiac surgery, particularly during the immediate postoperative period. Ventricular function, valvular abnormalities, and the presence and hemodynamic significance of pericardial effusions are easily and quickly assessed with echocardiography. However, in patients with mechanical circulatory support (MCS), there are several specific issues and conditions for which echocardiography can provide valuable information. Although some of these issues are common to all MCS devices, management of patients who have continuous flow devices may involve echocardiography more often both in the immediate postoperative phase and during long-term management. In contrast to pulsatile devices, which mostly fill passively, continuous flow devices actively decompress the left ventricle, and the degree of unloading is affected by pump speed, afterload, and preload. It is crucial to optimize device settings to obtain adequate decompression of the left ventricle without causing suction events. Suction events are the result of overdecompression of the left ventricle to the point where the septal and lateral walls become apposed. Suction events affect pump performance, lead to ventricular arrhythmias, and worsen right ventricular function by diminishing the septal contribution to right ventricular function.[1]

There should be a systematic approach to echocardiographic assessment of patients with left ventricular support. Often echocardiographic windows are limited, especially postoperatively. However, an adequate assessment can usually be achieved with apical four-chamber and five-chamber views alone. Assessment should include the degree of left ventricular decompression, assessment of right ventricular function, cannula position and angulation, and aortic regurgitation. Adequate left ventricular decompression can be judged by the reduction of the left ventricular end-diastolic dimension in the presence of minimal mitral regurgitation and infrequent or absent aortic valve opening (Fig. 14-1). Overdecompression can be determined by the degree that the interventricular septum is shifted left beyond the

midline. Right ventricular function is often difficult to quantitate by echocardiography and is often limited to a gross assessment, but the more dysfunctional right ventricular systolic function is at baseline, the less likely the patient would tolerate a septum that is shifted, even slightly, to the left.[2,3] The degree of tricuspid regurgitation and estimations of pulmonary arterial pressures are also useful in addition to the contractile status of the right ventricle.

The left ventricular apical cannula position and angulation should also be assessed if possible. Although a computed tomography (CT) scan is usually the best means to delineate the precise anatomic positioning of the cannula, echocardiography is often the first screening tool.[4] Sometimes the left ventricular apical cannula may be positioned too deeply into the ventricular cavity or is positioned near a papillary muscle, the chordal apparatus, or prominent trabeculae, or has lateral or septal angulation. A cannula that is not aligned with the central axis of the left ventricle may result in poor filling or, in the case of continuous flow devices, may increase the likelihood of a suction event. Lastly, the degree of aortic regurgitation, if any, should be noted. Worsening of aortic regurgitation results in inadequate effective forward flow because much of the pump output delivered to the ascending aorta regurgitates through the aortic valve, into the left ventricle, and then back into the pump creating a blind loop of blood flow.[5]

In the setting of left ventricular support, right ventricular function is crucial to maintaining pump flow. Right ventricular dysfunction is quite common in patients who have advanced heart failure, especially in the setting of pulmonary hypertension from chronic elevations of left ventricular filling pressures.[6] Right ventricular function may become further compromised after MCS by worsening pulmonary hypertension from acute lung injury, persistently elevated right atrial pressures, or ischemia secondary to compromise of bypass grafts to the right coronary artery. Right ventricular failure after left ventricular assist device (LVAD) implantation leads to a high degree of morbidity and mortality.[7–9]

Right ventricular failure is an important postoperative complication, and diagnosis

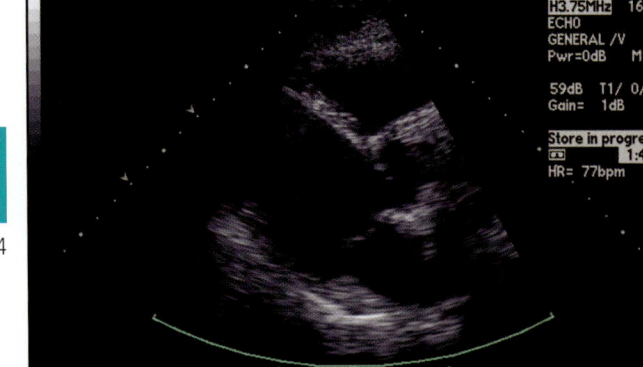

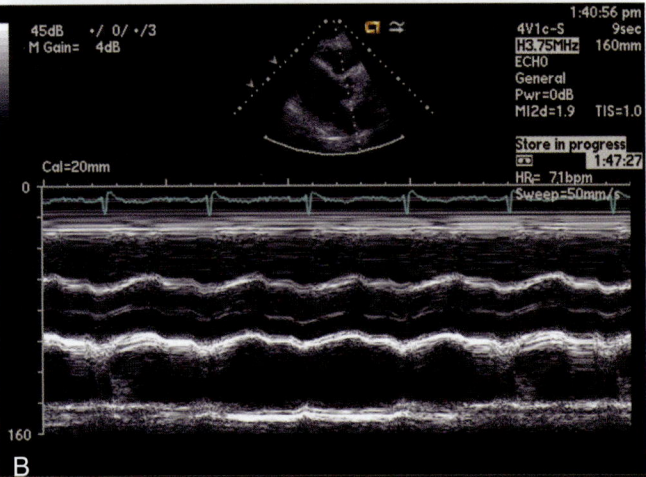

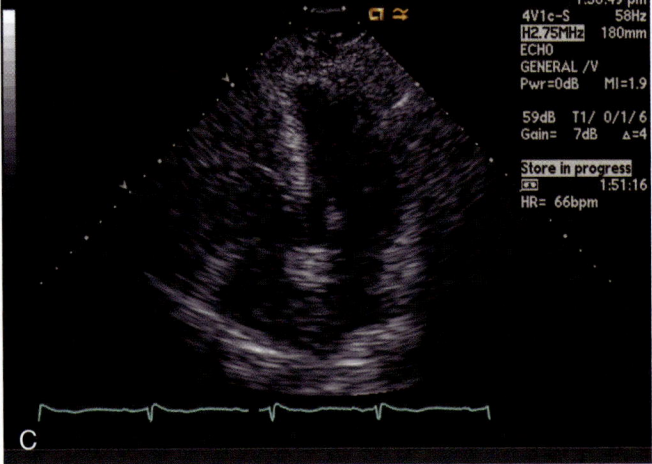

FIGURE 14-1 Echocardiographic assessment of adequate ventricular decompression. **A,** Parasternal long axis view with left ventricular end-diastolic dimension of 5 cm. **B,** M-mode through the aortic valve with little aortic valve excursion during systole. **C,** Apical four-chamber view with interventricular septum near the midline.

and treatment of right ventricular failure can be aided by timely echocardiography. The clinical scenario of right ventricular dysfunction after LVAD implantation is typically marked by high right atrial pressures and low pump flows despite adequate pump speeds and occurs in the setting of right ventricular insults such as pulmonary hypertension or acute lung injury. Although echocardiography is relatively poor at quantifying right ventricular function, it can confirm the clinical suspicion by showing a dysfunctional right

ventricle in conjunction with a poorly filled left ventricle. Echocardiography can also be used to monitor the effect of interventions for right ventricular failure, such as increased inotropy, volume removal, therapy for pulmonary hypertension, or altering pump speed.

Suction events are often heralded by nonsustained ventricular arrhythmias and may be noted by suction detection algorithms, such as in the HeartMate II device (Thoratec Corp, Pleasanton, CA).[4] Suction events can occur in numerous settings: after increasing the speed of the device; with volume loss in the setting of overdiuresis, bleeding, or dehydration from emesis, diarrhea, or insensible losses; sudden decreases in afterload, such as with aggressive treatment of hypertension; or some combination of these factors. Although echocardiography is not always needed to address the suction event, it can confirm the clinical suspicion by showing excessive leftward shift of the interventricular septum. The device speed can be adjusted under direct echocardiographic assessment to return the septum to a midline position, while maintaining adequate decompression of the left ventricle.

Given the rapidly changing hemodynamics immediately postoperatively with frequent alterations in preload, afterload, and right ventricular function, the pump speeds for continuous flow devices are typically set for adequate rather than maximal pump output. However, when the patient is stable, no longer receiving inotropes, and near euvolemia, the pump speed should be adjusted to achieve optimal flows with adequate decompression, but with a safety margin to avoid suction events. Although these adjustments can be made on a clinical basis alone, it is often useful to obtain a ramped speed study with echocardiography to determine the optimal pump speed (Fig. 14-2).[10] The patient first has a baseline study to assess end-diastolic dimension, degree of mitral regurgitation, aortic valve opening, and position of the septum. During the ramped speed study, the speed can be turned up incrementally with repeated echocardiographic assessment until the septum begins to be shifted beyond the midline and into the left ventricular cavity, which would represent the speed at which a suction event may become more likely. The final pump speed is set below this threshold at a point where the septum is midline but the left ventricle is still adequately decompressed.

Obstruction to flow within the pump or its cannulas results in diminished pump performance. Although CT scans provide a more comprehensive assessment of the pump and cannula position for potential cannula kinking, compression, or thrombosis (Fig. 14-3), the initial screening for inadequate flows is often echocardiography. Significant external compression or kinking of the cannula can result in loss of Doppler flow signal in the cannula.[11] Color flow aliasing at the left ventricular apical inflow cannula in combination with abnormally elevated Doppler flow velocities at the inflow cannula may also be a sign of obstruction to flow. Pulsatile flow pumps with velocities greater than 2.3 m/sec at the inflow and greater than 2.1 m/sec at the outflow and continuous axial flow pumps with velocities greater than 2.0 m/sec at the inflow cannula may be abnormal and should prompt further investigation in the appropriate clinical setting.[5,12,13] Lastly, in the setting of a suspected embolic phenomenon, echocardiography may show intracavitary clot or circumferential clot around the left ventricular inflow cannula.

USE OF HEART FAILURE THERAPIES

In patients who receive ventricular assist devices (VADs) as a possible bridge to recovery, many clinicians may attempt to add evidence-based heart failure therapy in an attempt to maximize the chance of recovery; however, there is no evidence base to support the efficacy of such a strategy in this

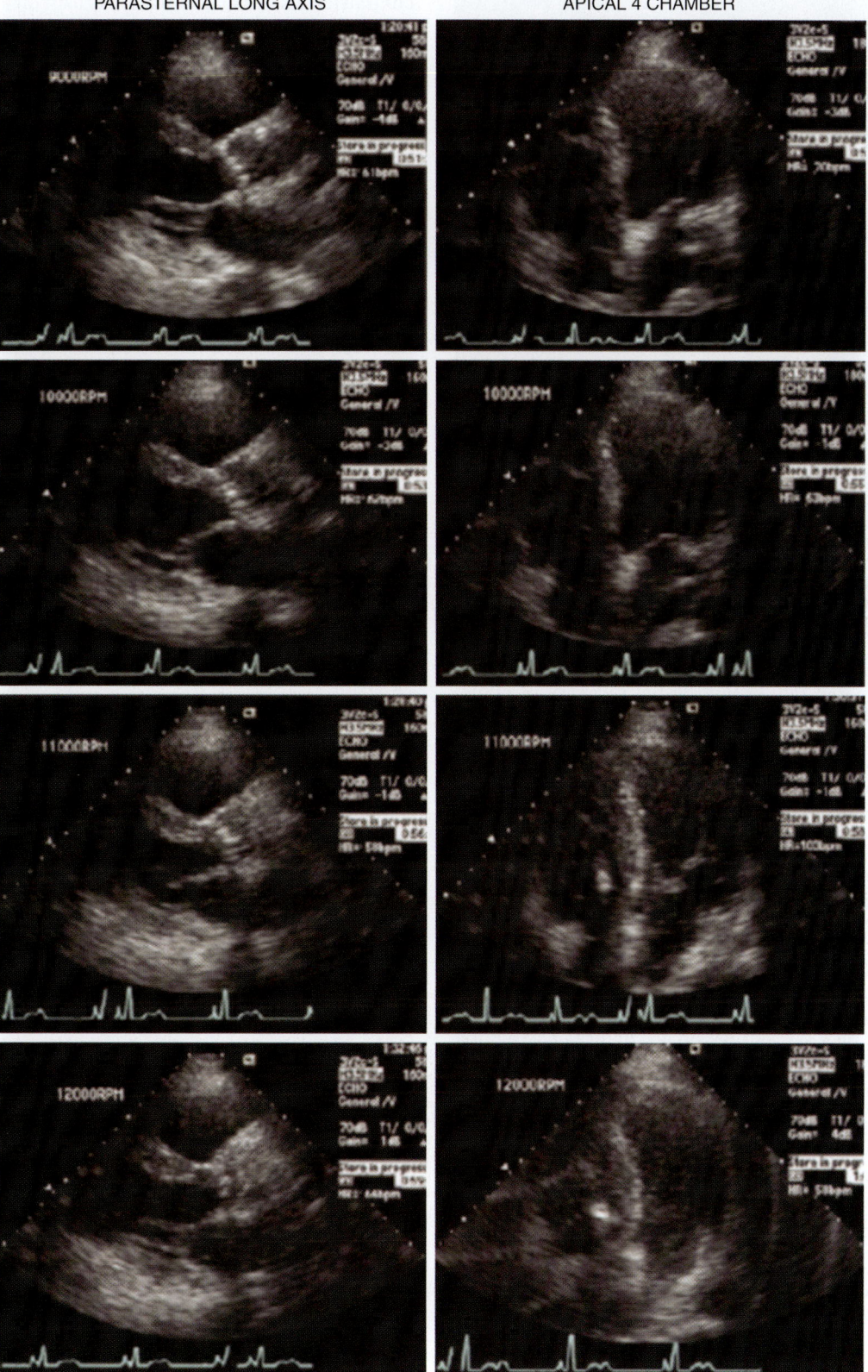

FIGURE 14-2 Echocardiography of patient during ramped speed study (9000 to 12,000 rpm) with a HeartMate II left ventricular assist device (LVAD). At increasing device speeds, there is a greater degree of left ventricular decompression, and the interventricular septum is progressively pulled toward the left ventricle. *(From Slaughter MS, Pagani FD, Rogers JG, et al. Clinical management of continuous-flow left ventricular assist devices in advanced heart failure. J Heart Lung Transplant. 2010;29:S1-S39.)*

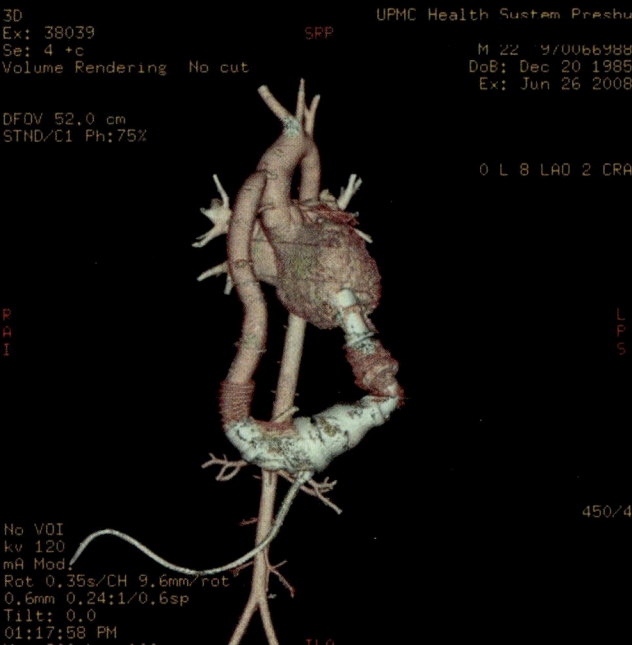

FIGURE 14-3 Three-dimensional computed tomography (CT) reconstruction of HeartMate II device.

setting. An increased rate of myocardial recovery in nonischemic myopathies using an aggressive heart failure–based regimen in addition to the beta$_2$ agonist clenbuterol[14] has been reported; however, clenbuterol is unavailable clinically outside of research protocols. In the setting of bridge to transplant (BTT) and destination therapy, there is no evidence of benefit in terms of outcome or recovery for any accepted heart failure therapy, alone or in combination.

MCS results in acute improvement to the heart failure state,[15] but volume overload typically persists until after discharge and in certain cases may become chronic if not aggressively treated. Numerous conditions may contribute to venous congestion, such as preoperative or postoperative right ventricular dysfunction, renal insufficiency, hypoalbuminemia, or inadequate unloading of the left ventricle owing to lack of optimization of VAD settings or mechanical obstruction to inflow or outflow. Most patients require diuretics at the time of discharge from the hospital after the implantation procedure. Over time, however, after euvolemia is achieved, diuretic use may be decreased or discontinued.

As patients recover after MCS, hypertension is very common, particularly if it was present before implantation. Apart from the long-term benefit of proper hypertension management in general, the increased afterload from hypertension can affect VAD performance and longevity. Pumps produce less flow and less ventricular unloading in the setting of hypertension. With pulsatile pumps, hypertension increases stress on the pneumatic or mechanical drivers, which can increase mechanical wear. Flow in continuous flow pumps is highly afterload dependent: At a constant speed, there is less forward flow in the setting of higher blood pressures. If the blood pressure becomes chronically elevated, the left ventricle becomes persistently inadequately unloaded because of the reduction in forward flow. Among the first-choice drugs for post-MCS hypertension are angiotensin-converting enzyme inhibitors (ACEIs) and angiotensin II receptor blockers (ARBs) because of their afterload reduction and the widespread evidence of their beneficial effects in patients with diabetes and vascular disease, which are common comorbidities in patients undergoing MCS. ACEIs are usually favored over ARBs in such

circumstances mostly because of cost considerations. Renal insufficiency or hyperkalemia may limit the use or dosage of ACEIs and ARBs especially early postoperatively before full renal recovery. For additional antihypertensive control, beta blockers, calcium channel blockers, and alpha blockers may be used.

Beta blockers are useful adjuncts to ACEIs and ARBs for blood pressure control, but caution should be exercised initiating beta blockade in the setting of marginal right ventricular function, especially in the face of persistent volume overload. Beta blockade is also useful for rate control in the setting of atrial and ventricular tachyarrhythmias. There is no evidence base for the routine addition of aldosterone blockade after MCS, and it is typically rarely indicated other than as a means to limit potassium supplementation. Although the renal dysfunction that accompanies advanced heart failure usually improves after MCS,[16] many patients still have some degree of renal insufficiency and may be more susceptible to hyperkalemia in the face of routine use of aldosterone blockade as has been seen in populations with heart failure.[17] Nitrates and hydralazine are useful for afterload reduction in patients who cannot tolerate an ACEI or ARB because of renal insufficiency or hyperkalemia. There is little role for digoxin after MCS except in the setting of atrial fibrillation with rapid rates that affect pump performance and that is not responsive to other medical therapies.

BLOOD PRESSURE MEASUREMENT AND GOALS

Although blood pressure control is important as previously described, there has been no trial evidence for target blood pressure goals for patients on MCS. The INTERMACS (Interagency Registry for Mechanically Assisted Circulatory Support) definition of a hypertension adverse event is new-onset systolic blood pressure greater than 140 mm Hg or diastolic blood pressure greater than 90 mm Hg for pulsatile pumps and mean blood pressure greater than 110 mm Hg for continuous flow pumps. Given the prevalence of vascular disease and diabetes and the mechanical consequences of persistently elevated blood pressure on pulsatile devices, American Diabetes Association blood pressure recommendations (systolic blood pressure <130 mm Hg and diastolic blood pressure <80 mm Hg) are reasonable goals.[18]

As noted previously, blood pressure control for patients with continuous flow pumps is essential to maximize pump output and to ensure adequate decompression of the left ventricle. However, outpatient assessment of blood pressure, especially at home, is difficult because patients may have very little pulsatility, and the blood pressure can be very difficult to auscultate (Fig. 14-4). Clinics that care for patients with continuous flow devices must be equipped with a Doppler probe to assess blood pressure properly (Fig. 14-5). There is no evidence base for blood pressure targets with continuous flow pumps, but a mean blood pressure of 80 mm Hg or less is a reasonable goal.

ARRHYTHMIA MANAGEMENT

Implantable Cardioverter-Defibrillators and Pacemakers

Most patients who receive MCS also have an implantable cardioverter-defibrillator (ICD) alone or in combination with biventricular pacing. In the HeartMate II BTT trial, 76% of patients had an ICD, and in the HeartMate II destination therapy trial, 82% had an ICD.[15,19] In the absence of persistent ventricular arrhythmias, the defibrillator function of an ICD

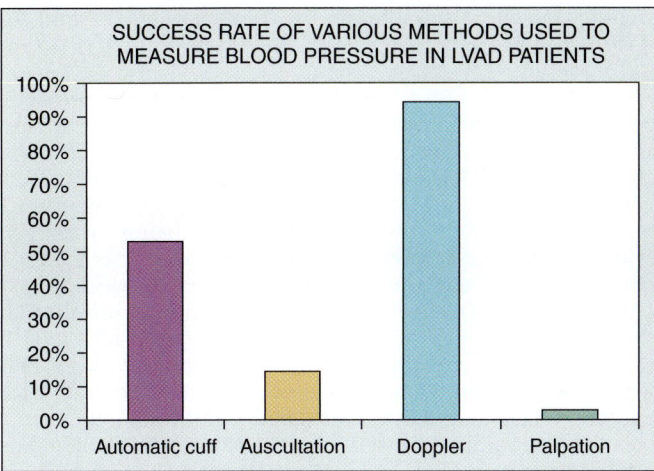

FIGURE 14-4 Successful blood pressure measurement in patients with continuous flow left ventricular assist devices (LVADs). Seventy measurements from 17 patients on continuous flow mechanical circulatory support (MCS) were compared with arterial line blood pressure. *(From Bennet MK, Roberts CA, Dordunoo D, et al. Ideal methodology to assess systemic blood pressure in patients with continuous-flow left ventricular assist devices. J Heart Lung Transplant 2010;29:593-594.)*

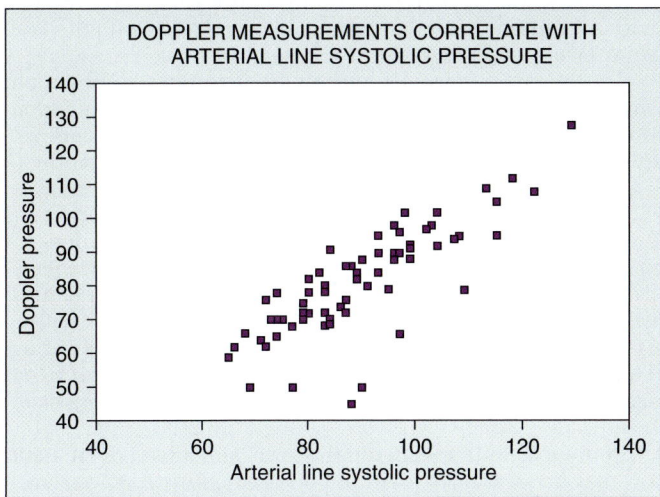

FIGURE 14-5 Correlation of blood pressure measurement by arterial line versus Doppler. *(From Bennet MK, Roberts CA, Dordunoo D, et al. Ideal methodology to assess systemic blood pressure in patients with continuous-flow left ventricular assist devices. J Heart Lung Transplant 2010;29:593-594.)*

should be turned back on postoperatively, and this should be confirmed before discharge from the implant hospitalization. The only patients who should routinely be considered for permanent inactivation of the defibrillator are patients who have biventricular support and are in persistent ventricular tachycardia or ventricular fibrillation. The functions of pacemakers or ICDs, such as backup pacing for bradycardia, biventricular pacing, antitachycardia pacing, and defibrillation, do not adversely affect most current generation pumps or their controlling systems. Rarely, some ICDs and pacemakers may have changes to their programming because of electromagnetic interference from the assist device. Device manufacturers often have a list of such pump-ICD interactions on their websites.

Patients who do not have an ICD before MCS are typically patients who receive MCS after presenting with acute myopathies or postcardiotomy failure. However, for patients who do not have an ICD before MCS, there are no clear data regarding the utility of placing an ICD before discharge, especially in the setting of primary prevention.

Atrial Fibrillation and Flutter

Both atrial fibrillation and atrial flutter are common with advanced heart failure, often persist after implantation, and new-onset atrial arrhythmias are frequent perioperatively. Rate control and adequate anticoagulation are the primary goals of therapy. Atrial arrhythmias may be more likely to occur or recur postoperatively in the setting of volume overload, inadequate decompression of the left or right ventricles, or right ventricular failure. When patients are rate controlled, the major impact of paroxysmal or persistent atrial arrhythmias is an increase in the goal international normalized ratio (INR) in devices that have target INRs less than 2. Poor rate control may cause right ventricular failure in the setting of marginal right ventricular function and poor LVAD filling.

For patients who have had long-standing atrial fibrillation before implantation, relief of the heart failure state may decrease atrial stretch enough to warrant an attempt at restoration of sinus rhythm. However, many patients have such substantial adverse remodeling to their atria that they are unlikely to maintain sinus rhythm even with normalization of hemodynamics. For patients with new-onset atrial fibrillation, it is reasonable to attempt cardioversion, either electrically or pharmaceutically, once they are no longer receiving inotropic support and their volume status has normalized. For patients who have had cardioversion in the setting of an antiarrhythmic, it is reasonable to continue the antiarrhythmic with appropriate follow-up, especially in the case of amiodarone. There is no known long-term advantage to an aggressive pursuit of sinus rhythm in the absence of uncontrolled ventricular rates aside from the anticoagulation requirements in patients with MCS. However, in the setting of atrial arrhythmias with poorly controlled ventricular rates, antiarrhythmics, cardioversion, and atrioventricular nodal ablation with permanent pacing (if an ICD or pacemaker is already in place) all are potential options.[20]

Ventricular Tachycardia and Fibrillation

In the immediate postoperative period, ventricular arrhythmias are also reasonably common. Such arrhythmias may precede MCS or be exacerbated by the postoperative state or by suction events. In the HeartMate II BTT trial, 56% of patients had history of ventricular arrhythmia, and postoperatively 42% had ventricular arrhythmias, most of which were in the first 30 days.[21] Beyond the first month after implantation, sustained ventricular arrhythmias are much less common. Occurrence of sustained ventricular tachycardia or ventricular fibrillation in the outpatient setting can manifest as palpitations, lightheadedness, or an appropriate ICD shock or be discovered on routine interrogation of the device. The effect of persistent ventricular arrhythmias on LVAD function is primarily through the effect of the tachycardia on right ventricular function. The more marginal the right ventricular function and the faster the ventricular rhythm, the more likely patients are to experience right ventricular dysfunction.

Right ventricular dysfunction usually results in underfilling of the left ventricle and hence the LVAD. Patients may experience hypotension and low flow alarms or, in patients with continuous flow pumps, an increased likelihood of suction events. Lastly, in contrast to LVADs, patients who have biventricular assist devices can usually tolerate persistent ventricular tachycardia or ventricular fibrillation without symptoms or a substantial change in hemodynamics. However, such patients may have compromised filling of the right ventricular assist device, a slightly higher long-term risk of thromboembolism, and no backup native heart function if support becomes interrupted through device failure or user error.

In the setting of ventricular arrhythmias, a screen for reversible causes such as electrolyte abnormalities, drugs that may prolong the QTc interval, or, more uncommonly, ischemia is reasonable. Causes of ventricular arrhythmias that are particular to MCS should be recognized, however. With the widespread adoption of continuous flow devices, clinicians have to be aware of the possibility of suction events, as a source for ventricular arrhythmias. Many ventricular arrhythmias that occur with suction events are not sustained but are rather recurrent episodes of premature ventricular contractions or short runs of ventricular tachycardia; however, the arrhythmias may become prolonged or even potentially sustained. In the setting of suction events, there should be a careful review of the patient and device parameters. Lastly, patients may experience new-onset ventricular tachycardia as a result of re-entry around the apical ventricular cannula. The treatment of ventricular tachycardia not related to suction events is otherwise as recommended for patients without MCS and includes beta blockade, antiarrhythmics, or cardioversion.[22] Reprogramming of the ICD may sometimes be necessary to avoid unnecessary or inappropriate shocks. Patients may require mapping and ablation if the rhythms are difficult to control pharmacologically.

Anticoagulation Goals and Bleeding Risks

Most devices, with the exception of the now rarely used HeartMate XVE, require long-term anticoagulation with warfarin. Patients typically have achieved their goal INR before being discharged home from the hospital after implantation; the goal INR ranges for various devices are shown in Table 14-1. It is crucial to have a reliable system to track the INR in all patients on MCS, to maintain a record of their goal level of anticoagulation, to ensure routine INR measurements, and to communicate the necessary changes to warfarin doses to maintain patients in their therapeutic range. Given the complexity of patients who receive MCS, the variety of potential devices, and patients' concomitant medical conditions, the outpatient anticoagulation is typically managed by the MCS team rather than using an anticoagulation clinic or outside physicians.

Goal INR ranges try to strike a balance between the potential risks of thromboembolism or pump thrombosis and bleeding risks. Pulsatile devices with mechanical valves such as the Thoratec paracorporeal ventricular assist device require warfarin with an INR range similar to mechanical heart valves. In contrast to most devices, the HeartMate XVE device does not have mechanical valves and has a textured volume displacement chamber that becomes endothelialized and does not require warfarin, only aspirin. However, with

smaller and more durable pumps available for BTT and for destination therapy, use of the HeartMate XVE has essentially ceased.

In contrast to the declining use of many of the previous generation pulsatile devices, there is increasing use of continuous flow devices such as the HeartMate II.[23] For the HeartMate II BTT trial, the goal INR was 2 to 3. With this goal INR, the rate of bleeding beyond 30 days that required 2 units or more of blood was 0.69 events per patient-year. The rates of hemorrhagic and ischemic strokes were less than 0.1 per patient-year, and the pump thrombosis rate was 0.02 per patient-year.[21] However, a review of 331 patients enrolled in the HeartMate II BTT trial and supported for at least 1 month revealed that thrombotic event rates increased with an INR less than 1.5, and hemorrhagic event rates increased with an INR greater than 2.5. Hemorrhagic and thrombotic events occurred at similar rates with an INR range of 1.5 to 2 versus 2 to 2.5 as seen in Figure 14-6.[24] Many centers have decreased their INR goals for the HeartMate II from 2.0 to 3.0 to 1.5 to 2.0. The postoperative transition from unfractionated heparin to warfarin may be another period where an intensive anticoagulation regimen may not be required for some pumps. A study of 418 patients who received a HeartMate II pump found no short-term increase in risk for thrombotic events and a lower short-term incidence of bleeding events requiring transfusion for patients who were transitioned to warfarin without unfractionated heparin compared with patients who were treated with heparin.[25]

There is no consensus on how frequently the INR should be monitored after the patient is discharged with a therapeutic INR. Monitoring of the INR may be weekly or more frequent until a dose that achieves a stable INR is determined. Thereafter the INR may be assessed monthly in the setting of clinical stability. The availability of home INR monitoring has not been established in patients on MCS but may allow for more frequent monitoring and more rigorous maintenance of INR in the therapeutic range. As in the setting of mechanical valves or atrial fibrillation, warfarin can be held in the setting of supratherapeutic INR values in the absence of bleeding. There is no role for and potential for harm with acute reversal of anticoagulation in the absence of clinically significant bleeding.

In devices with mechanical valves, an INR between 2 and 2.5 may require only a simple dose adjustment of warfarin; alternatively, patients with an INR substantially below the goal range could be treated with home administration of low-molecular-weight heparin, if feasible, or be admitted for heparin bridging. Patients frequently require invasive procedures for which they cannot be therapeutically anticoagulated with warfarin. Most patients are admitted and bridged with heparin, especially with devices requiring the most intense anticoagulation. Patients with continuous flow devices with lower therapeutic INR ranges, such as the HeartMate II, may be able to have many invasive procedures at the lower end of their therapeutic INR.

In the setting of clinically significant blood loss, warfarin may be held or reversed, with caution, if needed. Antiplatelet therapy can be continued in many cases but may also need to be stopped. Devices with higher INR ranges and mechanical valves are likely at the highest risk in these circumstances. Patients with extracorporeal pumps can have the pump housing inspected for clot if anticoagulation needs to be held, but clot that is not evident from visual inspection alone may still be present. Continuous flow devices may be at lower risk for thrombus than pulsatile devices in the setting of complete cessation of anticoagulation. There are cases of continuous flow pumps being managed for days to weeks without any warfarin in the setting of recurrent severe gastrointestinal bleeding. Such situations are the exception, but the risk of

TABLE 14-1	Anticoagulation for Permanent Devices		
Devices	Flow Type	INR Range	
Permanent Left Ventricular Support			
ABIOMED AB5000	Pulsatile	2.5-3.5	
HeartMate XVE	Pulsatile	No warfarin	
HeartMate II	Continuous	1.5-2.0	
HVAD	Continuous	2.0-3.0	
Jarvik 2000	Continuous	2.0-3.0	
MicroMed DeBakey	Continuous	2.0-3.0	
Thoratec PVAD/IVAD	Pulsatile	2.5-3.5	
Permanent Biventricular Support			
Thoratec PVAD	Pulsatile	2.5-3.5	
AbioCor	Pulsatile	2.5-3.5	
SynCardia CardioWest	Pulsatile	2.5-3.5	

INR, international normalized ratio; IVAD, intracorporeal ventricular assist device; PVAD, paracorporeal ventricular assist device.

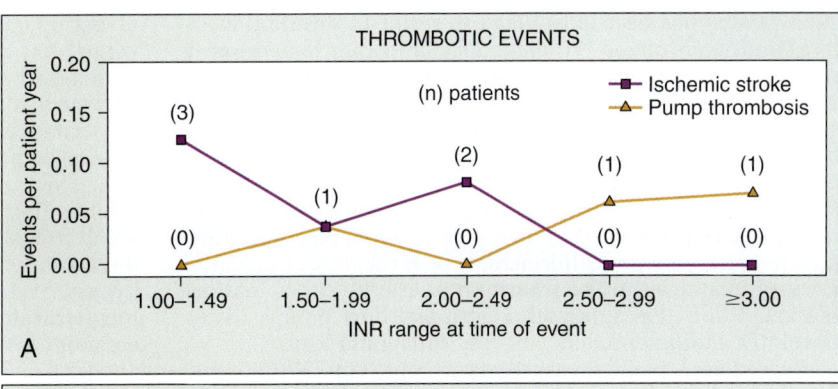

FIGURE 14-6 Thrombotic **(A)** and hemorrhagic **(B)** adverse events through 6 months. Patients are included only for their first event. INR, international normalized ratio; PRBC, packed red blood cells. *(From Boyle AJ, Russell SD, Teuteberg JJ, et al. Low thromboembolism and pump thrombosis with the HeartMate II left ventricular assist device: analysis of outpatient anti-coagulation. J Heart Lung Transplant. 2009;28:881-887.)*

bleeding must be balanced with the risk of thromboembolism or pump thrombosis for each patient, pump, and clinical setting.

Other concomitant medical conditions that may require anticoagulation at or above the level required for the VAD must be considered, such as atrial fibrillation, pulmonary embolism, low LVAD flows, or a mechanical valve.[4] Although some of these indications may be time limited, others may persist throughout the duration of MCS. Persistently low flows may be another situation where anticoagulation may need to be more intense because of the risk of thrombus formation from stasis.

ANTIPLATELET THERAPY

Many devices recommend aspirin, 81 mg/day or 325 mg/day, in addition to a warfarin regimen; however, the necessity of antiplatelet drugs, dosage, and frequency, has not been established. The variety of strategies for antiplatelet therapy can be seen from the HeartMate II BTT trial in Figure 14-7. The prevalence of aspirin resistance ranges widely in the literature from 5.5% to 60% and may be 55% in patients with heart failure.[26,27] In a small study of Thoratec LVADs, aspirin resistance was seen in 26% of patients and persisted weeks after the surgery in some patients.[28] Studies have also shown that markers of persistent platelet activation remain elevated for weeks

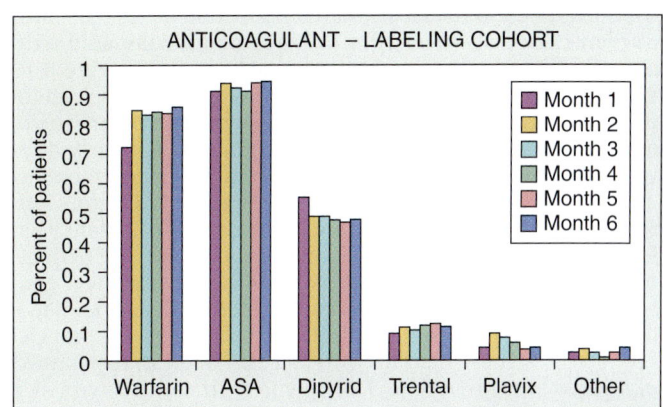

FIGURE 14-7 Antiplatelet therapy in the HeartMate II bridge to transplant trial. ASA, acetylsalicylic acid; Dipyrid, dipyridamole.

after implant surgery.[29] In small studies of patients with continuous flow devices, there have been similar observations of a prolonged elevation of inflammatory markers and impaired platelet function.[30,31]

Rates of significant gastrointestinal bleeding have been noted to be higher in patients with axial flow pumps than in patients with pulsatile pumps.[32] The high sheer stress of such pumps has been postulated to result in destruction of large multimers of von Willebrand factor leading to decreased platelet aggregation and leading to a picture of an acquired von Willebrand disease.[30,33,34] This situation is thought to be similar to the high sheer stress and resultant high rates of bleeding associated with aortic stenosis.[35,36] Although many cases of gastrointestinal bleeding are associated with arteriovenous malformations, it is unclear whether the decrease in platelet aggregation is responsible for more bleeding from occult arteriovenous malformations or if the lack of pulsatility itself may lead to the formation of arteriovenous malformations.[32,34,37,38] Patients with centrifugal flow pumps likely develop a similar deficiency of von Willebrand factor.

Regardless, platelet aggregation and von Willebrand factor activity are seen to return to normal after cardiac transplantation.[33] The evidence of impaired measures of platelet function and the development of an acquired von Willebrand syndrome has led some authors to question the utility of routine antiplatelet therapy in patients with axial flow pumps.[33]

When antiplatelet therapy is used, there is no consensus between the use of fixed dose antiplatelet therapy versus dosing based on platelet function or even the means by which one should assess platelet function if such a strategy is used.[30] As with the use of warfarin, one must also consider other coexisting medical considerations that may require antiplatelet therapy, such as drug-eluting stents, prior cerebrovascular accident, and peripheral vascular disease; such requirements may also be time limited or permanent.

NEUROLOGIC COMPLICATIONS AND RISKS

Neurologic adverse events continue to be a source of morbidity and mortality after MCS. A review of the INTERMACS database found that 14.1% of the deaths after a primary LVAD were attributed to a neurologic event. For patients who died less than 1 month after implantation, 11.6% of deaths were attributable to a neurologic event, whereas the 15.6% of the deaths after 1 month were attributable to a neurologic event.[39] The higher incidence of stroke in the early support period was also noted in the HeartMate II BTT population. The rates of events per patient-year for the first month compared with afterward were 0.37 versus 0.05 for ischemic stroke and 0.18 versus 0.03 for hemorrhagic stroke. The overall stroke rate in this trial was 8.9%, with ischemic strokes occurring more frequently. However, when a patient had a stroke, nearly 40% were fatal. Otherwise, the rate of transient ischemic attack was 2% and rate of other neurologic events was 5%.[15] Overall neurologic adverse event rates in the first year after implantation for primary LVADs was 2.87% or 164 events per 100 patient-months in INTERMACS. There were significantly fewer neurologic adverse events in the first year for patients who had a continuous flow versus a pulsatile LVAD (1.93% vs. 4.33%; $P < .0001$).[39] These data need to be considered in the context of a stroke rate of 1.4% to 3.5% per year in patients with systolic dysfunction who are not on MCS.[40]

The external surface of the inflow cannula, the cannulas, or components of the pump itself may be a source of embolism; however, patients who undergo MCS have numerous other potential sources of emboli. As noted earlier, atrial fibrillation and atrial flutter are common preoperatively, and intra-atrial thrombus may form and subsequently embolize. Another source of embolism may be from the aortic root. The outflow graft of an LVAD is anastomosed to the ascending aorta superior to the sinuses of Valsalva; this, in combination with a lack of or infrequent opening of the aortic valve, may result in an area of stasis in which thrombus may form. Intraventricular thrombus is also common before MCS and may be a source

of perioperative embolism.[41] Careful inspection of the left ventricular cavity for thrombus and being meticulous about its removal are critical to reducing the risk from this source. Although placing MCS off-pump avoids the potential risks associated with cardiopulmonary bypass, these risks must be weighed against the risk of missing significant thrombus that is not always visible on intraoperative transesophageal echocardiography. Perioperative neurologic events may also result from aortic atheroemboli as a result of manipulation of the ascending aorta or prolonged times on cardiopulmonary bypass.[42,43] Lastly, many patients may simply have a higher long-term stroke risk from pre-existing vascular disease of the aorta or carotid or vertebral arteries.

Strategies that may mitigate stroke risk are also crucial to optimize neurologic outcomes. Proper monitoring of warfarin and antiplatelet therapy is a critical first step in this process. Although some pumps may allow for INR goals less than 2, this goal may need to be reconsidered in the face of chronic or paroxysmal atrial fibrillation after MCS.[4] Adequate control of hypertension as noted previously is also an important long-term consideration for the prevention of neurologic adverse events whether the device is pulsatile or continuous flow. For continuous flow devices, setting the pump speed determines the degree of left ventricular unloading and determines the amount of aortic valve opening. Even at speeds below the threshold for suction events, the aortic valve may open rarely if at all. In such settings, stasis of blood between the aortic valve and outflow cannula can result in clot formation that can result in embolism. Many centers set pump speeds considering not only the degree of left ventricular decompression but also the frequency of aortic valve opening. A strategy of setting pump speeds that result in opening of the aortic valve every third cardiac systole may allow for better washing of the aortic root and may be reasonable but has not been validated.[41] The controller for the Jarvik 2000 pump has an algorithm to turn down pump speed intermittently to allow ventricular filling and aortic valve opening with flushing of the aortic root.

DRIVELINE MANAGEMENT

Although the incidence of driveline infection is lower with the current generation of continuous flow pumps, infection still occurs in about 14% of patients.[15,44] Education is the cornerstone to managing the driveline to minimize the occurrence of trauma and the risk of infection. Although the patient frequently does not change his or her own dressing, it is equally important that the patient is aware of the proper techniques for maintaining the driveline as the caregiver tasked with the dressing changes. Driveline dressing changes should be an integral part of the patient and caregiver education and a skill that is formally tested and observed before discharge. The exact protocol differs by institution but involves maintaining the sterility of the site using sterile dressings, proper handwashing, sterile gloves, and masks. The prior dressing is removed, and the site is gently cleaned and inspected for signs of drainage, discharge, bleeding, erythema, tenderness, and the integrity of tissue ingrowth (Fig. 14-8). A new sterile dressing is applied and secured in place. The frequency of driveline dressing changes also varies among institutions, but they generally should be performed more frequently in the setting of drainage or bleeding from the driveline.[45]

Driveline management begins in the operating room with careful consideration of the location of the driveline exit site, in particular, in an obese patient who may be more susceptible to infection.[46] The size of the patient and any physical or anatomic limitations should be considered in the driveline placement. The driveline should also not exit where it might

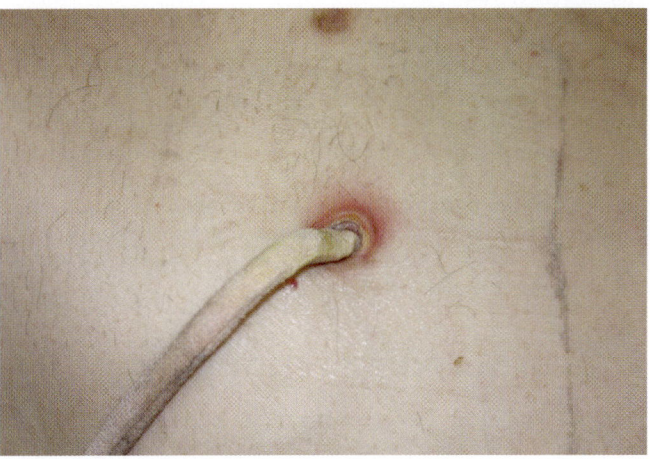

FIGURE 14-8 Infected driveline.

be subject to undue wear or trauma, such as near the patient's belt line. Postoperatively, the driveline not only should be dressed and inspected thoroughly with each dressing change but also should be secured in place distal to the skin exit site and beyond the driveline dressing with a device such as a Hollister tube drain holder (Fig. 14-9). This holder prevents movement of the driveline and limits tension on the driveline at the exit site if the controller is dropped or pulled unexpectedly. The use of abdominal binders may also be helpful in avoiding driveline trauma; however, they must be properly fitted and maintained because they may contribute to exit site injury if they are not properly maintained. Strict adherence to driveline protocol should be emphasized to care for the driveline site and avoid trauma to promote tissue ingrowth and maximize the chance of long-term freedom from driveline infection.

There should be a low threshold for the patient to return to the clinic to inspect and potentially obtain a culture of the driveline site if there is a clinical suspicion of an infection or trauma to the driveline exit site. For a true driveline infection, a prolonged course of intravenous antibiotics is often required. Inadequate treatment results in recurrent infections and may lead to infection of the pump pocket or may cause seeding of the device during episodes of bacteremia. Rarely, a patient with a severe driveline infection may require surgical revision of the site or, if a transplant candidate, urgent listing for transplantation.

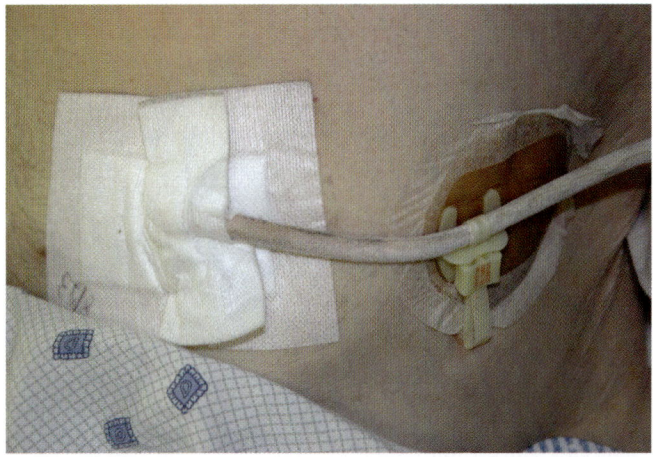

FIGURE 14-9 Driveline dressed and supported with a Hollister.

Before Implantation

Patient education should begin when a patient is referred to the MCS team. The proper approach to education should begin with an understanding of the patient's past medical history and current medical status, occupation, highest education level attained, family support, and living arrangements. Implant strategy (e.g., BTT, destination therapy) is also crucial to the education component; expectations of patients, families, and their support systems differ depending on the length and permanence of MCS. Education before implantation provides a comprehensive assessment of both the patient and his or her support system.

Ideally, implantation of MCS would be performed on an elective basis so that there would be an opportunity for education before implantation. The initial encounter should occur with both the patient and his or her support system present to discuss the reasons for MCS, the potential pumps that may be implanted, how the pumps function, and what to expect postoperatively. Patients should be shown the pump, controller, batteries, and location of the driveline exit site. The initial education also briefly covers what to expect during the postimplantation hospital stay and a general sense of the milestones that need to be achieved before discharge. Lastly, patients should be informed of the limitations that MCS would impose on their lifestyle.

Education before implantation should not be detail-focused but rather provide a general overview. Attempts at education, even on basic or general concepts, quickly allow for the assessment of not only the patient's cognitive and physical abilities (i.e., eyesight, colorblindness, hearing difficulties, motor skills) but also those of the support system and most critically allows early identification of postoperative barriers to education. Such barriers can be addressed to provide an effective and streamlined approach to education postoperatively, a more efficient marshaling of resources tailored to each patient's needs, and means to facilitate patient disposition.

There are limitations to education before implantation. Low cardiac output can affect a patient's ability to process the novelty or volume of the material presented. Patients and their support systems may still have anxiety related to the upcoming surgical procedure, and they may have difficulty fully focusing. An elective procedure provides for the time for numerous shorter sessions to overcome some of these issues, while providing an opportunity for the patient to become more comfortable with the MCS team. Lastly, the opportunity to speak with another patient who is currently on MCS, preferably with the same pump technology, is an extremely useful adjunct to the educational process before implantation.

After Implantation

The educational process after implantation should formally begin after the patient is discharged from the intensive care unit and is stable on the postoperative surgical floors. Although the patient can be expected to be debilitated, the patient ideally should be recovered to the point where he or she is beginning to engage actively with physical therapy. As with the education before implantation, the education after implantation should occur over several days to allow the patient and his or her support system to understand and process the information. However, planning for these sessions should begin as soon as the patient is transferred from the intensive care unit because it can be difficult to accommodate the schedules of both the MCS team and the patient's support system.

The initial education after implantation reviews some of the material from the educational sessions before implantation, such as the patient's need for the device, the basics of device function, and self-care. It is important that all educational sessions are accompanied by written material for reference during the session and for later review. Device-specific education on pump parameters, such as pump flow, rate, and power, is introduced, as is the importance of observing, recording, and assessing trends in these parameters. Non–device-related parameters, such as temperature, weights, and symptoms, and deviations that should prompt specific actions, such as contacting the MCS team, should also be reviewed. Patients are also provided with other important disease-specific information for future reference, such as anticoagulation, diet, exercise, and the changes to their prior medication regimen. Monitoring blood pressure is also an important general concept, and patients with nonpulsatile pumps should be familiarized with use of Doppler-based blood pressure assessment. The home environment is also reviewed for the presence of adequate and reliable power supply, presence of an adequate support system, and the location and type of local first responders.

The next major review is of the function of the device and its accessory components. The operation of the controller system is a major focus of this effort because the controller is the source of device alarms. Each alarm must be reviewed along with the proper response to each alarm. Demonstrations of these alarms using a mock loop not only can better serve to show the alarms but also provide patients with an opportunity for hands-on troubleshooting. The patient and caregivers are provided with device-specific handbooks to enable them to review device components and alarm conditions. Another critical portion of the controller is understanding, manipulating, and managing the connections of the controller to both the pump and the external power supply and batteries.

The means by which a controller is replaced and the circumstances that require a controller change are reviewed. The initial teaching sessions can take place on a mock circuit so that the important components of each step can be emphasized and then repeated by the patient. Changing the device from a fixed external power source to batteries and back again is also demonstrated. Because this is the most common interaction in the device-patient interface, this procedure is repeatedly reviewed and tested.

Driveline dressing changes are also reviewed with the patient, caregivers, and appropriate home nursing care agencies. Although most patients are unable to change their own dressings, it is still important that they are familiar with the entire process to ensure maintenance of a clean and sterile site. Early signs and symptoms of a driveline infection and center-specific driveline management protocols are reviewed. Driveline management is reviewed in more detail subsequently.

Certification of Device Knowledge

The final sessions before discharge should ensure the patient and his or her support system adequately understand the device and its accessories and their function and exhibit an ability to troubleshoot common problems.[47] Each device has a separate written test and assessment of hands-on device management, such as changing power sources and completing a controller change successfully. The patient and family members must successfully pass both the written and the practical components of the competency test to be certified for discharge. In the event of difficulties for either the

patient or caregivers passing these tests, remedial training sessions are required to address the learner's specific needs. Documentation of these tests, the participants, their results, and any remediation are essential components of the educational process. Rarely, the patient may be incapable of passing the competencies and may need to be discharged with a family member who is trained in case of an emergency. Otherwise, the patient may need to be discharged to a VAD-trained rehabilitation or skilled nursing facility until he or she can master the operation of the device or family members can provide sufficient support.

ROLE OF SUPPORT SYSTEM

Family members or direct caregivers function as the first point of contact for the patient in case of emergency. However, many patients return to communities that have never had a patient on MCS, and the MCS center needs to ensure that the local first responders are adequately trained on the device to allow them to assess the patient properly, contact the appropriate personnel in the implanting center, and transport them safely if needed.[48,49] Before discharge, members of the MCS team should meet and educate the local emergency department staff, emergency medical services (EMS) providers, home care staff, and cardiac rehabilitation staff as applicable.

For the above-mentioned care providers, a brief overview of the patient's medical condition, device, lack or presence of pulsatility, VAD dressings, alarms, MCS center contact information, and device patient booklets are provided. Bringing a device and even a mock loop often facilitates this educational process. The emergency department staff and EMS providers are instructed about which signs and symptoms would occur to make the patient contact EMS for transport to either the local emergency department or back to the hospital where the implantation was performed. Basic device functions, alarms, and common device-related adverse events are also reviewed. Local EMS staff may also be encouraged to visit the VAD patient voluntarily, to review the patient's equipment setup and become familiar with the patient and associated supplies. Lastly, the local power utilities should be contacted to inform them that a patient is being discharged home on MCS so that the patient can receive priority in the event of a loss of service.

If a patient requires home care, an agency willing to accept a patient with MCS must be identified and provided with specific criteria for assessing patients and management of the driveline or cannula sites. Home care nurses can be invited to the hospital where the implantation was performed to meet the patient, to obtain proper training and become familiar with the device. Discharge to a skilled nursing facility or rehabilitation services is also occasionally required. These facilities require more intensive training than community first responders. Training sessions should be provided for all staff members, who must then take and pass a written and practical test before the patient can be transferred. In facilities with many staff members or large staff turnover, it is helpful to identify key staff members who can act as "superusers" and provide ongoing training and competency testing to the other workers.

Discharging patients with MCS to the community requires a significant infrastructure and multidisciplinary teamwork. Open communication between the hospital where the implantation was performed, the patient, and community health care providers is essential.[50,51] Formalizing processes and providing written instruction and information reduce misunderstandings between the multiple parties involved in patient care. The MCS nurse coordinator usually serves as the interface between the implantation center and the patient's support system and their local community services.

REHABILITATION

Many patients with prolonged heart failure have considerable debilitation and loss of muscle mass; this is further exacerbated by the surgery and recovery period required after MCS. Early inpatient physical therapy is crucial to begin the process of rehabilitation or to identify patients who may benefit from more intensive inpatient rehabilitation after discharge.[47] Physical therapy should be continued after discharge home either with visiting therapists or with a cardiac rehabilitation center. Many rehabilitation centers require training on the device to be comfortable in designing a program for and supervising patients on MCS. After formal rehabilitation programs are completed, all patients should be encouraged to maintain routine aerobic exercise throughout the duration of support.

REFERENCES

1. Kormos RL, Teuteberg JJ, Pagani FD, et al. Right ventricular failure in patients with the HeartMate II continuous-flow left ventricular assist device: incidence, risk factors, and effect on outcomes. *J Thorac Cardiovasc Surg*. 2010;139:1316–1324.
2. Farrar DJ. Ventricular interactions during mechanical circulatory support. *Semin Thorac Cardiovasc Surg*. 1994;6:163–168.
3. Farrar DJ, Compton PG, Hershon JJ, et al. Right heart interaction with the mechanically assisted left heart. *World J Surg*. 1985;9:89–102.
4. Slaughter MS, Pagani FD, Rogers JG, et al. Clinical management of continuous-flow left ventricular assist devices in advanced heart failure. *J Heart Lung Transplant*. 2010;29:S1–S39.
5. Horton SC, Khodaverdian R, Chatelain P, et al. Left ventricular assist device malfunction: an approach to diagnosis by echocardiography. *J Am Coll Cardiol*. 2005;45:1435–1440.
6. Miller LW, Lietz K. Candidate selection for long-term left ventricular assist device therapy for refractory heart failure. *J Heart Lung Transplant*. 2006;25:756–764.
7. Kavarana MN, Pessin-Minsley MS, Urtecho J, et al. Right ventricular dysfunction and organ failure in left ventricular assist device recipients: a continuing problem. *Ann Thorac Surg*. 2002;73:745–750.
8. Ochiai Y, McCarthy PM, Smedira NG, et al. Predictors of severe right ventricular failure after implantable left ventricular assist device insertion: analysis of 245 patients. *Circulation*. 2002;106:I-198–I-202.
9. Farrar DJ, Hill JD, Pennington DG, et al. Preoperative and postoperative comparison of patients with univentricular and biventricular support with the Thoratec ventricular assist device as a bridge to cardiac transplantation. *J Thorac Cardiovasc Surg*. 1997;113:202–209.
10. Myers TJ, Frazier OH, Mesina HS, et al. Hemodynamics and patient safety during pump-off studies of an axial-flow left ventricular assist device. *J Heart Lung Transplant*. 2006;25:379–383.
11. Kirkpatrick JN, Wiegers SE, Lang RM. Left ventricular assist devices and other devices for end-stage heart failure: utility of echocardiography. *Curr Cardiol Rep*. 2010;12:257–264.
12. Scalia GM, McCarthy PM, Savage RM, et al. Clinical utility of echocardiography in the management of implantable ventricular assist devices. *J Am Soc Echocardiogr*. 2000;13:754–763.
13. Catena E, Milazzo F, Montorsi E, et al. Left ventricular support by axial flow pump: the echocardiographic approach to device malfunction. *J Am Soc Echocardiogr*. 2005;18:1422.
14. Birks EJ, Tansley PD, Hardy J, et al. Left ventricular assist device and drug therapy for the reversal of heart failure. *N Engl J Med*. 2006;355:1873–1884.
15. Pagani FD, Miller LW, Russell SD, et al. Extended mechanical circulatory support with a continuous-flow rotary left ventricular assist device. *J Am Coll Cardiol*. 2009;54:312–321.
16. Kamdar F, Boyle A, Liao K, et al. Effects of centrifugal, axial, and pulsatile left ventricular assist device support on end-organ function in heart failure patients. *J Heart Lung Transplant*. 2009;28:352–359.
17. Juurlink DN, Mamdani MM, Lee DS, et al. Rates of hyperkalemia after publication of the Randomized Aldactone Evaluation Study. *N Engl J Med*. 2004;351:543–551.
18. Executive summary: standards of medical care in diabetes—2009. *Diabetes Care*. 2009;32(suppl 1):S6–S12.
19. Slaughter MS, Rogers JG, Milano CA, et al. Advanced heart failure treated with continuous-flow left ventricular assist device. *N Engl J Med*. 2009;361:2241–2251.
20. Fuster V, Ryden LE, Cannom DS, et al. ACC/AHA/ESC 2006 Guidelines for the Management of Patients with Atrial Fibrillation: a report of the American College of Cardiology/American Heart Association Task Force on Practice Guidelines and the European Society of Cardiology Committee for Practice Guidelines (Writing Committee to Revise the 2001 Guidelines for the Management of Patients With Atrial Fibrillation): developed in collaboration with the European Heart Rhythm Association and the Heart Rhythm Society. *Circulation*. 2006;114:e257–e354.
21. Miller LW, Pagani FD, Russell SD, et al. Use of a continuous-flow device in patients awaiting heart transplantation. *N Engl J Med*. 2007;357:885–896.
22. Zipes DP, Camm AJ, Borggrefe M, et al. ACC/AHA/ESC 2006 Guidelines for Management of Patients With Ventricular Arrhythmias and the Prevention of Sudden Cardiac Death: a report of the American College of Cardiology/American Heart Association Task Force and the European Society of Cardiology Committee for Practice Guidelines (writing committee to develop Guidelines for Management of Patients With Ventricular Arrhythmias and the Prevention of Sudden Cardiac Death): developed in collaboration with the European Heart Rhythm Association and the Heart Rhythm Society. *Circulation*. 2006;114:e385–e484.
23. Holman WL, Pae WE, Teutenberg JJ, et al. INTERMACS: interval analysis of registry data. *J Am Coll Surg*. 2009;208:755–761.
24. Boyle AJ, Russell SD, Teuteberg JJ, et al. Low thromboembolism and pump thrombosis with the HeartMate II left ventricular assist device: analysis of outpatient anti-coagulation. *J Heart Lung Transplant*. 2009;28:881–887.
25. Slaughter MS, Naka Y, John R, et al. Post-operative heparin may not be required for transitioning patients with a HeartMate II left ventricular assist system to long-term warfarin therapy. *J Heart Lung Transplant*. 2010;29:616–624.
26. Gasparyan AY, Watson T, Lip GY. The role of aspirin in cardiovascular prevention: implications of aspirin resistance. *J Am Coll Cardiol*. 2008;51:1829–1843.
27. Mason PJ, Jacobs AK, Freedman JE. Aspirin resistance and atherothrombotic disease. *J Am Coll Cardiol*. 2005;46:986–993.
28. Houel R, Mazoyer E, Boval B, et al. Platelet activation and aggregation profile in prolonged external ventricular support. *J Thorac Cardiovasc Surg*. 2004;128:197–202.
29. Dewald O, Schmitz C, Diem H, et al. Platelet activation markers in patients with heart assist device. *Artif Organs*. 2005;29:292–299.
30. Steinlechner B, Dworschak M, Birkenberg B, et al. Platelet dysfunction in outpatients with left ventricular assist devices. *Ann Thorac Surg*. 2009;87:131–137.
31. Radovancevic R, Matijevic N, Bracey AW, et al. Increased leukocyte-platelet interactions during circulatory support with left ventricular assist devices. *ASAIO J*. 2009;55:459–464.
32. Crow S, John R, Boyle A, et al. Gastrointestinal bleeding rates in recipients of nonpulsatile and pulsatile left ventricular assist devices. *J Thorac Cardiovasc Surg*. 2009;137:208–215.
33. Klovaite J, Gustafsson F, Mortensen SA, et al. Severely impaired von Willebrand factor-dependent platelet aggregation in patients with a continuous-flow left ventricular assist device (HeartMate II). *J Am Coll Cardiol*. 2009;53:2162–2167.
34. Geisen U, Heilmann C, Beyersdorf F, et al. Non-surgical bleeding in patients with ventricular assist devices could be explained by acquired von Willebrand disease. *Eur J Cardiothorac Surg*. 2008;33:679–684.
35. Warkentin TE, Moore JC, Anand SS, et al. Gastrointestinal bleeding, angiodysplasia, cardiovascular disease, and acquired von Willebrand syndrome. *Transfus Med Rev*. 2003;17:272–286.
36. Warkentin TE, Moore JC, Morgan DG. Aortic stenosis and bleeding gastrointestinal angiodysplasia: is acquired von Willebrand's disease the link? *Lancet*. 1992;340:35–37.
37. Letsou GV, Shah N, Gregoric ID, et al. Gastrointestinal bleeding from arteriovenous malformations in patients supported by the Jarvik 2000 axial-flow left ventricular assist device. *J Heart Lung Transplant*. 2005;24:105–109.
38. Veyradier A, Balian A, Wolf M, et al. Abnormal von Willebrand factor in bleeding angiodysplasias of the digestive tract. *Gastroenterology*. 2001;120:346–353.
39. Kirklin JK, Naftel DC, Kormos RL, et al. Second INTERMACS annual report: more than 1,000 primary left ventricular assist device implants. *J Heart Lung Transplant*. 2010;29:1–10.
40. Pullicino PM, Halperin JL, Thompson JL. Stroke in patients with heart failure and reduced left ventricular ejection fraction. *Neurology*. 2000;54:288–294.
41. John R, Kamdar F, Liao K, et al. Low thromboembolic risk for patients with the HeartMate II left ventricular assist device. *J Thorac Cardiovasc Surg*. 2008;136:1318–1323.
42. Clark RE, Brillman J, Davis DA, et al. Microemboli during coronary artery bypass grafting: genesis and effect on outcome. *J Thorac Cardiovasc Surg*. 1995;109:249–257.
43. Moazami N, Roberts K, Argenziano M, et al. Asymptomatic microembolism in patients with long-term ventricular assist support. *ASAIO J*. 1997;43:177–180.
44. Zierer A, Melby SJ, Voeller RK, et al. Late-onset driveline infections: the Achilles' heel of prolonged left ventricular assist device support. *Ann Thorac Surg*. 2007;84:515–520.
45. Chinn R, Dembitsky W, Eaton L, et al. Multicenter experience: prevention and management of left ventricular assist device infections. *ASAIO J*. 2005;51:461–470.
46. Raymond AL, Kfoury AG, Bishop CJ, et al. Obesity and left ventricular assist device driveline exit site infection. *ASAIO J*. 2010;56:57–60.
47. Wilson SR, Givertz MM, Stewart GC, et al. Ventricular assist devices the challenges of outpatient management. *J Am Coll Cardiol*. 2009;54:1647–1659.
48. MacIver J, Ross HJ, Delgado DH, et al. Community support of patients with a left ventricular assist device: the Toronto General Hospital experience. *Can J Cardiol*. 2009;25:e377–e381.
49. Seemuth SC, Richenbacher WE. Education of the ventricular assist device patient's community services. *ASAIO J*. 2001;47:596–601.
50. Drews TN, Loebe M, Jurmann MJ, et al. Outpatients on mechanical circulatory support. *Ann Thorac Surg*. 2003;75:780–785.
51. El-Menyar AA. Multidisciplinary approach for circulatory support in patients with advanced heart failure. *Expert Rev Cardiovasc Ther*. 2009;7:259–262.

Psychosocial and Quality-of-Life Issues in Mechanical Circulatory Support

Kathleen L. Grady and Mary Amanda Dew

The use of mechanical circulatory support (MCS) as a therapy for end-stage heart failure is associated with a number of psychosocial considerations for both patients and their families. These considerations span the process of care: they encompass factors including evaluation, informed consent, and decision-making before implantation; health-related quality of life (HRQOL) and behavioral outcomes during and after MCS implantation; and end-of-life concerns. Like many other medical interventions, the success of MCS is ultimately judged by its ability not only to prolong life, but to maximize psychosocial and physical well-being. Hence, it is critical for health care providers and researchers alike to understand the key psychosocial issues that emerge at each step in the process of MCS intervention, as well as the empirical evidence available regarding them. Better understanding of the issues and related evidence is important for improved education of patients and their families when MCS is a treatment option. It is also important for the development and evaluation of new strategies to maximize psychosocial outcomes in patients receiving MCS.

This chapter discusses relevant psychosocial issues across the process of MCS intervention, organized according to the model depicted in Figure 15-1. We consider the issues from the perspective of providing better clinical care, and we note research findings that usefully inform this care. In the final section of the chapter, we delineate the most pressing clinical and research concerns that must be addressed in future work on psychosocial factors in MCS. Throughout the chapter, although we consider many psychosocial factors that are relevant to use of MCS in all age groups, our primary focus is on adult populations because of the increasing use of MCS in adults, particularly for extended periods.

PREIMPLANTATION CONSIDERATIONS

Whether patients receive MCS is determined by a variety of medical and psychosocial factors. Medical indications for MCS are discussed elsewhere in this volume; we review here the range of psychosocial factors that appear to influence access to

and patient preferences for this treatment. Then, among patients undergoing evaluation for MCS, we delineate the psychosocial issues that must be assessed in determining eligibility for bridge or destination MCS implantation, and we discuss procedures for ensuring patient and family informed consent for this treatment.

Disparities in Access to Mechanical Circulatory Support

Disparities in access to health care, including organ transplantation, have received extensive documentation; there are enduring disparities based on ethnicity, sex, geographic region, and socioeconomic status.[1-3] Emerging evidence suggests that similar psychosocial disparities exist for access to MCS. Some disparities have reflected the limitations of MCS technology. For example, the larger fully implantable pulsatile devices that predominated in the 1990s and early 2000s were not compatible with female patients' typically smaller body habitus. Thus, the proportion of MCS recipients who are women have under-represented the proportion of women with the end-stage disease who could benefit from this therapy.[4]

There are additional psychosocial disparities in access to MCS that are less easily explained by barriers in MCS technology. Joyce and colleagues[5] provided the first comprehensive analysis of a range of such factors. They examined a large national database on interventions used for patients admitted to U.S. hospitals from 2002 to 2003 with diagnoses of congestive heart failure or cardiogenic shock. Patients younger than 18 years of age and older than 85 years were excluded, as were those with diagnoses that represented clear contraindications to MCS implantation. They found that, even after controlling for severity of medical comorbidities, patients who were older than 65 years of age, female, and African American were less likely to receive MCS. In addition, there were marked geographic variations, with patients from the western U.S. showing an increased likelihood of receiving MCS relative to all other regions.

The Joyce study[5] showed that the ethnic and regional variations in MCS did not vary according to patient medical factors, or by

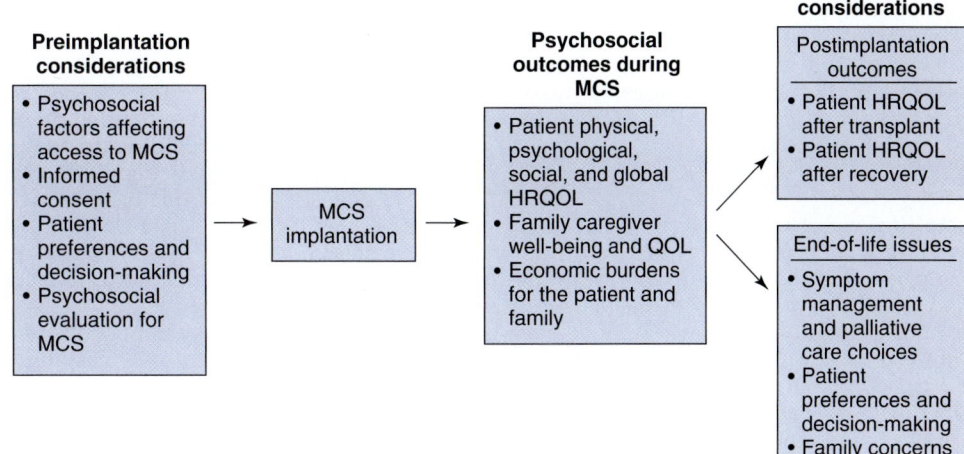

FIGURE 15-1 Psychosocial factors at each stage of the mechanical circulatory support (MCS) process. HRQOL, health-related quality of life; QOL, quality of life.

whether, for example, patients were admitted to academic versus nonacademic centers for care. Being admitted to an academic center was associated with a greater rate of MCS implantation and, in fact, African Americans were more likely to be admitted to academic medical centers. However, African Americans remained less likely than European Americans to receive MCS, even at academic centers. Interestingly, neither insurance status nor mean income in the communities where patients resided affected their likelihood of receiving MCS. Neither characteristic affected the association of ethnicity with receipt of MCS.

Similar to what has been observed in organ transplantation, it is likely that the ethnic group disparities noted by Joyce and colleagues[5] reflect a combination of referral practices and biases, as well as patient preferences for care. We address patient preferences later; we note here that further work is needed to delineate the underlying causes of unequal access to MCS so that appropriate steps can be taken to reduce or eliminate them.

Informed Consent

Impact on Patients

Informing patients with advanced heart failure and their families about therapeutic options necessarily includes discussing the patient's current medical condition, risks, benefits, need for self-management, effect on lifestyle, costs, caregiver burden, and end-of-life considerations for each option. Conversations to inform patients about their current medical condition would include a discussion of the patient's severity and prognosis of heart failure, presence and severity of comorbidities, and the current treatment plan. For patients who are hospitalized with acute heart failure, the treatment plan may include intravenous diuretics, nitrates, and use of inotropes, whereas refractory cardiogenic shock may require intra-aortic balloon pumping or short-term percutaneous or extracorporeal support.[6,7] Outpatient management may include additional cardiac risk stratification and further optimization of medical therapy,[8] along with assessment of comorbidities and potential referrals to other medical specialists and psychologists or social workers to address concurrent psychosocial, behavioral, environmental, and financial problems.

The option of continuing with medical therapy typically includes discussing advanced heart failure and its natural history, that is, the trajectory of end-stage heart failure and poor prognosis, likelihood of increasing symptom burden and declining functional status, poor quality of life, caregiver burden, future optimal medical management with the availability of concurrent supportive care (including palliative care and hospice), the potential for frequent hospital readmissions, costs, and advance care planning.[9] It is important that patients understand the risks and benefits of medical therapy, as well as the plan for continued care. It is important for patients and families to talk with members of the multidisciplinary team, including cardiologists, surgeons, ventricular assist device coordinators, the palliative care and hospice teams, social worker, and others.

When discussing the option of MCS, it is important to discuss benefits and risks for the specific device being recommended for implantation (overall and specific to the hospital where the device will be implanted) and the implantation strategy (for example, as a bridge to heart transplantation [BTT] or destination therapy [DT]). Potential benefits of improvement in survival, quality of life, and function need to be balanced with possible risks, including device-related adverse events such as bleeding, stroke, and infections, as well as concurrent or new comorbid conditions.[10–12] Although to some extent the risks will always be patient specific, the results from large published trials should be included in these discussions. In addition, potential symptoms, including fatigue, anxiety, depression, pain, and difficulty sleeping, need to be discussed with patients.[13] Length of hospitalization, recovery, and hospital readmission after MCS implantation are also important topics.[10] Regarding implantation strategy, patients need to understand that a given strategy might change after surgery. For example, patients who receive an implant as BTT and experience a serious, irreversible device-related complication may be removed from the waiting list for heart transplantation, and the MCS device would remain in place until the end of the patient's natural life. On the other hand, patients may receive MCS as DT, but exclusions to transplantation may be reversed with device therapy, and listing for transplantation may then become an option. Finally, a discussion of device durability and the option of device replacement, if medically beneficial and desirable, is important at the time of initial implantation.[14]

Discussions regarding self-management and changes in lifestyle should include the topics of device management and troubleshooting, dressing changes, permitted activities (e.g., return to work and home management), and activities that may not be permitted (e.g., immersion in water such as swimming, and driving). In addition, following a "heart healthy" diet and being active, including participating in a formal rehabilitation program or home exercise program, are important topics of discussion. Furthermore, patients need to learn about important safety issues in the home environment and community such as power supply, telephone services, and a plan for urgent/emergent return to the hospital. Costs associated with MCS implantation (including at the time of implantation and after discharge) are also important topics of discussion with patients and their families when deciding on therapeutic options.

Impact on Family and Caregivers

The lifestyle changes may impose burden on caregivers as well. It is expected that patients on MCS will have primary caregivers in order to be discharged from the hospital. Most caregiving for patients with major chronic illnesses is performed by family members.[15] Many device programs require that a device-trained person remain close to the patient at all times, which may impose stress and financial strain if the device-trained person is also employed. Also, additional caregiver burden may occur if patients on MCS suffer an adverse event, such as a stroke, with a permanent neurologic deficit. Thus, caregivers also need to be engaged in conversation when options are chosen so that they can learn about the significant commitment to care for which they may become responsible, including dressing changes, troubleshooting device malfunction, driving to follow-up appointments and tests, and initiating plans for emergency return to the hospital for device-related complications. Caregivers also need to be informed that they may experience psychological sequelae, including depression, anxiety, and post-traumatic stress disorder.[16,17]

End of Life

Discussing end of life is difficult, but necessary, in the context of MCS options. When and how much information to share about end of life is individualized and based on patient characteristics (including patient preferences and goals), clinical risk factors (e.g., high surgical risk), and implant strategy. For example, a less detailed discussion of end of life may be undertaken for patients receiving MCS as BTT, whereas more information may be appropriate for patients who receive implantation as a bridge to candidacy (BTC) or especially as DT. An end-of-life conversation, at the appropriate time, includes a discussion of anticipated end-of-life trajectories, availability of hospice, and device deactivation.[10,18]

In addition to discussing options with members of the MCS team, it may be helpful for patients to talk with other patients who have received MCS, preferably the same device as that being recommended to the patient. Participation in support groups is also highly encouraged. Written information or videos regarding device management, troubleshooting, and dressing change procedures, as well as illustrations of the device are important educational supplements during the informed consent process. Patients also may want to see the actual hardware and accessories. Discussions about treatment options require verification of patient and family understanding of relevant information.

Patient Preferences and Decision Making

Patient decision making regarding MCS implantation is based on the "process" of informed consent that ideally includes the components identified previously. Decision making may take time as patients consider their diagnosis, prognosis, treatment options, and effect on future survival and quality of life. The process may be complicated if the patient's level of acuity and cognitive capacity preclude decision making. This is a less-than-ideal situation because the burden on the family may be high, especially if expected patient outcomes are poor. Families may be faced with decisional conflict and uncertainty about the course of action to take, especially if there are high risks and the potential for poor patient outcomes. If possible, insertion of a short-term percutaneous or extracorporeal device as a bridge to longer-term MCS or transplantation would provide time to stabilize the patient, evaluate the next steps, and allow the family, and possibly the patient, time to consider options.[7] Advance directives can provide guidance for family members who must make emergent decisions regarding treatment options on behalf of a critically ill family member.[14] Appointment of a surrogate decision maker before surgery may prove important if patients lose the capacity for decision making after surgery.[18]

Furthermore, after being fully informed of all available therapeutic options, some patients with advanced heart failure may choose medical therapy, which may be viewed as a refusal of lifesaving therapy. Patients with decision-making capacity who understand the risks and benefits of medical therapy and the consequences of refusing MCS device implantation are, of course, permitted to make this choice.[19] Understanding patient values, preferences, goals, culture, and background may help to clarify the patient's choice of medical therapy.[9] Consultation with bioethics, social work, and psychiatry may be helpful to patients and families as they consider options.[19] Furthermore, health care professionals may have trouble with this choice and see it as conflicting with their own ethics of providing care. An ethics consultation not only can be helpful for the patient and family but can help reassure health care professionals that they have done their job and that the patient may legitimately decide to refuse treatment (i.e., it is not because the patient is depressed or unable to make a competent decision).

Current State of the Literature on Patient Preferences and Decision Making

Decision making by patients with advanced heart failure has received some examination in the literature, although not always directly in the context of MSC issues. In a recent study, ambulatory patients with heart failure overestimated their life expectancy compared with model-based predictions for survival, using the Seattle Heart Failure Model.[20] Furthermore, greater disease severity (i.e., higher New York Heart Association [NYHA] class and lower ejection fraction) was independently related to overestimation of life expectancy. Reasons for this discordance in patient with heart failure versus model estimations of survival were not clear, but may have included inadequate communication between clinicians and patients, patient-specific factors (e.g., hope and optimism), and language or cultural barriers.[20] The researchers suggested that a better understanding of prognosis and life expectancy may be important to decision making about advanced cardiac therapies, including MCS. Many patients with advanced heart failure may not have had the severity of their prognosis discussed, and discussions during consideration for MCS may be startling and affect their ability to comprehend the limited alternative options available and their poor prognosis.

Beyond estimates of survival time, patients with advanced heart failure have been queried regarding their preferences for quality versus quantity of life.[21–24] The implication of preference-based studies is that patient preferences would, in turn, influence their decisions about treatment. Stanek and colleagues[21] determined that more patients with heart failure (67% NYHA class III to IV) preferred improvement in symptoms rather than longer survival as the therapeutic outcome. Likewise, Lewis and coworkers[22] reported that patients favored better perceived health versus survival time with greater severity of heart failure (i.e., lower peak oxygen consumption, higher functional class, and higher jugular venous distention).

MCS was examined as a specific treatment option in only two studies on decision making. Using the standard gamble technique, Moskowitz and colleagues[24] elicited preferences from patients with a BTT left ventricular assist device (LVAD) before LVAD implant, during LVAD support, and after heart transplantation. Before LVAD implantation, patients with end-stage heart failure were willing to accept up to a 45% chance of dying in return for undergoing a treatment designed to return them to full health; however, within 3 months of implant, they were only willing to assume a mortality risk of up to 19% to improve health.[24] In short, they became more satisfied with their health and less willing to accept risks to improve it further. Using a treatment tradeoff tool, MacIver and associates[23] determined treatment preferences among patients with NYHA class II and IV heart failure. In rank order, patients preferred oral inotropes, LVAD implantation, and medical management, which did not differ by NYHA class. Only three patients were introduced to DT LVADs as a treatment option.[23] This is an important limitation of this study. Unfortunately, there are no studies of patient preferences in the current era where application of MCS as a long-term alternative to transplantation, or DT, is the predominant strategy.

An understanding of patient decision making can also be gained through examining regret after having made a treatment decision. Regret is "remorse or distress over a decision."[25] Grady and colleagues[26,27] examined regret in patients who underwent ventricular assist device (VAD) implantation. Patients were asked "if you had to do it all over again, would you decide to have a VAD implant knowing what you know now?" The vast majority of patients at 2 weeks[26] and 1 month[27] after VAD implantation responded "yes" (87% and 91%, respectively). It is unknown if patients experience regret and if it is related to HRQOL in the longer term after VAD implantation. Given the significant impact of VAD implantation on the daily lives of patients (especially patients receiving DT VAD), regret is an important area of study.

Psychosocial Evaluation for Mechanical Circulatory Support

Earlier we addressed the issue of psychosocial disparities in access to MCS—that is, the issue of who is entitled to receive consideration for device implantation. Although disparities in *access* are inherently unfair and unethical, MCS programs must legitimately weigh psychosocial as well as medical factors for each candidate for MCS therapy to appropriately *select* patients who are mostly likely to benefit from device implantation, as either BTT, BTC, or DT. Psychosocial factors must also be examined to determine whether psychological, behavioral, or other psychosocial interventions might usefully be offered to patients to increase their chances of favorable outcomes after MCS implantation.

Surprisingly, the specific components of the psychosocial evaluation have received relatively little attention in the MCS literature. This omission is noteworthy given the extensive scrutiny that other medical factors have received as potential criteria for the selection of optimal candidates for MCS.[28,29] In general, it has been proposed that the factors typically evaluated in potential transplantation candidates also be included in the evaluation of candidates for MCS.[29,30] Thus, important elements to be assessed are listed in Table 15-1 and include lifetime history of psychiatric disorders; history and current substance use or abuse; past and current level of adherence to medical regimens; cognitive capacity and ability to understand what will be required for care with an MCS; social history and current status, including financial circumstances; the availability of a primary family caregiver and general support from the family; and personal expectations of and knowledge about MCS.

TABLE 15-1	Components of the Psychosocial Evaluation of Candidates for Mechanical Circulatory Support (MCS)
Component	**Areas Addressed**
Mental health history and current status	Mood and anxiety disorders; suicidal ideation or past attempts; psychosis; personality disorders; treatment history
Substance use history and current status	Quantity, frequency, and recency of use of alcohol, tobacco, and other substances; symptoms of abuse or dependence; treatment and rehabilitation history
Adherence history and current status	Adherence to components of previous treatment regimens for heart disease or other chronic health conditions (e.g., taking medications, completing medical procedures and routine evaluations, adhering to lifestyle recommendations regarding diet and exercise)
Cognitive functioning and capacity	Orientation in person, time, and place; appearance and affect; insight into health condition; cognitive status (e.g., attention and concentration, memory, visuospatial skills); ability to understand what will be required for care during MCS and (if relevant) after transplantation
Social history and current status	Employment and financial circumstances; marital status; living arrangements; coping strategies for managing health issues; religious beliefs and orientation; concurrent stressors (work-related, home-related, other)
Family caregiver availability and general family supports	Presence of a family member to provide care and assistance on a daily basis; emotional supportiveness of family or close friends; understanding by family of patient's health situation
Personal expectations and knowledge about MCS and (if relevant) transplantation	Perceptions of medical condition; perceptions of health-related impairments in daily life; expectations and understanding of the risks and benefits of MCS; understanding of the transplant process (if relevant)

Of these elements, psychiatric and substance use history, cognitive status, medical adherence history, and the presence of a family caregiver are most often noted as important for team decisions about patients' eligibility for MCS, as well as for decisions about whether specific psychosocial interventions should be offered. With respect to eligibility, for example, presence of a family caregiver and availability of other supports from the family and friends are essential for guaranteeing that patients can be safely discharged to home after device implantation, and patients must be free from cognitive impairments (or have adequate caregiver support to overcome any impairments) that would limit their understanding of basic MCS functioning and maintenance.[29,31] Caution is required if potential candidates have cognitive impairments that render them unable to learn the device alarms, because this creates a significant dependence on the presence of the caregiver and increases the risk for significant complications due to lack of understanding.

An important distinction, however, in considering psychosocial factors as eligibility criteria concerns whether patients are being considered for BTT, BTC, or DT. If MCS is to be used for BTT, the psychosocial criteria used for transplantation candidacy would clearly be relevant, albeit with some modifications. For example, a greater emphasis is typically placed on ensuring the availability of a family caregiver during the period of MCS, compared with the family caregiver requirements usually demanded for transplantation eligibility. In addition, although abstinence from substance use is often considered important for MCS eligibility, the duration requirement imposed is likely to be less than that typically applied for transplantation candidates, most often because of the urgent need for MCS. The duration requirement might instead affect whether the MCS device is implanted as BTT rather than BTC. Thus, if a patient were unable to meet transplantation eligibility criteria regarding duration of abstinence at the time of the MCS psychosocial evaluation, or needed to demonstrate an enduring ability to adhere to treatment requirements, the psychosocial evaluation might result in a patient receiving MCS as BTC rather than BTT. Then, once the duration criteria were met, the patient might transition to BTT. This might also be the case for patients receiving MCS emergently and for whom a full psychosocial evaluation to determine eligibility for eventual transplantation cannot immediately be undertaken. In this regard, it is noteworthy that among the 157 patients entered into the Interagency Registry for Mechanically Assisted Circulatory Support (INTERMACS) database through December, 2007 as BTC rather than BTT at the time of implantation, 38% (n = 60) were considered not yet eligible for transplantation due to psychosocial factors (including current substance use in almost half of these cases, n = 28).[32]

Patients who are being considered for DT, however, may require a somewhat different approach in the application of any psychosocial criteria. These individuals are, by definition, not candidates for heart transplantation. Thus, the psychosocial criteria applied for heart transplantation eligibility—which evolved in response to the need to maximize the utility of scarce donor organs—may be only partially relevant. Because MCS devices are not in short supply (as are donor organs for heart transplantation), it has been argued that there may be few compelling reasons to deny patients DT based on, for example, factors related to continued substance use, or permanent cognitive disability—factors that would generally preclude transplantation candidacy.[14] For patients being considered for DT, the goal of applying psychosocial criteria should be to determine that patients are able, when drawing on the full range of resources that can be mustered for them, to live with MCS at home. A complication, however, in "relaxing" the application of psychosocial criteria for DT patients is the reality that some of these patients may ultimately move toward transplantation, becoming potential transplantation candidates. Under such circumstances, patients would require a re-evaluation of their psychosocial eligibility for transplantation, and the psychosocial standards more typically applied for transplantation candidacy then would become relevant.

PSYCHOSOCIAL OUTCOMES DURING MECHANICAL CIRCULATORY SUPPORT

Psychosocial outcomes in the field of cardiac replacement therapy encompass all the components of patient HRQOL.[33] HRQOL is multifaceted and encompasses physical functional well-being, emotional and social functioning, as well as global quality-of-life perceptions. In the following, we consider evidence regarding patient HRQOL and also summarize evidence concerning family caregiver well-being and quality of life. Finally, the economic burdens experienced by patients and their families are important issues to address insofar as the financial costs associated with MCS ultimately may affect access to this treatment and preferences for it versus other intervention strategies.

Patient Health-Related Quality of Life

Physical Functional Health-Related Quality of Life

Over the past 15 to 20 years, there has been consistent evidence that both objective measures (e.g., exercise capacity) and subjective measures of physical functioning (e.g., perceived functional status) improve during MCS. The bulk of the evidence comes from anecdotal reports and small case series.[34–38] However, a growing number of larger-scale single- or multi-site studies also indicate that once patients have recovered from the immediate effects of implantation, the majority become fully ambulatory, are discharged from the hospital, and are able to engage in routine activities of daily living.[11–13,39–42] Regardless of whether they received implantation as BTT or DT, they showed marked improvements over their preimplantation baseline in functional status (e.g., NYHA class; distance traveled in the 6-minute walk test) and physiologic parameters (e.g., mean oxygen consumption levels, resting cardiac output, and mean arterial pressure).[11,12,41–48] Among patients receiving MCS implantation as BTT, objectively assessed functional status, as well as their perceptions of physical well-being, are better than those of heart transplantation candidates not requiring MCS.[39] Similar advantages are seen in patients on DT compared with individuals who receive optimal medical management rather than DT.[42,46] MCS patients' perceptions of their physical functioning have been found to be indistinguishable from perceptions among transplant recipients,[39,49] and their objectively assessed functional capacity can improve to resemble capacity levels observed in heart transplant recipients.[44]

An important issue is whether and how patients' physical functional HRQOL continues to change over time after implantation. Among patients receiving MCS as BTT, Grady and coworkers[26] found reductions in self-reported bothersome physical symptoms as early as 2 weeks postimplantation, and several studies have documented sustained or continued gains in patients' overall physical functioning and satisfaction with physical status across the first year postimplantation.[13,39,50,51] Although few empirical studies have followed patients with BTT therapy beyond the first year, one report found that both patients implanted with continuous flow as well as pulsatile devices showed physical functional improvements throughout a 2-year observation period.[12]

Patients receiving DT appear to show continued benefits over time as well. Thus, in the REMATCH (Randomized Evaluation of Mechanical Assistance for the Treatment of Congestive Heart Failure) study, transplant-ineligible patients randomized to receive MCS as DT (rather than receiving optimal medical management) showed physical functional status gains even by the first month postimplantation despite the occurrence of adverse events such as bleeding and infection.[52] These gains continued and were maintained at 1 year postimplantation, relative to patients receiving medical management.[42] The gains were observed despite the level of severity of illness at the time of implantation, with patients on MCS requiring inotropic therapy at the time of randomization doing as well as other patients on MCS in terms of physical functional gains.[53]

Despite clear evidence of physical functional HRQOL benefits, the functional status of patients receiving MCS remains impaired, on average, relative to normative, "healthy" populations.[42,49] Furthermore, patients on MCS report significant physical functional difficulties and concerns in some areas. They frequently describe the onset of new physical symptoms after implantation, arising primarily as a result of device-related complications or linked to features of the devices they receive. Among the most common complications are infections,[54,55] which frequently lead to rehospitalizations, and the physical deconditioning and functional decline that result during extended hospital stays. The impact of complications such as infections can be particularly great because of the weakened state, including malnutrition, in patients on MCS even before implantation. Other complications such as stroke can lead to pronounced and permanent physical disability.[12,56,57] Patients report significant worries about the risk for these complications and resulting physical impairments,[16,58,59] and these worries increase with time postimplantation.[59] With respect to device-related symptoms, patients frequently report pain at the driveline exit site, difficulties sleeping due to the position of the driveline, and concerns about ability to engage in sexual activity due to worries about disrupting the positioning of the driveline.[16,59,60] In addition, despite general improvements in many areas of physical functioning from preimplantation to postimplantation, some areas do not show marked changes. For example, Grady and colleagues[26,50] found that sleep difficulties persisted from preimplantation to postimplantation.

Finally, it is important to note that studies reporting improvements in physical functional HRQOL over time focus on the subset of patients who are able to provide ongoing data on HRQOL. The risk for morbidities and mortality in patients on MCS remains high, with the rates of some complications (e.g., device malfunction) increasing over time.[54,61] However, the marked increase in durability of the current generation of MCS devices should markedly reduce the frequency of device dysfunction and failure. Patients who remain too ill or become too ill to provide HRQOL data are not captured in most studies' analyses, and thus physical functional HRQOL levels described among patients at 1 to 2 years postimplantation may be biased.[13,47] It is likely that the most accurate conclusion from work to date is that physical functional HRQOL *can* show dramatic and sustained gains over time among patients on MCS, although this potential may not be achieved in all patients. Continued advances in MCS technology and patient medical management strategies may ensure that increasing proportions of patients experience these gains. With regard to patient management in particular, the provision of uniform insurance coverage for cardiac rehabilitation program participation after MCS device implantation is essential.

Psychological Health-Related Quality of Life

Psychological HRQOL encompasses emotional well-being as well as cognitive functioning. HRQOL in this domain improves with MCS, although the improvements are less consistently observed than in the physical functioning domain. With respect to emotional well-being, some studies of patients receiving BTT and DT have noted that average levels of depressive and anxiety-related symptoms show significant reductions from before to after device implantation.[39,42] These improvements in psychological well-being have been observed despite differences in patients' severity of illness at the time of device implantation.[53] Among the subset of patients who remain well enough to be reassessed over time, the improvements in distress levels appear to continue or are at least maintained during the first year of MCS.[13,42] Among patients on BTT MCS, once they recover from the initial effects of device implantation, their emotional well-being is better than average levels observed among heart transplantation candidates who do not require MCS.[39] Their psychological HRQOL appears similar to average levels in heart transplant recipients,[39,49] but is lower than normative levels in healthy populations.[49] Patients who receive MCS as DT show considerably lower levels of distress by 1 year postimplantation than do patients receiving optimal medical management without MCS.[42]

Nevertheless, the likelihood of emotional well-being benefits related to MCS is strongly linked to factors such as the occurrence of significant adverse events during MCS, as well as the ability to be discharged to an outpatient setting. The impact of these factors on psychological HRQOL appears to be more pronounced than their impact on physical functional HRQOL. Patients who are able to live for extended periods outside of the hospital have a considerably more favorable psychological profile than those requiring extended inpatient care.[39,50] However, regardless of care setting, depressive and anxiety symptoms appear to rise as adverse events and complications mount,[35,62,63] and anxiety symptoms are strongly linked to worries over the potential for adverse events or recurrences of those events.[35,59,64] The presence of a diagnosable psychiatric disorder, including mood and anxiety disorders, is common in patients on MCS, with the majority experiencing at least one episode of disorder during MCS.[62,65,66] Commonly reported psychological stressors include concerns about device malfunction and failure.[16,58,59]

The sensitivity of psychological HRQOL to adverse events and complications postimplantation may explain why some studies have failed to note strong preimplantation to postimplantation improvements in patients' emotional well-being.[26,50] The risk of potentially devastating adverse events (and in BTT patients, the uncertainty regarding whether and when transplantation will occur) may also account for findings that the majority of patients on MCS require treatment with psychotropic medications and other psychological and behavioral interventions for mental health problems.[60,62,66]

Although there is little empirical work past the first 1 to 2 years of MCS in patients receiving either BTT or DT, case reports and small case series indicate that as the duration of MCS lengthens, patients whose emotional well-being improved initially during MCS may go on to show pronounced declines in psychological status. These declines appear closely linked to physical health declines.[35,65,67] Tigges-Limmer and colleagues[63] report the suicide of a patient on MCS at approximately 3 years postimplantation after a period of marked deterioration in his physical health, and despite intensive psychiatric treatment.

Cognitive functioning is also an integral component of psychological HRQOL in patients on MCS, and cognitive status has an important impact on patients' ability to function independently. Although there is considerable evidence that cognitive impairments are common in patients with end-stage heart disease, including those awaiting heart transplantation, there has been relatively little documentation of how cognitive functioning is affected by receipt of MCS.[68] However, because neurologic events during MCS remain relatively prevalent and can be devastating, patients receiving MCS are at risk for new, irreversible cognitive impairments. Whether these impairments are linked to the MCS per se or are complications associated with any cardiac surgery can be difficult to determine. Nevertheless, new cognitive impairments remain problematic in the MSC population.

It is therefore noteworthy that Petrucci and associates[69] observed statistically significant, although mild, improvements in several domains of cognitive functioning across the first 6 months in patients receiving BTT MCS: their performance in visual memory, executive function, visual spatial perception, and processing speed improved, and there were no significant declines in any test in any domain evaluated. These results are encouraging, although they must be tempered by the fact that, as noted earlier, patients who were too ill could not be reassessed. Thus, the findings may reflect the levels of cognitive functioning that are attainable in the absence of major neurologic insult.

Social functioning has presented assessment challenges in patients on MCS, perhaps because of the wide array of activities and concerns encompassed within this domain. Rather than systematic assessment, the literature is characterized by anecdotal and relatively general comments that patients receiving MCS are able to perform regular activities of daily living, engage in various leisure activities (e.g., going to restaurants, gardening, engaging in sports), travel, return to work or school, or otherwise have an "active lifestyle."[38,70–72]

Among the few studies attempting to quantify levels of social functioning, receipt of MCS is not uniformly associated with improved self-reported ability to interact with family and friends, or ability to engage in work and leisure pursuits.[26,39] In fact, Grady and coworkers[26] found that satisfaction with socioeconomic areas of life (e.g., ability to work) declined from preimplantation to 2 weeks after device implantation. Instead, the most important determinant of whether social functioning HRQOL improvements are observed during MCS appears to be postimplantation discharge from the hospital. Thus, the patients receiving BTT therapy studied by Grady and colleagues[50] showed marked improvements with hospital discharge in their satisfaction with socioeconomic well-being, and they reported less stress related to socioeconomic concerns, and less stress in relationships with family and friends. Dew and colleagues[39] also noted social functioning benefits with hospital discharge, although the benefits were less pronounced than those observed in physical functional and psychological HRQOL domains. Morales and coworkers[73] reported that 30% to 40% of their discharged patients on MCS returned to work or school, were able to resume driving, and resumed sexual activity during the next several months.

By the end of the first year of MCS, social functioning HRQOL may be less likely to show sustained gains than other HRQOL domains. For example, Grady and colleagues[13] observed that although satisfaction with socioeconomic areas of life remained stable, satisfaction with interpersonal relationships declined somewhat, and patients reported increased limitations in their ability to engage in social interactions.

Despite a more variable pattern of social functioning gains compared with other HRQOL domains, outpatients with MCS appear to have social functioning levels that are generally similar to those of transplant recipients[39,49] and better than those of transplantation candidates not requiring MCS.[39] For example, Dew and colleagues[39] found that outpatients receiving BTT therapy restricted their social interactions less, felt less of a burden to their family, and spent less time in their room than BTT inpatients or other transplant candidates residing at home who did not require MCS.

Several qualitative investigations provide added insights into the social functioning issues faced by patients who return home with MCS. Patients emphasize the importance of structuring their daily lives so as to maintain a sense of control over their general ability to function and interact with others, and they focus on normalizing their lives through specific routines and activities.[64] Many patients dislike the need to rely on others for assistance to engage in daily activities and wish that they could achieve more complete independence during MCS.[58,64] Whether patients feel able to return to sexual activity is an important source of concern,[60] and body image—including distress over one's surgical scars and seeing the device driveline—is also an important issue as patients attempt to return to daily activities and interactions with others.[58,64]

Global Health-Related Quality of Life

Particularly in recent clinical trials and large series of patients on MCS, only global indices, rather than domain-specific evaluations of HRQOL, are reported. Thus, patients may either be asked to complete multi-item measures that include items reflecting the full range of HRQOL (usually in the context of living with heart disease), and then a global score is computed. Alternatively, patients may be asked simply to rate their overall HRQOL. Either way, the result is a composite view that has the advantage of reflecting the "big picture" from the patient's perspective, but that has the disadvantage of not allowing for the identification of specific areas that might be uniquely problematic for patients on MCS.

Keeping this caveat in mind, it is noteworthy that global HRQOL perceptions generally have been found to show (1) improvements from preimplantation to postimplantation in patients receiving both BTT and DT[26,41,42,47,51,74]; (2) improvements over time during MCS, at least during the first several years of support[11,12,47,75]; and (3) advantages relative to equally ill patients who did not receive MCS.[42,74] Despite these positive changes, global HRQOL in patients on MCS appears poorer than that observed in transplant recipients.[39] However, the overall improvements in global perceptions with MCS remain striking and are sufficiently large to be considered clinically significant.[47]

Given evidence that there are important HRQOL domain-specific limitations and concerns linked to MCS, it is essential to supplement global HRQOL information with specific examination of patient self-reports in the separate physical functional, psychological, and social domains. In addition, the factors that may contribute to global HRQOL perceptions may differ from those that are the strongest determinants of domain-specific HRQOL. For example, Dew and coworkers[59] found that the important correlates of physical functional HRQOL (e.g., sleep disruptions related to the MCS device) were not significant correlates of patients' perceived global HRQOL. Interestingly, one report found that among the separate HRQOL domains, psychological well-being was the strongest contributor to global HRQOL.[27] However, psychological HRQOL did not fully account for variability in global perceptions, and other factors (e.g., African American ethnicity) also increased the likelihood of better global HRQOL perceptions.[27]

Family Caregiver Well-Being and Quality of Life

The impact of MCS extends well beyond the patient to encompass the primary family caregiver as well as other family members. Given family caregivers' role in assisting and providing emotional support to MCS recipients, it is important to understand both the benefits and burdens experienced by family members in order to develop educational strategies and to implement interventions to minimize strain on the family. Unfortunately, there has been very little examination of how family caregivers manage responsibilities in assisting patients on MCS, or of caregiver quality-of-life outcomes in general. In the only two empirical studies to date, family caregivers to outpatients on MCS were found to experience more burden related to caregiving tasks and time commitment entailed in caregiving, than did caregivers to several other patient groups (including inpatients receiving MCS, transplantation candidates residing at home who did not require MCS, and heart transplant recipients).[39,76] It is noteworthy that although outpatients on MCS themselves reported that they were less of a burden to their families than did other patient groups, their caregivers perceived their own caregiving burden to be greater than the burden levels reported by caregivers to the other patient groups.[39] Nevertheless, caregiver self-reported physical well-being did not worsen from before to after the patient on MCS was discharged from the hospital.[39] Anecdotally, these caregivers also reported benefits associated with having the patient at home and assisting with care, including a deepening of their relationship with the patient.

Like patients on MCS, family caregivers voice ongoing worries and concerns about living with MCS. In fact, the prevalence of concerns appears to be greater among caregivers than among the patients, particularly with regard to risks for infection, stroke, and device malfunction.[16,59,76] Worries that patients are experiencing ongoing pain and discomfort also appear common.[16]

Two qualitative analyses suggest that caregivers simultaneously face burdens and benefits during the patient's MCS.[17,77] Burden related to caregiving and responsibility for the well-being of the patient was observed to be a predominant and overwhelming factor in caregivers' lives early during MCS. Some of this burden was task related; other components involved fear and anxiety about the patient and about the caregiver's ability to provide assistance. As time elapsed after implantation, caregivers reported in both studies that they developed stronger feelings of mastery of daily tasks and adaptation to life with MCS, and they began to have more hope and optimism about the future, particularly after heart transplantation. It is noteworthy that these qualitative investigations, like the empirical studies of caregivers, have focused exclusively on caregivers to patients receiving BTT therapy. Whether or not feelings such as optimism about the future would be as common in caregivers to patients receiving DT is unknown.

Economic Burdens for the Patient and Family

Given the prevalence of heart failure in the United States, it is not surprising that the economic burden of heart failure is substantial.[78] In 2007, estimated direct and indirect costs of heart failure in the United States were $33.2 billion.[79] These costs were estimated to increase to $39.2 billion in 2010.[78] Importantly, costs and resource use increase significantly as death approaches. In a study conducted from 1998 to 2001, Russo and associates[80] estimated that patients with advanced heart failure expended an average of $156,168 during the last 2 years of life, with approximately 50% expended during the last 6 months of life. The expenditures during the last 6 months of life for patients with end-stage heart failure were two- to four-fold higher than reported costs for other terminal conditions.

For patients whose heart failure progresses and who become more refractory to medical therapies, other options, including heart transplantation and MCS, are considered increasingly often. MCS is an expensive technology. Mean costs reported from the REMATCH trial for the initial implant hospitalization were $210,187 ± $193,295 per patient, with an annual average readmission cost per patient of $105,326.[31] Implant hospitalization costs were significantly lower for survivors versus nonsurvivors in REMATCH, and complications (e.g., sepsis, infection, and bleeding) were found to be significant predictors of cost. Studies focusing on pulsatile pump implantation published since REMATCH have demonstrated lower hospital costs and shorter average lengths of stay compared with REMATCH findings.[81] Lower post–REMATCH era costs also favored survivors versus nonsurvivors. Cost data from use of potentially more durable second-generation pumps have yet to be reported.

The costs of this expensive technology have societal implications in both the United States and worldwide. Issues of feasibility have been raised in countries with national health care plans.[82] European countries, with their mix of public and private health systems, have variability in reimbursement models for VAD implantation.[83] Capitation and rigorous cost controls vary by country. Importantly, in this current world of cost containment, public acceptance, equitable access, and equitable distribution of cost are important, given that whether through insurance premiums, fees, or higher taxes, the costs of new technologies will ultimately be paid by the people of any given society. Thus, introducing new and expensive technologies must be considered carefully in light of the fact that health care systems, and societies in general, have finite resources.

As advances occur in use of this technology, MCS may become more cost effective. Improvements in patient selection, device design, and perioperative/postoperative care may contribute to reduced costs of future MCS therapy. Effective selection criteria can contribute to reduced costs of care through their positive effects on postimplantation outcomes (i.e., improved survival, reduced complications, and improved quality of life). The U.S. Centers for Medicare and Medical Services (CMS) has developed "acceptance criteria" as part of the Joint Commission advanced disease-specific care certification requirements for VAD DT (Box 15-1).[84] Lietz and colleagues[28] developed a composite preoperative risk score to estimate 90-day probability of in-hospital mortality after pulsatile LVAD implantation. The most important predictors of in-hospital mortality were poor nutrition, hematologic abnormalities, markers of end-organ or right ventricular dysfunction, and lack of inotropic support. Given that survivors of MCS device implantation consume fewer resources, these findings provide guidance for MCS patient selection, improving patient outcomes, and providing more cost-effective care. Demonstrating superior cost effectiveness of MCS is complicated by the lower cost with medical therapy where death is more likely, and therefore a less expensive alternative.

MCS design improvements may contribute to reduced costs through their ability to reduce the incidence of morbidities such as infection, bleeding, and neurologic events, as well as mortality. A DT trial of a second-generation continuous flow LVAD, compared with a first-generation pulsatile LVAD, demonstrated significantly improved 2-year survival rates free from disabling stroke and reoperation to repair or replace the device.[12] In addition, survival rates were significantly better and major adverse events (i.e., infection, right heart failure, respiratory failure, renal failure, and cardiac arrhythmia) were significantly lower in patients who received the continuous flow versus pulsatile flow pumps. These improvements in technology have important implications for cost effectiveness.

Finally, systematic perioperative and postoperative management of patients on MCS may contribute to improved outcomes and lower costs. In an effort to standardize care of patients receiving DT MCS, DT programs are required to be Joint Commission certified under CMS's national coverage determination. Certification is granted after an on-site review that looks at the program's commitment to excellence in providing disease-specific services in a comprehensive manner.[84] The Joint Commission's commitment to excellence also involves meeting center volume requirements.

BOX 15-1   Requirements Specific to Ventricular Assist Device Destination Therapy

Acceptance Criteria
- Patients who have an anticipated survival benefit
- Patients with New York Heart Association functional classification class IV heart failure symptoms that have failed to respond to optimal medical management
- Patients with a demonstrated functional limitation with a peak oxygen consumption of 14 mL/kg/min or less
- Patients with a continued need for intravenous inotropic therapy
- Patients who have been evaluated for heart transplant and were not selected as candidates

Lietz and colleagues[85] reported that although center volume did not independently predict 1-year survival after LVAD implantation, after adjusting for preoperative risk score, institutional experience and a systematic approach to care may affect outcomes. Improved outcomes in turn may contribute to enhanced cost effectiveness. In addition, guidelines for best practice with MCS have been published, which can help improve care in these patients and likely reduce cost.[86]

In addition, cost issues specific to patients and caregivers deserve comment. As mentioned earlier, it is imperative to discuss costs (both inpatient and outpatient) with patients and families before implant. Depending on insurance and governmental coverage plans, many patients and families may not be able to bear the economic burden of MCS. Discussion of potential cost and the individual patient's insurance coverage for MCS is greatly aided by a knowledgeable social worker or financial clearance officer of the program. After implantation, patients and families may experience significant stress and burden, including caregiver burden if family members are expected to function as caregivers, yet must also work.

Also specific to patients and caregivers, interventions that have focused on enhancing the self-care capacity of patients with heart failure have been linked to a reduction in heart failure hospitalizations and all-cause hospitalizations.[87,88] Another study demonstrated that patient self-care was related to direct heart failure inpatient costs.[89] Evidence of this relationship has not been found in the MCS literature. However, strategies to enhance patient and family MCS self-management contribute to safe (and perhaps early) discharge to the community and may also reduce the incidence of hospital readmission, which would ultimately contribute to more cost savings.[73,90] An understanding of the relationship between MCS patient and caregiver self-management and costs of care are needed.

POSTIMPLANTATION AND END-OF-LIFE CONSIDERATIONS

Compared with the expansion of the range of psychosocial issues considered before and during MCS, relatively little attention has been directed to outcomes beyond the period of MCS or at the terminal phases of such support. For patients receiving BTT therapy or for patients who are able to recover and found not to require transplantation, outcomes after explantation comprise a critical component of the cost–benefit analysis of MCS. For all patients on MCS, psychosocial issues that arise at the end of life also deserve careful attention, not only from the standpoint of preparing patients and their families, but in order to educate health professionals about issues of concern in this patient population.

Postimplantation Outcomes

Patient Health-Related Quality of Life after Transplantation

Two psychosocial issues have been considered in patients transplanted after MCS. The first concerns whether transplantation is linked to further domain-specific and global HRQOL changes: although heart transplantation itself has positive impact on HRQOL, does it offer further benefits to patients on MCS who have recovered from device implantation and already attained significant HRQOL gains? During the first several weeks after transplantation, patients on MCS appear to show little additional HRQOL benefit in either physical or psychological domains.[51] However, by 1 to 3 months post-transplantation, objective assessments of physical functional capacity (e.g., exercise duration) appear to exceed those observed in those same patients at similar time points after MCS implantation.[91] At 3 months post-transplantation, Grady and colleagues[50] found that former patients on MCS reported experiencing fewer distressing physical symptoms, less physical functional disability, and more satisfaction with their physical and emotional well-being than they had at 3 months after MCS implantation. Despite these improvements, transplantation did not appear to be linked to improvements in social functioning in these patients (e.g., ability to engage in interactions with others; satisfaction with social and economic circumstances), and transplantation was associated with heightened self-reported stress related to self-care activities and hospital and clinic visits.[50] The authors speculated that the new and relatively frequent medical procedures required post-transplantation (e.g., endomyocardial biopsies, right-heart catheterizations), plus a new medication and behavioral regimen, may have contributed to patients' greater perceived stress in these areas. In patients formerly on MCS, qualitative studies also note a shift in focus after transplantation from daily life with heart failure to the need to learn new routines for the longer-term future.[64]

A second important psychosocial issue for post-transplantation HRQOL outcomes in patients on MCS concerns how these patients' outcomes compare with those of other transplant recipients who did not require MCS. During the first year post-transplantation, Dew and coworkers[92] found that patients who had required MCS before transplantation and those who had not required MCS showed similar and significant improvements in physical functional status (e.g., sleep, mobility, ambulation, number of somatic complaints). Emotional well-being (e.g., depressive, anxiety, anger symptoms) was stable or improved in both groups. However, the post-transplantation cognitive status of patients on MCS was significantly poorer, and patients on MCS were less likely to return to employment. Social HRQOL (e.g., interpersonal activities/involvement, role function) showed a mixed pattern of effects. Cognitive impairment explained much of the association between MCS and post-transplantation employment; patients with greater cognitive impairment were less likely to return to work.

Additional studies examining rates of a full range of mood and anxiety disorders as well as psychiatric symptoms have also found no evidence that MSC recipients' post-transplantation outcomes are poorer than those of heart recipients who never required MSC.[92,93] Interestingly, Bunzel and associates[16] observed that no former patients on MCS developed post-traumatic stress disorder (PTSD) after transplantation, but that over one fourth of the spouses of the patients on MCS developed PTSD. However, without any non-MCS comparison group of heart recipients and caregivers, it is difficult to infer that stressors related to MCS led to caregiver PTSD, and there may have been other transplantation-related factors that triggered this disorder. PTSD has been observed in other samples of caregivers to heart transplant recipients—at about the same rate as observed by Bunzel and colleagues[16]—regardless of whether the recipients had required MCS.[94] Nevertheless, their study points to the need for a better understanding of caregiver as well as patient outcomes as they move from MCS to transplantation.

Patient Health-Related Quality of Life after Recovery from Mechanical Circulatory Support

The same psychosocial concerns about post-transplantation outcomes are relevant to patients on MCS who recover sufficiently that their device can be explanted. To date, however, there has been very limited consideration of this group—most likely because recovery and explantation remain rare.[55] One report of a small case series of explanted patients found that their HRQOL showed very few impairments.[95] A second study could not identify clear differences between explanted patients and either heart recipients or patients who continued on MCS.[49] It is difficult to reach conclusions in the absence of larger studies of the recovery population. A qualitative report noted that explanted patients were particularly likely to appreciate the greater independence they now experienced in their daily lives, and they felt that the sense of uncertainty experienced during the period of MCS had been removed.[64] Quality-of-life concerns or benefits among caregivers to these individuals have not yet been identified.

End-of-Life Considerations

Symptom Management and Palliative Care Choices

When patients experience adverse events after device implantation and are nearing the end of life, it is reasonable to initiate a referral to the palliative care team. The focus of palliative care is on improving quality of life through prevention and relief of suffering by treatment of symptoms and physical and psychosocial issues.[10] Thus, if a catastrophic complication of MCS occurs, palliative care team members can play a more prominent role in patient management, including symptom relief and providing patient comfort measures and supportive care, as well as helping family members with coping and anticipatory grief counseling, and initiating a conversation about elective device deactivation to allow for a natural death.[19,96]

Patient Preferences/Decision Making and Family Concerns

When therapies prolong life but do not reverse the underlying medical condition, the American Medical Association has concluded that the therapy may be withdrawn if it serves the best interests of the patient.[97] Withdrawal of life-sustaining therapy is "the cessation and removal of an ongoing medical therapy with the explicit intent not to substitute an equivalent alternative treatment; it is fully anticipated that the patient will die following the change in therapy."[98] Withdrawal of life-sustaining therapy (i.e., device deactivation) is discussed with patients and families as part of the consent process, as previously described, and again when the prognosis and burden of continued device use outweigh the benefits.[10,18] Conversations with patients and families about device deactivation should include informing them about the patient's current condition and prognosis, alternatives to withdrawal of MCS, and the anticipated consequences of device deactivation (i.e., death).[96] The decision to withdraw treatment belongs ultimately to the patient or a surrogate, if the patient is no longer capable of making informed decisions to withdraw treatment.[99] Bioethicists, social workers, psychiatrists, and the hospice team may be helpful to patients and families as they consider device withdrawal, especially when there are differences of opinion about whether to withdraw MCS between patients and families or among family members.[19]

The actual deactivation of the device, which is often done in the hospital but may be done at home, should be performed when the patient and family have made their decision and are ready to proceed. In addition, the MCS team and unit staff, if the patient is hospitalized, should be in agreement with the plan for device deactivation. It can be difficult for health care professionals to face these patient and family decisions. This might especially be the case if the patient has decided that the burden of care outweighs the benefits, but the care providers may not yet see it this way or question the patient's capacity to make this decision. Any conflict among staff about the plan should be discussed among staff with the goal of reaching agreement and formulating a plan to proceed.[100] Bioethicists may be helpful to this process through educating and reassuring staff that an ethical choice has been made. Deactivation is performed by staff who are trained in MCS and know how to stop the device, silence alarms, monitor the patient's condition until death, and disconnect the equipment, as well as provide comfort and support to the family.[96] A debriefing among staff after device deactivation may help individuals deal with their feelings about MCS withdrawal.[100] Institutions may consider developing hospital policies surrounding device withdrawal in collaboration with MCS and hospice teams and bioethicists.

CONCLUSIONS AND FUTURE CLINICAL AND RESEARCH DIRECTIONS

MCS, as a therapeutic option, generally improves HRQOL in patients from before to after implantation, but can nonetheless be adversely affected by many other factors, including complications associated with MCS. Understanding "life on a device" provides clinicians with important information with which to educate patients and their families during the informed consent process. After MCS, studies of HRQOL have provided information regarding benefits and potential risk factors for poor HRQOL outcomes that can guide clinicians in developing strategies to improve outcomes.

The literature on decision making and psychosocial outcomes regarding MCS is limited and, at times, based on opinion rather than data. There is almost no literature on the decision-making process regarding MCS. Furthermore, MCS HRQOL outcomes have been described primarily in patients on BTT therapy who have received first-generation devices. The few reports on continuous-flow pumps have typically provided findings that are broad overviews, with little information on domain-specific HRQOL. End of life on MCS has been discussed in the literature, most commonly through case studies. Clearly, opportunities abound for the future study of decision making regarding MCS, psychosocial evaluation for MCS, HRQOL during and in the long term after implantation, and end-of-life considerations.

REFERENCES

1. Smedley BD, Stith AY, Nelson AR, eds. *Unequal Treatment: Confronting Racial and Ethnic Disparities in Health Care* [2002 report]. Washington, DC: National Academies Press; 2003.
2. Mensah GA, Mokdad AH, Ford ES, et al. State of disparities in cardiovascular health in the United States. *Circulation.* 2005;111:1233–1241.
3. Dew MA, DiMartini AF. Transplantation. In: Friedman HS, ed. *The Oxford Handbook of Health Psychology.* New York: Oxford University Press (in press).
4. Shumway S. Transplant and ventricular assist devices: gender differences in application and implementation. *J Thorac Cardiovasc Surg.* 2004;127:1253–1255.
5. Joyce DL, Conte JV, Russell SD, et al. Disparities in access to left ventricular assist device therapy. *J Surg Res.* 2009;152:111–117.
6. Pang PS, Komajda M, Gheorghiade M. The current and future management of acute heart failure syndromes. *Eur Heart J.* 2010;31:784–793.
7. Gregoric ID, Jacob LP, La Francesca S, et al. The TandemHeart as a bridge to a long-term axial-flow left ventricular assist device (bridge to bridge). *Tex Heart Inst J.* 2008;35:125–129.
8. Jessup M, Abraham WT, Casey DE, et al. 2009 focused update: ACCF/AHA guidelines for the diagnosis and management of heart failure in adults: a report of the American College of Cardiology Foundation/American Heart Association Task Force on Practice Guidelines: developed in collaboration with the International Society for Heart and Lung Transplantation. *Circulation.* 2009;119:1977–2016.
9. Goodlin SJ, Hauptman PJ, Arnold R, et al. Consensus statement: palliative and supportive care in advanced heart failure. *J Card Fail.* 2004;10:200–209.
10. Rizzieri AG, Verheijde JL, Rady MY, et al. Ethical challenges with the left ventricular assist device as a destination therapy. *Philos Ethics Humanit Med.* 2008;3:20.
11. Pagani FD, Miller LW, Russell SD, et al. Extended mechanical circulatory support with a continuous-flow rotary left ventricular assist device. *J Am Coll Cardiol.* 2009;54:312–321.
12. Slaughter MS, Rogers JG, Milano CA, et al. Advanced heart failure treated with continuous-flow left ventricular assist device. *N Engl J Med.* 2009;361:2241–2251.
13. Grady KL, Meyer PM, Dressler D, et al. Longitudinal change in quality of life and impact on survival after left ventricular assist device implantation. *Ann Thorac Surg.* 2004;77:1321–1327.
14. Dudzinski DM. Ethics guidelines for destination therapy. *Ann Thorac Surg.* 2006;81:1185–1188.
15. Farran C. Family caregiving intervention research: where have we been? Where are we going? *J Gerontol Nurs.* 2001;27:38–45.
16. Bunzel B, Laederach-Hofmann K, Wieselthaler G, et al. Mechanical circulatory support as a bridge to heart transplantation: what remains? Long-term emotional sequelae in patients and spouses. *J Heart Lung Transplant.* 2007;26:384–389.

17. Casida J. The lived experience of spouses of patients with a left ventricular assist device before heart transplantation. *Am J Crit Care*. 2005;14:145–151.
18. Bramstedt KA, Wenger NS. When withdrawal of life-sustaining care does more than allow death to take its course: the dilemma of left ventricular assist devices. *J Heart Lung Transplant*. 2001;20:544–548.
19. Bramstedt KA, Nash PJ. When death is the outcome of informed refusal: dilemma of rejecting ventricular assist device therapy. *J Heart Lung Transplant*. 2005;24:229–230.
20. Allen LA, Yager JE, Funk MJ, et al. Discordance between patient-predicted and model-predicted life expectancy among ambulatory patients with heart failure. *JAMA*. 2008;299:2533–2542.
21. Stanek EJ, Oates MB, McGhan WF, et al. Preferences for treatment outcomes in patients with heart failure: symptoms versus survival. *J Card Fail*. 2000;6:225–232.
22. Lewis EF, Johnson PA, Johnson W, et al. Preferences for quality of life or survival expressed by patients with heart failure. *J Heart Lung Transplant*. 2001; 20:1016–1024.
23. MacIver J, Rao V, Delgado DH, et al. Choices: a study of preferences for end-of-life treatments in patients with advanced heart failure. *J Heart Lung Transplant*. 2008;27:1002–1007.
24. Moskowitz AJ, Weinberg AD, Oz MC, et al. Quality of life with an implanted left ventricular assist device. *Ann Thorac Surg*. 1997;64:1764–1769.
25. Brehaut JC, O'Connor AM, Wood TJ, et al. Validation of a decision regret scale. *Med Decis Making*. 2003;23:281–292.
26. Grady KL, Meyer P, Mattea A, et al. Improvement in quality of life outcomes 2 weeks after left ventricular assist device implantation. *J Heart Lung Transplant*. 2001;20:657–669.
27. Grady KL, Meyer P, Mattea A, et al. Predictors of quality of life at 1 month after implantation of a left ventricular assist device. *Am J Crit Care*. 2002;11:345–352.
28. Lietz K, Long JW, Kfoury AG, et al. Outcomes of left ventricular assist device implantation as destination therapy in the post-REMATCH era: implications for patient selection. *Circulation*. 2007;116:497–505.
29. Miller LW, Lietz K. Candidate selection for long-term left ventricular assist device therapy for refractory heart failure. *J Heart Lung Transplant*. 2006;25:756–764.
30. Eshelman AK, Mason S, Nemeh H, et al. LVAD destination therapy: applying what we know about psychiatric evaluation and management from cardiac failure and transplant. *Heart Fail Rev*. 2009;14:21–28.
31. Oz MC, Gelijns AC, Miller L, et al. Left ventricular assist devices as permanent heart failure therapy: the price of progress. *Ann Surg*. 2003;238:577–583 discussion 583–575.
32. Kirklin JK, Naftel DC, Stevenson LW, et al. INTERMACS database for durable devices for circulatory support: first annual report. *J Heart Lung Transplant*. 2008;27:1065–1072.
33. Cupples S, Dew MA, Grady KL, et al. Report of the Psychosocial Outcomes Workgroup of the Nursing and Social Sciences Council of the International Society for Heart and Lung Transplantation: present status of research on psychosocial outcomes in cardiothoracic transplantation: review and recommendations for the field. *J Heart Lung Transplant*. 2006;25:716–725.
34. Drews T, Loebe M, Jurmann M, et al. Outpatients on biventricular assist devices. *Thorac Cardiovasc Surg*. 2001;49:296–299.
35. Faggian G, Santini F, Franchi G, et al. Insights from continued use of a Novacor Left Ventricular Assist System for a period of 6 years. *J Heart Lung Transplant*. 2005;24:1444.
36. Myers TJ, Catanese KA, Vargo RL, et al. Extended cardiac support with a portable left ventricular assist system in the home. *ASAIO J*. 1996;42:M576–M579.
37. Siegenthaler MP, Martin J, van de Loo A, et al. Implantation of the permanent Jarvik-2000 left ventricular assist device: a single-center experience. *J Am Coll Cardiol*. 2002;39:1764–1772.
38. Westaby S, Banning AP, Saito S, et al. Circulatory support for long-term treatment of heart failure: experience with an intraventricular continuous flow pump. *Circulation*. 2002;105:2588–2591.
39. Dew MA, Kormos RL, Winowich S, et al. Quality of life outcomes in left ventricular assist system inpatients and outpatients. *ASAIO J*. 1999;45:218–225.
40. Frazier OH, Rose EA, Oz MC, et al. Multicenter clinical evaluation of the HeartMate vented electric left ventricular assist system in patients awaiting heart transplantation. *J Thorac Cardiovasc Surg*. 2001;122:1186–1195.
41. Miller LW, Pagani FD, Russell SD, et al. Use of a continuous-flow device in patients awaiting heart transplantation. *N Engl J Med*. 2007;357:885–896.
42. Rose EA, Gelijns AC, Moskowitz AJ, et al. Long-term mechanical left ventricular assistance for end-stage heart failure. *N Engl J Med*. 2001;345:1435–1443.
43. Allen JG, Weiss ES, Schaffer JM, et al. Quality of life and functional status in patients surviving 12 months after left ventricular assist device implantation. *J Heart Lung Transplant*. 2010;29:278–285.
44. de Jonge N, Kirkels H, Lahpor JR, et al. Exercise performance in patients with end-stage heart failure after implantation of a left ventricular assist device and after heart transplantation: an outlook for permanent assisting? *J Am Coll Cardiol*. 2001;37:1794–1799.
45. Haft J, Armstrong W, Dyke DB, et al. Hemodynamic and exercise performance with pulsatile and continuous-flow left ventricular assist devices. *Circulation*. 2007;116(suppl 11):I8–I15.
46. Rogers JG, Butler J, Lansman SL, et al. Chronic mechanical circulatory support for inotrope-dependent heart failure patients who are not transplant candidates: results of the INTrEPID Trial. *J Am Coll Cardiol*. 2007;50:741–747.
47. Rogers JG, Aaronson KD, Boyle AJ, et al. Continuous flow left ventricular assist device improves functional capacity and quality of life of advanced heart failure patients. *J Am Coll Cardiol*. 2010;55:1826–1834.
48. Sharples LD, Cafferty F, Demitis N, et al. Evaluation of the clinical effectiveness of the Ventricular Assist Device Program in the United Kingdom (EVAD UK). *J Heart Lung Transplant*. 2007;26:9–15.
49. Wray J, Hallas CN, Banner NR. Quality of life and psychological well-being during and after left ventricular assist device support. *Clin Transplant*. 2007;21:622–627.
50. Grady KL, Meyer PM, Dressler D, et al. Change in quality of life from after left ventricular assist device implantation to after heart transplantation. *J Heart Lung Transplant*. 2003;22:1254–1267.
51. Miller K, Myers TJ, Robertson K, et al. Quality of life in bridge-to-transplant patients with chronic heart failure after implantation of an axial flow ventricular assist device. *Congest Heart Fail*. 2004;10:226–229.
52. Richenbacher WE, Naka Y, Raines EP, et al. Surgical management of patients in the REMATCH trial. *Ann Thorac Surg*. 2003;75(suppl 6):S86–S92.
53. Stevenson LW, Miller LW, Desvigne-Nickens P, et al. Left ventricular assist device as destination for patients undergoing intravenous inotropic therapy: a subset analysis from REMATCH (Randomized Evaluation of Mechanical Assistance in Treatment of Chronic Heart Failure). *Circulation*. 2004;110:975–981.
54. Genovese EA, Dew MA, Teuteberg JJ, et al. Incidence and patterns of adverse event onset during the first 60 days after ventricular assist device implantation. *Ann Thorac Surg*. 2009;88:1162–1170.
55. Kirklin JK, Naftel DC, Kormos RL, et al. Second INTERMACS annual report: more than 1,000 primary left ventricular assist device implants. *J Heart Lung Transplant*. 2010;29:1–10.
56. Lazar RM, Shapiro PA, Jaski BE, et al. Neurological events during long-term mechanical circulatory support for heart failure: the Randomized Evaluation of Mechanical Assistance for the Treatment of Congestive Heart Failure (REMATCH) experience. *Circulation*. 2004;109:2423–2427.
57. Pae WE, Connell JM, Boehmer JP, et al. Neurologic events with a totally implantable left ventricular assist device: European LionHeart Clinical Utility Baseline Study (CUBS). *J Heart Lung Transplant*. 2007;26:1–8.
58. Chapman E, Parameshwar J, Jenkins D, et al. Psychosocial issues for patients with ventricular assist devices: a qualitative pilot study. *Am J Crit Care*. 2007;16:72–81.
59. Dew MA, Kormos RL, Winowich S, et al. Human factors issues in ventricular assist device recipients and their family caregivers. *ASAIO J*. 2000;46:367–373.
60. Samuels LE, Holmes EC, Petrucci R. Psychosocial and sexual concerns of patients with implantable left ventricular assist devices: a pilot study. *J Thorac Cardiovasc Surg*. 2004;127:1432–1435.
61. Hunt SA. Mechanical circulatory support: new data, old problems. *Circulation*. 2007;116:461–462.
62. Shapiro PA, Levin HR, Oz MC. Left ventricular assist devices: psychosocial burden and implications for heart transplant programs. *Gen Hosp Psychiatry*. 1996;18(suppl 6):30S–35S.
63. Tigges-Limmer K, Schonbrodt M, Roefe D, et al. Suicide after ventricular assist device implantation. *J Heart Lung Transplant*. 2010;29:692–694.
64. Hallas C, Banner NR, Wray J. A qualitative study of the psychological experience of patients during and after mechanical cardiac support. *J Cardiovasc Nurs*. 2009; 24:31–39.
65. Baba A, Hirata G, Yokoyama F, et al. Psychiatric problems of heart transplant candidates with left ventricular assist devices. *J Artif Organs*. 2006;9:203–208.
66. Petrucci R, Kushon D, Inkles R, et al. Cardiac ventricular support: considerations for psychiatry. *Psychosomatics*. 1999;40:298–303.
67. Marcus P. Left ventricular assist devices: psychosocial challenges in the elderly. *Ann Thorac Surg*. 2009;88:e48–e49.
68. Cupples SA, Stilley CS. Cognitive function in adult cardiothoracic transplant candidates and recipients. *J Cardiovasc Nurs*. 2005;20(suppl 5):S74–S87.
69. Petrucci RJ, Wright S, Naka Y, et al. Neurocognitive assessments in advanced heart failure patients receiving continuous-flow left ventricular assist devices. *J Heart Lung Transplant*. 2009;28:542–549.
70. Siegenthaler MP, Westaby S, Frazier OH, et al. Advanced heart failure: feasibility study of long-term continuous axial flow pump support. *Eur Heart J*. 2005;26:1031–1038.
71. Helman DN, Addonizio LJ, Morales DL, et al. Implantable left ventricular assist devices can successfully bridge adolescent patients to transplant. *J Heart Lung Transplant*. 2000;19:121–126.
72. Potapov EV, Jurmann MJ, Drews T, et al. Patients supported for over 4 years with left ventricular assist devices. *Eur J Heart Fail*. 2006;8:756–759.
73. Morales DL, Argenziano M, Oz MC. Outpatient left ventricular assist device support: a safe and economical therapeutic option for heart failure. *Prog Cardiovasc Dis*. 2000;43:55–66.
74. Park SJ, Tector A, Piccioni W, et al. Left ventricular assist devices as destination therapy: a new look at survival. *J Thorac Cardiovasc Surg*. 2005;129:9–17.
75. Sharples LD, Dyer M, Cafferty F, et al. Cost-effectiveness of ventricular assist device use in the United Kingdom: results from the evaluation of ventricular assist device programme in the UK (EVAD-UK). *J Heart Lung Transplant*. 2006;25:1336–1343.
76. Williams DL, Shapiro PA, Weinberg AD, et al. Quality of life and caregiver burden in LVAD, heart transplant, and heart failure patients. *J Heart Lung Transplant*. 1996;15:S54.
77. Baker K, Flattery M, Salyer J, et al. Caregiving for patients requiring left ventricular assistance device support. *Heart Lung*. 2010;39:196–200.
78. Lloyd-Jones D, Adams R, Carnethon M, et al. Heart disease and stroke statistics—2009 update: a report from the American Heart Association Statistics Committee and Stroke Statistics Subcommittee. *Circulation*. 2009;119:e21–e181.
79. Rosamond W, Flegal K, Friday G, et al. Heart disease and stroke statistics—2007 update: a report from the American Heart Association Statistics Committee and Stroke Statistics Subcommittee. *Circulation*. 2007;115:e69–e171.
80. Russo MJ, Gelijns AC, Stevenson LW, et al. The cost of medical management in advanced heart failure during the final two years of life. *J Card Fail*. 2008;14:651–658.
81. Miller LW, Nelson KE, Bostic RR, et al. Hospital costs for left ventricular assist devices for destination therapy: lower costs for implantation in the post-REMATCH era. *J Heart Lung Transplant*. 2006;25:778–784.
82. Carrier M. Left ventricular assist device: can Canada afford this? *Can J Cardiol*. 2005;21:1166–1168.
83. Bieniarz MC, Delgado R. The financial burden of destination left ventricular assist device therapy: who and when? *Curr Cardiol Rep*. 2007;9:194–199.
84. The Joint Commission. Disease-Specific Care Certification Guide. Oakbrook Terrace, IL: The Joint Commission; 2010.
85. Lietz K, Long JW, Kfoury AG, et al. Impact of center volume on outcomes of left ventricular assist device implantation as destination therapy: analysis of the Thoratec HeartMate Registry, 1998 to 2005. *Circ Heart Fail*. 2009;2:3–10.

86. Slaughter MS, Pagani FD, Rogers JG, et al. Clinical management of continuous-flow left ventricular assist devices in advanced heart failure. *J Heart Lung Transplant.* 2010;29(suppl 4):S1–S39.

87. McAlister FA, Stewart S, Ferrua S, et al. Multidisciplinary strategies for the management of heart failure patients at high risk for admission: a systematic review of randomized trials. *J Am Coll Cardiol.* 2004;44:810–819.

88. Jovcic A, Holroyd-Leduc JM, Straus SE. Effects of self-management intervention on health outcomes of patients with heart failure: a systematic review of randomized controlled trials. *BMC Cardiovasc Disord.* 2006;6:43.

89. Lee C, Carlson B, Riegel B. Heart failure self-care improves economic outcomes, but only when self-care confidence is high. *J Card Fail.* 2007;13:S75.

90. Grady K, Shinn J. Care of patients with circulatory assist devices. In: Moser D, Riegel B, eds. *Cardiac Nursing: A Companion to Braunwald's Heart Disease.* St. Louis: WB Saunders; 2008:977–997.

91. Jaski BE, Lingle RJ, Kim J, et al. Comparison of functional capacity in patients with end-stage heart failure following implantation of a left ventricular assist device versus heart transplantation: results of the experience with left ventricular assist device with exercise trial. *J Heart Lung Transplant.* 1999;18:1031–1040.

92. Dew MA, Kormos RL, DiMartini AF, et al. Prevalence and risk of depression and anxiety-related disorders during the first three years after heart transplantation. *Psychosomatics.* 2001;42:300–313.

93. Dew MA, Myaskovsky L, Switzer GE, et al. Profiles and predictors of the course of psychological distress across four years after heart transplantation. *Psychol Med.* 2005;35:1215–1227.

94. Dew MA, Myaskovsky L, DiMartini AF, et al. Onset, timing and risk for depression and anxiety in family caregivers to heart transplant recipients. *Psychol Med.* 2004;34:1065–1082.

95. Birks EJ, Tansley PD, Hardy J, et al. Left ventricular assist device and drug therapy for the reversal of heart failure. *N Engl J Med.* 2006;355:1873–1884.

96. Wiegand DL, Kalowes PG. Withdrawal of cardiac medications and devices. *AACN Adv Crit Care.* 2007;18:415–425.

97. American Medical Association. *Opinion 2.20. Withholding or withdrawing life-sustaining medical treatment.* AMA Code of Medical Ethics, Council on Ethical and Judicial Affairs of the American Medical Association. Available at www.ama-assn.org/ama/pub/physician-resources/medical-ethics/code-medical-ethics/opinion220.page; Accessed 12.06.11.

98. Prendergast TJ, Claessens MT, Luce JM. A national survey of end-of-life care for critically ill patients. *Am J Respir Crit Care Med.* 1998;158:1163–1167.

99. *Deciding to Forego Life-Sustaining Treatment: A Report on the Ethical, Medical, and Legal Issues in Treatment Decisions.* Washington, DC: U.S. Government Printing Office; 1983.

100. MacIver J, Ross HJ. Withdrawal of ventricular assist device support. *J Palliat Care.* 2005;21:151–156.

CHAPTER **16**

Mechanical Circulatory Support in Pediatrics

Peter D. Wearden and Elizabeth D. Blume

There has been much progress in the field of mechanical circulatory support for children since the first reported use of cardiopulmonary bypass in children in the 1950s. Gibbon[1] and Lillehei and colleagues[2] reported cardiopulmonary support for pediatric heart surgery in 1953. Kirklin and others[3] were the first group to developed a pump oxygenator using a much smaller priming volume. A number of major improvements allowing surface cooling and shorter pump times came in the 1970s followed by the description of deep hypothermic circulatory arrest in infants by Casteneda and colleagues[4] and Barratt-Boyes.[5] Over the next several decades, incremental improvements in cardiopulmonary bypass technology and operative techniques contributed to a significant reduction in mortality rates associated with pediatric cardiac surgery. The early use of adult ventricular support devices in children demonstrated encouraging outcomes. Key technical challenges remain, however, and pumps designed exclusively for children are under development. The field of pediatric mechanical support continues to grow rapidly, and outcomes and pediatric-specific challenges are important to understand and critically evaluate.

HEART FAILURE IN CHILDREN

Severe heart failure is a rare condition in children.[6] The overall incidence of congenital heart disease is estimated at 8 per 1000 live births[6] and the incidence of cardiomyopathy is estimated at 0.58 per 100,000 children.[7,8] Only a fraction of children diagnosed with either form of heart disease eventually progresses to advanced heart failure necessitating mechanical support. Similar to adults, the high mortality associated with pediatric end-stage heart disease stems from directly related sequelae, such as low cardiac output, respiratory failure, malignant arrhythmias, stroke, thromboembolism, irreversible end-organ dysfunction, and infection.[9]

Overall survival of infants born with severe forms of congenital heart disease has improved dramatically over the last few decades. In a study of the multiple-cause mortality files compiled by the National Center for Health Statistics of the Centers for Disease Control and Prevention, Boneva and colleagues[10] reviewed all death certificates filed in the United States. From 1979 through 1997, mortality from heart defects (all ages) declined 39%, from 2.5 to 1.5 per 100,000 population. Of the 5822 deaths in the last 2 years of the study, 51% were among infants and 7% among children 1 to 4 years of age. Over time, the age at death has increased for every congenital heart defect, as more palliated infants are surviving into adolescence and adulthood.[10] This will become an important factor as these patients survive longer, with more complicated anatomic and medical needs.

Heart transplantation has become the standard of care for children with end-stage heart disease secondary to cardiomyopathy or congenital heart disease. Although survival has steadily improved after pediatric heart transplantation,[11,12] waiting list mortality continues to be a problem.[13–18] In the current era,[13] in data analyzed from the United Network for Organ Sharing (UNOS), more than 1 in 5, or 500 children died on the heart transplantation waiting list before a suitable donor heart could be identified. The vast majority of these deaths occurred in children weighing less than 20 kg (Fig. 16-1). In this analysis, Almond and associates[13] found that factors such as extracorporeal membrane oxygenation (ECMO) support, ventilator support, listing status 1A, congenital heart disease, dialysis, and nonwhite race were independent risk factors associated with waiting list mortality (Fig. 16-2). These data indicate that children generally survived to transplantation if they could be stabilized with medical therapy alone. Given that most waiting list deaths occurred in the smallest patients, the data suggest that currently available circulatory support options for infants and toddlers who require bridge to transplantation are inadequate in the United States at present. In response to the clinical need, changes in the field of mechanical support for children over the last 5 years have been dramatic. Support from industry, the National Institutes of Health (NIH), and the U.S. Food and Drug Administration (FDA), working closely with clinicians and engineers, has led to significant advances in the field.

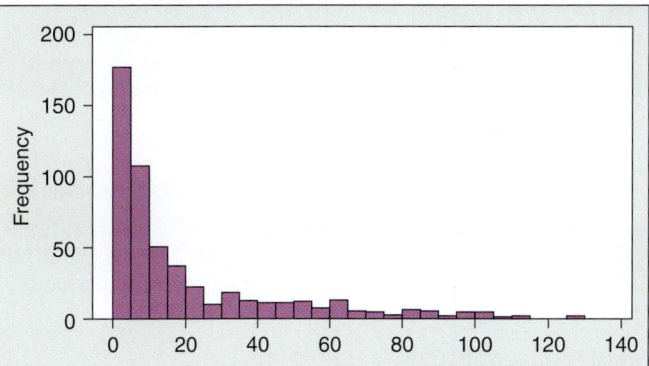

FIGURE 16-1 Pediatric heart transplantation waiting list mortality rates by weight of the recipient. United Network for Organ Sharing (UNOS) analysis from the current era revealed that one in five children die waiting for a suitable organ donor. Most of these deaths occur in children weighing less than 20 kg. *(From Almond CS, Thiagarajan RR, Piercey GE, et al. Waiting list mortality among children listed for heart transplantation in the United States. Circulation. 2009;119:717-727.)*

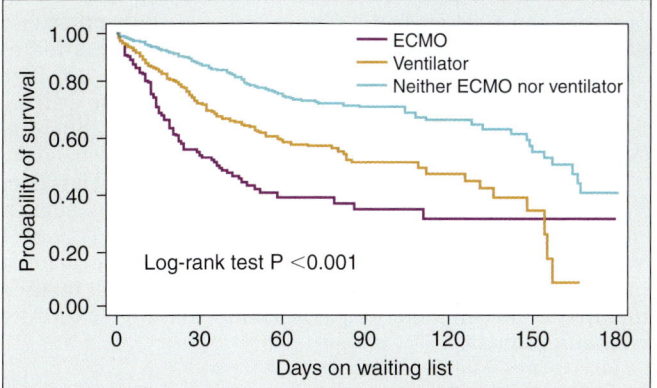

FIGURE 16-2 Survival rates for children listed status 1A, according to level of support. Extracorporeal membrane oxygenation (ECMO) and ventilator support were found to be independent risk factors for death while waiting for a donor organ in this United Network for Organ Sharing (UNOS) analysis. *(From Almond CS, Thiagarajan RR, Piercey GE, et al. Waiting list mortality among children listed for heart transplantation in the United States. Circulation. 2009;119:717-727.)*

CURRENT DEVICES FOR PEDIATRIC CARDIAC SUPPORT

Extracorporeal Membrane Oxygenation

Extracorporeal membrane oxygenation remains the most common method of mechanical circulatory support for pediatric patients (Box 16-1). In the past 30 years, development and improvements in ECMO technology have advanced it from a "heroic" therapy to one that is commonly used in

BOX 16-1 Advantages of Extracorporeal Membrane Oxygenation for Pediatric Mechanical Circulatory Support

1. Rapidity of deployment
2. Ease of setup
3. Ability to provide respiratory support
4. Extensive experience at many centers
5. Flexible cannulation options (neck, sternum, groin)

most pediatric cardiac intensive care units. This mechanical support is used to maintain cardiorespiratory function until other cardiopulmonary derangements have been adequately treated,[19–22] as a bridge to transplantation,[23–26] or as a bridge to long-term device placement. Techniques supporting only pulmonary function (i.e., venovenous), as well as both cardiac output and lung function (i.e., venoarterial), are well described and management strategies to optimize outcome are well reported and beyond the scope of this text. In pediatric populations, this support is frequently used for patients with potentially treatable pulmonary or cardiac disease. Advantages of ECMO include the rapidity and ease of setup, the ability to provide both respiratory and cardiac support, and the reliable history and extensive experience.

Historically, the initial use of ECMO in pediatric patients was for primary respiratory failure, with Bartlett and colleagues achieving the first successful use in 1975.[27] In the ensuing years, ECMO was used with increasing frequency in neonates with various forms of respiratory distress and insufficiency, with survival rates greater than 50% and normal growth and development in the majority of survivors.[28,29]

Subsequently, several randomized, controlled trials were conducted to examine the efficacy of ECMO for neonatal respiratory failure, all of which demonstrated a superior outcome for those patients treated with ECMO compared with standard medical therapy of the time.[30,31] Perhaps the most definitive study, published in 1996 from ECMO centers in the United Kingdom, randomized 185 patients at 5 centers to ECMO or conventional medical therapy and demonstrated a survival advantage for ECMO of 70% to 41%, causing the investigators to halt the study before enrollment of the projected 300 patients.[32]

These successes in treating pediatric respiratory failure are critical to understand in the context of pediatric cardiac support for two reasons. First, ECMO results appear to be different in children than in adults. In the early 1970s, before Bartlett's initial reports, there had been anecdotal reports of ECMO use in adult patients with respiratory distress, and an NIH trial was initiated. The trial was halted after the enrollment of a limited number of patients in both treatment arms (conventional and ECMO) because of a 90% mortality rate in both groups. It was concluded that ECMO afforded no survival benefit in this group.[33] The reasons for the differences observed in ECMO success in adult and pediatric patients are clearly multifactorial. One issue may be the difference in "end-stage" disease in adults compared with children. In children, these processes tend to have a very rapid onset and equally rapid recovery. Neonatal respiratory distress, as opposed to adult respiratory failure, often lends itself to effective medical treatment (i.e., surfactant). In addition, complicating comorbidities, common in adults, are frequently absent in children, somewhat simplifying their care. These treatment successes in pediatric respiratory failure suggest that if one could support the child without injuring the lung, and address the underlying etiology of lung failure, use of ECMO would be successful. *This conclusion highlights the need for pediatric-specific investigations of new devices, secondary to differences between the etiology and onset of heart failure in children and adults.* The second reason early neonatal respiratory ECMO success is important is because it likely altered the course of development of mechanical cardiac support in children. With clinicians encouraged by its success in the area of respiratory support, ECMO for cardiac support became increasingly common. Although this period marked a rapid increase in efforts to develop adult ventricular assist devices (VADs), there was little supported research in pediatric device development.

Shortly thereafter, the first descriptions of pediatric ECMO support for primary cardiac failure began to be published,[34–37] mostly in the postcardiotomy patients. Survival rates for all pediatric patients supported for cardiac indications were near 50%, with significant complications of bleeding, thrombosis, and neurologic injury.[38-40] In 1992, Del Nido and colleagues[19] described the use of ECMO in 33 patients for cardiac support after cardiac surgery. Eleven of these patients were placed on support after cardiac arrest and an average of 65 minutes of cardiopulmonary resuscitation (CPR). Those patients supported in this "rescue" fashion had a 64% early survival rate and 55% long-term survival rate despite the relatively lengthy duration of CPR.[19] In addition, survival in this group was similar to that of the entire group. These findings led most centers with significant volumes of pediatric cardiac surgery to develop "rapidly deployed" ECMO units.[41,42]

In addition to its use as an extension of CPR, ECMO continues to be the mainstay of mechanical support for children who cannot be weaned from cardiopulmonary bypass and those with low cardiac output postcardiotomy or pulmonary hypertension; at some centers, it is used as a bridge to transplantation.[43] Generally, this therapy has been reserved for patients in the most extreme situations where all nonmechanical means of support have been exhausted, and it is necessary to interpret outcomes data in this light. The only potential contraindications to ECMO support are severe neurologic injury, prematurity and small size (<2 kg), bleeding, irreversible disease, and noncardiac structural and chromosomal abnormalities.[44] According to the most recent data from the Extracorporeal Life Support Organization (ELSO) registry,[45] the annual number of cardiac runs, and percentage of all patients supported by ECMO for primary cardiac failure have increased steadily since 1985 (Fig. 16-3). Considering the extreme circumstances faced by most of these patients before initiation of ECMO support, it should come as no surprise that survival remains essentially unchanged from the initial reports, with only 39% of neonatal patients and 47% of pediatric patients surviving to hospital discharge (see Fig. 16-3). Average support times have consistently ranged from 150 to 160 hours over the most recent period. In addition, the incidences of mechanical, hemorrhagic, and neurologic complications all exceed 30%.[45] Several centers have examined their use and outcomes of ECMO support after cardiotomy (Table 16-1).[46] The rate of use ranged from 1.8% to 5.4% of cardiac patients, with survival rates from 35% to 61%. It is likely that these survival rates, which are better than those in the ELSO registry as a whole, reflect individual center expertise and volume.

It is clear that the presence of residual hemodynamic lesions frequently prohibits weaning from ECMO and

TABLE 16-1	Use and Outcomes of Extracorporeal Membrane Oxygenation (ECMO) Support after Cardiotomy		
Author	Study Period	Number Needing ECMO (%) of Cardiopulmonary Cases Needing ECMO	Survival Rate (%)
Walters III	1984-1994	66 (3.0)	57.6
Jaggers	1994-1999	35 (3.4)	61
Aharon	1997-2000	50 (4.0)	50
Kolovos	1995-2000	74 (2.2)	50
Chaturvedi	1992-2001	81 (2.5)	49
Morris	1995-2001	89 (3.4)	40
Thourani	2002-2004	17 (1.8)	35

Adapted from Salvin JW, Laussen PC, Thiagarajan RR. Extracorporeal membrane oxygenation for postcardiotomy mechanical cardiovascular support in children with congenital heart disease. *Paediatr Anaesth.* 2008;18:1157-1162.

increases the risk of death. Those patients with otherwise normal end-organ function may be considered candidates for cardiac transplantation. The use of ECMO as a bridge to transplantation has been associated with a high waiting list mortality rate (see Fig. 16-2) and a survival to hospital discharge of less than 50%.[23,24,26,47-49]

In general, successful support has been for periods of less than 2 weeks. Even more troubling is that the post-transplantation survival rate has been reported[50] to be as low as 67% at 1 year and 52% at 5 years, significantly less than pediatric heart transplant recipients as a whole, with risk factors that include impaired renal function, fungal infection, and high exposure to blood products.

Early Left Ventricular Assist Device Centrifugal Pump Experience

In addition to pulmonary function, ECMO can support both the right and left heart using a single cannulation strategy of systemic venous and systemic arterial cannulation. In the current era, most centers still therefore rely on ECMO for all patients needing rapid or postcardiotomy support. Although many pediatric patients requiring ECMO support for cardiac indications need both right and left heart support, or

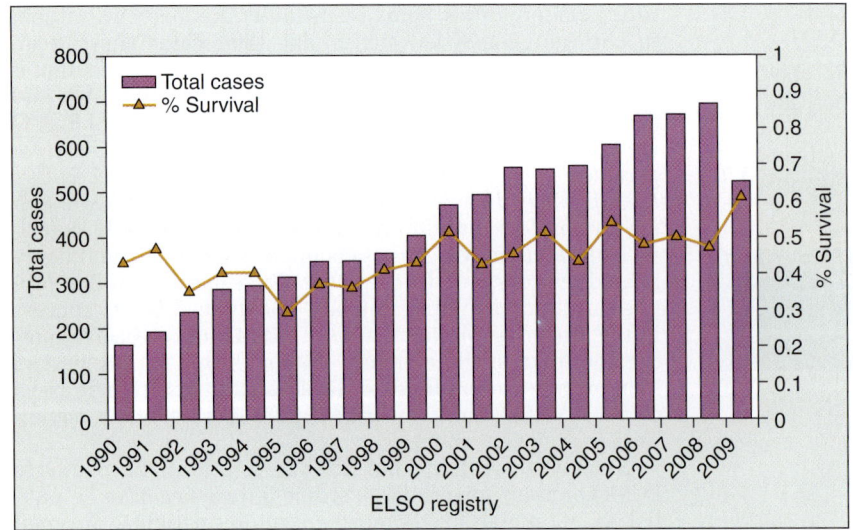

FIGURE 16-3 Survival by year for pediatric cardiac extracorporeal membrane oxygenation (ECMO). ECMO use continues to increase as more centers gain experience with the technology for failure to wean from cardiopulmonary bypass, for treatment of acute decompensated heart failure, and as an extension to cardiopulmonary resuscitation. Overall survival rates, however, have remained relatively steady. ELSO, Extracorporeal Life Support Organization. *(Adapted from Extracorporeal Life Support Organization. Extracorporeal Life Support Organization Registry Report. Ann Arbor, MI: University of Michigan; 2010.)*

pulmonary support necessitating an oxygenator, some do not. Recognizing this, several investigators have proposed the use of standard centrifugal and roller pumps in a VAD configuration to support postcardiotomy patients.[51–54] The Melbourne group, in examining 116 patients supported from 1989 to 2005, observed a probability of weaning patients from VAD support of 66% and a probability of hospital discharge of 43% with a median support time of 75 hours.[55] Ungerleider and associates[56] examined their use of primarily roller pumps to support 23 patients after the stage I Norwood procedure. The patients were enrolled in the protocol before surgery and supported as a matter of routine regardless of operative course. They reported a survival rate to hospital discharge of 87%, "easier" intensive care unit care, and a 22% incidence of complications. The hospital discharge survival rate reported in this study exceeds that generally reported for the stage I Norwood procedure.[54,56]

It is therefore clear that ECMO outcomes in children are generally better than those observed in adults, that it can be rapidly deployed, and can be lifesaving at times. It is, however, equally clear that unchanged survival rates since 1985, high incidences of complications, and the relative inability to support children for longer than 2 weeks leave significant room for improvement. Over the same period of the development of ECMO technology for children, ever-improving VAD technologies were being developed for long-term adult cardiac support. This technology is being re-examined for its potential applicability to children.

Adult Devices in Pediatric Patients

As "adult" VADs became available over the past 20 years, they have been increasingly used in adolescents. Although covered in detail elsewhere in this text (see Chapter 8, Types of Left Ventricular Assist Devices), VADs can be grouped broadly into two separate categories, pulsatile and continuous-flow pumps. Pulsatile pumps were the first VADs developed for use in patients. These devices function much like the heart in that there is a reservoir that must fill with blood, which is then ejected from the reservoir either pneumatically or electrically. Continuous-flow pumps, on the other hand, do not have periods of filling (diastole) and ejection (systole); rather, the flow is continuous, much like an ECMO machine. Pulsatile pumps are larger than continuous-flow pumps because of the need for a blood reservoir. As a result, these pumps are mostly paracorporeal when used in all but the largest of pediatric patients. They are approved for use only in patients with a body surface area greater than 1.5 m². They also usually require a larger cannula because a larger volume of blood must be forced through the cannula in a shorter time than in a continuous-flow pump. For these reasons, these pumps could be used only in older children.

In contrast to the ECMO experience, outcomes for older children placed on VADs are better and have continued to improve. Initial, smaller, single-center studies[56–59] and device registry data[58,60] report approximately a 60% to 70% successful bridge to transplantation in pediatric patients supported with a VAD. Improved outcomes over time (Fig. 16-4)[60,61] may be related to increasing experience with the surgical techniques and perioperative care, better patient selection, earlier introduction of support before irreversible end-organ injury develops, and the application and development of device technology over time.

The first outcomes for these patients have been at least as promising as the adult data. The Pediatric Heart Transplant Study (PHTS) investigators[60] examined the PHTS database, comprising patients younger than 18 years of age listed at 23 North American centers. In the 10 years between 1993 and 2003, 2375 patients were listed for transplantation and enrolled in the database. Of these patients, 99 (4%) received

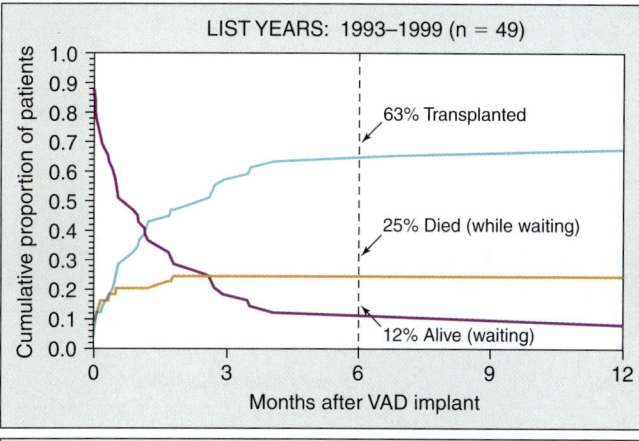

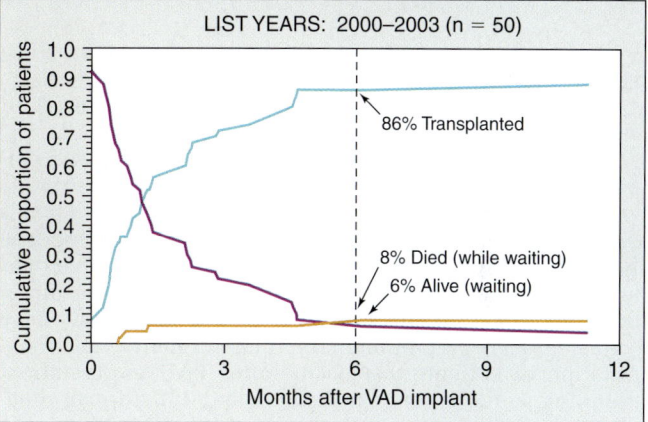

FIGURE 16-4 Improved survival over time in pediatric ventricular assist device (VAD) outcomes. Competing outcomes risk is shown for the early era **(A)** and the later era **(B)** for children receiving "adult" VADs. The analysis shows improved outcomes with a significant era effect for survival to transplantation. (*From Blume ED, Naftel DC, Bastardi HJ, et al. Outcomes of children bridged to heart transplantation with ventricular assist devices: a multi-institutional study. Circulation. 2006;113:2313-2319.*)

VAD implantation before transplantation, in increasing numbers each year of the study. The average age of the patients receiving a VAD was 13.3 years, compared with 4.8 years for those not receiving VAD implantation. Similar discrepancies were noted in body surface area (1.5 m² VAD vs. 0.67 m² non-VAD) and weight (56 kg vs. 20 kg). Virtually all of the patients receiving a VAD were implanted with some form of a pulsatile device. The probabilities of successful bridge to transplantation were 85%, 80%, and 76% at 1 month, 3 months, and 6 months of age (Fig. 16-5). The diagnosis of congenital heart disease, younger age, and smaller body surface area were increased risk factors for death while waiting. Importantly, the post-transplantation survival rate was not significantly different between patients who had or had not been supported with a VAD.

Hill and Reinhartz[60] analyzed 209 patients from the Thoratec registry with a mean age of 14.5 years, mean weight of 57 kg, and mean body surface area of 1.6 m², demonstrating the use of VAD technology primarily in larger adolescents. The mean duration of VAD support was 44 days, with a survival rate to recovery or transplantation of 68.4%. The Pittsburgh group reported on 18 patients supported with pulsatile pumps from 1990 to 2005 and observed 3 deaths and a 77% survival rate to transplantation. The survival rate 6 months after transplantation was 93% and remained at 83% at 1 and 5 years post-transplantation. The average duration of support was 57 days.[62]

These data showed a significant improvement over ECMO as a bridge to transplantation in pediatric patients,

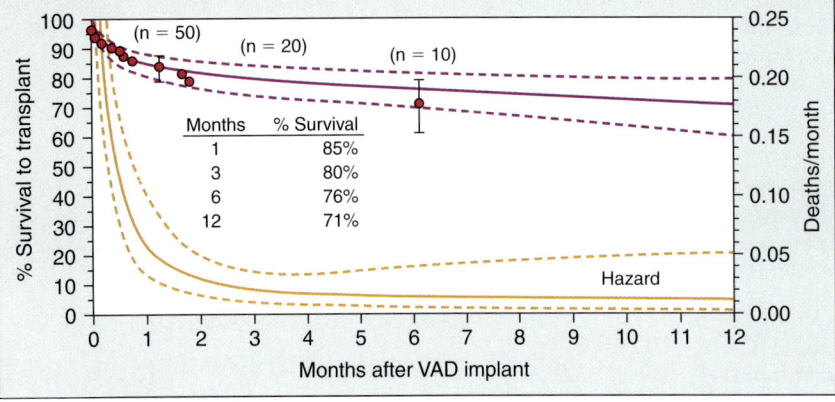

Months	% Survival
1	85%
3	80%
6	76%
12	71%

FIGURE 16-5 Survival to transplantation after "adult" ventricular assist device (VAD) implantation in children. Percentage survival to transplantation for children bridged with a VAD is shown. The hazard risk for death while waiting shows an early risk for these patients, with a small but constant late-phase risk. (*From Blume ED, Naftel DC, Bastardi HJ, et al. Outcomes of children bridged to heart transplantation with ventricular assist devices: a multi-institutional study.* Circulation. *2006;113:2313-2319.)*

at least in those patients large enough to receive an adult pulsatile VAD. Overall, support duration in this early pediatric experience was significantly shorter than for their adult counterparts. In addition, compared with ECMO, the children supported with "adult" VADs have improved survival rates post-transplantation, similar to those of patients who received inotropic support alone.[60] The reasons for this are most likely multifactorial. The inflammatory response seen with ECMO may be less with VAD therapy, which does not include an oxygenator. In addition, the patient population may be different in that the ECMO group may have a greater degree of pulmonary injury. Finally, the rehabilitation of patients that occurs after VAD implantation, including ambulation, extubation, and nutritional rehabilitation, contributes to improved health status going into transplantation.

Most recently, as outlined elsewhere (see Chapter 21), the manner by which adult patients are supported has transitioned to a greater use of continuous-flow pumps, particularly the HeartMate II (Thoratec Corporation, Pleasanton, CA), either as long-term bridge to transplantation or as destination therapy. When this pump was compared in a randomized fashion with the HeartMate XVE (Thoratec), a pulsatile pump, in a destination therapy population, it was found to have a significantly greater rate of "survival free from disabling stroke and reoperation to repair or replace the left ventricular assist device (LVAD; 62% vs. 7%)" with a one year survival of 68% vs 58% for the pulsatile pump. Improved rates of survival and durability were accompanied by significantly greater improvements in quality of life and functional capacity in patients receiving a continuous-flow pump.[63] In light of this improved pump performance, it is not surprising that there has been a recent report of this pump's use in pediatric patients.[64,65] The CentriMag (Levitronix LLC, Waltham, MA) is a molded plastic, fully magnetically levitated, centrifugal, extracorporeal pump primarily used as a "bridge to decision" or for temporary right heart support in adult patients[66] that has also seen use in small numbers of pediatric patients.[67,68] A pump based on the same design but optimized for a smaller priming volume and flow rates is commercially available in Europe.[69] Other continuous-flow pumps that have seen sporadic use in pediatric patients include the Impella catheter pump (Abiomed Corporation, Danvers, MA),[70] the VentrAssist LVAD (Ventracor Corporation, Sydney, Australia),[71] the TandemHeart (CardiacAssist Technologies, Inc., Pittsburgh, PA),[72] and the DeBakey VAD Child (MicroMed Corporation, Houston, TX). Approved by the FDA as a Humanitarian Use Device (HUD), the DeBakey VAD Child (Fig. 16-6)[73] has seen very limited use (<10 patients) because of its capability of providing left-sided support only, mixed early results, and lack of approval for children with a body surface area less than 0.7 m².[74,75]

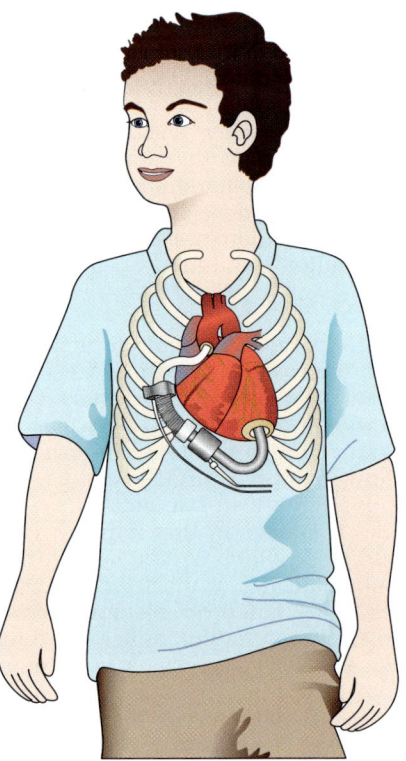

FIGURE 16-6 The DeBakey VAD Child was the first device for children approved by the U.S. Food and Drug Administration (FDA). (*Courtesy of MicroMed Corporation, Houston, TX.*)

Pediatric Mechanical Support Devices

Berlin Heart EXCOR

The Berlin Heart EXCOR (Berlin Heart AG, Berlin, Germany) is a paracorporeal pulsatile, pneumatically compressed volume displacement pump, similar to the volume displacement pumps discussed previously. It is available in 10-, 25-, 30-, 50-, and 60-mL blood chamber sizes (Fig. 16-7). Use of customized polyurethane valves has allowed the manufacture of smaller blood pump sizes than are available with "adult" pumps, which use commercially available mechanical valves. Its first reported successful use as a bridge to transplantation occurred in 1990.[76] It has now seen worldwide use in more than 800 patients in 109 centers, with a median age at implantation of 2 years and a mean duration on device support of 68 days. The longest support time has been 476 days (personal communication). The experience at the Berlin Heart Institute (Berlin, Germany) has been extensively reported.[77–79] A total

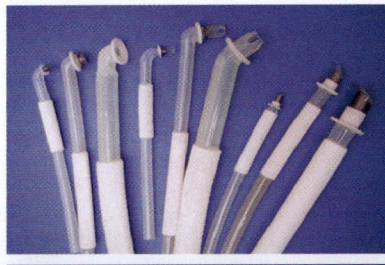
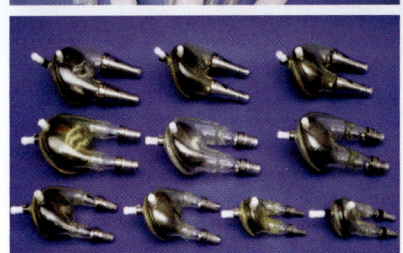
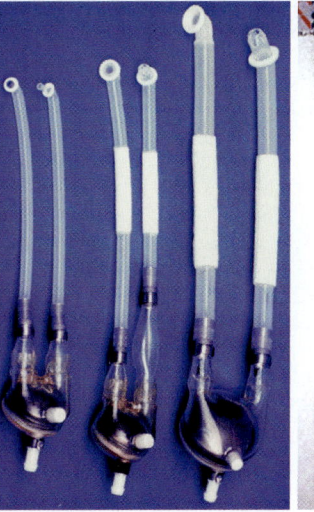
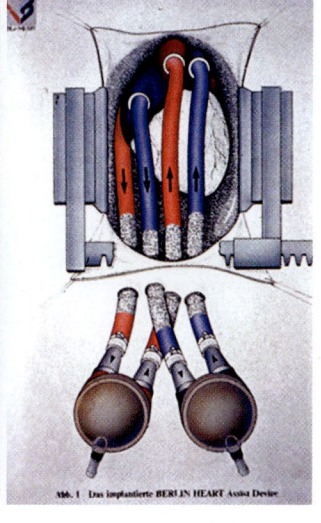

FIGURE 16-7 The Berlin Heart EXCOR device has five blood chamber sizes (10, 25, 30, 50, and 60 mL) and multiple cannula options to span the pediatric age group. *(Courtesy of Robert Kroslowitz, Berlin Heart, Inc., Berlin, Germany.)*

of 74 pediatric patients were supported there from 1990 to 2006, with a mean age of 7.6 years (range 2 days to 17 years) and a mean support time of 36 days. Fifteen percent of these patients were weaned from the device, with 43% receiving a heart transplant; 41% of the children died during VAD support. The group notes significant improvement from the year 2000 onward, with a 74% survival rate to transplantation or discharge despite a younger patient population. The authors also note that changes in their decision-making process from earlier to later in the experience included earlier implementation of support before the development of irreversible organ failure, improvements in cannula design, apical rather than atrial cannulation of the left ventricle, and improvements in the anticoagulation protocol.

The device was first used in North America in 2001, and by 2004 had begun to see widespread use. In 2008, the FDA approved the device for an Investigational Device Exemption (IDE) trial at up to 10 centers. The IDE trial included two study arms for smaller and larger patients. As of this writing (2010), enrollment has been completed in both arms and the device remains available under a Continuing Use Exemption from the FDA. Because of the investigational nature of the device pending FDA approval, few data are currently available regarding North American outcomes, although several single-center reports (Table 16-2) have been made. The Toronto group reported on 15 patients with a mean age of 8.8 years and weight of 31.1 kg. The average duration of support was 29 days, and three patients had previously been placed on ECMO. Of the 15 patients, 14 received biventricular VAD support. Two patients (13%) died while on VAD support.[80] Another report examined nine patients with a median age of 1.7 years and a

median weight of 9.4 kg. All of these patients received biventricular VAD support for an average of 35 days. ECMO support had been used in 33% before placement of VADs. There was one death, with the other eight undergoing successful transplantation.[81] A third report described a single-center experience with 17 children, only 4 of whom required biventricular VAD support. The median age was 1.8 years and the median weight 10 kg. One third of these patients had been on ECMO before initiation of support with the Berlin Heart. There were four deaths (29%), three while on support and one after transplantation. Specifically regarding the smallest patients, two recent publications examined use of the Berlin Heart EXCOR in patients weighing less than 10 kg, with mixed results. In one Italian series, 10 patients were implanted from 2002-2010 (median age 10.4 months, median weight 6.4 kg). Biventricular VADs were used in 30% and the average support time was 61 days. The mortality rate was 40%, with one child still awaiting transplantation.[82] A second study from Great Ormond Street Hospital (London) reported the results of 11 patients treated from 2004 to 2009. In this group, the median weight was 8.0 kg and the average age 12.3 months. Mean support time was 27 days. Ten of 11 (91%) were successfully transplanted. The group further notes that these results are comparable with those in their patients weighing greater than 10 kg.[83]

Although limited, these data are very encouraging and exceed the results of patients supported with ECMO. Results of the large North American IDE trial are eagerly anticipated. These early reports, however, suggest that the North American experience will benefit from the earlier European experience, with less of a "learning curve."

Pediatric Device Initiatives

With increased use of the Berlin Heart in North America, the U.S. Department of Health and Human Services identified pediatric mechanical circulatory support as a critical unmet need for pediatric patients. Because of the relatively small numbers of children requiring support compared with the adult market, company investment was lacking. This prompted the development of a $22 million National Heart, Lung and Blood Institute (NHLBI) initiative, the Pediatric Mechanical Circulatory Support Program, to promote research and development of mechanical support devices specifically for small children. These awards (2004-2009) led to significant scientific advances culminating in the development of five novel pediatric circulatory support devices. These include a smaller version of the Jarvik 2000 (Jarvik Heart, New York) continuous-flow pump; a smaller pulsatile pump based on the Pierce-Donachy design of the Thoratec PVAD (Penn State Pediatric VAD; Pennsylvania State University–Hershey

TABLE 16-2	Berlin Heart Single-Center Experiences			
Author, Year	No.	Mean Age	Support Duration (days)	Survive to Transplant (%)
Humpl, 2010[3]	15	8.8 yr	29	87
Gandhi, 2008	9	1.7 yr	35	89
Stanford, 2009	17	1.8 yr	57	76
Brancaccio, 2010	10	10 mo	61	60
Karimora, 2010	11	12 mo	27	91
Fan, 2010	56	12 mo	55	81 (30 days)
				51 (1 yr)

From Fan Y, Weng YG, Xiao YB, et al. Outcomes of ventricular assist device support in young patients with small body surface area. *Eur J Cardiothorac Surg.* 2011;39:699-704.

TABLE 16-3 | **Pediatric Mechanical Circulatory Support Devices under Development (2010)**

Device	Size/Age	Cardiac Output (L/min)	Priming Volume (mL)	Support Duration (mo)	Oxygen Delivery?	Implantable?	Pulsatile Flow?
Impella Pediatric (AbioMed)	3-10 kg	0.5-1.5	0	0.25-0.50		Yes	Yes
pCAS (Ension)	2-12 kg	0.7-2.0	105	0.5	Yes		Yes
PediPL (University of Maryland/ Levitronix)	3.5-25 kg	3.0	<100	1	Yes		†
Syncardia Pediatric VAD	3-9 kg	1.2-1.4	10	1		Yes	Yes
PediVAS (Levitronix)	<20 kg	3.0	14	1			†
TinyPump (Tokyo Medical & Dental University)	3.5-15 kg	0.1-2.0	5	1		Yes	
PedM-Pump (MC3)	<25 kg	2.5	35	1	Yes		Yes
PediPump (Perfusion Solutions)	>15 kg	3.0	0.6	1		Yes	
Pediatric Synergy VAD (Circulite)	Infant Child	0.3-1.5 1.5-3.0	1.75	>3		Yes	
Ultramag Pediatric VAS (Levitronix)	Neonate–adults	0.5-6	7.5	6			†
PediaFlow (Pittsburgh)	Neonate–2 yr	0.3-1.5	0.5	6		Yes	
Penn State Pediatric VAD	Infant Child	0.7-1.6 1.6-3.3	10 25	6		Yes	Yes
Jarvik Pediatric 2000	Infant–25 kg	0.25-4.0	1	120		Yes	

Courtesy Tim Baldwin, PhD.
†Potential development.

Medical Center, Hershey, PA); an adult catheter-based pump modified for extracardiac, intrapericardial use (Cleveland Clinic PediPump; Cleveland, OH); an implantable, fully magnetically levitated mixed flow pump (PediaFlow; University of Pittsburgh, Pittsburgh, PA); and a paracorporeal integrated pump oxygenator (Ension pCAS; Ension, Inc., Pittsburgh, PA). All of these pumps have seen successful animal experimentation but have not yet been used in children.

The continuation of the Pediatric Mechanical Circulatory Support Program is the NHLBI Pumps for Kids, Infants, and Neonates (PumpKIN) program (2010). The PumpKIN program is funding four projects to move these devices into the preclinical and IDE trial phases in the next 3 to 5 years. The devices currently funded under this initiative include the PediaFlow, the pediatric Jarvik 2000, and the Ension pCAS. A second integrated pump oxygenator device (Levitronix LLC) was also funded. These programs and the Berlin Heart IDE trial have resulted in an explosion of interest in the field of pediatric mechanical circulatory support (Table 16-3).

In addition to device development, the NIH has recognized the importance of rigorous data collection after approval of a device. INTERMACS (Interagency Registry for Mechanically Assisted Circulatory Support) has been a pivotal development for this field. Although there are limited data currently in the registry because of the lack of a pediatric-approved device, data definitions and adverse events have been standardized for children, and these should be important for future data collection in the U.S. device experience.

MANAGEMENT OF PEDIATRIC PATIENTS RECEIVING CARDIAC ASSIST DEVICE THERAPY

Cardiac support in children presents particular challenges beyond those seen in adults. Because of their size, devices must be smaller than those used in adults, which adds to the complexity. In addition, whereas the majority of adults in need of these services have normal cardiac and arteriovenous anatomy, the anatomy in children can be highly complex. To compound this, the number of children requiring these devices is far smaller than the number of adults, leaving the learning curve for each device and each center to extend over many months to years.

Indications for Mechanical Circulatory Support in Children

As mentioned previously, the general indications for cardiac support in children are bridge to transplantation or bridge to recovery. Currently, the destination therapy used in adult patients is unlikely to become a common indication in children without the design of devices allowing for growth and improved long-term (i.e., years) reliability. There may be a role for destination therapy, however, in older pediatric patients and adults with complex congenital heart disease for whom heart transplantation is not an option secondary to chronic medical conditions. It is possible in this group that destination therapy will improve end-organ function, allowing some patients to move forward with transplantation.

Heart failure in children most often presents in a very acute fashion, leaving little time for a prolonged decision-making process. Acute pediatric heart failure (Box 16-2) most

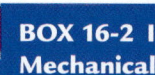

BOX 16-2 Indications for Short-Term Mechanical Circulatory Support in Children

Acute myocarditis
Post-transplant
   Graft failure
   Acute rejection
Intractable arrhythmia
Pulmonary hypertensive crisis
Inability to wean from cardiopulmonary bypass
Acute decompensated heart failure (dilated cardiomyopathy)

commonly arises after cardiotomy, induced by cardiopul-monary bypass and ischemic cardiac arrest, or as an exac-erbation of pre-existing myocardial dysfunction. The second group comprises patients who have not undergone recent cardiotomy and includes patients with structurally normal hearts presenting with acute myocarditis or decompensated cardiomyopathy. The last group of patients are those with an acute change in congenital heart disease with long-standing myocardial dysfunction.[84] Because of the short-term nature of successful ECMO support, initiation of mechanical circu-latory support was historically reserved for those patients in extremis with fulminant cardiovascular collapse and impend-ing cardiac arrest, and often only after cardiac arrest. Because ECMO allows for the rapid initiation of biventricular support, it is still most often used for these extreme situations. It also continues be used in situations where a short duration of sup-port (i.e., days) is generally expected. Timing the interven-tion before complete collapse is likely to result in improved survival. Chaturvedi and colleagues[85] described 81 patients placed on ECMO at Great Ormond Street Hospital. Those patients placed on ECMO in the operating room had a 64% survival rate, compared with a 29% survival rate for those placed on ECMO in the cardiac intensive care unit. Although a selection bias cannot be excluded here, the data do suggest that earlier intervention may better allow for cardiac recov-ery.[85] Early initiation of support may avoid the traditional use of pharmacologic agents (catecholamines) that increase myo-cardial oxygen demands while also increasing the workload of the heart (systemic and pulmonary vascular resistance). These effects are exacerbated further by an increased heart rate. These additional stresses can compound the ongoing myocardial injury. Mechanical support, by its nature, "off-loads" the heart, reducing myocardial work while maximiz-ing myocardial oxygen delivery. These benefits are enhanced by the frequent ability to wean the patient from pharmaco-logic support.[84] Other conditions that still benefit from the initiation of ECMO support include acute myocarditis, intrac-table arrhythmias, and pulmonary hypertension.

Myocarditis

Patients with fulminant myocarditis present a unique decision-making dilemma. In one large, multi-institutional database study, pediatric patients presenting with myocardi-tis had an average length of hospital stay of 14.4 days and a mortality rate of 7.8%. Mechanical ventilation was required in 37.5% including 32.2% of the patients who survived, with 40% requiring vasoactive medicines. Only 7.4% of all 216 patients required ECMO. Survivors received ECMO only 4.5% of the time, whereas 41.2% of those children who died were placed on ECMO.[86] Although the authors suggest that ECMO should be reserved only for those patients who have failed other therapies, one must wonder if earlier ECMO support might not benefit a greater number of patients. Enthusiasm for earlier ECMO support must, however, be tempered by the high incidence of complications with ECMO support. An examination of the ELSO registry from 1995 to 2006 found 260 (1.3%) ECMO runs in 255 pediatric patients for myo-carditis.[87] The median age and weight for these patients were 17 months and 11 kg. Seventy-three percent were decannu-lated from ECMO and 61% survived to hospital discharge. Of the 70 patients who died on ECMO or had support with-drawn, irreversible organ failure was recorded as the rea-son in 83%. The duration of ECMO support did not differ between survivors and nonsurvivors. Of patients, 15% were supported for greater than 2 weeks, with 47% of them surviv-ing to hospital discharge, and 6% of patients were supported for greater than 3 weeks, with 33% surviving to hospital dis-charge. ECMO complications included bleeding (27%), brain injury (21%), renal injury (36%), infectious complications (15%), and pulmonary hemorrhage (11%). All of these com-

plications except infection occurred significantly more often in nonsurvivors.[87]

Post-Transplantation

Another cohort of patients that still may benefit from short-term ECMO support are patients with primary graft failure or acute onset of rejection after heart transplantation. The benefits of ECMO in this patient population are the ability to support pulmonary function as well as both sides of the heart; many of these patients have some degree of pulmonary hypertension and pulmonary dysfunction from long-standing left heart failure. In one series, 28 of 310 (9%) patients under-going pediatric heart transplantation required postopera-tive ECMO support for early graft failure. Only 54% of these patients survived. The average length of support was 2.8 days for survivors and 4.8 days for nonsurvivors. In survivors, graft function was comparable with that in patients not requiring ECMO, although there was an increased incidence of rejec-tion episodes. All of the patients surviving ECMO were alive at 3 years, yet only 46% were alive at a mean follow-up of 8.1 years.[88] These data are comparable with other reports of the use of ECMO in pediatric patients after heart transplan-tation.[89–91] The overall survival rate of 54% is, however, no better than that for other pediatric postcardiotomy patients, suggesting the possible need for early transition to VAD sup-port if prompt recovery of the cardiac allograft is not seen.

Arrhythmia

Arrhythmia per se seems to be a relatively uncommon indication for pediatric ECMO support, comprising less than 4% of patients in several large series of pediatric ECMO interventions.[92,93] However, this number may be under-reported in patients where a supraven-tricular arrhythmia exacerbates underlying marginal cardiac per-formance in the postoperative period. This patient population would seem to be ideal candidates for rapidly deployed ECMO, presuming the arrhythmia is rapidly brought under control.[94]

ECMO remains a commonly used modality for pediatric circulatory support in situations calling for the rapid deploy-ment of short-term support for a likely recoverable problem. These conditions include delayed recovery postcardiotomy or post-transplantation, as a continuation of CPR, and in the setting of myocarditis or arrhythmia. There is also likely a slowly resolving bias for the use of ECMO in younger patients because of the lack of availability of acceptable long-term support devices. The more widespread availability of the Berlin Heart EXCOR in North America, as well as the bur-geoning interest in long-term pediatric support, has led to an ongoing refinement of the decision-making process to initi-ate support in many centers. The need to make this decision within a relatively short window of opportunity can be com-plicated by the inability to distinguish an acute myocarditis from a more long-standing cardiomyopathy, as well as by the relatively short waiting list times for pediatric heart trans-plantation. This leaves the clinician weighing the patient's ability to recover, or at least wait for a heart transplant while being managed with conventional therapy, against the risks of a rapid collapse requiring emergency resuscitation, versus the risks of VAD placement and its associated complications. Therefore, in contradistinction to the adult literature, ECMO is a precursor, if not required indication, for pediatric VAD placement. In published series of pediatric patients receiving a VAD, 6% to 53% of patients have been supported on ECMO before VAD implantation,[77,80–83,95] with some suggesting that the modalities are complementary.[96] The Berlin Heart Institute has argued, fairly conclusively, that the early implementation of VAD support, before end-organ deterioration, leads to sig-nificantly better outcomes.[77,97,98] In pediatric patients there is a relative lack of reliable, objective data to aid in decision making. It does appear, however, that evidence of renal or hepatic injury, which may be considered contraindications to

VAD placement in adult patients, is not prohibitive in pediatric patients.[62,99] In fact, evidence of end-organ injury should be considered a relative indication for VAD placement in the pediatric population.

At least for the near future, then, indications for initiation of mechanical support will need to be individualized based on each patient's clinical course. ECMO would seem warranted for those patients who acutely collapse or who have a condition thought to be rapidly reversible over the course of days (e.g., arrhythmia, post-cardiotomy or post-transplantation, myocarditis). The projected inability to wean from ECMO in days (<1 week) and the absence of contraindications (e.g., severe neurologic injury, unrecoverable concomitant illness) should be considered an indication for ECMO. In those patients not requiring emergent ECMO support, the clinician should consider the need for intubation due to cardiac failure; escalating or high doses of inotropic support; poor peripheral perfusion as evidenced by acidosis or base deficit, low mixed venous saturation, and cool extremities; and the onset of end-organ failure (renal or hepatic failure; Box 16-3).

The authors consider any of these to be strong relative indications for the initiation of VAD support, which should be balanced only against the possibility that the patient could recover in a matter of days.

Biventricular versus Left Ventricular Assist Device Support

In two large adult series, the need for biventricular support ranged from 16% to 24% in patients receiving VADs. The requirement for biventricular support was clearly associated with an increase in mortality in both studies.[100,101] The use of biventricular support appears to be far more common in the pediatric population. In larger patients, Blume and colleagues observed its use 39% of the time,[61] the Pittsburgh group reported 56%,[62] and the Thoratec registry, 50%.[99] The association between biventricular VAD support and worse outcomes seen in adults, however, was not observed. The latest series with the Berlin Heart also noted a much greater reliance on biventricular support, with incidences ranging from 82% to 100% in three studies.[80,81,102] This difference may be due to the nature of pediatric versus adult heart failure, with heart failure in children affecting both chambers and resulting in increased pulmonary vascular resistance. It is intuitive that biventricular support might magnify certain risks over LVAD support alone in pediatric patients. Most notably, bleeding and infectious complications may increase because of the necessity of placing more equipment and having more exit sites from a small pediatric patient. The Berlin Heart Institute pointed to the decreased reliance on biventricular support, from 68% to 33%, as their experience progressed as one reason for their significantly improved outcomes.[77] The authors note that a transition from left atrial to left ventricular apex helped to decrease pulmonary vascular resistance. Hetzer and colleagues[79] noted that of 121 European pediatric EXCOR implants, the survival rate for LVADs was 71%,

versus 59% for biventricular VADs. At this time, most centers place an LVAD and attempt to wean from cardiopulmonary bypass. Once the patient is weaned and on LVAD support, right ventricular function and geometry are monitored in the operating room by transesophageal echocardiography, invasive pulmonary artery monitoring, and right ventricular or central venous pressure, as is gas exchange and lung compliance. Any evidence of poor right ventricular function is treated with nitric oxide and inotropes; continued deterioration necessitates placement of a right ventricular assist device (RVAD). Uncontrolled arrhythmia also requires placement of biventricular support. Intensive care unit management is somewhat different with biventricular VADs versus LVAD only. Usually no inotropes are required, nor is pharmacologic or electrical control of the heart rhythm. With LVAD use alone, careful attention must be paid to right ventricular filling to ensure adequate filling of the LVAD. Central venous pressure should initially be closely monitored. The echocardiogram should be followed for tricuspid regurgitation and estimation of right ventricular/pulmonary artery pressure. Right ventricular filling and function may be negatively affected by pericardial effusion as well as compression of the right ventricle by the LVAD outflow cannula. With biventricular VAD support, the RVAD settings generally are made to ensure slightly less flow than for the LVAD to avoid a fluid load to the lungs.

Need for Respiratory Support

The need for pulmonary support in addition to cardiac support should be viewed as a relative indication for ECMO and as a relative contraindication to VAD implantation. Situations may develop where improved gas exchange is necessary. This most often is accomplished by concomitant ECMO cannulation, either centrally or peripherally. If a venoarterial cannulation strategy is used, it may raise unique problems with VAD filling, necessitating a greater measure of anticoagulation. Extracorporeal centrifugal pumps, such as the Levitronix CentriMag or PediVAS, Jostra RotaFlow (MAQUET, Inc., Rastatt, Germany), or Medtronic (Minneapolis, MN) Biomedicus pumps, lend themselves to the "splicing" of an oxygenator into the VAD circuit tubing.[103] This increases the clotting risk and should lead to higher levels of anticoagulation. Other novel techniques have been used to place a gas exchange membrane within an existing VAD circuit.[104,105]

Congenital Heart Disease

Long-term mechanical support of congenital heart disease presents significant clinical challenges and is associated with significantly worse outcomes than for cardiomyopathy patients.[61,99] The reasons for this are likely multifactorial. Many of these patients are not placed on support until after one or more failed operations, and frequently in the immediate postcardiotomy period. Many of these patients also have intracardiac communications, mixed circulations, or single-ventricle presentations, which can make the use of VADs quite difficult. In patients with dual-ventricle physiology, all intracardiac shunts should be closed at the time of VAD implantation to avoid desaturation or pulmonary overcirculation. There have been multiple case reports of single VAD implantation to support a single-ventricle patient. These include patients with systemic-to-pulmonary shunts,[106,107] cavopulmonary or Glenn anastamoses,[108,109] and total cavopulmonary or Fontan anastamoses.[110-115] Many of these cases have been compiled by Christina and colleagues.[116] It has recently been proposed experimentally and demonstrated clinically that completion of a cavopulmonary anastomosis in adult patients requiring biventricular support may hasten the ability to wean RVAD support in the context of a marginal right

BOX 16-3 Consideration for Long-Term Ventricular Assist Device Support

1. Need for intubation owing to cardiac failure
2. Escalating high-dose inotropic support
3. Poor peripheral perfusion
4. Evidence of end-organ dysfunction (renal, hepatic)
5. Inability to wean from extracorporeal membrane oxygenation in 72 to 96 hours (without contraindication to ventricular assist device)

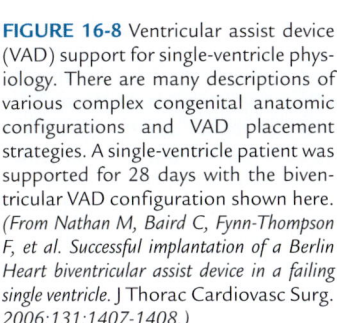

FIGURE 16-8 Ventricular assist device (VAD) support for single-ventricle physiology. There are many descriptions of various complex congenital anatomic configurations and VAD placement strategies. A single-ventricle patient was supported for 28 days with the biventricular VAD configuration shown here. *(From Nathan M, Baird C, Fynn-Thompson F, et al. Successful implantation of a Berlin Heart biventricular assist device in a failing single ventricle. J Thorac Cardiovasc Surg. 2006;131:1407-1408.)*

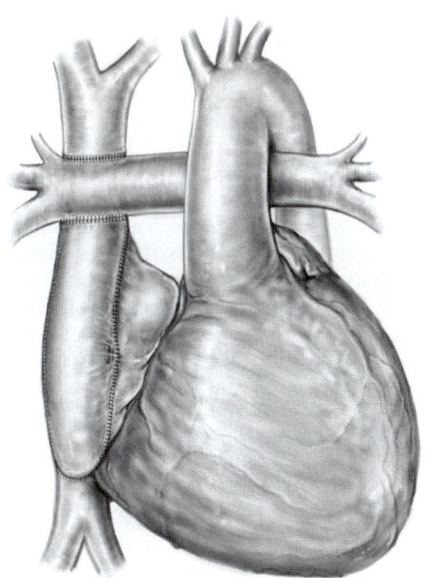

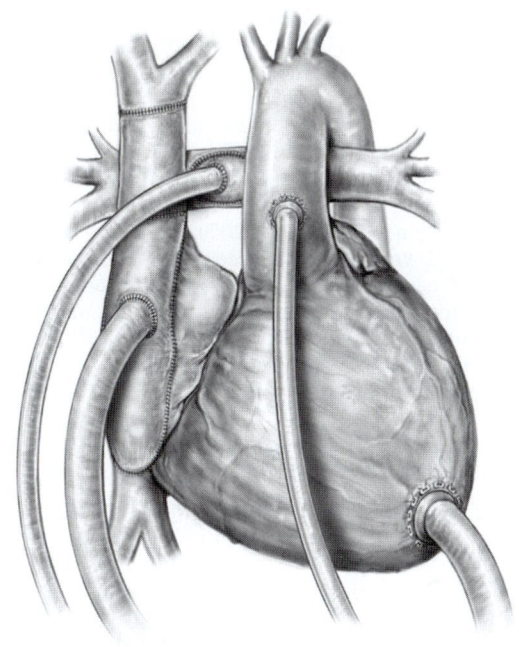

ventricle.[117,118] Generally, this support has been accomplished with pulsatile VADs for patients requiring more than days of supports, although the newer continuous-flow pumps likely will lend themselves to this application as well (Fig. 16-8).

Elevated Pulmonary Vascular Resistance

Many patients with long-standing heart failure from congenital heart disease present with markedly elevated pulmonary vascular resistance and may be considered "untransplantable." A period of LVAD support and maximal medical manipulation of the pulmonary vascular resistance may significantly lower this resistance. Repeat catheterization may then show these patients to be candidates for heart transplantation.[81,119]

Adult Congenital Heart Disease

Adults with congenital heart disease represent a larger population than children with congenital heart disease, and represent an increasing proportion of heart transplant recipients. These patients face a higher mortality rate and higher risk of retransplantation. These patients are also likely to have longer mean waiting times and significantly higher pulmonary vascular resistances.[109,120,121] It is therefore likely that increasing numbers of these patients will require VAD implantation before heart transplantation. These patients are most likely to have single-ventricle physiology, as well as dextrotransposition of the great arteries (d-TGA) or congenitally corrected (levo-) transposition (l-TGA). Both adult and pediatric patients with single-ventricle physiology have been supported with VADs, as noted previously. Consideration may be given to either common atrial or ventricular cannulation depending on residual ventricular function and the risk of thromboembolism. At least in the reported cases, single systemic ventricular VAD support appears to be adequate to support both the systemic and pulmonary circulations.

Patients with both l-TGA and d-TGA corrected by an atrial switch procedure (Senning or Mustard) are susceptible to failure of the systemic morphologic right ventricle, necessitating heart transplantation. VADs have generally been designed for implantation in an apex-forming left ventricle. These patients present challenges in the implantation of the ventricular cannula owing to the different anatomy of the right compared with the left ventricle and the fact that the left ventricle does not form an apex. Adjustments also need to be made to the orientation of the pump because the systemic ventricle may

be anterior (d-TGA) or more posterior and with dextrorotation (l-TGA), and the great vessels situated differently than in normal anatomy. Both pulsatile[122–126] and continuous-flow pumps have been used for this application.[127,128] Many of these authors offer nuanced descriptions of the implantation technique in their reports.

Adverse Events

In a 2005 report from the International Society for Heart and Lung Transplantation Mechanical Circulatory Support Database, the following adverse events, among others, were reported as percentages of all patients: infection (32.5%), bleeding (27.8%), and neurologic dysfunction (14%).[129] Not surprisingly, early series of pediatric patients relying on "adult" devices had similar findings. Data from the Thoratec registry included a 52% incidence of infectious complications, a 33% incidence of bleeding events, and a 27% incidence of neurologic events, which were comparable to incidences for adult patients in this registry.[99] Similarly, the Pittsburgh group reported a 22% incidence of bleeding requiring reoperation, a 39% incidence of infection, and a 28% incidence of neurologic events.[62] In 2006, Blume and coworkers[61] reported a 41% infection rate, a 31% incidence of reoperation for bleeding, and a 13% incidence of stroke. From these data, it would appear that infectious complications and possibly neurologic events occur more frequently in pediatric patients. The incidence of neurologic events at the Berlin Heart Institute appears to be between 6% and 15%, with a 23% incidence of "thromboembolic complications."[130] Reoperation for bleeding in their series occurred between 20% and 23.5% of the time depending on the period being reported. Because the EXCOR is translucent, accumulation of thrombotic material can be followed over time and "pump changes" performed if necessary. These blood pump changes can provide a surrogate measure of the level of anticoagulation and potential for thrombotic events. In the Berlin Heart series there were 35 pump changes in 68 patients, although it is not clear how many patients received more than one pump change.[77] The Arkansas group reported on 17 patients and saw a 30% incidence of bleeding and a 41% incidence of neurologic complications, two of which were fatal.[102] In eight patients, the Stanford group saw only a 13% incidence of bleeding complications, no device-related infections, device exchange in 50% of patients, and a 63% incidence of neurologic events, most of which were explained by embolism or hemorrhage.[95] Gandhi and colleagues, in nine patients receiving biventricular VAD EXCOR implantation, had no bleeding, neurologic, or thromboembolic events, but a 44% incidence of infection and a 56% incidence of pump change.[81] Humpl and associates in Toronto reported on 15 patients and noted a 20% reoperation rate for bleeding, a 20% incidence of neurologic symptoms, and a 20% incidence of pump changes.[80] The large variability of these results is likely due to the small size of each of these studies, as well as variability in management strategies, duration of support, and learning curves between institutions. All of these data do suggest, however, that the incidence of complications in children will not be greater, and perhaps will be lower than that seen in adults.

Anticoagulation

Children have unique physiologic issues that affect the dosing, metabolism, and complications of most drugs. In addition, few drugs have been studied as extensively in the pediatric population as they have been in the adult population. These factors present unique challenges for anticoagulation of pediatric patients. Marked differences exist in both the procoagulation and anticoagulation pathways between children and adults. These differences also continually change until adulthood. Andrew and colleagues examined these differences in premature and term infants in the first 6 months of life and in children 1 and 16 years of age.[131–133] In infants, contact and vitamin K–dependent factors are at 70% of the levels found in the adult population. The coagulation inhibitors antithrombin III and proteins C and S are also low at birth. In newborns and children to 16 years of age, the capacity to generate thrombin is both decreased and delayed, although these change are less notable in older children. Various genetic mutations, including the prothrombotic mutations factor V Leiden and the prothrombin gene; deficiencies of antithrombin, protein C, and protein S; as well as hyperhomocysteinemia and dysfibrogenemia, may also affect the infant patient.[134] All of these changes may alter the therapeutic effects of anticoagulation in children.[135] Central venous catheters are recognized as the single greatest risk factor for the development of thromboses in children.[136–138] Central venous catheters are associated with 90% of neonatal venous thromboses and over 66% of childhood thromboses.[137,139] Infection also plays a significant role in prothrombotic processes in children.[134] Neonatal platelets are hyporeactive to thrombin, epinephrine/adenosine diphosphate, and thromboxane,[140] whereas the bleeding time is decreased because of increased red cell size and hematocrit and increased levels of von Willebrand factor. It follows that the placement of a significant surface area of artificial material into the bloodstream of a critically ill child, while simultaneously administering anticoagulants, would significantly alter the incidence of thrombosis and bleeding.

Anticoagulation for pediatric mechanical circulatory support has traditionally involved management with heparin while on ECMO. Monitoring was generally done by activated clotting time, and the incidences of bleeding and thrombotic complications both remain greater than 30% for ECMO support. Management of anticoagulation for long-term support devices presents a unique set of challenges. In both adult and pediatric patients with long-term devices, greater focus has been placed on the ongoing platelet activation that occurs in mechanical circulatory support.[141] It is also recognized to be advantageous to switch from a continuous intravenous infusion (i.e., heparin) to anticoagulants that are dosed intermittently (i.e., warfarin, low-molecular-weight heparin, antiplatelet agents) because this aids in patient mobility and decreases infectious risks. Oral management of coagulation with warfarin is difficult because of variable intake and absorption of the drug in children unable to take pills or with frequent gastrointestinal issues. Vitamin K is present in many formula preparations as well, which can alter dosing because the dietary intake rapidly changes in a growing child. For these reasons, low-molecular-weight heparin may be a more acceptable substitute in children, although it does require twice-daily subcutaneous injections.

The group at the Berlin Heart Institute has described the changes in their anticoagulation regimen over time.[130,142] At the present time, they divide their anticoagulation protocol into stages. In the preoperative period, no antiplatelet agents are administered and heparin is used as warranted for patients with heart failure. In the intraoperative period, heparin is use for cardiopulmonary bypass and is fully reversed with protamine at the end of implantation. In the first 8 hours after surgery, no anticoagulation is administered. After 8 hours, in the absence of bleeding, heparin therapy is initiated at a low dose and gradually titrated upward. Days later, once platelet function and count have normalized, what the group refers to as antiplatelet aggregation (aspirin) and antiplatelet adhesion (dipyridamole) drugs are administered. In the late postoperative period, the transition is made to warfarin (or low-molecular-weight heparin). Using the "newer" strategy, they were able to demonstrate slight reductions in bleeding and thrombotic complications. These incidences remained at 38% (bleeding) and 22% (thrombotic), however.[130] The North American IDE trial has largely followed this regimen.

The Berlin Heart Institute group also retrospectively compared the use of blood products in their patients receiving ECMO and those receiving a VAD. Patients with a VAD received 4.3 mL/kg/day of platelets compared with 24.6 mL/kg/day in patients on ECMO. Striking differences were also seen in packed red blood cells (17.2 mL/kg/day vs. 60.3 mL/kg/day) and plasma (8.5 mL/kg/day vs. 46.9 mL/kg/day).[143] Although it is difficult to draw many conclusions from a nonrandomized study of very different patient populations, most would agree that the consumption of blood products is much greater in patients on ECMO.

With the advent of antiplatelet agents in the management of these patients, the laboratory regulation of anticoagulation also increased in complexity. Commonly used laboratory tests such as prothrombin and partial thromboplastin time do not measure platelet function, and although the activated clotting time does, this test was designed for high levels of anticoagulation. Although a number of different tests have been explored for the measurement of platelet function and aggregation in the adult VAD and interventional cardiology literature, the sole test routinely used for platelet function measurement in the pediatric VAD population is the thromboelastogram[144]; it is a requirement for the Berlin Heart IDE trial.

Other Management Issues

Other management issues include anesthesia for other procedures while on mechanical support. One group examined 29 anesthesia cases in 11 patients with the Berlin Heart EXCOR and found these patients to be particularly sensitive to reductions in systemic vascular resistance because of the fixed nature of the cardiac output.[145] Not surprisingly, pediatric VAD support was associated with the development of increased human leukocyte antigen (HLA) sensitization,[146] but this was not associated with changes in the short- or medium-term outcomes of heart transplantation. Last, because the field has lacked the capacity for longer-term support until recently, the capacity of the failing pediatric myocardium to recover with support remains largely untested. One group examined serial biopsy specimens from four patients treated with VADs and found that even short-term VAD therapy resulted in reverse remodeling of the myocardium.[147] This exciting possibility will require the development of VAD weaning protocols to predict better which patients can undergo VAD explantation.

CONCLUSION

As survival with severe forms of palliated congenital heart disease continues to improve, and heart failure management strategies allow for long-term survival of children with heart disease, the end-stage heart failure population in pediatrics in expanding. Mechanical support options for this group of patients has been limited in the past. Over the last few years, coordinated efforts between regulatory agencies, the NIH, clinicians, and advocacy groups have produced a rapidly changing environment for mechanical circulatory support in children. Understanding the differences between the pediatric end-stage patient and the adult is critical to assess outcomes. Financial analyses and cost studies should be included in the next generation of device studies. In addition, the pediatric-specific issues of anticoagulation and neurodevelopmental outcomes will be critical to assess with scientific rigor. Pediatric-specific device development and registry data collection will continue, and the next decade in this field will be exciting and challenging.

REFERENCES

1. Gibbon Jr JH. Application of a mechanical heart and lung apparatus to cardiac surgery. *Minn Med*. 1954;37:171–185; passim.
2. Lillehei CW, Varco RL, Cohen M, et al. The first open heart corrections of tetralogy of Fallot: a 26–31 year follow-up of 106 patients. *Ann Surg*. 1986;204:490–502.
3. Kirklin JW, Dushane JW, Patrick RT, et al. Intracardiac surgery with the aid of a mechanical pump-oxygenator system (Gibbon type): report of eight cases. *Proc Staff Meet Mayo Clin*. 1955;30:201–206.
4. Castaneda AR, Lamberti J, Sade RM, et al. Open-heart surgery during the first three months of life. *J Thorac Cardiovasc Surg*. 1974;68:719–731.
5. Barratt-Boyes BG. Complete correction of cardiovascular malformations in the first two years of life using profound hypothermia. In: Barratt-Boyes BG, Neutze JM, Harris EA, eds. *Heart Disease in Infancy*. Edinburgh: Churchill Livingstone; 1973:25–36.
6. Keane J, Lock J, Fyler D, eds. *Nadas' Pediatric Cardiology*. 2nd ed. Philadelphia: Saunders Elsevier; 2006.
7. Lipshultz SE, Sleeper LA, Towbin JA, et al. The incidence of pediatric cardiomyopathy in two regions of the United States. *N Engl J Med*. 2003;348:1647–1655.
8. Nugent AW, Daubeney PE, Chondros P, et al. The epidemiology of childhood cardiomyopathy in Australia. *N Engl J Med*. 2003;348:1639–1646.
9. Rosenthal D, Chrisant MR, Edens E, et al. International Society for Heart and Lung Transplantation: practice guidelines for management of heart failure in children. *J Heart Lung Transplant*. 2004;23:1313–1333.
10. Boneva RS, Botto LD, Moore CA, et al. Mortality associated with congenital heart defects in the United States: trends and racial disparities, 1979–1997. *Circulation*. 2001;103:2376–2381.
11. Boucek MM, Aurora P, Edwards LB, et al. Registry of the International Society for Heart and Lung Transplantation: tenth official pediatric heart transplantation report—2007. *J Heart Lung Transplant*. 2007;26:796–807.
12. United Network for Organ Sharing. Available at www.unos.org; Accessed 21.01.2008.
13. Almond CS, Thiagarajan RR, Piercey GE, et al. Waiting list mortality among children listed for heart transplantation in the United States. *Circulation*. 2009;119:717–727.
14. Mah D, Singh TP, Thiagarajan RR, et al. Incidence and risk factors for mortality in infants awaiting heart transplantation in the USA. *J Heart Lung Transplant*. 2009;28:1292–1298.
15. McGiffin DC, Naftel DC, Kirklin JK, et al. Predicting outcome after listing for heart transplantation in children: comparison of Kaplan-Meier and parametric competing risk analysis. Pediatric Heart Transplant Study Group. *J Heart Lung Transplant*. 1997;16:713–722.
16. Mital S, Addonizio LJ, Lamour JM, et al. Outcome of children with end-stage congenital heart disease waiting for cardiac transplantation. *J Heart Lung Transplant*. 2003;22:147–153.
17. Morrow WR, Naftel D, Chinnock R, et al. Outcome of listing for heart transplantation in infants younger than six months: predictors of death and interval to transplantation. The Pediatric Heart Transplantation Study Group. *J Heart Lung Transplant*. 1997;16:1255–1266.
18. Nield LE, McCrindle BW, Bohn DJ, et al. Outcomes for children with cardiomyopathy awaiting transplantation. *Cardiol Young*. 2000;10:358–366.
19. del Nido PJ, Dalton HJ, Thompson AE, et al. Extracorporeal membrane oxygenator rescue in children during cardiac arrest after cardiac surgery. *Circulation*. 1992;86(suppl 5):II300–II304.
20. Kulik TJ, Moler FW, Palmisano JM, et al. Outcome-associated factors in pediatric patients treated with extracorporeal membrane oxygenator after cardiac surgery. *Circulation*. 1996;94(suppl 9):II63–II68.
21. Raithel SC, Pennington DG, Boegner E, et al. Extracorporeal membrane oxygenation in children after cardiac surgery. *Circulation*. 1992;86(suppl 5):II305–II310.
22. Walters III HL, Hakimi M, Rice MD, et al. Pediatric cardiac surgical ECMO: multivariate analysis of risk factors for hospital death. *Ann Thorac Surg*. 1995;60:329–336.
23. del Nido PJ, Armitage JM, Fricker FJ, et al. Extracorporeal membrane oxygenation support as a bridge to pediatric heart transplantation. *Circulation*. 1994;90:II66–II69.
24. Fiser WP, Yetman AT, Gunselman RJ, et al. Pediatric arteriovenous extracorporeal membrane oxygenation (ECMO) as a bridge to cardiac transplantation. *J Heart Lung Transplant*. 2003;22:770–777.
25. Gajarski RJ, Mosca RS, Ohye RG, et al. Use of extracorporeal life support as a bridge to pediatric cardiac transplantation. *J Heart Lung Transplant*. 2003;22:28–34.
26. Kirshbom PM, Bridges ND, Myung RJ, et al. Use of extracorporeal membrane oxygenation in pediatric thoracic organ transplantation. *J Thorac Cardiovasc Surg*. 2002;123:130–136.
27. Bartlett RH, Gazzaniga AB, Huxtable RF, et al. Extracorporeal circulation (ECMO) in neonatal respiratory failure. *J Thorac Cardiovasc Surg*. 1977;74:826–833.
28. Bartlett RH, Andrews AF, Toomasian JM, et al. Extracorporeal membrane oxygenation for newborn respiratory failure: forty-five cases. *Surgery*. 1982;92:425–433.
29. Bartlett RH, Gazzaniga AB, Huxtable RH, et al. Extracorporeal membrane oxygenation (ECMO) in newborn respiratory failure: technical consideration. *Trans Am Soc Artif Intern Organs*. 1979;25:473–475.
30. Bartlett RH, Roloff DW, Cornell RG, et al. Extracorporeal circulation in neonatal respiratory failure: a prospective randomized study. *Pediatrics*. 1985;76:479–487.
31. O'Rourke PP, Crone RK, Vacanti JP, et al. Extracorporeal membrane oxygenation and conventional medical therapy in neonates with persistent pulmonary hypertension of the newborn: a prospective randomized study. *Pediatrics*. 1989;84:957–963.
32. UK Collaborative ECMO Trial Group. UK collaborative randomised trial of neonatal extracorporeal membrane oxygenation. *Lancet*. 1996;348:75–82.
33. Zapol WM, Snider MT, Hill JD, et al. Extracorporeal membrane oxygenation in severe acute respiratory failure: a randomized prospective study. *JAMA*. 1979;242:2193–2196.
34. Bartlett RH, Gazzaniga AB, Wetmore NE, et al. Extracorporeal membrane oxygenation (ECMO) in the treatment of cardiac and respiratory failure in children. *Trans Am Soc Artif Intern Organs*. 1980;26:578–581.
35. Hardesty RL, Deeb GM, Griffith BP, et al. Clinical experience with pediatric microporous oxygenator for profound hypothermia. *Arch Surg*. 1980;115:1355–1358.
36. Hardesty RL, Griffith BP, Debski RF, et al. Extracorporeal membrane oxygenation: successful treatment of persistent fetal circulation following repair of congenital diaphragmatic hernia. *J Thorac Cardiovasc Surg*. 1981;81:556–563.
37. Trento A, Estner SM, Griffith BP, et al. Massive hemoptysis in patients with cystic fibrosis: three case reports and a protocol for clinical management. *Ann Thorac Surg*. 1985;39:254–256.
38. Kanter KR, Pennington G, Weber TR, et al. Extracorporeal membrane oxygenation for postoperative cardiac support in children. *J Thorac Cardiovasc Surg*. 1987;93:27–35.
39. Klein MD, Shaheen KW, Whittlesey GC, et al. Extracorporeal membrane oxygenation for the circulatory support of children after repair of congenital heart disease. *J Thorac Cardiovasc Surg*. 1990;100:498–505.
40. Weinhaus L, Canter C, Noetzel M, et al. Extracorporeal membrane oxygenation for circulatory support after repair of congenital heart defects. *Ann Thorac Surg*. 1989;48:206–212.
41. Duncan BW, Ibrahim AE, Hraska V, et al. Use of rapid-deployment extracorporeal membrane oxygenation for the resuscitation of pediatric patients with heart disease after cardiac arrest. *J Thorac Cardiovasc Surg*. 1998;116:305–311.
42. Jacobs JP, Ojito JW, McConaghey TW, et al. Rapid cardiopulmonary support for children with complex congenital heart disease. *Ann Thorac Surg*. 2000;70:742–749; discussion 749–750.
43. Hines MH. ECMO and congenital heart disease. *Semin Perinatol*. 2005;29:34–39.
44. Van Meurs KP, Hintz SR, Sheehan AM. ECMO for neonatal respiratory failure. In: Van Meurs K, Lally K, Peek G, et al., eds. *ECMO: Extracorporeal Cardiopulmonary Support in Critical Care*. 3rd ed. Ann Arbor, MI: Extracorporeal Life Support Organization; 2005:273–295.
45. Extracorporeal Life Support Organization. *Extracorporeal Life Support Organization Registry Report*. Ann Arbor, MI: University of Michigan; 2010.
46. Salvin JW, Laussen PC, Thiagarajan RR. Extracorporeal membrane oxygenation for postcardiotomy mechanical cardiovascular support in children with congenital heart disease. *Paediatr Anaesth*. 2008;18:1157–1162.
47. Alsoufi B, Al-Radi OO, Gruenwald C, et al. Extra-corporeal life support following cardiac surgery in children: analysis of risk factors and survival in a single institution. *Eur J Cardiothorac Surg*. 2009;35:1004–1011.
48. Ishino K, Weng Y, Alexi-Meskishvili V, et al. Extracorporeal membrane oxygenation as a bridge to cardiac transplantation in children. *Artif Organs*. 1996;20:728–732.
49. Pollock-BarZiv SM, McCrindle BW, West LJ, et al. Competing outcomes after neonatal and infant wait-listing for heart transplantation. *J Heart Lung Transplant*. 2007;26:980–985.
50. Levi D, Marelli D, Plunkett M, et al. Use of assist devices and ECMO to bridge pediatric patients with cardiomyopathy to transplantation. *J Heart Lung Transplant*. 2002;21:760–770.
51. del Nido PJ, Duncan BW, Mayer Jr JE, et al. Left ventricular assist device improves survival in children with left ventricular dysfunction after repair of anomalous origin of the left coronary artery from the pulmonary artery. *Ann Thorac Surg*. 1999;67:169–172.
52. Karl TR, Sano S, Horton S, et al. Centrifugal pump left heart assist in pediatric cardiac operations: indication, technique, and results. *J Thorac Cardiovasc Surg*. 1991;102:624–630.
53. Kesler KA, Pruitt AL, Turrentine MW, et al. Temporary left-sided mechanical cardiac support during acute myocarditis. *J Heart Lung Transplant*. 1994;13:268–270.
54. Shen I, Ungerleider RM. Routine use of mechanical ventricular assist following the Norwood procedure. *Semin Thorac Cardiovasc Surg Pediatr Card Surg Annu*. 2004;7:16–21.

55. Karl TR, Horton SB, Brizard C. Postoperative support with the centrifugal pump ventricular assist device (VAD). *Semin Thorac Cardiovasc Surg Pediatr Card Surg Annu.* 2006;83–91.
56. Ungerleider RM, Shen I, Yeh T, et al. Routine mechanical ventricular assist following the Norwood procedure: improved neurologic outcome and excellent hospital survival. *Ann Thorac Surg.* 2004;77:18–22.
57. Arabía FA, Tsau PH, Smith RG, et al. Pediatric bridge to heart transplantation: application of the Berlin Heart, Medos and Thoratec ventricular assist devices. *J Heart Lung Transplant.* 2006;25:16–21.
58. Coskun O, Parsa A, Weitkemper H, et al. Heart transplantation in children after mechanical circulatory support: comparison of heart transplantation with ventricular assist devices and elective heart transplantation. *ASAIO J.* 2005;51:495–497.
59. Kaczmarek I, Sachweh J, Groetzner J, et al. Mechanical circulatory support in pediatric patients with the Medos assist device. *ASAIO J.* 2005;51:498–500.
60. Hill JD, Reinhartz O. Clinical outcomes in pediatric patients implanted with Thoratec ventricular assist device. *Semin Thorac Cardiovasc Surg Pediatr Card Surg Annu.* 2006;115–122.
61. Blume ED, Naftel DC, Bastardi HJ, et al. Outcomes of children bridged to heart transplantation with ventricular assist devices: a multi-institutional study. *Circulation.* 2006;113:2313–2319.
62. Sharma MS, Webber SA, Morell VO, et al. Ventricular assist device support in children and adolescents as a bridge to heart transplantation. *Ann Thorac Surg.* 2006;82:926–932.
63. Slaughter MS, Rogers JG, Milano CA, et al. Advanced heart failure treated with continuous-flow left ventricular assist device. *N Engl J Med.* 2009;361:2241–2251.
64. Blume ED, Rosenthal DN, Chen JM, et al. Outcomes of children implanted with ventricular assist device therapy: analysis of the Interagency Registry for Mechanical Circulatory Support (INTERMACS). *J Heart Lung Transplant.* 2010;29:S34.
65. Owens WR, Bryant 3rd R, Dreyer WJ, et al. Initial clinical experience with the HeartMate II ventricular assist system in a pediatric institution. *Artif Organs.* 2010;34:600–603.
66. John R, Long JW, Massey HT, et al. Outcomes of a multicenter trial of the Levitronix CentriMag ventricular assist system for short-term circulatory support. *J Thorac Cardiovasc Surg.* 2011;141:932–939.
67. Hirata Y, Charette K, Mosca RS, et al. Pediatric application of the Thoratec CentriMag BIVAD as a bridge to heart transplantation. *J Thorac Cardiovasc Surg.* 2008;136:1386–1387.
68. Kouretas PC, Kaza AK, Burch PT, et al. Experience with the Levitronix CentriMag in the pediatric population as a bridge to decision and recovery. *Artif Organs.* 2009;33:1002–1004.
69. Dasse KA, Gellman B, Kameneva MV, et al. Assessment of hydraulic performance and biocompatibility of a maglev centrifugal pump system designed for pediatric cardiac or cardiopulmonary support. *ASAIO J.* 2007;53:771–777.
70. Andrade JG, Al-Saloos H, Jeewa A, et al. Facilitated cardiac recovery in fulminant myocarditis: pediatric use of the Impella LP 5.0 pump. *J Heart Lung Transplant.* 2009;29:96–97.
71. Ruygrok PN, Esmore DS, Alison PM, et al. Pediatric experience with the VentrAssist LVAD. *Ann Thorac Surg.* 2008;86:622–626.
72. Ricci M, Gaughan CB, Rossi M, et al. Initial experience with the TandemHeart circulatory support system in children. *ASAIO J.* 2008;54:542–545.
73. U.S. Food and Drug Administration. *DeBakey VAD Child Left Ventricular Assist System—H030003.* Available at www.accessdata.fda.gov/cdrh_docs pdf3/H030003a.pdf.
74. Fraser Jr CD, Carberry KE, Owens WR, et al. Preliminary experience with the MicroMed DeBakey pediatric ventricular assist device. *Semin Thorac Cardiovasc Surg Pediatr Card Surg Annu.* 2006;109–114.
75. Padalino MA, Ohye RG, Chang AC, et al. Bridge to transplant using the MicroMed DeBakey ventricular assist device in a child with idiopathic dilated cardiomyopathy. *Ann Thorac Surg.* 2006;81:1118–1121.
76. Warnecke H, Berdjis F, Hennig E, et al. Mechanical left ventricular support as a bridge to cardiac transplantation in childhood. *Eur J Cardiothorac Surg.* 1991;5:330–333.
77. Hetzer R, Alexi-Meskishvili V, Weng Y, et al. Mechanical cardiac support in the young with the Berlin Heart EXCOR pulsatile ventricular assist device: 15 years' experience. *Semin Thorac Cardiovasc Surg Pediatr Card Surg Annu.* 2006:99–108.
78. Hetzer R, Dandel M, Knosalla C. Left ventricular assist devices and drug therapy in heart failure. *N Engl J Med.* 2007;356:869–870; author reply 871–862.
79. Hetzer R, Potapov EV, Stiller B, et al. Improvement in survival after mechanical circulatory support with pneumatic pulsatile ventricular assist devices in pediatric patients. *Ann Thorac Surg.* 2006;82:917–924; discussion 924–915.
80. Humpl T, Furness S, Gruenwald C, et al. The Berlin Heart EXCOR Pediatrics: the SickKids experience 2004-2008. *Artif Organs.* 2010;34:1082–1086.
81. Gandhi SK, Huddleston CB, Balzer DT, et al. Biventricular assist devices as a bridge to heart transplantation in small children. *Circulation.* 2008;118(suppl 14):S89–S93.
82. Brancaccio G, Amodeo A, Ricci Z, et al. Mechanical assist device as a bridge to heart transplantation in children less than 10 kilograms. *Ann Thorac Surg.* 2010;90:58–62.
83. Karimova A, Van Doorn C, Brown K, et al. Mechanical bridging to orthotopic heart transplantation in children weighing less than 10 kg: feasibility and limitations. *Eur J Cardiothorac Surg.* 2011;39:304–309.
84. Cohen G, Permut L. Decision making for mechanical cardiac assist in pediatric cardiac surgery. *Semin Thorac Cardiovasc Surg Pediatr Card Surg Annu.* 2005;41–50.
85. Chaturvedi RR, Macrae D, Brown KL, et al. Cardiac ECMO for biventricular hearts after paediatric open heart surgery. *Heart.* 2004;90:545–551.
86. Klugman D, Berger JT, Sable CA, et al. Pediatric patients hospitalized with myocarditis: a multi-institutional analysis. *Pediatr Cardiol.* 2009;31:222–228.
87. Rajagopal SK, Almond CS, Laussen PC, et al. Extracorporeal membrane oxygenation for the support of infants, children, and young adults with acute myocarditis: a review of the Extracorporeal Life Support Organization registry. *Crit Care Med.* 2009;38(2):382–387.
88. Tissot C, Buckvold S, Phelps CM, et al. Outcome of extracorporeal membrane oxygenation for early primary graft failure after pediatric heart transplantation. *J Am Coll Cardiol.* 2009;54:730–737.
89. Bae JO, Frischer JS, Waich M, et al. Extracorporeal membrane oxygenation in pediatric cardiac transplantation. *J Pediatr Surg.* 2005;40:1051–1056 discussion 1056–1057.
90. Fenton KN, Webber SA, Danford DA, et al. Long-term survival after pediatric cardiac transplantation and postoperative ECMO support. *Ann Thorac Surg.* 2003;76:843–846 discussion 847.
91. Galantowicz ME, Stolar CJ. Extracorporeal membrane oxygenation for perioperative support in pediatric heart transplantation. *J Thorac Cardiovasc Surg.* 1991;102:148–151 discussion 151–142.
92. Delmo Walter EM, Stiller B, Hetzer R, et al. Extracorporeal membrane oxygenation for perioperative cardiac support in children: I. Experience at the Deutsches Herzzentrum Berlin (1987-2005). *ASAIO J.* 2007;53:246–254.
93. Thourani VH, Kirshbom PM, Kanter KR, et al. Venoarterial extracorporeal membrane oxygenation (VA-ECMO) in pediatric cardiac support. *Ann Thorac Surg.* 2006;82:138–144 discussion 144–135.
94. Walker GM, McLeod K, Brown KL, et al. Extracorporeal life support as a treatment of supraventricular tachycardia in infants. *Pediatr Crit Care Med.* 2003;4:52–54.
95. Malaisrie SC, Pelletier MP, Yun JJ, et al. Pneumatic paracorporeal ventricular assist device in infants and children: initial Stanford experience. *J Heart Lung Transplant.* 2008;27:173–177.
96. Imamura M, Dossey AM, Prodhan P, et al. Bridge to cardiac transplant in children: Berlin Heart versus extracorporeal membrane oxygenation. *Ann Thorac Surg.* 2009;87:1894–1901 discussion 1901.
97. Potapov EV, Stiller B, Hetzer R. Ventricular assist devices in children: current achievements and future perspectives. *Pediatr Transplant.* 2007;11:241–255.
98. Stiller B, Weng Y, Hubler M, et al. Pneumatic pulsatile ventricular assist devices in children under 1 year of age. *Eur J Cardiothorac Surg.* 2005;28:234–239.
99. Reinhartz O, Keith FM, El-Banayosy A, et al. Multicenter experience with the Thoratec ventricular assist device in children and adolescents. *J Heart Lung Transplant.* 2001;20:439–448.
100. Deng MC, Edwards LB, Hertz MI, et al. Mechanical circulatory support device database of the international society for heart and lung transplantation: third annual report—2005. *J Heart Lung Transplant.* 2005;24:1182–1187.
101. Holman WL, Pae WE, Teutenberg JJ, et al. INTERMACS: interval analysis of registry data. *J Am Coll Surg.* 2009;208:755–761; discussion 761–752.
102. Rockett SR, Bryant JC, Morrow WR, et al. Preliminary single center North American experience with the Berlin Heart pediatric EXCOR device. *ASAIO J.* 2008; 54:479–482.
103. Huang SC, Chi NH, Chen CA, et al. Left ventricular assist for pediatric patients with dilated cardiomyopathy using the Medos VAD cannula and a centrifugal pump. Artif Organs. 2009;33:1032–1037.
104. Camboni D, Philipp A, Haneya A, et al. Serial use of an interventional lung assist device and a ventricular assist device. *ASAIO J.* 2010;56:270–272.
105. Wermelt JZ, Honjo O, Kilic A, et al. Use of a pulsatile ventricular assist device (Berlin Heart EXCOR) and an interventional lung assist device (Novalung) in an animal model. *ASAIO J.* 2008;54:498–503.
106. Matsuda H, Taenaka Y, Ohkubo N, et al. Use of a paracorporeal pneumatic ventricular assist device for postoperative cardiogenic shock in two children with complex cardiac lesions. *Artif Organs.* 1988;12:423–430.
107. Pearce FB, Kirklin JK, Holman WL, et al. Successful cardiac transplant after Berlin Heart bridge in a single ventricle heart: use of aortopulmonary shunt as a supplementary source of pulmonary blood flow. *J Thorac Cardiovasc Surg.* 2009;137:e40–e42.
108. Chu MW, Sharma K, Tchervenkov CI, et al. Berlin Heart ventricular assist device in a child with hypoplastic left heart syndrome. *Ann Thorac Surg.* 2007;83:1179–1181.
109. Irving C, Parry G, O'sullivan J, et al. Cardiac transplantation in adults with congenital heart disease. *Heart.* 2010;96:1217–1222.
110. Calvaruso DF, Ocello S, Salviato N, et al. Implantation of a Berlin Heart as single-ventricle by-pass on Fontan circulation in univentricular heart failure. *ASAIO J.* 2007;53(6):e1–e2.
111. Cardarelli MG, Salim M, Love J, et al. Berlin Heart as a bridge to recovery for a failing Fontan. *Ann Thorac Surg.* 2009;87:943–946.
112. Frazier OH, Gregoric ID, Messner GN. Total circulatory support with an LVAD in an adolescent with a previous Fontan procedure. *Tex Heart Inst J.* 2005;32:402–404.
113. Morris CD, Gregoric ID, Cooley DA, et al. Placement of a continuous-flow ventricular assist device in the failing ventricle of an adult patient with complex cyanotic congenital heart disease. *Heart Surg Forum.* 2008;11:E143–E144.
114. Newcomb AE, Negri JC, Brizard CP, et al. Successful left ventricular assist device bridge to transplantation after failure of a Fontan revision. *J Heart Lung Transplant.* 2006;25:365–367.
115. Wheeler DS, Dent CL, Manning PB, et al. Factors prolonging length of stay in the cardiac intensive care unit following the arterial switch operation. *Cardiol Young.* 2008;18:41–50.
116. Christina JV, Ivan MR, David BR, et al. The use of ventricular assist devices in pediatric patients with univentricular hearts. *J Thorac Cardiovasc Surg.* 2011;141:588–590.
117. Martin JP, Allen JG, Weiss ES, et al. Glenn shunt facilitated weaning of right ventricular mechanical support. *Ann Thorac Surg.* 2009;88:e16–e17.
118. Succi GM, Moreira LF, Leirner AA, et al. Cavopulmonary anastomosis improves left ventricular assist device support in acute biventricular failure. *Eur J Cardiothorac Surg.* 2009;35:528–533.
119. Liden H, Haraldsson A, Ricksten SE, et al. Does pretransplant left ventricular assist device therapy improve results after heart transplantation in patients with elevated pulmonary vascular resistance? *Eur J Cardiothorac Surg.* 2009;35:1029–1034; discussion 1034–1025.
120. Karamlou T, Hirsch J, Welke K, et al. A United Network for Organ Sharing analysis of heart transplantation in adults with congenital heart disease: outcomes and factors associated with mortality and retransplantation. *J Thorac Cardiovasc Surg.* 2010;140:161–168.
121. Patel ND, Weiss ES, Allen JG, et al. Heart transplantation for adults with congenital heart disease: analysis of the United Network for Organ Sharing database. *Ann Thorac Surg.* 2009;88:814–821; discussion 821–812.

122. George I, Xydas S, Mancini DM, et al. Effect of clenbuterol on cardiac and skeletal muscle function during left ventricular assist device support. *J Heart Lung Transplant.* 2006;25:1084–1090.

123. Gregoric ID, Kosir R, Smart FW, et al. Left ventricular assist device implantation in a patient with congenitally corrected transposition of the great arteries. *Tex Heart Inst J.* 2005;32:567–569.

124. Stewart AS, Gorman RC, Pocchetino A, et al. Left ventricular assist device for right side assistance in patients with transposition. *Ann Thorac Surg.* 2002;74(3):912–914.

125. Sugiura T, Kurosawa H, Shin'oka T, et al. Successful explantation of ventricular assist device for systemic ventricular assistance in a patient with congenitally corrected transposition of the great arteries. *Interact Cardiovasc Thorac Surg.* 2006;5:792–793.

126. Wiklund L, Svensson S, Berggren H. Implantation of a left ventricular assist device, back-to-front, in an adolescent with a failing Mustard procedure. *J Thorac Cardiovasc Surg.* 1999;118:755–756.

127. Jouan J, Grinda JM, Bricourt MO, et al. Non-pulsatile axial flow ventricular assist device for right systemic ventricle failure late after Senning procedure. *Int J Artif Organs.* 2009;32:243–245.

128. Joyce DL, Crow SS, John R, et al. Mechanical circulatory support in patients with heart failure secondary to transposition of the great arteries. *J Heart Lung Transplant.* 2010;29:1302–1305.

129. Deng MC, Edwards LB, Taylor DO. et al. Mechanical circulatory support device database of the International Society for Heart and Lung Transplantation: third annual report 2005. *J Heart Lung Transplant.* 2005;24:1182–1187.

130. Drews T, Stiller B, Hubler M, et al. Coagulation management in pediatric mechanical circulatory support. *ASAIO J.* 2007;53:640–645.

131. Andrew M, Paes B, Milner R, et al. Development of the human coagulation system in the healthy premature infant. *Blood.* 1988;72:1651–1657.

132. Andrew M, Paes B, Milner R, et al. Development of the human coagulation system in the full-term infant. *Blood.* 1987;70:165–172.

133. Andrew M, Vegh P, Johnston M, et al. Maturation of the hemostatic system during childhood. *Blood.* 1992;80:1998–2005.

134. Hoppe C, Matsunaga A. Pediatric thrombosis. *Pediatr Clin North Am.* 2002;49:1257–1283.

135. Revel-Vilk S, Chan A, Bauman M, et al. Prothrombotic conditions in an unselected cohort of children with venous thromboembolic disease. *J Thromb Haemost.* 2003;1:915–921.

136. Andrew M, Marzinotto V, Pencharz P, et al. A cross-sectional study of catheter-related thrombosis in children receiving total parenteral nutrition at home. *J Pediatr.* 1995;126:358–363.

137. Massicotte MP, Dix D, Monagle P, et al. Central venous catheter related thrombosis in children: analysis of the Canadian Registry of Venous Thromboembolic Complications. *J Pediatr.* 1998;133(6):770–776.

138. Nowak-Göttl U, Dubbers A, Kececioglu D, et al. Factor V Leiden, protein c, and lipoprotein (a) in catheter-related thrombosis in childhood: a prospective study. *J Pediatr.* 1997;131:608–612.

139. Monagle P, Adams M, Mahoney M, et al. Outcome of pediatric thromboembolic disease: a report from the Canadian Childhood Thrombophilia Registry. *Pediatr Res.* 2000;47:763–766.

140. Monagle P, Chan A, Massicotte P, et al. Antithrombotic therapy in children: the Seventh ACCP Conference on Antithrombotic and Thrombolytic Therapy. *Chest.* 2004;126(suppl 3):645S–687S.

141. Houel R, Mazoyer E, Boval B, et al. Platelet activation and aggregation profile in prolonged external ventricular support. *J Thorac Cardiovasc Surg.* 2004;128:197–202.

142. Stiller B, Lemmer J, Schubert S, et al. Management of pediatric patients after implantation of the Berlin Heart EXCOR ventricular assist device. *ASAIO J.* 2006;52:497–500.

143. Stiller B, Lemmer J, Merkle F, et al. Consumption of blood products during mechanical circulatory support in children: comparison between ECMO and a pulsatile ventricular assist device. *Intensive Care Med.* 2004;30:1814–1820.

144. Seibel K, Berdat P, Boillat C, et al. Hemostasis management in pediatric mechanical circulatory support. *Ann Thorac Surg.* 2008;85:1453–1456.

145. Cave DA, Fry KM, Buchholz H. Anesthesia for noncardiac procedures for children with a Berlin Heart EXCOR Pediatric Ventricular Assist Device: a case series. *Paediatr Anaesth.* 2010;20:647–659.

146. O'Connor MJ, Menteer J, Chrisant MR, et al. Ventricular assist device-associated anti-human leukocyte antigen antibody sensitization in pediatric patients bridged to heart transplantation. *J Heart Lung Transplant.* 2010;29:109–116.

147. Mohapatra B, Vick 3rd GW, Fraser Jr CD, et al. Short-term mechanical unloading and reverse remodeling of failing hearts in children. *J Heart Lung Transplant.* 2010;29:98–104.

CHAPTER 17

Myocardial Recovery with Use of Ventricular Assist Devices

Emma J. Birks and Leslie W. Miller

Heart failure (HF) is characterized by a process known as remodeling, which clinically usually entails progressive enlargement of the ventricle, reduction in contractility, and an increase in intracardiac pressures. These changes are associated with cellular, structural, and functional changes in the myocardium. The remodeling process previously was considered largely irreversible once HF has been present for a period of time (years), although modest improvements were shown with several oral HF medications. However, patients with chronic advanced HF who are supported with a left ventricular assist device (LVAD) that provides near-total unloading of the ventricle can show a near-normalization of nearly all structural abnormalities of the myocardium, or "reverse remodeling." Despite this significant reversal of structural changes in most patients after a period of support, only a small percentage of patients have shown sufficient improvement in myocardial function to allow the device to be removed (recovery). Reverse remodeling does not equate with recovery. However, many patients who have had the device weaned have had sustained recovery (years) and can return to a normal quality of life without requiring transplantation.

One long-term goal of mechanical circulatory support (MCS) is to learn the molecular mechanisms involved in remodeling to develop new targets and strategies to induce significant reverse remodeling and durable recovery without the device. As noted previously, abundant data show near-normalization of multiple key components of myocardial structure, beta receptors, calcium handling proteins, and metabolic substrates as well as increased myocardial contractility, which collectively suggest that recovery should be possible in more patients who are supported with an LVAD for a period of time. One more recent study suggested that combining LVAD support with adjuvant drug therapy, specifically the combinations of five oral HF drugs and the novel beta-2 adrenergic receptor agonist, clenbuterol, was associated with a 70% recovery rate, which was evident for more than 3 years of follow-up.[1] This area of myocardial recovery from chronic HF is a new, exciting, and developing field. However, many controversial and challenging questions persist: Can chronic HF really reverse? Is there a state of irreversibility? How can clinicians test for recovery? Is the recovery sustainable? What are the markers and predictors of recovery? This chapter addresses these questions and presents the data available on the concept of myocardial recovery with LVAD support.

HISTORY OF RECOVERY AND DEVICE EXPLANTATION

LVADs provide profound pressure and volume unloading of the left ventricle while restoring systemic blood flow. In 1994, Frazier and colleagues[2,3] were the first to describe improvement in a study of 18 patients supported with the pneumatic vented electric HeartMate device (Thoratec Corp, Pleasanton, CA). Of the patients, 12 had nonischemic etiology, and 6 had ischemic etiology of HF. The investigators found that in all cases LVAD support resulted in a significant reduction in the cardiothoracic ratio (from 0.65 to 0.55, $P < .003$), a decrease in left ventricular end-diastolic dimensions (from 7.0 to 5.5 cm, $P < .05$), and a 43% improvement in left ventricular ejection fraction from baseline by echocardiography.[2,3] These patients also showed improved hemodynamics, including a reduction in pulmonary capillary wedge pressure (PCWP) and improvement in cardiac index. Histologic examination showed the mean area of attenuated myocytes to be reduced from 60% to 21% from the time of implantation compared with after MCS. This was the first report suggesting that significant improvement of cardiac function was possible with LVAD support.

Levine and colleagues[4,5] measured the end-diastolic pressure-volume relationship (EDPVR) at the time of cardiac transplantation in patients treated with medical therapy and patients bridged with LVAD support. EDPVRs of hearts from medically treated patients were shifted toward markedly larger volumes. In contrast, EDPVRs of hearts from LVAD-supported patients were similar to EDPVRs of normal hearts technically unsuitable for transplantation (Fig. 17-1). This study suggested that chronic hemodynamic unloading of sufficient magnitude and duration can result in reversal

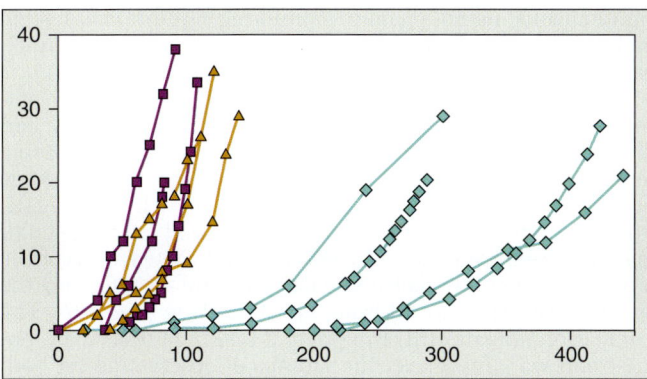

FIGURE 17-1 Graph showing end-diastolic pressure-volume relationship (EDPVRs) of hearts from medically treated patients with end-stage idiopathic cardiomyopathy (♦), patients with heart failure (HF) after prolonged left ventricular assist device (LVAD) support (▲), and normal subjects (■). EDPVRs of hearts from medically treated patients were shifted far to the right of the normal hearts, whereas EDPVRs from the LVAD groups were close to normal. x axis, volume in milliliters; y axis, pressure in mm Hg. *(From Levine HR, Oz MC, Chen JM, et al. Reversal of chronic ventricular dilation in patients with end-stage cardiomyopathy by prolonged mechanical unloading.* Circulation. *1995;91:2717-2723.)*

of chamber enlargement and normalization of cardiac structure (as indexed by the EDPVR) even in the most advanced stages of HF.

The first report of actual recovery and device explantation with a period of LVAD support was in a small series of five patients with advanced nonischemic HF (three with idiopathic dilated cardiomyopathy and two with postpartum cardiomyopathy). In three of these patients, the LVAD was removed electively after the patient showed recovery of myocardial function. In the other two patients, it was removed because of device malfunction. One patient died of a noncardiac cause 10 days after LVAD removal, but the other four patients remained alive and well 35, 33, 14, and 2 months after LVAD removal.[6]

Several subsequent reports showed recovery rates between 5% and 10% and impressive transplant-free survival rates near 70% 5 years after explantation (Table 17-1). One of the largest series by Farrar and coworkers[7] reported the results from the large multicenter Thoratec Registry, showing that 22 of 281 (8.1%) patients with nonischemic etiologic factors underwent explantation, with 17 of the 22 (70%) patients

alive and well (16 in New York Heart Association [NYHA] class I and 1 in class II) at latest follow-up. These patients had 86% and 77% transplant-free survival rates at 1 year and 5 years (see Table 17-1). Of the remaining five patients, two died and three underwent transplantation. Approximately 50% of the patients had proven myocarditis or postpartum cardiomyopathy as the cause of HF, a finding that has been true of several patients who have had recovery with LVAD support.

Another large series was reported by Mancini and associates,[8] who observed in a retrospective review of 111 patients with LVAD support as bridge to transplant (BTT) (46% of whom had dilated cardiomyopathy) that only 5 of the 111 patients (4.5% overall, but 9% of patients with nonischemic etiology) had sufficient myocardial recovery for the device to be explanted. Four of these five patients had nonischemic cardiomyopathy. Only one of the five patients who underwent explantation remained alive and well with maintained left ventricular function after 15 months of follow-up; one patient died as a result of HF 3 months after explantation, one patient had sudden death, and two patients required LVAD reimplantation. These authors argued that significant recovery occurred in only a small percentage of patients and primarily in patients with nonischemic causes of HF. This study slowed the belief that recovery was very likely.

Although myocardial recovery had been shown in patients with chronic HF, the success was limited almost entirely to younger patients with short duration of HF and most with suspected or proven myocarditis, which is generally considered a more acute and inflammatory condition with a greater likelihood of recovery. Sustained recovery in patients with chronic HF (years of established treatment) still needed to be shown. However, no one had done any active intervention to promote recovery or performed any systematic testing to show possible recovery.

A high success of device removal and sustained recovery was reported by the Berlin group, who updated their series in numerous reports over a 10-year period.[10-12] Their initial report showed that all of the first five patients who underwent explantation had sustained normal function for 51 to 592 days. By 2004, 32 of 131 (24%) patients with nonischemic HF had device explantation and had an impressive survival rate of 78.3 ± 8.1% 5 years after device explantation. HF recurred in the first 3 years in 14 of the 31 patients whose devices were explanted (31.3%), but only 2 patients died from HF after explantation. The other 12 patients with recurrent HF underwent successful transplantation. The patients

TABLE 17-1	Published Series Reporting Recovery of Native Left Ventricular Function as Defined by Successful Explantation of the Device*				
Study	No. Overall Patients	No. Nonischemic Patients	No. (%) Recovered Overall	No. (%) Nonischemic Patients Recovered	Sustainability
Mancini et al[8]	111	51	5 (4.5%)	4/51 (7.8%)	1/5 no recurrence at 15-mo follow-up
Farrar et al[7]		271		22 (8.1%)	86% and 77% transplantation-free survival at 1-yr and 5-yr follow-up
Simon et al[9]	154	74	10 (6.4%)	8/74 (11%)	80% alive and free from transplant at 1.6 ± 1.1 yr
Dandel et al[12]		131		32 (24.4%)	69.4% and 58.2% freedom from recurrent HF at 3 yr and 5 yr
Dandel et al[13]		188	81	35 (18.5%)	Postexplant 5-yr and 10-yr transplant-free survival 76.2 ± 8.1% and 70.7 ± 9.2%; 5 yr post explant 61.3 ± 9% probability from freedom HF recurrence
Maybaum et al[14]	67	37	6 (9%)	5/37 (13.5%)	Only 6-mo follow-up but no deaths or transplants in explanted patients

*The period of follow-up is variable.

HF, heart failure.

whose devices were explanted had 69.4% and 58.2% freedom from recurrence of HF at 3 years and 5 years. Several risk factors were identified that were associated with recurrence of HF after explantation, including a pre-explantation ejection fraction (EF) less than 45%; end-diastolic diameter (EDD) greater than 55 mm; and history of HF greater than 5 years. Among patients who did not have these risk factors, none had HF recurrence during the first 3 years after explantation.By 2008,[13] the Berlin group reported 81 patients weaned from LVADs, biventricular ventricular assist devices (VADs), and right VADs that had been implanted for terminal HF. The investigators analyzed patients older than 14 years who had received an LVAD for nonischemic cardiomyopathy (excluding patients with myocarditis) and identified 35 of 188 (18.5%) patients who were able to undergo device explantation, all of whom underwent the procedure as a BTT indication.[13] Of the 35 patients, 30 had the device explanted electively, and in 5 it was precipitated by pump-related complications. There were no established criteria to define recovery and suggest safety in removing the device. In eight of the electively weaned patients, the LVAD was removed with a subnormal EF (30% to 44%) and left ventricular end-diastolic diameters (LVEDDs) (56 to 60 mm) before explantation. However, the overall 5- and 10-year survival rates after LVAD removal (including post-transplant survival for patients with HF recurrence) were 79.1 ± 7.1% and 75.3 ± 7.7%. At the end of the 5th post-weaning year, these patients had a 61.3 ± 9.0% probability of freedom from HF recurrence. The authors showed that if the patient remained stable 1 year after explantation, the probability of freedom from HF recurrence at the end of 5 and 10 years after LVAD explantation was 84.2 ± 8.4% and 61.8 ± 11.4%. An important observation in their series was that patients with long-term weaning stability had a shorter history of HF, were younger, and required a shorter duration of support. One potentially important difference in the approach of the Berlin group was to begin to reduce pump speed and flow to examine native heart function 1 month after implantation, but as with all published reports on recovery, there was no standardized use of an oral HF drug regimen in these patients.

The only prospective serial observation of the natural history of LVAD support on ventricular size or function is a multicenter study of 67 patients with both ischemic and nonischemic etiologies (37 with nonischemic cardiomyopathy and 30 with ischemic cardiomyopathy) who had an LVAD placed for refractory HF by a group of investigators at eight LVAD centers, called the LVAD Working Group.[14] All patients received a HeartMate XVE device, which minimized the potential confounding effect of various types of support. The patients were to be placed on a regimen of oral HF drugs including angiotensin-converting enzyme inhibitor (ACEI), beta blocker, digoxin, angiotensin II receptor blocker, and aldosterone inhibitors if tolerated after implantation. No target doses of the HF medications were defined, and investigators managed drug selection and dosing by personal preference rather than by protocol. As a result, the maximum doses achieved were highly variable among patients, or the drugs were not given, and no conclusion could be reached regarding the potential benefit of routine use of background oral HF drug therapy.

The device that was used, the Thoratec HeartMate XVE, could be turned off from automatic pumping and hand pumped four to five times per minute to allow examination of the natural history of native heart function over time. Not all of the centers in this study were experienced with "pump-off" studies, and they were not performed in all of the patients. Some patients had an echocardiogram at reduced, rather than zero, LVAD support (15 minutes after reducing the LVAD flow to 4 L/min). Patients with an EF greater than 40% at reduced or zero LVAD support underwent dobutamine echocardiography with simultaneous hemodynamic monitoring. Additional testing included cardiopulmonary exercise tests that were performed on full pump support in a subset of patients at one site.

The echocardiograms were read by a core laboratory and showed that there was a fair amount of recovery of native cardiac function after 1 month of support, with EF increasing from a mean of 17% before LVAD implantation to an average of 34% (P <.001), reverse remodeling with reduction of LVEDD from 7.1 cm to 5.1 cm (P <.001) (Fig. 17-2), and left ventricular mass reduced from 320 g to 194 g (P <.001). However, over the next 4 months, the ventricle enlarged again in size, and the ejection fraction reduced from 30% to 22% at 4 months. The number of patients still supported at that time was small, but the trend was linear over the months of observation for both endpoints of EF and LVEDD supporting a decline, not improvement, in native cardiac function despite total unloading over time. Peak VO$_2$ improved on LVAD support (13.7 ± 4.2 mL/kg/min vs. 18.9 ± 5.5 mL/kg/min at 30 days vs. 120 days; P <.001). Only six (9%) subjects underwent explantation for myocardial recovery, but there were no protocol-specified explantation criteria. This study serves as the one observational data set that showed that the ventricle dilates over time after the first month and the EF declines and suggested that prolonged MCS per se did not lead to myocardial recovery.

POSSIBLE EXPLANATIONS OF THE LOW RATE OF MYOCARDIAL RECOVERY

The aforementioned studies showed that reverse remodeling sufficient to allow device removal could occur after LVAD support, but the frequency was low, and the sustainability of this recovery was variable. However, most programs were bridging their patients to transplantation without even testing for recovery. There was still no clear answer as to the rate of recovery that is possible or its durability.

Role of Atrophy with No Mechanical Work of the Ventricle

The atrophy of skeletal muscle observed with isolation and lack of mechanical work is a well-described sequela of many limb injuries, which require plaster cast immobilization. It seemed logical that cardiac muscle "atrophy" would be a possible consequence of a period of LVAD myocardial unloading, and lack of preload and mechanical work of the ventricle may partially explain the lack of durability of myocardial recovery observed.[14] It was hypothesized that to achieve consistent successful device explantation, regression of myocardial pathologic hypertrophy should be followed by attempts to block or reduce the amount of disuse atrophy that occurred.[15]

Studies of isolated myocytes obtained at the time of LVAD implantation compared with samples after a period of unloading verified previous observations of a marked increase in cell mass when the patient has refractory HF that regresses almost completely after a period of support to often lower than normal volume (Fig. 17-3). Investigators[16] observed that prolonged mechanical unloading resulted in reduction to lower than normal cell volume and concluded that it caused actual atrophy of the heart and individual myocytes. This hypothesis was dramatically illustrated in a study[17] that examined the effect of 48 to 72 hours of passive mechanical ventilation and diaphragm movement in patients with brain death about to become organ donors. Biopsy specimens of the diaphragm obtained at the time of organ retrieval served as the study group and were compared with an age-matched cohort who underwent elective abdominal surgery and agreed to diaphragm biopsy as the control group. Despite a very short period of only passive movement of the diaphragm, there was a 50% reduction in diaphragmatic muscle mass

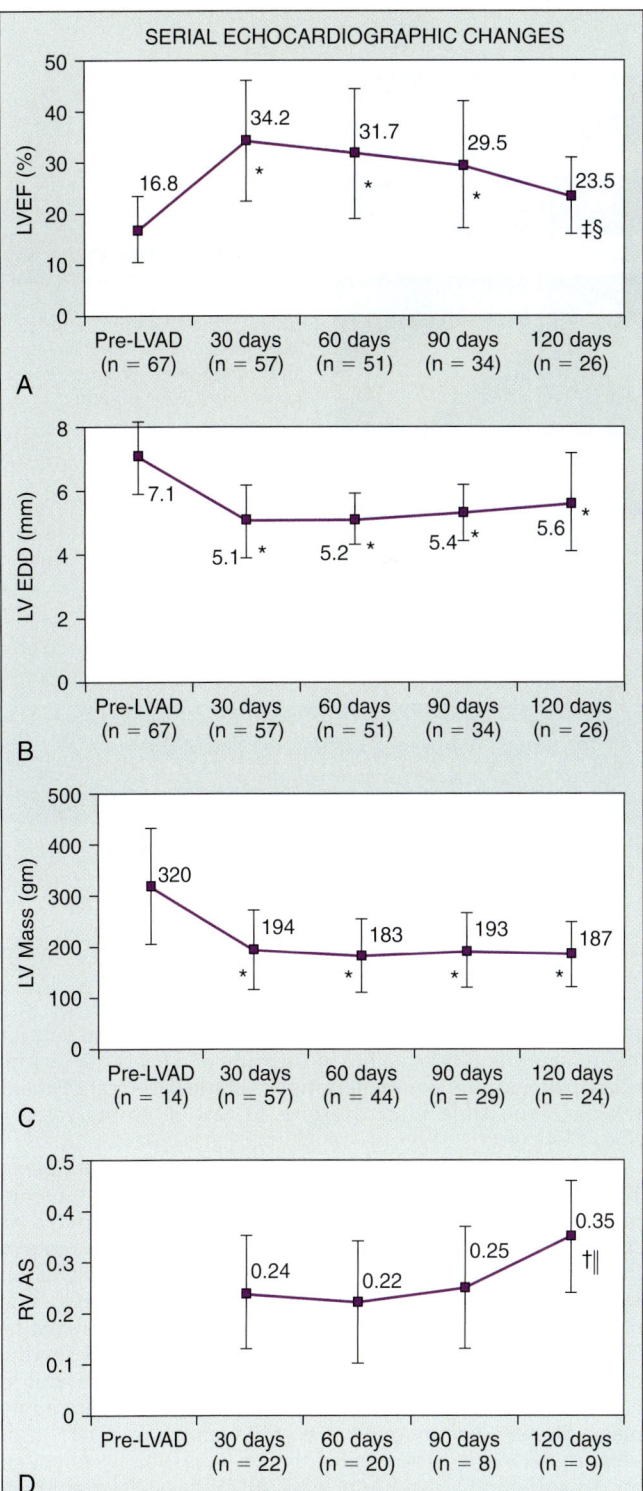

cross-sectional area by careful histologic analysis compared with control patients. These studies support the concept that skeletal muscle atrophy can be induced by lack of mechanical work and that this atrophy can occur quite rapidly and may be progressive over time.

Role of Reloading the Ventricle

Intermittently decreasing the pump speed to allow reduced withdrawal of blood from the ventricle to allow increased preload and sufficient contractility to open the aortic valve and increase myocardial work might be an alternative way to retrain the left ventricle and cause physiologic hypertrophy in the future. Patients may benefit from defined periods of significantly reduced LVAD support, such as during sleep hours, with additional interposed reductions throughout the day by computer-designed programs of reduced support. This concept is already in place to some degree with the Jarvik ILS (Intermittent Low Speed) device (Heart, Inc, Manhattan, NY) and is likely to undergo clinical evaluation to examine the potential improvement in native ventricular function with increased mechanical work over time.

TESTING FOR MYOCARDIAL RECOVERY

Regular testing of myocardial function is essential during the recovery process. Most of the described weaning protocols have not assessed the true native myocardial function because they were based on measurements taken while the device was operating at full support. Echocardiographic studies, cardiopulmonary exercise testing, and right and left heart catheterization methods have been described without clinical problems, with the pump turned off or essentially off (see later), and can be performed regularly to monitor and detect recovery. To date, very few programs have given any oral HF drugs or used any other methods to promote myocardial recovery after LVAD implant. Starting ACEIs, angiotensin II inhibitors, beta blockers, and aldosterone antagonists has been shown to reduce the heart size, improve myocardial function, and increase the rate of recovery.

Differences in Volume Displacement versus Continuous Flow Left Ventricular Assist Device Support

There has been almost total replacement of volume displacement, pulsatile flow design LVADs with the newer second-generation and third-generation continuous flow designs. (See Chapter 8 on types of LVADs and Chapter 21 for results of clinical trials.) The question has been raised as to whether, despite superior outcomes with the continuous flow design, there is similar or reduced left ventricular unloading. This question becomes potentially more significant when recovery and device explantation is the goal. Left ventricular wall stress (i.e., PCWP) has been thought to be the most important stimulus for activation of all the downstream adverse compensatory mechanisms triggered by perturbations in left ventricular function leading to the HF phenotype. Maximal reduction of wall stress seems a potentially important goal.

The data available suggest that continuous flow pumps might achieve less reduction in left ventricular end-diastolic pressure than the pulsatile flow pumps, but the ability to adjust pump speed and left ventricular decompression suggests that this too is variable. The secondary induction of significant ventricular arrhythmias with excessive speeds and reduction in left ventricular size owing to physical contact of the left ventricular wall with the inlet cannula of the device may limit continuous flow pumps as well.

FIGURE 17-2 Serial echocardiographic changes. **A-C,** Left ventricular ejection fraction (LVEF) **(A)**, left ventricular end-diastolic diameter (LV EDD) **(B)**, and left ventricular (LV) mass **(C)** were significantly improved compared with before left ventricular assist device (LVAD) implantation. **D,** Right ventricular area shortening (RVAS) was improved at 120 days versus measurements at 30 days and 60 days of support. Comparisons with pre-LVAD: *$P<0.001$. Comparisons with 30-day values: †$P<0.05$, ‡$P<0.01$. Comparisons with 60-day values: §$P<0.05$, ‖$P<0.01$. (From Maybaum S, Mancini D, Xydas S, et al. Cardiac improvement during mechanical circulatory support a prospective multicentre study of the LVAD Working group. Circulation. 2007;115:2497-2505.)

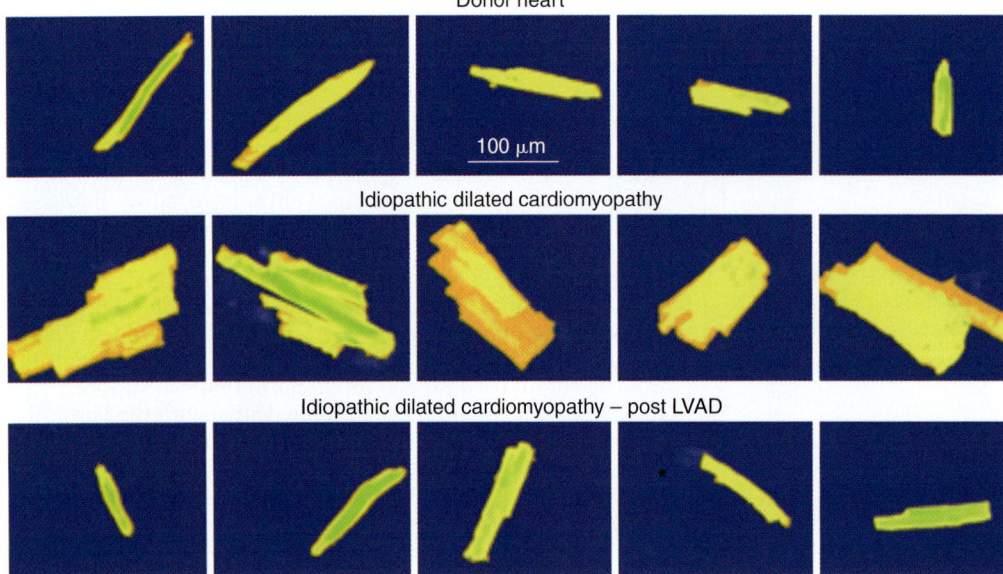

Donor heart

100 μm

Idiopathic dilated cardiomyopathy

Idiopathic dilated cardiomyopathy – post LVAD

FIGURE 17-3 Isolated cardiac myocytes—*top panel* from donor heart, *middle panel* from patient with heart failure at the time of left ventricular assist device (LVAD) implantation, and *bottom panel* from recovered patient after LVAD support.

Very few data are available to show the potential benefit of altering pump speed and design in programmed reductions, such as at night, that might help enhance preload and potential work of the ventricle and avoid atrophy. Several groups have conducted hemodynamic comparisons of patients with either type of pump, but few patients have had support with both types of pumps for a direct comparison in the individual patient. These data suggest that left ventricular unloading is better with a pulsatile flow device. It will be important to correlate the incidence of recovery and the data from molecular and histologic examinations of explanted hearts to begin to assess the relative importance of the two different types of support. The almost total change to continuous flow pumps based on superior outcomes and patient preference of the smaller, silent continuous flow pump may make this comparison obsolete, shifting the focus to methods of adjusting the continuous flow pumps to maximize left ventricular unloading.

ASSESSMENT OF MYOCARDIAL RECOVERY

In most LVAD centers, LVADs are implanted either as a BTT or as destination therapy, and the underlying myocardial function is not tested. Patients are unlikely to show or to have a very high rate of recovery. Wider testing is likely to reveal more recovery and increased rates of explantation. One of the main reasons for the low reported overall incidence of recovery in patients with chronic HF is probably the lack of belief that these patients can recover and lack of testing for it.

Achieving myocardial recovery depends critically on a safe, accurate, and reproducible method of monitoring myocardial recovery during the period of limited or no LVAD support. It is important to perform echocardiographic, functional, and hemodynamic tests before deciding whether to explant the pump from the patient. Box 17-1 lists the variables in the Berlin studies most associated with the ability to wean or remove an LVAD.

A method was developed at Harefield Hospital[18] for off-pump echocardiographic assessment of patients on the pulsatile flow HeartMate XVE pump (see Box 17-1), which consisted of acutely stopping the LVAD (with hand pumping three bursts every 15 seconds to prevent stagnation of blood

BOX 17-1 Factors Correlated with Recovery to Allow Left Ventricular Assist Device Explantation[13]

Duration of heart failure <5 years
Younger age
Left ventricular end-diastolic diameter <5.5 with pump off
Ejection fraction >45% with pump off

within the pump) and taking measurements of several peripheral hemodynamics (e.g., blood pressure and heart rate) while echocardiographic parameters were obtained both at rest and whenever possible after exercise to test inotropic reserve (Fig. 17-4).

Box 17-2 details the protocol in which patients are given 10,000 units of unfractionated heparin 5 minutes before pump cessation. Pneumatic hand pumping is instituted as soon as the HeartMate XVE device is switched off at a rate of three hand pumps every 15 seconds to avoid blood stagnation within the pump. Pneumatic hand pumping is stopped while taking hemodynamic and echocardiographic measurements. Hemodynamic assessments are done at baseline with the device on; immediately after LVAD discontinuation; and at 5, 10, and 15 minutes after device cessation. Echocardiographic measurements are obtained at baseline and at 5 and 15 minutes after device cessation. If device cessation is tolerated for 15 minutes, a 6-minute walk (6MW) test is performed with repeat measurements afterward to determine the inotropic reserve. Echocardiographic measurements include left ventricular end-systolic diameter (LVESD), LVEDD, and EF. Simultaneous hemodynamic measurements include systolic blood pressure, diastolic blood pressure, mean arterial pressure (MAP), and heart rate. During the off-pump periods, patients are closely observed for symptoms such as dizziness, sweating, or palpitations. Box 17-3 lists the criteria for LVAD explantation based on the above-described evaluation.

This was the first time that these pumps had been turned completely off, and in a large reported series from Harefield[18] none of the patients tested showed any short-term or long-term adverse effects after the testing, including the patients who eventually recovered and the patients who did not recover;

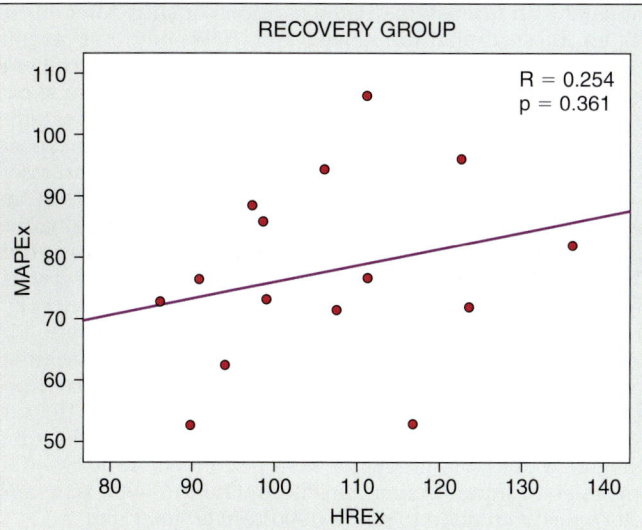

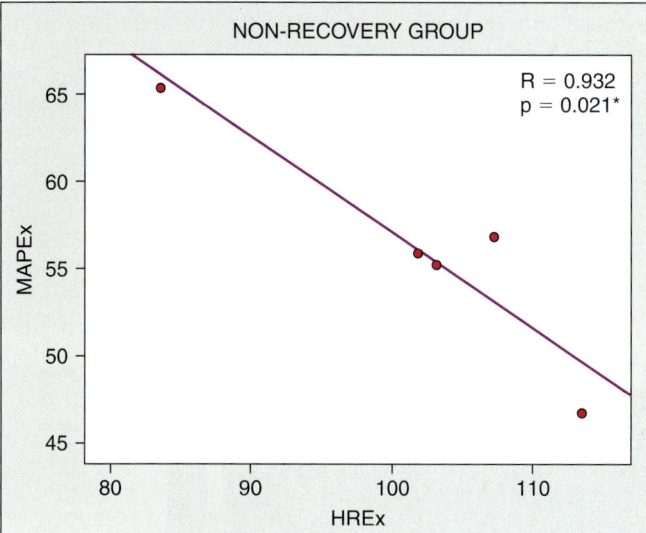

FIGURE 17-4 *Top panel,* Recovery group showing no correlation between the heart rate (HREx) and mean arterial pressure (MAPEx) after the 6-minute walk (6MW) test, suggesting that the increase in heart rate (HR) was independent of the mean arterial pressure (MAP) change and a true inotropic reserve response. *Bottom panel,* Nonrecovered group showing a significantly negative correlation between HREx and MAPEx after the 6MW test, suggesting the increase in the HR was compensatory for MAP reduction. *(From George RS, Yacoub MH, Tasca G, et al. Hemodynamic and echocardiographic responses to acute interruptions of left ventricular assist device support—relevance to assessment of myocardial recovery. J Heart Lung Transplant. 2007;26:967-973.)*

in particular, no thromboembolic complications were seen. Initial device discontinuation was tolerated in 97.6% of cases with no adverse effects.[18] There was no correlation between the heart rate and MAP after the 6MW in the recovered group, suggesting that the increase in heart rate was independent of the MAP change, which suggests a true inotropic reserve response. In contrast, the nonrecovered group showed a significantly negative correlation between heart rate and MAP after the 6MW, suggesting that the increase in heart rate was compensatory for MAP reduction (see Fig. 17-4).

During these "off-pump" tests in all LVAD conditions, EF was significantly higher in the patients who subsequently recovered compared with the patients who did not. Similarly, the recovered group showed a significant increase in EF after the 6MW compared with the 15-minute off-pump test, suggesting the presence of inotropic reserve, but there was no

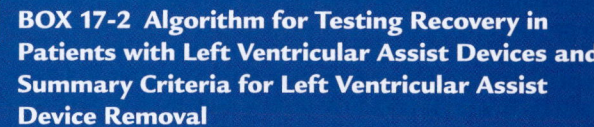

BOX 17-2 Algorithm for Testing Recovery in Patients with Left Ventricular Assist Devices and Summary Criteria for Left Ventricular Assist Device Removal

Heparin bolus of 10,000 units if INR <2.0
Baseline blood pressure
Baseline echocardiographic dimension (left and right ventricles, parasternal, and four-chamber view)
Gradual reduction in pump support to off (HeartMate XVE) or minimal support (6000 rpm; HeartMate II)
Serial blood pressure checks every 5 minutes or with change in symptoms
If asymptomatic and stable blood pressure for 15 minutes *and*
If ejection fraction >40% by surface echocardiogram
    Exercise tolerance test to peak capacity or target heart rate with echocardiographic assessment of ejection fraction and dimensions
If VO_2 >16 mL/kg/min or 65% *and* ejection fraction >45%, left ventricular end-diastolic diameter <5.5 cm
Right heart catheterization (with or without exercise)

BOX 17-3 Explantation Criteria

Stable blood pressure with pump off or on minimal support for >30 minutes
Ejection fraction >45% on no or minimal support for 15 minutes; two studies 1 month apart
Left ventricular end-diastolic diameter <5.5 cm; 2 studies 1 month apart
VO_2 >16 mL/kg/min or >65% predicted (reaching RER >1.1)
Pulmonary capillary wedge pressure <14 mm Hg
Cardiac index >2.5 L/min/m²

RER, respiratory exchange rate.

significant change in EF in the nonrecovered group. Both ventricular dimensions, LVESD and LVEDD, increased significantly in diameter after 5 minutes of device cessation in both groups. In the recovered group, these dimensions did not change at 15-minutes off-pump or after 6MW. In contrast, the LVEDD continued to increase in the nonrecovered group, which was statistically significant compared with LVEDD at 5 minutes off-pump

Inotropic reserve was defined as change in hemodynamics and echocardiograph parameters after the 6MW test but without any infusion with inotropic agents. Both the systolic blood pressure and the pulse pressure decreased significantly within 5 minutes after turning the pump off in the nonrecovered group. In contrast, an improvement was noted in systolic blood pressure and pulse pressure in the recovered group as well as a significant increase in EF and maintenance of LVESD and LVEDD. These improvements suggest that inotropic reserve was preserved in the recovered group. In the nonrecovered group, there was also an increase in heart rate along with reduced MAP, which appeared to be compensatory for the decrease in MAP (and a significant increase in LVEDD).

Identifying predictive factors that correlate with possible recovery and device explantation has always been challenging and difficult. The best predictor of recovery was stable or increased MAP (60 mm Hg) and pulse pressure measured after the pump was off for 15 minutes and after the 6MW, which were strong predictors for recovery with high sensitivity and specificity. An EF 53% or greater after the 6MW was the strongest predictor of recovery with sensitivity and specificity of 93% and 80% (receiver operating characteristic curve area = 0.82). Except for the EF, none of the echocardiographic or hemodynamic parameters measured with the device on full support predicted recovery. This study showed that switching off the HeartMate XVE LVAD was safe and an effective method for monitoring myocardial recovery.

It is well recognized that stopping the LVAD could result in blood regurgitating from the ascending aorta into the outflow graft in diastole (i.e., "reverse flow"). In patients supported with pulsatile flow devices such as the HeartMate XVE, this regurgitant volume is of no significance because of the presence of a one-way valve at the inflow cannula obstructing blood from reaching the left ventricle; retrograde loading of the left ventricle does not occur. Left ventricular loading secondary to cessation of the HeartMate XVE device is a physiologic response that reveals the true underlying function of the native left ventricle. In contrast to the pulsatile flow LVADs, acute interruption of new second-generation continuous flow devices does not provide an accurate assessment of the underlying left ventricular function because of the absence of the one-way valve system resulting in significant regurgitant flow. Reducing the speed of continuous flow devices, such as the HeartMate II LVAD, results in the regurgitant volume flowing from the outflow graft toward the rotor of the pump. Because reverse flow occurs in diastole, analogous to the coronary circulation, it is assumed that the degree of flow would be inversely proportional to the speed of the device. Should the regurgitant volume reach the left ventricle, assessment of the native left ventricular function would be unreliable. It is important to identify a speed of running each pump at which there is no forward or back flow so that the underlying myocardial function could be safely and effectively assessed.

The HeartMate II LVAD is currently the most commonly used continuous flow device. George and colleagues[19] prospectively studied flow across the HeartMate II LVAD in patients with idiopathic dilated cardiomyopathy. After ensuring an international normalized ratio (INR) of 2.0 or greater, left ventricular echocardiographic parameters and peripheral hemodynamics were measured serially at three device speed settings: the baseline speed of the device; 15 minutes after reducing the speed to 6000 rpm; and after reducing the speed to 5000 or 4000 rpm. The LVAD flow pattern was also assessed by positioning a pulsed wave Doppler sample volume at the inflow cannula in the best possible window. Peak velocities in the forward direction ($Vmax_f$) and the reverse direction ($Vmax_r$) were assessed by measuring the distances between the baseline and the peak of the positive and negative spectra (Fig. 17-5). The changing velocities over the flow period in both the forward and the reverse directions were determined by tracing (integrating) the areas under the Doppler curve from the leading edges of the velocity spectrum to obtain the forward velocity time integral (VTI_f) and reverse velocity time integral (VTI_r). Measurements were performed at the baseline speed, at 15 minutes after speed reduction to 6000 rpm, and after speed reduction to either 5000 rpm or 4000 rpm.

No adverse incidents were noted when the speed was reduced in patients from their baseline to 4000 rpm in all patients tested with no symptoms or thromboembolic complications. Hence, assessment of the native myocardium through speed reduction of the HeartMate II LVAD seems to be safe. Reducing the speed to less than 6000 rpm did not have a significant effect on LVEDD, LVESD, fractional shortening (FS), or EF, and suggests that there is no need to reduce the speed of the device to less than 6000 rpm in the assessment of the native left ventricle. As the LVAD speed is reduced to 6000 rpm, the blood volume through the inflow cannula decreases significantly, but further reductions in the LVAD speed did not change the inflow cannula blood volume significantly,

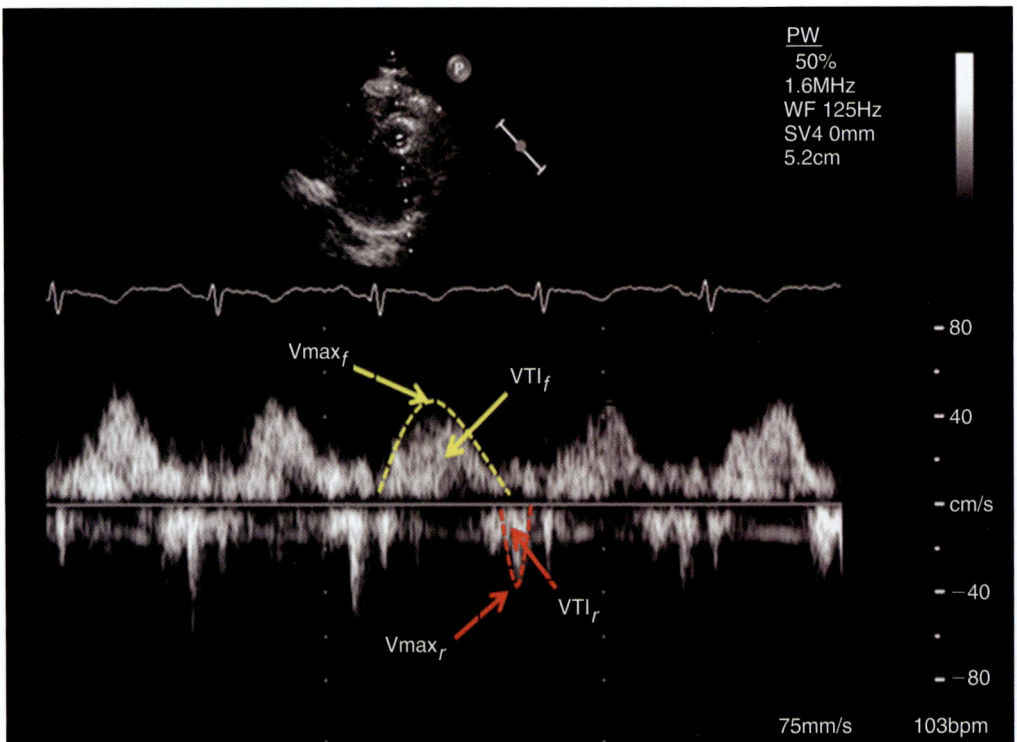

FIGURE 17-5 Measurements taken from pulsed wave Doppler to quantify the forward and reverse flows. The positive spectrum represents forward flow and is occurring in systole, whereas the negative spectrum represents the reverse flow and is occurring in diastole. The spectra were quantified by measuring the peak velocity and their time integral. $Vmax_f$, forward peak velocity; VTI_f, forward velocity time integral; $Vmax_r$, reverse peak velocity; VTI_r, reverse velocity time integral. *(From George RS, Yacoub MH, Tasca G, et al. Hemodynamic and echocardiographic responses to acute interruptions of left ventricular assist device support—relevance to assessment of myocardial recovery. J Heart Lung Transplant. 2007;26:967-973.)*

confirming that speeds less than 6000 rpm are not needed to assess the underlying left ventricular function and that this testing was safe. Myers and coworkers[20] reported that patients with Jarvik 2000 devices who had larger regurgitant flows did not tolerate discontinuation compared with patients who did not have larger regurgitant flows.

Other groups have relied on assessing patients while the device is on or after reducing the speed of the device.[21–23] However, these weaning protocols do not reliably assess the true myocardial response to device cessation because the contribution of the device to the circulation remains significant. These protocols subsequently provide only a rough estimate of the underlying myocardial function.

Patients who tolerate LVAD flow reduction to minimal levels should undergo exercise testing with continuous monitoring of several clinical, hemodynamic, and echocardiographic parameters to provide a more robust method to assess the true underlying function and inotropic reserve. This method allows assessment of the true capacity of the unaided myocardium to support the circulation and to respond to increased demand through loading and exercise.

Several investigators have reported more sophisticated echocardiographic parameters to assess recovery potential. Ferrari and colleagues[24] used a minimally invasive method to determine the predictive power of Emax, the slope of the left ventricular end-systolic pressure-volume relationship, and an afterload-independent and preload-independent index of left ventricular contractility. Contractile reserve, also known as inotropic reserve, refers to the objective quantification of left ventricular contractility after either a pharmacologic or physiologic stress and is reduced in patients with ischemic or nonischemic cardiomyopathy.[25–28] Contractile reserve is tested in the 6MW test described earlier. However, different indices have been used to determine contractile reserve. The most frequently used is the absolute change in EF after dobutamine infusion,[22,23,29,30] although there is an inability to distinguish abnormalities in contractility from alterations in preload or afterload. Conventionally, an absolute increase in the EF by 5% during dobutamine infusion compared with resting indicates preservation of contractile reserve with a strong correlation to prognosis.[29,30]

By recording the hemodynamic response with the use of dobutamine stress echocardiography, Khan and coworkers[22,23] evaluated 16 patients with increasing doses of dobutamine (from 5 μg/kg/min to 40 μg/kg/min). Hemodynamics and two-dimensional echocardiography were performed at each dose level. Dobutamine stress separated the study population into two groups: patients who had favorable responses to dobutamine (9 of 16) and patients who had unfavorable responses (i.e., experienced hemodynamic deterioration; 7 of 16). Favorable dobutamine responses were characterized by improved cardiac index, improved force-frequency relationship in the left ventricle (dP/dt), improved left ventricular EF, and decreased left ventricular end-diastolic dimension. All nine favorable responders underwent LVAD explantation, and six survived for more than 12 months. Dobutamine stress echocardiography with hemodynamic assessment is also a useful tool in assessing physiologic improvement in myocardial function of patients with LVAD support.

Cardiopulmonary exercise testing, both with the patient on full LVAD support and with the pump reduced to a speed at which there is no net forward or backward flow, is also an important part of the recovery testing process of underlying myocardial function. In the Harefield recovery protocol (see subsequently), patients have a cardiopulmonary exercise test twice during the same day with at least 4 hours of rest between tests. During the first (morning) test, the LVAD is on full support. If the INR is greater than 2 during the second (afternoon) test, the speed of the device (HeartMate II LVAD in this case) is reduced to 6000 rpm. If the INR is less than 2,

10,000 units of unfractionated heparin is given 10 minutes before pump speed reduction. The pump speed is reduced manually in decrements of 1000 rpm, and measurements are taken after pump speed reduction to 6000 rpm. During the pump speed reduction and during the cardiopulmonary exercise test with reduced device support, the patients are closely observed for symptoms, and measurements at rest and at peak exercise of the modified Bruce protocol are undertaken. After cardiopulmonary exercise testing with reduced LVAD support and 5 minutes of resting recovery measurements, the speed of the LVAD is returned to its previously defined optimal settings. Mancini and colleagues[8] also performed hemodynamic and metabolic measurements both at rest and at peak exercise (cycling) with optimal and reduced LVAD support without reported complications.

Cardiac power output (CPO) is a novel, central hemodynamic measure that has been suggested to be a direct and possibly the best indicator of overall cardiac function.[31] CPO is calculated as MAP × cardiac output/451, where MAP = [(systolic blood pressure − diastolic blood pressure)/3] + diastolic blood pressure. By incorporating both pressure and flow domains of the cardiovascular system, cardiac power output is an integrative and unique measure of cardiac pumping capability. Resting and peak exercise cardiac power output has been shown to be a powerful predictor of prognosis and mortality in patients with chronic HF and patients with cardiogenic shock.[32–37] Patients with a peak CPO less than 2 watts have a considerably higher mortality rate than patients with a peak CPO greater than 2 watts. Jakovljevic and associates[38] more recently tested CPO in patients with an LVAD and with a continuous flow LVAD reduced to a level at which there is no forward or back flow during cardiopulmonary exercise testing and found cardiac power output to be a useful and predictive marker of recovery.

Before device explantation, other important data to obtain to determine if the patient is sufficiently recovered for explantation are data obtained from right and left heart cardiac catheterization. Important measurements to obtain include right atrial pressures, pulmonary artery pressure, PCWP, left ventricular end-diastolic pressure, and cardiac output (both thermodilution and Fick). It is important to obtain these measurements both with the device on and at the speed at which there is no contribution from the device for 15 minutes. A left ventriculogram after the LVAD has been at low speed for 15 minutes also shows ventricular function well. To verify minimal contribution from the device at the speed at which the hemodynamics have been measured, a pigtail catheter can be placed in the outflow conduit of the device and dye can be injected to ensure there is no significant forward or backward flow in diastole (Fig. 17-6).

The first important step to increase the rate of myocardial recovery is active testing for it. Second, active promotion of recovery is important. Using a VAD as a platform to induce myocardial recovery and combining the unloading with other therapies to maximize recovery might lead further to a significant increase in the rate of recovery.

OPTIMIZING MYOCARDIAL RECOVERY

Until the mid-1990s, little was known about the pathophysiology of cardiac hypertrophy.[39] Two types of hypertrophy are induced by different stimuli and mechanisms.[40,41] Isoproterenol (a beta-1 and beta-2 agonist) and norepinephrine lead to pathologic myocardial hypertrophy, whereas thyroxine and exercise training produce the physiologic type.[42]

Pathologic myocardial hypertrophy, as seen in pressure overload and after catecholamine administration, involves re-expression of proteins as fetal isoforms. RNA molecular markers of gene expression are often used to differentiate the

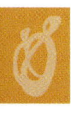

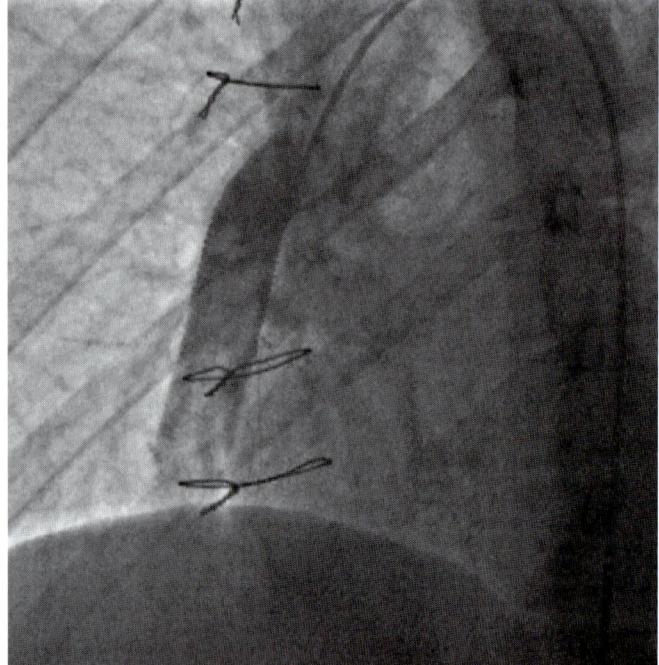

FIGURE 17-6 Pigtail catheter in the outflow conduit of the device with dye injected to ensure there is no significant forward or backward flow in diastole.

pathologic condition from the physiologic condition. In rat heart models, these markers comprise sarcomeric α-actins, cardiac myosin heavy chains (MHCs), and atrial natriuretic factor (ANF).[39] Cardiac α-actin is the usual predominant type of sarcomeric α-actin, but in pathologic hypertrophy, skeletal α-actin is induced instead. Similarly, MHC isoform expression also changes. Downregulation of SERCA2 and PLB also occurs along with increased interstitial collagen that may result in impaired cardiac function.[43–45]

Physiologic myocardial hypertrophy is defined as increased left ventricular mass with normal systolic and diastolic left ventricular function, normal relaxation times (consistent with normal expression of SERCA2 and PLB), normal morphology, extracellular structure (left ventricular collagen concentration and morphology) and gene expression (SERCA2 and PLB mRNA), and left ventricular re-expression of ANF mRNA (nonspecific molecular marker of left ventricular hypertrophy) but without contractile protein isoform switching from cardiac to skeletal α-actin to β-MHC.[39,40,46] Clenbuterol induces this type of myocardial hypertrophy, which can be summarized morphologically as the induction of hypertrophy associated with improved function, functionally as enhanced systolic and diastolic function, histochemically through prevention of increased fibrosis, and molecularly by physiologic gene expression.[39,46,47]

Clenbuterol as an Adjunctive Agent to Induce Cardiac Hypertrophy

Clenbuterol, a novel, selective, beta-2 adrenergic receptor agonist, is a potent synthetic pharmacologic analogue to epinephrine and is used clinically in treatment of asthma and obstructive airways disease. It was initially used in the meat industry to increase muscle bulk and subsequently was prescribed in horses with croup or the equine equivalent of asthma. The realization that it induced significant nonselective skeletal muscle hypertrophy led to its use and abuse as a performance-enhancing drug by eight athletes at the 1992 Barcelona Olympic Games for its "anabolic" properties, despite not being a steroid.

There was considerable subsequent dispute about the mechanism of action of clenbuterol.[39,48] In animal models, clenbuterol induces *skeletal* muscle hypertrophy.[39] Investigators showed that long-term beta-2 agonist administration induced slow-to-fast fiber–type transition resulting in an increase in greater, faster contractions with increased stroke power and reduced contraction and relaxation times.[49,50] It induces insulin-like growth factor 1 through which skeletal muscle hypertrophy is mediated. A trend toward increased fast isoforms of myosin heavy chain and SERCA has been observed.[49] Clenbuterol also inhibits and reverses skeletal muscle atrophy caused by denervation, disuse, endotoxemia, and cachexia.[51–54] Atrophic skeletal muscles are more sensitive to clenbuterol and can respond to doses sufficiently low to avoid general skeletal or cardiac hypertrophy.[52]

Other groups have reported consistent beneficial functional effects of beta-2 adrenergic overexpression in mouse hearts[55] and that the beneficial effect of beta-2 cardiac receptors is prolonged.[56] In addition, beta receptor mediated apoptosis has been shown to be selectively associated with beta-1 rather than beta-2 receptors.[57] One study showed that overexpression of beta-2 receptors potentiated the functional recovery of unloaded failing hearts, consistent with its use below.[58] Because most negative effects of beta stimulation seem to be beta-1 receptor mediated, administration of beta-1 antagonists in conjunction with beta-2 agonists such as clenbuterol seems safe and appropriate. Other investigators showed that clenbuterol induced nerve regeneration.[59]

In 2004, Terracciano and colleagues[60] showed that the use of clenbuterol in the below-described combination therapy induced an increase in sarcoplasmic reticulum Ca^{2+} content and prolonged the action potential (although patients had received the whole protocol). They also identified in experimental models that long-term administration of clenbuterol induced changes in Ca^{2+} regulation, energy metabolism, and organ and cellular hypertrophy in rat hearts. Investigating the mechanisms involved at the molecular and cellular level showed that clenbuterol induced development of cellular and organ hypertrophy (cardiac hypertrophy identified by echocardiography); increased Ca^{2+} transients and sarcoplasmic reticulum Ca^{2+} content without changes in the rate of Ca^{2+} decline in isolated ventricular myocytes; increased expression of SERCA2a, PLB, and Na^+/Ca^{2+} exchanger; and increased oxidative carbohydrate use in the heart.[61]

The increased Ca^{2+} transients generate larger contractions and can be explained by the increased Ca^{2+} content. The increased contractility at the cellular level was not observed at the organ level, but this could relate to the possibility that optimal cardiac performance was already present because normal animals were studied. In HF, the Ca^{2+} transients are reduced in size and have a slower decline, acting as a possible basis for systolic and diastolic dysfunction. Restoring Ca^{2+} content has been shown to reverse Ca^{2+} dysregulation. Clenbuterol also increases the carbohydrate (rather than fatty acid) contribution to cardiac oxidative metabolism after long-term treatment. This observation may represent a beneficial adaptive change to the different metabolic environment of HF because glucose and pyruvate are better substrates for cardiac cells under stress. Experiments have shown that unloading a rat heart leads to myocardial atrophy (Fig. 17-7).

Infusion of clenbuterol into a rat via a minipump leads to an increase in cell surface area along with prolongation of the action potential, increased calcium transient amplitude, increased sarcoplasmic reticulum content, and increased SERCA expression (Fig. 17-8).[61] Animal models have also shown that when unloading is combined with clenbuterol administration in a HF model, an improvement in myocardial function occurs; this does not happen if clenbuterol is given

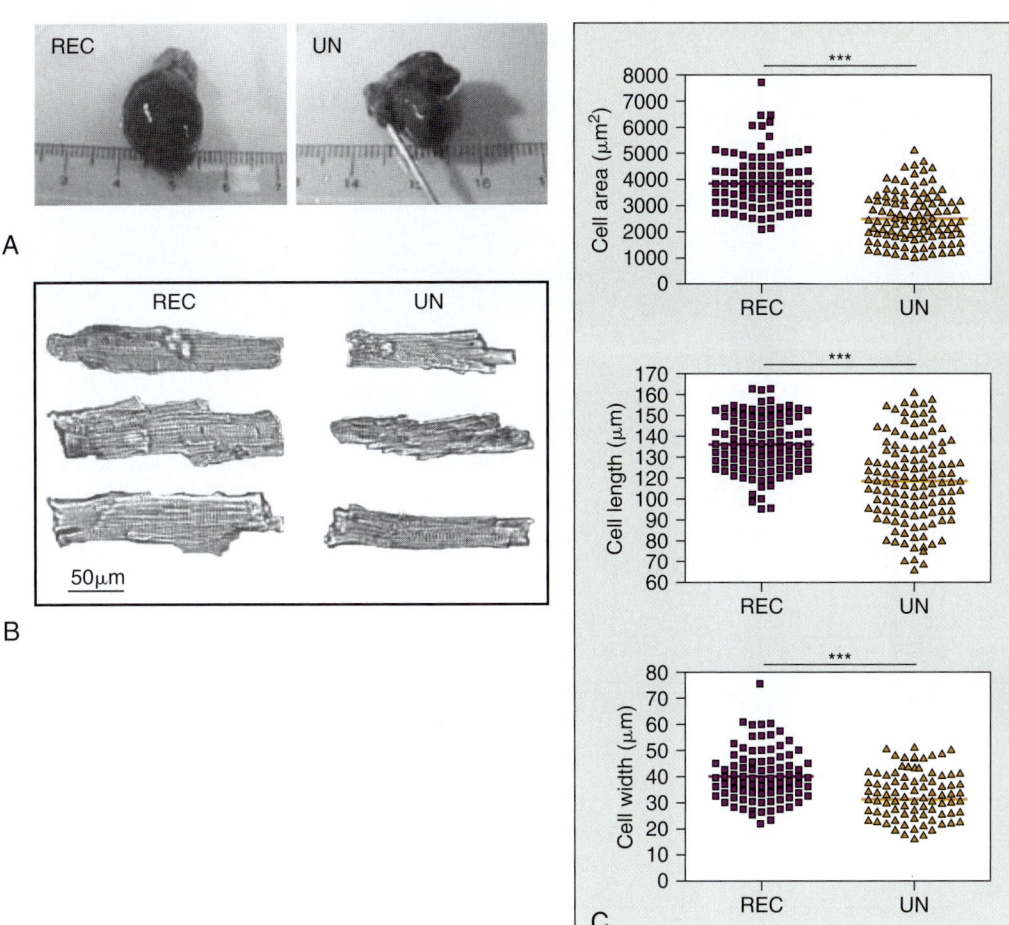

FIGURE 17-7 A, Control recipient (REC) rat hearts and hearts unloaded (UN) by heterotopic heart transplantation showing unloading induced atrophy. **B,** Representative cardiac myocytes showing unloading induced atrophy. **C,** Reduction in cell area, length, and width. *(From Terracciano CM, Hardy J, Birks EJ, et al. Clinical recovery from end-stage heart failure using a left ventricular assist device and pharmacological therapy correlates with increased sarcoplasmic reticulum calcium content but not with regression of cellular hypertrophy. Circulation. 2004;109:2263-2265.)*

without unloading (Fig. 17-9). Some data suggest that acute administration of clenbuterol might impair myocardial function and that long-term administration of clenbuterol may be beneficial to cardiac function.

This body of evidence suggested that clenbuterol treatment in association with mechanical unloading and multidrug reverse remodeling therapy could be beneficial in advanced HF. The induction of cardiac hypertrophy with preserved ventricular function in vivo and without fibrosis, which is characteristic of infusion of catecholamines, may have a role in preventing disuse atrophy in completely unloaded hearts. This improved contractility without fibrosis is often referred to as physiologic hypertrophy (Fig. 17-10).[61] In addition, the ability of clenbuterol to induce skeletal hypertrophy may be beneficial because many patients with severe HF have structural and functional cachexia of skeletal muscles. In skeletal muscle, clenbuterol induces variable degrees of hypertrophy in the same organism, which may relate to heterogeneous beta-2 receptor density in different muscles.[53] The antagonist propranolol has shown varying degrees of blockade, suggesting that other mechanisms may also be involved.[62]

Clenbuterol use in stimulated cardiac myocyte culture has no effect on cell morphology, in contrast to isoproterenol, which does cause change and induced skeletal α-actin in myocytes, a recognized feature of pathologic hypertrophy.[39] Other mechanisms may also be involved because there is some evidence that myocardial beta-2 receptors operate through a different pathway to beta-1 receptors.[39,63]

Prospective Studies of the Harefield Recovery Protocol

A strategy was developed at Harefield Hospital that combines LVAD mechanical unloading with specific pharmacologic interventions in an attempt to maximize the incidence of recovery in patients with dilated cardiomyopathy and improve the durability of recovery in these patients after explantation.[15] This protocol systematically and regularly tests underlying cardiac function in patients with the pump off, or essentially off, at regular intervals to assess response to treatment and guide therapy. This regimen consists of an LVAD combined with drugs known to enhance reverse remodeling, followed by the use of clenbuterol.

Phase I

The strategy is divided into two phases. The pharmacologic interventions of the first phase of therapy are designed to act on component parts of the myocardium with the aim of reversing pathologic hypertrophy, remodeling, and normalizing cellular metabolic function. In the first phase of the pharmacologic intervention, oral HF drugs are initiated immediately after weaning of inotropic support when there is adequate end-organ recovery and titrated to the following maximum doses: lisinopril, 40 mg daily; carvedilol, 25–50 mg three times daily; spironolactone, 25 mg daily; digoxin, 125 μg daily; and losartan, 100 mg daily. Patients have simultaneous increases in ACEIs, beta-1 and beta-2 blockers, aldosterone

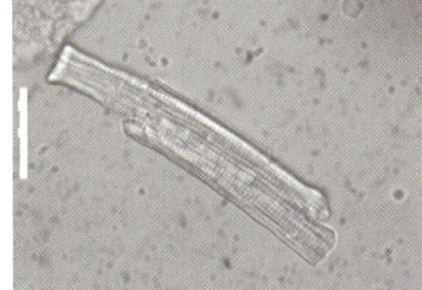
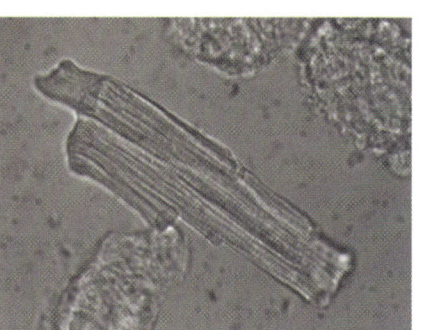

Saline | Clenbuterol

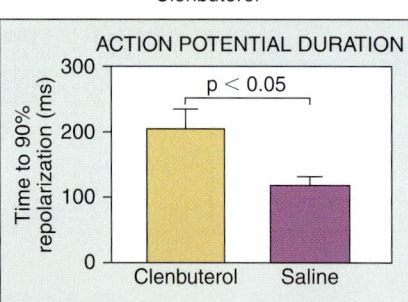
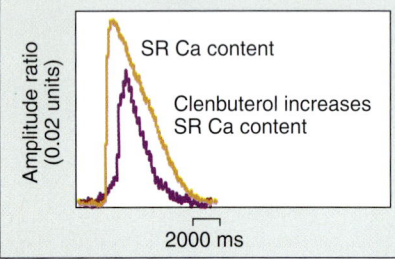
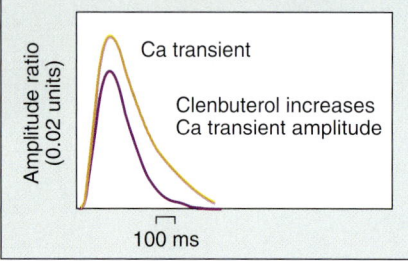
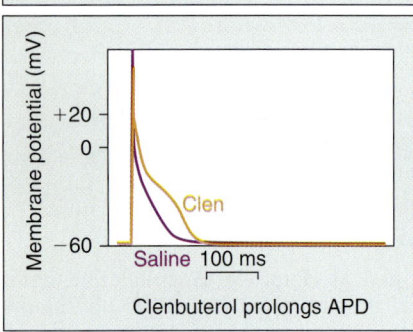

FIGURE 17-8 *Top,* Isolated cardiac myocytes from the left ventricle showed increased cell area in clenbuterol (Clen)-treated rats compared with control. *Middle left,* Action potentials recorded from cardiac myocytes isolated from Clen-treated and control animals (saline). Cells were stimulated at 1 Hz using a pulse of 1.2 nA current (5 msec). *Middle right,* Action potential duration was increased in myocytes from the Clen-treated group. *Bottom,* Sarcoplasmic reticulum (SR) Ca²⁺ content was monitored by changes in indo-1 fluorescence induced by rapid application of 20 mM of caffeine. Caffeine application was preceded by a train of stimulation at 1 Hz followed by 1 second of rest. In the Clen-treated group, caffeine elicited a larger indo-1 transient suggesting a larger SR Ca²⁺ content compared with control. *P* <.01 versus saline. *(From Soppa GK, Smolenski RT, Latif N, et al. Effects of chronic administration of clenbuterol on function and metabolism of adult rat cardiac muscle. Am J Physiol. 2005;288:1468-1476.)*

inhibitors, and angiotensin II antagonists, but the ACE and angiotensin II inhibition are the greatest priority in increasing the therapy (Table 17-2).

The rationale of the first phase of this regimen is to combine mechanical unloading with drugs known to enhance reverse remodeling. Patients often do not tolerate large doses of ACEIs, beta blockers, aldosterone antagonists, and angiotensin II inhibitors while in severe HF because of renal failure or hypotension. However, once patients achieve good cardiac output and adequate blood pressure and renal function from LVAD support they tolerate HF drugs well. ACE and angiotensin II inhibition is a crucial part of this strategy and is used (along with the aldosterone antagonist) to reduce fibrosis.

The specific benefits of neurohormonal inhibition by using ACEIs with VAD support have also been shown by Klotz and colleagues.[64–67] These authors showed prolonged mechanical hemodynamic unloading to increase myocardial tissue levels of angiotensin II with concomitant increases in collagen cross-linking and elevation in myocardial stiffness.[64] Elevated serum levels of angiotensin II can be reduced by blocking the

renin-angiotensin-aldosterone system with an ACEI.[65] Klotz and colleagues examined the myocardium of patients before and after LVAD support in two groups of patients who had and had not had ACEI therapy during LVAD support. After LVAD, tissue angiotensin II levels were significantly reduced in the ACEI group but increased in control subjects. Similarly, cross-linked collagen decreased during LVAD support in the ACEI group. Left ventricular mass and myocardial stiffness were lower in the ACEI group. Myocardial tissue levels of total, soluble, and insoluble cross-linked collagen significantly increased during LVAD support in the control group. ACEI therapy during LVAD support reduced tissue angiotensin II concentration and decreased total and cross-linked collagen and myocardial stiffness.[66]

The same group also investigated paired left ventricular myocardial samples obtained from 20 patients before and after LVAD support with and without ACEI therapy and found pre-LVAD renin levels to be 100 times greater than normal.[67] In patients not receiving ACEIs, LVAD support, by normalizing blood pressure, reversed this situation. Cardiac aldosterone

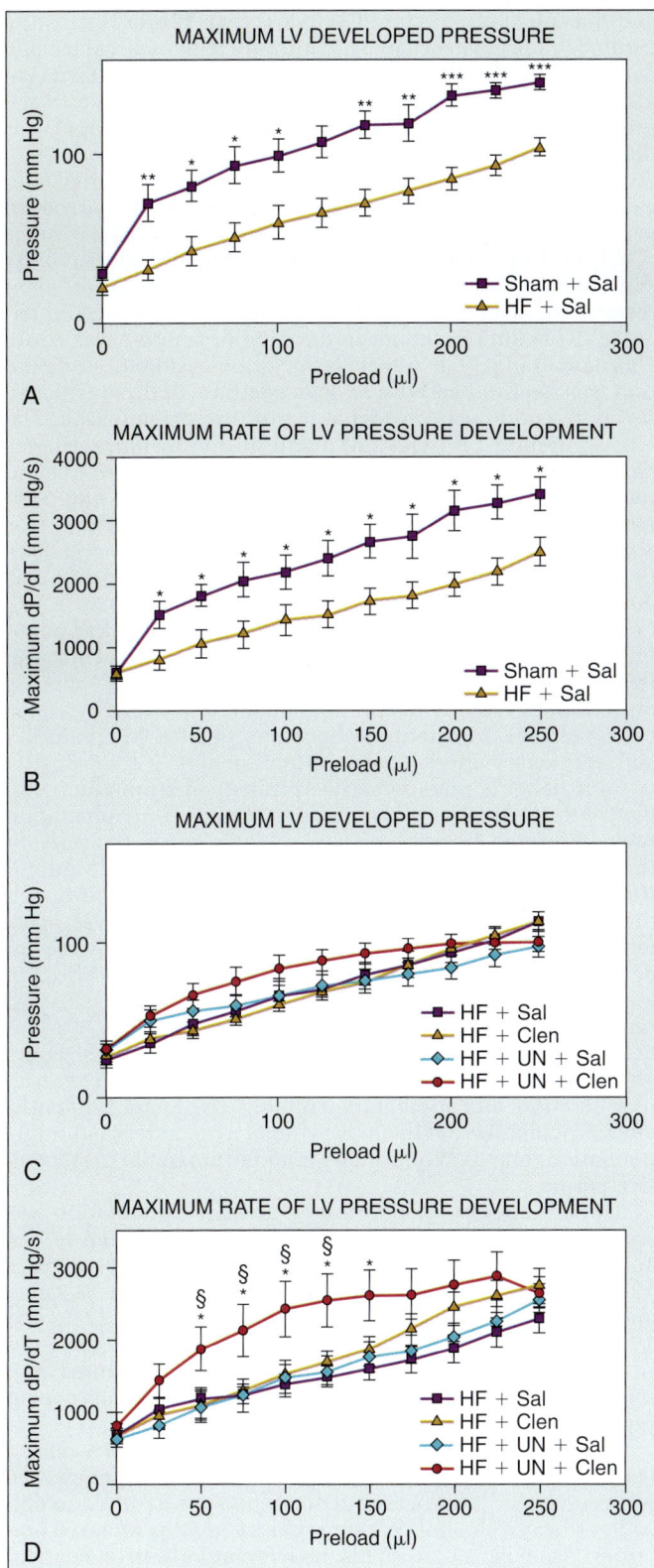

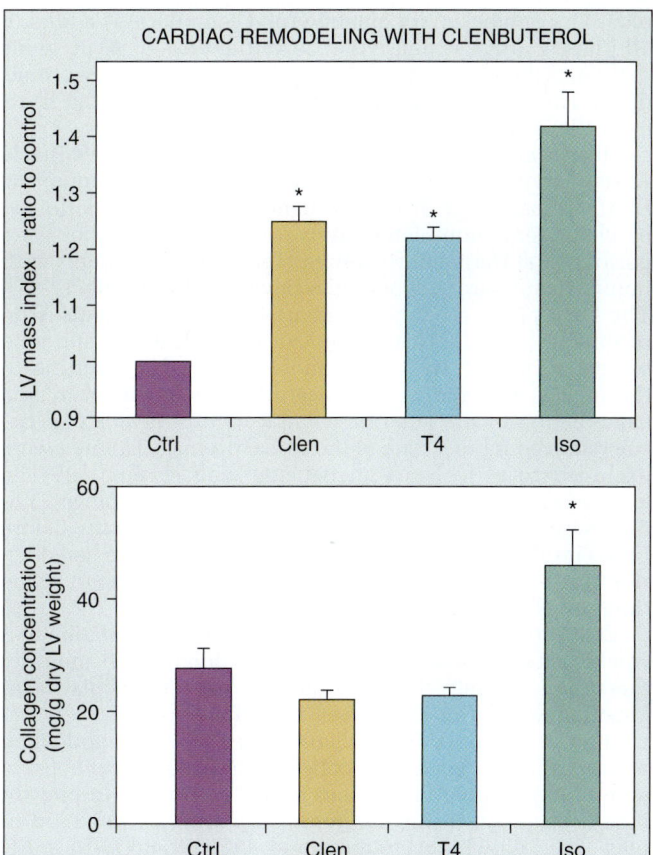

FIGURE 17-10 Effect of clenbuterol on left ventricular (LV) mass and collagen concentration in an animal model. *(From Soppa GK, Smolenski RT, Latif N, et al. Effects of chronic administration of clenbuterol on function and metabolism of adult rat cardiac muscle. Am J Physiol. 2005;288:1468-1476.)*

TABLE 17-2	Target Doses of Phase I Therapy in the Harefield Study	
Drug	**Dose**
Lisinopril	40 mg daily
Carvedilol	25–50 mg three times daily
Spironolactone	25 mg daily
Digoxin	125 µg daily
Losartan	100 mg daily

* p < 0.05; HF + UN + Clen vs HF + UN + Sal

§ p < 0.05; HF + UN + Clen vs HF + Sal

FIGURE 17-9 A and **B,** Pressure-volume relationship of sham operated and heart failure (HF) groups showing a reduced left ventricular (LV) developed pressure **(A)** and dP/dT_{max} **(B)** of failing hearts treated with saline. **C** and **D,** The combination of clenbuterol treatment and mechanical unloading did not affect the LV developed pressure **(C)** but improved dP/dT_{max} **(D,** *red line)* (**P <.05, **P <.01, ***P <.001 HF + Sal vs. Sham + Sal; §P <.05 HF + UN + Sal vs. HF + UN + Clen.) (From Soppa GK, Smolenski RT, Latif N, et al. Effects of chronic administration of clenbuterol on function and metabolism of adult rat cardiac muscle. Am J Physiol. 2005;288:1468-1476.)*

decreased in parallel with cardiac renin. Cardiac norepinephrine increased sevenfold, possibly owing to the increase in angiotensin II. ACEI therapy prevented these changes; renin and aldosterone remained high, and no increase in norepinephrine occurred. Although left ventricular unloading lowers renin and aldosterone, it allows cardiac angiotensin generation to increase and to activate the sympathetic nervous system. ACEIs prevent this.

Phase II: Inwitiation of Clenbuterol

The second stage of pharmacologic therapy was instituted after maximal regression in the LVEDD had been achieved while the LVAD was in place. When the LVEDD measured with the pump at 6000 rpm for 15 minutes was less than 60 mm, the initial nonselective beta blocker carvedilol was switched to a beta-1 selective adrenergic receptor blocker (e.g., bisoprolol or metoprolol), leaving beta-2 receptors unblocked for clenbuterol. Clenbuterol is added to all phase I drugs as phase II at an initial dose of 40 μg twice daily and then titrated to a target dose of 700 μg three times daily. The dose was adjusted to maintain the resting heart rate at less than 100 beats/min.

HeartMate XVE Volume Displacement Left Ventricle Assist Device. Using the Harefield strategy of combining LVAD unloading with reverse remodeling therapy followed by clenbuterol administration, two prospective studies were performed at Harefield Hospital in London[1,68] in patients with non-ischemic cardiomyopathy receiving an LVAD (Fig. 17-11). The first prospective study consisted of 20 patients who received a pulsatile HeartMate XVE LVAD as a BTT and who became clinically stable 4 or more weeks after insertion of the device. Patients with myocarditis proven on histologic examination of the large transmural core of myocardial tissue removed for insertion of the apical drainage cannula were excluded so as to focus on patients with chronic HF. The average age of the patients was 37.6 ± 13.7 years (range 15 to 57 years), and the mean duration of HF symptoms before LVAD implantation was 4.5 ± 4.5 years. All patients had deteriorating NYHA class IV HF despite inotropic support at the time of VAD implantation.

Echocardiography was performed before implantation and weekly after implantation for the first month and monthly thereafter. During the first month, measurements were obtained when the LVAD was on. After week 4, measurements were obtained both when the device was on and when it was off (after the administration of 10,000 units of heparin and hand-pumping three times every 15 seconds to prevent blood stagnation inside the pump) at 5 minutes and 15 minutes. The following were measured: LVEDD and LVESD, EF, and left atrial diameter. The inflow valve of the LVAD was also assessed for evidence of regurgitation.

If the LVAD could be stopped for 20 minutes with no symptoms experienced by the patient, a 6MW test was performed, with repeated echocardiographic measurements to determine inotropic reserve. When the patients were able to walk 450 m in 6 minutes while the device was off, with no deterioration of the echocardiographic measurements, cardiopulmonary exercise tests were performed monthly with the device on and repeated with it off.

Cardiac catheterization was performed before implantation and before explantation. Right-sided and left-sided pressures and cardiac output were measured (with the device on and off for 15 minutes), and a left ventriculogram was obtained (with the device off). Explantation was considered if the following criteria were met (measured with the LVAD off for 15 minutes): LVEDD less than 60 mm, LVESD less than 50 mm, and left ventricular EF greater than 45%; a left ventricular end-diastolic pressure (or PCWP) less than 12 mm Hg; resting cardiac index greater than 2.8 L/min/m²; and maximal oxygen consumption (VO₂ max) with exercise greater than 16 mL/kg/min and increase in minute ventilation (V_E) relative to the production of carbon dioxide (VCO_2) (V_E/VCO_2 slope) less than 34.

Lisinopril, spironolactone, and losartan were restarted after explantation, but clenbuterol was discontinued. Carvedilol was restarted in place of bisoprolol.

Of the 15 patients who received a complete course of the combination therapy (see Fig. 17-11), 11 (73%) had sufficient recovery to meet the explantation criteria. For patients undergoing explantation, the mean duration of support was 320 ± 186 days (range, 63 to 603 days). In one patient, explantation was required because of device failure. In three patients, severe infection was present at the time of explantation. The left ventricular EF (with the pump off for 15 minutes) was 64 ± 8% before explantation compared with 12 ± 6% before implantation (P = .001), the LVEDD was 55.9 ± 8.3 mm compared with 75.1 ± 16.3 mm (P = .002), and the LVESD was 39.6 ± 6.5 mm compared with 66.9 ± 16.3 mm (P = 0.002). Before explantation, the VO₂ max (with the pump off) was 20.7 ± 6.1 mL/kg/min, with a VE/VCO₂ slope of 32.5 ± 7.9. Cardiac catheterization before explantation (with the pump off) showed mean right atrial pressure of 5.6 ± 3.4 mm Hg, PCWP of 9.0 ± 4.1 mm Hg (compared with 23.8 ± 9.7 mm Hg on inotropic therapy before implantation; P = .004), cardiac output of 5.4 ± 1.2 L/min, cardiac index of 2.8 ± 0.7 L/min/m², and pulmonary artery oxygen saturation of 66.9 ± 4.8%.

Four patients underwent heart transplantation after completing the full course of combination therapy. Transplantation was performed because of lack of myocardial recovery in three patients and the development of appreciable mitral, tricuspid, and aortic regurgitation in one patient. Although the numbers were too small for meaningful analysis, age, left ventricular dimensions, and the duration of HF were not determinants of recovery. Of five patients with a LVEDD of greater than 80 mm, four recovered. The actuarial survival rate 1 year and 4 years after explantation was 90.9% and 81.8%. One patient died of intractable arrhythmia 24 hours after explantation without evidence of deteriorating ventricular function, and another died of lung carcinoma 27 months after explantation. Of the four patients who underwent transplantation, one died of primary graft failure in the perioperative period.

The minimum period of follow-up after explantation was approximately 4 years (range 1519 to 2058 days; mean 1799 ± 153 days). At a mean follow-up of 59 ± 5 months, EF was 64 ± 12%, LVEDD was 59.4 ± 12.1 mm, LVESD was 42.5 ± 13.2 mm, and mean VO₂ max was 26.3 ± 6.0 mL/kg/min (Figs. 17-12 and 17-13). An asymptomatic decline in the EF to 30% occurred in one patient 45 months after explantation. He underwent implantation of a biventricular pacemaker, with a subsequent increase in EF to 45%.

All surviving patients continued to be in NYHA class I except one, in whom severe HF recurred, with progressive left ventricular dilation and reduction of the EF after an episode of heavy alcohol consumption 21 months after explantation (see Fig. 17-12). This patient underwent successful transplantation 33 months after explantation. Among the surviving patients, the cumulative rate of freedom from recurrence of HF 1 year and 4 years after explantation was 100% and 88.9% (Fig. 17-14).

Among the patients whose devices were successfully explanted, hemodynamic testing 1 year after explantation showed PCWP of 9.5 ± 6.2 mm Hg, left ventricular end-diastolic pressure of 9.3 ± 5.5 mm Hg, cardiac output of 4.9 ± 2.1 L/min, cardiac index of 2.4 ± 1.2 L/min/m², and pulmonary artery oxygen saturation of 73.5 ± 32%. The quality of life as assessed by the Minnesota Living with Heart Failure

OUTCOME

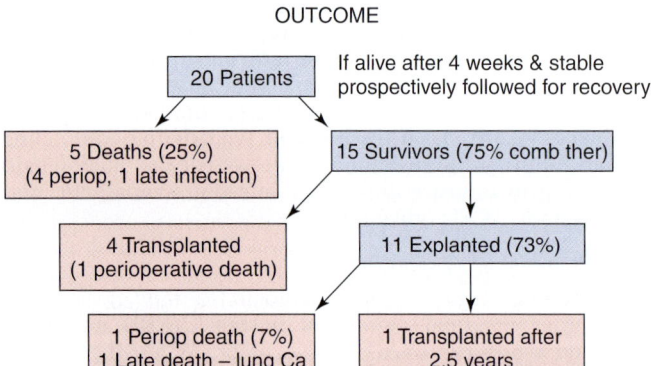

FIGURE 17-11 Flow diagram of outcome of Harefield study. *(From Birks EJ, George RS, Hedger M, et al. Left ventricular assist device and drug therapy for the reversal of heart failure. N Engl J Med. 2006;355:1873-1884.)*

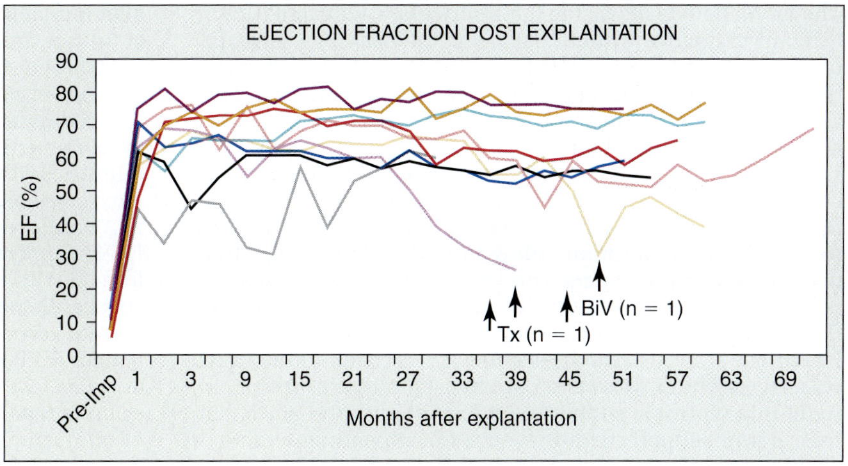

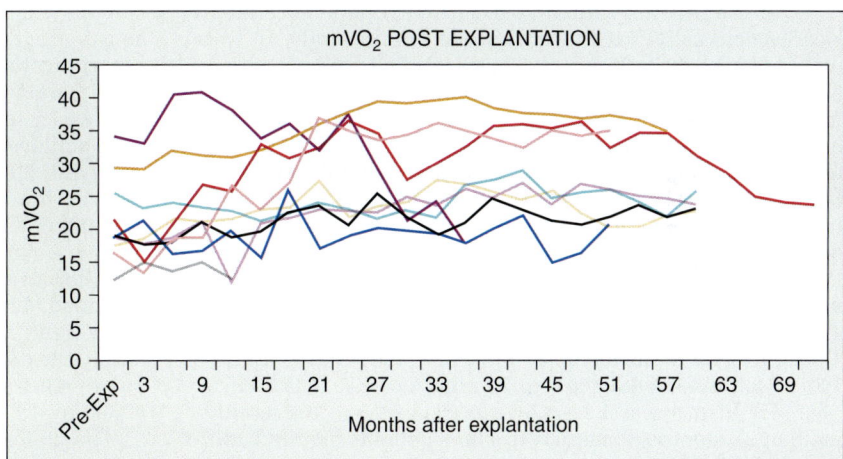

FIGURE 17-12 Ejection fraction (EF) before implantation and after explantation. BiV, biventricular pacing; Tx, transplantation. *(From Birks EJ, George RS, Hedger M, et al. Left ventricular assist device and drug therapy for the reversal of heart failure.* N Engl J Med. *2006;355:1873-1884.)*

FIGURE 17-13 Maximal oxygen consumption (VO$_2$ Max) with exercise before and after explantation in patients with explantation of the HeartMate I device. *(From Birks EJ, George RS, Hedger M, et al. Left ventricular assist device and drug therapy for the reversal of heart failure.* N Engl J Med. *2006;355:1873-1884.)*

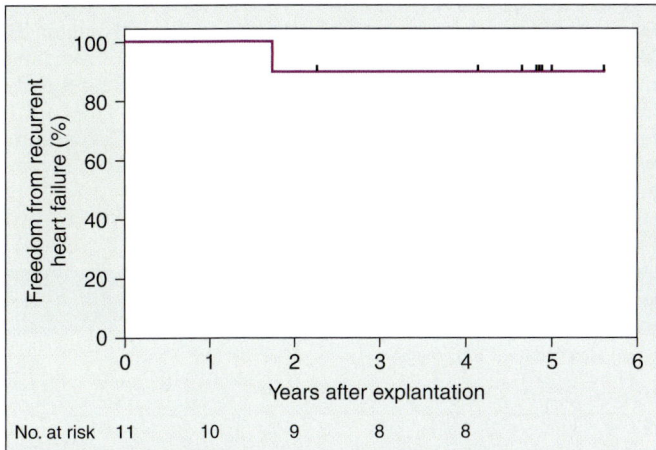

FIGURE 17-14 Cumulative rate of freedom from recurrence of heart failure (HF) among the surviving patients who underwent explantation of a HeartMate I device. *(From Birks EJ, George RS, Hedger M, et al. Left ventricular assist device and drug therapy for the reversal of heart failure.* N Engl J Med. *2006;355:1873-1884.)*

Score in these patients at 3 years was near-normal. The longest follow-up is of a patient 10 years after explantation.

HeartMate II Continuous Flow Left Ventricular Assist Device. Although pulsatile flow volume displacement devices provide excellent hemodynamic support and improved survival, they have many constraints, including the need for extensive surgical dissection; the presence of a large-diameter lead, which is more prone to infection; an audible pump; the need for a medium to large body habitus; and limited long-term durability. These limitations resulted in a transition to the use of rotary devices. These devices are continuous flow pumps that are smaller and quieter and usually have a less traumatic surgical implantation procedure. They have only one moving part, the rotor, and are more durable.

The hydrodynamic characteristics of pulsatile flow and continuous flow VADs vary markedly, and it is unknown whether the latter are as effective in promoting myocardial recovery. With continuous flow devices, the characteristics of unloading are different, testing of underlying myocardial function is more complex, and optimizing medication is likely to be more difficult because of reduced pulse pressure.

There was now sufficient evidence to show that sustained recovery could occur from chronic HF after support with pulsatile flow pumps. The next question was whether the profound pressure and volume unloading of the left ventricle, which causes unloading and myocardial recovery, that occurs with LVAD was specific to the pulsatile flow pumps or whether recovery can also occur with continuous flow pumps. Theoretically, continuous flow pumps might unload less, but they unload continuously, whereas the pulsatile flow pumps are asynchronous with the cardiac cycle and might intermittently load the ventricle.

Of the 15 patients originally receiving the combination therapy in the original Harefield study, 1 had a HeartMate II continuous flow pump, which was explanted 9 years ago. The patient remains alive and well with good functional capacity and ventricular function. The protocol was subsequently successfully applied to a few patients with the Jarvik 2000 device and chronic HF, one of which had familial cardiomyopathy.[69,70]

CH 17

The Jarvik device sits inside the ventricular cavity and is more difficult to remove without damaging the heart or ventricular function; the graft was ligated, and the device was left inside the ventricle without any adverse sequelae for the patients. One patient is alive and well 5 years after ligation of the graft and discontinuation of the device.[70]

A second trial with the Harefield Recovery Protocol was conducted between February 2006 and January 2009 in 20 prospective patients with dilated nonischemic cardiomyopathy receiving a continuous flow pump as BTT.[68] The study used the same drug regimen and protocol as in the first study (see Table 17-2) with only the substitution of the pulsatile flow HeartMate XVE LVAD for the newer continuous flow HeartMate II LVAD. The indication for insertion of the LVAD was severe HF unresponsive to intensive medical treatment, including inotropic support with or without intra-aortic balloon pump support, with evidence of (impending or actual) multiorgan failure owing to low cardiac output. None of the patients had histologic evidence of acute myocarditis.

Of the 20 patients with dilated cardiomyopathy receiving a HeartMate II as BTT who were enrolled in the study, 16 were men. Mean age was 35.2 ± 12.6 years, and all patients were in NYHA class IV with decompensating HF. Patients were receiving a mean of two inotropes, seven (35%) had intra-aortic balloon pump support, two were ventilated, and two had hemofiltration devices. Four patients required prior bridging support because they were considered too sick for initial implantation with a long-term device, three with a Levitronix device, and one with extracorporeal membrane oxygenation. Preoperative cardiac index was 1.39 ± 0.43 L/min/m², PCWP was 31.5 ± 5.7 mm Hg, pulmonary artery saturation was 43.7 ± 12.6%, creatinine was 1.8 ± 1.0 mg/dL, and bilirubin was 2.8 ± 1.5 mg/dL. Echocardiography showed preoperative LVEDD 71.7 ± 8.9 mm, LVESD 65.7 ± 7.7 mm, and EF 14.6 ± 6.6%. Mean HF history was 3.2 ± 3.5 years (range 1.5 to 132 months, median 21 months) (Table 17-3). Three patients required additional right VAD (Levitronix Centrimag) support for 24.3 ± 9.1 days. The cohort was followed until all patients underwent explantation, underwent transplantation, or remained listed at study termination, with all patients whose devices were explanted being at least 8 weeks postexplantation.[69] At the end of phase I therapy, 16 patients reached the criteria to receive clenbuterol (end-diastolic diameter was <60 mm with the pump at 6000 rpm for 15 minutes).

As with the first study with the pulsatile flow VAD, echocardiograms were performed before implantation and monthly

after implantation. Measurements were obtained with the LVAD at full speed initially, followed by reduction of the pump speed to 6000 rpm if the INR was greater than 2 (if INR was <2 10,000 units of intravenous heparin was given first). The study was stopped if the patient became symptomatic. Echocardiographic measurements and images were repeated after 5 minutes and 15 minutes (with the pump at 6000 rpm). Measurements included left ventricular diameters in systole and diastole and EF. The LVAD inflow was also assessed for regurgitation. If reduction of LVAD support was tolerated for 15 minutes, a 6MW test was performed with the device still at 6000 rpm, followed by repeated echocardiographic measurements to determine the left ventricular response to exercise and inotropic reserve. When the patient achieved a 6MW distance of 450 m, a cardiopulmonary exercise test was performed monthly with the device on and again at 6000 rpm (if the INR was >2; otherwise 10,000 units of intravenous heparin was given) (see Box 17-2).

Right and left heart cardiac catheterization was performed before implantation and explantation. Explantation was considered when the same criteria as mentioned previously were achieved with the LVAD at 6000 rpm for 15 minutes. These criteria were considered the minimum for explantation, and if the parameters were still improving, the combination therapy was continued until the maximum improvement had been achieved in each patient.

Of the 20 patients, 12 (60%) showed sufficient recovery to meet the above-described explantation criteria and were explanted. One patient became lost to follow-up, did not receive a significant drug or testing protocol, and was admitted after an out-of-hospital arrest and died. If this patient is excluded, 12 (63.2%) of 19 patients recovered sufficiently to allow pump removal. For patients undergoing device explantation, the duration of LVAD support was 286 ± 97 days (range 193 to 439). Actuarial survival after explantation was 83.3% at 30 days, 1 year, 2 years, and 3 years.

The cohort was followed until all patients were 8 weeks postexplantation, had undergone transplantation, or were listed for transplantation (Fig. 17-15). After a mean follow-up of 430.7 ± 337.1 days (range 56 to 1112 days), all 10 surviving explanted patients remained in NYHA class I with mean EF 58.1 ± 13.8%, LVEDD 59.0 ± 9.3 mm, LVESD 4.2 ± 10.7 mm, and mVO₂ 22.6 ± 5.3 mL/kg/min. Mean creatinine was 1.3 ± 0.5 g/dL, and bilirubin was 1.1 ± 0.4 mg/dL (see Table 17-3). The cumulative freedom from death and recurrence of HF in the patients who underwent explantation was 83.3% at 30 days, 1 year, and 3 years (Fig. 17-16).

TABLE 17-3	Baseline Demographic, Clinical, Echocardiographic, and Laboratory Data of Patients in Harefield HeartMate I and HeartMate II Prospective Recovery Studies and the U.S. HARP Recovery Study		
	Harefield HeartMate I Recovery Study	Harefield HeartMate II Recovery Study	U.S. HARP Study
Total no. patients	20	20	17
Mean age (range)	37.6 ± 13.7 yr (15-57 yr)	35.2 ± 12.6 yr (16-58 yr)	48 yr (31-60 yr)
Sex	16 men, 4 women	16 men, 4 women	15 men, 2 women
Race	19 white, 1 black	17 white, 3 black	8 white, 6 black, 3 Hispanic
HF history	4.5 ± 4.6 yr	3.2 ± 3.5 yr	7.2 ± 4.3 yr (1-16.5 yr)
Baseline			
LVEDD (cm)			
EF			
Sodium			
BUN/creatinine			
Inotrope-dependent (%)			

BUN, blood urea nitrogen; EF, ejection fraction; HF, heart failure; LVEDD, left ventricular end-diastolic diameter.

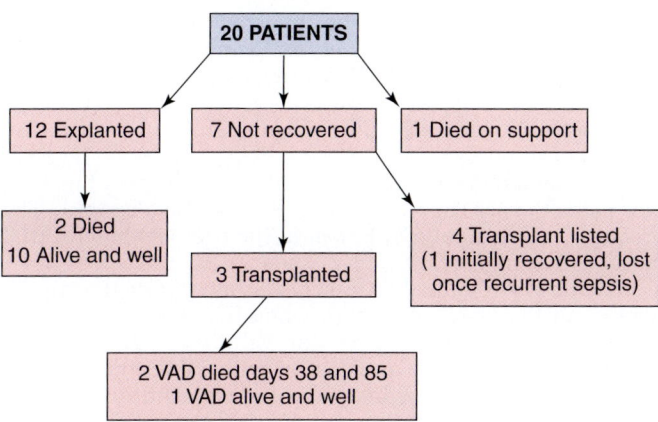

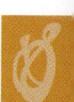

FIGURE 17-15 Outcomes for patients enrolled in the Harefield II study using the HeartMate II left ventricular assist device (LVAD). *(From Birks EJ, George RS, Hedger M, et al. Reversal of severe heart failure using a continuous flow left ventricular assist device and pharmacologic therapy: A prospective study.* Circulation. *2011; 123:381-390.)*

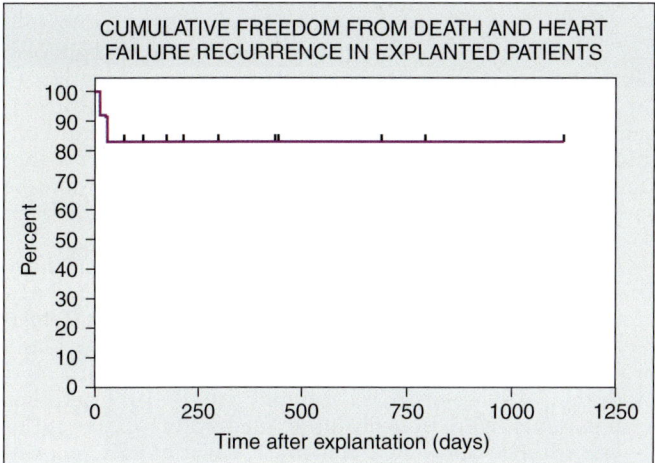

FIGURE 17-16 Durability of recovery—freedom from death or heart failure (HF) recurrence in patients with explantation of HeartMate II device. *(From Birks EJ, George RS, Hedger M, et al. Myocardial recovery from advanced heart failure using HeartMate II LVAD combined with drug therapy: early results from a prospective study.* J Heart Lung Transplant. *2009;28:2S.)*

This prospective study[68] showed that reversal of severe HF secondary to nonischemic cardiomyopathy can be achieved in a high proportion of patients using continuous flow pumps combined with aggressive pharmacologic therapy. The rate and durability of recovery in this series using this strategy is significantly higher than previously reported. It is unclear what role clenbuterol plays in the success of the combination therapy because it is initiated after the heart is mostly reverse remodeled and there is already significant improvement in myocardial function. However, there are no reports of this sustained dramatic improvement in EF with any medical therapy alone. Clenbuterol is likely to improve myocardial function further and, more importantly, to improve the durability of recovery by causing physiologic hypertrophy.

U.S. Harefield Recovery Protocol Study. The success of the Harefield study in showing the highest percentage of patients able to be weaned from MCS and have durable preserved ventricular function brought substantial enthusiasm for the potential of clenbuterol to induce recovery in association with use of an LVAD and an aggressive multidrug regimen of oral HF medications shown to be associated with some degree of positive remodeling in patients with HF. It also brought a

degree of skepticism based primarily on the unprecedented success and inclusion of some patients who had a relatively short duration of HF. The skeptics suggested that many patients with acute HF have a form of myocarditis and a good chance of spontaneous recovery without the protocol, even though each patient had a large transmural piece of the ventricle excised at the time of VAD implant to insert the cannula for left ventricular drainage, and none of the samples revealed any evidence of myocarditis or inflammation or reversible disease. All patients were enrolled before LVAD implantation, and four patients receiving a HeartMate XVE device died of complications of severe HF shock post-operatively before receiving clenbuterol, reflecting the severity of HF at the time of enrollment in these patients who had an average EF of 15% on multiple inotropes. In the HeartMate II study, four patients required prior bridging with a short-term device because they were not well enough to receive a HeartMate II device directly; 35% were on a balloon pump and a mean of two inotropes each with end-organ dysfunction.

There was enough interest in the Harefield results that a multicenter U.S. trial was initiated using this protocol to try to duplicate the results. The U.S. Harefield Recovery Protocol (HARP) trial was a multicenter trial with clinical research organization based at the University of Michigan. In response to the aforementioned criticisms on the duration of HF in the Harefield study, strict protocol requirements included documentation of treatment of established HF (with documented absence of significant coronary artery disease) for at least 1 year, and patients needed to be considered candidates for BTT LVAD therapy to be eligible for enrollment. The protocol was essentially the same protocol used in the two Harefield Recovery studies and included the phase I uptitration to maximal recommended doses of an ACEI, beta blocker, angiotensin receptor blocker, aldosterone I, and digitalis until the reduction in LVEED afforded by the LVAD had plateaued at less than 6.0 cm (see Table 17-3). At that time, clenbuterol was started and uptitrated by protocol to target doses. See the previous section for details.

Patients gave informed consent to be withheld from being on the United Network for Organ Sharing (UNOS) active heart transplant waiting list for 6 months after LVAD implantation to evaluate adequately the potential for sufficient myocardial recovery. The patients otherwise were managed exactly as the Harefield study with phase I drugs before the introduction of clenbuterol. However, during the period of recruitment for this trial, the HeartMate II device became widely used in the United States, and implantation of HeartMate I devices dramatically decreased. The U.S. protocol had been designed for the HeartMate I device only because it was thought that the Harefield protocol should be tested exactly as in the initial publication from Harefield, which had included offloading with the pulsatile flow HeartMate I device because at the time the HeartMate II study had not been performed. As a result, recruitment was very slow.

Many of the patients experienced complications from the HeartMate I device and had to be withdrawn from the trial. There were 17 patients enrolled in the U.S. study: 15 men and 2 women, including 8 whites, 6 blacks, and 3 Hispanics. Mean age was 48 years (range 31 to 60 years). The mean HF duration was 7.2 years (median 8.0 years and range 1 to 16.5 years). The demographics of the U.S. study cohort are shown in Table 17-3 compared with the Harefield cohort studied with the XVE device. A reduction in LVEDD and increase in EF was seen by the end of phase I of the trial (Figs. 17-17 and 17-18); EF increased from 21% before VAD implantation to 40% at the end of phase I, and LVEDD decreased from 75 mm to 56 mm.

Overall, many patients dropped out of the study because of investigator decision, owing to a VAD-related complication or severe right ventricular failure. The near-total conversion

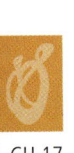

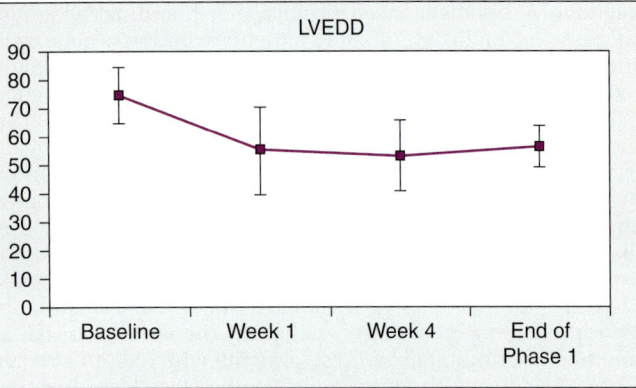

FIGURE 17-17 Reduction in left ventricular end-diastolic diameter (LVEDD) after phase I therapy in the HARP trial (unpublished data).

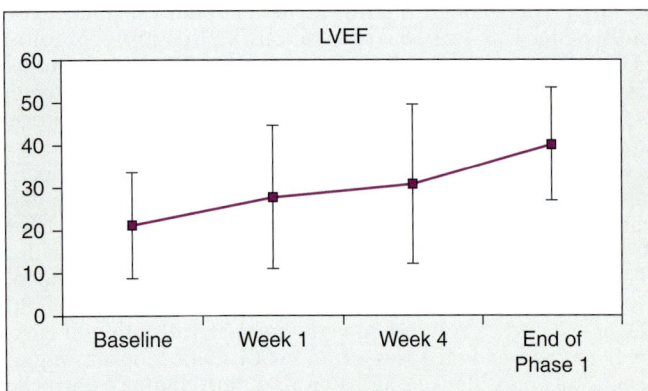

FIGURE 17-18 Increase in left ventricular ejection fraction (LVEF) after phase I therapy in the HARP trial (unpublished data).

from a large pulsatile volume displacement pump such as the HeartMate XVE to the much smaller and silent continuous flow HeartMate II made enrollment during the latter half of the study very difficult. Nine patients were withdrawn from the study, five before receiving any clenbuterol (because of right HF, two abdominal perforations, one device complication, and one subdural bleed) and four after receiving some clenbuterol (two because of pump failure and pump exchange, one driveline infection, and one owing to the investigator leaving). Consequently, only a few patients reached target clenbuterol doses. One patient died of a cerebral hemorrhage during the study before receiving a dose of clenbuterol. Two patients were successfully recovered on the LVAD (15%); only one underwent explantation and remained free of HF at 6 months of follow-up.

Reasons for Differences in Outcomes U.S. versus Harefield Studies. Many potentially important observations have been made from the Harefield study, and the basic science data are currently being analyzed. The most obvious differences between the original Harefield and U.S. studies were the logistics and the demographics of the two cohorts (see Table 17-3). The Harefield cohort was mainly white with an average age of 32, whereas the U.S. trial had 40% African Americans with an average age of 48 years. One explanation of the importance of these differences is the increasing awareness of the reduction in stem cell effectiveness with age. The significantly younger age in the Harefield cohort may have played an important role in the findings based on the increasing body of evidence that suggests that a potentially significant mechanism involved in the response to clenbuterol may be mobilization of native cardiac or peripheral stem cells. This mechanism is based on significant upregulation of the potent stem cell

mitogen SDF-1 in patients who show recovery of left ventricular function and LVAD weaning and removal (see Chapter 20 on molecular responses to LVAD therapy). Another potential explanation for the percentage of the patients in the Harefield study who did not respond to clenbuterol is the 30% frequency of the polymorphism for low expression of the beta-11 and beta-2 receptors initially reported by Liggett,[55] making the patients very unlikely to respond to a beta agonist. The frequency of this polymorphism in the U.S. clenbuterol trial is being investigated.

The nearly identical 65% success rate reported again by Birks and the Harefield group using the HeartMate II continuous flow pump supports the validity of the hypothesis that clenbuterol in association with LVAD therapy and a multidrug oral HF regimen can induce significant recovery of ventricular function. A phase II study was planned for the U.S. trial that would switch from the pulsatile flow HeartMate XVE pump to the contemporary continuous flow HeartMate II LVAD and allow direct comparison of the second Birks study with this device. However, the planned second phase of the U.S. study using the HeartMate II device was halted because of lack of adequate supply of the oral formulation of clenbuterol. The oral tablet form is only 20 µg, and the target dose for the study was 2100 µg, or 100 tablets/day, which was difficult for reliable drug compliance. Clenbuterol has pleiotropic effects beyond stimulation of insulin-like growth factor and SDF-1, and the scientific evidence about the mechanisms of action of clenbuterol continues to be explored. One significant question is whether clenbuterol could be used at an earlier stage of HF and be shown to halt or alter HF progression. Further studies are being planned.

The Texas Heart Institute and other investigators have also recovered numerous patients with chronic dilated cardiomyopathy who were supported with the HeartMate II device (Frazier OH: personal communication, 2010). Many of these patients did not undergo explantation until after more than 2 years of LVAD support. The Berlin group has five patients who underwent explantation of the InCor device (Berlin Heart AG, Berlin).[71] Theoretically, continuous flow pumps might unload the ventricle less effectively than pulsatile flow devices, particularly if the pump speed is suboptimal. However, the continuous flow pumps unload continuously, whereas the pulsatile flow pumps are asynchronous with the cardiac cycle and might intermittently load the ventricle. Data from several centers suggest that continuous flow pumps can unload enough to recover patients with chronic HF sufficiently to have the device explanted.

QUALITY OF LIFE AFTER LEFT VENTRICULAR ASSIST DEVICE EXPLANTATION

Quality of life, or "the functional effect of an illness and its consequent therapy upon a patient, as perceived by the patient," is also extremely important. Long-term quality of life was assessed in patients who had had their LVAD explanted because of myocardial recovery (bridge to recovery [BTR]) and compared with the quality of life of patients who underwent BTT and patients who underwent direct transplantation.[72] The study comprised 72 patients—14 BTR patients (3.6 ± 1.9 years since LVAD removal); 29 BTT patients (3.3 ± 2.3 years since transplantation); and 29 transplantation patients (3.8 ± 0.6 years since transplantation). The total quality-of-life SF-36 score was higher in the BTR group compared with both the BTT and the transplantation groups. In all but two of the domains of the SF-36 questionnaire,

the scores were significantly better in the BTR group compared with both the BTT and the transplantation groups. The Physical Health Dimension score tended to be better in the BTR group compared with both the BTT and transplantation groups. Similarly, the Mental Health Dimension score was significantly better in the BTR group compared with both the BTT and the transplantation groups. In the longer term, BTR patients appear to have a better quality of life than both BTT and transplantation patients.

This study showed that BTR patients had a better quality of life compared with both BTT and transplanted patients who did not require LVAD support. The improved quality of life in the BTR group could be related to better renal function, lack of immunosuppression-related complications, absence of rejection, less infection, and lack of coronary disease. There is now a substantial body of evidence to show that myocardial recovery from chronic HF can occur. It is reproducible and has now been shown in several different centers and with several different devices. Durability of myocardial recovery has also been shown, and patients have a good quality of life. More recent studies have shown that the frequency and degree of recovery can be enhanced by combining drug therapy aimed to promote reverse remodeling and durability of recovery with LVAD support. Additionally, more reliable and durable devices are becoming available, providing more opportunity for promoting and testing for recovery.

SUMMARY AND NEXT STEPS TO ENHANCE RATE OF RECOVERY

The ability to recover the cardiac ventricle with the assistance of VADs to completely unload the heart has been an area of interest for many years. Unfortunately, the percentage of patients who have been able to have an LVAD removed successfully and sustain good ventricular function for a prolonged period (months to years) has been very low—approximately 5% to 20%—with the success reported primarily in younger patients with nonischemic etiology and typically acute HF from etiologies such as myocarditis, where the natural history of recovery is quite high.

The concept of inducing myocardial recovery with MCS has not previously undergone rigorous investigation in terms of use of protocols, such as employing aggressive oral HF drug therapy to target doses during support or sophisticated and systematic weaning attempts to judge and assess for recovery. One of the main reasons for the low reported overall incidence of recovery in patients with chronic HF is probably the lack of belief that these patients can recover and lack of testing for it. The answer to whether myocardial recovery is possible with periods of MCS used to be unknown because the question had never been studied in a rigorous manner. However, now there is no doubt from the data that myocardial recovery can occur; however, most programs do not test for it or promote it. Widespread testing of myocardial function with the contribution of the pump reduced ideally to effectively no contribution in all patients with dilated cardiomyopathy is the next desired step.

VADs can be used as a platform for recovery by adding additional novel strategies such as clenbuterol and soon possibly stem cells and gene therapy. A multicenter SCCOR study has just started using a protocol that included injecting bone marrow–derived mesenchymal stem cells into the myocardium at the time of VAD implantation. Using these strategies, it may be possible to increase the rate of recovery further. In the future, it is likely that most patients with nonischemic HF who receive a VAD will undergo an aggressive attempt to induce recovery. Patients with an ischemic etiology or who do not respond to attempts at recovery will

stay on the device for a prolonged period, and patients who develop VAD-related complications will undergo transplantation. It is likely that VADs will be used in the future as a platform to promote myocardial recovery in combination with drugs, stem cells, or gene therapy.

The number of usable donor hearts has been declining, necessitating an alternative approach for these patients. Patients who can be explanted because of myocardial recovery avoid the need for immunosuppression and its associated complications and spare the donor heart for another individual. Even if patients should decompensate and require transplantation at a later stage, this approach is likely to extend their overall life span considerably. LVADs are being increasingly implanted in patients with advanced HF with improving survival and reduced complication rates. An increasing number of patients in the future are likely to have these devices implanted as an alternative to transplantation, and all patients with nonischemic dilated cardiomyopathy are candidates for recovery. Some data suggest that patients with shorter duration of HF and younger age (<45 years old) may be most likely to show long-term recovery with a period of LVAD support. Recovery will be an important goal for the field of MCS in the future.

REFERENCES

1. Birks EJ, Tansley PD, Hardy J, et al. Left ventricular assist device and drug therapy for the reversal of heart failure. *N Engl J Med.* 2006;355:1873–1884.
2. Frazier OH, Radovancevic B, Abou-Awdi NL, et al. Ventricular remodelling after prolonged ventricular unloading "heart rest" experience with the HeartMate left ventricular assist device (abstract). *J Heart Lung Transplant.* 1994;13(Pt 2):77.
3. Frazier OH, Benedict CR, Radovancevic B, et al. Improved left ventricular function after chronic left ventricular unloading. *Ann Thorac Surg.* 1996;62:675–682.
4. Levine HR, Oz MC, Chen JM, et al. Reversal of chronic ventricular dilation in patients with end-stage cardiomyopathy by prolonged mechanical unloading. *Circulation.* 1995;91:2717–2720.
5. Levine HR, Oz MC, Cantanese KA, et al. Transient normalisation of systolic and diastolic function after support with a left ventricular assist device in a patient with dialed cardiomyopathy. *J Heart Lung Transplant.* 1996;15:840–842.
6. Frazier OH, Myers TJ. Left ventricular assist system as a bridge to myocardial recovery. *Ann Thorac Surg.* 1999;68:734–741.
7. Farrar DJ, Holman WR, McBride LR, et al. Long-term follow-up of Thoratec ventricular assist device bridge-to-recovery patients successfully removed from support after recovery of ventricular function. *J Heart Lung Transplant.* 2002;21:516–521.
8. Mancini DM, Beniaminovitz A, Levin H, et al. Low incidence of myocardial recovery after left ventricular assist device implantation in patients with chronic heart failure. *Circulation.* 1998;98:2383–2389.
9. Simon MA, Kormos RL, Murali S, et al. Myocardial recovery using ventricular assist devices: prevalence, clinical characteristics, and outcomes. *Circulation.* 2005;112(suppl 9):I-32–I-36.
10. Muller J, Wallukat G, Weng YG, et al. Weaning from mechanical cardiac support in patients with idiopathic dilated cardiomyopathy. *Circulation.* 1997;96:542–549.
11. Loebe M, Hennig E, Muller J, et al. Long-term mechanical circulatory support as a bridge to transplantation, for recovery from cardiomyopathy, and for permanent replacement. *Eur J Cardiothorac Surg.* 1997;11(suppl):S18–S24.
12. Dandel M, Weng Y, Siniawski H, et al. Long-term results in patients with idiopathic dilated cardiomyopathy after weaning from left ventricular assist devices. *Circulation.* 2005;112(suppl 9):I-37–I-45.
13. Dandel M, Weng Y, Siniawski H, et al. Prediction of cardiac stability after weaning from left ventricular assist devices in patients with idiopathic dilated cardiomyopathy. *Circulation.* 2008;118(suppl 1):S94–S105.
14. Maybaum S, Mancini D, Xydas S, et al. Cardiac improvement during mechanical circulatory support a prospective multicentre study of the LVAD Working group. *Circulation.* 2007;115:2497–2505.
15. Yacoub MH. A novel strategy to maximize the efficacy of left ventricular assist devices as a bridge to recovery. *Eur Heart J.* 2001;22:534–540.
16. Oriyanhan W, Tsuneyoshi H, Nishina T, et al. Determination of optimal duration of mechanical unloading for failing hearts to achieve bridge to recovery in a rat heterotopic heart transplantation model. *J Heart Lung Transplant.* 2007;26:16–23.
17. Levine S, Nguyen T, Taylor N, et al. Rapid disuse atrophy of diaphragmatic fibers in mechanically ventilated humans. *N Engl J Med.* 2008;358:1245–1253.
18. George RS, Yacoub MH, Tasca G, et al. Haemodynamic and echocardiographic responses to acute interruption of left ventricular assist device support—relevance to assessment of myocardial recovery. *J Heart Lung Transplant.* 2007;26:967–973.
19. George RS, Sabharwal NK, Webb C, et al. Echocardiographic evaluation of flow across HeartMate II axial flow LVADs at varying low speeds (abstract). *J Heart Lung Transplant.* 2009;28:2S.
20. Myers TJ, Frazier OH, Mesina HS, et al. Hemodynamics and patient safety during pump-off studies of an axial-flow left ventricular assist device. *J Heart Lung Transplant.* 2006;25:379–383.

21. Slaughter M, Silver M, Farrar D, et al. A new method of monitoring recovery and weaning the Thoratec LVAD. *Ann Thorac Surg.* 2001;71:215–218.

22. Khan T, Delgado RM, Radovancevic B, et al. Dobutamine stress echocardiography predicts myocardial improvement in patients supported by left ventricular assist devices (LVADs): hemodynamic and histologic evidence of improvement before LVAD explantation. *J Heart Lung Transplant.* 2003;22:137–146.

23. Khan T, Okerberg K, Hernandez A, et al. Assessment of myocardial recovery using dobutamine stress echocardiography in LVAD patients. *J Heart Lung Transplant.* 2001;20:202–203.

24. Ferrari G, Górczynska K, Mimmo R, et al. Mono and bi-ventricular assistance: their effect on ventricular energetics. *Int J Artif Organs.* 2001;24:380–391.

25. Nagaoka H, Kubota S, Iizuka T, et al. Relation between depressed cardiac response to exercise and autonomic nervous activity in mildly symptomatic patients with idiopathic dilated cardiomyopathy. *Chest.* 1996;109:925–932.

26. Ypenburg C, Sieders A, Bleeker GB, et al. Myocardial contractile reserve predicts improvement in left ventricular function after cardiac resynchronization therapy. *Am Heart J.* 2007;154:1160–1165.

27. Bax JJ, Poldermans D, Schinkel AFL, et al. Perfusion and contractile reserve in chronic dysfunctional myocardium: relation to functional outcome after surgical revascularization. *Circulation.* 2002;106(suppl I):I-14–I-18.

28. Chaudhry FA, Tauke JT, Alessandrini RS, et al. Prognostic implications of myocardial contractile reserve in patients with coronary artery disease and left ventricular dysfunction. *J Am Coll Cardiol.* 1999;34:730–738.

29. Kobayashi M, Izawa H, Cheng XW. Dobutamine stress testing as a diagnostic tool for evaluation of myocardial contractile reserve in asymptomatic or mildly symptomatic patients with dilated cardiomyopathy. *J Am Coll Cardiol Cardiovasc Imaging.* 2008;1:718–726.

30. Otasevic P, Popovic ZB, Vasiljevic JD, et al. Relation of myocardial histomorphometric features and left ventricular contractile reserve assessed by high-dose dobutamine stress echocardiography in patients with idiopathic dilated cardiomyopathy. *Eur J Heart Fail.* 2005;7:49–56.

31. Cotter G, Williams SG, Vered Z, et al. Role of cardiac power in heart failure. *Curr Opin Cardiol.* 2003;18:215–222.

32. Tan LB. Cardiac pumping capability and prognosis in heart failure. *Lancet.* 1986;13:1360–1363.

33. Fincke R, Hochman JS, Lowe AM, et al. Cardiac power is the strongest hemodynamic correlate of mortality in cardiogenic shock: a report from the shock trial registry. *J Am Coll Cardiol.* 2004;44:340–348.

34. Mendoza DD, Cooper HA, Panza JA. Cardiac power output predicts mortality across a broad spectrum of patients with acute cardiac disease. *Am Heart J.* 2007;153:366–370.

35. Roul G, Moulichon ME, Bareiss P, et al. Prognostic factors of chronic heart failure in NYHA class II or III: value of invasive exercise haemodynamic data. *Eur Heart J.* 1995;16:1387–1398.

36. Tan LB, Littler WA. Measurement of cardiac reserve in cardiogenic shock: implication for prognosis and management. *Br Heart J.* 1990;64:121–128.

37. Williams SG, Cooke GA, Wright DJ, et al. Peak exercise cardiac power output: an indicator of cardiac function strongly predictive of prognosis in chronic heart failure. *Eur Heart J.* 2001;22:1496–1503.

38. Jakovljevic DG, George RS, Donovan G, et al. Comparison of cardiac power output and exercise performance in patients with left ventricular assist devices, explanted (recovered) patients, and those with moderate to severe heart failure. *Am J Cardiol.* 2010;105:1780–1785.

39. Petrou M, Wynne DG, Boheler KR, et al. Clenbuterol induces hypertrophy of the latissimus dorsi muscle and heart in the rat with molecular and phenotypic changes. *Circulation.* 1995;92(suppl 9):II-483–II-489.

40. Scheuer J, Buttrick P. The cardiac hypertrophic responses to pathologic and physiologic loads. *Circulation.* 1987;75(1 Pt 2):I-63–I-68.

41. Morgan HE, Baker KM. Cardiac hypertrophy: mechanical, neural, and endocrine dependence. *Circulation.* 1991;83:13–25.

42. Bersohn MM, Scheuer J. Effects of physical training on end-diastolic volume and myocardial performance of isolated rat hearts. *Circ Res.* 1977;40:510–516.

43. Wong K, Boheler KR, Petrou M, et al. Pharmacological modulation of pressure-overload cardiac hypertrophy: changes in ventricular function, extracellular matrix, and gene expression. *Circulation.* 1997;96:2239–2246.

44. Stein B, Bartel S, Kirchhefer U, et al. Relation between contractile function and regulatory cardiac proteins in hypertrophied hearts. *Am J Physiol.* 1996;270(6 Pt 2):H2021–H2028.

45. Weber KT, Brilla CG. Pathological hypertrophy and cardiac interstitium: fibrosis and renin-angiotensin-aldosterone system. *Circulation.* 1991;83:1849–1865.

46. Wong K, Boheler KR, Bishop J, et al. Clenbuterol induces cardiac hypertrophy with normal functional, morphological and molecular features. *Cardiovasc Res.* 1998;37:115–122.

47. Hon JK, Yacoub MH. Bridge to recovery with the use of left ventricular assist device and clenbuterol. *Ann Thorac Surg.* 2003;75(suppl 6):S36–S41.

48. Beckett AH. Clenbuterol and sport. *Lancet.* 1992;340:1165.

49. Petrou M, Clarke S, Morrison K, et al. Clenbuterol increases stroke power and contractile speed of skeletal muscle for cardiac assist. *Circulation.* 1999;99:713–720.

50. Zeman RJ, Peng H, Etlinger JD. Clenbuterol retards loss of motor function in motor neuron degeneration mice. *Exp Neurol.* 2004;187:460–467.

51. Maltin CA, Reeds PJ, Delday MI, et al. Inhibition and reversal of denervation-induced atrophy by the beta-agonist growth promoter, clenbuterol. *Biosci Rep.* 1986;6:811–818.

52. Maltin CA, Hay SM, McMillan DN, et al. Tissue-specific responses to clenbuterol: temporal changes in protein metabolism of striated muscle and visceral tissues from rats. *Growth Regul.* 1992;2:161–166.

53. Maltin CA, Delday MI, Watson JS, et al. Clenbuterol, a beta-adrenoceptor agonist, increases relative muscle strength in orthopaedic patients. *Clin Sci (Lond).* 1993;84:651–654.

54. Delday MI, Maltin CA. Clenbuterol increases the expression of myogenin but not myoD in immobilized rat muscles. *Am J Physiol.* 1997;272(5 Pt 1):E941–E944.

55. Liggett SB. Pharmacogenetics of beta-1- and beta-2-adrenergic receptors. *Pharmacology.* 2000;61:167–173.

56. Liggett SB, Tepe NM, Lorenz JN, et al. Early and delayed consequences of beta(2)-adrenergic receptor overexpression in mouse hearts: critical role for expression level. *Circulation.* 2000;101:1707–1714.

57. Zaugg M, Xu W, Lucchinetti E, et al. Beta-adrenergic receptor subtypes differentially affect apoptosis in adult rat ventricular myocytes. *Circulation.* 2000;102:344–350.

58. Tevaearai HT, Eckhart AD, Walton GB, et al. Myocardial gene transfer and overexpression of beta2-adrenergic receptors potentiates the functional recovery of unloaded failing hearts. *Circulation.* 2002;106:124–129.

59. Frerichs O, Fansa H, Ziems P, et al. Regeneration of peripheral nerves after clenbuterol treatment in a rat model. *Muscle Nerve.* 2001;24:1687–1691.

60. Terracciano CM, Hardy J, Birks EJ, et al. Clinical recovery from end-stage heart failure using left-ventricular assist device and pharmacological therapy correlates with increased sarcoplasmic reticulum calcium content but not with regression of cellular hypertrophy. *Circulation.* 2004;109:2263–2265.

61. Soppa GK, Smolenski RT, Latif N, et al. Effects of chronic administration of clenbuterol on function and metabolism of adult rat cardiac muscle. [erratum in *Am J Physiol Heart Circ Physiol.* 2005;288:H2546]. *Am J Physiol Heart Circ Physiol.* 2005;288:H1468–H1476.

62. Maltin CA, Delday MI, Hay SM, et al. Propranolol apparently separates the physical and compositional characteristics of muscle growth induced by clenbuterol. *Biosci Rep.* 1987;7:51–57.

63. Kuznetsov V, Pak E, Robinson RB, et al. Beta 2-adrenergic receptor actions in neonatal and adult rat ventricular myocytes. *Circ Res.* 1995;76:40–52.

64. Klotz S, Foronjy RF, Dickstein ML, et al. Mechanical unloading during left ventricular assist device support increases left ventricular collagen cross-linking and myocardial stiffness. *Circulation.* 2005;112:364–374.

65. Tang WH, Vagelos RH, Yee YG, et al. Neurohormonal and clinical responses to high- versus low-dose enalapril therapy in chronic heart failure. *J Am Coll Cardiol.* 2002;39:70–78.

66. Klotz S, Jan Danser AH, Foronjy RF, et al. The impact of angiotensin-converting enzyme inhibitor therapy on the extracellular collagen matrix during left ventricular assist device support in patients with end-stage heart failure. *J Am Coll Cardiol.* 2007;49:1166–1174.

67. Klotz S, Burkhoff D, Garrelds IM, et al. The impact of left ventricular assist device-induced left ventricular unloading on the myocardial renin-angiotensin-aldosterone system: therapeutic consequence. *Eur Heart J.* 2009;30:805–812.

68. Birks EJ, George RS, Hedger M, et al. Myocardial recovery from advanced heart failure using the HeartMate II LVAD combined with drug therapy: early results from a prospective study (abstract). *J Heart Lung Transplant.* 2009;28:2S.

69. Haj-Yahia S, Birks EJ, Rogers P, et al. Midterm experience with the Jarvik 2000 axial flow left ventricular assist device. *J Thorac Cardiovasc Surg.* 2007;134:199–203.

70. George RS, Khaghani C, Bowles CT, et al. Sustained myocardial recovery 5 years after in situ disconnection of a Jarvik 2000 device. *J Heart Lung Transplant.* 2010;29:587–588.

71. Komoda T, Komoda S, Dandel M, et al. Explantation of INCOR left ventricular assist device after myocardial recovery. *J Card Surg.* 2008;23:642–647.

72. George RS, Yacoub MH, Bowles CT, et al. Quality of life after removal of left ventricular assist device for myocardial recovery. *J Heart Lung Transplant.* 2008;27:165–172.

CHAPTER **18**

Regenerative Therapy as an Adjunct to Mechanical Support

Marc S. Penn

Mechanical support for patients with chronic heart failure has evolved significantly over the past decades from the concept of complete replacement of the heart to adjunctive support. The success of mechanical support instead of replacement has progressed sufficiently to bring destination left ventricular assist device placement into reality. The concept and data for these advances are discussed in great detail in other chapters of this book. Over the past decade, biologic-based strategies to prevent and treat left ventricular dysfunction have grown in parallel with advances in mechanical support of the heart. The most common form of biologic intervention for the purpose of regenerating cardiac function in chronic heart failure is cellular therapy. We are now a decade beyond the first reports of cell-based therapies for the treatment of chronic heart failure.[1,2] More recently, preclinical studies of stem cell–based therapies have identified several novel targets for gene transfer[3–5] that are now entering clinical populations for study. Many of the great science fiction writers suggested that true advancement was not the creation of mechanical beings, but the fusion of mechanical devices with living tissue. In that spirit, many today are contemplating the integration of mechanical support with biologic therapy as a strategy to restore cardiac function in chronic heart failure. The goal of this chapter is to review the current understanding and state of cell-based therapies and gene transfer for the treatment of chronic heart failure and discuss how these treatment strategies could interface with, or be integrated into, mechanical support.

CELL THERAPY FOR THE TREATMENT OF CARDIAC DYSFUNCTION

Perhaps the earliest form of cell therapy for the treatment of cardiac dysfunction was cardiac myoplasty (cardiomyoplasty), in which the heart was wrapped in skeletal muscle that was then paced to augment the intrinsic contractility of the weakened heart.[6–8] Studies of hearts from patients who died or underwent cardiac myoplasty revealed engraftment of skeletal muscle in the epicardial layers of the heart.[9,10] We now realize that the ingrowth of skeletal cells into the myocardium was due to skeletal myoblasts.[11] Skeletal myoblasts are progenitor cells in skeletal muscle that are committed to differentiating into skeletal muscle after injury. These early findings led to the development of autologous skeletal myoblasts as a treatment for chronic heart failure.[12–14]

The early preclinical and clinical studies with skeletal myoblasts taught us a great deal and laid the groundwork for the stem cell–based studies that followed. We learned that exogenous cells could engraft into the heart and that the engraftment of skeletal myoblasts could lead to clinical benefit, including inducing reverse remodeling of the left ventricular remodeling.[4,15,16] We further learned the importance of mechanical coupling of exogenous cells to the cellular milieu of the heart.[17] Skeletal myoblasts do not integrate into the electrical syncytium of the myocardium, and have been shown in animal studies to induce slow conduction[18] and increase the risk of re-entrant rhythm,[19] and to increase premature ventricular contractions and ventricular tachycardia in patients.[13]

In May 2001, two seminal articles were published on the potential role of bone marrow–derived stem cells in myocardial repair in the setting of acute myocardial infarction.[20,21] These data clearly demonstrated that bone marrow–derived stem cells migrate or home to the area of myocardial damage within the first 48 hours after acute myocardial infarction, leading to vessel growth, decreased infarct size, and improved cardiac function. These studies differ in whether there is growth of new cardiac myocytes or myocardial regeneration in response to bone marrow–derived stem cell engraftment.

After the release of preclinical data, the feasibility of exogenous cell delivery of skeletal myoblasts to the myocardium by percutaneous or direct surgical injection was demonstrated, which led to the rapid initiation of phase I clinical trials of bone marrow–derived stem cell therapy in patients with chronic heart failure. From the release of rodent data in May 2001, it was less than 18 months before the first clinical data, from the TOPCARE-AMI (Transplantation of Progenitor Cells and Regeneration Enhancement in Acute Myocardial Infarction) study, were published. Since then, dozens of clinical trials[22] have been undertaken in the setting of acute myocardial infarction,[23–28] chronic ischemia,[29] and chronic heart failure.[1,30,31] Beyond the clinical trials, our understanding of the process of stem cell–based myocardial repair has been greatly advanced through both basic and preclinical studies.

Perhaps the most pertinent concept to have emerged in the field of stem cell–based myocardial repair is that there are as yet no absolutes, only generalizations, for each of which there are data to the contrary. Thus, although open-mindedness is necessary, generalizations are a useful tool to understand where the field is, how it may proceed, and how to translate its results to clinical populations.

Generalizations about stem cell therapy include the following:
- Multiple adult stem cell populations tested lead to improved cardiac function when delivered in the peri-infarct period.[32–36]
- The benefits associated with adult stem cell engraftment are due to paracrine factor release leading to:
  - Increased vascular density in the infarct border zone.[32,37,38]
  - Decreased infarct size.[33,39]
  - Recruitment of cardiac stem cells.[5,40]
- Adult stem cells do not induce significant cardiogenesis.[3,20,33,41,42]
- Regeneration of cardiac myocytes will likely involve the use of embryonic stem cells or induced pluripotent stem cells.[43–46]
- Both autologous and allogeneic stem cell sources appear to have benefit.[28,32,39]

Stem cell types that have been delivered in the peri-infarct period in preclinical models include autologous or syngeneic bone marrow mononuclear cells, mesenchymal stem cells,[33,47,48] multipotent adult progenitor cells,[32] CD34+ hematopoietic stem cells,[20,35] and cardiac stem cells[49] (Table 18-1). Allogeneic stem cells that have been used in preclinical and clinical studies in the peri-infarct period include mesenchymal stem cells[28,39] and multipotent progenitor cells.[32] Human stem cells that have been studied in immune-deficient rodent models include human umbilical cord–derived stem cells[34] and adipose-derived mesenchymal stem cells.[48] In all cases, positive results have been observed, and by modulating dose (number of cells) and route of delivery, equivalent results can be obtained from all cell sources.

Given the potential for equivalent results from many different adult stem cell populations, how will the field choose relevant adult stem cells to move forward? Ultimately, the distinguishing feature of any given adult stem cell population is derived from how it can be implemented clinically. For example, if one of the benefits of stem cell therapy is to decrease inflammation, then delivery of stem cells before the onset of inflammation is critical. However, only allogeneic stem cells are readily available and deliverable at the time of primary percutaneous coronary intervention in patients with ST-elevation acute myocardial infarction. Bone marrow mesenchymal stem cells, multipotent adult progenitor cells, and potentially the more recently identified amniotic sack–derived mesenchymal stem cells may be the cells of choice because they can be used in an allogeneic strategy and "off the shelf." Both mesenchymal stem cells and multipotent adult progenitor cells have been delivered to patients in the peri-infarct period with evidence of safety and some efficacy.[28]

Conversely, other cell populations may be better suited or optimal in the setting of open heart surgery. Previous teaching suggested that the heart was terminally differentiated, but recently a cardiac stem cell has been identified by several investigators. Based on relative dosing of stem cells in preclinical trials, it would appear that cardiac stem cells may be the most potent of all the adult stem cells.[49] If true, then cardiac stem cells may be the best cells for use as an adjunct to open heart surgery in the setting of coronary grafting, valve surgery, or left ventricular assist device implantation (Fig. 18-1). Just as adipose-derived stem cells can be rapidly harvested from adipose tissue, it may become possible rapidly to isolate cardiac stem cells from the left atrial appendage in the operating room in sufficient numbers to allow for delivery during surgery. If the cardiac stem cell number is inadequate, the cells can be isolated during surgery and infused percutaneously after expansion, as is being done in the SCIPIO (Cardiac Stem Cell Infusion in Patients with Ischemic Cardiomyopathy) trial (ClinicalTrials.gov—NCT00474461). In the setting of mechanical support, cardiac stem cells could be obtained through myocardial biopsy, isolated and propagated, and then introduced at the time of assist device implantation. Similarly, cardiac stem cells can be isolated from myocardial tissue obtained at the time of assist device implantation and delivered by percutaneous catheter, through multiple infusions over time through the assist device, or during a subsequent surgery (see Fig. 18-1).

TABLE 18-1	Stem Cell Types of Interest in Cardiovascular Regenerative Therapies That Have Entered Clinical Trials		
Cell Type	**Potential Sources**	**Clinical Indications Studied**	**Comments**
Bone marrow mononuclear cells (BMMNC)	Bone marrow	AMI, CHF, and CLI	Autologous Mixed cell population
AC133+	Bone marrow	CHF	Delivered peri-CABG
CD34+	Bone marrow Cellular pheresis	AMI, chronic ischemia, CLI	
Mesenchymal stem cells (MSC)	Bone marrow Adipose Placenta	Bone marrow used in AMI; ongoing CHF trials	Allogeneic cell source AMI trial delivered cells IV
Multipotent progenitor cells (MPC)	Bone marrow	Ongoing trials	Allogeneic cell source STRO3 bright
Multipotent adult progenitor cell (MAPC)	Bone marrow	Completed AMI trial	Allogeneic cell source AMI trial used percutaneous adventitial delivery
Cardiac stem cells	Autologous atrial tissue	Ongoing CHF trial	Cells delivered percutaneously some time after OHS
Cardiospheres	Autologous myocardial biopsy	Ongoing CHF trial	

AMI, acute myocardial infarction; CABG, coronary artery bypass grafting; CHF, congestive heart failure; CLI, critical limb ischemia; IV, intravenously; OHS, open heart surgery

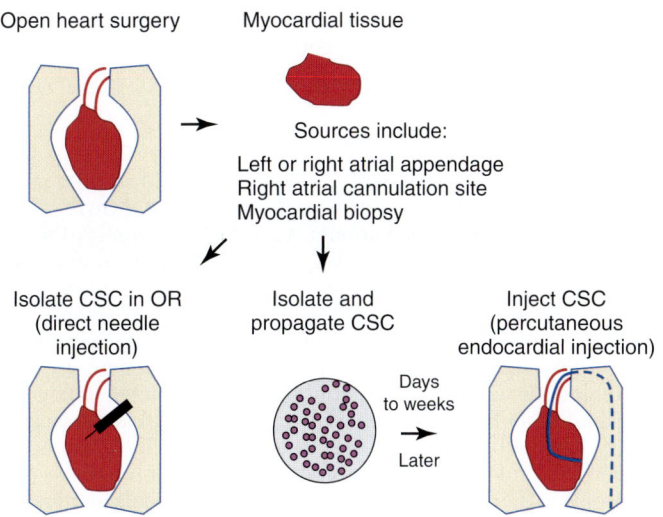

FIGURE 18-1 Schematic representation of potential protocols for cardiac stem cell (CSC) delivery in patients who undergo open heart surgery. OR, operating room.

Two other variables that could be potentially important in the eventual choice between allogeneic or autologous stem cell sources for the prevention and treatment of cardiac dysfunction are aging and comorbidities. There is growing evidence that aging and comorbidities contribute to stem cell dysfunction over time. In particular, the loss of insulin-like growth factor-1 expression appears to be a critical factor associated with stem cell dysfunction with aging.[50–52] Similarly, cellular function appears depressed in stem cells derived from patients with chronic diseases such as diabetes with coronary artery disease (renal failure and dialysis) and chronic heart failure.[53] Eventually we will need to determine if stem cell function can been restored during ex vivo expansion. If not, then allogeneic stem cells derived from young, healthy donors may be preferred.

Germane to the focus of this chapter, there are far fewer clinical data in the setting of nonischemic or idiopathic cardiomyopathy than acute myocardial infarction. Table 18-2 is a list of many of the clinical trials that have enrolled patients with chronic heart failure, and reveals that the majority of these trials demonstrated some benefit. Several clinical studies are ongoing to determine the effects of bone marrow mononuclear cells, as in the FOCUS (Autologous Bone Marrow Mononuclear Cells for Patients with Chronic Ischemic Heart Disease and Left Ventricular Dysfunction) trial being executed by the National Heart, Lung and Blood Institute–funded Cardiovascular Cell Therapy Research Network, as well as of specific populations of mesenchymal stem cells to be delivered percutaneously (POSEIDON [Percutaneous Stem Cell Injection Delivery Effects on Neomyogenesis] study; Clinicaltrials.gov—NCT01087996), during open heart surgery (PROMETHEUS [Prospective Randomized Study of Mesenchymal Stem Cell Therapy in Patients Undergoing Cardiac Surgery] study), or surgically as a stand-alone procedure (Cardiac Repair Cell Treatment of Patients with Heart Failure Due to Dilated Cardiomyopathy [IMPACT-DCM]; Clinicaltrials.gov—NCT00765518). There is also an open but currently not enrolling trial to determine the Effect of Intramyocardial Injection of Mesenchymal Precursor Cells on Heart Function in People Receiving an LVAD (Clinicaltrials.gov—NCT00927784), the results of which will bear directly on the topic of this text.

Cardiac Regeneration

At this time there are no published clinical data for the delivery of significant numbers of cardiac myocytes to treat patients with chronic heart failure. Perhaps the closest ongoing clinical trial involves the delivery of autologous cardiospheres to patients with chronic heart failure (CADUCEUS [Cardiosphere-Derived Autologous Stem Cells to Reverse Ventricular Dysfunction] Clinicaltrials.gov—NCT00893360). The evidence to date suggests that the benefits associated with adult stem cell therapy in patients with ischemic heart failure are associated with improvement in the biology and contractile function of the infarct border zone.[54–56] Thus, ultimately the delivery of cardiac myocytes to restore cardiac contractility will likely require the delivery of scaffolds that allow the transplanted cardiac myocytes to integrate with the remaining viable myocardial tissue and replace areas of significant scar (Fig. 18-2). The discovery of induced pluripotent stem cells offers the potential to generate autologous cardiac myocytes that could be used in the future to construct contractile networks for implantation into patients with chronic heart failure.[46,57,58]

In summary, stem cell therapy has made significant advancements in the past decade and all the data to date suggest that there is significant potential for the use of adult stem cells to prevent and treat cardiac dysfunction. That said, it is clear that there is a significant amount of research yet to be

TABLE 18-2	Stem Cell Transplantation in Heart Failure or Ischemic Cardiomyopathy				
Study	No. Patients	Cell Type	Delivery Method	Left Ventricular Function	Comments
Tse[75]	8	BMNC	NOGA, intramyocardial	Unchanged	Improvement in target wall motion by MRI
Seiler[76]	21	Stem cells mobilized from BM	GM-CSF, intracoronary dose, then subcutaneously ×2 wk	Unchanged	Decreased ischemia, improved coronary collateral circulation
Assmus[30]	75	CPC or BMNC	Intracoronary	Improvement with BMNC	
Perin[1]	21	BMNC	NOGA, intramyocardial	Improved	
Fuchs[77]	10	BMNC	Intramyocardial, percutaneous	Improved	
van Ramhorst[78]	50	BMNC	Intramyocardial, percutaneous	3% increase in left ventricular function	Reduction in ischemia by SPECT and improved CCS angina score
FOCUS[79]	87	BMNC	NOGA, intramyocardial	—	Ongoing enrollment

BM, bone marrow; BMNC, blood mononuclear cell; CCS, Canadian Cardiovascular Society; CPC, cardiac progenitor cell; GM-CSF, granulocyte-macrophage colony-stimulating factor; MRI, magnetic resonance imaging; SPECT, single photon emission computed tomography.

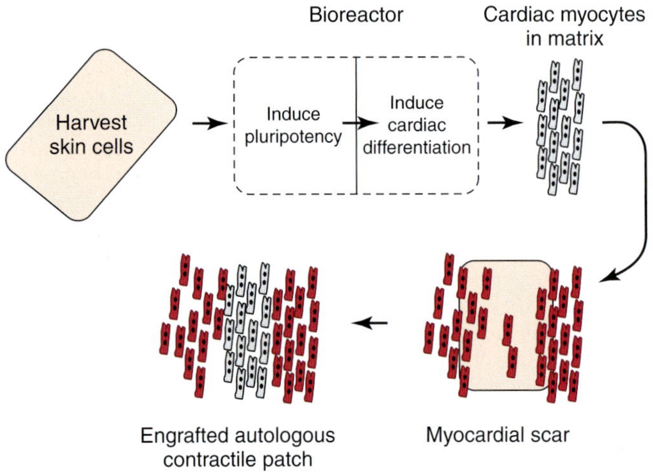

Bioreactor

Cardiac myocytes in matrix

Harvest skin cells

Induce pluripotency

Induce cardiac differentiation

Engrafted autologous contractile patch

Myocardial scar

FIGURE 18-2 Process of generation of custom biologic contractile networks that are integrated into matrices before delivery.

done to define the relevant biology and optimize the clinical translation of stem cell therapy to treat cardiac dysfunction. There are multiple potential points at which stem cell therapy and mechanical assist devices can intersect and there is great interest in the field to exploit these points of intersection. Perhaps the best data on the biology of engraftment, survival, differentiation, and efficacy of stem cell therapies can be garnered by implanting stem cells at the time of assist device implantation and studying the resulting tissue at the time of heart explant for transplantation.[59] Similarly, from the device point of view, using assist devices to support the patient until the development of successful techniques for myocardial regeneration that can potentially lead to permanent recovery of function would greatly increase the population of patients that might benefit from a mechanical device approach.

GENE TRANSFER FOR THE TREATMENT OF CARDIAC DYSFUNCTION

There has been significant excitement over the past 2 decades about the potential for gene transfer as a strategy to improve outcomes in patients with cardiovascular disease. The early work focused on mechanisms of angiogenesis in an attempt to improve outcomes with chronic myocardial ischemia. The focus of these potential therapies was on constructs that induced the expression of gene products, including vascular endothelial growth factor and fibroblast growth factor, to induce vascular growth. These vectors were delivered as plasmid and adenoviral constructs. Importantly, the clinical studies in this era demonstrated safety when clinical protocols were adhered to with respect to patient selection and dosing. Unfortunately, to date gene transfer has not shown great benefit and is not an approved treatment for any cardiovascular disease. The goal of this section is to look at where we have been, where we are, and where we may go in the future of cardiovascular gene transfer, with an eye toward how the growing acceptance of left ventricular assist devices may provide the safest and most effective platform for approaching gene transfer, both as a means to increase the frequency of explant of the assist device and as an adjunct to destination therapy. Finally, the potential for combined cell and gene transfer will be discussed, specifically as it relates to use in the left ventricular assist device population. It should be noted that in virtually all cases gene transfer is currently being pursued to minimize the need for left ventricular assist device implantation; however, given the extent to which some genes of

interest optimize remodeling, the combination of gene transfer with device implantation could offer significant clinical benefit.

Where We Have Been

As stated previously, the early forays into cardiovascular gene transfer focused on strategies to induce vascular growth, typically for claudication or patients with coronary artery disease beyond hope of catheter-based revascularization. There are many potential reasons for the lack of demonstrated efficacy leading to the fact that there is not routine use of gene transfer at this time. These include inappropriate dosing, inadequate targets for therapeutic response, inappropriate genetic vectors, difficult clinical populations, and the risks associated with gene transfer (Table 18-3). Further challenging the field is the lack of clearly defined end points that indicate clinically meaningful responses. Understanding the ramifications of each of these can be useful in the design of new strategies and protocols for moving cardiovascular gene transfer forward in the near and long term.

Dosing for gene transfer is a complex interaction between the number of injections, the concentration of the injectate, the uptake of the genetic vector by local cells, the activity of the promoter regulating gene expression, and the processing and stability of the transcribed gene product. The most common promoter implemented in cardiovascular gene transfer studies to date is the cytomegalovirus promoter. This promoter has high activity in mammalian cells, with long-term expression in most species other than mouse. The level of expression can be enhanced through the addition of cytomegalovirus enhancer introns. The cytomegalovirus promoter can be silenced by excessive methylation. In strategies where the goal is to minimize noncardiac expression of gene product, the cardiac-specific α-myosin heavy chain promoter can be used. Although use of this promoter limits expression to cardiac myocytes and cardiac stem cell populations, in our hands it also decreases the overall expression of an injected vector by 26-fold (Table 18-4). The overall amount of the final protein generated using either

TABLE 18-3	Difficulties with Earlier Gene Transfer Trials to Treat Cardiac Disorders
Difficulty	**Possible Resolution**
Gene of interest	Novel targets have been generated through studies with stem cells and furthering of knowledge on changes in myopathic tissue
Genetic vectors	Advances in knowledge of viral vectors and enhancer elements
Gene dosing	Commercially available plasmid production eliminates constraints of plasmid generation
Vector delivery	New catheter systems for engaging tissue and mapping myocardium have been developed
Adverse effects of viral vectors	Vectors that induce less inflammation and have tropism for cardiac myocytes

TABLE 18-4	Relative Luciferase Expression after Gene Transfer to the Rodent Myocardium*	
	Enhancer Element	
Promoter	**None**	**RU5**
CMV	26	258
α-MHC	1	155

Data represent fold increase of peak expression over α-MHC promoter without enhancer element.

TABLE 18-5	Relative Luciferase Expression after Gene Transfer to the Rodent Myocardium as a Function of Dose*			
Dose	10	50	100	500
Expression	1	10.9	58.1	73.6

*The vector contained the cytomegalovirus promoter without RU5 enhancer element. Data represent fold increase of peak expression over 10-μg injection.

of these promoters can be enhanced through the inclusion of the 5′-UTR (untranslated region) enhancer element RU5; although the degree of enhancement appears to depend on the activity of the promoter (see Table 18-4). The RU5 enhancer element does not alter gene transcription; rather, it enhances translation of messenger RNA to protein.

Beyond the design of the plasmid, the amount of DNA delivered is critical. As seen in Table 18-5, we observed a clear response of myocardial luciferase expression as a function of dose of plasmid DNA injected in the rodent heart. However, injections of these amounts of plasmid did not lead to significant luciferase expression in the porcine myocardium. Figure 18-3 shows a summary of the dosing strategy of plasmid DNA in previous clinical trials. We have recently found that this dose of plasmid DNA does not result in significant protein expression in the porcine myocardium. These findings led us to re-evaluate efficacious plasmid delivery to injured myocardium. We found that volume of injectate, concentration of plasmid, and other similar parameters can greatly affect plasmid delivery and protein expression. These data suggest that one reason for the lack of clinical efficacy in prior plasmid-based cardiovascular gene transfer studies may have been significant underdosing of plasmid.

Although gene dosing may have limited the success of earlier cardiovascular gene transfer studies, the targets of therapy may have contributed to long-term success as well. The majority of the early trials were focused on inducing angiogenesis, most commonly by targeting vascular endothelial growth factor (VEGF) or fibroblast growth factor. With respect to VEGF, several obstacles were encountered, including the multiple isoforms of VEGF, that VEGF delivery did not result in the formation of arterioles, and that the vascular memory of the tissue was not altered by VEGF overexpression. The lack of change in tissue vascular memory meant that once the VEGF signal was turned off, there was regression of the new vasculature. Strategies were implemented in an attempt to overcome these limitations of the earlier targets. For example, angiopoietin was added to VEGF in an attempt to induce the growth of more mature vessels. Although many of these types of strategies showed promise in preclinical studies, fibroblast growth factor-1 as a potential therapy for critical limb ischemia is the only early strategy that is still being pursued.[60,61]

Where We Are

There has been a resurgence more recently in cardiovascular gene therapy, particularly for chronic heart failure. Part of this resurgence is based on a deeper understanding of the biology of chronic heart failure, and the identification of novel targets for gene transfer. Many of the new targets have been generated from results in the last decade of work on myocardial repair. In particular, the implementation of exogenous stem cell therapies has led to the identification of multiple novel factors as well as a deeper understanding of the mechanisms of myocardial repair in general. Potential targets for cardiovascular gene transfer are depicted in Figure 18-4.

FIGURE 18-3 **A** and **B**, Distribution of parameters of injectate concentration (**A**) and DNA (**B**) injected per site versus the number of injections given in pivotal porcine studies of cardiovascular gene transfer. The size of the globe represents the relative total amount of DNA injected in the study. *(Courtesy Juventas Therapeutics, Inc., Cleveland, OH.)*

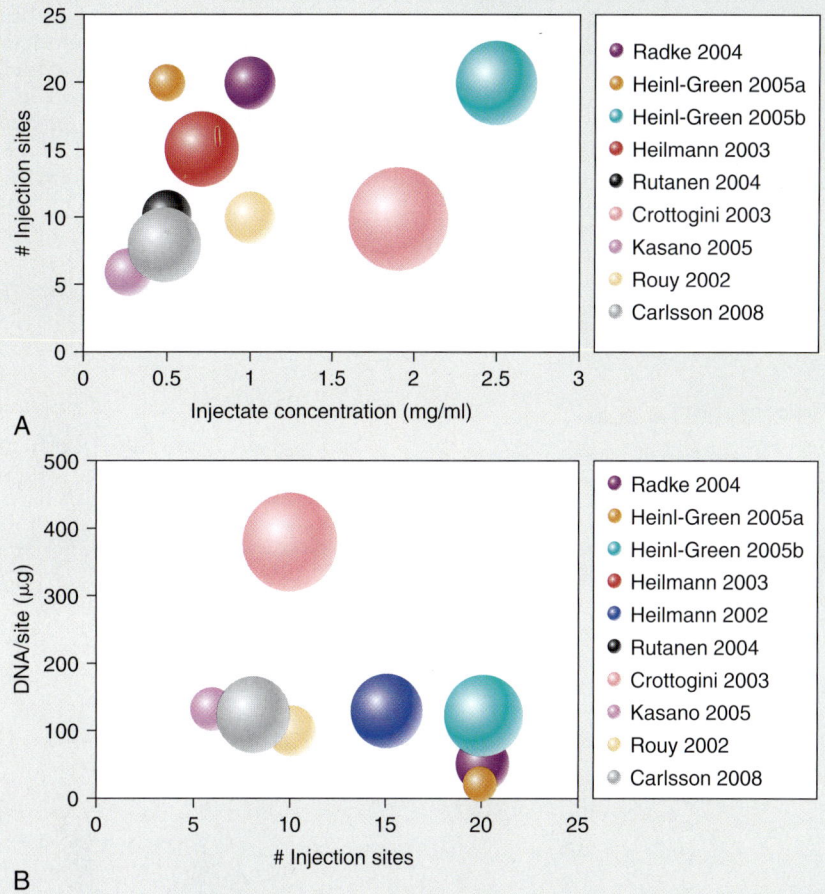

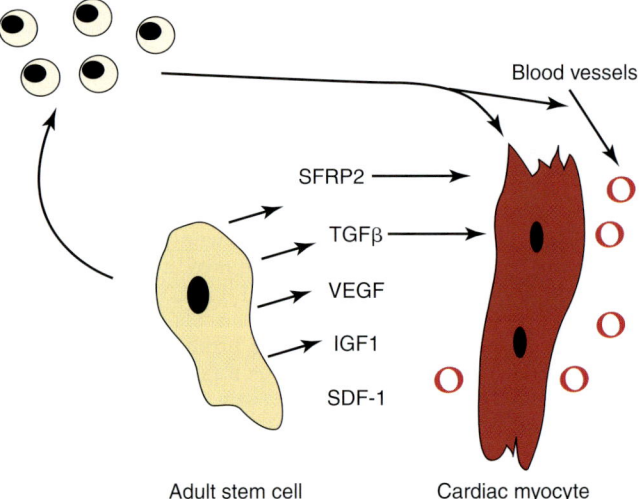

FIGURE 18-4 Schematic representation of possible target mechanisms associated with adult stem cell engraftment in myocardial tissue. SFRP2, secreted frizzled-related protein 2; TGFβ, transforming growth factor-beta; VEGF, vascular endothelial growth factor; IGF, insulin growth factor; SDF, stromal cell–derived growth factor.

Adult stem cell therapy does not appear to be convincingly able to induce regeneration of lost cardiac myocytes; rather, it would appear that the stem cells optimize left ventricular remodeling and cardiac myocyte function. Two examples of cardiovascular gene transfer that are now under investigation in clinical populations of chronic heart failure are re-establishment of stem cell homing with stromal cell–derived factor-1 (SDF-1) and increased cardiac myocyte contractility with sarcoplasmic reticulum Ca^{2+} ATPase (SERCA2a).

Secreted Soluble Factors

The initiation of clinical trials with SDF-1 is a direct reflection of the growing understanding of stem cell–mediated cardiac repair. It is becoming increasingly clear that although the delivery of stem cells to induce cardiac repair may offer

significant benefit, as depicted in Figure 18-5, the paracrine factors released by the stem cells could be therapeutic themselves. Said a different way, in the 1990s we performed gene transfer with genes we thought the heart wanted (e.g., VEGF, fibroblast growth factor-1), but in the next generation of cardiovascular gene therapy we will deliver what the stem cells have taught us the heart needs.

SDF-1 was identified as the myocardial factor responsible for the recruitment of stem cells to the heart after an acute myocardial infarction.[3,62] Consistent with the hypothesis that stem cell–based repair is clinically inefficient not because of the lack of stem cells, but because of dysregulated expression of key molecular signals responsible for orchestrating stem cell–based cardiac repair, the SDF-1 signal lasts less than 1 week. Our group and several others have demonstrated that prolonging the SDF-1 signal results in prolonged stem cell recruitment to the heart, decreased cardiac myocyte death, and improved overall cardiac remodeling and function (see Fig. 18-5).[33,42,63,64] We have similarly shown that re-establishment of SDF-1 signaling months after an acute myocardial infarction results in remodeling of the left ventricle and improved cardiac function.[3,4] Cardiac myocytes in the infarct border zone express the SDF-1 receptor CXC chemokine receptor type 4 (CXCR4), the expression of which has negative inotropic effects.[65] Several mechanisms appear to be involved in this process, including recruitment of cardiac stem cells to the infarct border zone, neovascularization of the infarct and infarct border zone, and the long-term downregulation of cardiac myocyte CXCR4 expression.

Although SDF-1 has been brought to the forefront for cardiovascular gene transfer in patients with chronic heart failure, it should also be noted that its expression has also been shown to be upregulated and thought to be critical in the response to left ventricular assist device implantation.[66] Furthermore, the upregulation of SDF-1 in response to left ventricular assist device implantation with or without clenbuterol has been shown to be associated with successful device explant. How upregulation of myocardial SDF-1 expression could alter cardiac remodeling and function is depicted in Figure 18-3.

We have shown using both cell-based gene transfer and direct plasmid injection that the expression of SDF-1 for a period of 14 days at a time remote from acute myocardial infarction is sufficient to induce left ventricular remodeling.[4] This approach has been validated in a porcine model of

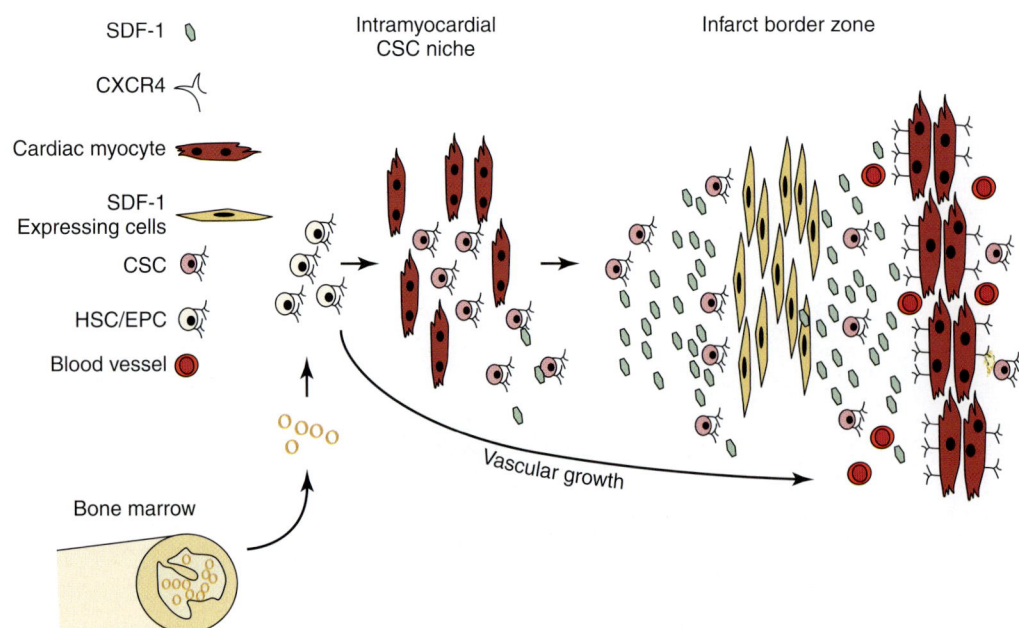

FIGURE 18-5 Schematic representation of the targets and effects of stromal cell–derived factor-1 (SDF-1) overexpression at a time remote from acute myocardial infarction. CSC, cardiac stem cell.

chronic heart failure and is the topic of an open-label phase I clinical trial in patients with New York Heart Association class III chronic heart failure. Preclinical studies in the porcine heart suggested that earlier cardiovascular gene transfer studies may have been significantly underdosed. This SDF-1 plasmid trial is studying a total of 5, 15, and 30 mg of plasmid DNA equally divided among 15 intraventricular injections.

Intracellular Targets

Paracrine factor expression and the definition of molecular targets identified through stem cell therapy have suggested multiple potential targets for cardiovascular gene transfer. Similarly, careful molecular biology and preclinical studies have demonstrated targets that directly address the loss of contractile function of cardiac myocytes in failing human hearts. The best developed of these targets and the focus of recent clinical studies is SERCA2a. SERCA2a is responsible for calcium handling in cardiac myocytes. The loss of SERCA2a in cardiac myocytes isolated from patients with chronic heart failure has suggested that abnormal calcium handling is a key factor in abnormal cardiac contractility. In pioneering work, Roger Hajjar and colleagues have developed novel gene transfer protocols that allow for the long-term expression of SERCA2a in cardiac myocytes in patients with chronic heart failure. Because SERCA2a upregulation must be persistent for sustained benefit, novel strategies for gene transfer needed to be implemented (Fig. 18-6). Thus, in contrast to earlier attempts at cardiovascular gene transfer, these clinical trials are using an adeno-associated virus (AAV) that leads to integration of the gene into the transduced cells (see Fig. 18-6). This variant of the original studies using pure adenovirus seems very safe and nontoxic. Intracoronary infusion of the AAV vector in these patients has demonstrated the ability to achieve meaningful levels of gene transfer. As AAV vectors with different degrees of cardiac tropism are developed, systemic gene delivery to target organs could become a reality. Most exciting, the early results from a recent phase II study (CUPID [Calcium Up-Regulation by Percutaneous Administration of Gene Therapy in Cardiac Disease] trial) demonstrated decreases in biomarkers of heart failure, left ventricular end-systolic volume, and heart failure admissions in patients who received high-dose SERCA2a:AAV1 compared with control subjects (Fig. 18-7).

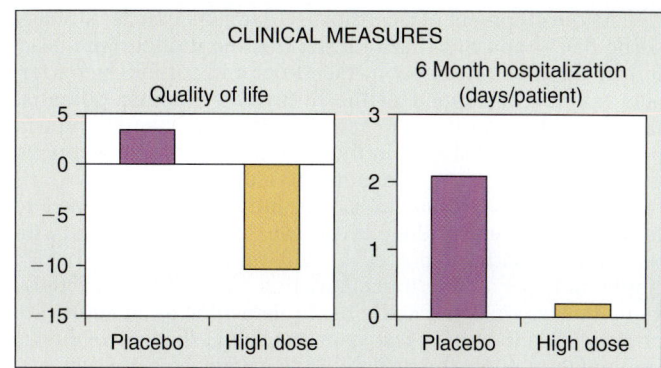

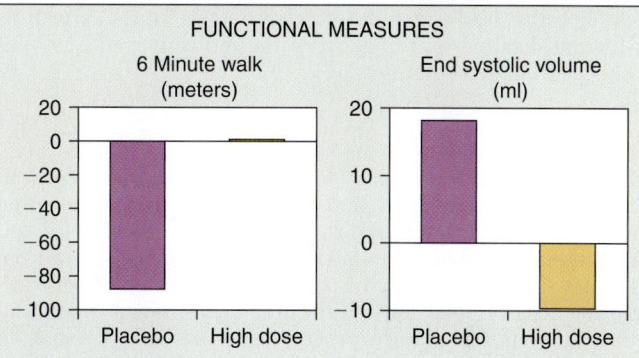

FIGURE 18-7 Results of the phase II CUPID trial: adeno-associated virus (AAV)-SERCA2a delivery to patients with chronic heart failure. *(Hajjar R: Presented at the annual meeting of the Heart Failure Association of the European Society of Cardiology, Berlin, May 2010.)*

Although these results are exciting, it should be noted nearly 50% of the adult population has antibodies to the AAV1 vector. Previous exposure can limit the efficacy of AAV1 vectors, ultimately limiting the number of patients who can receive this potentially efficacious therapy; however, it is hoped that ongoing studies will identify novel AAV vectors that have increased cardiac tropism to which the population as a whole has limited exposure.

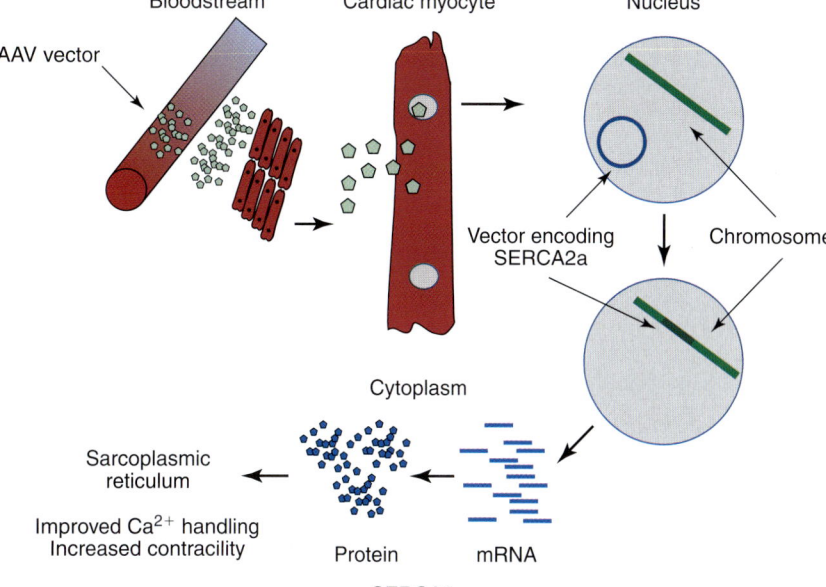

FIGURE 18-6 Steps involved from the delivery of adeno-associated virus (AAV) vector encoding SERCA2a into the bloodstream until SERCA2a is delivered to the sarcoplasmic reticulum.

The development of a cardiovascular gene transfer strategy using SDF-1 and SERCA2a for the treatment of chronic heart failure demonstrates how intracellular and soluble factor targets may be developed in the future. Many other potential targets, such as periostin,[67-69] phospholambam,[70] and thymosin β4,[71-73] can be developed in the future based on the technical and clinical findings of ongoing clinical studies.

Each of these strategies is currently being developed to treat patients early in the clinical course of chronic heart failure, thus obviating the need for left ventricular assist device implantation or cardiac transplantation. That said, both of these gene transfer strategies could be implemented as an adjunct to device implantation. In fact, gene transfer at the time of device implantation offers the real ability to optimize vector delivery, which could lead to greater efficacy in the future as well as allowing detailed examination of the molecular and cellular changes from gene therapy.

Where We May Go

Patients with chronic heart failure who need left ventricular assist device support and implantation offer interesting opportunities for gene transfer and the combination of cellular therapy and gene transfer. The opportunities arise from the fact that the majority of patients with chronic heart failure eventually need left ventricular assist device implantation; thus, as the disease progresses, plans can be made to generate custom biologic therapies that can be deployed at the time of device implantation. After implantation, the heart can be supported by the assist device while these custom biologics mature to the point where they can reliably support the myocardium in the absence of mechanical assistance. In addition, the mechanical unloading produced by the left ventricular assist device may enhance the benefit of gene therapy by partially reversing the adverse effects of high chamber pressures and low cardiac output, and prove synergistic if not additive.

Previously we have proposed a three-phase development path for cardiovascular regenerative medicine (Fig. 18-8). In phase 1 (adult stem cell phase) and phase 2 (paracrine factor phase), true myocardial regeneration would not occur because there are few data suggesting that adult stem cells can regenerate lost cardiac myocytes.[33,41] Phase 1 would include the REPAIR-AMI (Reinfusion of Enriched Progenitor Cells and Infarct Remodeling in Acute Myocardial Infarction) trials and others like it[24]; phase 2 would include the SDF-1 trial discussed previously. We proposed that in phase 3 true cardiac regeneration would occur by implementing embryonic stem cells or, more likely now, inducible pluripotent stem cells (see Fig. 18-2). Clearly, gene transfer as well as many other facets of tissue engineering will play meaningful parts in cardiac regeneration.

Figure 18-4 shows schematically how cardiovascular gene transfer can be implemented to develop custom biologics for availability at the time of left ventricular assist device implantation. As they progress in their symptoms, autologous cells can be obtained from patients. After placement in a bioreactor, these cells can be manipulated to enter into a pluripotent state and then differentiated into cardiac myocytes. Because of the marked decline in function with advanced age and chronic disease that is typical of patients with heart failure, current focus has moved from use of autologous cells to allogeneic mesenchymal stem cells, which do not express MHC antigens and thus do not require immunosuppression. Young donors can be used as a more ideal source of cells for carrying genes. Potential strategies to induce dedifferentiation and redifferentiation could include protein,[74] plasmid, or cell-penetrating peptide[54] delivery of critical factors to minimize genetic manipulation of the therapeutic cell and any long-term oncogenic risk.

More recent data suggest that the simple injection of stem cells that differentiate into cardiac myocytes in vivo does not result in the generation of large areas of myocardial tissue.[55] Thus, after generation of patient-specific cardiac myocytes it will likely be necessary to engraft these cells on biomaterials that will aid in generation of contractile networks that will optimally contract after integration into the native myocardium. The addition of these contractile networks could benefit from and result in greater improvements associated with surgical left ventricular remodeling at the time of assist device implantation.

Engineered cells for implantation are another form of custom biologics associated with gene transfer at the time of assist device implantation. One possibility in this regard is the generation of cells containing an inducible gene expression cassette. In this case, the gene could be turned on through the administration of tetracycline, steroids, or other small molecules that induce expression of the engineered construct. Through these means we could develop a system that allows the physician to induce or enhance, for example:

- Vascular growth in patients who develop ischemia after left ventricular assist device implantation.
- Gene expression to optimize or respond to the degree of left ventricular remodeling.
- Gene expression at the time of stem cell infusion to induce or optimize stem cell engraftment.

Summary

Significant excitement surrounded the potential for cardiovascular gene transfer to improve the outcomes of patients with cardiovascular disease. Although this approach has not yet realized any clinical successes, the ongoing clinical development of several gene transfer strategies offers significant hope that this approach will improve patient outcomes in the future. To demonstrate proof-of-concept and clinical feasibility, many of the current clinical trials focus on patients with chronic heart failure who do not need left ventricular assist devices, in the hope that we will be able in the future to prevent the need for mechanical assistance and heart transplantation in many of these patients. That said, as reviewed previously, the combination of gene transfer, cell therapy, and mechanical assistance shows great promise to truly regenerate myocardial tissue. Critical in this process will be the fact that there is significant access to the myocardium at the time of left ventricular assist device implantation, as well as mechanical support of the heart while the biologics integrate and mature before having to take on a mechanical load. Successful development and implementation of these therapies will require multidisciplinary expertise and support, but ultimately they offer great hope for patients with severe left ventricular dysfunction and chronic heart failure.

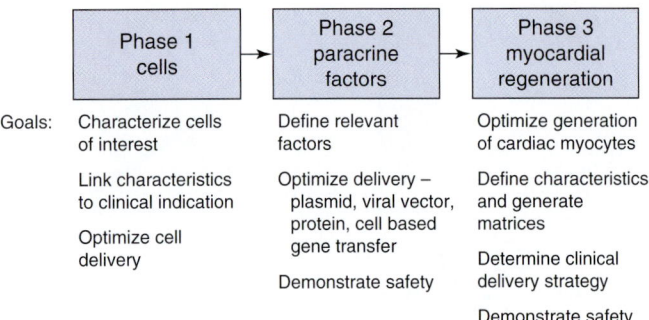

FIGURE 18-8 Proposed three-phase development plan for cardiovascular regenerative therapies.

REFERENCES

1. Perin EC, Dohmann HF, Borojevic R, et al. Transendocardial, autologous bone marrow cell transplantation for severe, chronic ischemic heart failure. *Circulation*. 2003;107:2294–2302.
2. Stamm C, Kleine HD, Westphal B, et al. CABG and bone marrow stem cell transplantation after myocardial infarction. *Thorac Cardiovasc Surg*. 2004;52:152–158.
3. Askari A, Unzek S, Popovic ZB, et al. Effect of stromal-cell-derived factor-1 on stem cell homing and tissue regeneration in ischemic cardiomyopathy. *Lancet*. 2003;362:697–703.
4. Deglurkar I, Mal N, Mills WR, et al. Mechanical and electrical effects of cell-based gene therapy for ischemic cardiomyopathy are independent. *Hum Gene Ther*. 2006;17:1144–1151.
5. Urbanek K, Rota M, Cascapera S, et al. Cardiac stem cells possess growth factor-receptor systems that after activation regenerate the infarcted myocardium, improving ventricular function and long-term survival. *Circ Res*. 2005;97:663–673.
6. Moreira LF, Bocchi EA, Stolf NA, et al. Dynamic cardiomyoplasty in the treatment of dilated cardiomyopathy: current results and perspectives. *J Card Surg*. 1996;11:207–216.
7. Bocchi EA, Moreira LF, de Moraes, et al. Effects of dynamic cardiomyoplasty on regional wall motion, ejection fraction, and geometry of left ventricle. *Circulation*. 1992;86:II231–II235.
8. Jatene AD, Moreira LF, Stolf NA, et al. Left ventricular function changes after cardiomyoplasty in patients with dilated cardiomyopathy. *J Thorac Cardiovasc Surg*. 1991;102:132–138.
9. Chiu RC, Kochamba G, Walsh G, et al. Biochemical and functional correlates of myocardium-like transformed skeletal muscle as a power source for cardiac assist devices. *J Card Surg*. 1989;4:171–179.
10. Misawa Y, Mott BD, Lough JO, et al. Pathologic findings of latissimus dorsi muscle graft in dynamic cardiomyoplasty: clinical implications. *J Heart Lung Transplant*. 1997;16:585–595.
11. Menasché P, Hagege AA, Vilquin JT, et al. Autologous skeletal myoblast transplantation for severe postinfarction left ventricular dysfunction. *J Am Coll Cardiol*. 2003;41:1078–1083.
12. Menasché P. Skeletal myoblasts and cardiac repair. *J Mol Cell Cardiol*. 2008;45:545–553.
13. Menasché P, Alfieri O, Janssens S, et al. The Myoblast Autologous Grafting in Ischemic Cardiomyopathy (MAGIC) trial: first randomized placebo-controlled study of myoblast transplantation. *Circulation*. 2008;117:1189–1200.
14. Smits PC, van Geuns RJ, Poldermans D, et al. Catheter-based intramyocardial injection of autologous skeletal myoblasts as a primary treatment of ischemic heart failure: clinical experience with six-month follow-up. *J Am Coll Cardiol*. 2003;42:2063–2069.
15. Askari A, Goldman CK, Forudi F, et al. VEGF-expressing skeletal myoblast transplantation induces angiogenesis and improves left ventricular function late after myocardial infarction. *Mol Ther*. 2002;5:S162.
16. Dowell JD, Rubart M, Pasumarthi KB, et al. Myocyte and myogenic stem cell transplantation in the heart. *Cardiovasc Res*. 2003;58:336–350.
17. Reinecke H, MacDonald GH, Hauschka SD, et al. Electromechanical coupling between skeletal and cardiac muscle. Implications for infarct repair. *J Cell Biol*. 2000;149:731–740.
18. Fouts K, Fernandes B, Mal N, et al. Electrophysiological consequence of skeletal myoblast transplantation in normal and infarcted canine myocardium. *Heart Rhythm*. 2006;3:452–461.
19. Mills WR, Mal N, Kiedrowski MJ, et al. Stem cell therapy enhances electrical viability in myocardial infarction. *J Mol Cell Cardiol*. 2007;42:304–314.
20. Kocher AA, Schuster MD, Szabolcs MJ, et al. Neovascularization of ischemic myocardium by human bone-marrow-derived angioblasts prevents cardiomyocyte apoptosis, reduces remodeling and improves cardiac function. *Nat Med*. 2001;7:430–436.
21. Orlic D, Kajstura J, Chimenti S, et al. Transplanted adult bone marrow cells repair myocardial infarcts in mice. *Ann N Y Acad Sci*. 2001;938:221–229.
22. Abdel-Latif A, Bolli R, Tleyjeh IM, et al. Adult bone marrow-derived cells for cardiac repair: a systematic review and meta-analysis. *Arch Intern Med*. 2007;167:989–997.
23. Assmus B, Schachinger V, Teupe C, et al. Transplantation of Progenitor Cells and Regeneration Enhancement in Acute Myocardial Infarction (TOPCARE-AMI). *Circulation*. 2002;106:3009–3017.
24. Schachinger V, Erbs S, Elsasser A, et al. Intracoronary bone marrow-derived progenitor cells in acute myocardial infarction. *N Engl J Med*. 2006;355:1210–1221.
25. Janssens S, Dubois C, Bogaert J, et al. Autologous bone marrow-derived stem-cell transfer in patients with ST-segment elevation myocardial infarction: double-blind, randomised controlled trial. *Lancet*. 2006;367:113–121.
26. Penn MS. Stem-cell therapy after acute myocardial infarction: the focus should be on those at risk. *Lancet*. 2006;367:87–88.
27. Traverse JH, Henry TD, Vaughn DE, et al. Rationale and design for TIME: a phase II, randomized, double-blind, placebo-controlled pilot trial evaluating the safety and effect of timing of administration of bone marrow mononuclear cells after acute myocardial infarction. *Am Heart J*. 2009;158:356–363.
28. Hare J, Traverse J, Henry T, et al. A randomized, double-blind, placebo-controlled, dose-escalation study of intravenous adult human mesenchymal stem cells (Prochymal) following acute myocardial infarction. *J Am Coll Cardiol*. 2009;54:2277–2286.
29. Losordo DW, Schatz RA, White CJ, et al. Intramyocardial transplantation of autologous CD34+ stem cells for intractable angina: a phase I/IIa double-blind, randomized controlled trial. *Circulation*. 2007;115:3165–3172.
30. Assmus B, Honold J, Schachinger V, et al. Transcoronary transplantation of progenitor cells after myocardial infarction. *N Engl J Med*. 2006;355:1222–1232.
31. Ichim TE, Solano F, Lara F, et al. Combination stem cell therapy for heart failure. *Int Arch Med*. 2010;3:5.
32. Van't HW, Mal N, Huang Y, et al. Direct delivery of syngeneic and allogeneic large-scale expanded multipotent adult progenitor cells improves cardiac function after myocardial infarct. *Cytotherapy*. 2007;9:477–487.
33. Zhang M, Mal N, Kiedrowski M, et al. SDF-1 expression by mesenchymal stem cells results in trophic support of cardiac myocytes after myocardial infarction. *FASEB J*. 2007;21:3197–3207.
34. Leor J, Guetta E, Feinberg MS, et al. Human umbilical cord blood-derived CD133+ cells enhance function and repair of the infarcted myocardium. *Stem Cells*. 2006;24:772–780.
35. Orlic D, Kajstura J, Chimenti S, et al. Bone marrow cells regenerate infarcted myocardium. *Nature*. 2001;410:701–705.
36. Zuba-Surma EK, Kucia M, Dawn B, et al. Bone marrow-derived pluripotent very small embryonic-like stem cells (VSELs) are mobilized after acute myocardial infarction. *J Mol Cell Cardiol*. 2008;44:865–873.
37. Rota M, Padin-Iruegas ME, Misao Y, et al. Local activation or implantation of cardiac progenitor cells rescues scarred infarcted myocardium improving cardiac function. *Circ Res*. 2008;103:107–116.
38. Tillmanns J, Rota M, Hosoda T, et al. Formation of large coronary arteries by cardiac progenitor cells. *Proc Natl Acad Sci U S A*. 2008;105:1668–1673.
39. Amado LC, Saliaris AP, Schuleri KH, et al. Cardiac repair with intramyocardial injection of allogeneic mesenchymal stem cells after myocardial infarction. *Proc Natl Acad Sci U S A*. 2005;102:11474–11479.
40. Unzek S, Zhang M, Mal N, et al. SDF-1 recruits cardiac stem cell like cells that depolarize in vivo. *Cell Transplant*. 2007;16:879–886.
41. Murry CE, Soonpaa MH, Reinecke H, et al. Haematopoietic stem cells do not transdifferentiate into cardiac myocytes in myocardial infarcts. *Nature*. 2004;428:664–668.
42. Tang YL, Zhu W, Cheng M, et al. Hypoxic preconditioning enhances the benefit of cardiac progenitor-cell therapy for treatment of myocardial infarction by inducing CXCR4 expression. *Circ Res*. 2009;104:1209–1216.
43. Laflamme MA, Chen KY, Naumova AV, et al. Cardiomyocytes derived from human embryonic stem cells in pro-survival factors enhance function of infarcted rat hearts. *Nat Biotechnol*. 2007;25:1015–1024.
44. Nelson TJ, Chiriac A, Faustino RS, et al. Lineage specification of Flk-1+ progenitors is associated with divergent Sox7 expression in cardiopoiesis. *Differentiation*. 2009;77:248–255.
45. Faustino RS, Behfar A, Perez-Terzic C, et al. Genomic chart guiding embryonic stem cell cardiopoiesis. *Genome Biol*. 2008;9:R6.
46. Nelson TJ, Martinez-Fernandez A, Yamada S, et al. Induced pluripotent reprogramming from promiscuous human stemness related factors. *Clin Transl Sci*. 2009;2:118–126.
47. Toma C, Pittenger MF, Cahill KS, et al. Human mesenchymal stem cells differentiate to a cardiomyocyte phenotype in the adult murine heart. *Circulation*. 2002;105:93–98.
48. Cai L, Johnstone BH, Cook TG, et al. IFATS collection: human adipose tissue-derived stem cells induce angiogenesis and nerve sprouting following myocardial infarction, in conjunction with potent preservation of cardiac function. *Stem Cells*. 2009;27:230–237.
49. Bearzi C, Rota M, Hosoda T, et al. Human cardiac stem cells. *Proc Natl Acad Sci U S A*. 2007;104:14068–14073.
50. Leri A, Kajstura J, Li B, et al. Cardiomyocyte aging is gender-dependent: the local IGF-1-IGF-1R system. *Heart Dis*. 2000;2:108–115.
51. Torella D, Rota M, Nurzynska D, et al. Cardiac stem cell and myocyte aging, heart failure, and insulin-like growth factor-1 overexpression. *Circ Res*. 2004;94:514–524.
52. Mayack SR, Shadrach JL, Kim FS, et al. Systemic signals regulate ageing and rejuvenation of blood stem cell niches. *Nature*. 2010;463:495–500.
53. Vasa M, Fichtlscherer S, Aicher A, et al. Number and migratory activity of circulating endothelial progenitor cells inversely correlate with risk factors for coronary artery disease. *Circ Res*. 2001;89:E1–E7.
54. Bian J, Popovic ZB, Benejam C, et al. Effect of cell-based intercellular delivery of transcription factor GATA4 on ischemic cardiomyopathy. *Circ Res*. 2007;100:1626–1633.
55. Tsuji H, Miyoshi S, Ikegami Y, et al. Xenografted human amniotic membrane-derived mesenchymal stem cells are immunologically tolerated and transdifferentiated into cardiomyocytes. *Circ Res*. 2010;106:1613–1623.
56. Penn MS, Mayorga ME. Searching for understanding with the cellular lining of life. *Circ Res*. 2010;106:1554–1556.
57. Kuzmenkin A, Liang H, Xu G, et al. Functional characterization of cardiomyocytes derived from murine induced pluripotent stem cells in vitro. *FASEB J*. 2009;23:4168–4180.
58. Moretti A, Bellin M, Jung CB, et al. Mouse and human induced pluripotent stem cells as a source for multipotent Isl1+ cardiovascular progenitors. *FASEB J*. 2010;24:700–711.
59. Pagani FD, DerSimonian H, Zawadzka A, et al. Autologous skeletal myoblasts transplanted to ischemia-damaged myocardium in humans. Histological analysis of cell survival and differentiation. *J Am Coll Cardiol*. 2003;41:879–888.
60. Baumgartner I, Chronos N, Comerota A, et al. Local gene transfer and expression following intramuscular administration of FGF-1 plasmid DNA in patients with critical limb ischemia. *Mol Ther*. 2009;17:914–921.
61. Nikol S, Baumgartner I, Van BE, et al. Therapeutic angiogenesis with intramuscular NV1FGF improves amputation-free survival in patients with critical limb ischemia. *Mol Ther*. 2008;16:972–978.
62. Abbott JD, Huang Y, Liu D, et al. Stromal cell-derived factor-1alpha plays a critical role in stem cell recruitment to the heart after myocardial infarction but is not sufficient to induce homing in the absence of injury. *Circulation*. 2004;110:3300–3305.
63. Cheng Z, Ou L, Zhou X, et al. Targeted migration of mesenchymal stem cells modified with CXCR4 gene to infarcted myocardium improves cardiac performance. *Mol Ther*. 2008;16:571–579.
64. Jin DK, Shido K, Kopp HG, et al. Cytokine-mediated deployment of SDF-1 induces revascularization through recruitment of CXCR4+ hemangiocytes. *Nat Med*. 2006;12:557–567.
65. Pyo RT, Sui J, Dhume A, et al. CXCR4 modulates contractility in adult cardiac myocytes. *J Mol Cell Cardiol*. 2006;41:834–844.

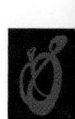

66. Barton PJ, Felkin LE, Birks EJ, et al. Myocardial insulin-like growth factor-I gene expression during recovery from heart failure after combined left ventricular assist device and clenbuterol therapy. *Circulation.* 2005;112:I46–I50.

67. Shimazaki M, Nakamura K, Kii I, et al. Periostin is essential for cardiac healing after acute myocardial infarction. *J Exp Med.* 2008;205:295–303.

68. Oka T, Xu J, Kaiser RA, et al. Genetic manipulation of periostin expression reveals a role in cardiac hypertrophy and ventricular remodeling. *Circ Res.* 2007;101:313–321.

69. Litvin J, Blagg A, Mu A, et al. Periostin and periostin-like factor in the human heart: possible therapeutic targets. *Cardiovasc Pathol.* 2006;15:24–32.

70. Del Monte F, Harding SE, Dec GW, et al. Targeting phospholamban by gene transfer in human heart failure. *Circulation.* 2002;105:904–907.

71. Bock-Marquette I, Saxena A, White MD, et al. Thymosin beta4 activates integrin-linked kinase and promotes cardiac cell migration, survival and cardiac repair. *Nature.* 2004;432:466–472.

72. Bock-Marquette I, Shrivastava S, Pipes GC, et al. Thymosin beta4 mediated PKC activation is essential to initiate the embryonic coronary developmental program and epicardial progenitor cell activation in adult mice in vivo. *J Mol Cell Cardiol.* 2009;46:728–738.

73. Srivastava D, Saxena A, Michael DJ, et al. Thymosin beta4 is cardioprotective after myocardial infarction. *Ann N Y Acad Sci.* 2007;1112:161–170.

74. Behfar A, Zingman LV, Hodgson DM, et al. Stem cell differentiation requires a paracrine pathway in the heart. *FASEB J.* 2002;16:1558–1566.

75. Tse HF, Kwong YL, Chan JK, et al. Angiogenesis in ischaemic myocardium by intramyocardial autologous bone marrow mononuclear cell implantation. *Lancet.* 2003;361:47–49.

76. Seiler C, Pohl T, Wustmann K, Hutter D, et al. Promotion of collateral growth by granulocyte-macrophage colony-stimulating factor in patients with coronary artery disease: a randomized, double-blind, placebo-controlled study. *Circulation.* 2001;104:2012–2017.

77. Fuchs S, Dib N, Cohen BM, et al. A randomized, double-blind, placebo-controlled, multicenter pilot study of the safety and feasibility of catheter-based intramyocardial injection of AdVEGF121 in patients with refractory advanced coronary artery disease. *Catheter Cardiovasc Interv.* 2006;68:372–378.

78. van Ramshorts J, Bax JJ, Beeres SL, et al. Intramyocardial bone marrow cell injection for chronic myocardial ischemia: a randomized controlled trial. *JAMA.* 2009;301:1997–2004.

79. Willerson JT, Perin EC, Ellis SG, et al. Intramyocardial injection of autologous bone marrow mononuclear cells for patients with chronic ischemic heart disease and left vantricular dysfunction (First Mononuclear Cells injected in the US [FOCUS]): Rationale and design. *Am Heart J.* 2010;60:215–223.

Biologic Responses to the Interface Between Device and Circulation

Bleeding and Thrombosis with Mechanical Circulatory Support

Joshua R. Woolley, Robert L. Kormos, and William R. Wagner

Ventricular assist devices (VADs) present a unique challenge regarding blood biocompatibility compared with other medical devices in that blood contacts a large surface area with complex flow fields for an extended time. Other chronic devices such as stents or grafts may have surface areas that are orders of magnitude smaller with favorable flow conditions, whereas similar-sized devices, such as membrane oxygenators, are intended for acute use in the presence of substantial anticoagulation. In contrast, the blood in a patient with a VAD must come in extensive contact with artificial surfaces for months or years while the patient is simultaneously being weaned to the lowest allowable levels of anticoagulation for chronic use. In light of these challenging circumstances, it is not surprising that many of the biologic complications such as thrombosis, thromboembolism, and bleeding encountered with the first implants during the mid-1980s are still problematic today. These complications contributed to a dampening of the initial enthusiasm for application of these devices to patients with heart failure, and remain problematic for clinicians and device designers.[1,2]

This chapter provides an overview of blood biocompatibility in the setting of VADs. A brief review of blood interaction with materials is followed by a discussion of the special constraints these interactions present to VAD designers. We also present some of the tools clinicians, researchers, and manufacturers are using to investigate and minimize complications. The goal of this chapter is to build a frame of reference regarding the extent and severity of these complications, as well to provide an appreciation for the complexity of the underlying processes contributing to these problems in this challenging patient population.

The first VADs mimicked the biphasic flow of the natural heart and served as effective bridges to transplantation for patients with heart failure waiting for donor organs.[3] The volume displacement needed for pulsatile flow required these VADs be large,

preventing implant in smaller patients. The introduction of rotary blood pumps decreased the size and power requirements and increased the mechanical life of VADs, expanding the eligible patient population and increasing their overall quality of life.[4] The use of sophisticated computational fluid dynamic modeling programs and of magnetic levitation to eliminate bearings improved the blood path through the pumps, helping to improve hemocompatibility. However, even with these technological advancements, all patients with VADs are still vulnerable to hemostatic complications such as thrombosis, thromboemboli, and bleeding (Fig. 19-1).[5]

Thromboembolic rates in patients with VADs can be difficult to define and compare, with reported rates varying substantially between specific VADs and institutions. Early reports and investigational device studies may have different levels of reporting that could distort cross-comparisons. Goldstein combined "embolic stroke, transient ischemic attack, and peripheral embolism" into the single parameter of "thromboembolic event"[6]; in contrast, Miller and colleagues reported separately on ischemic stroke, hemorrhagic stroke, transient ischemic attack, "other neurologic," and "peripheral nonneurologic thromboembolic event."[4] The combination of careful standardized assessment and reporting of potential thromboembolic events across centers would provide a better framework for comparative studies between devices and patient management protocols. A related situation is found in the reporting of bleeding rates.[4,7]

Given this need, INTERMACS (Interagency Registry for Mechanically Assisted Circulatory Support), a voluntary national patient registry for U.S. Food and Drug Administration (FDA)–approved devices, was formed as a centralized source for VAD implant information, including detailed adverse event definitions and rates. INTERMACS provides standardized definitions for suspected neurologic or bleeding events (Box 19-1).

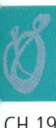
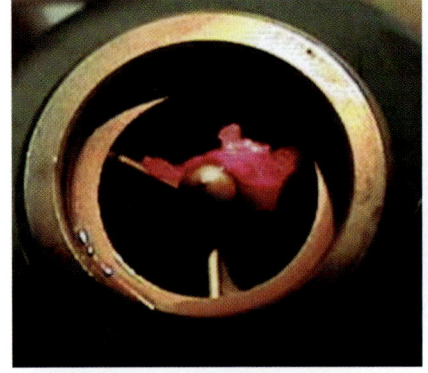

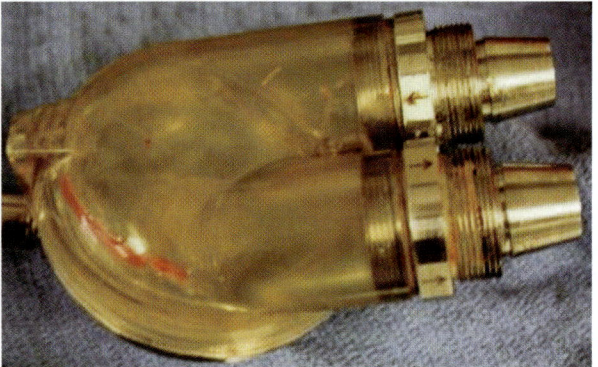

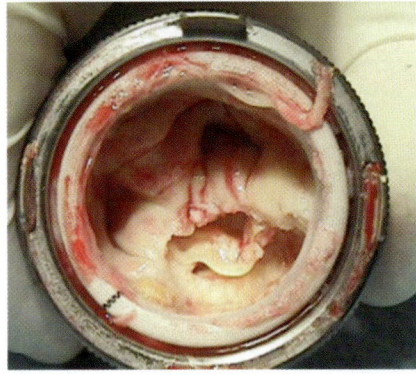

FIGURE 19-1 Thrombosis in ventricular assist devices (VADs). *Clockwise from upper left:* Partial occlusion of a rotary pump by thrombus on the inlet stator blades and bearing; polyurethane blood sac with thrombus on the far wall near the outlet valves; partial occlusion and disruption of inflow trileaflet valve. *(Courtesy of Robert Kormos, MD, University of Pittsburgh, Pittsburgh, PA.)*

 Box 19-1   INTERMACS Definitions of Neurologic Dysfunction and Major Bleeding Episode Adverse Events

Neurologic Dysfunction

Any new, temporary or permanent, focal or global neurologic deficit ascertained by a standard neurologic examination (administered by a neurologist or other qualified physician and documented with appropriate diagnostic tests and consultation note). The examining physician distinguishes between a transient ischemic attack, which is fully reversible within 24 hours (and without evidence of infarction), and a stroke, which lasts longer than 24 hours (or <24 hours if there is evidence of infarction). The NIH Stroke Scale (for patients >5 years old) must be readministered at 30 days and 60 days following the event to document the presence and severity of neurologic deficits. Each neurologic event must be subcategorized as:

1. Transient ischemic attack (acute event that resolves completely within 24 hours with no evidence of infarction)
2. Ischemic or hemorrhagic cardiovascular accident or cerebrovascular accident (event that persists >24 hours or <24 hours associated with infarction on an imaging study)
   In addition, for patients younger than 6 months, either of the following:
3. New abnormality on head ultrasound
4. Electroencephalogram positive for seizure activity with or without clinical seizure

Major Bleeding Episode

Episode of suspected internal or external bleeding that results in one or more of the following:

1. Death
2. Reoperation
3. Hospitalization
4. Transfusion of red blood cells as follows
   During first 7 days after implant
   Adults (≥50 kg): ≥4 units packed red blood cells within any 24-hour period during first 7 days after implant
   Children (<50 kg): ≥20 mL/kg packed red blood cells within any 24-hour period during first 7 days after implant
   More than 7 days after implant
   Any transfusion of packed red blood cells after 7 days following implant with the investigator recording the number of units given (record number of units given per 24-hour period)

Note: Hemorrhagic stroke is considered a neurologic event and not as a separate bleeding event.
From INTERMACS User's Guide. Manual of Operations 10/30/08. Version 2.3, updated 5/5/09. Available from http://www.uab.edu/ctsresearch/intermacs/Document%20 Library/Site%20Users%20Guide%20v2.3%20update%2006052009.pdf. Accessed July 5, 2011.

In addition to reporting each adverse event, institutions participating in INTERMACS must provide information on aspects surrounding the event, such as date and location of patient during onset, contributing factors, event type and severity, anticoagulation therapy, and mortality, among other details.[8] Based on these definitions, INTERMACS investigators reported that 18% of patients with a VAD experience neurologic dysfunction and 35% have bleeding complications (420 patients).[9] In addition, biventricular support presents an especially challenging situation because twice the artificial surface is implanted into typically the sickest of such patients. INTERMACS reports substantially higher bleeding rates for pulsatile biventricular support compared with only left VAD (LVAD) support (55% vs. 35%); interestingly, neurologic complications are slightly lower for biventricular support (16% vs. 18%), illustrating the challenge clinicians face in attempting to predict risk factors for adverse events (465 LVADs, 128 biventricular VADs).[10]

Outside of INTERMACS, other researchers and institutions have reported bleeding and thrombotic adverse event rates in the literature. Given the different flow fields and shear stresses in each type of pump, one would expect that pulsatile and rotary pumps may have different rates of adverse events. The Thoratec (Pleasanton, CA) pulsatile internal pneumatic VAD (IVAD) was reported to have stroke rate of 8% and bleeding rate of 46% (with 33% requiring reoperation; 39 patients in the study).[11] Miller and colleagues reported on a multicenter study of the HeartMate II rotary LVAD in which 11% of patients experienced hemorrhagic or ischemic strokes (0.18 events/patient year), 2% had pump thrombosis, and 41% of patients had bleeding requiring reoperation (a slight increase in thromboembolic complications over the pulsatile Thoratec IVAD; 133 patients).[4] Furthermore, in an illustration of differences between implant centers, John and colleagues also reported on the HeartMate II but in a single-center setting; only 3% experienced stroke and 15% had bleeding that required reoperation (a significant reduction in adverse event rates compared with both previous reports; 47 patients).[12]

As clinicians become more familiar with these patients and devices, improvements in event rates owing to progress in patient anticoagulant management have also been reported in the literature. Long and associates demonstrated decreases in adverse event rates through refined patient management and preimplantation screening; a new patient management protocol provided by the manufacturer addressed patient selection, wound care, nutrition, and perioperative and postoperative care. Long and colleagues continued to show that for patients implanted with the pulsatile HeartMate XVE, neurologic dysfunction (0.15 vs. 0.39 events/patient year) and bleeding (0.15 vs. 0.46 events/patient-year) were reduced under the new protocol compared with previously published values that were collected during early use of this device (42 patients).[7,13]

The introduction of impeller-levitation technology (no internal bearings; single moving part) and improved fluid dynamics design for VADs have not been able to eliminate these complications. For one such pump, the Ventracor (Chatswood, New South Wales, Australia) LVAD, reported complications (33 patients) were stroke in 24% (0.48 events/patient year), thrombosis or thromboembolism in 15%, and hemorrhage in 24% (0.48 events/patient year).[14] These relatively high complication rates remain troubling for clinicians, especially when compared with similar heart failure populations that do not receive VAD support but remain on optimal medical therapy. Rogers and colleagues followed patients on optimal medical therapy for a length of time comparable with VAD implantation and found that 11% experienced stroke while 0% experienced bleeding (18 patients).[15] Similarly, Rose and coworkers found neurologic dysfunction at a rate of 0.09 events/patient year and no bleeding events (61 patients).[7] A meta-analysis by Witt and colleagues found that only 5% of

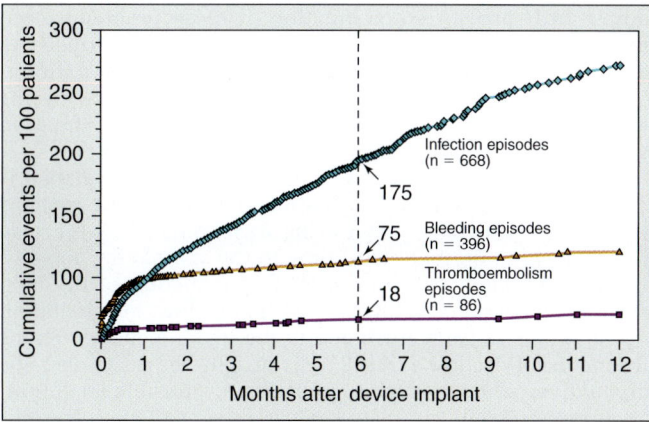

FIGURE 19-2 Neurologic adverse events and bleeding from INTERMACS; notice the preponderance of thromboembolism and bleeding incidents in the first 30 days of support. *(From Deng MC, Edwards LB, Hertz MI, et al. Mechanical circulatory support device database of the International Society for Heart and Lung Transplantation: third annual report—2005.* J Heart Lung Transplant. *2005;241182-1187.)*

patients with heart failure experience ischemic stroke within the first 5 years of diagnosis.[16]

Regardless of the pump or institution, studies suggest that patients are most at risk for thromboembolism and bleeding events during the first 30 days of VAD implantation (Fig. 19-2).[4,6,7,17] Refinement of anticoagulation protocols and increased experience with this patient population has helped to reduce the quantity and severity of these events, but these are still high enough to give pause to referring clinicians regarding the effectiveness of this technology. In addition, thromboembolic events causing neurologic damage are frequently seen as especially pernicious complications because of their often sudden onset and debilitating nature. The INTERMACS database shows that neurologic adverse events are the primary cause in 18% of deaths while on device, whereas surgical bleeding accounts for only 3%.[9] Clearly, more investigation into changes in the hemostatic state of these unique patients postimplantation is warranted, and may enable clinicians to advance the management of this population and improve outcomes in morbidity and mortality.[18,19]

VIRCHOW'S TRIAD APPLIED TO VENTRICULAR ASSIST DEVICES

Thrombogenicity is a material characteristic that may be used interchangeably to describe the localized formation of blood clots, the systemic damage inflicted by embolization of a clot, or the destruction or consumption of blood components resulting in a relative reduction in the ability of blood to function normally.[20] Each of these facets of thrombogenicity may contribute to the failure of a medical device to function properly with the host. A device may trigger a "stabilized" local thrombus formation that is well anchored to the substrate; however, it is difficult to accurately predict the location and size of adherent thrombus and an ill-placed clot may completely undermine the function of the device (e.g., incomplete valve seal, stent occlusion). In addition, a material may resist thrombus adherence but still cause embolism through transient clot formation; hence, there are reports of in vivo material evaluations demonstrating "clean" surfaces but producing end-organ infarcts.[21] Furthermore, some devices exhibit a continual destruction or removal of blood cells or proteins resulting in a hemostatic imbalance that may contribute to adverse events (e.g., consumptive coagulopathy from oxygenator circuits, anemia from hemolysis). Often a

device will present a combination of these problems, confounding attempts to improve the device or even properly to isolate the offending processes. Note, however, that a thrombogenic device may cause seemingly opposite adverse events within the same host—namely, unregulated clot formation and uncontrolled bleeding.

In a healthy individual without an implant, a balance is maintained between the coagulation and fibrinolytic systems to prevent severe blood loss during vessel puncture while also re-establishing normal blood flow to the vessel after repair.[22] In 1856, Virchow proposed that the interaction of the constitution of the blood, interrupted blood flow, and irritation of the blood vessel contributed to the phenomena of venous thrombosis (Virchow's triad).[23] His insight helped to describe qualitatively the underlying processes responsible for thrombus formation and to isolate key variables that could be optimized by researchers to minimize thrombogenicity in medical procedures. However, when artificial surfaces are introduced, this balance may be disrupted by the body's interaction with the foreign matter, resulting in unregulated reactions that may be difficult to remedy.[24–27] Virchow's triad still provides the framework for medical device design and assessment, with an expanded focus on the composition of the blood and subtle changes to the other variables to reflect a more general application to artificial and organic surfaces. Blood coagulation in the setting of artificial surfaces involves three areas of interdependence: the blood (platelets, the coagulation cascade, fibrinolysis), the flow over the material, and the blood-contacting material.[22] The following is a brief discussion of each variable as it relates to VAD thrombosis and hemostasis.

Blood: The Delicate Balance

At first contact with blood, artificial surfaces very quickly undergo protein adsorption, forming a layer over the material almost instantly. This dynamic protein layer is thermodynamically driven by the Vroman effect, where smaller, diffusible proteins initially adsorb to the material surface and are gradually displaced by less diffusible proteins with higher affinity for the surface.[28] All subsequent blood interactions with the device then involve the plasma proteins with the most affinity for the material, and not the material surface itself. The shear forces of the flowing blood on the surface will further influence the Vroman effect; a setting of high shear stress (e.g., arterial flow) may remove all low-affinity proteins that may be present on the same material in a low-shear milieu (e.g., venous flow, recirculation zones). This adds substantial complexity to predicting device thrombogenicity because the same material may have different adsorbed proteins depending on the flow through the device.[24]

Platelets adhere to artificial surfaces through the binding of platelet surface receptors with adsorbed plasma proteins; in particular, glycoprotein (GP) Ib adheres to adsorbed von Willebrand factor, whereas GP IIb/IIIa adheres to adsorbed fibrinogen, fibronectin, and von Willebrand factor.[29,30] This process is driven by the shear force of the blood such that at lower wall shear rates (<1000 s^{-1}), binding depends on GP IIb/IIIa, whereas at higher shear rates the tethering shifts to GP Ib.[29] Adherent platelets become activated, resulting in the release of the contents of internal vesicles (α- and dense granules) into the extracellular environment, formation of pseudopodia, exposure of phosphatidylserine (a negatively charged phospholipid), and binding with other platelets to form aggregates. Dense granules contain platelet activation agonists such as adenosine diphosphate, calcium ions, and serotonin that help to recruit passing platelets to the site of injury and solidify the platelet aggregate. The phospholipid surface of the deposited platelet mass provides a catalytic surface for the cleavage of prothrombin to thrombin; thrombin then is a potent platelet activator and serves as a positive feedback agent for the growing thrombus. In addition, there is a growing body of literature suggesting that regions of high shear stress may induce low-level activation in the platelet, causing the formation of tendrils that then bind to adsorbed proteins or adherent platelets to form aggregates.[31]

Blood coagulation involves the serial proteolytic cleavage of circulating plasma proteins converging in the activation of prothrombin to thrombin. Of particular importance for artificial materials is the intrinsic system of the coagulation cascade leading to the common pathway. The negatively charged surface of the deposited platelets provides a favorable environment for the anchoring of plasma proteins involved in the initial steps of the intrinsic system. The formation of the platelet plug may help to reduce the flow of blood through the area of insult, allowing the coagulation proteins to form a local gradient to aid in the rapid development of the thrombus.

The fibrinolytic system regulates clot formation through the degradation of excess fibrin mesh, allowing flow to return to normal to the region of insult after healing. Plasminogen is the principal fibrinolytic agent and is incorporated into the fibrin mesh during clot formation. During healing, plasminogen activators (e.g., tissue plasminogen activator and urokinase) are released by cells near the injury and the fibrin mesh is disassembled.[22]

Not only are VADs ambitious for the amount of surface area exposed to the blood and the length of time implanted, these devices are reserved for implantation into some of the very sickest patients. Patients with VADs often have conditions that predispose them to blood clots (e.g., coagulopathies, fibrillation, ischemia) before VAD placement, and the artificial device may unfortunately serve to aggravate the issue. In addition, 44% of patients undergo implantation after critical cardiogenic shock, which characteristically magnifies extreme inflammation and hypercoagulation.[9] Postoperative patient management is difficult and frequently includes administration of blood products and varying levels of anticoagulation. The effects of surgery and postoperative care on the blood cells can last for weeks before reaching steady state. In short, the hemostatic state of the patient with a VAD represents one of the most challenging environments in which to place a medical device.

As stated previously, postoperative bleeding and adverse neurologic events generally occur during the first month of implantation. Bleeding may be broadly defined by a combination of chest tube drainage, blood products required, and reoperation for hemorrhage. A number of mechanisms contribute to difficulties in patient management during this early postoperative period. The highly invasive surgical procedure is associated with blood loss, hemodilution, coagulation protein consumption, and platelet activation.[32] The dynamic hemostatic state of these patients immediately after implantation often drives clinicians to balance the anticoagulation regimen delicately to ensure proper inhibition of thrombosis while preventing over-anticoagulation (and associated bleeding).[33–35]

Some reports have shown that the traditional measures of anticoagulation such as activated partial thromboplastin time (aPTT) and international normalized ratio (INR) are not predictive of observed thromboembolic events.[36] Difficulties with keeping a patient's INR in range while on warfarin (and the poor outcomes associated with highly variable INR values) have been studied.[37] In an effort to find more descriptive indices of a patient's hemostatic state (and possibly predictors of adverse events), researchers and clinicians have investigated circulating biomarkers of thrombosis and fibrinolysis. Joshi and colleagues measured INR, aPTT, and prothrombin fragment F1.2 (a protein cleaved when prothrombin is converted to thrombin) in patients with a VAD daily before discharge, then weekly thereafter. The investigators found that an elevation of F1.2 was a significant predictor of neurologic events, whereas INR and aPTT were not.[36] In addition, Wilhelm and coworkers found increasing levels of plasma F1.2 coincided with an increase in cranial microembolic signals measured using transcranial Doppler.[38] Global platelet activation has been investigated through measurement of plasma levels of proteins released from platelet α-granules (platelet factor 4 and β-thromboglobulin).[39,40] Individual interrogation of platelet activation state has been performed by flow cytometry through measurement of surface expression of CD62P and CD63 (both cell receptors are found in platelet α-granules and are expressed on activation).[38,41] These reports suggest that platelet activation levels in patients with a VAD rise after implantation and continue to be elevated through the duration of support. D-dimer has been targeted as a potential indicator of thrombus formation because it is a byproduct of fibrin degradation.[39,42] Platelet response to stimulation,[43,44] circulating thrombin-antithrombin III complex,[40] plasminogen activator inhibitor-1,[44] monocyte-platelet aggregates,[38] and monocyte expression of tissue factor,[45] among others, have also been targeted to help assess the patient's coagulation state as well as predict adverse events.

Although the hemostatic state of patients with a VAD is often varied and dynamic, anticoagulation protocols are surprisingly uniform across institutions and devices, based on heparin in the perioperative and immediate postoperative period, and chronic warfarin administration supplemented with acetylsalicylic acid or dipyridamole as additional antiplatelet agents.[4,11,14,15,39,46,47] Advances in individualized therapy may help significantly reduce the occurrence of adverse events through patient-specific regimens. Platelet genotyping and platelet function testing for detection of hyperresponsiveness or hyporesponsiveness to anticoagulation or antiplatelet agents have been increasingly used for other cardiac procedures (e.g., stent and valve placements)[48,49]; however, consensus on the utility and robustness of this approach has not yet been achieved.[50] Another approach to tailored medicine is systems biology modeling of patient-specific blood response to activating factors and pharmaceutical agents. Several complex coagulation models are being developed (reviewed by Diamond[51]) that allow for user input of values such as coagulation factor concentrations and platelet response to known agonist concentrations. Patient-specific data may be obtained (for individualization of the model) by high-throughput blood screening using microfluidics blood analysis. The result is a powerful tool that may be able to diagnose blood defects or predict the effectiveness of anticoagulant and antiplatelet agents. However, further progress needs to be made regarding robustness of the models, computational capabilities, and clinical implementation before the potential of this technology is realized.[52,53]

Flow: Complex Flow Fields with a Non-Newtonian Fluid

As described earlier, blood flow controls the rate at which blood cells and proteins contact the device wall through diffusion and convection.[54] Flow fields and shear stresses in VADs vary dramatically between different types of pumps and even in different regions in the same pump. The shear forces of the blood help to determine the composition of adsorbed proteins and resultant thrombus. Areas of recirculation in a pump may trap platelets, increasing their exposure time to the artificial surface while also increasing the local concentrations of agonists released from previously adherent platelets. High-shear regions in a pump may become problematic as passing platelets are transiently activated by the shear and deposit on pump seams and bearings that under low-shear flow may have been free from thrombus. In contrast, areas of uninterrupted laminar flow at moderate shear stresses may increase

the hemocompatibility of the device by reducing platelet exposure time to artificial surfaces and rapidly removing or diluting agonists from previously adherent platelets. Thus, the flow conditions within the VAD may enhance or exasperate the hemocompatibility of the pump surface, undermining even the best attempts at presenting an optimal surface to prevent platelet adhesion and activation.

Shear forces are substantially different between different VAD models depending on a myriad of factors, not the least of which is whether the pump is pulsatile or rotary. Pulsatile pumps are generally characterized as low-shear flow because of the slow filling of a large blood sac and then the gradual increase in pressure to dispel the fluid. However, this is true only when the shear stresses are averaged over an entire pump cycle; the biphasic nature of pulsatile pumps causes changing conditions that may result in transiently suboptimal flow conditions at localized regions in the pump. For example, shear stresses at the valves during systole will initially be very severe (a high-velocity nozzle during the opening of the valve) and then decrease greatly (fully open valve becomes a large-diameter tube), even resulting in recirculation and stasis zones near the valves once they close during diastole.[55] Pulsatile pumps often operate with a "residual volume" of blood that is unable to be completely dispelled from the blood sac during diastole because of the pump's geometric constraints. This residual volume of blood is inevitably exposed to the pump surface for a relatively long time and may become a nidus for platelet deposition or bulk-phase aggregate formation. Although most pulsatile pumps are designed such that the fluid rotationally fills the pump sac (to discourage stasis in the pump during the transition from diastole to systole), this solution is imperfect and unable to completely remove the flow disturbances that occur during transitions in biphasic flow conditions (Fig. 19-3).[55,56] These disturbances in flow may dislodge adherent thrombi or break off aggregates, sending emboli downstream with possibly catastrophic results.

Rotary VADs are different from pulsatile pumps in that the blood continuously flows through the pump at a relatively constant rate. Rotary VADs use a spinning impeller to move the blood forward; depending on the VAD, this impeller may be supported by bearings in the flow field or magnetic suspension. The blade tips of the spinning impeller in rotary VADs present regions of consistently high shear stress that gradually decreases toward the center of the flow field. These high-shear regions vary between pumps (often depending on the width of the gap between the impeller blades and pump housing, among other factors) but are usually supraphysiologic.[57] Leverett and colleagues described a relationship between cell exposure time and shear stress that helps to define the hemolysis threshold for blood cells (Fig. 19-4)[58]; as such, many researchers attempt to design pump operation within this limit, but this is often not possible. However, despite continuously exposing blood to high-shear regions, these pumps have not experienced the hemolysis that was a concern during development.[59] Studies have suggested that laminar flow through the pump allows a cell-free boundary layer to form, which then experiences most of the high shear while pushing the cells toward the lower-shear regions, effectively excluding the cells from high shear stresses. For pumps that require bearings, this area has typically required special design to limit stasis at the bearing site and reduce blood damage from friction, leading to crushing of cells and local heat generation. Thrombus forming at pump bearings has been especially problematic because it poses not only a biologic threat of embolization, but a mechanical threat to the pump because of abnormal bearing wear or unexpected power consumption (limiting the accuracy of flow estimation and reducing battery life). Magnetically levitated impellers are not free from problems, however, because the slightest thrombus formation on

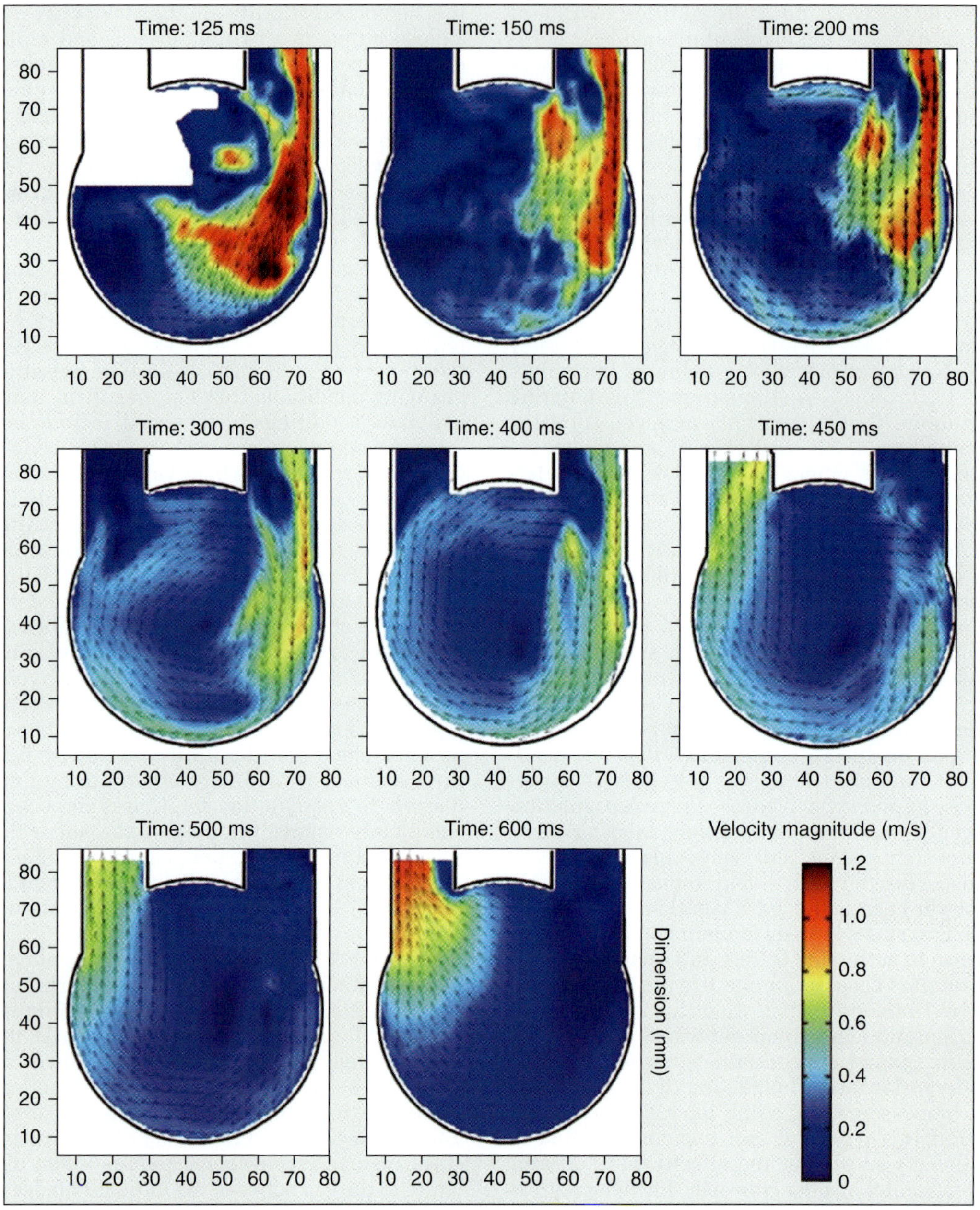

FIGURE 19-3 Particle image velocimetry (a computational fluid dynamics tool) of a pulsatile ventricular assist device (VAD) at the onset of pump systole. Note the initial high velocity at the opening of each valve, followed by very low velocity caused by recirculation and stasis. *(From Hochareon P, Manning KB, Fontaine AA, et al. Fluid dynamic analysis of the 50 cc Penn State artificial heart under physiological operating conditions using particle image velocimetry.* J Biomech Eng. *2004;126:585-593.)*

an impeller blade may disrupt the delicate magnetic balance and cause the impeller to crash into the pump housing.

Computational fluid dynamics (CFD) is the mathematical simulation of fluid flow in which a programmer is able to import a technical drawing of a VAD and model varying conditions of blood flow.[60] CFD has emerged as a powerful tool for designers to visualize the effects of pump changes during development and identify potentially problematic flow fields in silico.[61] CFD allows for the in silico manipulation of design of the pump in order to optimize targeted design parameters and predict pump performance prior to fabrication.[62,63] However, the non-Newtonian nature of blood increases the difficulty of predicting flow through even the simplest medical devices, whereas VADs present some of the most complex flow geometries in medicine. In addition, research is still ongoing concerning which parameters of the pump design are most important during optimization.[64]

Material Surface: The Interface between Body and Machine

In addition to their differing fluid dynamics, pulsatile and rotary VADs usually contain different blood-contacting surfaces because of the material design requirements specific to each pump. Despite these differences, the various materials are selected for relative blood biocompatibility, meaning relative resistance to thrombotic deposition and a lack of hemolytic activity. The blood sac in many pulsatile VADs is composed of a durable elastomer incorporating a manufacturer-specific nonthrombogenic molecular component at the surface. For example, the Thoratec pneumatic VAD contains an inflow cannula and blood sac composed of a proprietary polymer consisting of polyurethane blended with a biocompatible surface modifier (Thoralon) intended to reduce thrombogenicity.[65]

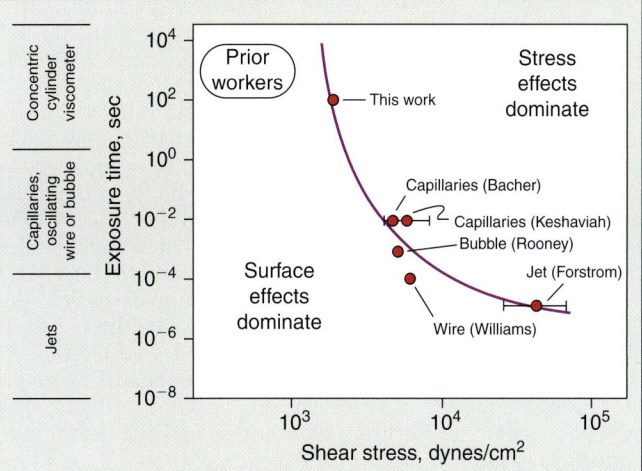

FIGURE 19-4 Original curve from the study of Leverett and colleagues suggesting the shear stress limits to red blood cells before lysis; the "safe zone" for red blood cells is beneath the curve. *(From Leverett LB, Hellums J D, Alfrey CP, et al. Red blood cell damage by shear stress.* Biophys J. *1972;12:257-273.)*

application in future medical devices. Interestingly, this technology has not been successfully translated to rotary VADs, possibly owing to their low tolerances and clearance requirements that are not compatible with the inability to control the thickness of the pseudointima layer.

The pump housing and impeller found in rotary VADs require hard materials that can be easily manufactured and are able to withstand mechanical wear. Some manufacturers use hard polymers (e.g., polycarbonate in the Levitronix [Waltham, MA] CentriMag) or coatings (e.g., diamond-like carbon coating on the Ventracor VentrAssist[70]) to improve thrombogenicity, but most rotary VADs use a highly polished titanium alloy (TiAl$_6$V$_4$) as the blood-contacting material (e.g., Thoratec HeartMate II; Jarvik 2000 [Jarvik Heart, Inc., New York]; HeartWare [Framingham, MA] HVAD).[70] TiAl$_6$V$_4$ excels at the aforementioned material properties; it also is nonmagnetic, which allows it to be incorporated into pumps that are magnetically suspended or controlled.

TiAl$_6$V$_4$ produces an oxide layer that helps to make this material relatively inert to thrombus formation. However, the tolerance of blood to this material appears to be proportional to the width of the oxide layer, which may vary in vivo; in addition, titanium without the oxide layer is relatively thrombogenic and has exhibited problems with general biocompatibility compared with other surfaces.[71] One area of improvement being explored by researchers is the development of long-lasting coatings applied to the blood-contacting surfaces in pumps. Synthetic phospholipid polymers have been studied extensively for their ability to mimic cell surfaces to prevent platelet activation and adhesion.[72,73] Polymers containing phosphorylcholine groups appear to be especially promising for reducing thrombogenicity, in particular the covalent attachment of 2- methacryloyloxyethylphosphorylcholine (MPC) to titanium alloys[74-76] (Fig. 19-5). Polyethylene glycol (PEG) coatings have also been extensively studied because of the remarkable resistance of PEG to protein adsorption (and hence platelet adhesion).[77] However, PEG is typically adsorbed onto the titanium surface, resulting in a weak coating; the flow rates experienced under normal pump operation may lead to a relatively quick removal of the coating, exposing the thrombogenic titanium. Another limiting factor with the application of this technology is the prohibitive

The biocompatibility strategy pursued by the HeartMate XVE VAD is in stark contrast to that of other pulsatile and rotary VADs. Rather than using blood-contacting surfaces that do not support platelet deposition, the inside of the HeartMate XVE contains on one side a stationary titanium wall covered in sintered 50- to 75-μm titanium microspheres and on the other side a pusher-plate covered by a roughly textured Biomer polyurethane diaphragm.[66] These thrombogenic surfaces encourage the formation of a highly organized clot that firmly anchors and matures into a "pseudointima" composed of platelets, monocytes, lymphocytes, fibroblasts, and in some cases endothelial cells.[67,68] This biologic blood interface has allowed many patients to be effectively weaned from all anticoagulant medications except aspirin with few thromboembolic events.[69] Although mechanical problems and size considerations have caused a decline in the rate of HeartMate XVE implantation, the challenge to traditional paradigms by this device will continue to be studied by researchers for

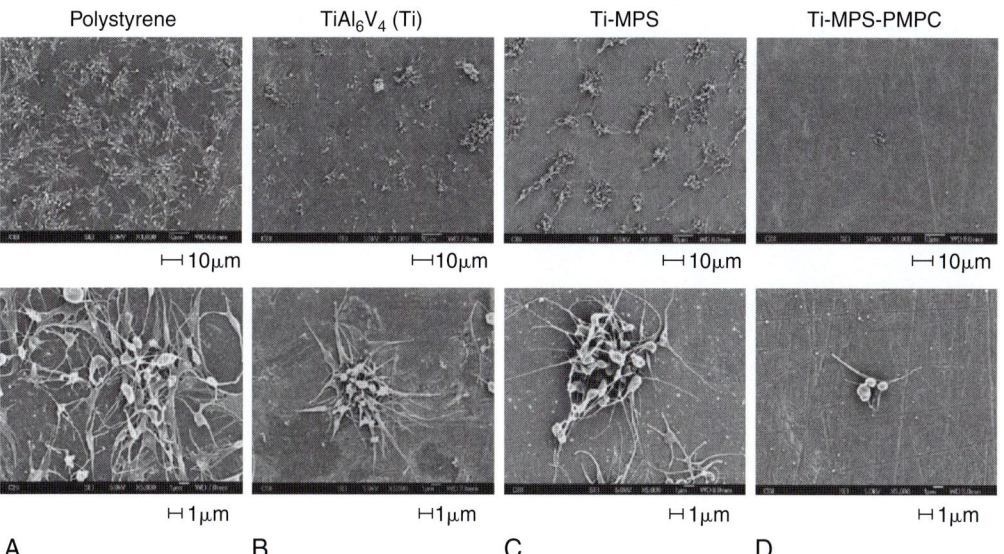

FIGURE 19-5 Reduction of platelet adhesion to a titanium substrate after application of a phosphorylcholine polymer (methacryloyloxyethylphosphorylcholine [MPC]) as shown by scanning electron micrographs of the surface after contact with sheep blood. **A,** Polystyrene positive control. **B,** TiAl$_6$V$_4$. **C,** Titanium just before attachment of MPC (as a control surface). **D,** MPC-coated titanium. *(From Ye SH, Johnson CA Jr, Woolley JR, et al. Surface modification of a titanium alloy with a phospholipid polymer prepared by a plasma-induced grafting technique to improve surface thromboresistance.* Colloids Surf B Biointerfaces. *2009;74:96-102.)*

costs for FDA approval (if necessary) or third-party licensing (if patented by other manufacturers). Regardless, the short-comings and uniform use of titanium as the primary blood-contacting material in rotary VADs provide an opportunity for great strides to be made in reducing thrombotic events through investment in this area of research.

THROMBOSIS MODELING: APPLICATION OF VIRCHOW'S TRIAD TO PREDICT DEVICE PERFORMANCE

Advances in computing power and mathematical modeling have allowed for recent attempts by researchers to develop a tool for predicting thrombus formation in silico during the design of medical devices.[78-80] Complex modeling of the inter-action between blood constituents, flow fields, and blood-contacting surfaces involves a concerted, balanced effort to advance both the accuracy of the numerical simulations and the experimental methods necessary for providing input val-ues and validating outcomes.[81] The success of such a tool could greatly reduce the cost of developing a VAD while pos-sibly improving the performance of the device. VAD design typically consists of a trial-and-error methodology to reduce the thrombogenicity of the pump; often many design gen-erations are necessary owing to the discovery of unforeseen thrombogenic areas with each consecutive round of test-ing, driving up the cost of the product (Fig. 19-6). Even after

multiple design iterations and expensive preclinical ani-mal testing, clinical trials free of thrombotic events are not ensured.[82,83] As discussed previously, progress in VAD CFD research has helped to elucidate some of the nonphysiologic flow fields present in mechanical valves and rotating impel-lers; if these results are combined with experimental deter-minations of protein and platelet interactions with given materials, it may be possible to define a predictive numerical relationship between the flowing blood and the VAD.[84,85] One form the mathematical model may take is that of a map of the probability and location of thrombus formation in the VAD.[78] Researchers could then use this information to design out the "hot spots" predicted in the model, optimizing the pump in silico for a fraction of the cost of previous design methods.[86] Although the accuracy of the current models still needs to be refined, this area of research will be vital to decreasing adverse events and improving outcomes as VAD technology continues to evolve.

CONCLUSIONS

Technological innovation in mechanical circulatory support has greatly improved the lives of people with end-stage heart failure. New devices and advances in peripheral equipment have expanded the eligible patient population, making this therapy now routine in some institutions. Despite mechani-cal progress, some of the same problems experienced with the first implants are still confounding clinicians today. Thrombosis, thromboembolism, and bleeding remain major complications plaguing patients with VADs and are persis-tent partly because of their multifactorial nature. Tools such as blood biomarkers, individualized anticoagulation therapy, CFD, platelet-resistant coatings, and thrombosis modeling may help to decrease the amount of adverse events experi-enced with this technology while positioning it at the fore-front of heart failure support and transplantation medicine.

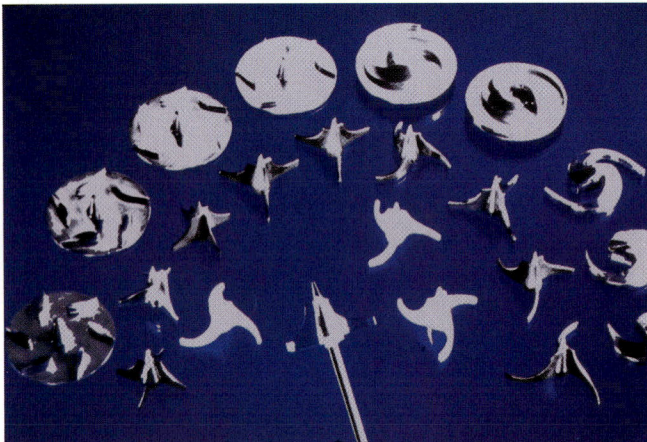

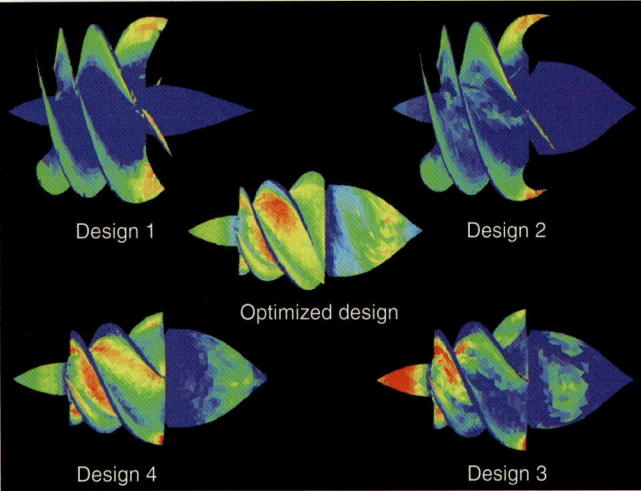

Design 1   Design 2

Optimized design

Design 4   Design 3

FIGURE 19-6 *Top,* Results from a trial-and-error method of impeller design by a ventricular assist device (VAD) manufacturer. *Bottom,* Computational fluid dynamics optimization of a VAD impeller before fabrication. *(Top, Courtesy of K. Butler, Nimbus, Inc.; Bottom, Courtesy of James Antaki, PhD.)*

REFERENCES

1. Argenziano M, Oz MC, Rose EA. The continuing evolution of mechanical ventricular assistance. *Curr Probl Surg.* 1997;34:317–386.
2. Goldstein DJ, Oz MC, Rose EA. Implantable left ventricular assist devices. *N Engl J Med.* 1998;339:1522–1533.
3. Guy TS. Evolution and current status of the total artificial heart: the search continues. *ASAIO J.* 1998;44:28–33.
4. Miller LW, Pagani FD, Russell SD, et al. Use of a continuous-flow device in patients awaiting heart transplantation. *N Engl J Med.* 2007;357:885–896.
5. Wagner WR, Schaub RD, Sorensen EN, et al. Blood biocompatibility analysis in the set-ting of ventricular assist devices. *J Biomater Sci Polym Ed.* 2000;11:1239–1259.
6. Goldstein DJ. Worldwide experience with the MicroMed DeBakey Ventricular Assist Device as a bridge to transplantation. *Circulation.* 2003;108(suppl 1):II272–II277.
7. Rose EA, Gelijns AC, Moskowitz AJ, et al. Long-term mechanical left ventricular assis-tance for end-stage heart failure. *N Engl J Med.* 2001;345:1435–1443.
8. INTERMACS. *Manual of Operations, Version 2.3.* Available at www.uab.edu/ctsresearch/intermacs/manuals.htm; 2008.
9. Kirklin J. INTERMACS annual report 2008. Presented at the 28th Annual Meeting and Scientific Sessions of the International Society of Heart and Lung Transplantation, Boston; April 9–12, 2008. Available at www.intermacs.org.
10. Kormos R. *Early neurological adverse events (NAE) after pulsatile VAD implantation in 455 patients: incidence, severity and outcome.* Presented at the 29th Annual Meeting and Scientific Sessions of the International Society of Heart and Lung Transplantation, Paris; April 22–25, 2009. Available at www.intermacs.org.
11. Slaughter MS, Tsui SS, El-Banayosy A, et al. Results of a multicenter clinical trial with the Thoratec Implantable Ventricular Assist Device. *J Thorac Cardiovasc Surg.* 2007;133:1573–1580.
12. John R, Kamdar F, Liao K, et al. Improved survival and decreasing incidence of adverse events with the HeartMate II left ventricular assist device as bridge-to-transplant therapy. *Ann Thorac Surg.* 2008;86:1227–1234; discussion 1234–1235.
13. Long JW, Kfoury AG, Slaughter MS, et al. Long-term destination therapy with the HeartMate XVE left ventricular assist device: improved outcomes since the REMATCH study. *Congest Heart Fail.* 2005;11:133–138.
14. Esmore D, Kaye D, Spratt P, et al. A prospective, multicenter trial of the VentrAssist left ventricular assist device for bridge to transplant: safety and efficacy. *J Heart Lung Transplant.* 2008;27:579–588.
15. Rogers JG, Butler J, Lansman SL, et al. Chronic mechanical circulatory support for inotrope-dependent heart failure patients who are not transplant candidates: results of the INTrEPID Trial. *J Am Coll Cardiol.* 2007;50:741–747.

16. Witt BJ, Gami AS, Ballman KV, et al. The incidence of ischemic stroke in chronic heart failure: a meta-analysis. *J Card Fail.* 2007;13:489–496.

17. Lazar RM, Shapiro PA, Jaski BE, et al. Neurological events during long-term mechanical circulatory support for heart failure: the Randomized Evaluation of Mechanical Assistance for the Treatment of Congestive Heart Failure (REMATCH) experience. *Circulation.* 2004;109:2423–2427.

18. Mussivand T. Neurological dysfunction associated with mechanical circulatory support: complications that still need attention. *Artif Organs.* 2008;32:831–834.

19. Mussivand T. Mechanical circulatory support devices: is it time to focus on the complications, instead of building another new pump? *Artif Organs.* 2008;32:1–4.

20. Sefton MV, Gemmell CH, Gorbet MB. What really is blood compatibility? *J Biomater Sci Polym Ed.* 2000;11:1165–1182.

21. Hoffman AS, Cohn D, Hanson SR, et al. Application of radiation-grafted hydrogels as blood-contacting biomaterials. *Radiat Physics Chemistry (1977).* 1983;22:267–283.

22. Gorbet MB, Sefton MV. Biomaterial-associated thrombosis: roles of coagulation factors, complement, platelets and leukocytes. *Biomaterials.* 2004;25:5681–5703.

23. Lowe GD. Virchow's triad revisited: abnormal flow. *Pathophysiol Haemost Thromb.* 2003;33:455–457.

24. Basmadjian D, Sefton MV, Baldwin SA. Coagulation on biomaterials in flowing blood: some theoretical considerations. *Biomaterials.* 1997;18:1511–1522.

25. Gemmell CH, Ramirez SM, Yeo EL, et al. Platelet activation in whole blood by artificial surfaces: identification of platelet-derived microparticles and activated platelet binding to leukocytes as material-induced activation events. *J Lab Clin Med.* 1995;125:276–287.

26. Gemmell CH, Yeo EL, Sefton MV. Flow cytometric analysis of material-induced platelet activation in a canine model: elevated microparticle levels and reduced platelet life span. *J Biomed Mater Res.* 1997;37:176–181.

27. Sefton MV, Sawyer A, Gorbet M, et al. Does surface chemistry affect thrombogenicity of surface modified polymers? *J Biomed Mater Res.* 2001;55:447–459.

28. Vroman L. Effect of absorbed proteins on the wettability of hydrophilic and hydrophobic solids. *Nature.* 1962;196:476–477.

29. Jackson SP. The growing complexity of platelet aggregation. *Blood.* 2007;109:5087–5095.

30. Savage B, Saldivar E, Ruggeri ZM. Initiation of platelet adhesion by arrest onto fibrinogen or translocation on von Willebrand factor. *Cell.* 1996;84:289–297.

31. Nesbitt WS, Westein E, Tovar-Lopez FJ, et al. A shear gradient-dependent platelet aggregation mechanism drives thrombus formation. *Nat Med.* 2009;15:665–673.

32. Livingston ER, Fisher CA, Bibidakis EJ, et al. Increased activation of the coagulation and fibrinolytic systems leads to hemorrhagic complications during left ventricular assist implantation. *Circulation.* 1996;94(suppl 9):II227–II234.

33. Meuris B, Arnout J, Vlasselaers D, et al. Long-term management of an implantable left ventricular assist device using low molecular weight heparin and antiplatelet therapy: a possible alternative to oral anticoagulants. *Artif Organs.* 2007;31:402–405.

34. Sandner SE, Zimpfer D, Zrunek P, et al. Low molecular weight heparin as an alternative to unfractionated heparin in the immediate postoperative period after left ventricular assist device implantation. *Artif Organs.* 2008;32:819–822.

35. Spanier T, Oz M, Levin H, et al. Activation of coagulation and fibrinolytic pathways in patients with left ventricular assist devices. *J Thorac Cardiovasc Surg.* 1996;112:1090–1097.

36. Joshi A, Magder LS, Kon Z, et al. Association between prothrombin activation fragment (F1.2), cerebral ischemia (S-100beta) and international normalized ratio (INR) in patients with ventricular assisted devices. *Interact Cardiovasc Thorac Surg.* 2007;6:323–327.

37. Butchart EG, Payne N, Li HH, et al. Better anticoagulation control improves survival after valve replacement. *J Thorac Cardiovasc Surg.* 2002;123:715–723.

38. Wilhelm CR, Ristich J, Kormos RL, et al. Measurement of hemostatic indexes in conjunction with transcranial Doppler sonography in patients with ventricular assist devices. *Stroke.* 1999;30:2554–2561.

39. Koster A, Loebe M, Hansen R, et al. Alterations in coagulation after implantation of a pulsatile Novacor LVAD and the axial flow MicroMed DeBakey LVAD. *Ann Thorac Surg.* 2000;70:533–537.

40. Himmelreich G, Ullmann H, Riess H, et al. Pathophysiologic role of contact activation in bleeding followed by thromboembolic complications after implantation of a ventricular assist device. *ASAIO J.* 1995;41:M790–M794.

41. Dewald O, Schmitz C, Diem H, et al. Platelet activation markers in patients with heart assist device. *Artif Organs.* 2005;29:292–299.

42. Wang IW, Kottke-Marchant K, Vargo RL, et al. Hemostatic profiles of HeartMate ventricular assist device recipients. *ASAIO J.* 1995;41:M782–M787.

43. Etz C, Welp H, Rothenburger M, et al. Analysis of platelet function during left ventricular support with the Incor and Excor system. *Heart Surg Forum.* 2004;7:E423–E427.

44. Majeed F, Kop WJ, Poston RS, et al. Prospective, observational study of antiplatelet and coagulation biomarkers as predictors of thromboembolic events after implantation of ventricular assist devices. *Nat Clin Pract Cardiovasc Med.* 2009;6:147–157.

45. Wilhelm CR, Ristich J, Kormos RL, et al. Monocyte tissue factor expression and ongoing complement generation in ventricular assist device patients. *Ann Thorac Surg.* 1998;65:1071–1076.

46. Haj-Yahia S, Birks EJ, Rogers P, et al. Midterm experience with the Jarvik 2000 axial flow left ventricular assist device. *J Thorac Cardiovasc Surg.* 2007;134:199–203.

47. Pae WE, Connell JM, Boehmer JP, et al. Neurologic events with a totally implantable left ventricular assist device: European LionHeart Clinical Utility Baseline Study (CUBS). *J Heart Lung Transplant.* 2007;26:1–8.

48. Breet NJ, van Werkum JW, Bouman HJ, et al. Comparison of platelet function tests in predicting clinical outcome in patients undergoing coronary stent implantation. *JAMA.* 2010;303:754–762.

49. Damani SB, Topol EJ. The case for routine genotyping in dual-antiplatelet therapy. *J Am Coll Cardiol.* 2010;56:109–111.

50. Gurbel PA, Tantry US, Shuldiner AR, et al. Genotyping one piece of the puzzle to personalize antiplatelet therapy. *J Am Coll Cardiol.* 2010;56:112–116.

51. Diamond SL. Systems biology to predict blood function. *J Thromb Haemost.* 2009;7(suppl 1):177–180.

52. Kitano H. Systems biology: a brief overview. *Science.* 2002;295:1662–1664.

53. Vodovotz Y, Csete M, Bartels J, et al. Translational systems biology of inflammation. *PLoS Comput Biol.* 2008;4:e1000014.

54. Sakariassen KS, Muggli R, Baumgartner HR. Measurements of platelet interaction with components of the vessel wall in flowing blood. *Methods Enzymol.* 1989;169:37–70.

55. Deutsch S, Tarbell JM, Manning KB, et al. Experimental fluid mechanics of pulsatile artificial blood pumps. *Annu Rev Fluid Mech.* 2006;38:65–86.

56. Hochareon P, Manning KB, Fontaine AA, et al. Fluid dynamic analysis of the 50 cc Penn State artificial heart under physiological operating conditions using particle image velocimetry. *J Biomech Eng.* 2004;126:585–593.

57. Wu ZJ, Antaki JF, Burgreen GW, et al. Fluid dynamic characterization of operating conditions for continuous flow blood pumps. *ASAIO J.* 1999;45:442–449.

58. Leverett LB, Hellum JD, Alfrey CP, et al. Red blood cell damage by shear stress. *Biophys J.* 1972;12:257–273.

59. Kameneva MV, Burgreen GW, Kono K, et al. Effects of turbulent stresses upon mechanical hemolysis: experimental and computational analysis. *ASAIO J.* 2004;50:418–423.

60. Behbahani M, Behr M, Arora D, et al. A review of computational fluid dynamics analysis of blood pumps. *Eur J Appl Mathematics.* 2009;20:363–397.

61. Antaki JF, Ghattas O, Burgreen GW, et al. Computational flow optimization of rotary blood pump components. *Artif Organs.* 1995;19:608–615.

62. Burgreen GW, Antaki JF, Griffith BP. A design improvement strategy for axial blood pumps using computational fluid dynamics. *ASAIO J.* 1996;42:M354–M360.

63. Burgreen GW, Antaki JF, Wu ZJ, et al. Computational fluid dynamics as a development tool for rotary blood pumps. *Artif Organs.* 2001;25:336–340.

64. Kim NJ, Diao C, Ahn KH, et al. Parametric study of blade tip clearance, flow rate, and impeller speed on blood damage in rotary blood pump. *Artif Organs.* 2009;33:468–474.

65. Farrar DJ, Litwak P, Lawson JH, et al. In vivo evaluations of a new thromboresistant polyurethane for artificial heart blood pumps. *J Thorac Cardiovasc Surg.* 1988;95:191–200.

66. Menconi MJ, Pockwinse S, Owen TA, et al. Properties of blood-contacting surfaces of clinically implanted cardiac assist devices: gene expression, matrix composition, and ultrastructural characterization of cellular linings. *J Cell Biochem.* 1995;57:557–573.

67. Frazier OH, Baldwin RT, Eskin SG, et al. Immunochemical identification of human endothelial cells on the lining of a ventricular assist device. *Tex Heart Inst J.* 1993;20:78–82.

68. Rafii S, Oz MC, Seldomridge JA, et al. Characterization of hematopoietic cells arising on the textured surface of left ventricular assist devices. *Ann Thorac Surg.* 1995;60:1627–1632.

69. Slater JP, Rose EA, Levin HR, et al. Low thromboembolic risk without anticoagulation using advanced-design left ventricular assist devices. *Ann Thorac Surg.* 1996;62:1321–1327; discussion 1328.

70. Sin DC, Kei HL, Miao X. Surface coatings for ventricular assist devices. *Expert Rev Med Devices.* 2009;6:51–60.

71. Schaub RD, Kameneva MV, Borovetz HS, et al. Assessing acute platelet adhesion on opaque metallic and polymeric biomaterials with fiber optic microscopy. *J Biomed Mater Res.* 2000;49:460–468.

72. Ishihara K, Fukumoto K, Iwasaki Y, et al. Modification of polysulfone with phospholipid polymer for improvement of the blood compatibility. Part 2: protein adsorption and platelet adhesion. *Biomaterials.* 1999;20:1553–1559.

73. Ishihara K, Fukumoto K, Iwasaki Y, et al. Modification of polysulfone with phospholipid polymer for improvement of the blood compatibility. Part 1: surface characterization. *Biomaterials.* 1999;20:1545–1551.

74. Ye SH, Johnson Jr CA, Woolley JR, et al. Covalent surface modification of a titanium alloy with a phosphorylcholine-containing copolymer for reduced thrombogenicity in cardiovascular devices. *J Biomed Mater Res A.* 2009;91:18–28.

75. Snyder TA, Tsukui H, Kihara S, et al. Preclinical biocompatibility assessment of the EVAHEART ventricular assist device: coating comparison and platelet activation. *J Biomed Mater Res A.* 2007;81:85–92.

76. Ye SH, Johnson Jr CA, Woolley JR, et al. Surface modification of a titanium alloy with a phospholipid polymer prepared by a plasma-induced grafting technique to improve surface thromboresistance. *Colloids Surf B Biointerfaces.* 2009;74:96–102.

77. Hansson KM, Tosatti S, Isaksson J, et al. Whole blood coagulation on protein adsorption-resistant PEG and peptide functionalised PEG-coated titanium surfaces. *Biomaterials.* 2005;26:861–872.

78. Bluestein D, Chandran KB, Manning KB. Towards non-thrombogenic performance of blood recirculating devices. *Ann Biomed Eng.* 2010;38:1236–1256.

79. Goodman PD, Barlow ET, Crapo PM, et al. Computational model of device-induced thrombosis and thromboembolism. *Ann Biomed Eng.* 2005;33:780–797.

80. Goubergrits L. Numerical modeling of blood damage: current status, challenges and future prospects. *Expert Rev Med Devices.* 2006;3:527–531.

81. Xenos M, Girdhar G, Alemu Y, et al. Device Thrombogenicity Emulator (DTE) - Design optimization methodology for cardiovascular devices: a study in two bileaflet MHV designs. *J Biomech.* 2010;43:2400–2409.

82. Dowling RD, Etoch SW, Stevens KA, et al. Current status of the AbioCor implantable replacement heart. *Ann Thorac Surg.* 2001;71(suppl 3):S147–S149; discussion S183–4.

83. Dowling RD, Gray Jr LA, Etoch SW, et al. Initial experience with the AbioCor implantable replacement heart system. *J Thorac Cardiovasc Surg.* 2004;127:131–141.

84. Hund SJ, Antaki JF. An extended convection diffusion model for red blood cell-enhanced transport of thrombocytes and leukocytes. *Phys Med Biol.* 2009;54:6415–6435.

85. Sorensen EN, Burgreen GW, Wagner WR, et al. Computational simulation of platelet deposition and activation: I. Model development and properties. *Ann Biomed Eng.* 1999;27:436–448.

86. Antaki JF, Ricci MR, Verkaik JE, et al. PediaFlow™ maglev ventricular assist device: a prescriptive design approach. *Cardiovasc Eng.* 2010;1:104–121.

Cellular, Molecular, Genomic, and Functional Changes That Occur in the Failing Heart in Response to Mechanical Circulatory Support

Jennifer L. Hall and Guillermo Torre-Amione

The term *cardiac remodeling* has been used to describe the changes that occur in the myocardium after cardiac injury, typically manifested by progressive dilation of the cardiac ventricle, with reduced systolic function, increased wall stress, and accompanying histologic and molecular changes in the failing myocardium. Remodeling is measured in a variety of ways depending on the unique technique, marker, or property of the myocardium of interest. For example, imaging techniques describe changes in ventricular size, volume, and the degree of hypertrophy as markers of remodeling. From a histologic and molecular standpoint, the definition of remodeling in human myocardium has been more difficult to study because obtaining samples of myocardial tissue at different stages of the process has always been challenging. Remodeling from a molecular and genomic perspective has been measured using gene expression arrays and real-time quantitative polymerase chain reaction. Genomic studies have not identified one or two definitive markers of remodeling, but rather signaling networks or pathways that undergo changes in response to remodeling.

The field of mechanical circulatory support offers the unique opportunity to study failing human myocardium at two different stages of the illness and analyze the molecular changes induced by ventricular unloading. Failing human myocardium obtained at the time of left ventricular assist device (LVAD) implantation represents myocardium at a point of maximal "stress" and can be compared with a myocardial sample obtained at the time of LVAD removal, which represents myocardium after a prolonged period of chronic unloading or "rest." The changes that occur after LVAD support, including reduction in ventricular size and volume as well as histologic, genomic, and molecular changes, are described as *reverse remodeling* (Fig. 20-1).

Although many markers of the failing phenotype appear to improve or normalize after mechanical unloading, these changes infrequently result in sustainable cardiac improvement sufficient to support circulation after removal of the device. This area represents a focus for future work and understanding.

The ability to compare failing human myocardium before and after mechanical unloading of the failing human heart has provided us with the unique opportunity to identify markers or elements of the reverse remodeling process that may be essential in preventing disease progression or enhancing the ability of failing myocardium to improve sufficiently to support the circulation, as well as to identify potential new targets for therapy. The variable time of LVAD support and varying severity and etiology of heart failure (HF) at the time of LVAD implantation, plus the modest number of paired samples that have been examined to date, have limited the strength of some conclusions, but new insights into the remodeling process have nevertheless been gained.

This chapter describes reverse remodeling at the histologic, molecular, and genomic levels and the impact of those changes on myocardial function. We also discuss the implications of those changes for preventing the progression of HF.

CELLULAR, MOLECULAR, AND GENOMIC EVIDENCE OF REVERSE REMODELING

Myocyte Size and the Matrix

Myocyte Size

The most consistent and earliest finding to be described in the response of failing myocardium to chronic mechanical unloading is the reduction in myocyte size after LVAD support.[1] In a single-center study of 18 patients in which paired myocardial samples were studied, it was found that myocyte size was reduced from 33 to 24 μ. Normal myocyte size in a group of normal control subjects was 17 μ (Fig. 20-2). Although in all cases LVAD support resulted in a reduction of myocyte size, the degree of reduction did

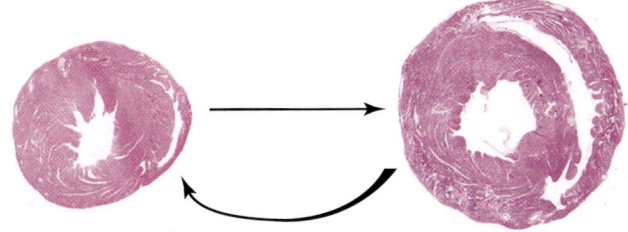

FIGURE 20-1 Reverse remodeling. Heart failure results from progressive dysfunction that occurs in the myocardium secondary to the degree of initial injury and to the neurohormonal and hemodynamic changes that continuously injure the failing heart. Prolonged mechanical support decreases the hemodynamic forces and improves the systemic responses involved in disease progression. As a result, histologic and structural changes occur that are generically referred to as *reverse remodeling*.

259

CH 20

Cellular, Molecular, Genomic, and Functional Changes That Occur in the Failing Heart in Response to Mechanical Circulatory Support

collagen type I, and collagen type III have been shown to be reduced in response to LVAD support (Fig. 20-3).[2] The major disadvantage of this approach is that the individual performing the analysis may be affected by bias. In particular, major areas of scar may not be counted and only the intramyocardial collagen measured. An alternative strategy has been the quantification of myocardial collagen by measuring hydroxyproline content in the soluble and insoluble collagens. When measured in this manner, total and cross-linked collagen increased after LVAD support; this finding was also associated with increases in chamber and myocardial stiffness.[3] Matrix biology is affected by matrix metalloproteinase, inflammatory cytokines, and underlying etiology. Thus, the response of the matrix of the failing heart to LVAD support may be a critical component to clinical recovery, but this is not yet fully understood. It is becoming clear that matrix biology plays an important role in diastolic heart disease. DNA variants in matrix genes, epigenetic changes, or altered microRNA (miRNA) expression resulting in HF may have a significant impact on how the failing heart responds to LVAD support.

not reach levels that were comparable with the normal control samples. The study also determined the effect of duration of LVAD support on the reduction of myocyte cell size; it was found that the longer the LVAD support, the greater the reduction in myocyte size.[2]

Matrix

In association with changes in myocyte size, a number of investigators using different techniques have studied the changes that occur in collagen content. The analysis of collagen content has been controversial because of the different techniques used to measure it. One strategy to determine collagen content uses a semiquantitative approach based on immunohistochemistry. Using this technique, total collagen,

Contractility in Individual Myocytes and Isolated Trabecular Preparations

There is evidence of early mechanical improvement in failing hearts treated with LVADs.[4–11] These early findings were important in showing that contractile performance of myocytes is partially recovered in response to LVAD therapy. Myocyte contractile performance was significantly greater in isolated myocytes from failing human hearts post-LVAD support compared with failing human hearts without LVAD support (Table 20-1).[5] Improvements in the magnitude of

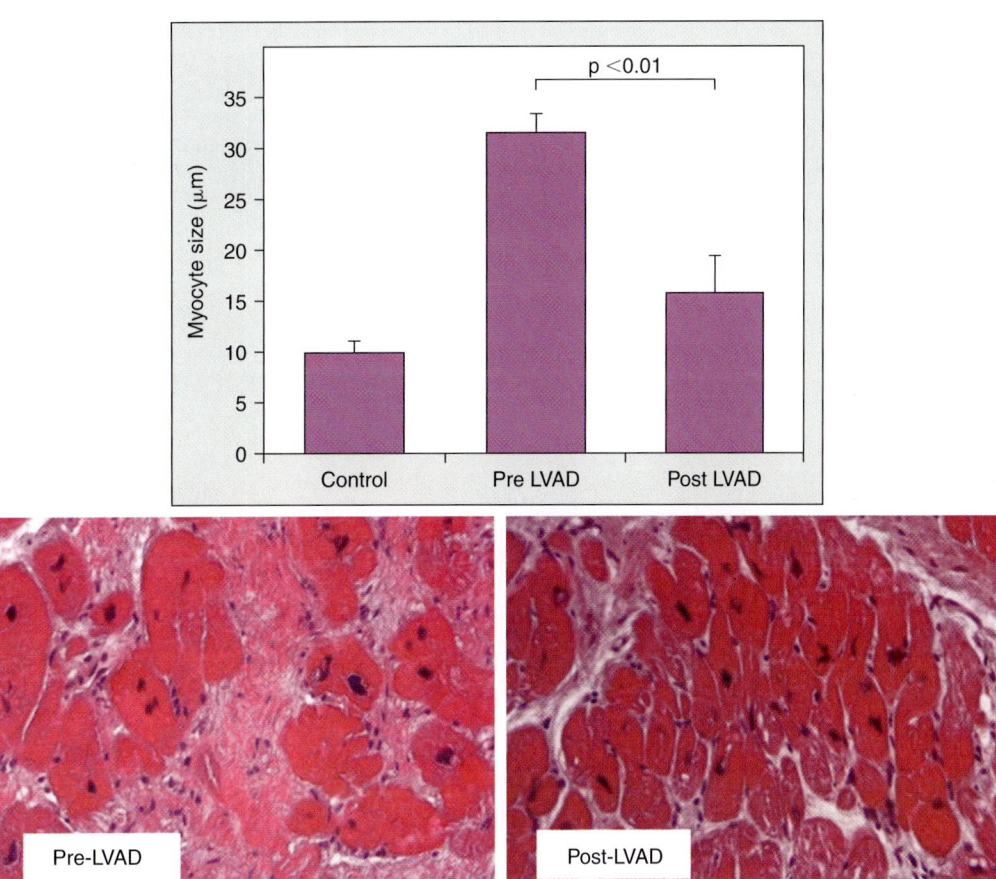

FIGURE 20-2 Myocyte size is reduced in response to left ventricular assist device (LVAD) support (*upper left* and *bottom left*); *n* = 4 control subjects and *n* = 6 patients with end-stage cardiomyopathy before and after LVAD support. Histograms are mean ± SE. (Original magnification ×20.)

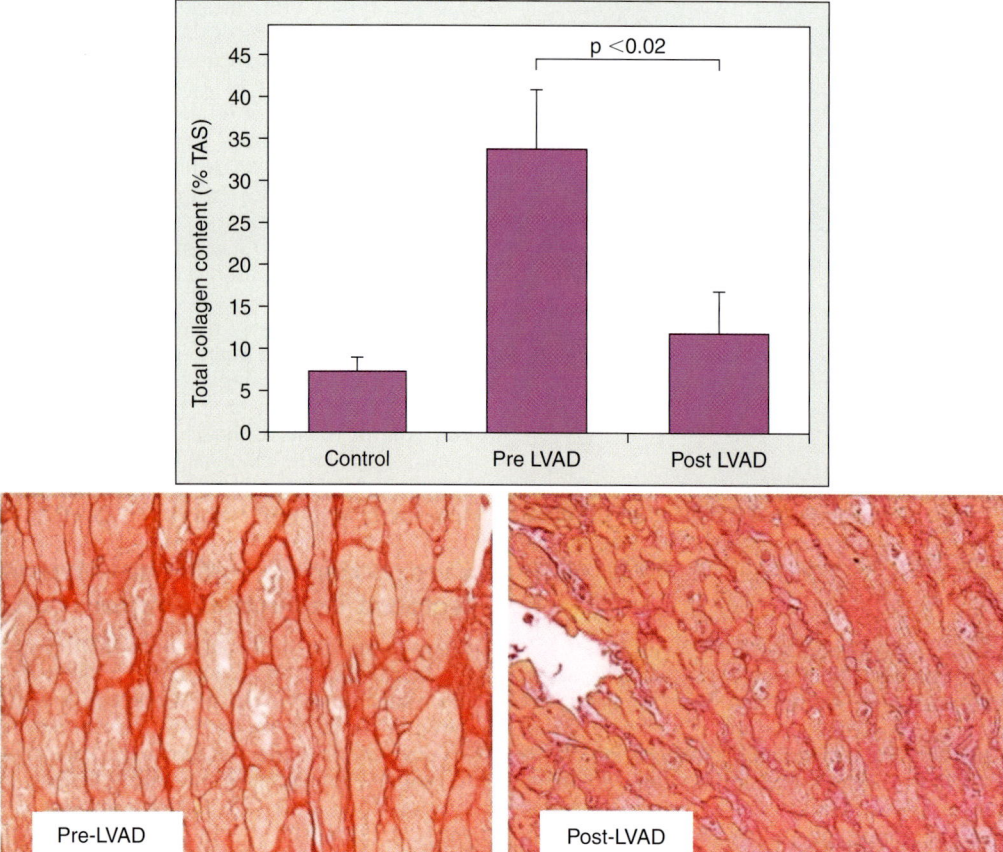

FIGURE 20-3 Total collagen is reduced in response to left ventricular assist device (LVAD) support; *n* = 4 control subjects and *n* = 6 patients with end-stage cardiomyopathy. Histograms are mean ± SE. (Original magnification ×20.)

shortening were seen in response to beta-adrenergic agonists (Table 20-2).[5] Basal relaxation was also improved in myocytes after LVAD support, but relaxation rates in response to isoproterenol were not improved (see Table 20-2).[5] This was confirmed in isolated trabecular preparations in a separate study (Fig. 20-4).[10] These improvements in developed tension were accompanied by increased beta-adrenergic receptor density (Fig. 20-5).[10] It is of interest that although developed tension is improved with the LVAD, resting tension remained significantly impaired.

TABLE 20-1	Contractile Characteristics Are Improved in Myocytes after Support with a Left Ventricular Assist Device (LVAD)		
	Stimulation Frequency (Hz)		
	0.2	**0.5**	**1.0**
Magnitude of shortening in HF myocytes (*n* = 13), % RCL	8.31 ± 0.70	7.59 ± 0.53	5.72 ± 0.46
Magnitude of shortening in HF-LVAD myocytes (*n* = 13), % RCL	10.31 ± 0.99*	10.18 ± 1.03*	8.72 ± 1.01*

*Significant differences (*P* <.05) between the HF and the HF-LAVD myocytes.
HF, heart failure; RCL, resting cell length.
From Dipla K, Mattiello JA, Jeevanandam V, et al. Myocyte recovery after mechanical circulatory support in humans with end-stage heart failure. *Circulation.* 1998;97:2316-2322.

TABLE 20-2	Isoproterenol Response on Contractile Parameters			
Contractile Parameter	**Disease Group**	**Baseline**	**Isoproterenol**	**Delta Scores**
Magnitude of shortening, % RCL	HF	6.43 ± 0.73	8.92 ± 0.78*	2.49 ± 0.58‡
	HF-VAD	7.63 ± 0.88	12.56 ± 1.01*†	4.93 ± 1.42
Time to 50% relaxation, sec	HF	1.28 ± 0.19	0.95 ± 0.16	0.32 ± 0.15
	HF-VAD	0.70 ± 0.07†	0.53 ± 0.03	0.17 ± 0.08

*Significant difference (*P* <.0125) between baseline and isoproterenol (paired *t* test).
†Significant difference (*P* <.0125) between HF and HF-VAD myocytes (*t* test for independent samples).
‡Significant difference (*P* <.05) between HF and HF-VAD myocytes on the delta scores (*t* test for independent samples).
HF, heart failure; RCL, resting cell length.; VAD, ventricular assist device.
From Dipla K, Mattiello JA, Jeevanandam V, et al. Myocyte recovery after mechanical circulatory support in humans with end-stage heart failure. *Circulation.* 1998;97:2316-2322.

Beta-Adrenergic Signaling

More recent work assessed beta-adrenergic signaling pathways in an unbiased analysis using a gene chip platform in six paired heart samples from patients who achieved recovery and explantation of their device.[12,13] A novel combination therapy consisting of an LVAD combined with pharmacologic therapy including the selective beta-2 agonist

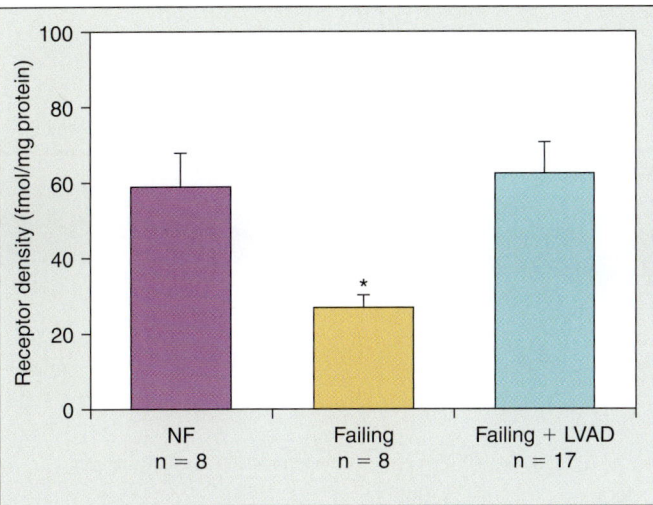

FIGURE 20-4 Beta-adrenergic receptor density in nonfailing (NF) hearts, failing hearts without LVAD, and failing hearts with LVAD. *P <0.05 vs. NF. *(From Ogletree-Hughes ML, Stull LB, Sweet WE, et al. Mechanical unloading restores β-adrenergic responsiveness and reverses receptor downregulation in the failing human heart. Circulation. 2001;104:881-886.)*

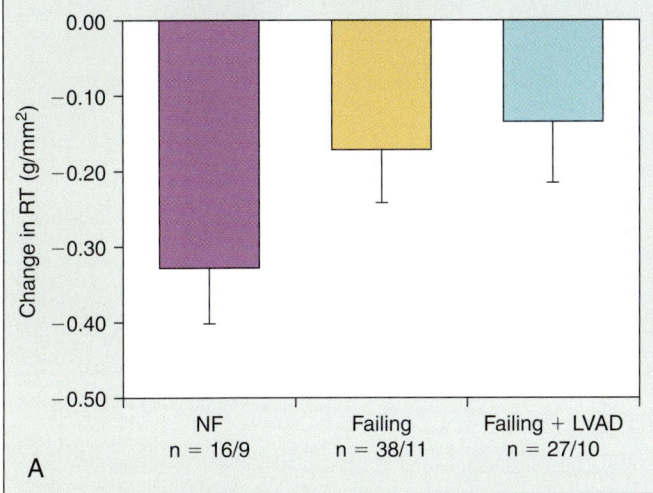

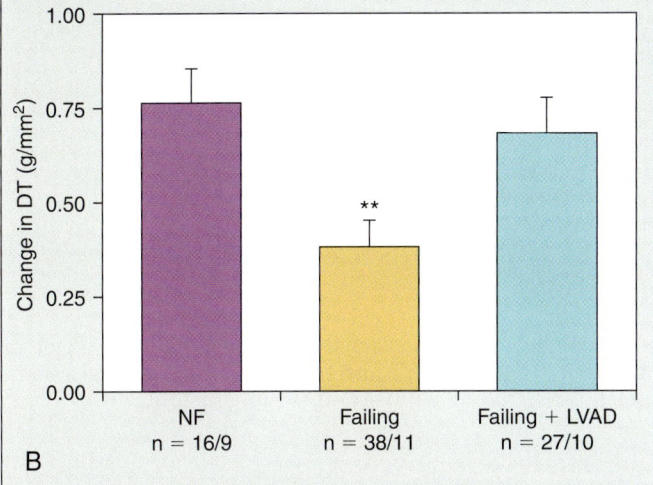

FIGURE 20-5 Data (mean ± SE) showing changes in response of isolated trabecular muscles to 1 μmol of isoproterenol from baseline. **A,** Change in resting tension (RT). **B,** Change in developed tension (DT). LVAD, left ventricular assist device; NF, nonfailing. *(From Ogletree-Hughes ML, Stull LB, Sweet WE, et al. Mechanical unloading restores β-adrenergic responsiveness and reverses receptor downregulation in the failing human heart. Circulation. 2001;104:881-886.)*

261

CH 20

Cellular, Molecular, Genomic, and Functional Changes That Occur in the Failing Heart in Response to Mechanical Circulatory Support

clenbuterol has shown promise in restoring ventricular function in patients with HF.[12] The aim of this study was to identify common genes and signaling pathways whose expression was associated with reversal of HF and restoration of ventricular function and whose expression was likely different from all patients who exhibited little or no recovery, suggesting important control genes for remodeling. Microarray analysis was performed on six paired human heart samples harvested at the time of LVAD implant and at the time of LVAD removal for recovery of ventricular function. Follow-up data show that the improvements in ventricular function have been maintained for an average of 3.8 years after LVAD removal.[12]

This data set represented the first description of signaling pathways associated with the functional recovery of end-stage human HF and the identification of new targets in the human heart that are modified by this combination therapy.[13] Analyzing the gene expression profiles from these patients resulted in the identification of pathways significantly enriched with genes whose expression was statistically different between HF and recovery. Instead of looking at one gene at a time, this analysis used a network approach with the goal of identifying networks that are altered in the process of recovery from HF.[13] Put simply, one imports gene lists into the Ingenuity database and the program overlays these genes into several described networks to identify the best overall fit. As seen in Figure 20-6, significant changes in genes in the beta-adrenergic signaling pathway in recovered hearts included Rap guanine nucleotide exchange factor 4 (EPAC2), protein kinase, regulatory, type I alpha (PKAr, downregulated 1.5-fold), phosphodiesterase 1A (PDE1A), phosphodiesterase 3B (PDE3B), and calcineurin A (PPP3CA/PP2B).[13] Using specific cut points to define statistically significant changes in gene expression may be somewhat misleading because even moderate changes "upstream" in a pathway may be sufficient to alter important molecular signaling events that affect clinical phenotypes.

Calcium-Handling Genes

An overview of the functional effects of LVAD support on calcium handling is shown in Figure 20-7. A clinical characteristic of HF is impairment of relaxation. The reported improvements in basal relaxation rate with the LVAD have not been definitively linked to changes in calcium handling. Elegant functional experiments have been carried out to assess calcium transients and expression of calcium-handling proteins.[4,14] In a study by Chaudhary and colleagues,[4] myocytes from hearts supported with an LVAD exhibited a faster decay in both early and late stages of the $[Ca^{2+}]_i$ transient compared with myocytes from failing hearts not supported with an LVAD. The same findings were seen in recovered patients. An increase in RNA expression of the Na^+/Ca^{2+} exchanger was identified in this study from recovered patients.[14] In the study with nonrecovered patients, changes were not measured at the RNA level and no changes were detected at the protein level of the Na^+/Ca^{2+} exchanger,[4] so the faster decay times in the $[Ca^{2+}]_i$ transients remained unexplained. These studies identifying the degree of restoration of calcium-handling proteins may be one approach to defining cardiac recovery and guiding the timing of LVAD removal.

Expanding on these findings, work by Terracciano and colleagues showed the greatest improvements in action potential duration and sarcoplasmic reticulum calcium content in individuals who achieved clinical recovery with LVAD implantation and pharmacologic therapy (Fig. 20-8).[15] These findings help distinguish contractile and molecular differences in myocytes from hearts that achieve clinical recovery versus those that achieve partial recovery.[15] These findings also

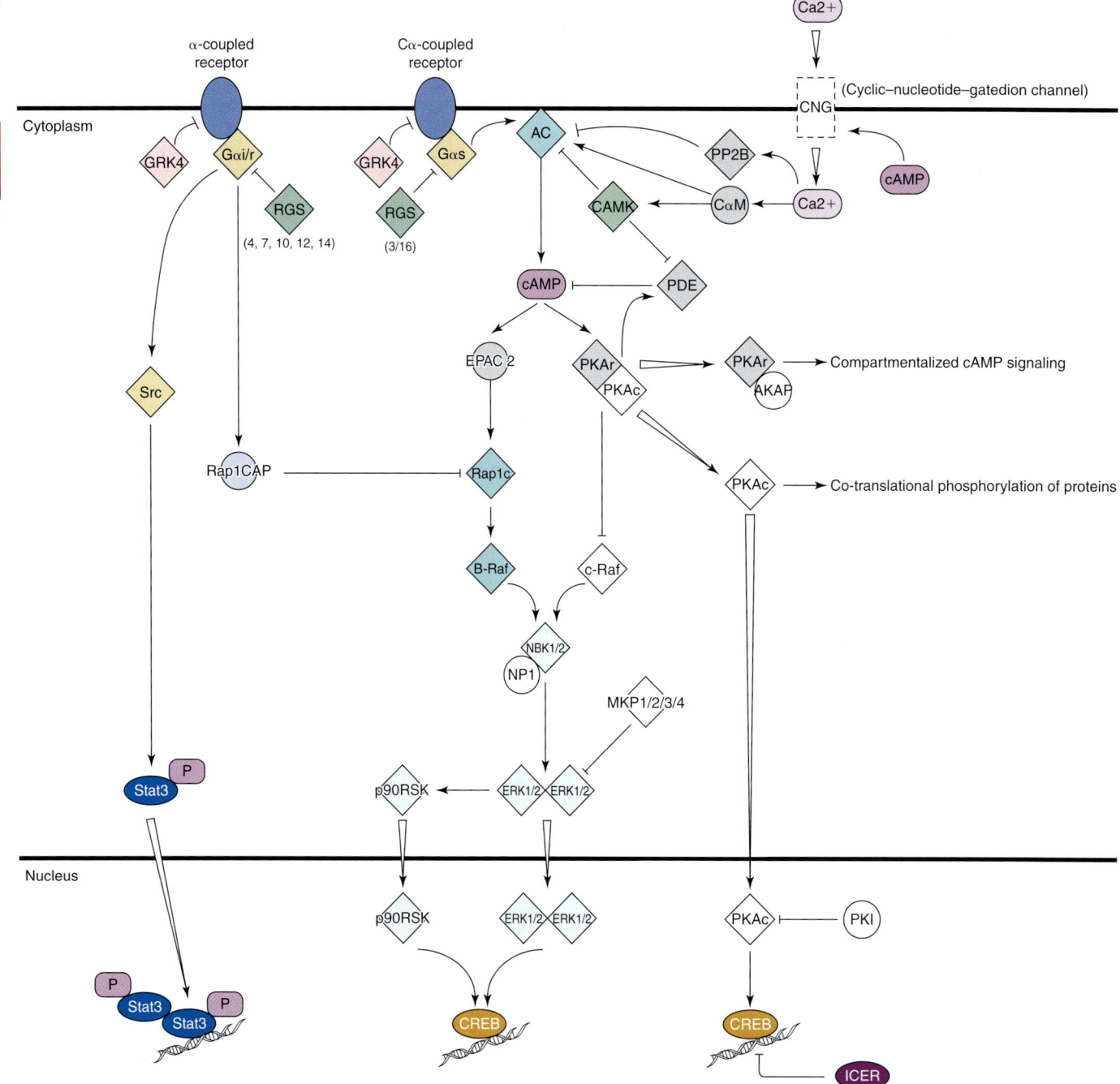

FIGURE 20-6 Identification of genes in the cyclic adenosine monophosphate (cAMP)–mediated signaling pathway whose expression was altered with recovery of myocardial function. *Shaded symbols* represent genes whose expression was significantly altered in explanted versus implanted samples. *(From Hall JL, Birks EJ, Grindle S, et al. Molecular signature of recovery following combination left ventricular assist device [LVAD] support and pharmacologic therapy. Eur Heart J. 2007;28:613-627.)*

point toward calcium-handling genes and miRNA or other post-transcriptional mechanisms that regulate sarcoplasmic reticulum calcium as prime targets for pharmacologic therapy in the treatment of HF.

One potential target for pharmacologic therapy is EPAC2. A significant decrease in expression of the calcium-regulating gene EPAC2 was identified post-LVAD support in 11 recovered hearts (Fig. 20-9).[13] This decrease in EPAC2 expression was unique to recovered hearts because the pattern was not found in nonrecovered hearts (see Fig. 20-9).[13] EPAC2 has been shown to tether cyclic adenosine monophosphate (cAMP) to mitogen-activated protein kinase (MAPK), to reg-

ulate calcium-mediated signaling through nuclear factor of activated T cells (NFAT), and to play an instrumental role in metabolic signaling pathways involving insulin.

Cytoskeleton Proteins

Myocardial recovery has also been associated with a specific pattern of changes in sarcomeric, nonsarcomeric, and membrane-associated proteins.[16] These changes are highlighted in Figure 20-10. Specifically, microarray analysis was performed on paired samples (pre-LVAD and post-LVAD) and analyzed with reference to sarcomeric and nonsarcomeric cytoskeletal

263

CH 20

Cellular, Molecular, Genomic, and Functional Changes That Occur in the Failing Heart in Response to Mechanical Circulatory Support

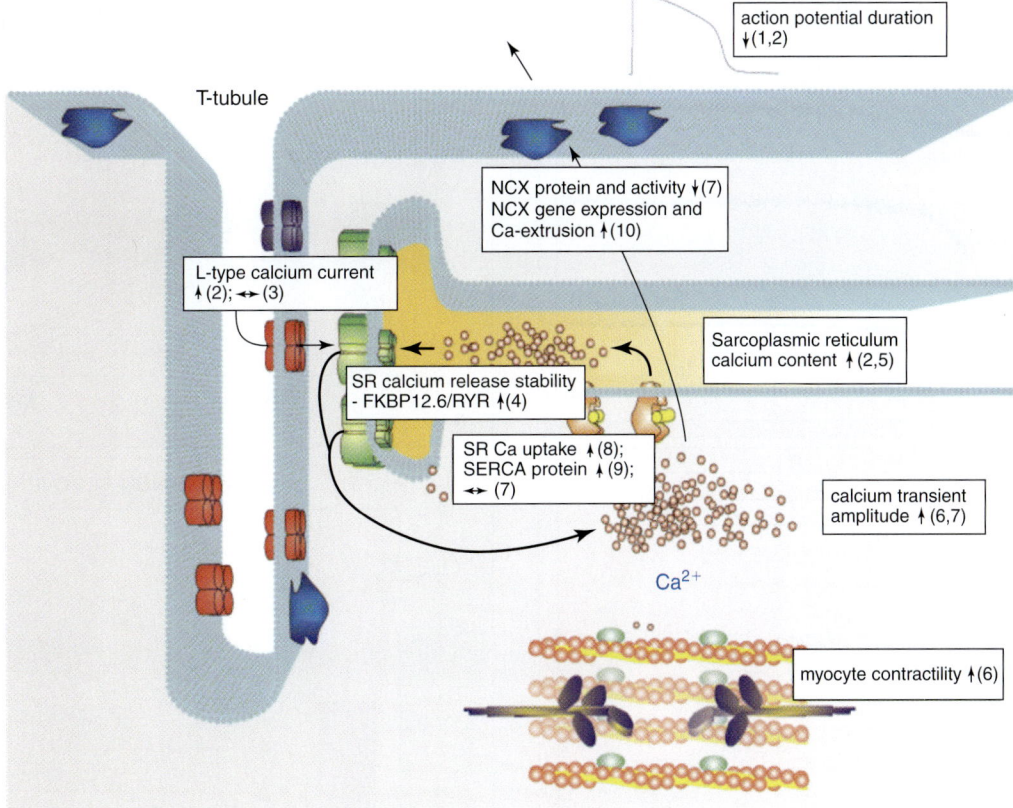

FIGURE 20-7 Calcium handing after left ventricular assist device (LVAD) support. This figure summarizes the work to date in the LVAD literature. *(1)* Harding and colleagues,[6] 2001; *(2)* Terracciano and colleagues,[15] 2004; *(3)* Chen and colleagues,[55] 2002; *(4)* Marx and colleagues,[56] 2000; *(5)* Terracciano and colleagues,[57] 2003; *(6)* Dipla and colleagues,[5] 1998; *(7)* Chaudhary and colleagues,[4] 2004; *(8)* Frazier and Myers,[58] 1999; *(9)* Heerdt and colleagues,[7] 2000; *(10)* Terracciano and colleagues,[14] 2007. *(From Terracciano CM, Koban MU, Soppa GK, et al. The role of the cardiac Na+/Ca2+ exchanger in reverse remodeling: relevance for LVAD-recovery. Ann N Y Acad Sci. 2007;1099:349-360.)*

proteins.[16] Unique changes in transcription levels of sarcomeric and nonsarcomeric proteins are listed in Table 20-3.

Experimental HF models suggest that a final common pathway for contractile dysfunction may result from changes in the integrity, quantity, and function of dystrophin.[17] Indeed, in humans with either ischemic or nonischemic cardiomyopathy, there is a selective abnormality in the amino-terminal end of dystrophin. In a single-center study in which pre-LVAD and post-LVAD samples were compared in terms of the integrity and quantity of dystrophin, it was found that in the pre-LVAD sample, there was selective disruption in the quantity and integrity of the amino-terminal end of dystrophin; this abnormality was partly reconstituted after LVAD support. This finding was consistent with the experimental and hypothetical observation of the importance of dystrophin expression as a final common pathway to explain the contractile defect in HF (Fig. 20-11).[18]

Integrins

There is a growing body of evidence that integrins are bidirectional signaling molecules that play a role in mechanotransduction by mediating mechanical (stretch) signals from the extracellular matrix through protein kinase cascades that provoke changes in gene expression, including those involved in the hypertrophic response. These data suggest that the integrin pathway may play a key role at the molecular and cellular levels in the processes of reverse remodeling and subsequent functional recovery in these patients. Figure 20-12 summarizes changes in the integrin signaling pathway that occurred in the recovery cohort

from Harefield Hospital (Harefield, United Kingdom) that received an LVAD plus pharmacologic therapy that included the beta-2 agonist clenbuterol.

Metabolic Protein Changes

In addition to the finding that the process of recovery was associated with cAMP, calcium-handling genes, and integrin signaling, several new targets were identified in an unbiased microarray approach, including those that regulate metabolism. Arginine:glycine amidinotransferase (AGAT), a rate-limiting enzyme in the creatine synthesis pathway, was significantly downregulated after unloading in the recovered hearts, returning to normal levels in direct contrast to the upregulation of AGAT in patients with HF compared with donor hearts.[13,19] These changes in AGAT messenger RNA (mRNA) levels suggest a response to HF that involves elevated local creatine synthesis.[13,19] The mechanisms leading to induced AGAT expression are unknown but may be a response to the depletion of the local creatine pool, which we and others have shown to be a feature of HF.

Unbiased Microarray Approaches

Using the same unbiased microarray approach, an analysis of 19 paired patient samples before and after LVAD support in a cohort of individuals who underwent transplantation (i.e., did not achieve full recovery) revealed 22 genes that

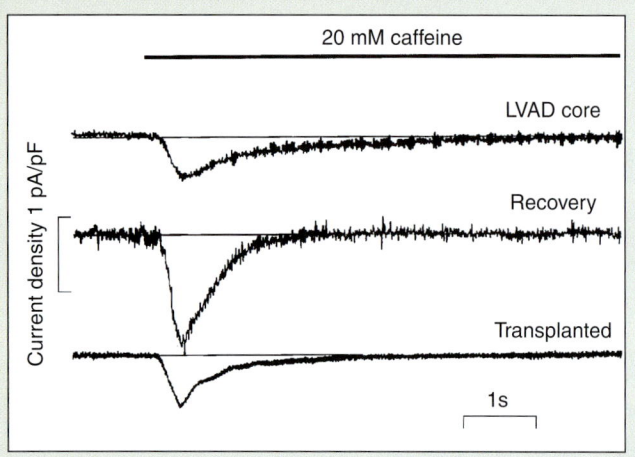

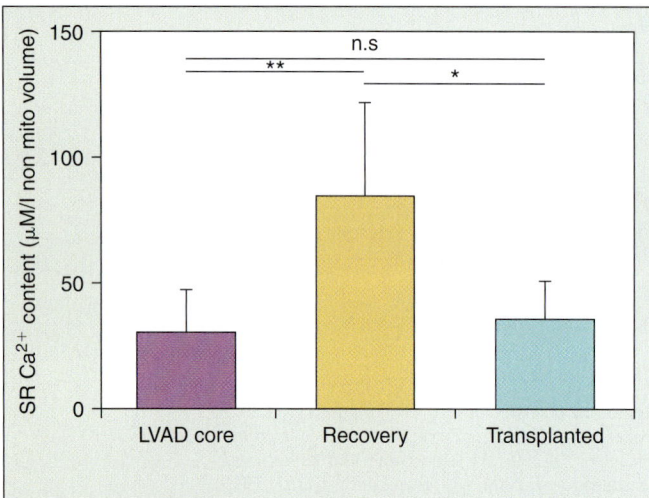

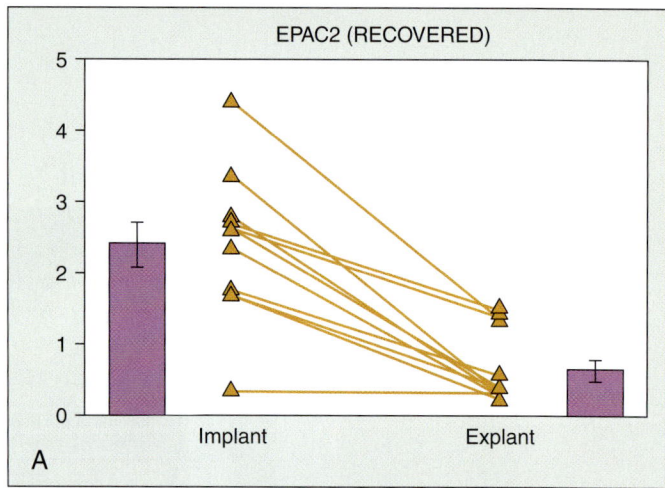

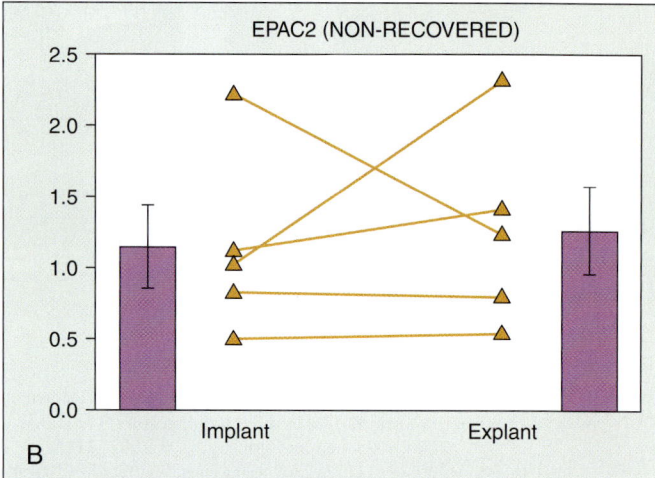

FIGURE 20-8 Sarcoplasmic reticulum calcium (SR Ca^{2+}) content from myocytes isolated from left ventricular assist device (LVAD) cores and tissue from explanted hearts (recovery) and transplanted hearts (no recovery). *(From Terracciano CM, Hardy J, Birks EJ, et al. Clinical recovery from end-stage heart failure using left-ventricular assist device and pharmacological therapy correlates with increased sarcoplasmic reticulum calcium content but not with regression of cellular hypertrophy. Circulation. 2004;109:2263-2265.)*

FIGURE 20-9 A, Messenger RNA levels for EPAC2 are significantly reduced in recovered hearts after left ventricular assist device (LVAD) support (*n* = 11; *P* < .01). **B,** No significant differences were seen in nonrecovered hearts (*n* = 5; *P* NS). *(From Hall JL, Birks EJ, Grindle S, et al. Molecular signature of recovery following combination left ventricular assist device [LVAD] support and pharmacologic therapy. Eur Heart J. 2007;28:613-627.)*

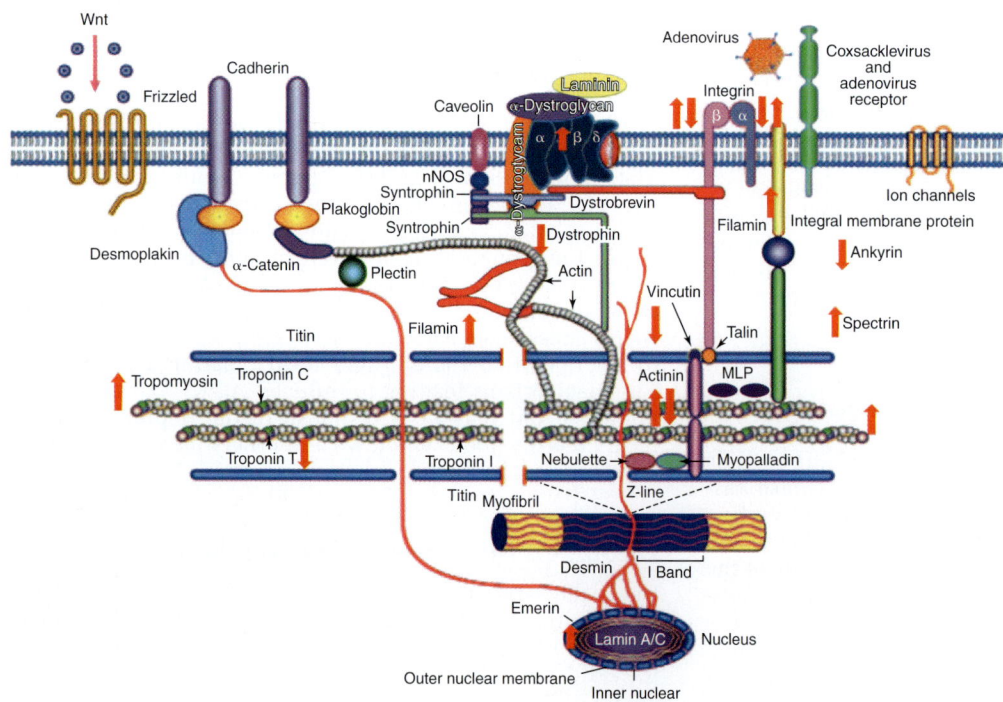

FIGURE 20-10 Changes in the cytoskeletal pathway occurring only in recovered patients. *(From Birks EJ, Hall JL, Barton PJR, et al. Gene profiling changes in cytoskeletal proteins during clinical recovery after left ventricular-assist device support. Circulation. 2005;112[9 Suppl]:I57-I64; adapted from Towbin JA, Bowles NE. Dilated cardiomyopathy: a tale of cytoskeletal proteins and beyond. J Cardiovasc Electrophysiol. 2006;17:919-926.)*

TABLE 20-3	Unique Transcript Changes in Sarcomeric and Nonsarcomeric Proteins in Individuals Who Achieved Recovery after Mechanical Support	
Target	After Left Ventricular Assist Device Implantation	Class
Lamin A/C	Increase	Nonsarcomeric
Spectrin	Increase	Nonsarcomeric
Beta-actin	Increase	Sarcomeric
Alpha-tropomyosin	Increase	Sarcomeric
Alpha-1-actinin	Increase	Sarcomeric
Alpha-filamin	Increase	Sarcomeric
Troponin-T3	Decrease	Sarcomeric
Alpha-2-actinin	Decrease	Sarcomeric
Vinculin	Decrease	Sarcomeric

From Birks EJ, Hall JL, Barton PJR, et al. Gene profiling changes in cytoskeletal proteins during clinical recovery after left ventricular-assist device support. *Circulation.* 2005;112(9 Suppl):I-57-I-64.

were significantly downregulated and 85 genes that were upregulated.[20] Included in this list were a host of genes not previously characterized as changing in response to reverse remodeling, including those governing vascular organization, Forkhead family genes, and genes governing the angiotensin-insulin signaling axis. LVAD support also led to a significant reduction in GATA-4 binding protein, a critical mediator of hypertrophy and remodeling in the mouse and rat heart. This analysis also identified a significant correlation in expression between Forkhead box 03A and Ang II type 1 receptor.[20]

The paired design of the study and the stringent approach to data analysis, leading to a false discovery rate of less than 1%, most likely decreases the potential variability induced by age, sex, length of time on support, or pharmacologic-dependent differences that clearly play a role in the transcriptome pattern. The mean age of the patients was 51 ± 2 years. The 19 pairs included 4 women and 15 men. Our analysis also confirmed the significance of a set of genes identified and reconfirmed by real-time quantitative polymerase chain reaction in an earlier analysis of a subset of seven nonischemic pairs included in this analysis; these genes included FOX03A, metallothionein IH, GADD45, connexin 43, and transmembrane 4 superfamily 1.[21] A head-to-head comparison of the genes shared in common between this analysis of 8 nonischemic patients and an earlier report by Chen and colleagues[21] of 7 nonischemic pairs revealed a list of 25 genes that notably also included neuropilin-1, stromal cell–derived factor-1 (SDF-1), CD163 antigen, tumor necrosis factor (TNF) superfamily member 10, and metallothioneins 1X, 1L, and 2A.

MicroRNA

MicroRNAs constitute one of the more abundant classes of molecules that regulate genes in animals. They are small, endogenous, noncoding RNAs.[22] Many of these miRNAs have been shown to inhibit post-transcriptional processing.[22,23] At least 80% of human miRNAs are conserved in fish.[23] This high degree of conservation suggests an important regulatory role for miRNA.

Recent work by Matkovich and colleagues suggests that adding miRNA profiling to mRNA profiling enhances the ability of mRNA profiles to categorize the clinical status of HF before and after biomechanical unloading.[24] The results of this study confirmed three earlier identified miRNAs associated with HF (miR-24, miR-125b, and miR-195).[24,25] In

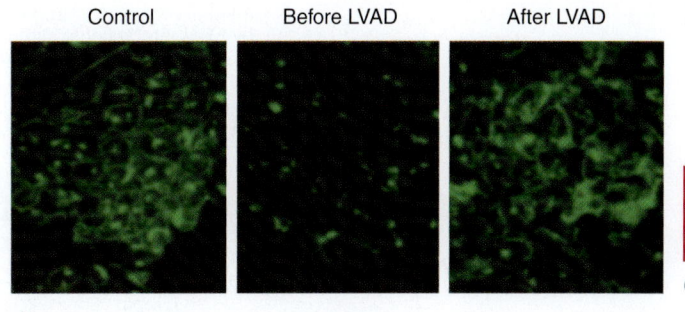

Control   Before LVAD   After LVAD

A

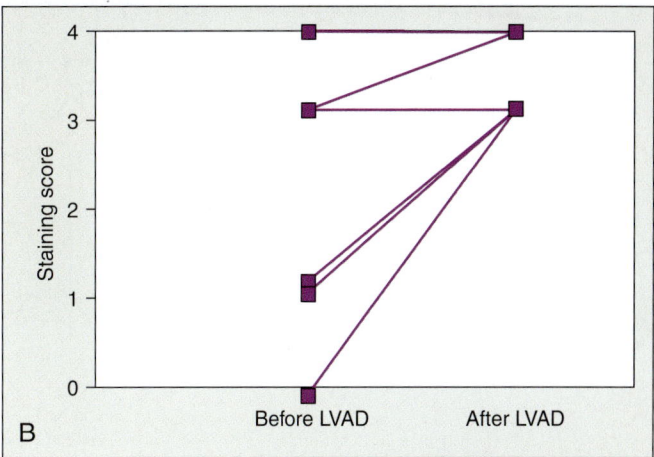

B

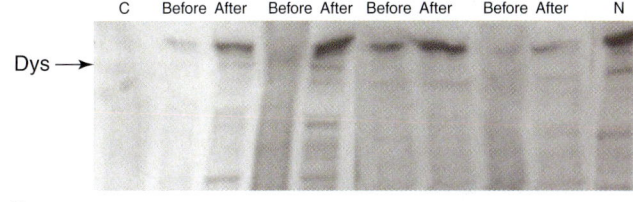

C

FIGURE 20-11 Dystrophin expression is increased in hearts after left ventricular assist device (LVAD) support. **A,** Immunohistochemical staining with the N-terminal–specific antibody to dystrophin on heart sections of a non-failing heart *(left)* and paired samples from a patient with end-stage cardiomyopathy before *(middle)* and after *(right)* LVAD support. **B** and **C,** Staining scores for immunohistochemistry **(B)** and Western blotting **(C)** for dystrophin before and after LVAD support in individual paired samples. C, a negative control protein extracted from 293 cells that did not express dystrophin. *(From Vatta M, Stetson SJ, Perez-Verdia A, et al. Molecular remodelling of dystrophin in patients with end-stage cardiomyopathies and reversal in patients on assistance-device therapy.* Lancet. *2002;359:936-941.)*

addition, Matkovich and coworkers extended earlier work in mouse models[25,26] showing that miR-21, miR-23a, and miR-199a-3p were also regulated in human HF.[24] One of the most exciting findings of the study by Matkovich and colleagues was the reversibility of the miRNAs with LVAD support. Table 20-4 lists the miRNAs that normalize after LVAD support.

Factors That Influence Gene Expression

Because the subjects' clinical conditions, medications, sex, and age cannot be controlled in the experimental analysis of human samples, particularly those obtained during LVAD support, the samples studied may have unique genetic or histologic differences that result from those covariables. To this end, a number of studies have been reported and it is important to keep them in mind to understand fully the observations obtained from the analysis of paired myocardial samples in LVAD-supported patients.

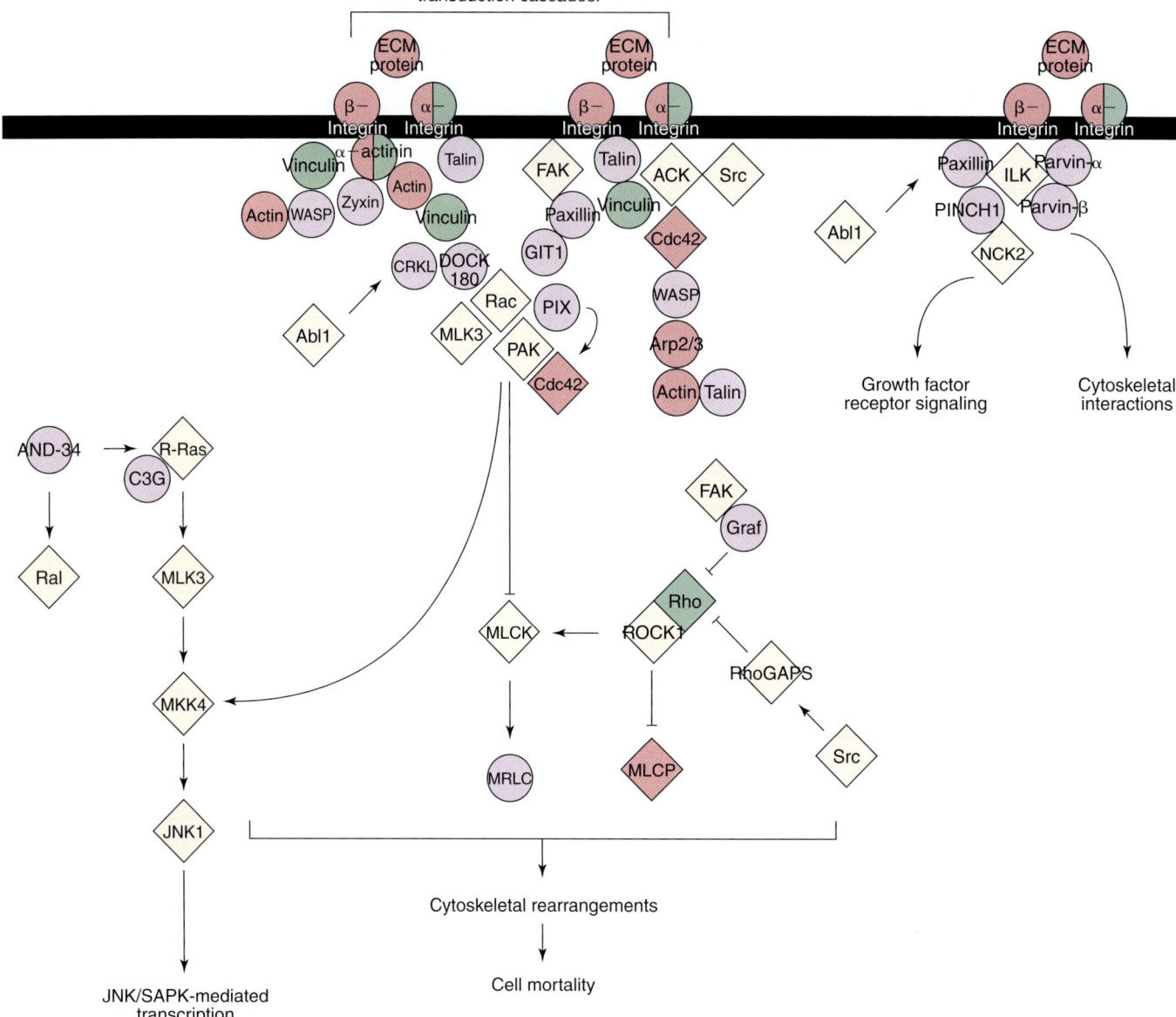

FIGURE 20-12 Gene expression changes in the beta-integrin signaling pathway in the recovered group. Gene expression changes were significantly different at the receptor level (beta-integrins). The differential expression of beta-integrin receptors is associated with the differential expression of genes distal to the receptor, including vinculin (downregulated in the recovered group, where *green* indicates downregulation after left ventricular assist device support), a gene previously shown to play a role in heart failure, and the Rho family member cdc42. (*From Birks EJ, Hall JL, Barton PJR, et al. Gene profiling changes in cytoskeletal proteins during clinical recovery after left ventricular-assist device support. Circulation. 2005;112[9 Suppl]:I-57-I-64.*)

Earlier work by Blaxall and colleagues[27] and more recent work from Kittleson and associates[28] suggested that the underlying etiology of HF in patients receiving mechanical support played an important role in gene expression patterns. The underlying etiology and accompanying gene expression profiles were also analyzed in the 19-pair compendium of pre-LVAD/post-LVAD matched samples described previously.[20] The age, length of time on support, left ventricular ejection fraction (LVEF), and medications were not significantly different between etiology cohorts. As expected, the gene list of statistically significant genes in each cohort included a subset of different genes, reconfirming the previous observations by Blaxall and colleagues

highlighting the differences among patients with nonischemic, ischemic, and acute myocardial infarction etiologies. A Venn diagram revealed that when analyzed as separate groups with a strict cutoff of $P < .005$, only one gene with an unidentified function was found in common to all three etiologically distinct cohorts: PARP7. Although it is clear that the underlying etiology is an important variable, most analyses to date have been weakened by the loss of power in each cohort owing to small sample sizes. A number of investigators have tested the influence of additional covariates on gene expression in HF, including sex, age, and support time.[29–31] These studies provided early evidence that support time does not affect abundance or directional-

TABLE 20-4 | MicroRNAs That Normalize after Ventricular Assist Device Support*

Name	Fold Change			P Value		
	Failing vs. Nonfailing	Post-LVAD vs. Nonfailing	Post-LVAD vs. Failing	Failing vs. Nonfailing	Post-LVAD vs. Nonfailing	Post-LVAD vs. Failing
miR-27b	3.15	1.14	−4.75	2.60E-04	.270	.0620
miR-30a-5p	3.06	1.07	−2.85	4.76E-04	.566	.0821
miR-30c	3.31	1.32	−2.51	1.24E-04	.105	.0853
miR-30d	2.96	1.23	−2.40	6.47E-04	.211	.116
miR-103	3.54	1.20	−2.94	1.24E-04	.156	.0834
miR-130a	3.06	1.36	−2.26	6.80E-04	.127	.270
miR-378	3.60	1.20	−3.00	6.25E-05	.153	.0544
let-7f	4.84	1.18	−4.11	1.50E-06	.211	.00543

*Ten hearts supported by a ventricular assist device, 80% male, 40% ischemic, average support time 1.7 months, type of device not disclosed.
LVAD, left ventricular assist device.
From Matkovich SJ, Van Booven DJ, Youker KA, et al. Reciprocal regulation of myocardial microRNAs and messenger RNA in human cardiomyopathy and reversal of the microRNA signature by biomechanical support. *Circulation.* 2009;119:1263-1271.

CH 20

Cellular, Molecular, Genomic, and Functional Changes That Occur in the Failing Heart in Response to Mechanical Circulatory Support

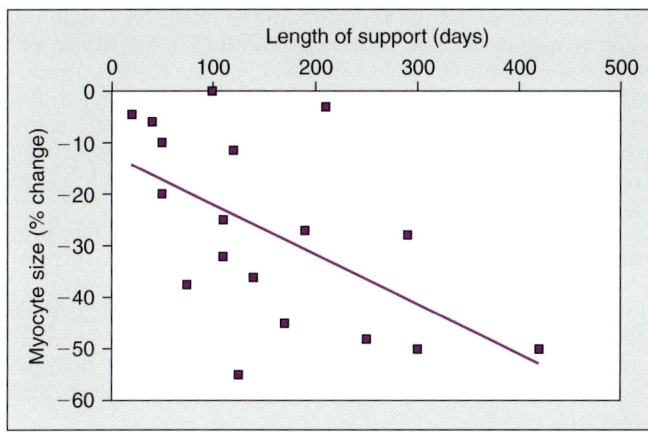

FIGURE 20-13 Effect of length of left ventricular assist device (LVAD) support on myocyte size. Myocyte sizes at the time of LVAD implantation and at LVAD removal were obtained. The percentage change was calculated and plotted against duration of LVAD support.

ity of a significant number of transcripts compared using two different statistical models.[31] However, in particular, the effect of length of support on histologic change as defined by change in myocyte size and collagen content has been studied, and it does appear that the longer the time of support, the greater the reduction in myocyte size (Fig. 20-13).[2]

Other important variables are the effect of age and sex; it appears that women older than 55 years of age may have unique variances in genetic expression.[30] More work needs to be done in this area to further identify the role of covariates in the response of patients to LVAD therapy and the underlying biochemical, molecular, genetic, and functional changes that accompany these responses.

Genes and Proteins Associated with Recovery

A major factor in the significance of the observed genetic changes is the clinical response seen in the myocardium of the particular subject treated with LVAD support and, more important, the ability to compare these genetic changes with myocardial and clinical function. Genetic changes associated with recovery of function leading to device removal are more likely to be of greater significance than those that are not. For example, in a very early study of patients who underwent LVAD placement, it was found that intramyocardial concentration of TNF-α decreased significantly (Fig. 20-14). More important, four of the eight patients studied underwent LVAD removal in association with significant improvement in myocardial function. In this cohort of patients, there was greater reduction in intramyocardial TNF content than in patients who underwent cardiac transplantation and did not demonstrate myocardial improvement.[32] This observation was important because it set a precedent for what was possible, but clearly the small number of patients and the technical difficulties associated with the measurements are another set of confounding variables that affect interpretation of the data.

Finally, there seems to be a growing consensus that left ventricular unloading in patients with end-stage HF and LVAD support improves myocardial structure and function, including improved beta-adrenergic responsiveness and myocyte contractility. Several working groups have defined changes in gene expression that occur with LVAD support that may be important in improving beta-adrenergic responsiveness and calcium handling, including partial restoration of beta receptor density and altered regulation of the genes in G-protein–regulated signaling and calcium handling. However, partial restoration of these changes in gene expression may be sufficient to improve the level of ventricular function, yet not sufficient for recovery of native cardiac function, allowing explantation of the device and freedom from recurrent HF. A gene expression profile analysis using gene chips with 199 myocardial samples from failing, LVAD-supported and nonfailing human hearts demonstrated that the majority of transcriptional changes accompanying morphologic and functional alterations in the heart were modest.[33] However, we are learning that modest changes, particularly in transcription factors and regulatory points, may be sufficient to trigger changes in contraction, action potentials, calcium handling, and other intermediate phenotypes that are important for myocardial recovery, vascularization of the heart, or matrix formation/degradation.

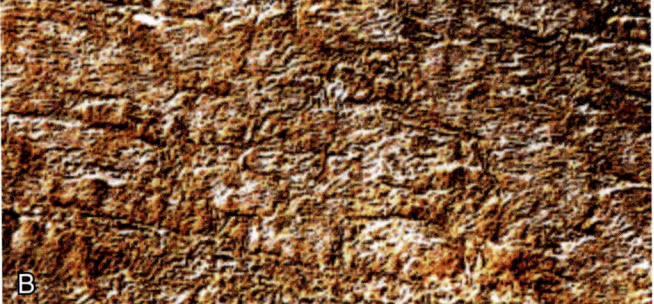

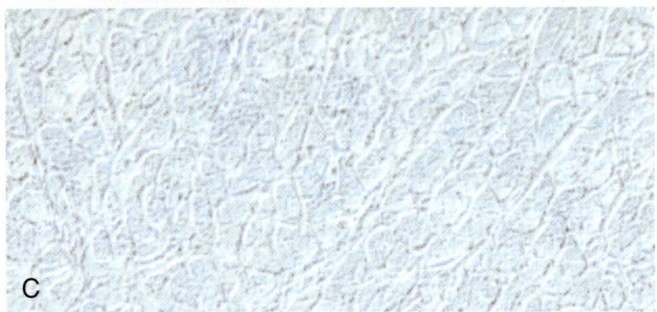

FIGURE 20-14 Decreased expression of intramyocardial tumor necrosis factor (TNF) after left ventricular assist device (LVAD) support. Data for normal myocardium **(A)**, failing myocardium at time of LVAD implant **(B)**, and failing myocardium after LVAD support **(C)** are shown. All myocardial tissue sections were stained for TNF-α and developed with a brown reagent. There is increased TNF expression in failing myocardium at the time of LVAD implantation and a profound reduction in expression after LVAD support. *(From Torre-Amione G, Stetson SJ, Youker KA, et al. Decreased expression of tumor necrosis factor-α in failing human myocardium after mechanical circulatory support: a potential mechanism for cardiac recovery.* Circulation. *1999;100:1189-1193.)*

IMPACT OF REVERSE REMODELING ON CARDIAC FUNCTION

It is germane to this discussion to note that myocardial recovery of function is not a unique virtue of mechanical circulatory support, and that indeed major changes in function are observed among patients with severe forms of cardiomyopathies that present in an acute form or are of recent onset. For example, in the IMAC (Inflammatory Mediators in Acute Cardiomyopathy) study, where patients with nonischemic, new-onset cardiomyopathies were treated with modern pharmacologic therapy, the proportion of patients after the initial observation who deteriorated to the point at which they either died or needed an LVAD or transplant was 15%. The mean ejection fraction for the remaining population at the study onset was 22%, which improved to 40% at 6 months.[34] The natural history of acute nonischemic cardiomyopathy is such that a high probability of recovery exists. Because the natural history of patients who present with acute nonischemic cardiomyopathy is associated with a high frequency of improvement, the impact of LVAD support in the recovery of myocardial function in these patients cannot be separated

from that of the natural course of the illness.[35,36] In addressing the phenomenon of reverse remodeling and the impact of mechanical circulatory support on myocardial function, we focus on patients who have a long duration of illness and are chronically ill so that one can study the true effect of chronic unloading and not the natural history of acute cardiomyopathy.

To this end, the maximal expression of myocardial recovery is the ability to remove the LVAD because of an improvement in myocardial function sufficient to support the circulation. The first major report documenting that device removal was possible came from the Berlin Heart Institute, wherein patients with nonischemic dilated cardiomyopathy underwent LVAD implantation for progressive deterioration in functional status. After prolonged mechanical support, 5 of 16 patients showed improvement and normalization of ventricular function at low levels of LVAD support, prompting the clinical decision to remove the devices.[37] In an expanded version of a similar patient cohort, the 5-year survival rate after device removal was 78.3%. In the same study, markers of subsequent HF were long HF duration (>5 years), off-pump left ventricular end-diastolic diameter greater than 55 mm, or an LVEF lower than 45%.[38]

These early reports demonstrating the possibility of device removal were reproduced at other institutions. One study at the Texas Heart Institute reported on the experience with six patients who underwent LVAD explanation. In that study, the major determinant for device removal was the ability to maintain adequate filling pressures after pump stoppage.[39] In the other, from Harefield Hospital in the United Kingdom, recovery of function was associated with aggressive pharmacologic therapy using standard drugs as well as clenbuterol, a beta agonist that may enhance recovery.[40]

These observations document that in some patients, prolonged mechanical circulatory support leads to sufficient myocardial recovery to permit device removal. A gene expression analysis was completed on the Harefield cohort with follow-up analysis on individual targets, as discussed earlier; however, additional studies are needed to define myocardial functional improvement at the genomic, histologic, and molecular levels.

To address these questions in a systematic way, a prospective observational study was conducted among six large U.S. institutions, with the objective of evaluating cellular, functional, and clinical changes after LVAD support in the same cohort of patients. The study group was known as the LVAD Working Group and included researchers from Columbia University, the Texas Heart Institute, Cleveland Clinic, the University of Michigan, the University of Minnesota, and the Methodist DeBakey Heart Center/Baylor College of Medicine. In this study, paired myocardial samples were collected prospectively, as well as a number of clinical variables, including clinical history and functional class, serial echocardiograms, and exercise cardiopulmonary tests, in an attempt to define correlations between cellular, hemodynamic, and clinical variables. Among the important observations from this study was, first, an almost universal reduction in markers of hypertrophy as measured by changes in cell size, collagen, and myocardial TNF-α (Fig. 20-15). These changes were seen in 95% of the samples studied. Second, only a few patients (6 of 67) showed sustained improvement in LVEF fraction that permitted device removal, when the device was set to function at the lowest possible level of support. The mean ejection fraction before LVAD implantation was 19%, and improved to 40% at 60 days. Of interest, when patients were supported for longer periods, there appeared to be a negative effect, with LVEF decreasing to 25% at 120 days. Third, there was a substantial improvement in functional class over time. At 120 days, peak VO_2 was 18.9 mL/kg/min.[9]

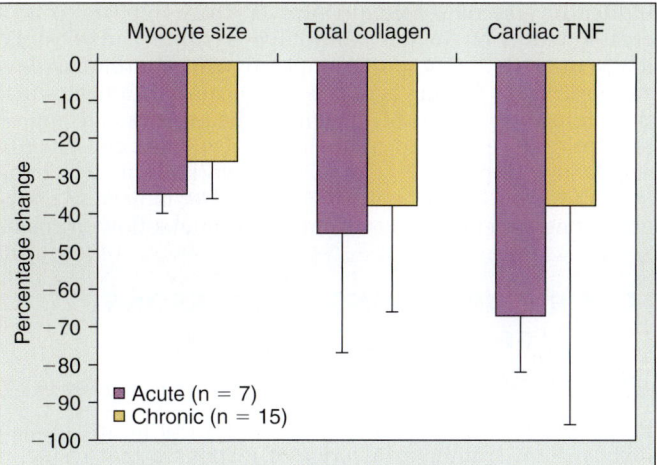

FIGURE 20-15 Reduction in markers of hypertrophy. Measurements at left ventricular assist device (LVAD) implantation and after LVAD removal were obtained for each of the parameters tested. Percentage change from baseline was calculated and plotted. As shown, there is reduction in myocyte size, collagen content, and intramyocardial tumor necrosis factor (TNF).

These observations suggest that cellular normalization in the failing myocardial phenotype may be a largely universal response to mechanical unloading; however, the translation of histologic improvement into recovery of contractile function as measured by echocardiography occurs at a much lower frequency—and device removal to an even lesser degree. In other words, it is clear that reverse remodeling as measured by histologic changes, molecular markers, or echocardiographic parameters is not commensurate with myocardial recovery. More important, myocardial recovery may occur to varying degrees but not sufficiently to allow device removal, at least with current technology and pharmacologic therapy.

Effect of Left Ventricular Assist Device Support on Right Ventricular Histology and Function

An important but often overlooked aspect of LVAD therapy is the effect of LVAD support on the function of the failing right ventricle. From a clinical standpoint, the presence of right ventricular failure after LVAD support varies depending on the population studied, but if one looks at registry data, the proportion of patients receiving an LVAD who subsequently require an RVAD is approximately 10%.[41] If we use these data as the sole parameter for defining right ventricular failure, it is clear that most patients selected for LVAD therapy do not have overt right ventricular failure. However, the right ventricle in these patients is not normal.

When right ventricular histologic markers from normal control subjects were compared with right ventricular samples from patients with chronic HF undergoing heart transplantation, it was found that total collagen content and myocardial TNF content were increased, whereas the change in myocyte cell size was insignificant. After LVAD support, the structural abnormalities observed in the right ventricle normalized.[42] Consistent with this observation is the finding that abnormal expression of dystrophin is also seen in the failing right ventricle, and that after chronic LVAD therapy dystrophin expression normalizes.[43]

Other myocardial parameters have been studied in the right ventricle. Studies in isolated left and right ventricular trabeculae obtained from LVAD-supported patients demonstrated improvement in force generation after beta-adrenergic stimulation. Consistent with this physiologic finding is the observation that LVAD-treated patients had higher myocardial beta-adrenergic receptor densities in both the left and right ventricles.[44,45]

What are the mechanisms by which the right ventricle fails and the potential mechanisms by which chronic left ventricular unloading affects right ventricular function? Two plausible explanations are worth discussing: first, hemodynamic effects, and second, alterations in the neurohormonal milieu.

Chronic HF leads to a persistent increase in the left ventricular end-diastolic pressure, which in turn raises pulmonary artery pressure and creates a state of chronic pressure and volume load on the right ventricle. Effective LVAD therapy decreases left ventricular end-diastolic pressure and pulmonary artery pressure, reducing pressure and volume load on right ventricle.[46] These effects can be seen more dramatically in patients who appear to have "fixed pulmonary hypertension," generically defined as a transpulmonary gradient greater than 15 mm Hg or a pulmonary vascular resistance greater than 4 Wood units. Chronic LVAD support in this group of patients also leads to normalization of pulmonary pressures, creating a state in which the right ventricle is no longer subjected to the effects of pressure and volume.[47] The reversal of pulmonary hypertension among patients with severe HF requires time, but neither the frequency nor the definite time course for this phenomenon is known. However, it is clear that chronic left ventricular unloading affects the failing right ventricle by normalizing the hemodynamic forces that affect right ventricular myocardial structure and function.

The systemic neurohormonal response associated with HF is also deactivated after LVAD support. Epinephrine and norepinephrine, natriuretic peptide, and cytokine levels all tend to decrease over time. These peptides have unique and direct hypertrophic effects that, after their deactivation, may lead to a reversal in cell hypertrophy.[48–50] The influence of these trophic factors on the failing right ventricle has not been directly tested, but the observation that regression of hypertrophy occurs in some studies in the absence of major hemodynamic findings supports a potential role of humoral mediators in this process.

Electrophysiologic Improvements

Electrophysiologic disturbances are important manifestations of HF, resulting in part from abnormalities in myocyte action potential shape and duration.[51] The prolongation of the action potential seen in HF may be a compensatory response that initially results in increased Ca^{2+} flux with a positive inotropic result, but later becomes maladaptive owing to a decreased Ca^{2+} response.[52] The question of whether the cellular and structural changes observed with LVAD unloading affect the electrophysiologic responses of the heart has not been extensively investigated. Comparisons of the electrophysiologic characteristics of myocytes from the explanted hearts of transplant recipients who had prior LVAD support with myocytes from unsupported transplant recipients indicated improved function in the LVAD-supported hearts.[44] The magnitude of myocyte contraction was significantly higher in the LVAD-supported hearts and the time to maximal contraction and the action potential duration at 50% repolarization (APD_{50}) were decreased, indicating superior electrophysiologic function.

More recently, a retrospective analysis of LVAD-supported patients was undertaken that compared paired electrocardiographic findings before and after LVAD support. It was found that there was a decrease in heart rate (107 beats/min vs. 91 beats/min) as well as a reduction in QT intervals corrected for heart rate (479 ± 10 msec vs. 445 ± 9 msec).[45] A comparison of myocytes from LVAD-supported hearts with myocytes from unsupported hearts showed that the APD_{50} was

CH 20

Cellular, Molecular, Genomic, and Functional Changes That Occur in the Failing Heart in Response to Mechanical Circulatory Support markedly lower in the previously supported cells (863 ± 37 msec vs. 529 ± 154 msec). The changes observed in this study add to the body of work documenting not only the cellular changes but the functional effects that may be consistent with recovery of cardiac function.

FAILING MYOCARDIAL RESPONSE TO PULSATILE VERSUS CONTINUOUS FLOW MECHANICAL SUPPORT

Most of the experimental work on changes in myocardial structure and function has come from studies of patients supported with pulsatile pumps. However, the use of continuous flow pumps has surpassed and supplanted pulsatile support. There are clear differences in how these two types of devices produce hemodynamic unloading, and it may not be an appropriate comparison to assume continuous flow support produces the same changes as those induced by pulsatile support.

Few studies have compared the histologic and cellular responses to pulsatile and continuous flow support. The more consistent findings are shown in Figure 20-16, which demonstrates that if one looks at myocyte size, collagen content, or myocardial TNF expression, there seems to be no difference in the biologic response to mechanical unloading.[46] In other words, both pulsatile and continuous-flow devices

induce reverse remodeling. However, there appears to be a greater reduction in left ventricular systolic and diastolic loads in pulsatile support compared with continuous-flow support.[53] This finding is of interest because it indicates that the biologic response of the failing heart does not appear to require the profound unloading that is most consistently achieved with pulsatile pumps. More work needs to be done in defining the directional changes in other molecular markers among patients supported on a continuous-flow regimen.

FUTURE DIRECTIONS AND LESSONS FROM LEFT VENTRICULAR ASSIST DEVICE RESEARCH

Prolonged mechanical circulatory support of failing human myocardium stimulates a series of responses that result in profound structural and biochemical changes consistent with at least partial reversal of the failing phenotype. The primary importance of these observations is that by analyzing the changes induced, we may uncover mechanisms suggesting new pathways for treatment of HF. Second, we may determine targets of therapy that in the context of LVAD support might further stimulate recovery of function. To this end, the use of LVAD support to stimulate recovery needs greater work and a deeper understanding of the signaling pathways associated with recovery. Third, we may develop strategies that improve the ability to identify patients who will benefit from LVAD support, as well as those who likely will not benefit. For example, Levy and colleagues tested the ability of the Seattle Heart Failure Model to risk-stratify patients for LVAD therapy.[54] This model was able to estimate 1-year survival for high-risk patients deciding between medical therapy and LVAD support with an accuracy of 0.73.[54] The addition of genetic markers to predictive models such as this one may further strengthen their predictive ability, although this has not been successful in other areas of cardiovascular medicine.

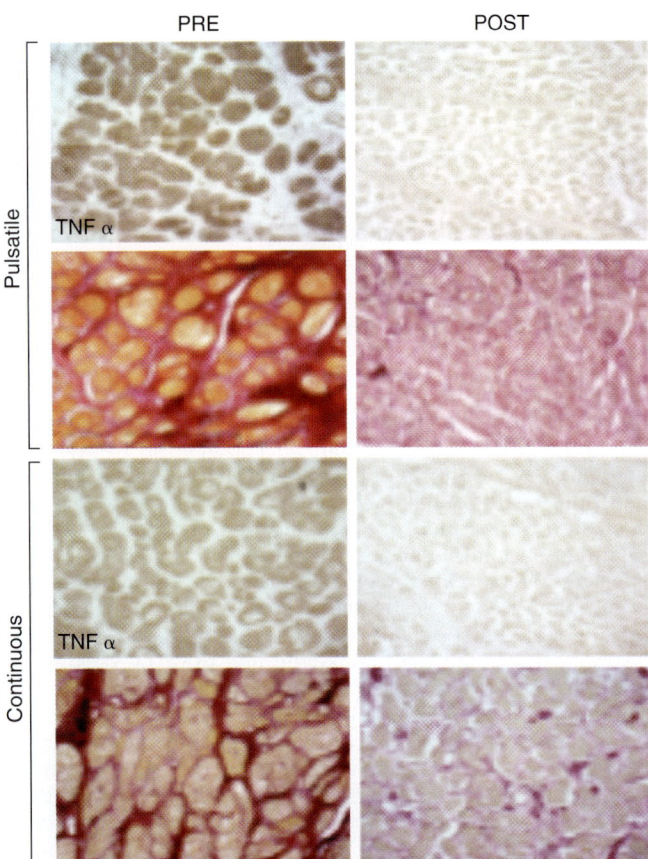

FIGURE 20-16 Differences between pulsatile and continuous-flow left ventricular assist device (LVAD) support. Paired myocardial samples from a patient supported with pulsatile LVAD and from another patient supported with continuous-flow LVAD are shown. Paired myocardial tissue sections from each patient were stained for collagen content with picrosirius red and for tumor necrosis factor-α (TNF-α). Pre-LVAD support samples showed higher collagen (indicated by red staining) and TNF expression (brown). Staining intensity for both markers decreased with both types of LVAD support.

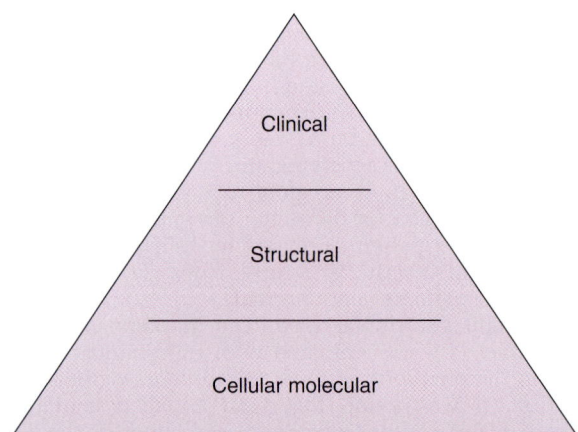

FIGURE 20-17 The pyramid of reverse remodeling. Left ventricular assist device (LVAD) support produces major hemodynamic and volume changes that stimulate the process of reverse remodeling. Changes that are almost universal after LVAD support include reduction in myocyte size; decrease in intercellular collagen content; and deactivation of various cytokines, including tumor necrosis factor-α (TNF-α). These changes occur in more than 90% of the samples studied. At the functional level, defined by improvement in contractility as measured by echocardiography, improvement is observed in approximately 30% of LVAD-supported patients. At the clinical level, and the most pertinent test of myocardial recovery, is the ability to remove the LVAD and maintain adequate function secondary to sufficient myocardial recovery. This is a low-frequency event, seen in less than 10% of LVAD-treated patients.

Finally, it is important to recognize that although myocardial improvement at the histologic, cellular, and molecular levels is prevalent, these improvements rarely result in restoration of function sufficient to achieve device removal and sustainable recovery (Fig. 20-17). Strategies to augment myocardial function during LVAD support and the identification of key signals that link structure and function are targets of ongoing investigation.

REFERENCES

1. Scheinin SA, Capek P, Radovancevic B, et al. The effect of prolonged left ventricular support on myocardial histopathology in patients with end-stage cardiomyopathy. *ASAIO J.* 1992;38:M271–M274.
2. Bruckner BA, Stetson SJ, Perez-Verdia A, et al. Regression of fibrosis and hypertrophy in failing myocardium following mechanical circulatory support. *J Heart Lung Transplant.* 2001;20:457–464.
3. Klotz S, Foronjy RF, Dickstein ML, et al. Mechanical unloading during left ventricular assist device support increases left ventricular collagen cross-linking and myocardial stiffness. *Circulation.* 2005;112:364–374.
4. Chaudhary KW, Rossman EI, Piacentino III V, et al. Altered myocardial Ca^{2+} cycling after left ventricular assist device support in the failing human heart. *J Am Coll Cardiol.* 2004;44:837–845.
5. Dipla K, Mattiello JA, Jeevanandam V, et al. Myocyte recovery after mechanical circulatory support in humans with end-stage heart failure. *Circulation.* 1998;97:2316–2322.
6. Harding JD, Piacentino III V, Gaughan JP, et al. Electrophysiological alterations after mechanical circulatory support in patients with advanced cardiac failure. *Circulation.* 2001;104:1241–1247.
7. Heerdt PM, Holmes JW, Cai B, et al. Chronic unloading by left ventricular assist device reverses contractile dysfunction and alters gene expression in end-stage hf. *Circulation.* 2000;102:2713–2719.
8. Margulies KB. Reversal mechanisms of left ventricular remodeling: lessons from left ventricular assist device experiments. *J Card Fail.* 2002;8(suppl 6):S500–S505.
9. Maybaum S, Mancini D, Xydas S, et al. Cardiac improvement during mechanical circulatory support: a prospective multicenter study of the LVAD Working Group. *Circulation.* 2007;115:2497–2505.
10. Ogletree-Hughes ML, Stull LB, Sweet WE, et al. Mechanical unloading restores β-adrenergic responsiveness and reverses receptor downregulation in the failing human heart. *Circulation.* 2001;104:881–886.
11. Zafeiridis A, Jeevanandam V, Houser SR, et al. Regression of cellular hypertrophy after left ventricular assist device support. *Circulation.* 1998;98:656–662.
12. Birks EJ, Tansley PD, Hardy J, et al. Left ventricular assist device and drug therapy for the reversal of heart failure. *N Engl J Med.* 2006;355:1873–1884.
13. Hall JL, Birks EJ, Grindle S, et al. Molecular signature of recovery following combination left ventricular assist device (LVAD) support and pharmacologic therapy. *Eur Heart J.* 2007;28:613–627.
14. Terracciano CM, Koban MU, Soppa GK, et al. The role of the cardiac Na+/Ca2+ exchanger in reverse remodeling: relevance for LVAD-recovery. *Ann N Y Acad Sci.* 2007;1099:349–360.
15. Terracciano CM, Hardy J, Birks EJ, et al. Clinical recovery from end-stage heart failure using left-ventricular assist device and pharmacological therapy correlates with increased sarcoplasmic reticulum calcium content but not with regression of cellular hypertrophy. *Circulation.* 2004;109:2263–2265.
16. Birks EJ, Hall JL, Barton PJR, et al. Gene profiling changes in cytoskeletal proteins during clinical recovery after left ventricular-assist device support. *Circulation.* 2005;112(suppl 9):I57–I64.
17. Towbin JA, Bowles NE. Dilated cardiomyopathy: a tale of cytoskeletal proteins and beyond. *J Cardiovasc Electrophysiol.* 2006;17:919–926.
18. Vatta M, Stetson SJ, Perez-Verdia A, et al. Molecular remodelling of dystrophin in patients with end-stage cardiomyopathies and reversal in patients on assistance-device therapy. *Lancet.* 2002;359:936–941.
19. Cullen ME, Yuen AH, Felkin LE, et al. Myocardial expression of the arginine:glycine amidinotransferase gene is elevated in heart failure and normalized after recovery: potential implications for local creatine synthesis. *Circulation.* 2006;114(suppl 1):I16–I20.
20. Hall JL, Grindle S, Han X, et al. Genomic profiling of the human heart before and after mechanical support with a ventricular assist device reveals alterations in vascular signaling networks. *Physiol Genomics.* 2004;17:283–291.
21. Chen Y, Park S, Li Y, et al. Alterations of gene expression in failing myocardium following left ventricular assist device support. *Physiol Genomics.* 2003;14:251–260.
22. Saunders MA, Liang H, Li WH. Human polymorphism at microRNAs and microRNA target sites. *Proc Natl Acad Sci U S A.* 2007;104:3300–3305.
23. Lim LP, Glasner ME, Yekta S, et al. Vertebrate microRNA genes. *Science.* 2003; 299:1540.
24. Matkovich SJ, Van Booven DJ, Youker KA, et al. Reciprocal regulation of myocardial microRNAs and messenger RNA in human cardiomyopathy and reversal of the microRNA signature by biomechanical support. *Circulation.* 2009;119:1263–1271.
25. van Rooij E, Sutherland LB, Liu N, et al. A signature pattern of stress-responsive microRNAs that can evoke cardiac hypertrophy and heart failure. *Proc Natl Acad Sci U S A.* 2006;103:18255–18260.
26. Tatsuguchi M, Seok HY, Callis TE, et al. Expression of microRNAs is dynamically regulated during cardiomyocyte hypertrophy. *J Mol Cell Cardiol.* 2007;42:1137–1141.
27. Blaxall BC, Tschannen-Moran BM, Milano CA, et al. Differential gene expression and genomic patient stratification following left ventricular assist device support. *J Am Coll Cardiol.* 2003;41:1096–1106.
28. Kittleson MM, Ye SQ, Irizarry RA, et al. Identification of a gene expression profile that differentiates between ischemic and nonischemic cardiomyopathy. *Circulation.* 2004;110:3444–3451.
29. Boheler KR, Volkova M, Morrell C, et al. Sex- and age-dependent human transcriptome variability: implications for chronic heart failure. *Proc Natl Acad Sci U S A.* 2003;100:2754–2759.
30. Fermin D, Barac A, Lee S, et al. Sex and age dimorphism of myocardial gene expression in nonischemic human heart failure. *Circ Cardiovasc Genet.* 2008;1:117–125.
31. Huang X, Pan W, Park S, et al. Modeling the relationship between LVAD support time and gene expression changes in the human heart by penalized partial least squares. *Bioinformatics.* 2004;20:888–894.
32. Torre-Amione G, Stetson SJ, Youker KA, et al. Decreased expression of tumor necrosis factor-α in failing human myocardium after mechanical circulatory support: a potential mechanism for cardiac recovery. *Circulation.* 1999;100:1189–1193.
33. Margulies KB, Matiwala S, Cornejo C, et al. Mixed messages: transcription patterns in failing and recovering human myocardium. *Circ Res.* 2005;96:592–599.
34. McNamara DM, Holubkov R, Starling RC, et al. Controlled trial of intravenous immune globulin in recent-onset dilated cardiomyopathy. *Circulation.* 2001;103:2254–2259.
35. Farrar DJ, Holman W, McBride L, et al. Long-term follow-up of Thoratec ventricular assist device bridge-to-recovery patients successfully removed from support after recovery of ventricular function. *J Heart Lung Transplant.* 2002;21:516–521.
36. Simon MA, Kormos RL, Murali S, et al. Myocardial recovery using ventricular assist devices: prevalence, clinical characteristics, and outcomes. *Circulation.* 2005;112(suppl 9):I32–I36.
37. Müller J, Wallukat G, Weng YG, et al. Weaning from mechanical cardiac support in patients with idiopathic dilated cardiomyopathy. *Circulation.* 1997;96:542–549.
38. Dandel M, Weng Y, Siniawski H, et al. Long-term results in patients with idiopathic dilated cardiomyopathy after weaning from left ventricular assist devices. *Circulation.* 2005;112(suppl 9):I37–I45.
39. Khan T, Delgado RM, Radovancevic B, et al. Dobutamine stress echocardiography predicts myocardial improvement in patients supported by left ventricular assist devices (LVADs): hemodynamic and histologic evidence of improvement before LVAD explantation. *J Heart Lung Transplant.* 2003;22:137–146.
40. Birks EJ, Latif N, Owen V, et al. Quantitative myocardial cytokine expression and activation of the apoptotic pathway in patients who require left ventricular assist devices. *Circulation.* 2001;104(12 suppl 1):I233–I240.
41. Kirklin JK, Naftel DC, Kormos RL, et al. Second INTERMACS annual report: more than 1,000 primary left ventricular assist device implants. *J Heart Lung Transplant.* 2010;29:1–10.
42. Küçüker SA, Stetson SJ, Becker KA, et al. Evidence of improved right ventricular structure after LVAD support in patients with end-stage cardiomyopathy. *J Heart Lung Transplant.* 2004;23:28–35.
43. Vatta M, Stetson SJ, Jimenez S, et al. Molecular normalization of dystrophin in the failing left and right ventricle of patients treated with either pulsatile or continuous flow-type ventricular assist devices. *J Am Coll Cardiol.* 2004;43:811–817.
44. Barbone A, Holmes JW, Heerdt PM, et al. Comparison of right and left ventricular responses to left ventricular assist device support in patients with severe heart failure: a primary role of mechanical unloading underlying reverse remodeling. *Circulation.* 2001;104:670–675.
45. Klotz S, Barbone A, Reiken S, et al. Left ventricular assist device support normalizes left and right ventricular beta-adrenergic pathway properties. *J Am Coll Cardiol.* 2005;45:668–676.
46. Thohan V, Stetson SJ, Nagueh SF, et al. Cellular and hemodynamics responses of failing myocardium to continuous flow mechanical circulatory support using the DeBakey-Noon left ventricular assist device: a comparative analysis with pulsatile-type devices. *J Heart Lung Transplant.* 2005;24:566–575.
47. Torre-Amione G, Southard RE, Loebe MM, et al. Reversal of secondary pulmonary hypertension by axial and pulsatile mechanical circulatory support. *J Heart Lung Transplant.* 2010;29:195–200.
48. Kuhn M, Voss M, Mitko D, et al. Left ventricular assist device support reverses altered cardiac expression and function of natriuretic peptides and receptors in end-stage heart failure. *Cardiovasc Res.* 2004;64:308–314.
49. Milting H, EL Banayosy A, Kassner A, et al. The time course of natriuretic hormones as plasma markers of myocardial recovery in heart transplant candidates during ventricular assist device support reveals differences among device types. *J Heart Lung Transplant.* 2001;20:949–955.
50. Thompson LO, Skrabal CA, Loebe M, et al. Plasma neurohormone levels correlate with left ventricular functional and morphological improvement in LVAD patients. *J Surg Res.* 2005;123:25–32.
51. Tomaselli GF, Marban E. Electrophysiological remodeling in hypertrophy and heart failure. *Cardiovasc Res.* 1999;42:270–283.
52. Wickenden AD, Kaprielian R, Kassiri Z, et al. The role of action potential prolongation and altered intracellular calcium handling in the pathogenesis of heart failure. *Cardiovasc Res.* 1998;37:312–323.
53. Akhter SA, D'Souza KM, Malhotra R, et al. Reversal of impaired myocardial beta-adrenergic receptor signaling by continuous-flow left ventricular assist device support. *J Heart Lung Transplant.* 2010;29:603–609.
54. Levy WC, Mozaffarian D, Linker DT, et al. Can the Seattle heart failure model be used to risk-stratify heart failure patients for potential left ventricular assist device therapy? *J Heart Lung Transplant.* 2009;28:231–236.
55. Chen X, Piacentino III V, Furukawa S, et al. L-type Ca^{2+} channel density and regulation are altered in failing human ventricular myocytes and recover after support with mechanical assist devices. *Circ Res.* 2002;91:517–524.
56. Marx SO, Reiken S, Hisamatsu Y, et al. PKA phosphorylation dissociates FKBP12.6 from the calcium release channel (ryanodine receptor): defective regulation in failing hearts. *Cell.* 2000;101:365–376.
57. Terracciano CM, Harding SE, Adamson D, et al. Changes in sarcolemmal Ca entry and sarcoplasmic reticulum Ca content in ventricular myocytes from patients with end-stage heart failure following myocardial recovery after combined pharmacological and ventricular assist device therapy. *Eur Heart J.* 2003;24:1329–1339.
58. Frazier OH, Myers TJ. Left ventricular assist system as a bridge to myocardial recovery. *Ann Thorac Surg.* 1999;68(suppl 2):734–741.

CHAPTER **21**

Results of Clinical Trials to Date

Joseph G. Rogers and Francis D. Pagani

Disclosures: Dr. Pagani is a principal site investigator for clinical trials evaluating the HeartMate II (Thoratec Corporation, Pleasanton, CA), DuraHeart (Terumo Cardiovascular Corporation, Ann Arbor, MI), and HVAD (HeartWare Corporation, Miami, FL) devices. Dr. Rogers is a consultant for Thoratec Corporation.

OVERVIEW OF CLINICAL TESTING OF MECHANICAL CIRCULATORY SUPPORT DEVICES AND DEVELOPMENT OF INDICATIONS FOR USE

In 1976, the U.S. Congress passed the Medical Device Amendments Act, giving the U.S. Food and Drug Administration (FDA) the authority to preapprove the use of medical devices in the United States. This landmark act changed the landscape of clinical device testing in the United States and gave regulatory oversight to the FDA over the processes of clinical evaluation and testing of mechanical circulatory support (MCS) devices in the United States. This influence on testing of MCS devices shaped, in part, the early patient populations studied in clinical trials evaluating MCS devices and, importantly, influenced the development of the treatment paradigms of bridge to recovery (BTR), bridge to transplantation (BTT), and destination therapy (DT), indications now used in clinical practice.

Early clinical trials of temporary extracorporeal MCS devices were quite simplistic and focused largely on the efficacy of a temporary MCS device to sustain life until the time of cardiac recovery in cases where medical therapy was thought futile. The earliest clinical scenario studied was postcardiotomy shock, where failure to wean from cardiopulmonary bypass as a result of myocardial injury sustained during a cardiac surgical operation was uniformly fatal if the patient was not rescued with a temporary MCS device. This pattern of clinical use of temporary MCS devices established the concept and indication of BTR, where a temporary MCS device would support the circulation until the time of cardiac recovery. A robust experience with temporary MCS devices in the postcardiotomy setting led to expansion of the use of temporary MCS devices to non-postcardiotomy settings, including cardiogenic shock caused by myocardial infarction, fulminant or acute myocarditis, or acute cardiac allograft dysfunction in the setting of heart transplantation. As smaller, partial-support, percutaneously placed, temporary MCS device designs came into clinical evaluation, prospective, randomized comparison with the intra-aortic balloon pump was used in several clinical trial designs.

The development of durable, implantable MCS devices was initially conceived for the permanent support of the heart as an alternative to heart transplantation. However, FDA concerns for the long-term performance and safety of durable, implantable MCS devices largely restricted the initial use of clinical testing of implantable MCS devices to patients eligible for heart transplantation, and not as a permanent therapy. This strategy was thought to provide additional safety to patients in that transplantation could provide a potential backup to failed durable, implantable MCS therapy. This bias by clinicians and the FDA to limit the population to transplant-eligible patients set the early stage for what has become the BTT indication and formed a regulatory pathway by which most durable, implantable MCS devices are initially evaluated today.

The early clinical evaluation of implantable MCS devices was performed without the complexity and medical standard of a randomized, controlled trial design owing to the perceived life-saving value of implantable MCS devices by physicians, the ethical dilemma of withholding this therapy in patients at risk of imminent death, and difficulty of blinding treatment arms. Inclusion of a historical or contemporaneous, nonrandomized, observational control group became commonplace to justify a single-arm, nonrandomized, observational approach to the study of implantable MCS devices. As device designs evolved and the acuity of illness of patients selected for implantable MCS devices lessened, the futility of medical therapy became less apparent, and the need for more rigorous clinical evaluation of implantable MCS devices became more obvious. More sophisticated analysis and assessment of efficacy parameters and of serious adverse events were incorporated into clinical trial designs, but uniform definitions of adverse events, that would allow side-by-side comparisons of the devices, were several years away. Primary or secondary outcomes, including assessment of functional capacity, quality of life, and neurocognitive evaluation, became important components of the full evaluation of the benefit and efficacy of MCS devices. As more data were accumulated on implantable MCS device performance, efficacy, and frequency of serious adverse advents through industry registries, the ability of the FDA to set benchmarks that implantable MCS devices must achieve for regulatory approval resulted in the comparison of investigational, durable MCS devices with a performance goal or measure for BTT indication. This type of trial design is now frequently used for testing durable MCS devices for BTT indication.

Confidence in the ability of implantable MCS devices to provide long-term support, obtained through the BTT experience, prompted further expansion of indications for MCS devices as a permanent alternative to heart transplantation in patients considered non–transplant eligible, termed *destination therapy*. The process to evaluate implantable MCS devices for DT led to the first use of a prospective, randomized, controlled clinical trial design comparing an MCS device (HeartMate VE; Thoratec Corporation, Pleasanton, CA) with optimal medical management in the historic REMATCH (Randomized Evaluation of Mechanical Assistance for the Treatment of Congestive Heart Failure) trial.[1] Today, the regulatory pathway for DT requires new technology to be compared with FDA-approved technology through prospective, randomized clinical trial designs and is exemplified by the HeartMate II Pivotal Trial for DT indication.[2] Clinical evaluation of implantable MCS devices in novel patient populations that extend current indications will require randomization against established therapy. For example, the REVIVE-IT (Randomized Evaluation of VAD Intervention before Inotrope Therapy) pilot trial will be a National Institutes of Health, National Heart, Lung and Blood Institute (NHLBI)–sponsored, prospective, randomized, nonblinded trial design evaluating the use of ventricular assist device (VAD) therapy compared with optimal medical therapy in a cohort of ambulatory non–inotrope-dependent patients with less advanced heart failure than studied in the REMATCH trial.

Another important milestone in the advance of MCS therapy was the development of the NHLBI-sponsored national registry, INTERMACS (Interagency Registry for Mechanically Assisted Circulatory Support) evaluating the use of implantable MCS devices. INTERMACS is a mandated registry of all patients in the United States receiving implantation of FDA-approved, durable MCS devices. The development of INTERMACS has added flexibility to clinical trial designs by providing the ability to use a prospective, nonrandomized observational control cohort of patients receiving FDA-approved MCS devices in INTERMACS for comparison with investigational devices. This process of comparison gives investigators the ability to stratify risk for appropriate comparison of control and treatment groups and is a method now incorporated into the clinical evaluation of durable, implantable MCS devices for BTT indication. Importantly, INTERMACS also provides the ability to obtain critical data on MCS device performance in the postmarket phase.

The paradigms of BTR, BTT, and DT are now integrated into the processes by which MCS devices are evaluated and used by clinicians for patient care, regulatory agencies for monitoring of use, and insurance payers for reimbursement. Thus, an understanding of the clinical trial evaluation of all MCS devices is necessarily shaped by this perspective. These paradigms do not consistently describe all clinical situations and realities of patient care, and it is likely that the indications for MCS therapy will continue to evolve in the future for the treatment of advanced heart failure. This evolution will require more complex clinical trial designs for MCS device evaluation.

CLINICAL TRIALS EVALUATING MECHANICAL CIRCULATORY SUPPORT DEVICES AS BRIDGE TO HEART TRANSPLANTATION

Pulsatile Pumps

Heart transplantation has remained the most successful therapy for patients with advanced heart failure.[3] However, persistent limitations in the availability of donors have driven the development of durable, implantable MCS devices as a means to sustain critically ill patients awaiting transplantation. These devices have become an established treatment option for patients with advanced heart failure as a BTT.[4] The successful clinical use of implantable MCS devices for BTT therapy was first reported by Hill and colleagues in 1986 who described the successful use of the pneumatically actuated Pierce-Donachy paracorporeal ventricular assist device (PVAD).[4,5] The paracorporeal design of the Pierce-Donachy VAD permitted flexible support options for the right or left ventricle, or both, but required tethering to a large drive console that limited patient mobility and potential for hospital discharge (Fig. 21-1). The Pierce-Donachy VAD, later to become the Thoratec PVAD (Thoratec Corporation, Pleasanton, CA), underwent early clinical evaluation in a multicenter, prospective, single-arm, observational, FDA-sponsored study in 29 patients (average age, 36 years) for BTT indication.[6] Of patients, 21 (72%) survived to transplantation after 8 hours to 31 days of MCS. Biventricular support was required in 14 (48%); 15 patients required left ventricular assist device (LVAD) support only. Of the 21 patients who subsequently underwent heart transplantation, 20 (95%) survived to hospital discharge after a median of 31 days. At follow-up, ranging from 7 to 39 months, 19 patients remained alive. The successful clinical evaluation of the Thoratec PVAD led to FDA approval for the BTT indication in 1992. Subsequent device improvements included the development of a small, portable pneumatic drive console permitting hospital discharge (Fig. 21-2).[7,8] Although the Thoratec PVAD remains in clinical use today for BTT, its paracorporeal design has limited its preference by clinicians for general use. To overcome this limitation, the Thoratec intracorporeal ventricular assist device (IVAD), based on a significant redesign of the Thoratec PVAD, was developed to move from an external paracorporeal design to an implantable design (Fig. 21-3).[9] This design change required clinical validation through an FDA-approved, multicenter, prospective, nonrandomized clinical trial performed by Slaughter and colleagues in 39 patients for the BTT indication from October 2001 to June 2004.[10] The study cohort was compared with a historical observational control group consisting of 100 patients undergoing implantation of the Thoratec PVAD, previously submitted to the FDA as part of the regulatory approval process for that device. The study cohort consisted of 28 men and 11 women with a mean age of 48 years (range 16 to 71 years) and a mean body surface area of $1.9\,m^2$ (range 1.3 to $2.4\,m^2$). Twenty-four patients (62%) required support with an LVAD alone and 15 (38%) required biventricular support, similar to the earlier Thoratec PVAD experience. Indications included BTT ($n = 30$) and postcardiotomy failure ($n = 9$). Eighteen patients were discharged after a mean duration of 96 days. There were no VAD failures. Complications included 13 cases of bleeding requiring re-exploration (33.3%), 1 embolic and 2 hemorrhagic strokes (7.7%), 5 driveline infections (12.8%), and 2 pocket infections (5%). The rate of support to successful outcomes was 70% for BTT and 67% for postcardiotomy recovery, versus historical results for the Thoratec PVAD of 69% for BTT and 48% for postcardiotomy recovery. This experience led to FDA approval of the Thoratec IVAD for BTT in 2006. There have

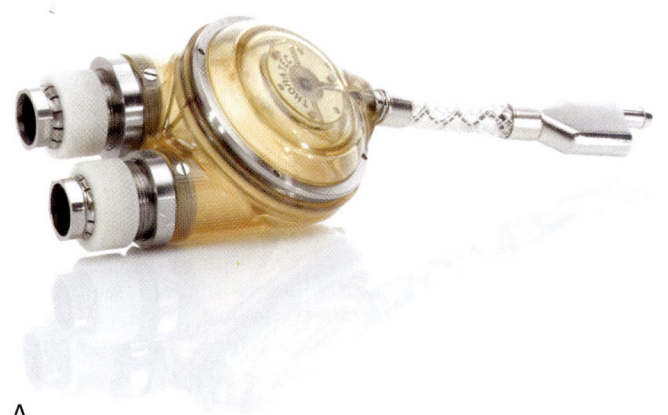

A

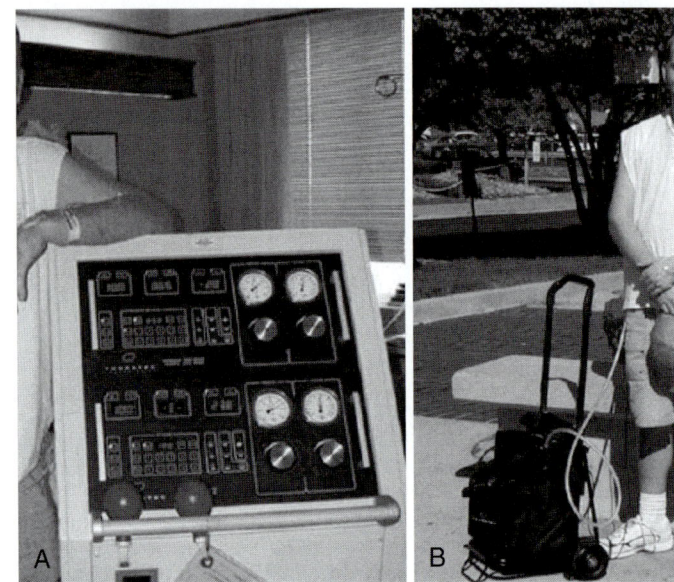

A   B

FIGURE 21-2 **A,** Original Thoratec dual-drive console permitted limited patient mobility and required in-hospital patient management. **B,** Thoratec TLC-II portable driver allows outpatient management and increased patient mobility. *(From Slaughter MS, Sobieski MA, Martin M, et al. Home discharge experience with the Thoratec TLC-II portable driver. ASAIO J. 2007;53:132-135.)*

Left side   Right side

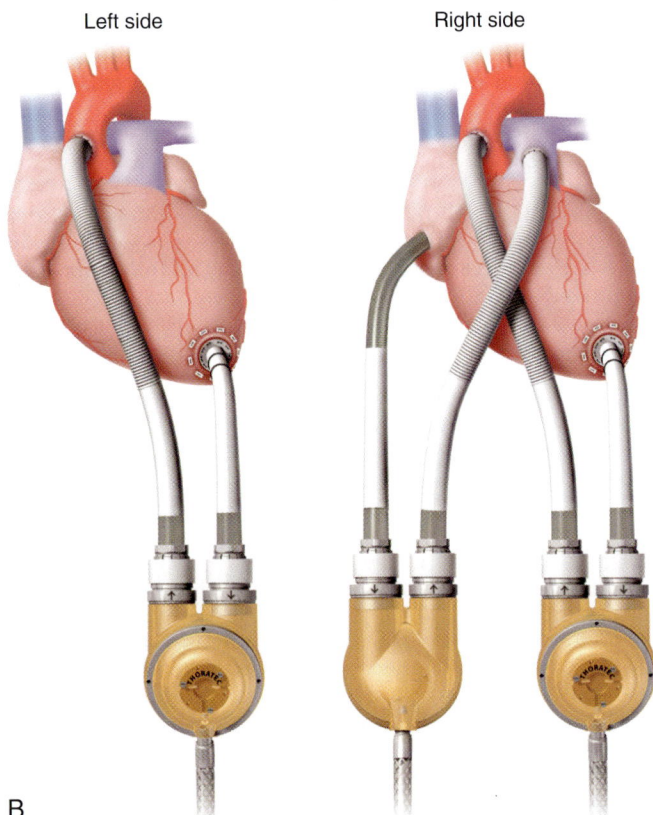

B

FIGURE 21-1 A, Thoratec paracorporeal ventricular assist device (PVAD) is a paracorporeal, pneumatically actuated ventricular assist device (VAD) designed for right-sided, left-sided, or biventricular support. **B,** Thoratec PVAD in left ventricular assist *(left side)* and biventricular assist configuration *(right side).*

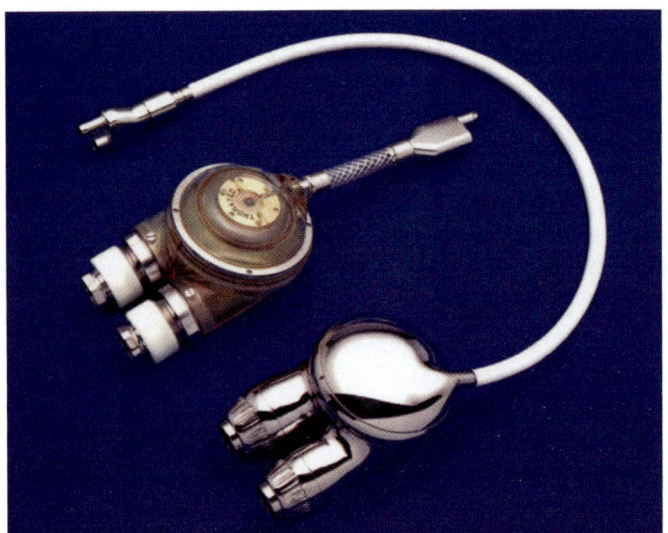

FIGURE 21-3 Thoratec intracorporeal ventricular assist device (IVAD) *(lower right corner)* beside Thoratec paracorporeal ventricular assist device (PVAD). The Thoratec IVAD is an implantable version of the Thoratec PVAD.

been no trials directly comparing the performance of these devices to new MCS device technology.

During the early 1980s and concurrent with the development of the Pierce-Donachy PVAD or Thoratec PVAD, other durable MCS device designs, dedicated exclusively to left ventricular support, were being developed for implantation with the intent of long-term use. These durable, implantable MCS devices included the Novacor LVAD (World Heart Corporation, Oakland, CA), first implanted in 1984, and the HeartMate IP1000 LVAD (Thoratec Corporation), implanted in 1988.[11-13] The Novacor LVAD was the first use of an electrically actuated, pulsatile, implantable LVAD that permitted "hands-free," untethered mobility (Fig. 21-4).[4] The HeartMate IP1000 was an implantable, pneumatically actuated, pulsatile

device that used a unique textured blood-contacting surface that promoted cellular ingrowth on the surface, creating a pseudo-endothelium, with the result that the patient required only antiplatelet therapy with aspirin, eliminating the need for anticoagulation therapy with warfarin (Fig. 21-5).[4] The HeartMate IP1000, although an implantable device, still required pneumatic actuation with a large portable drive console that precluded hospital discharge. Despite this limitation, the HeartMate IP1000 was generally favored by clinicians over the Novacor LVAD because of the benefits of its sintered surface. In 1994, nearly 6 years after its first implant in a patient, the HeartMate IP1000 became the first durable, implantable MCS device approved for BTT after completion of a multicenter clinical trial.[14,15] The multicenter clinical

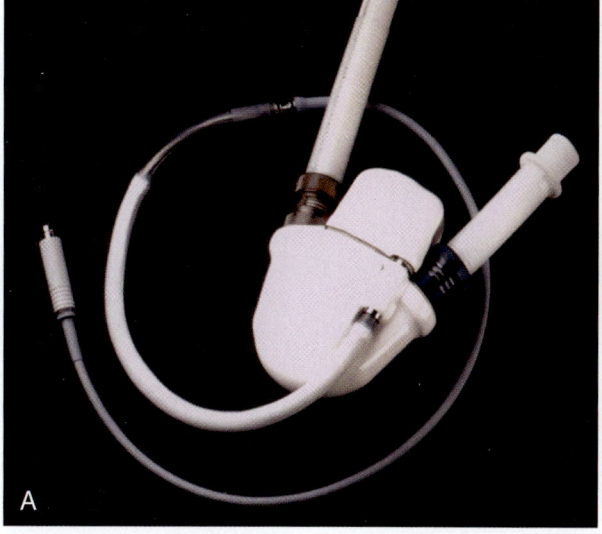 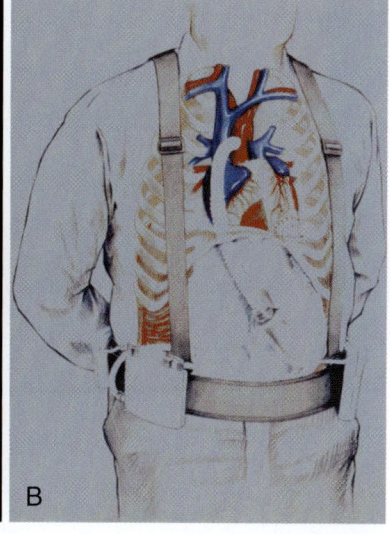

FIGURE 21-4 **A,** World Heart Novacor left ventricular assist device (LVAD). The Novacor LVAD is an implantable, electrically actuated pulsatile pump designed for long-term support. **B,** Novacor LVAD implanted in its preperitoneal position below the diaphragm and showing the percutaneous line and external wearable components, including batteries and controller.

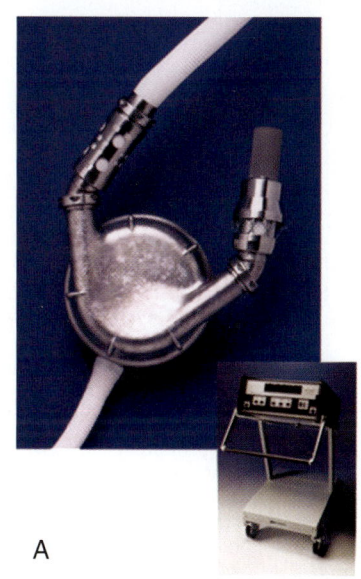 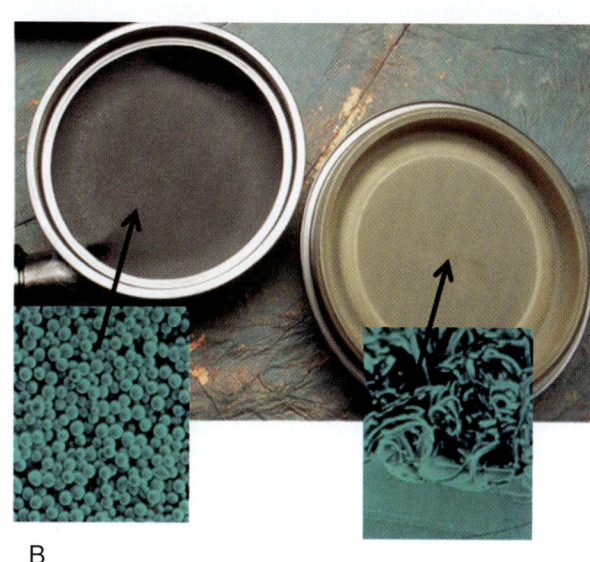

FIGURE 21-5 **A,** Thoratec HeartMate IP1000 is an implantable, pulsatile LVAD requiring a mobile but large drive console for pneumatic actuation of the pump's internal pusher plate. **B,** The internal surfaces of the pump are coated with sintered titanium microspheres on the pump housing and integrally textured polyurethane on the flexible diaphragm covering the pusher plate. These surfaces create a pseudoendothelium that is resistant to thrombus formation.

A

B

evaluation of the HeartMate IP1000 for BTT was performed by Frazier and colleagues in 34 patients.[14,15] The trial represented the first comparison of durable MCS device outcomes with a cohort of patients receiving medical therapy alone. Efficacy and safety of the device in the study cohort were compared with six nonrandomized patients who met inclusion criteria but did not receive a device and were supported by optimal medical management with intra-aortic balloon pump (IABP) as a BTT. Of the 34 patients receiving LVAD support, 22 (65%) survived to heart transplantation, with 80% (17 of 22) surviving to hospital discharge after transplantation. This compared with a survival to transplantation of 50% (3 patients) in the control group. However, overall mortality for the control cohort, including heart transplantation, was 100% (6 of 6 patients) within 77 days of having met the LVAD inclusion criteria, confirming the extremely poor prognosis in these patients and the benefit of durable, implantable MCS therapy. The HeartMate IP1000 is largely of historical interest now, having been replaced by device designs with electrical actuation that eliminate the need for a large pneumatic drive console, permitting hospital discharge.

The Thoratec HeartMate VE and XVE represented the next major redesign of the HeartMate IP1000 that required extensive prospective clinical evaluation by the FDA. The HeartMate VE was a pulsatile, electrically actuated, implantable LVAD evaluated for BTT.[16] The HeartMate XVE is the current generation of the original VE model (Fig. 21-6). The importance of the HeartMate VE design was that it incorporated an electrical power source consisting of two external batteries rather than the pneumatic actuation of the HeartMate IP1000, which allowed much greater patient mobility. Frazier and colleagues conducted a prospective, nonrandomized, multicenter clinical evaluation of the HeartMate VE at 24 centers in the United States in 280 transplant candidates (232 men, 48 women; median age, 55 years; range, 11 to 72 years) for the BTT indication.[16] It was the largest clinical trial for evaluation of a durable MCS device performed at that time. The study cohort was compared with a nonrandomized, historical control cohort of 48 patients (40 men, 8 women; median age 50 years; range 21 to 67 years) listed for heart transplantation but not receiving VAD therapy. The study cohort and control cohort were similar in terms of age, sex, and distribution of patients by diagnosis. Mean support duration in the study cohort was 112 days (range 1 to 691 days), with 54 patients supported for longer than 180 days. Serious device-related events included bleeding in 31 patients (11%), infection in

CH 21

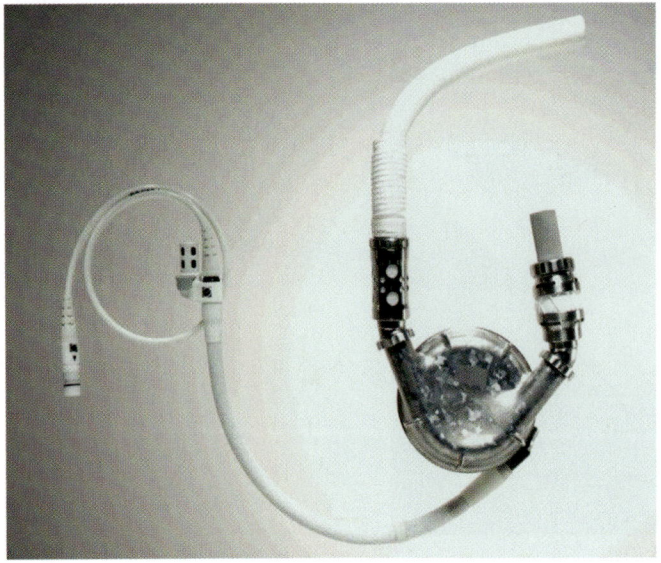

FIGURE 21-6 Thoratec HeartMate XVE is an implantable, pulsatile, electrically actuated left ventricular assist device (LVAD).

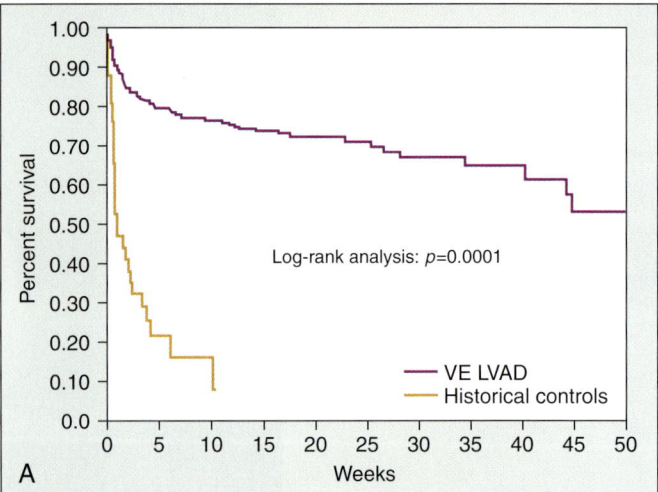

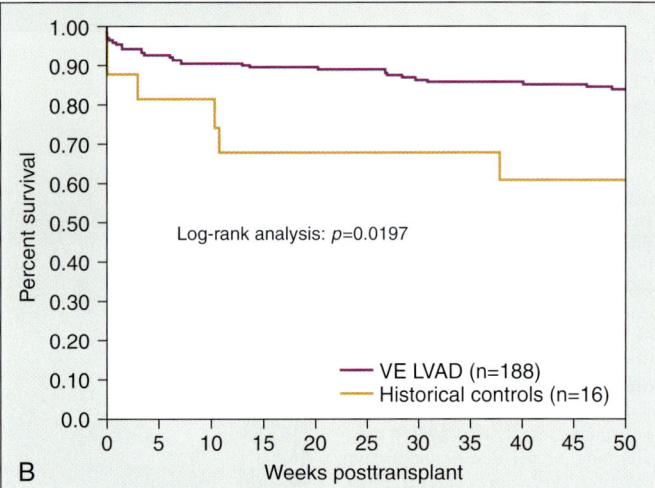

FIGURE 21-7 A, Kaplan-Meier survival estimate of the probability of survival to transplantation for patients receiving the HeartMate VE left ventricular assist device (LVAD) versus nonrandomized, historical control subjects. **B,** Kaplan-Meier survival estimate of the probability of 1-year posttransplantation survival for patients receiving the HeartMate VE LVAD versus nonrandomized, historical control subjects. *(From Frazier OH, Rose EA, Oz MC, et al. Multicenter clinical evaluation of the HeartMate vented electric left ventricular assist system in patients awaiting heart transplantation. J Thorac Cardiovasc Surg. 2001;122:1186-1195.)*

113 (40%), neurologic dysfunction in 14 (5%), and thromboembolic events in 17 (6%). Twenty-nine percent (82 of 280) of patients receiving the HeartMate VE died before heart transplantation, compared with 67% of control subjects (32 of 48; $P < .001$). Overall, 71% (198 of 280) of the study cohort survived, with 67% (188 of 280) receiving heart transplantation and 4% (10 of 280) undergoing elective device explantation. One-year post-transplantation survival of the study cohort receiving LVAD therapy was superior to that of the control cohort (84% [158 of 188] vs. 63% [10 of 16]; log rank analysis $P = .0197$) (Fig. 21-7).

The HeartMate VE was approved for BTT in 1998. The HeartMate XVE, a modification of the HeartMate VE device, included design enhancements to the internal diaphragm, inflow and outflow valve housing, and percutaneous lead. This device was incorporated into clinical practice without the need for formal clinical evaluation and replaced the HeartMate VE device.[17,18] One of the major limitations of the HeartMate VE and XVE design was the limited reliability and durability of the inflow valve and internal motor bearings, leading to the need for device replacement or change in over 50% by 2 years (Fig. 21-8).[19] The HeartMate XVE is now rarely used in clinical practice, having been almost entirely replaced by the newer generation of continuous-flow rotary pumps.

Although the Novacor device was the subject of an FDA-approved clinical trial before the introduction of the HeartMate VE device, the HeartMate VE device became the more frequently used device of the era.[20] The major asset of the Novacor device design was its long-term mechanical reliability and durability compared with other pulsatile device designs of the time (i.e., HeartMate XVE and HeartMate IP). However, limitations in the inflow conduit design resulted in a high rate of thromboembolic events leading to stroke.[21] Subsequent modifications to materials in the inflow conduit decreased rates of stroke.[21] The Novacor LVAD was approved by the FDA for BTT in 1998 and underwent further clinical evaluation for DT (see section on Clinical Trials Evaluating Mechanical Circulatory Support Devices for Destination Therapy [Permanent Pump Implantation]). However, manufacture of the device was halted in 2007 and it is no longer available for clinical use.

A randomized clinical trial comparing durable, implantable MCS devices with medical therapy for BTT has not been performed because of the perceived efficacy of VAD therapy and the ethical concerns regarding withholding this therapy in a critically ill population at risk of imminent death (estimated 6-month mortality >75%).[16] Robust and consistent historical outcomes data on more than 500 MCS pulsatile devices accumulated in an industry-sponsored registry (Thoratec Corporation), gathered from both premarket, FDA-sponsored clinical trials and postmarket surveillance and spanning 10 years of use with the Thoratec PVAD, HeartMate IP1000, HeartMate VE, and Thoratec IVAD devices, have permitted the establishment of benchmarks for evaluation of subsequent devices.[6,8,16] These benchmarks, or performance measures, have been generally defined as the cumulative percentage of patients meeting the following successful endpoints: (1) survival on device support to transplantation, (2) survival on device support until myocardial recovery, or (3) alive on device support at 180 days while remaining eligible for heart transplantation. The last criterion of 180 days of support was defined based on the average duration of support observed in the aforementioned trials until transplantation. The historical data support a performance measure of approximately 70% of patients obtaining a successful outcome as defined by the aforementioned criteria. This performance measure was subsequently used by the FDA to evaluate clinical efficacy and safety of the next generation of durable, implantable MCS devices for BTT.

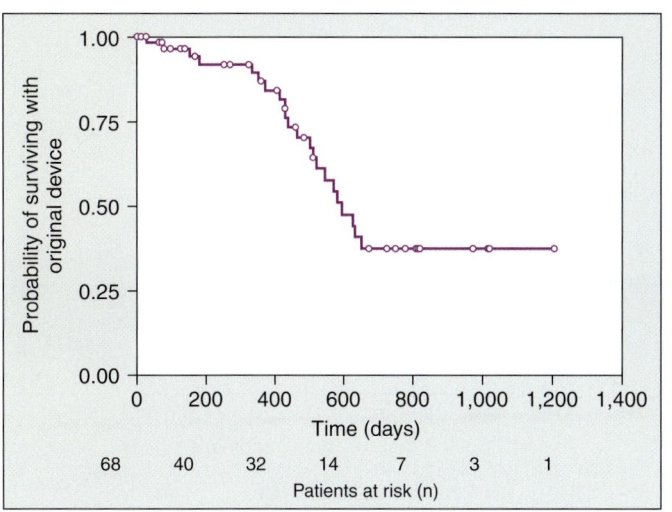

FIGURE 21-8 Freedom from left ventricular assist device (LVAD) replacement. A product-limit estimate curve plotting the probability of being free of device replacement versus time (days) on the HeartMate VE device. Patients were censored (circles) when they died or if, at the last date of follow-up, they had not undergone a device replacement. (From Dembitsky WP, Tector AJ, Park S, et al. Left ventricular assist device performance with long term circulatory lessons from the REMATCH trial. Ann Thorac Surg. 2004;78:2123-2130.)

Continuous-Flow MCS Devices with Axial Design

Until recently, first-generation pulsatile volume-displacement devices have been the mainstay of VAD therapy for BTT, with more than 12,000 devices implanted worldwide. However, significant limitations in their design preclude their practical use for extended MCS. These limitations included a large pump size, requirement for extensive surgical dissection for implantation, the need for a large body habitus of the recipient, the presence of a large-diameter percutaneous lead for venting air, and audible pump operation. A critical limitation of the most commonly used implantable pulsatile pump, the HeartMate XVE, was the high incidence of reoperation for device exchange because of malfunction secondary to failure of the inflow valve or internal pump bearings.[17-19]

The development of continuous-flow rotary pump technology represents an innovative design that is likely the single most important advance in the field of MCS. Continuous-flow device technology has now largely replaced the first-generation pulsatile pump designs. Continuous-flow rotary pumps have the advantage of smaller size and the potential for greater mechanical reliability, having simplified the pumping mechanism to a single moving part (Fig. 21-9). In addition, noiseless operation represents a significant advance in patient satisfaction. Reports from clinical trials of newer, axial-design continuous-flow pumps have demonstrated efficacy in providing hemodynamic support and improvements in functional capacity and quality of life.[22]

The HeartMate II (Thoratec Corporation) is a continuous-flow axial rotary pump representative of the second generation of LVAD technology in clinical use in the United States (see Fig. 21-9)[22]; it has undergone extensive clinical evaluation.[22,23] The HeartMate II Pivotal Trial for BTT was an FDA-approved, prospective, nonrandomized, multicenter study of 133 patients with end-stage heart failure who were on a waiting list for heart transplantation and received implantation of the HeartMate II device. The primary endpoint was a composite of the proportions of patients who, at 180 days, had undergone transplantation, had cardiac recovery, or had ongoing MCS with the HeartMate II while remaining eligible for transplantation. The study also assessed functional status and quality of life as well as frequency of serious adverse events.

Of the 133 patients receiving support with the HeartMate II device, the principal outcomes were observed in 100 patients (75%). The median duration of support was 126 days (range 1 to 600 days). The survival rates during support were 75% at 6 months and 68% at 12 months (Fig. 21-10).[22] At 3 and 6 months, device support with the HeartMate II was associated with significant improvement in functional status (according to the New York Heart Association [NYHA] class and results of a 6-minute walk test) and in quality of life (according to both the Minnesota Living with Heart Failure and Kansas City Cardiomyopathy questionnaires; Figs. 21-11 and 21-12).[24] Major adverse events included postoperative bleeding, stroke, right heart failure, and percutaneous lead infection. Pump thrombosis occurred in two patients (Table 21-1).

This, the first report of a clinical trial of the new continuous-flow LVAD, demonstrated the efficacy and safety of an innovative device design in providing effective hemodynamic support for a period of at least 6 months in patients awaiting heart transplantation, with improved functional status and quality of life. Further, this study demonstrated that hemodynamic support with a continuous-flow device, which has a significantly lower pulse pressure than the older pulsatile devices, preserved long-term end-organ function.[25] A historical comparison of adverse events using identical definitions of patients supported by a continuous-flow pump with a similar cohort of patients supported by pulsatile devices

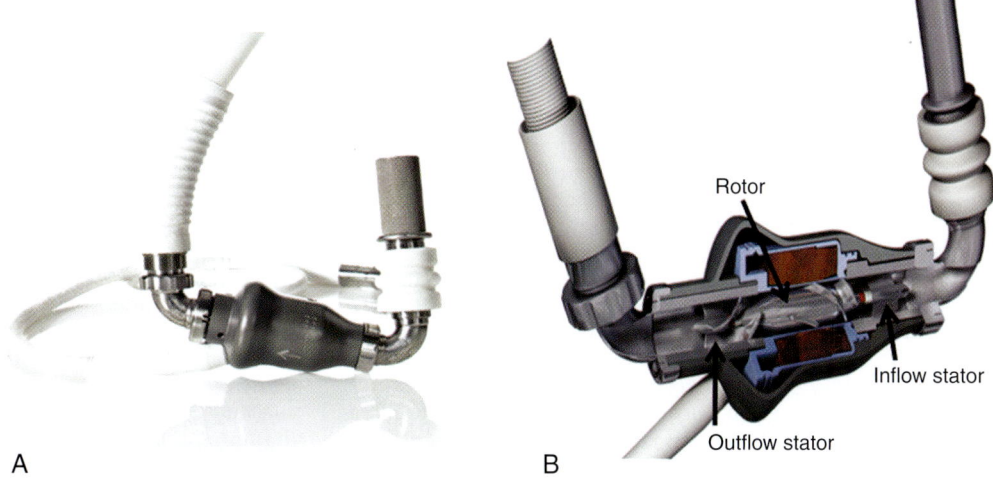

FIGURE 21-9 A, Thoratec HeartMate II is a continuous-flow rotary pump with axial design representative of the second generation of left ventricular assist device (LVAD) technology in clinical use in the United States. B, Diagram showing the internal rotor suspended on bearings within the inflow and outflow stators. The internal rotor is the only moving part in the HeartMate II.

A

B

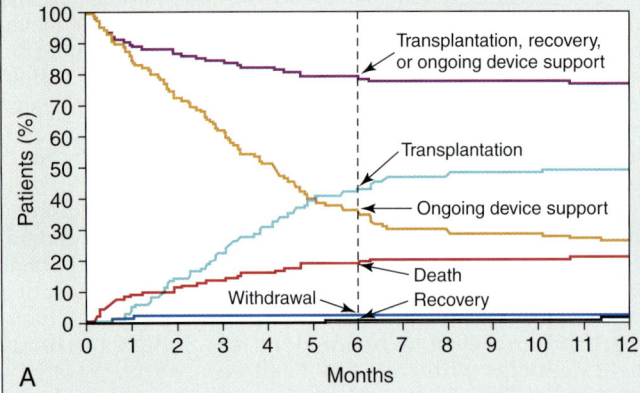

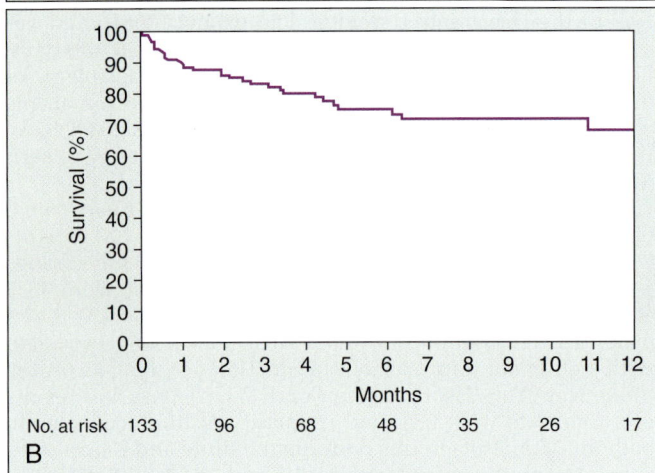

FIGURE 21-10 Outcomes for 133 patients after implantation of the continuous-flow left ventricular assist device (LVAD). **A,** All outcomes over time. After 6 months of mechanical circulatory support (MCS), the outcomes were as follows: 56 patients had undergone heart transplantation (42%); 48 continued to receive MCS (36%), 5 of whom were ineligible for transplantation; 25 had died while receiving MCS (19%); 3 had withdrawn from the study (2%); and 1 had had recovery of ventricular function after explantation of the device (1%). A total of 105 patients (79%) had undergone transplantation, had undergone explantation of the device with recovery of ventricular function, or continued to receive MCS. **B,** Kaplan-Meier analysis of survival for patients who continued to receive MCS, with data censored for heart transplantation and recovery of ventricular function. Withdrawal from the study was counted as a death. *(From Miller LW, Pagani FD, Russell SD, et al. Use of a continuous flow device in patients awaiting heart transplantation. N Engl J Med. 2007;357:885-896.)*

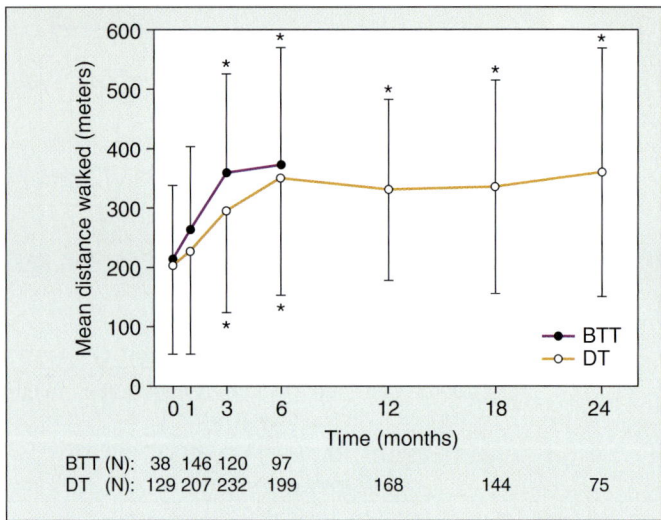

FIGURE 21-11 Submaximal exercise performance after HeartMate II implantation. Mean 6-minute walk distances in the bridge to transplantation (BTT) and destination therapy (DT) trials are shown over time. Ascertainment of baseline 6-minute walk distance was limited to patients able to ambulate. The number of observations (*N*) at each time point is shown at the bottom of the figure. *$P <.05$ compared with baseline. *(From Rogers JG, Aaronson KD, Boyle AJ, et al; HeartMate II Investigators. Continuous flow left ventricular assist device improves functional capacity and quality of life of advanced heart failure patients. J Am Coll Cardiol. 2010;55:1826-1834.)*

demonstrated a significant reduction in major complications with the new continuous-flow design (Fig. 21-13). After this initial report of 133 patients, a follow-up evaluation was conducted in an additional 148 patients undergoing device support with the HeartMate II through a continued-access protocol approved by the FDA during their review of the longer-term data from the original cohort of 133 patients.[23] In an extended, 18-month follow-up report of 281 patients evaluated for BTT therapy with the HeartMate II, 222 (79%) patients met the primary endpoint and either received a transplant, recovered cardiac function and underwent device explantation, or remained alive with ongoing LVAD support.[23] At 18 months, 157 (55.8%) patients had received a heart transplant, 58 (20.6%) remained alive with ongoing LVAD support, 56 (19.9%) patients died, 7 (2.5%) patients recovered cardiac function and underwent device explantation, and 3 (1%) patients were withdrawn from the study after device explantation and exchange for another type of LVAD (Fig. 21-14). The overall survival rate for the patients who continued on LVAD support was 82% (95% confi-

dence interval [CI] 77% to 87%) at 6 months, 73% (95% CI 66% to 80%) at 1 year, and 72% (95% CI 65% to 79%) at 18 months. Of the 157 patients who received a transplant, post-transplantation survival was equal to that in patients not supported by an LVAD in the ISHLT (International Society for Heart and Lung Transplantation) Registry, with survival rates of 96% at 30 days and 86% at 1 year. Notably, the HeartMate II Pivotal Trial for the BTT indication demonstrated a significant improvement in survival and successful study endpoints in the continued-access protocol cohort over the original primary cohort, demonstrating the importance of experience and improved patient selection in device therapy (Fig. 21-15). The primary causes of death were sepsis, stroke, and right heart failure (Table 21-2). Bleeding requiring transfusion and surgery were the most common adverse events in the study, followed by stroke, localized infection not related to the device, infection associated with the percutaneous lead, and pre-peritoneal pump pocket infection and right heart failure. There were no mechanical failures of the pumping mechanism. The freedom from device replacement for all causes, including infection, device thrombosis, and percutaneous lead failure, was 92% (95% CI 88% to 97%) at 18 months (Fig. 21-16).[23] Hepatic (total bilirubin, serum aspartate aminotransferase, and serum alanine aminotransferase) and renal (blood urea nitrogen) function significantly improved from baseline to 6 months, but changes in serum creatinine were not statistically significant.[25]

A very important aspect of the HeartMate II Pivotal Trial was the depth of assessment of the functional improvement and quality-of-life benefits associated with VAD therapy. Functional assessments using the 6-minute walk and NYHA functional classification were performed for patients remaining on device support up to 6 months. Of 109 patients with paired values at baseline and 6 months, only 14 of 109 (13%) were able to perform a 6-minute walk test at baseline, compared with 97 (89%) after 6 months of support. There was significant improvement in distance walked between baseline and 6 months, with over 50% of patients experiencing an improvement in the 6-minute walk distance of over 200 m. The improvement in 6-minute walk distance and quality of

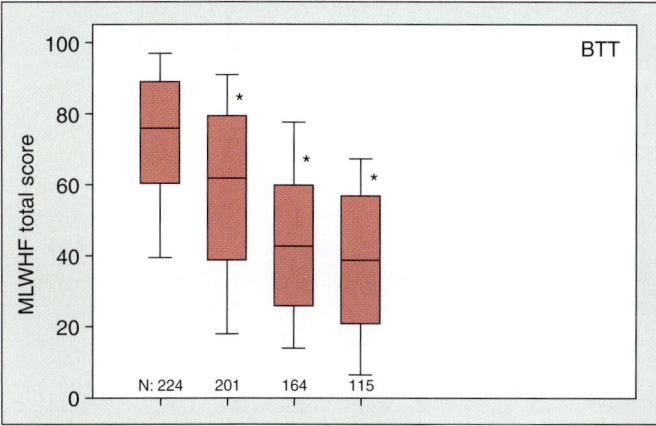

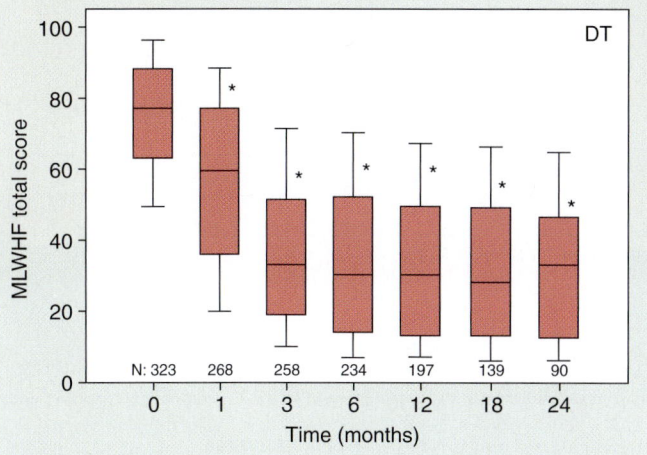

FIGURE 21-12 Changes in quality of life: Minnesota Living with Heart Failure (MLWHF) questionnaire results in the HeartMate II bridge to transplantation (BTT) and destination therapy (DT) clinical trials. Changes in quality of life assessed with the MLWHF questionnaire are shown. Lower values signify improved quality of life. Bars indicate 25th, 50th, and 75th percentiles, whiskers indicate 5th and 95th percentiles. *P <.05 compared with baseline. *(From Rogers JG, Aaronson KD, Boyle AJ, et al; HeartMate II Investigators. Continuous flow left ventricular assist device improves functional capacity and quality of life of advanced heart failure patients. J Am Coll Cardiol. 2010;55:1826-1834.)*

life associated with LVAD therapy, when placed into perspective with improvements seen with cardiac resynchronization therapy, is substantial and dramatic.[3,24,26] In addition, NYHA functional classification improved from 3.9 ± 0.3 at baseline (with 0% of patients in NYHA functional class I or II) to 1.8 ± 0.7 at 6 months (with 83% in functional class I or II). Quality of life as assessed by both the Minnesota Living with Heart Failure and the Kansas City Cardiomyopathy questionnaires was significantly improved at 6 months compared with baseline, with mean scores improving over 25 units, or 41% and 75%.

The introduction of continuous-flow technology into clinical practice was a milestone in the field of MCS therapy and led to significant improvements in survival and reduction of serious major adverse events, especially in the area of device malfunctions. Compared with pulsatile devices, continuous-flow technology demonstrated at least equal efficacy regarding hemodynamic support, ability to improve renal and hepatic function, rates of heart transplantation, and overall patient survival. Importantly, significantly fewer deaths were observed during late follow-up (6 to 18 months), suggesting that the incidences of major events contributing to deaths such as stroke, infection, and device malfunction were significantly lower. This late reduction in deaths had not been observed with pulsatile pumps.[1,16] Excellent late survival on LVAD support (12 to 18 months) was maintained in the absence of continuing high rates of attrition to heart transplantation, suggesting that significant complications were not treated with urgent transplantation; this can likely be attributed, in part, to the improved durability of the device and the markedly reduced need for replacement.

Several other CF pumps with axial design are in clinical evaluation in the United States. These include the Jarvik 2000 (Jarvik Heart, New York) and MicroMed DeBakey HeartAssist 5 (MicroMed Corporation, Houston, TX). The Jarvik 2000 is an axial-design continuous-flow rotary pump with the unique feature of having the pumping chamber located inside the left ventricle (Fig. 21-17).[27,28] The device design permits flexibility in surgical approach, including placement through a median sternotomy with a left ventricular apical-to-ascending aortic connection, or through a left thoracotomy incision with a left ventricular apical-to-descending aortic connection. The Jarvik 2000 is currently undergoing clinical

TABLE 21-1	Adverse Events in Original Study Cohort of 133 Study Patients in the HeartMate II Bridge to Transplant Pivotal Trial*								
	Overall			*0-30 Days*			*>30 Days*		
Event	Patients with Event (%)	No. Events	Event Rate per PY	Patients with Event	No. Events	Event Rate per PY	Patients with Event	No. Events	Event Rate per PY
Bleeding									
Requiring surgery	41 (31)	48	0.78	40	45	4.41	1	3	0.06
Requiring ≥2 units of packed red cells only	70 (53)	129	2.09	60	85	8.33	10	44	0.85
Ventricular arrhythmias†	32 (24)	49	0.79	24	26	2.55	8	23	0.45
Infection									
Local, not related to device	37 (28)	70	1.13	28	37	3.63	9	33	0.64
Sepsis	27 (20)	38	0.62	18	18	1.77	9	20	0.39
Percutaneous lead	18 (14)	23	0.37	0	0	0.00	18	23	0.45
Pump pocket	0	0	0.00	0	0	0.00	0	0	0.00
Respiratory failure	34 (26)	43	0.70	29	32	3.14	5	11	0.21
Renal failure	18 (14)	19	0.31	15	15	1.47	3	4	0.08
Right heart failure									
Need for right ventricular assist device	5 (4)	5	0.08	4	4	0.39	1	1	0.02
Need for extended inotropic support‡	17 (13)	17	0.28	12	12	1.18	5	5	0.10

TABLE 21-1 | **Adverse Events in Original Study Cohort of 133 Study Patients in the HeartMate II Bridge to Transplant Pivotal Trial*—Cont'd**

Event	Overall			0-30 Days			>30 Days		
	Patients with Event (%)	No. Events	Event Rate per PY	Patients with Event	No. Events	Event Rate per PY	Patients with Event	No. Events	Event Rate per PY
Stroke									
Ischemic	8 (6)	8	0.13	5§	5	0.49	3	3	0.06
Hemorrhagic	3 (2)	3	0.05	2	2	0.20	1	1	0.02
Spinal cord infarct	1 (1)	1	0.02	0	0	0.00	1	1	0.02
Transient ischemic attack	5 (4)	6	0.10	2	2	0.20	3	4	0.08
Psychological	9 (7)	11	0.18	6	6	0.59	3	5	0.10
Other neurologic	8 (6)	10	0.16	3	3	0.29	5	7	0.14
Peripheral non-neurologic thromboembolic event	9 (7)	9	0.15	8	8	0.78	1	1	0.02
Device replacement¶	5 (4)	5	0.08	3	3	0.29	2	2	0.04
Device thromboses‖	2 (2)	2	0.03	1	1	0.10	1	1	0.02
Complications of surgical implantation**	3 (2)	3	0.05	2	2	0.20	1	1	0.02
Hemolysis	4 (3)	4	0.06	3	3	0.29	1	1	0.02
Hepatic dysfunction	3 (2)	3	0.05	2	2	0.20	1	1	0.02

*The cumulative duration of device support was 61.7 patient-years (PY) overall, 10.2 PY for 0-30 days, and 51.5 PY for >30 days.

†This event required cardioversion or defibrillation.

‡The duration of support was for a period longer than 14 days or starting after day 14.

§All events occurred within the first 2 days after implantation.

¶Devices were replaced with another HeartMate II in two patients and with another left ventricular assist device in three patients.

‖These events occurred on day 24 and day 56.

**Complications included a surgical pledget that was trapped in the pump (day 1), a temporary right ventricular assist device that caused a kink in the outflow graft (day 15), and malpositioning of the inflow cannula (day 32).

From Miller LW, Pagani FD, Russell SD, et al. Use of a continuous-flow device in patients awaiting heart transplantation. *N Engl J Med*. 2007;357:885-896.

Event	HeartMate II Cohort* (92.4 pt yrs)		HeartMate VE BTT# (86.2 pt yrs)		Risk ratio (95% CI)
	# Events	Events/pt yr	# Events	Events/pt yr	
Stroke	17	0.18	38	0.44	0.42 (0.22-0.79)
Other neurologic event	19	0.21	58	0.67	0.31 (0.17-0.55)
Bleeding requiring surgery	65	0.70	127	1.47	0.48 (0.31-0.73)
Percutaneous lead infection	30	0.32	301	3.49	0.09 (0.06-0.15)
RHF requiring RVAD	10	0.11	26	0.30	0.36 (0.16-0.79)

FIGURE 21-13 Historical comparison of adverse events using identical definitions of patients supported with a continuous flow pump (HeartMate II) with a similar cohort of patients supported with a pulsatile device (HeartMate VE) showed significant reductions in major complications with the new continuous flow design. BTT, bridge to transplant; CI, confidence interval; RHF, right heart failure; RVAD, right ventricular assist device. *(From Thoratec Corporation FDA Advisory Panel Presentation, November 2007; Frazier OH, Rose EA, Oz MC, et al. Multicenter clinical evaluation of the HeartMate vented electric left ventricular assist system in patients awaiting heart transplantation.* J Thorac Cardiovasc Surg. *2001;122:1186-1195; Pagani FD, Miller LW, Russell SD, et al. Extended mechanical circulatory support with a continuous-flow rotary left ventricular assist device: HeartMate II Investigators.* J Am Coll Cardiol. *2009;54:312-321.)*

evaluation for BTT in the United States in an FDA-approved clinical trial. As of this writing, comprehensive published data from its pivotal trial are not available.

The MicroMed DeBakey HeartAssist 5 is another axial-design continuous-flow rotary pump (Fig. 21-18).[29] The device initially underwent U.S. clinical evaluation for BTT in an FDA-approved, multicenter, nonrandomized clinical trial in 2004. A significant rate of device thrombosis with the initial pump design resulted in a number of modifications, culminating in the current HeartAssist 5 model. Comprehensive published data from the FDA-approved Pivotal Trial for BTT are not currently available.

Continuous-Flow MCS Devices with Centrifugal Design

Although significant improvements in pump design have been realized with the second generation of continuous-flow rotary pumps (axial design), there remain a number of potential concerns with this technology. The use of contact bearings and stators to suspend the rotor offers a potential point of frictional wear that can result in device failure and need for device exchange (see Fig. 21-9). Second-generation pump technology also remains vulnerable to thrombus formation on the device rotor and bearing interface owing

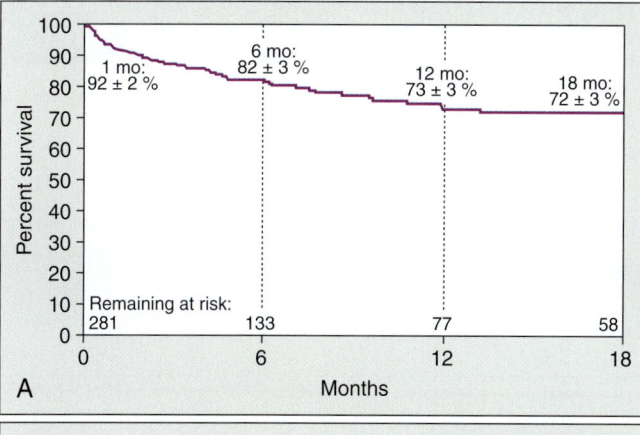

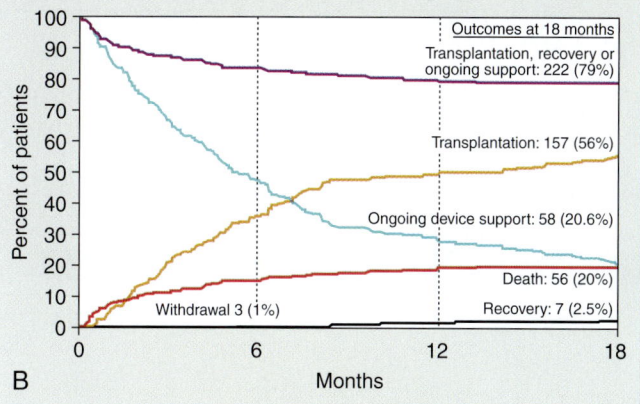

FIGURE 21-14 A, Survival analysis for patients who continued to receive support with the continuous-flow left ventricular assist device (LVAD) censored at the time of heart transplantation and device explantation for cardiac recovery. **B,** Competing outcomes analysis of patients undergoing implantation of the continuous flow LVAD for the first 18 months after device implantation. *(From Pagani FD, Miller LW, Russell SD, et al. Extended mechanical circulatory support with a continuous flow rotary left ventricular assist device: HeartMate II Investigators.* J Am Coll Cardiol. *2009;54:312-321.)*

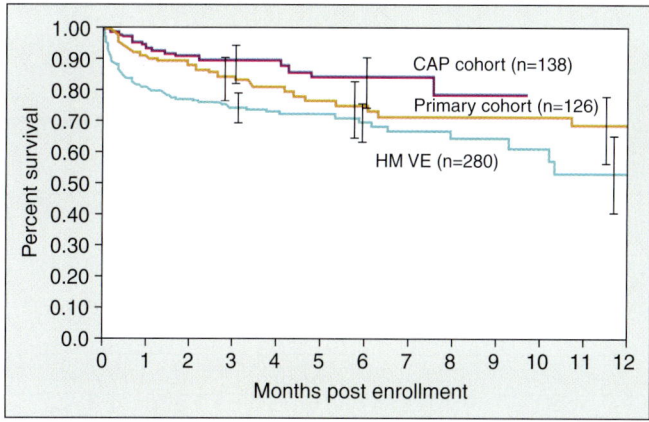

FIGURE 21-15 Kaplan-Meier survival estimate for patients receiving the HeartMate II continuous-flow device during the original FDA-sponsored clinical trial (primary cohort) compared with patients receiving the HeartMate II continuous-flow device during the continued-access protocol (CAP cohort) and patients receiving the HeartMate VE pulsatile device (HM VE—historical comparison). *(From Thoratec Corporation FDA Advisory Panel Presentation, November 2007; Frazier OH, Rose EA, Oz MC, et al. Multicenter clinical evaluation of the HeartMate vented electric left ventricular assist system in patients awaiting heart transplantation.* J Thorac Cardiovasc Surg. *2001;122:1186-1195; Miller LW, Pagani FD, Russell SD, et al. Use of a continuous-flow device in patients awaiting heart transplantation.* N Engl J Med. *2007;357:885-896.)*

to hemodynamic stasis and incomplete bearing wash.[23,29] However, the concern for development of thrombus on the rotor and bearing contact points has varied significantly with different second-generation rotary pumps.[29] The presence of stators to suspend and redirect blood flow also places an obstruction in the path of flow. Thrombosis resulting from blood stasis can be caused by blood flow disturbances and recirculating zones associated with the supports required by the contact bearing design. Clinical studies have documented the problem with device thrombus requiring device exchange or treatment with thrombolytic therapy, and have also shown a reduced but persistent risk of stroke.[23,29,30] A significant proportion of strokes reported during clinical trials with second-generation devices have occurred early after surgery and were associated with the implant procedure, likely representing air or particulate emboli from sources such as the left ventricular cavity rather than arising from device design. The proportion of strokes attributable to transient thrombus formation in the pump as opposed to thrombus formation in the heart is unknown. In addition, this technology still requires long-term antithrombotic therapy, which has been associated with an increase in the rate of hemorrhagic complications over that seen with pulsatile devices.

The designation *third-generation rotary pump* has generally been used to categorize continuous-flow rotary devices with an impeller or rotor suspended in the blood flow path using a noncontact bearing design (Fig. 21-19).[31,32] In most circumstances this design uses a "centrifugal" blood flow path and incorporates either magnetic or hydrodynamic levitation of the internal impeller. Continuous-flow pumps incorporating a centrifugal blood flow path and noncontact bearing design in clinical trial evaluation in the United States include the DuraHeart (Terumo Heart Corporation, Ann Arbor, MI), HVAD (HeartWare Corporation, Miami, FL), and Levacor (World Heart Corporation).

The VentrAssist (Ventracor Corporation, Sydney, Australia) is a third-generation continuous-flow pump with hydrodynamic bearing design that has undergone successful clinical evaluation in the United States with an FDA-approved, prospective, multicenter, single-arm study of 140 patients with end-stage heart failure awaiting heart transplantation (Fig. 21-20).[33–35] The primary endpoint of the study was survival to transplantation or listed for transplantation at 180 days after LVAD implantation. The primary hypothesis was to determine if the proportion of patients implanted with the VentrAssist LVAD and meeting the primary endpoint was noninferior to a performance measure of 75%. A total of 98 patients reached an endpoint at the prespecified interim analysis, with 77 (78.6%) reaching a successful outcome of transplantation or alive while remaining listed for transplantation at 180 days. This was the first U.S. trial to demonstrate the efficacy of the advanced, noncontact bearing, centrifugal design for durable, implantable MCS support. Despite the success of the VentrAssist device in the FDA-approved pivotal trial for BTT, device manufacturing was discontinued and this VAD is no longer available. Although the data were presented at several national and international forums, the results of this study have not been published.

The DuraHeart is a continuous-flow rotary pump of centrifugal, noncontact bearing design (Fig. 21-21).[36,37] The device uses active magnetic levitation of the impeller along with hydrodynamic bearings to support impeller levitation in case the magnetic levitation system fails. Clinical evaluation of the DuraHeart device was recently concluded in Europe and began in the United States in July 2008. The comprehensive trial data are unavailable at this time. The DuraHeart device has received European Union CE Mark (*Conformité Européenne*) approval based on the results of

TABLE 21-2	Adverse Events in 286 Patients Enrolled in the HeartMate II Bridge to Transplant Pivotal Trial including 133 Primary Cohort Patients and 153 Patients Entered through the Continued Access Protocol								
	Overall			*0-30 Days*			*> 30 Days*		
Cumulative Support Duration (Patient-Years)	*181.8*			*21.7*			*160.2*		
Adverse Event	**Patients with Event, n (%)**	**No. Events**	**Event Rate***	**Patients with Event, n (%)**	**No. Events**	**Event Rate***	**Patients with Event, n (%)**	**No. Events**	**Event Rate***
Bleeding									
Requiring surgery	72 (26)	82	0.45	67	72	3.32	10	10	0.06
Requiring ≥ 2 units packed red blood cells only	148 (53)	303	1.67	128	190	8.76	54	111	0.69
Ventricular arrhythmias†	56 (20)	72	0.40	37	41	1.89	23	31	0.19
Infection									
Local non–device-related infection	84 (30)	155	0.85	64	78	3.59	46	78	0.49
Sepsis	49 (17)	64	0.35	26	27	1.24	27	37	0.23
Percutaneous lead infection	41 (14)	56	0.31	2	2	0.09	39	54	0.34
Pump pocket infection	5 (2)	5	0.03	1	1	0.05	4	4	0.02
Respiratory failure	72 (26)	88	0.48	61	69	3.18	16	19	0.12
Renal failure	30 (11)	31	0.17	24	24	1.11	7	7	0.04
Right heart failure									
Need for right ventricular assist device	17 (6)	17	0.09	16	16	0.74	1	1	0.01
Need for extended inotropic support‡	36 (13)	37	0.20	28	29	1.34	8	8	0.05
Stroke									
Ischemic	15 (5)	16	0.09	8§	8	0.37	7	8	0.05
Hemorrhagic	9 (3)	9	0.05	4	4	0.18	5	5	0.03
Spinal cord infarct	1 (<1)	1	0.01	0	0	0.00	1	1	0.01
Transient ischemic attack	6 (2)	7	0.04	3	3	0.14	4	4	0.02
Psychological	16 (6)	18	0.10	13	13	0.60	3	5	0.03
Other neurologic	15 (5)	17	0.09	4	4	0.18	11	13	0.08
Peripheral non-neurologic thromboembolic event	18 (6)	25	0.14	16	22	1.02	3	3	0.02
Device replacement‖	12 (4)	12	0.07	4	4	0.18	8	8	0.05
Primary device thrombosis¶	4 (1)	4	0.02	2	2	0.09	2	2	0.01
Complications of surgical implantation**	3 (1)	3	0.02	2	2	0.09	1	1	0.01
Percutaneous lead wire damage	4 (1)	4	0.02	0	0	0.00	4	4	0.03
Lead and pump pocket infection	1 (0.4)	1	0.01	0	0	0.00	1	1	0.01
Hemolysis	11 (4)	11	0.06	6	6	0.28	5	5	0.03
Hepatic dysfunction	7 (2)	7	0.04	4	4	0.18	3	3	0.02

*Events per patient-year.
†Requiring cardioversion or defibrillation.
‡Longer than 14 days or starting after day 14.
§Five events within day 0-2.
‖Replaced with HeartMate II (*n* = 9) or other left ventricular assist devices (*n* = 3).
¶ Days 0, 24, 56, 123.
**Surgical pledget trapped in pump (day 1), temporary right ventricular assist device caused kink in left ventricular assist device outflow graft (day 15), or malposition of inflow cannula (day 31).
From Pagani FD, Miller LW, Russell SD, et al. Extended mechanical circulatory support with a continuous-flow rotary left ventricular assist device. HeartMate II Investigators. *J Am Coll Cardiol*. 2009;54:312-321.

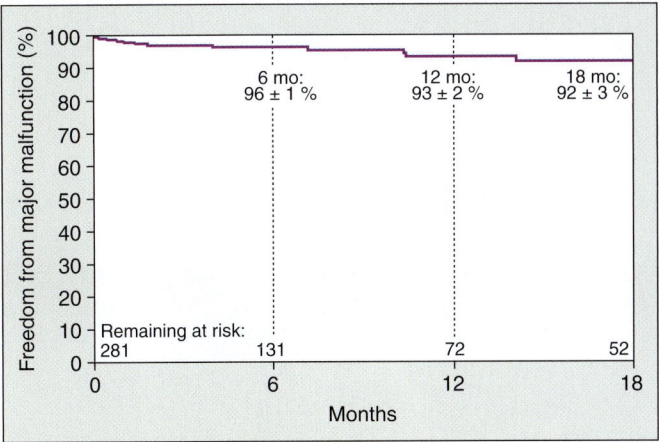

FIGURE 21-16 Kaplan-Meier analysis of the freedom from need for device replacement in the HeartMate II Bridge to Therapy Pivotal Trial. *(From Pagani FD, Miller LW, Russell SD, et al. Extended mechanical circulatory support with a continuous-flow rotary left ventricular assist device: HeartMate II Investigators. J Am Coll Cardiol. 2009;54:312-321.)*

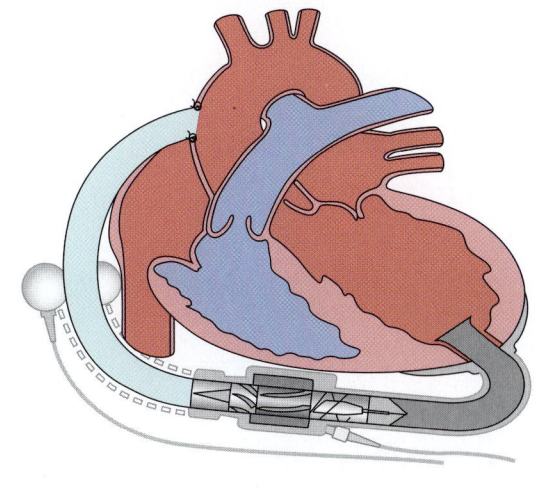

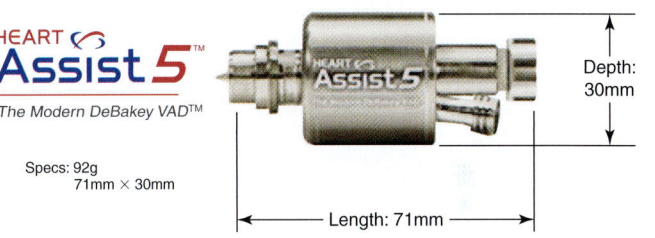

FIGURE 21-18 MicroMed DeBakey HeartAssist 5 is a continuous-flow rotary pump with axial design. *(From Thunberg CA, Gaitan B, Arabia FA, et al. Ventricular assist devices today and tomorrow. J Cardiothorac Vasc Anesth. 2010;24:656-680.)*

its European trial. A preliminary report of the European experience was presented at the meeting of the ISHLT in April 2008.[37] From January 2004 through September 2007, 35 patients with advanced heart failure (NYHA class IV, 14 ischemic, 5 female) who were eligible for heart transplantation underwent implantation of the DuraHeart device. Of patients, 14 (40%) underwent heart transplantation at 194 ± 146 days. There were 19 patients (54%) supported for at least 6 months and 7 (20%) patients supported for greater than 1 year. There were 14 patients (40%) alive with ongoing device support (330 ± 292) days. The Kaplan-Meier estimate of survival at 2 years was 78%.

The HVAD (HeartWare Corp., Framingham, MA) is a small continuous-flow rotary pump of centrifugal, noncontact bearing design (Fig. 21-22).[38,39] The unique feature of the HVAD is its small size, permitting implantation in the cardiac ventricle with the pump located within the pericardium and obviating the need to create a preperitoneal pump pocket. The HVAD has undergone clinical evaluation in Europe and Australia; clinical evaluation in the United States began in May 2008 and completed enrollment in March 2010. A continued-access protocol extension approved by the FDA to allow continued enrollment is now ongoing. A unique feature of the HVAD Pivotal Trial for BTT was the comparison of the device arm with a prospective, observational control arm accumulated

through the INTERMACS registry (see section on Mechanical Circulatory Support Device Outcomes in INTERMACS). There are no published data from U.S. trials, but the device has received European Union CE Mark approval based on the results of a 50-patient trial.

The Levacor (World Heart Corp., Salt Lake City, UT) is a continuous-flow rotary pump using total magnetic levitation and a noncontact bearing design (Fig. 21-23).[40] Clinical evaluation of the Levacor device was initiated in Europe and Canada with successful results reported in a BTR protocol.[41] Clinical evaluation in the United States began in 2010 with an FDA-approved, multicenter, prospective, single-arm trial for BTT. There are no published data from U.S. trials to date.

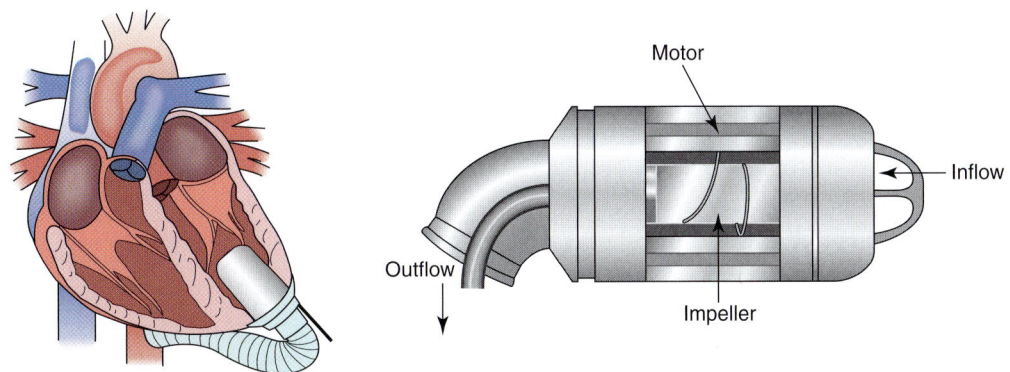

FIGURE 21-17 Jarvik 2000 is a continuous-flow rotary pump with axial design and the unique feature of having the pumping chamber located within the left ventricle. *(From Thunberg CA, Gaitan B, Arabia FA, et al. Ventricular assist devices today and tomorrow. J Cardiothorac Vasc Anesth. 2010;24:656-680.)*

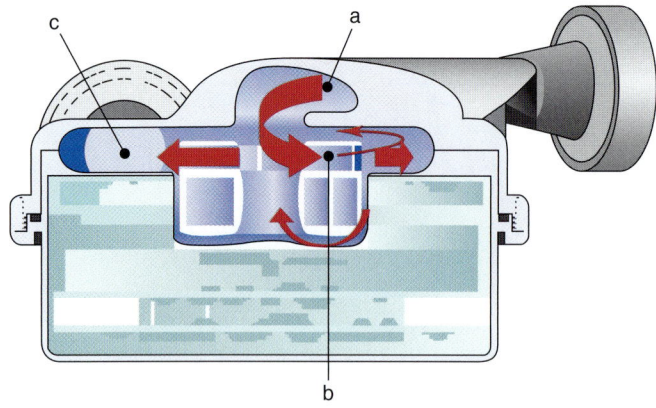

FIGURE 21-19 Example of a third-generation continuous-flow rotary pump with centrifugal design incorporating active magnetic levitation and coupling of the internal impeller with a bearingless drive system. Schematic diagram of the Thoratec HeartMate III: the main blood flow path from the inflow section *(a)*, blood flow path through the impeller and the backflow paths above the shroud and between the rotor and motor *(b)*, and outflow path *(c)*. The impeller is suspended in the blood using a magnetic field, obviating the need for bearing support. *(From Farrar DJ, Bourque K, Dague CP, et al. Design features, developmental status, and experimental results with the Heartmate III centrifugal left ventricular assist system with a magnetically levitated rotor. ASAIO J. 2007;53:310-315.)*

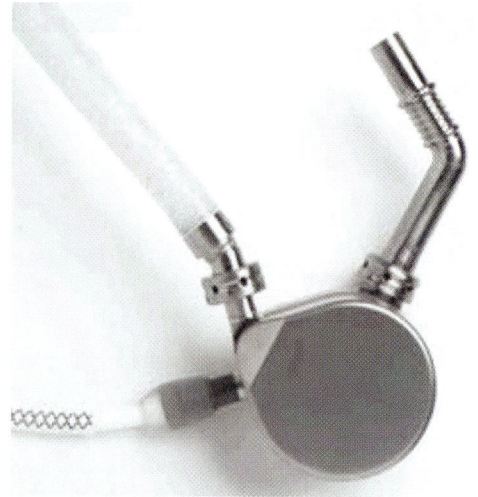

FIGURE 21-21 DuraHeart left ventricular assist device (LVAD) is a continuous-flow rotary pump with centrifugal and noncontact bearing design. The device has a displacement volume of $180 \, cm^3$ and a weight of $540 \, g$. Its external dimensions are 72 mm in width and 45 mm in height. The pumping unit consists of an upper housing with the levitation system, the impeller, and a bottom housing containing the external drive motor. The device is designed with active magnetic levitation of the impeller along with hydrodynamic bearings to support impeller levitation in case the magnetic levitation system fails. The impeller is rotated through magnetic coupling between permanent magnets embedded on the motor side of the impeller and an external drive motor that uses a bearing design. Three electromagnets and three position sensors are mounted in the upper housing. Tilting and axial displacements of the impeller are monitored and controlled using a three-degrees-of-freedom controller. The ferromagnetic ring on the opposite side of the impeller is levitated by the electromagnet, and position sensors control the impeller so that it is always positioned at the center of the blood chamber. Radial impeller movement is passively suspended with a bias flux through the electromagnetic rotor and drive magnet rotor.

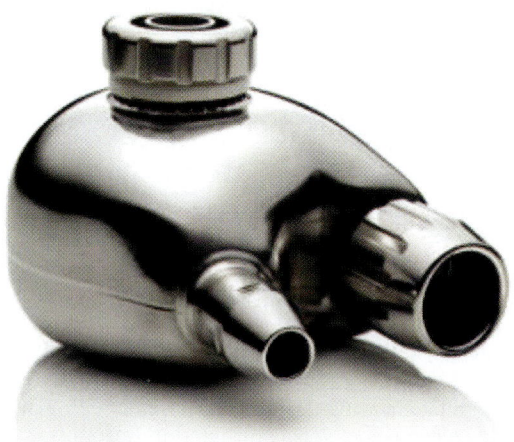

FIGURE 21-20 Ventracor VentrAssist left ventricular assist device (LVAD) is a continuous-flow rotary pump with noncontact bearing design. Impeller levitation inside the pump is achieved using hydrodynamic bearings.

Total Artificial Heart Technology

The CardioWest total artificial heart (TAH; Syncardia Corporation, Tucson, AZ) is a pneumatically actuated pump designed for orthotopic replacement of the native cardiac ventricles and all cardiac valves (Fig. 21-24).[42,43] The only clinical evaluation of this device was a large, prospective, nonrandomized trial conducted in five centers in 81 BTT patients at risk for imminent death from irreversible biventricular cardiac failure.[42] The study cohort was compared with a nonrandomized, observational control cohort of 35 patients. The primary study endpoints included the rates of survival to heart transplantation and survival after transplantation. The rate of survival to transplantation was 79% (95% CI 68% to 87%). Of the 35 patients in the control cohort who met the same entry criteria but did not receive the TAH, 46% (16) survived to transplantation (*P* <.001; Fig. 21-25). Overall, the 1-year survival rate among the patients who received the TAH was 70% compared

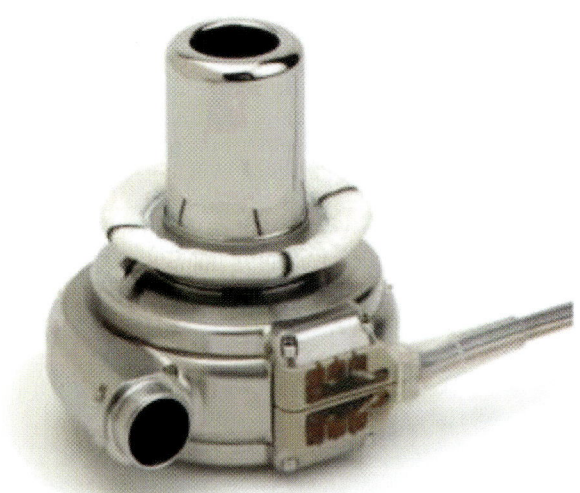

FIGURE 21-22 HeartWare HVAD left ventricular assist device (LVAD) is a small, continuous-flow rotary pump with centrifugal and noncontact bearing design. The unique feature of the HVAD is its small size. It has a displacement volume of 45 mL and weighs 145 g but has a flow capacity of up to 10 L/min. The impeller of the HVAD is suspended in place by a combination of passive magnetic and hydrodynamic bearing systems. The impeller suspension system uses a passive magnetic bearing for radial stiffness. Axial magnetic preload and hydrodynamic bearings on top of each impeller blade provide axial constraint. The magnetic bearing consists of a stack of rare earth ring magnets near the inside diameter of the impeller that repel the magnetic force of a similar stack of magnets inside the center post. The axial alignment of the center-post magnet stack is set to provide an axial force that pushes the impeller toward the forward housing (the assembly with the inflow cannula). Physical contact between the housing and the impeller is prevented by a thin blood film generated by the hydrodynamic bearings.

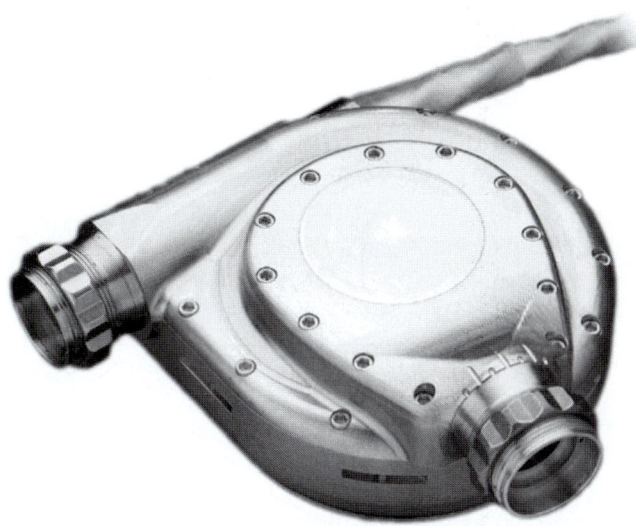

FIGURE 21-23 The Levacor left ventricular assist device (LVAD) is a continuous-flow rotary pump with centrifugal and noncontact bearing design. The pump is 35 mm high, is 75 mm in diameter, and weighs 440 g. The magnetic levitation system uses a combination of permanent magnets that provide passive levitation and a magnet coil that provides active levitation along one degree-of-freedom of movement of the impeller. The magnetic levitation of the rotor allows large fluid gaps compared with pumps with conventional bearings, resulting in lower shear stress on blood components.

with 31% among the control subjects (P <.001). After transplantation, 1-year and 5-year survival rates among patients who had received the TAH were 86% and 64%.

The CardioWest TAH was approved by the FDA for BTT in 2007. To date, there have been no randomized comparisons of the CardioWest TAH with biventricular assist technology. Importantly, the TAH demonstrated excellent survival to heart transplantation, comparable with that observed with use of VADs, despite the critical illness of the study cohort. The CardioWest TAH represents an alternative or possibly preferable device option in large patients with severe biventricular failure for whom the likelihood of myocardial recovery is extremely low. Development of new designs for the pneumatic drive console permit enhanced patient mobility and hospital discharge. A major limitation to the CardioWest TAH is the technical complexity of implant. In addition, TAH device malfunctions are generally fatal given the absence of the native heart to provide circulatory support in the setting of pump failure.

CLINICAL TRIALS EVALUATING MECHANICAL CIRCULATORY SUPPORT DEVICES FOR DESTINATION THERAPY (PERMANENT PUMP IMPLANTATION)

The limited availability of suitable donor hearts coupled with the residually high morbidity and mortality associated with advanced heart failure in patients ineligible for transplantation led to trials that investigated MCS as permanent therapy. The preliminary BTT experience suggested that prolonged MCS was not only feasible, but that patients were likely to experience survival and quality-of-life improvements relative to treatment with medical therapy. This enthusiasm was counterbalanced by the recognition that the age and comorbidities of DT patients might significantly differ from the BTT population, and the impact of these characteristics on VAD outcomes was unexplored. These factors converged to provide the rationale for clinical trials examining the role for mechanical circulatory support in nontransplant candidates.

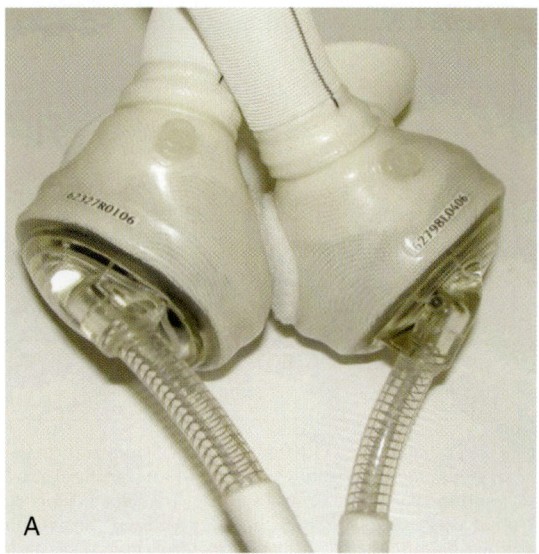

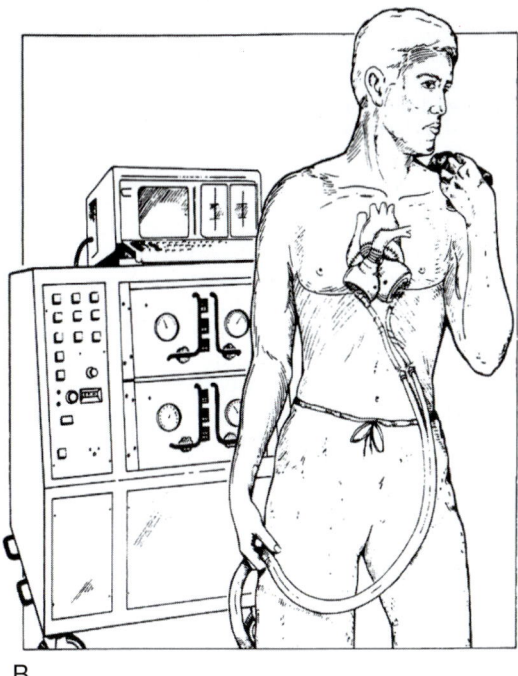

FIGURE 21-24 A, The Syncardia CardioWest total artificial heart (TAH) is a pneumatically actuated pump designed for orthotopic replacement of the native cardiac ventricles and valves. The pump weighs 160 g, has a maximal stroke volume of 70 mL, and is capable of delivering an output of 9 L/min. B, The standard driver for the Syncardia device allowed patients to be ambulatory but was typically limited to hospital use. A newer pneumatic driver that is smaller and enables hospital discharge is under investigation.

Pulsatile Pumps

The practical aspects of prolonged MCS in patients ineligible for transplantation was initially explored in a small pilot study that enrolled 21 patients at 5 sites.[44] The results of this trial were never published, but several patients were successfully supported in excess of 600 days. Based on these results, it was thought that a larger scale, randomized trial testing VAD therapy against optimal-medical therapy was feasible.

In 1998, the NHLBI funded the REMATCH trial.[1] REMATCH was a pivotal trial designed to assess morbidity, mortality, and functional outcomes in a homogeneous cohort of patients with advanced heart failure who were ineligible for cardiac transplantation. This study randomized patients with chronic

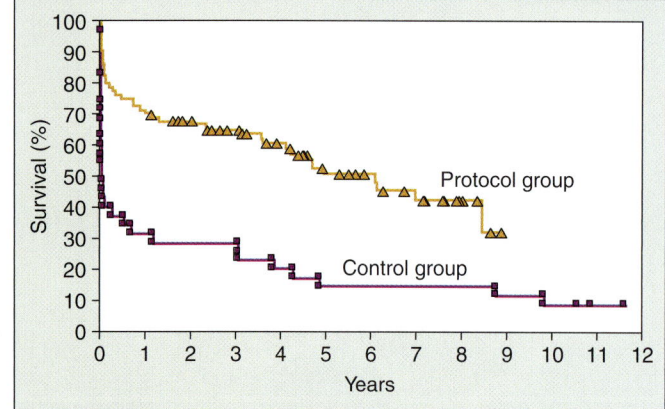

FIGURE 21-25 Overall survival rate from the time of study entry to the termination of the study among patients who received a total artificial heart (TAH) according to protocol, and the control subjects. The Kaplan-Meier curve for the control subjects extends 2.5 years beyond the curve of the patients in the protocol group because the recruitment of control subjects began in 1991 and recruitment of patients for the protocol group began in 1993. There was a large difference in the early mortality rate between the two groups, but the survival curves became parallel after transplantation. The symbols on each curve indicate the points at which data were censored. *(From Copeland JG, Smith RG, Arabia FA, et al; CardioWest Total Artificial Heart Investigators. Cardiac replacement with a total artificial heart as a bridge to transplantation. N Engl J Med. 2004;351:859-867.)*

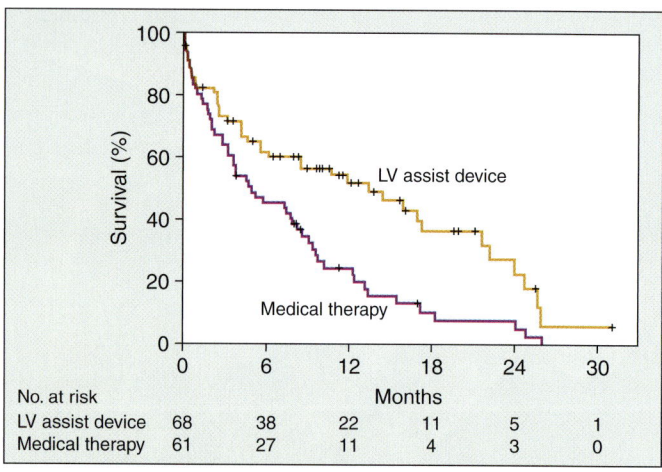

FIGURE 21-26 Kaplan-Meier analysis of survival in the group that received left ventricular (LV) assist devices and the group that received optimal medical therapy in the REMATCH trial. *Crosses* depict censored patients. Enrollment in the trial was terminated after 92 patients had died; 95 deaths had occurred by the time of the final analysis. *(From Rose EA, Gelijns AC, Moskowitz AJ, et al; Randomized Evaluation of Mechanical Assistance for the Treatment of Congestive Heart Failure [REMATCH] Study Group. Long-term mechanical left ventricular assistance for end-stage heart failure. N Engl J Med. 2001;345:1435-1443.)*

end-stage heart failure, NYHA class IV symptoms, an ejection fraction of 25% or less, and a maximal oxygen consumption of no more than 12 mL/kg/min (or dependence on continuous infusion inotropic therapy) to optimal medical therapy or the HeartMate VE LVAD. Contraindications to transplantation included advanced age, diabetes with end-organ dysfunction, chronic renal insufficiency (serum creatinine >2.5 mg/dL), or other comorbidities determined to preclude transplantation. The trial was conducted at 20 U.S. centers with expertise in medical and device therapies for advanced heart failure. Patient enrollment was monitored by a "gatekeeper" to ensure uniformity of the patient population, conformity to the inclusion and exclusion criteria, and the use of evidence-based therapies at baseline.

For study enrollment, 930 patients were screened, and 129 patients met inclusion criteria. REMATCH was an event-driven trial scheduled to enroll 140 patients or continue until 92 deaths occurred. At the time enrollment was halted, 68 patients had been randomly assigned to VAD and 61 patients had been randomly assigned to medical therapy. Baseline characteristics of the cohort included a mean age of 67 years, 20% women, and a mean ejection fraction of 17%. Marked hemodynamic derangements were present, including a mean pulmonary capillary wedge pressure of 24 mm Hg and a mean cardiac index of 2 L/min/m² despite the use of intravenous inotropic medications in nearly 70% of the overall cohort. Additional high-risk features of the study population included elevated serum creatinine and hyponatremia.

The REMATCH survival analysis is shown in Figure 21-26. Survival at 1 year (52% vs. 25%; P = .002) and 2 years (23% vs. 8%; P = .09) was superior in the VAD patients compared with the patients randomly assigned to medical therapy. The relative risk reduction for mortality was 0.52 (range 0.34 to 0.78; P = .001) at 12 months. The trial was analyzed by intent-to-treat despite an open access to crossover from the medical arm to receive a device at 1 year, which occurred in eight patients. The mode of death in nearly all of the patients in the medical therapy arm was heart failure, whereas patients with a VAD were more likely to die from infectious complications or device failure. The overall adverse event rate was higher

in the VAD cohort (risk ratio 2.35; 95% CI 1.86 to 2.95), with higher rates of bleeding, neurologic dysfunction, infections, thromboembolic complications, and renal failure.

Secondary endpoints of the trial included quality of life and patient functionality. VAD-treated patients had significant improvements in quality of life as measured by the SF-36 physical and emotional scores. The Minnesota Living with Heart Failure score was not different between groups. The median NYHA functional class at 1 year in the survivors was II in the VAD-treated patients versus IV in the patients on medical therapy.

The results of the REMATCH trial showed the feasibility of "long-term" MCS and led to FDA approval in 2002 of the HeartMate XVE for use in patients with advanced heart failure who were failing optimal medical therapy and were ineligible for transplantation. REMATCH also reinforced the impressively poor survival rate of advanced heart failure treated with contemporary medical therapy. Although the trial demonstrated improvements in mortality and quality of life in VAD-treated patients, the overall 2-year survival rate of 24% and the frequency of device-related complications and modest device durability limited the clinical application of the HeartMate XVE for DT.

After publication of the original REMATCH results, Park and colleagues analyzed the outcomes of the trial based on the era of enrollment (Fig. 21-27).[45] Despite more high-risk characteristics, patients enrolled in the latter half of the study had significantly higher 1- and 2-year survival rates than those enrolled early in the experience. A similar improvement in survival outcomes was seen in the postapproval registry, with a 56% 1-year survival rate.[46,47] Improved outcomes with VAD use and experience is a consistent observation that was also evident in the continued-access protocol cohort versus primary cohort in the HeartMate II BTT trial. Demonstration of improved survival outcomes in patients with preimplantation risk profiles that are similar to or worse than those enrolled in the initial randomized trial suggests that refinement of preoperative and postoperative management as well as greater experience with MCS are important factors in determining survival and functional improvement after VAD implantation.

In 2000, World Heart Corporation initiated a pilot trial of the pulsatile Novacor device for use as permanent support in nontransplantation candidates (see Fig. 21-4).[48] The

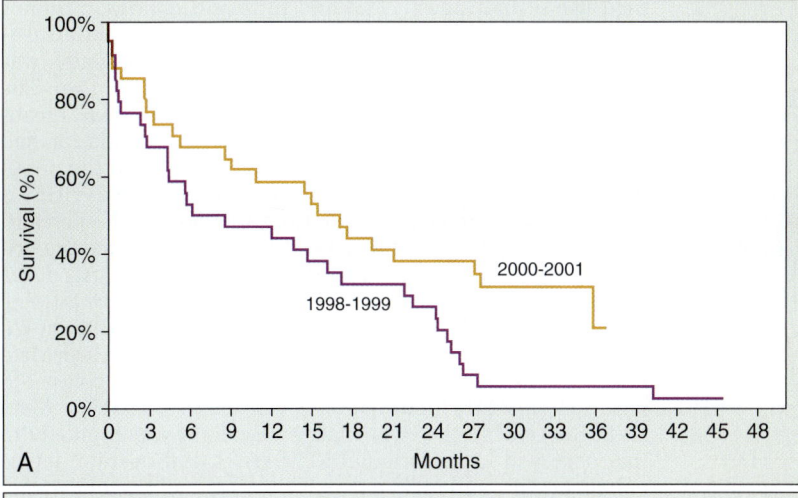

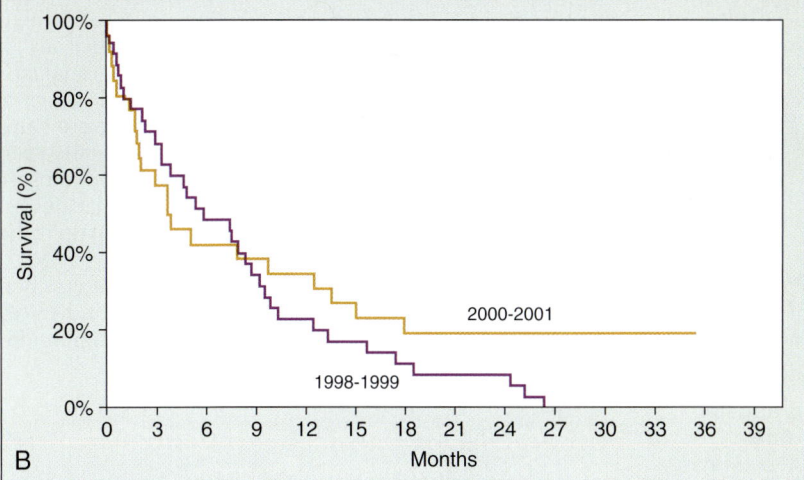

FIGURE 21-27 **A,** Kaplan-Meier survival curves for patients in the REMATCH trial receiving left ventricular assist devices (LVADs) enrolled in 1998-1999 and patients enrolled in 2000-2001 (*P* = .00293). **B,** Kaplan-Meier survival curves of patients in the REMATCH trial receiving optimal medical management enrolled in 1998-1999 and patients enrolled in 2000-2001 (*P* = .2551). *(From Park SJ, Tector A, Piccioni W, et al. Left ventricular assist devices as destination therapy: a new look at survival. J Thorac Cardiovasc Surg. 2005;129:9-17 [erratum appears in J Thorac Cardiovasc Surg. 2005;129:1464].)*

INTrEPID (Investigation of Nontransplant-Eligible Patients Who Are Inotrope Dependent) trial was a prospective, nonrandomized, controlled clinical trial comparing the Novacor LVAD with optimal medical therapy in patients with advanced heart failure. Patients enrolled in this trial had advanced heart failure requiring treatment with intravenous inotropic agents and required two attempts to wean the inotropes separated by at least 7 days.[48] A contemporaneous control group was comprised patients who met the inclusion and exclusion criteria but elected to be treated with medical therapy, had a mechanical aortic valve, or had insufficient financial resources for device implantation and follow-up.

INTrEPID patients were younger than the REMATCH population (mean age, 60 vs. 66 years), but other patient characteristics were similar, including the severity of left ventricular dysfunction and elevated filling pressures despite inotropic support. This cohort also had evidence of end-organ dysfunction, with elevated baseline blood urea nitrogen and creatinine and hyponatremia.

There were 81 patients screened, and 55 patients were enrolled (37 LVAD, 18 optimal medical therapy). The survival rates observed in the trial are shown in Figure 21-28. Patients treated with the VAD had a superior survival at 6 months (46% vs. 22%; *P* = .03) and 12 months (27% vs. 11%) than the patients treated with medical therapy. Stroke and infection were the primary causes of mortality in the VAD-treated patients, whereas progressive heart failure was the cause of death in the medical arm. NYHA functional class and quality-of-life scores improved more in the VAD-treated patients than the patients who remained on medical ther-

apy. Five LVAD patients and one medical therapy patient improved sufficiently while on therapy to qualify for heart transplantation.

The results of INTrEPID were thought sufficient to support a pivotal trial of the Novacor device for DT. The RELIANT (Randomized Evaluation of Novacor LVAD in a Non-Transplant Population) trial was designed to compare morbidity and mortality outcomes in patients randomized to the Novacor versus the HeartMate XVE. During the conduct of this trial, World Heart Corporation elected to focus on the development of a different technology platform and the Novacor device was phased out of clinical use before completion of the study.

Despite differences in trial design, INTrEPID confirmed many of the observations made in REMATCH. First, the role for medical therapy in patients with advanced heart failure is limited, with 1-year survival rates of only 10% to 20%. In addition, both trials demonstrated that medically treated patients are unlikely to experience meaningful improvement in symptoms or quality of life. Conversely, MCS was shown in both trials to improve survival, functional capacity, and quality of life. The cumulative experience from these studies provided a "proof-of-concept" that prolonged LVAD support of patients was feasible. The high early mortality rates seen in the VAD-treated patients focused additional analyses on the importance of patient selection. In addition, it was recognized that the development of VAD technology associated with fewer adverse events and enhanced durability coupled with improved postoperative and long-term management strategies would likely result in more acceptable long-term outcomes.

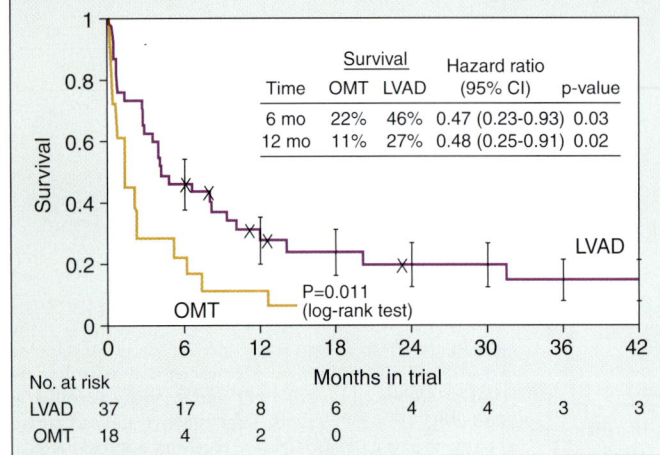

FIGURE 21-28 Survival at 6 months and 12 months in the INTrEPID trial shows an approximate 50% reduction in the risk of death at these time points. Kaplan-Meier survival curves are also shown. The *X* represents censoring at the time of transplantation. CI, confidence interval; LVAD, left ventricular assist device; OMT, optimal medical therapy. *(From Rogers JG, Butler J, Lansman SL, et al. Chronic mechanical circulatory support for inotrope-dependent heart failure patients who are not transplant candidates: results of the INTrEPID Trial. INTrEPID Investigators. J Am Coll Cardiol. 2007;50:741-747.)*

Continuous-Flow Pumps

The new generation of continuous-flow pumps with axial flow design were anticipated to provide hemodynamic benefits similar to those seen with the pulsatile pumps, but were expected to have superior durability with fewer adverse events. In light of these perceived benefits, the HeartMate II Destination Therapy Pivotal Trial was designed and initiated nearly simultaneously with the BTT Pivotal Trial study.

The HeartMate II DT Pivotal Trial randomized 200 patients with NYHA class IIIb to IV symptoms, ejection fraction less than 25%, and a maximal oxygen consumption not exceeding 14 mL/kg/min, or treatment with intravenous inotropic agents for at least 14 days, or an intra-aortic balloon pump for 7 days to receive a HeartMate II (*n* = 134) or a HeartMate XVE (*n* = 66).[2] The primary endpoint was a composite of survival to 24 months without disabling stroke or the need for an operation to repair or replace the device. The patient population was predominantly male, with a mean age of 62 years. This was a severely ill population as reflected by the relatively low use of baseline neurohormonal antagonists coupled with the high use of inotropes (77%) and intra-aortic balloon pumps (22%) in the study cohort. The mean ejection fraction was 17%, the mean pulmonary capillary wedge pressure was 24 mm Hg, and the mean cardiac index was 2 L/min/m². The mean serum sodium was 135 mmol/L and the mean creatinine was 1.6 mg/dL. Thus, the overall patient population had characteristics of advanced heart failure similar to the populations in previous trials performed with pulsatile devices.

There was a greater than fourfold increase in the percentage of HeartMate II patients who successfully reached the primary endpoint (46% vs. 11%; *P* <.001; Table 21-3). All of the components of the composite endpoint favored the HeartMate II (see Table 21-3).[2] Actuarial survival from the trial is shown in Figure 21-29. Patients randomly assigned to the HeartMate II had 1- and 2-year survival rates of 68% and 58% compared with 55% and 24% for the patients who received the HeartMate XVE. Survival in the HeartMate XVE cohort was identical to that observed in the original REMATCH trial despite device enhancements and more extensive patient management experience (see Fig. 21-29). All adverse events were less frequent in the HeartMate II patients, with significant reductions in sepsis, device-related infections, right heart failure, renal failure, and rehospitalizations. Changes in functional capacity, 6-minute walk distance, and quality-of-life scores were similar between groups, suggesting that the improvements seen in these metrics in VAD-supported patients are more closely linked to the favorable effects of increasing the cardiac output and lowering the left-sided filling pressures rather than the characteristics of blood flow.

The results of the HeartMate II DT Pivotal Trial resulted in FDA approval of this device in 2010 as the second LVAD indicated for long-term support of patients ineligible for transplantation.[24]

Continuous-Flow Device with Centrifugal Design for Destination Therapy

The VentrAssist centrifugal flow LVAD was tested in a DT trial with an innovative design of two distinct modules aimed at shortening the time to study completion. Module A randomized patients (2:1) without urgent need for MCS to receive a VentrAssist LVAD or to remain on medical therapy. At time points beyond 6 weeks after enrollment, patients in the medical therapy arm were reassessed for crossover to the LVAD arm of the trial and would receive the HeartMate XVE device. Patients with urgent need for MCS were enrolled in Module B, a randomized (2:1) assessment

TABLE 21-3	Primary Endpoint and Hazard Ratios, According to Treatment Group in the HeartMate II Pivotal Destination Therapy Trial*			
Endpoint	Continuous-Flow LVAD (*n* = 134), no. (% [95% CI])	Pulsatile-Flow (LVAD (*n* = 66), no. (% [95% CI])	Hazard Ratio (95% CI)	P Value
Survival free from disabling stroke and reoperation to repair or replace LVAD at 2 yr (primary composite endpoint)	62 (46 [38-55])	7 (11 [3-18])		<0.001
First event that prevented patient from reaching the primary endpoint				
Disabling stroke†	15 (11 [6-17])	8 (12 [4-20])	0.078 (0.33-1.82)	0.56
Reoperation to repair or replace pump‡	13 (10 [5-15])	24 (36 [25-48])	0.018 (0.09-0.37)	<0.001
Death within 2 yr after implantation	44 (33 [25-41])	27 (41[29-53])	0.59 (0.35-0.99)	0.048
Any	72 (54 [45-62])	59 (89 [82-97])	0.38 (0.27-0.54)	<0.001

*Hazard ratios were calculated with the use of Cox regression, and the *P* value for the primary endpoint with the use of Fisher's exact test.

†Disabling stroke was defined as stroke with a Rankin score of >3.

‡Reoperation to repair or replace pump included urgent heart transplantation or device explantation.

CI, confidence interval; LVAD, left ventricular assist device.

From Slaughter MS, Rogers JG, Milano CA, et al; HeartMate II Investigators. Advanced heart failure treated with continuous-flow left ventricular assist device. *N Engl J Med.* 2009;361:2241-2251.

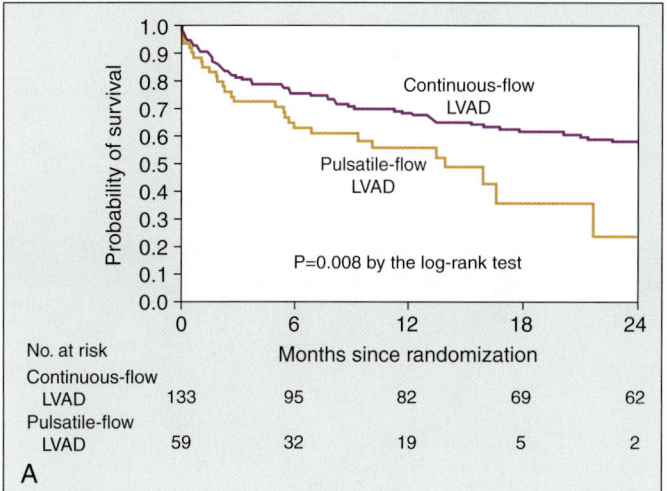

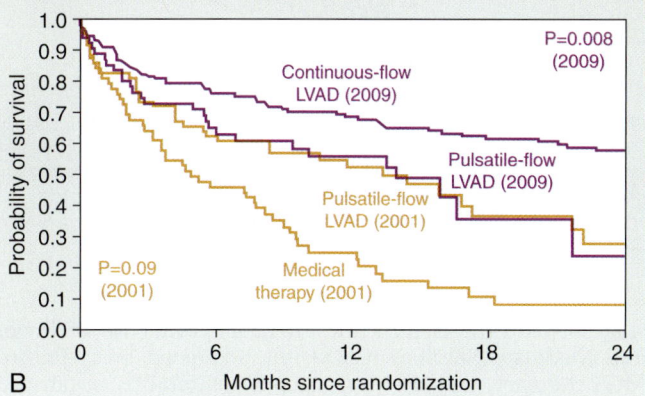

FIGURE 21-29 **A,** Kaplan-Meier estimates of survival from the as-treated analysis, according to treatment group. The data shown are for 192 patients who received a left ventricular assist device (LVAD). Of the 59 patients who had a pulsatile-flow LVAD, 20 had the device replaced during the study period, with 18 (31%) receiving a continuous-flow LVAD instead of another pulsatile-flow LVAD. By 2 years, only two patients had a pulsatile-flow LVAD, both of whom had replacement devices. **B,** Survival rates in two trials of LVADs as destination therapy (DT). The curves labeled 2009 are those reported by Slaughter and colleagues (2009), and the curves labeled 2001 were reported for the REMATCH trial. *(From Slaughter MS, Rogers JG, Milano CA, et al; HeartMate II Investigators. Advanced heart failure treated with continuous-flow left ventricular assist device. N Engl J Med. 2009;361:2241-2251; Rose EA, Gelijns AC, Moskowitz AJ, et al. Randomized Evaluation of Mechanical Assistance for the Treatment of Congestive Heart Failure [REMATCH] Study Group. Long-term mechanical left ventricular assistance for end-stage heart failure. N Engl J Med. 2001;345:1435-1443.)*

of the VentrAssist LVAD versus the HeartMate XVE pulsatile LVAD. Unfortunately, manufacture of the device was halted before completion of the trial and the results were not published.

CLINICAL TRIALS EVALUATING TEMPORARY EXTRACORPOREAL MECHANICAL CIRCULATORY SUPPORT DEVICES

The clinical evaluation of temporary MCS devices for refractory cardiogenic shock has generally not required randomized clinical trial design but has relied on the use of prospective, single-arm observations studies to validate device design, safety, and efficacy. It is accepted that patients with cardio-

genic shock refractory to conventional medical therapies are at risk of imminent death.

The TandemHeart pVAD (CardiacAssist Technologies, Inc., Pittsburgh, PA) is a percutaneous left atrial–to–femoral artery VAD (Fig. 21-30).[49–51] The pump is a low-speed continuous-flow pump using centrifugal design. The device is implanted percutaneously through the right femoral vein, requiring transseptal puncture with placement of the catheter into the left atrium. In a randomized comparison of IABP with the TandemHeart PVAD, Thiele and colleagues reported greater improvement in cardiac power index as well as other hemodynamic and metabolic variables with the Tandem Heart PVAD compared with IABP.[49,50] However, complications, including severe bleeding and limb ischemia, were encountered more frequently after support with the TandemHeart. The 30-day mortality rates were similar between the groups. The TandemHeart PVAD is approved by the FDA for temporary MCS for cardiogenic shock in patients refractory to optimal medical therapy and IABP.

The CentriMag VAD (Levitronix LLC, Waltham, MA) is an extracorporeal system composed of a centrifugal blood pump, a motor, a console, a flow probe, and a circuit that requires surgical implant (Fig. 21-31).[52–54] The device is based on a magnetically levitated "bearingless motor" design. The rotor located inside the upper pump housing is magnetically coupled to the lower motor housing to produce rotor levitation and spin, which combines the drive, the magnetic bearing, and the rotor function into a single unit. The motor generates the magnetic bearing force that levitates the rotor into the pump housing while also generating the torque necessary to produce the unidirectional flow. This device can produce flows of up to 10 L/min under normal physiologic conditions, with a priming volume of 31 mL. Single-center reports have

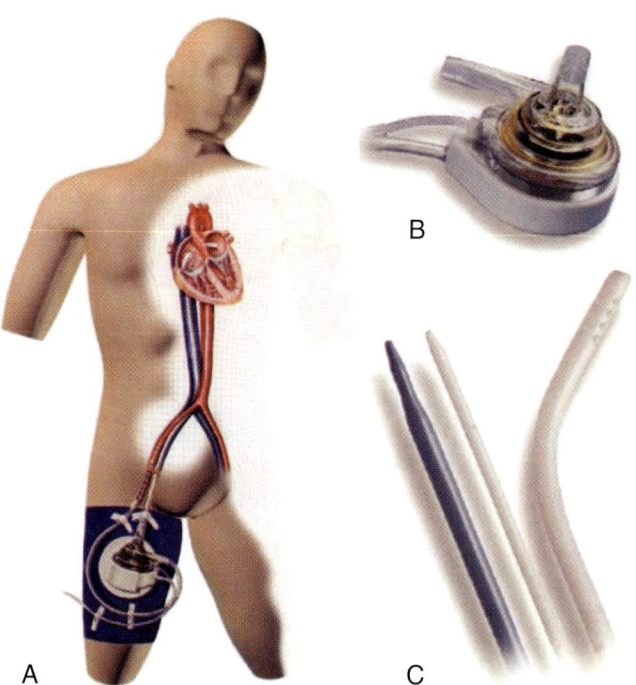

FIGURE 21-30 TandemHeart left ventricular assist device (LVAD) is a centrifugal pump with bearing support of the internal impeller that is designed for temporary mechanical circulatory support (MCS). **A,** Graphic of the percutaneously inserted device in place. Note the femoral venous transseptal and arterial cannula connected to the TandemHeart centrifugal pump. **B,** Close-up view of the centrifugal pump. **C,** Close-up view of the TandemHeart trans-septal cannula. *(From Pulido JN, Soon J, Charanjit S, et al. Percutaneous left ventricular assist devices: clinical uses, future applications, and anesthetic considerations. J Cardiothorac Vasc Anesth. 2010;24:478-486.)*

demonstrated successful use of the CentriMag device as BTR therapy or a bridge to durable, implantable MCS device. The CentriMag is approved by the FDA for short-term temporary support.

The Impella VAD (Abiomed Corporation, Danvers, MA) is a catheter-based, impeller-driven, microaxial-flow pump (Fig. 21-32).[55–58] The device is positioned across the aortic valve with the inlet port below the valve and outlet port above the valve. The device can be implanted through a percutaneous approach, or by a surgical approach through the femoral artery, axillary artery, or ascending aorta. The Impella LP2.5 is approved by the FDA for partial MCS for up to 6 hours. In a prospective, randomized clinical trial comparing the Impella LP2.5 with IABP, cardiac index was significantly increased in patients with the LP2.5 device compared with patients supported by IABP.[57] Overall mortality rates at 30 days were similar in both groups. Based on the results of the Impella LP2.5, the FDA has approved two similar but larger devices, the Impella 5.0, which is implanted by surgical cut down in the femoral artery, and the Impella LP, which is implanted by surgical thoracotomy. Both devices provide flows of up to 5 L/min for short-term support.

The Abiomed BVS5000 (Abiomed Corporation) is an extracorporeal VAD intended to provide left, right, or biventricular support (Fig. 21-33).[59–61] The Abiomed BVS5000 is approved by the FDA for short-term MCS support for bridge to myocardial recovery for cardiogenic shock due to postcardiotomy failure to wean, acute myocarditis, myocardial infarction, and acute allograft dysfunction after heart transplantation. In addition to the traditional BVS5000, a device with new blood pump and console designs, designated the AB5000, has been introduced and approved by the FDA for short-term support. The AB5000 design has now replaced the BVS5000 design for clinical use. The AB5000 blood pumps are connected to the patient in a paracorporeal configuration to enhance patient mobility and potential for hospital discharge.

MECHANICAL CIRCULATORY SUPPORT DEVICE OUTCOMES IN INTERMACS

INTERMACS is one of the largest available data repositories for the study of durable MCS outcomes intended for BTT or DT.[62] INTERMACS, an NHLBI-sponsored collabora-

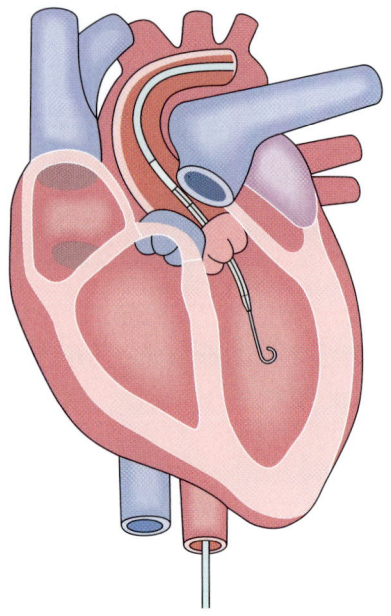

FIGURE 21-32 Impella ventricular assist device (VAD) is a catheter-based, impeller-driven, microaxial flow pump. The device is inserted percutaneously or by surgical placement through the femoral artery or ascending aorta and positioned across the aortic valve. *(From Thunberg CA, Gaitan B, Arabia FA, et al. Ventricular assist devices today and tomorrow. J Cardiothorac Vasc Anesth. 2010;24:656-680.)*

tion between the NHLBI, the FDA, the Center for Medicaid and Medicare Services (CMS), the advanced heart failure/MCS industry, and the professional community, began prospective patient enrollment and data collection on June 23, 2006. On March 27, 2009, CMS and the U.S. Department of Health and Human Services mandated that all U.S. hospitals approved for use of MCS for DT enter MCS patient data into a national database, INTERMACS, for all noninvestigative MCS devices approved by the FDA. The power of INTERMACS data stems from the mandatory data submission on all durable MCS devices in order to receive reimbursement from CMS, a formal process for adverse event adjudication, dedicated innovative electronic data submission,

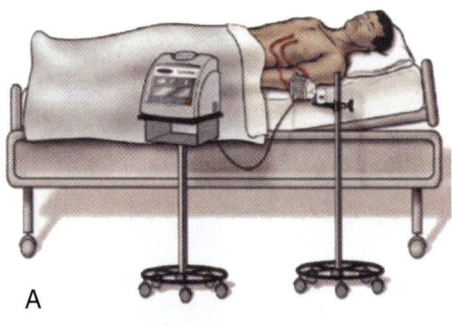

A

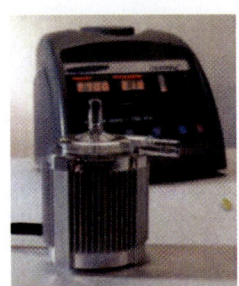

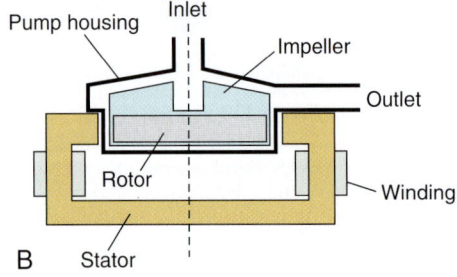

B

FIGURE 21-31 **A,** Levitronix CentriMag is a continuous-flow rotary pump with centrifugal and noncontact bearing design. The impeller is magnetically levitated. The CentriMag is connected to a free-standing power console located external to the patient. **B,** A floating rotor rests in the magnetic field of a stator with no mechanical contact, and electronic controls regulate the rotor position and speed. Blood flows through the inlet above the rotor and is directed by the centrifugal force of the spinning rotor through the outlet port.

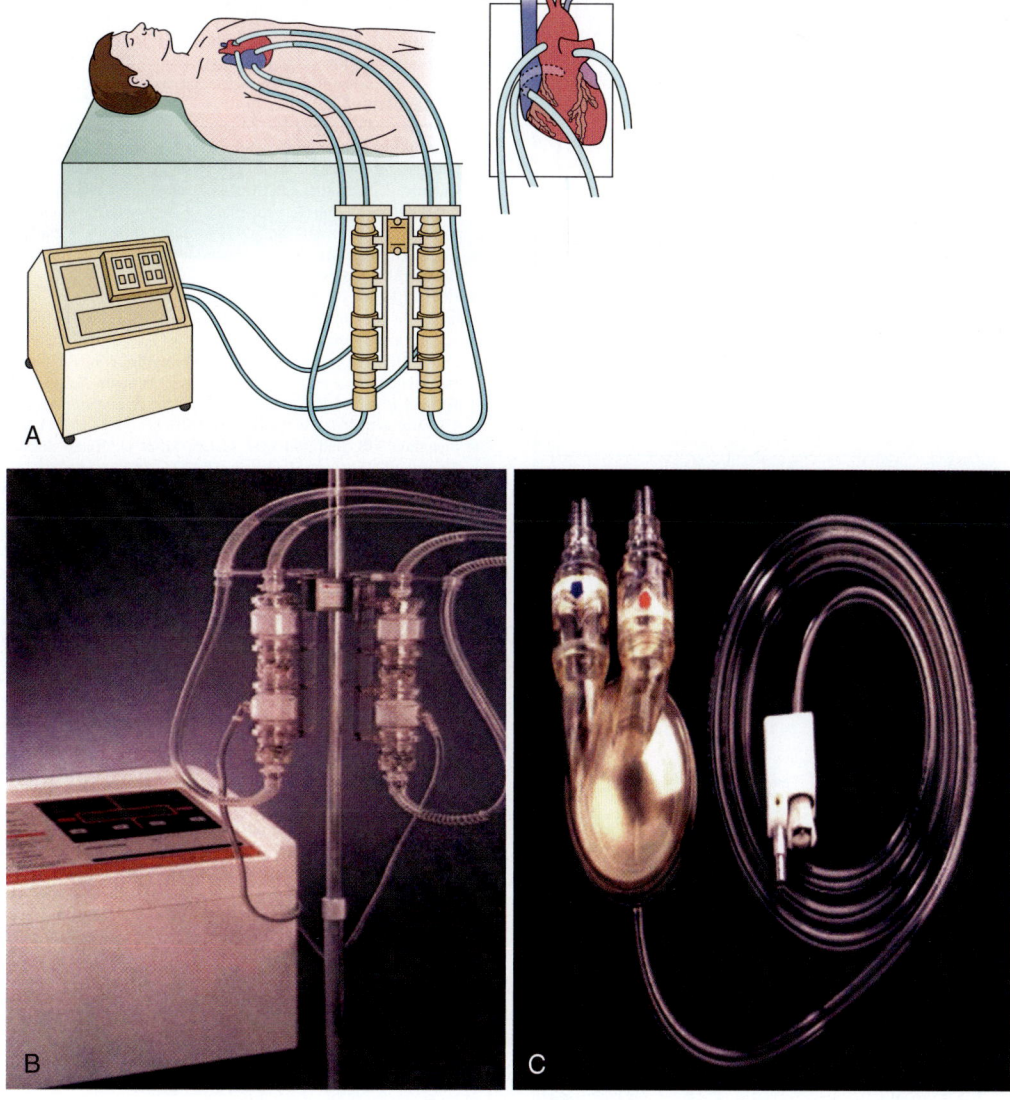

FIGURE 21-33 The Abiomed BVS5000 is an extracorporeal, pulsatile, short-term pump approved in the United States for temporary mechanical circulatory support (MCS). **A,** Extracorporeal biventricular support configuration. **B,** Pneumatic drive console with BVS 5000 blood pumps. **C,** FDA-approved redesign of the BVS 5000 blood pumps to a paracorporeal blood pump, AB 5000. *(Copyright ©ABIOMED, Danvers, MA.)*

data element design to create a template for comparison with medical therapy, rigorous data monitoring, hospital auditing through the United Network of Organ Sharing, and a formal process for data access and publications. Since the inception of INTERMACS, the ongoing evolution of strategies for device application and the types of available devices has continued to refine the landscape of MCS. The major limitation of the INTERMACS registry is the inability to enter patient information on investigative devices currently in evaluation in the United States. In the early experience of the INTERMACS registry, the only devices approved in the United States for DT or BTT therapy were pulsatile pumps such as the HeartMate XVE and the Thoratec pVAD and IVAD. After FDA approval of continuous-flow technology for clinical use in 2008 (Thoratec HeartMate II), data on current device technology began being entered into the registry in robust numbers. The most recent report from the INTERMACS registry reflects this dramatic switch from pulsatile to continuous-flow technology for MCS therapy and provides a basis for rigorous comparison of patient outcomes between the two different technologies.

In 2010, data on over 1000 patients receiving durable MCS therapy had been reported to INTERMACS.[62] The overall survival rates of patients undergoing primary implantation of a durable MCS device was approximately 75% at 1 year and 45% at 2 years (Fig. 21-34). Survival for patients undergoing primary implantation with an LVAD was superior to biventricular support or support after implantation of a TAH.

CONCLUSIONS

MCS therapy with durable, implantable devices is an established and viable treatment option for patients with advanced heart failure awaiting heart transplantation, as well as permanent therapy for patients ineligible for transplantation. Over the past decade there has been a transition from pulsatile pumps to continuous-flow pumps with axial and, more recently, centrifugal blood flow design. This transition to new technology has been associated with important enhancements in pump design contributing to significant improvements

SURVIVAL BY DEVICE TYPE

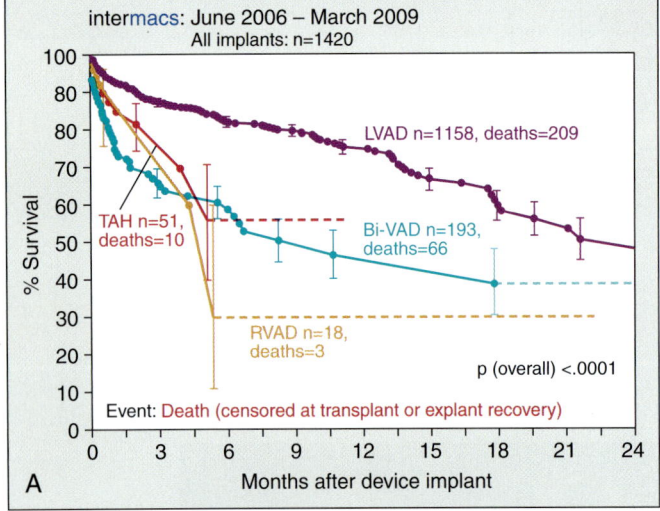

LVAD, left ventricular assist device; RVAD, right ventricular assist device; Bi-VAD, biventricular assist device; TAH, total artificial heart

INTERMACS LEVEL AT IMPLANT

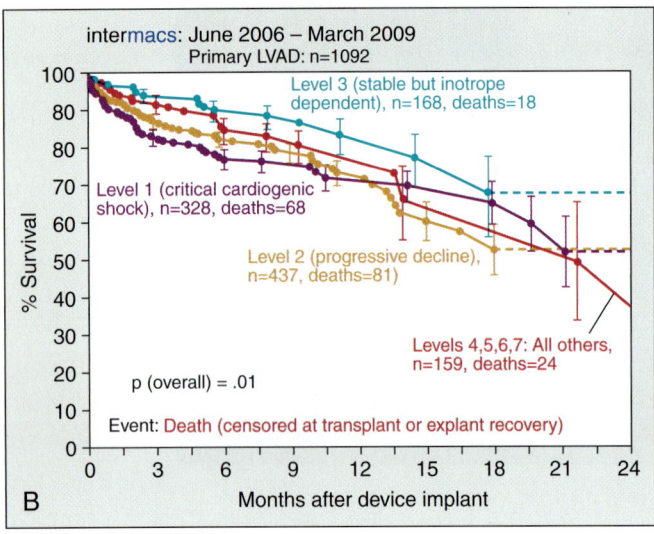

LVAD, left ventricular assist device;

FIGURE 21-34 Survival analysis of patients on mechanical circulatory support (MCS) entered into the INTERMACS Registry from June 2006 through September 2009 and stratified by device location **(A)** and acuity of illness **(B)**, as assessed using the INTERMACS Patient Profiles. Bi-VAD, biventricular ventricular assist device; LVAD, left ventricular assist device; RVAD, right ventricular assist device; TAH, total artificial heart. *(From Kirklin JK, Naftel DC, Kormos RL, et al. Second INTERMACS annual report: more than 1,000 primary left ventricular assist device implants.* J Heart Lung Transplant. *2010;29:1-10.)*

in patient survival and reduction in the occurrence of serious adverse events, particularly pump malfunction, device-related infection, and right heart failure. Bleeding, stroke, and thromboembolic events remain an important concern with VAD therapy. An improved understanding of the biology of the blood–device interface is necessary for optimal management of anticoagulation and device design to prevent these adverse events. Despite these limitations, new technology has led to dramatic increases in numbers of patients now referred for VAD therapy. Continuing improvements in device technology will, perhaps, lead to outcomes that may be comparable with heart transplantation for some patients, and to the clinical comparison of VAD therapy with heart transplantation and the investigation of VADs in patients with less advanced heart failure in clinical trials.

REFERENCES

1. Rose EA, Gelijns AC, Moskowitz AJ, et al. Randomized Evaluation of Mechanical Assistance for the Treatment of Congestive Heart Failure (REMATCH) Study Group. Long-term mechanical left ventricular assistance for end-stage heart failure. *N Engl J Med.* 2001;345:1435–1443.
2. Slaughter MS, Rogers JG, Milano CA, et al. HeartMate II Investigators. Advanced heart failure treated with continuous-flow left ventricular assist device. *N Engl J Med.* 2009;361:2241–2251.
3. Christie JD, Edwards LB, Aurora P, et al. The Registry of the International Society for Heart and Lung Transplantation: Twenty-sixth official adult lung and heart-lung transplantation report—2009. *J Heart Lung Transplant.* 2009;28:1031–1049.
4. Joyce LD, Noon GP, Joyce DL, et al. Mechanical circulatory support: a historical review. *ASAIO J.* 2004;50:x–xii.
5. Hill JD, Farrar DJ, Hershon JJ, Compton PG, et al. Use of a prosthetic ventricle as a bridge to cardiac transplantation for postinfarction cardiogenic shock. *N Engl J Med.* 1986;314:626–628.
6. Farrar DJ, Hill JD, Gray Jr LA, et al. Heterotopic prosthetic ventricles as a bridge to cardiac transplantation: a multicenter study in 29 patients. *N Engl J Med.* 1988;318:333–340.
7. Farrar DJ, Buck KE, Coulter JH, et al. Portable pneumatic biventricular driver for the Thoratec ventricular assist device. *ASAIO J.* 1997;43:M631–M634.
8. Slaughter MS, Sobieski MA, Martin M, et al. Home discharge experience with the Thoratec TLC-II portable driver. *ASAIO J.* 2007;53:132–135.
9. Reichenbach SH, Farrar DJ, Hill JD. A versatile intracorporeal ventricular assist device based on the Thoratec VAD system. *Ann Thorac Surg.* 2001;71(suppl 3):S171–S175.
10. Slaughter MS, Tsui SS, El-Banayosy A, et al. Results of a multicenter clinical trial with the Thoratec implantable Ventricular Assist Device. *J Thorac Cardiovasc Surg.* 2007;133:1573–1580. [erratum appears in *J Thorac Cardiovasc Surg.* 2007;134:A34].
11. Portner PM, Oyer PE, McGregor CGA, et al. First human use of an electrically-powered implantable ventricular assist system. *Artif Organs.* 1985;9:36 [abstract].
12. Starnes VA, Oyer PE, Portner PM, et al. Isolated left ventricular assist as bridge to cardiac transplantation. *J Thorac Cardiovasc Surg.* 1988;96:62–71.
13. McGee MG, Parnis SM, Nakatani T, et al. Extended clinical support with an implantable left ventricular assist device. *ASAIO Trans.* 1989;35:614–616.
14. Frazier O, Rose E, Macmanus Q, et al. Multicenter clinical evaluation of the Heart Mate 1000 IP left ventricular assist device. *Ann Thorac Surg.* 1992;53:1080–1090.
15. Frazier OH, Rose EA, McCarthy P, et al. Improved mortality and rehabilitation of transplant candidates treated with a long-term implantable left ventricular assist system. *Ann Surg.* 1995;222:327–336.
16. Frazier OH, Rose EA, Oz MC, et al. Multicenter clinical evaluation of the HeartMate vented electric left ventricular assist system in patients awaiting heart transplantation. *J Thorac Cardiovasc Surg.* 2001;122:1186–1195.
17. Dowling RD, Park SJ, Pagani FD, et al. HeartMate VE LVAS design enhancements and its impact on device reliability. *Eur J Cardiothorac Surg.* 2004;25:958–963.
18. Pagani FD, Long JW, Dembitsky WP, et al. Improved mechanical reliability of the HeartMate XVE left ventricular assist system. *Ann Thorac Surg.* 2006;82:1413–1419.
19. Dembitsky WP, Tector AJ, Park S, et al. Left ventricular assist device performance with long-term circulatory support: lessons from the REMATCH trial. *Ann Thorac Surg.* 2004;78:2123–2129.
20. Dagenais F, Portner PM, Robbins RC, et al. The Novacor left ventricular assist system: clinical experience from the Novacor registry. *J Card Surg.* 2001;16:267–271.
21. Mussivand T, Hetzer R, Vitali E, et al. Clinical results with an ePTFE inflow conduit for mechanical circulatory support. *J Heart Lung Transplant.* 2004;23:1366–1370.
22. Miller LW, Pagani FD, Russell SD, et al. Use of a continuous-flow device in patients awaiting heart transplantation. *N Engl J Med.* 2007;357:885–896.
23. Pagani FD, Miller LW, Russell SD, et al. Extended mechanical circulatory support with a continuous-flow rotary left ventricular assist device. HeartMate II Investigators. *J Am Coll Cardiol.* 2009;54:312–321.
24. Rogers JG, Aaronson KD, Boyle AJ, et al., HeartMate II Investigators. Continuous flow left ventricular assist device improves functional capacity and quality of life of advanced heart failure patients. *J Am Coll Cardiol.* 2010;55:1826–1834.
25. Russell SD, Rogers JG, Milano CA, et al., HeartMate II Clinical Investigators. Renal and hepatic function improve in advanced heart failure patients during continuous-flow support with the HeartMate II left ventricular assist device. *Circulation.* 2009;120:2352–2357.
26. Bristow MR, Saxon LA, Boehmer J, et al. Cardiac-resynchronization therapy with or without an implantable defibrillator in advanced chronic heart failure. *N Engl J Med.* 2004;350:2140–2150.
27. Frazier OH, Myers TJ, Jarvik RK, et al. Research and development of an implantable, axial-flow left ventricular assist device: the Jarvik 2000 heart. *Ann Thorac Surg.* 2001;71(suppl):S125–S132.
28. Siegenthaler MP, Frazier OH, Beyersdorf F, et al. Mechanical reliability of the Jarvik 2000 Heart. *Ann Thorac Surg.* 2006;81:1752–1758.
29. Goldstein DJ, Zucker M, Arroyo L, et al. Safety and feasibility trial of the MicroMed DeBakey ventricular assist device as a bridge to transplantation. *J Am Coll Cardiol.* 2005;45:962–963.
30. Jahanyar J, Noon GP, Koerner MM, et al. Recurrent device thrombi during mechanical circulatory support with an axial-flow pump is a treatable condition and does not preclude successful long-term support. *J Heart Lung Transplant.* 2007;26:200–203.
31. Takatani S. Progress of rotary blood pumps: Presidential Address, International Society for Rotary Blood Pumps, 2006, Leuven, Belgium. *Artif Organs.* 2007;31:329–344.
32. Farrar DJ, Bourque K, Dague CP, et al. Design features, developmental status, and experimental results with the Heartmate III centrifugal left ventricular assist system with a magnetically levitated rotor. *ASAIO J.* 2007;53:310–315.
33. Esmore D, Spratt P, Larbalestier R, et al. VentrAssist left ventricular assist device: clinical trial results and clinical development plan update. *Eur J Cardiothorac Surg.* 2007;32:735–744.

CH 21

34. Esmore DS, Kaye D, Salamonsen R, et al. First clinical implant of the VentrAssist left ventricular assist system as destination therapy for end-stage heart failure. *J Heart Lung Transplant.* 2005;24:1150–1154.

35. Boyle A, John R, Moazami N, et al. U.S. experience with a novel centrifugal LVAD in bridge to transplant (BTT) patients. *J Heart Lung Transplant.* 2009;28:S80–S81.

36. Nishinaka T, Schima H, Roethy W, et al. The DuraHeart VAD, a magnetically levitated centrifugal pump: the University of Vienna bridge to transplant experience. *Circ J.* 2006;70:1421–1425.

37. Nojiri C, Fey O, Jaschke F, et al. Long-term circulatory support with the DuraHeart mag-lev centrifugal left ventricular assist system for advanced heart failure patients eligible to transplantation: European experiences. *J Heart Lung Transplant.* 2008;27:S245 [abstract].

38. Wieselthaler GM, Strueber M, O'Driscoll GA, et al. Experience with the novel HeartWare HVAD with hydromagnetically levitated rotor in a multi-institutional trial. *J Heart Lung Transplant.* 2008;27:S245.

39. Tuzun E, Roberts K, Cohn WE, et al. In vivo evaluation of the HeartWare centrifugal ventricular assist device. *Texas Heart Inst J.* 2007;34:406–411.

40. Bearnson GB, Jacobs GB, Kirk J, et al. HeartQuest ventricular assist device magnetically levitated centrifugal blood pump. *Artif Organs.* 2006;30:339–346.

41. Pitsis AA, Visouli AN, Vassilikos V, et al. First human implantation of a new rotary blood pump: design of the clinical feasibility study. *Hellenic J Cardiol.* 2006;47:368–376.

42. Copeland JG, Smith RG, Arabia FA, et al. CardioWest Total Artificial Heart Investigators. Cardiac replacement with a total artificial heart as a bridge to transplantation. *N Engl J Med.* 2004;351:859–867.

43. Arabia FA, Copeland JG, Pavie A, et al. Implantation technique for the CardioWest total artificial heart. *Ann Thorac Surg.* 1999;68:698–704.

44. Skolnick A. Using ventricular assist devices as long-term therapy for heart failure. *JAMA.* 1998;279:1509–1510.

45. Park SJ, Tector A, Piccioni W, et al. Left ventricular assist devices as destination therapy: a new look at survival. *J Thorac Cardiovasc Surg.* 2005;129:9–17 [erratum appears in *J Thorac Cardiovasc Surg.* 2005;129:1464].

46. Long JW, Healy AH, Rasmusson BY, et al. Improving outcomes with long-term "destination" therapy using left ventricular assist devices. *J Thorac Cardiovasc Surg.* 2008;135:1353–1360.

47. Lietz K, Long JW, Kfoury AG, et al. Outcomes of left ventricular assist device implantation as destination therapy in the post-REMATCH era: implications for patient selection. *Circulation.* 2007;116:497–505.

48. Rogers JG, Butler J, Lansman SL, et al. Chronic mechanical circulatory support for inotrope-dependent heart failure patients who are not transplant candidates: results of the INTrEPID Trial. INTrEPID Investigators. *J Am Coll Cardiol.* 2007;50:741–747.

49. Thiele H, Sick P, Boudriot E, et al. Randomized comparison of intra-aortic balloon support with a percutaneous left ventricular assist device in patients with revascularized acute myocardial infarction complicated by cardiogenic shock. *Eur Heart J.* 2005;26:1276–1283.

50. Burkhoff D, Cohen H, Brunckhorst C, et al. A randomized multicenter clinical study to evaluate the safety and efficacy of the TandemHeart percutaneous ventricular assist device versus conventional therapy with intraaortic balloon pumping for treatment of cardiogenic shock. *Am Heart J.* 2006;152:469.e1–469.e8.

51. Pulido JN, Park SJ, Rihal CS. Percutaneous left ventricular assist devices: clinical uses, future applications, and anesthetic considerations. *J Cardiothorac Vasc Anesth.* 2010;24:478–486.

52. Thunberg CA, Gaitan B, Arabia FA, et al. Ventricular assist devices today and tomorrow. *J Cardiothorac Vasc Anesth.* 2010;24:656–680.

53. Haj-Yahia S, Birks EJ, Amrani M, et al. Bridging patients after salvage from bridge to decision directly to transplant by means of prolonged support with the CentriMag short-term centrifugal pump. *J Thorac Cardiovasc Surg.* 2009;138:227–230.

54. John R, Liao K, Lietz K, et al. Experience with the Levitronix CentriMag circulatory support system as a bridge to decision in patients with refractory acute cardiogenic shock and multisystem organ failure. *J Thorac Cardiovasc Surg.* 2007;134:351–358.

55. Jurmann MJ, Siniawski H, Erb M, et al. Initial experience with miniature axial flow ventricular assist devices for postcardiotomy heart failure. *Ann Thorac Surg.* 2004;77:1642–1647.

56. Thiele H, Smalling RW, Schuler GC. Percutaneous left ventricular assist devices in acute myocardial infarction complicated by cardiogenic shock. *Eur Heart J.* 2007;28:2057–2063.

57. Seyfarth M, Sibbing D, Bauer I, et al. A randomized clinical trial to evaluate the safety and efficacy of a percutaneous left ventricular assist device versus intra-aortic balloon pumping for treatment of cardiogenic shock caused by myocardial infarction. *J Am Coll Cardiol.* 2008;52:1584–1588.

58. Sassard T, Scalabre A, Bonnefoy E, et al. The right axillary artery approach for the Impella Recover LP 5.0 microaxial pump. *Ann Thorac Surg.* 2008;85:1468–1470.

59. Guyton RA, Schonberger J, Everts P, et al. Postcardiotomy shock: clinical evaluation of the BVS 5000 biventricular support system. *Ann Thorac Surg.* 1993;56:346–356.

60. Jett GK. Postcardiotomy support with ventricular assist devices: selection of recipients. *Semin Thorac Cardiovasc Surg.* 1994;6:136–139.

61. Gray LA, Champsaur GG. The BVS 5000 biventricular assist device: the worldwide registry experience. *ASAIO J.* 1994;40:M460–M464.

62. Kirklin JK, Naftel DC, Kormos RL, et al. Second INTERMACS annual report: more than 1,000 primary left ventricular assist device implants. *J Heart Lung Transplant.* 2010;29:1–10.

CHAPTER **22**

Design Challenges for Clinical Trials in Mechanical Circulatory Support*

Deborah D. Ascheim, Alan Moskowitz, Michael Parides, and
Annetine C. Gelijns

Clinical trials are a critical transition point between bench and bedside. In recent years, there has been an important shift toward more rigorous clinical trials demonstrating the value of device-based therapies. At the same time, finding the appropriate balance between promoting rigorous clinical evaluation and preserving the incentives for therapeutic innovation remains a major challenge for clinicians, policy makers, and industry alike. Increasing the rigor of clinical evaluation increases the time and costs of the development process of new therapies, whereas fostering innovation requires finding ways to accelerate this same process. The balancing act between innovation and evaluation has been especially challenging in the case of novel therapies for small patient populations or those with life-threatening conditions, such as children with hypoplastic left heart syndrome or adults with glioblastoma. But perhaps one of the most salient areas of recent debate about this tradeoff between evaluative rigor and fostering innovation can be found in the realm of mechanical circulatory assist devices.

First generation left ventricular assist devices (LVAD) were approved as a bridge to transplantation (BTT) in 1994, and, in 2002, they received U.S. Food and Drug Administration (FDA) approval for long-term implantation in patients with advanced heart failure who were ineligible for cardiac transplantation (destination therapy [DT]). The trials supporting approval demonstrated the value, and potential, of LVAD therapy, but also highlighted the need for improved devices that would address the significant side effects, such as bleeding, sepsis, and neurologic events, associated with this therapy.[1,2] Over subsequent years, there has been substantial innovation in devices and clinical management strategies. The first continuous-flow device (HeartMate II; Thoratec Corporation, Pleasanton, CA), which addressed several shortcomings of predicate devices, was approved for BTT in 2008 and for DT in 2010.[3,4] Several newer-generation LVADs, which may incorporate additional improvements, have entered, or are poised to enter, clinical trials in this country.

An effective development process, however, requires an adequate translational research infrastructure of patients, investigators, and financial resources. Yet, herein lies the problem. BTT is an "orphan indication" and the patient population that is currently being referred to LVAD therapy for long-term implantation still remains severely limited, despite the significant number of patients with end-stage heart failure who could, in principle, be eligible for treatment.[5] As a result, the increasing numbers of devices entering clinical trials have to compete for a limited patient population. This situation underscores the need for designing trials that minimize sample sizes.

In this chapter, we will explore the pros and cons of a range of clinical trial designs, particularly in terms of sample size, the strength of the resulting evidence, and their impact on the timeliness of trial completion. We discuss trials for the established indications of BTT and DT, as well as for the evolving application for less severely ill patients with heart failure.

BRIDGE TO TRANSPLANTATION

First-Generation Devices: Single-Arm Studies

Early failures with heart transplantation, before the development of modern immunosuppressive agents, led to a period in the 1970s when few transplantations were performed and interest in mechanical circulatory support grew.[6] Throughout the 1970s and 1980s, several first-generation LVADs were developed, characterized by the use of pulsatile flow and positive displacement. Early clinical application of these LVADs focused on the BTT population. As of the mid-1980s, clinical trials started, which were designed as single-arm, nonrandomized studies. At this time, there were ethical concerns regarding the use of a control arm. Mortality on the cardiac transplant waiting list was substantial and well established over nearly a decade of observation. Moreover, based on the ability

*Authors funded in part by National Heart Lung and Blood Institute Grant U01 HL088942.

of LVADs to support physiologic function, the magnitude of the effect size was expected to be large. As such, the clinical evaluation of early first-generation LVADs was based on fairly small single-arm studies.

The TCI (later Thoratec) pneumatic HeartMate IP and VE (vented electric) LVADs received FDA approval for the BTT indication in 1994 and 1998, respectively.[1,7] In the case of the HeartMate VE, the U.S. BTT study provided clinical data derived from a cohort of 86 implanted patients, of whom 74 met all eligibility criteria and were included in the survival analysis that formed the basis for FDA granting post marketing approval (PMA). The survival to transplantation for the HeartMate VE was 65%, and the major adverse events were infection (44%) and bleeding (44%). By comparison, the Novacor LVAS U.S. BTT study used a concurrent control group in a nonrandomized design.[1] This study formed the basis for FDA approval of the Novacor LVAS for BTT in 1998, the same day as the HeartMate VE BTT approval. The Novacor clinical data were derived from 191 patients, 156 of whom were implanted with the device. Of the implanted patients, all were included in the evaluation of adverse events, 129 who met all eligibility criteria were included in the CORE LVAS cohort, and of those, the 104 who reached the study endpoint as of the PMA submission date were included in the survival analysis. The concurrent control group comprised 35 patients who met all eligibility criteria, but were treated with standard approved therapy, "either because the device was unavailable, or they chose not to accept a device." Although a concurrent control arm provides contemporary outcomes for making the relevant comparison, the potential to constitute the control group with patients that have, at the start, a different likelihood of achieving the study outcome than patients in the experimental treatment arm (i.e., differences in relevant clinical characteristics) leaves this type of design open to bias. With this in mind, it is possible that unwillingness to accept device implantation among patients in the control arm of the Novacor study reflected the fact that control patients were in worse condition at enrollment than their experimental counterparts. If this was the case, contrasting the treatment and control arm outcomes would constitute a biased comparison. The reported rate of survival to transplantation in the LVAD arm was 78%, and the major adverse events were infection (66 ± 8%) and neurologic events (41 ± 8%).

Despite the limitations inherent in the early BTT trials, these two landmark studies defined the original benchmark for the BTT population to which subsequent devices have been compared: a prespecified minimum performance goal of 65%. These were critical first steps in the evolution of increasingly rigorous clinical trials to evaluate the safety and efficacy of VADs.

Continuous-Flow Devices: Randomized Trials or Objective Performance Criterion–Based Studies

To stimulate further innovation in the field, in 1994, the National Heart, Lung and Blood Institute (NHLBI) issued a request for proposals for innovative VAD systems. The goals of the initiative were to increase the application of VADs through smaller design, improved durability, and lower complications. This initiative led to the development of second-generation VADs, characterized by continuous-flow. One of the greatest challenges facing the design of trials for these devices was the size of the available study population. Interestingly, this small sample size is driven not by a low prevalence of advanced heart disease, but rather by the relatively low dissemination of technology. The extensive surgery required to use this type of device and the ongoing risks and

TABLE 22-1	Bridge to Transplant Sample Size Calculations under Various Survival Assumptions*	
Approved Device (%)	Experimental Device (%)	Sample Size (n)
70	75	2502
70	80	586
70	85	240
70	90	126

*Based on a two-sided .05 level test with 80% power.

lifestyle changes associated with its implantation have historically led clinicians to select an even more limited, extremely end-stage subgroup of pre-transplantation patients for LVAD implantation, further reducing an already small patient population of potential recipients.

In light of the small size of the population, randomized trials using a device-to-device comparison were deemed not feasible. Let us consider, for instance, what a clinical trial would look like if subsequent trials of LVADs for the BTT indication were required to incorporate an active control arm. To illustrate this point, assume, for example, that with iterative improvements in devices and clinical management, the marketed devices have a true success probability, or a survival to transplantation (π), of 70% and that the experimental device improves mortality over marketed devices by an absolute margin of 5%. Designing such a trial would require over 2500 patients to ensure that a two-sided test has 80% power to reject the null hypothesis.* Table 22-1 depicts sample size calculations under various assumptions about the treatment benefit of the experimental device.[8] Only when a new device has an expected survival to transplantation of 90%, which is unrealistically high for current-generation devices, will the sample size come into a feasible range of about 125 patients.

By designing trials that eliminate a concurrent control group and use point estimates from historical data instead, a so-called performance goal– or objective performance criterion–(OPC)–based study, the sample size is reduced by roughly 75% (because the control group has been eliminated and the performance goal is a fixed number, with no variability). Moreover, because newer devices are not expected to increase survival substantially but may offer other advantages such as fewer adverse events, these trials test noninferiority rather than superiority. In such a trial, the goal is to show with high probability that the experimental device is no worse than the predicate device by a prespecified (noninferiority) margin.

Usually, noninferiority trials require larger sample sizes, but this can be mitigated by using a wider noninferiority margin, which has the effect of reducing the sample size. For example, if we again assume that marketed devices have a 70% survival to transplantation and a noninferiority margin of 10%, a claim of noninferiority would require that the lower 95% confidence bound for the observed survival to transplantation exceed 60%. This means that the observed point estimate for survival to transplantation would need to be 68%. To ensure that the experimental device exceeds this threshold, with a high probability (at least 80%), the required sample size is approximately 120 patients.

Evolution of the Primary Endpoint: Setting the Objective Performance Criterion

The original OPC was based on the observations made during premarketing testing of the HeartMate VE and Novacor devices and a review of the current literature.[1,7,9–12] On the

---

*This is a test of $H_0:\pi = 70\%$ (null hypothesis) versus $H_1:\pi = 75\%$ (the alternative hypothesis).

basis of this original OPC, success required that devices meet a prespecified minimum performance goal of 65% survival to transplantation, and the trial was deemed positive if the observed lower one-sided 95% confidence bound for the success proportion exceeded the performance goal.

One significant limitation to the utility of this benchmark was that the original trials used survival to transplantation as the primary endpoint, which did not account for temporal and geographic variations in waiting times on the transplantation list. To account for this, the definition of success in BTT LVAD trials was extended to include survival to 180 days on LVAD support while remaining eligible for cardiac transplantation in addition to survival to transplantation. The first trial to use this endpoint was the HeartMate II BTT Trial that began enrollment in 2005.[13] This definition was modified slightly for the VentrAssist BTT Trial, where the primary endpoint was defined as survival to cardiac transplantation or to 180 days post-LVAD implantation *and listed for cardiac transplantation with Network for United Organ Sharing (UNOS) as Status 1A or 1B* (unpublished data, International Center for Health Outcomes & Innovation Research [InCHOIR], MSSM Data Coordinating Center). This seemingly minor modification to the definition of success required that the UNOS status listing reflect the patient's official national transplantation listing and not simply the judgment of the investigator alone.

In addition, both the primary endpoints for the HeartMate II and VentrAssist LVAD trials both included explantation for cardiac recovery. If explantation for recovery were not explicitly incorporated into the outcome measure, it would be challenging to distinguish it from any other reason for explants, such as a device replacement, in the context of an ongoing clinical trial. It is important to define a priori when an explant for recovery would be considered a success (e.g., the duration of support-free survival after LVAD explantation). An optimal trial design distinguishes an LVAD explant for recovery, defined as a success, from an explant for any other reason (considered a failure).

Evolution of Adverse Event Definitions in Bridge to Transplantation Trials

One of the significant limitations of the early LVAD studies was the lack of common nomenclature and definitions for adverse events. This impacted not only the ability of physicians and patients to make informed clinical decisions, but also the ability to create accurate pooled benchmarks of the safety profile as LVADs became approved for the BTT indication. To address this critical issue the clinical, scientific, and regulatory communities responded in collaboration to create a standardized registry for outcomes in the postmarketing period. This effort, INTERMACS (Interagency Registry for Mechanically Assisted Circulatory Support), began enrollment in the spring of 2006.[14] The registry was devised as a joint effort of the NHLBI, the Centers for Medicare and Medicaid Services (CMS), the FDA, clinicians, scientists, and industry representatives. Within the context of INTERMACS, a standardized set of adverse event classifications and definitions was created by harmonizing existing definitions from a number of completed and ongoing LVAD clinical trials. These adverse event classifications and definitions, with minor adjustments since 2006, have become the FDA-mandated standard for VAD trials initiated since 2006.

In addition to the evolution and standardization of adverse event definitions, adverse events in premarketing trials are now independently adjudicated by experts—which was not the case for the pivotal trials of the currently marketed devices—and the newer devices are, therefore, held to stricter standards.

Results from Continuous-Flow Device Bridge to Transplantation Trials

The HeartMate II multicenter, single-arm study enrolled 133 patients with end-stage heart failure who were on the waiting list for heart transplantation.[13] One hundred eighty days after device implantation, 75% of patients had reached the principal outcome, which included transplantation, cardiac recovery, or ongoing mechanical support while remaining eligible for transplantation. This device received FDA approval in 2008 for the BTT indication. Another rotary device, the VentrAssist LVAD, was evaluated in a prospective, multicenter, single-arm feasibility study of 28 patients. Eighty-six percent of patients survived to cardiac transplantation or were supported for 180 days post-LVAD implantation (unpublished data, InCHOIR). The outcomes of the prospective, multicenter, single-arm pivotal study, in which 137 patients were implanted with the VentrAssist as a bridge to cardiac transplantation, were similar to the earlier feasibility experience. Eighty-two percent of the 127 patients who had met the primary endpoint as of August 2009 survived to transplantation or to 180 days on support and listed as UNOS Status 1, without need for device replacement. Despite the promising outcomes of the patients enrolled in the VentrAssist Feasibility BTT Trial and the completion of enrollment of the Pivotal BTT Trial, the company was unable to remain solvent, and the clinical development program for this promising LVAD was terminated.

Although adopting OPC-based studies deals with the small size of the BTT population, the absence of a concurrent control group poses problems for data interpretation. This becomes particularly problematic in an area with active therapeutic innovation, ongoing changes in patient selection, and evolution of trial conduct. One major challenge, for example, is that the transplantation population has changed since the original HeartMate VE and Novacor premarketing trials—contemporary BTT patients may not be comparable in their risk profile to the patients from the original studies. Moreover, clinical management of patients with advanced heart failure and LVAD support has evolved, affecting the survival rates and adverse event profiles of patients receiving the current devices compared with historical control subjects. Another issue is the changing waiting times for donor hearts. Thus, although this design may offer precision in its estimates of treatment effect (e.g., narrow confidence intervals), those estimates are potentially biased by an unquantifiable amount because of unmeasured differences in patient comparison groups.

INTERMACS: Concurrent Controls?

Many of the aforementioned challenges can be addressed through the use of concurrent controls from INTERMACS.[14–16] For FDA-approved devices, INTERMACS can provide concurrent benchmarks of the baseline characteristics of BTT patients, their survival to transplantation rates and waiting times, and adverse event rates using standardized definitions. This dataset could also provide a comparison group that, through modeling, could be appropriately adjusted for risk factors. For instance, the recently completed ADVANCE (Evaluation of the HeartWare HVAD Left Ventricular Assist Device System for the Treatment of Advanced Heart Failure) BTT Trial of the HVAD (HeartWare, Inc., Framingham, MA) includes a control group from INTERMACS. The primary endpoint in this trial is survival to 180 days, which is defined as alive on the originally implanted HVAD or transplanted or explanted for recovery; the patient must survive 60 days postexplantation for recovery to be considered successful.[17]

LONG-TERM LEFT VENTRICULAR ASSIST DEVICE THERAPY TRIALS: CHALLENGES AND DESIGN OPTIONS

Setting the Stage: REMATCH Trial

The NHLBI-supported REMATCH (Randomized Evaluation of Mechanical Assistance for the Treatment of Congestive Heart Failure) trial established the indication for long-term LVAD use, or destination therapy (DT). This trial evaluated the efficacy and safety of implantation with an LVAD compared with optimal medical management in patients with chronic end-stage (stage D) heart failure. Compared with optimal medical management (n = 61), LVAD implantation (n = 68) was found to double the 1-year survival (from 25% to 51%) in this terminally ill population.[2] REMATCH illustrates some of the important ongoing challenges in the design and conduct of randomized trials of implantable devices in comparison with pharmaceutical trials. A major challenge in conducting randomized trials of new devices or procedures is that the comparison arm is often a very different treatment modality, unlike the comparison of two drugs. In REMATCH, for instance, the use of an LVAD was compared with pharmacologic therapy. Such vastly different treatment approaches may engender strong physician and patient preferences, which may make it harder to achieve equipoise or buy-in for randomization (especially in the case of a life-threatening condition). Moreover, compared with drug trials, blinding in a trial evaluating a device such as an LVAD often is not feasible, which affects the potential for observer bias, especially in the assessment of more subjective endpoints like quality of life or functional status. Efforts to minimize bias include both an independent (from the treating physicians) assessment of the patient's status (e.g., New York Heart Association [NYHA] class) and an independent analysis of these endpoints by core laboratories.

Another challenge, in comparison with pharmaceutical trials, in designing trials of novel procedures is dealing with the high level of incremental change that characterizes surgical innovation. By contrast, a drug generally does not undergo substantial changes as it moves through the phases of clinical trials. For example, in the aforementioned REMATCH trial, several changes were implemented, such as modification of the driveline, introduction of a locking screw ring to prevent detachment of the blood transport conduits to and from the pump, and a clinical protocol to prevent and manage driveline infections with antimicrobial agents and laminar flow operating rooms. Such modifications in the device or

clinical management can be accommodated in the design of clinical trials. With these variations in protocol, the predetermined sample size in the REMATCH trial did not change. If, however, the device design or clinical management change substantially alters the measures of outcome, additional patients may need to be recruited to satisfy specific subgroup analyses. Typical of trials of complex technologies, there was a learning curve phenomenon. If we compare patients enrolled in the first half of the trial with those enrolled in the second half, we see a significant improvement in survival in the LVAD arm (Fig. 22-1). Such improvement was not seen in the medical management arm. Moreover, we see a similar significant improvement over time in terms of the adverse event profile of LVAD-treated patients, with less driveline infections, postoperative bleeding, and sepsis.[18] One strategy to mitigate the effects of learning is to design a pilot trial or a run-in period that will not be counted in the final analysis. Another strategy is to prespecify an analytical plan that adjusts for experiential differences over the course of the trial, should these differences affect outcome.

Finally, an important challenge in designing the REMATCH trial, which remains an issue for advanced heart failure trials in general, is establishing control group event rates. The understanding of the predictors of survival in these patients is still limited, and the literature shows great variation in survival. In the design of the REMATCH trial, for instance, we assumed that the 2-year mortality rate for the target population would be approximately 75%, and presumed that the minimum benefit of LVAD therapy would be a reduction of mortality by at least a third.[19] However, we underestimated the mortality in the control arm patients, who were found to have a 1-year mortality rate of 75%. This observation makes the case for having randomized trials for evaluating new indications, when there is significant uncertainty regarding the outcomes in the control arm. If the REMATCH study had been designed as a single-arm study in which LVAD survival was compared with a performance goal of survival in medically managed patients (who we assumed had a much better survival than ultimately was found in the trial), the device would have been deemed unsuccessful.

Based on the REMATCH data, LVAD therapy was approved by the FDA for DT in 2002, and it received coverage approval by Medicare in 2003. The device was slowly adopted into clinical practice. In the first 4 years after Medicare reimbursement approval (2003-2007), some 400 patients were implanted with the HeartMate XVE. A major challenge in the design of DT trials of next-generation devices was the small number of DT patients being referred to LVAD therapy; such limited patient numbers make it difficult to complete trials in a timely manner. Thus, a fundamental design issue in DT LVAD trials is how one can design pivotal studies that can be conducted in a tractable time period. In particular, this situation raises the following questions: (1) What is the role of observational versus randomized trials? (2) If we conduct randomized trials, how can we reduce their sample size? (3) How can we design randomized trials that access a larger heart failure population?

Is There a Role for Nonrandomized Destination Therapy Trials?

The limited number of patients who were being referred for DT raised the question whether the FDA should allow nonrandomized trial designs and opt for OPC-type studies for evaluating LVADs in a DT population, similar to the REMATCH population, as was the case in BTT trials. A registry such as INTERMACS, with its standardized data collection procedures and outcome definitions, has substantial promise over time for the design of efficient premarketing studies. It may offer a means to eliminate the need for collecting a new

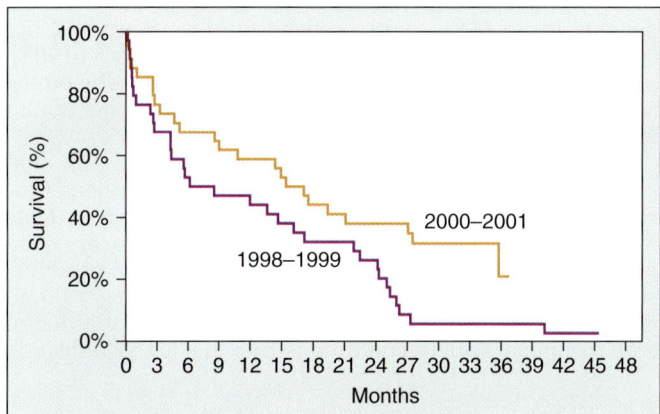

FIGURE 22-1 Kaplan-Meier survival curves for patients receiving left ventricular assist devices (LVADs) enrolled in the REMATCH trial in 1998-1999, and those enrolled in 2000-2001 (P = .00293).

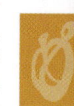

control group. It can provide an empirically derived OPC to facilitate a single-arm study. It can also generate a concurrent comparison group, adjusted for risk factors through multivariable risk modeling or propensity score-based matching. Finally, such studies may also stimulate enrollment by eliminating randomization. Random assignment may be a deterrent in a situation with strong physician and patient preferences, which is often the case with major surgical interventions for life-threatening diseases.

For DT, however, there was limited clinical experience on which to base an OPC. As of 2007, for instance, only 38 DT LVAD-treated patients had been entered in INTERMACS, with only limited follow-up data. Moreover, whereas we have seen important new risk score models for LVAD-treated patients, they are based on small datasets, not yet confirmed in the INTERMACS validation cohort or for newer pumps. The resulting uncertainty limits our ability to balance prognostic variables between comparison arms and, thus, to interpret how much of the difference in outcomes is due to treatment effect. This is exacerbated by the fact that stage D heart failure comprises a spectrum of patients and, as previous studies have shown, there is important variation and evolution in patient selection.[20] In addition, there are ongoing incremental device modifications as well as changes in patient management. Device-related management changes, for example, involve anticoagulation requirements for nonpulsatile pumps, and device-unrelated ones include beta blockers, aldosterone inhibitors, and biventricular pacing for patients with advanced heart failure. As such, the premarketing evaluation of newer-generation devices, which were in clinical development after the REMATCH trial, still required randomized, controlled trials. Clearly, the major strength of such trials is that they eliminate bias in the assigning patients to treatment arms, and thereby ensure equal constitution of comparison arms for known and unknown factors. This is especially important if treatment effects are small, and where treatment preferences are strong.

Device-to-Device Trials: Endpoint Selection and Trial Design

The REMATCH trial set the stage for the design of randomized trials of next-generation LVADs. Key considerations in planning these, and any, trials are the selection of the primary endpoint and the control group. Mortality remains a critical metric for comparison in these trials, whether alone or as part of a composite measure. In view of the significant survival benefit of LVAD therapy found in REMATCH, most DT trials of subsequent LVADs were to have an active device control arm (i.e., the FDA-approved predicate device, which at the time was the HeartMate XVE).

Superiority Trials

Novel devices, although offering potential improvements in the adverse event profile, are unlikely to offer major survival benefits over existing devices, which means that the hypothesized treatment effect will be small. As such, traditional superiority trials, based on device-to-device comparisons with survival as the primary endpoint, raise sample size issues. Assume, for example, that 2-year survival in the control arm (the marketed device) is 45%. This is not an unrealistic assumption because survival was nearly 40% for those patients enrolled in the second half of the REMATCH trial, and experienced LVAD centers are likely to have improved their outcomes with ongoing learning in the postmarketing setting.[18] If we then assume that a new device decreases mortality by a relative 10% (i.e., the hazard ratio [or instantaneous relative risk of death] $\theta = 0.90$), a sample size of nearly 4500 patients is required to ensure that a two-sided test has

TABLE 22-2	Destination Therapy Sample Size Calculations under Various Assumptions for the Relative Benefit of the Experimental Device*	
Relative Benefit (%)	Sample Size (N)	No. Deaths
10	4486	3783
20	1138	844
30	424	331
40	220	161
50	128	88

*Based on a two-sided .05 level test with 80% power.

80% power to reject the null hypothesis.* Table 22-2 shows sample size requirements under various assumptions for the mortality benefit of the experimental device, assuming 30 months of accrual and 18-month follow-up. Even if a new device decreases mortality by a relative 30%, which would bring the 2-year survival rate of its recipients close to 60%, the sample size of a well-powered trial would still need to be over 400 patients, which is a challenging sample size to accrue in this patient population.

Noninferiority Trials

What other design options exist to reduce sample size? One possibility is a noninferiority trial with a "liberal" specification of a noninferiority margin. If we choose a noninferiority margin of 30%, we can claim noninferiority for the new device if the lower one-sided 95% confidence bound for the hazard ratio exceeds 0.70.[†] The hazard ratio compares the mortality seen with the predicate device with that seen with the experimental device. Assuming no survival difference between the predicate and experimental devices, and a 2-year survival rate of 45% (with survival times following an exponential distribution), 196 deaths are required to provide at least 80% power to detect that the hazard ratio for death from any cause is at least 0.70. If accrual times are the same as described previously, 310 patients would need to be randomly assigned to observe 196 deaths.

Composite Endpoints

Another option is to use a composite endpoint, which may highlight the differences between comparison devices by combining survival with important adverse events for patients, such as stroke or device replacements.[21] Such an endpoint may increase the difference in event rates and, consequently, statistical power. A case in point is device replacement–free survival. In the REMATCH trial, for example, LVAD-treated patients had a 65% 2-year probability of replacement.[2] If a new device would improve device reliability by 30% to 50%, one would have a good chance of showing superiority on the basis of device replacement–free survival with about 300 or 200 patients.

The HeartMate II DT trial followed such a design. Two hundred patients were randomized to either the continuous-flow HeartMate II device or the approved pulsatile flow HeartMate XVE between March 2005 and May 2007. The primary composite endpoint was, at 2 years, survival free from disabling stroke (stroke with a modified Rankin scale rating >3) and reoperation to repair or replace the device. This trial found that treatment with a continuous-flow device significantly

---

*This will test H_0:$\theta = 1.0$ (the null hypothesis) versus H_1:$\theta = 0.90$ (the alternative hypothesis).

†To claim noninferiority under this design, the survival experience in the two arms has to be similar.

improved the probability of survival free from stroke and device failure at 2 years compared with a pulsatile device.[22]

An alternative option is to design a trial that compares LVAD therapy with "standard" medical care, under the assumption that such a trial may reduce barriers to randomization. We designed such a trial, in collaboration with Ventracor, Inc. (Sydney, Australia), to evaluate the VentrAssist LVAD in patients with stage D heart failure.

Left Ventricular Assist Device Therapy versus Standard Medical Care: Adaptive Trial Designs

After the REMATCH trial, most clinical investigators viewed the predicate device as the logical control arm. However, standard therapy for advanced heart failure comprises a spectrum of therapies, including various medications, resynchronization therapy, and LVAD therapy. Relative to the number of DT LVAD candidates (conservatively estimated to be 75,000 annually in the United States), LVADs were infrequently used for this indication (<650 during the period 2003-2007). The majority of patients with stage D heart failure in 2007 were treated with pharmacologic therapy, implanted cardioverter-defibrillators, and cardiac resynchronization therapy (i.e., biventricular pacing), without the use of LVAD therapy. The use of LVADs, and the timing of their implantation, depended heavily on clinical factors as well as the risk-benefit perceptions of both the practitioner and the patient. The way in which patients with heart failure were managed argued for evaluating a novel LVAD against both medical management strategies and the predicate LVAD; therefore, we designed a trial that included standard medical therapy as a control arm. The advantage of such a trial design is that it could increase enrollment because this trial also accesses the pool of patients who are interested in the experimental device (with its promise of lower side effects) but may not be interested in the commercially available device (i.e., the HeartMate XVE, which had a high probability of device failure by 2 years). The control group, because it reflected standard therapy, would provide results that are more generalizable.

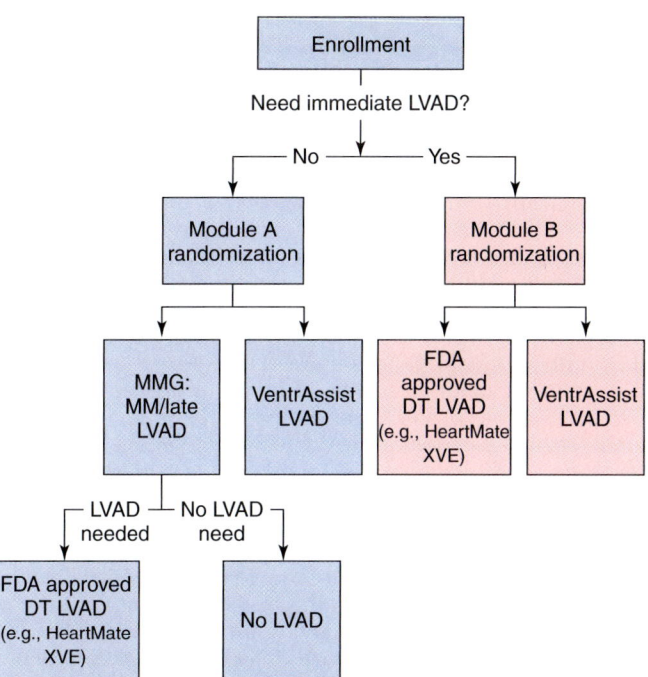

FIGURE 22-2 Ventracor destination therapy (DT) trial design schematic. LVAD, left ventricular assist device; MMG, medical management group.

Following discussions with the FDA, the ultimate trial design included two modules (see Fig. 22-2 for a schematic of the trial design). The first module randomly assigned patients to either the investigational LVAD or to continued medical management, which included, at the discretion of the treating physician and patient, any medical therapy considered optimal standard care in accordance with current medical practice guidelines, with the option of subsequent implantation of an FDA-approved LVAD. The intent was to stay within the REMATCH eligibility criteria but move toward a less acutely ill population. If a patient decompensated in the control arm, the physician and patient could opt for implantation of the FDA-approved DT LVAD. The trial stipulated that elective LVAD implantation should occur no sooner than 6 weeks after randomization, unless the patient decompensated despite maximal therapy, necessitating urgent LVAD implantation. An independent Event Adjudication Committee reviewed the compliance of these decisions with protocol-defined guidelines. Criteria for early LVAD implantation in the control arm included clinical decompensation of patients as defined by worsening end-organ perfusion: hemodynamic instability requiring increasing inotropic therapy, the need for intra-aortic balloon pump support, and the development of new refractory ventricular arrhythmias.

The second module provided a direct device-to-device comparison in patients who required "immediate" (within 14 days of enrollment) LVAD support; these patients were randomly assigned to either the investigational LVAD or an FDA-approved LVAD for the DT population. Patients in both experimental modules were randomized in a 2:1 ratio to receive either the investigational LVAD or the control therapy. In the first module, 180 patients were to be randomized, and in the second module, 45 patients were expected to be randomly assigned, although the plan was to continue randomization in this module until enrollment into the first module was completed.

Success of the trial was defined by the primary analysis of the first module, which assessed the superiority of the investigational LVAD to the standard therapy group with respect to the composite endpoint of disabling stroke (defined as a modified Rankin Scale rating of 4 or 5) or death from any cause. The sample size was determined based on the following assumptions: (1) time-to-event would be exponentially distributed with a constant hazard, (2) the 2-year event rate for patients randomly assigned to standard medical care would be 67%, and (3) patient accrual would occur uniformly for 24 months and follow-up would continue for an additional 18 months after the last patient is randomly assigned. A total of 180 patients, randomly assigned in a 2:1 allocation to the investigational LVAD or to standard therapy, would yield the required 103 events within the assumed accrual and follow-up periods and ensure at least 80% power (power would be approximately 82.5%) to detect a 46% reduction (hazard ratio of 0.54) in the risk of an event for the LVAD arm compared to standard therapy. This reduction in risk corresponded to an absolute reduction in the 2-year event rate of 22% for the investigational LVAD from 67% to 45%.

One risk of this trial design was that the proportions in the control arm receiving an LVAD would be vastly different than assumed and, therefore, the expected event rates would be different from expected. We therefore adopted an adaptive trial design, which called for a sample size re-estimation by an independent statistician if this was found to be the case.

This trial started enrolling in 2007, but before enrollment was completed the manufacturer of the LVAD went bankrupt. By comparison, the HeartMate II DT trial completed enrollment and its results led to FDA approval in early 2010. Currently, there are several additional continuous-flow devices in clinical development that will be ready to be evaluated in a DT population. Device-to-device trials would then compare these investigational devices with the FDA-approved LVAD, which is now the HeartMate II. Because the HeartMate II is a durable device, there is no longer an opportunity to reduce sample size through a composite endpoint that includes device replacement. As such, noninferiority trials that compare an investigational device with the predicate device will require sample sizes on the order of 450 patients. Even though the use of LVADs for DT is increasing, having several devices competing for a relatively limited patient population will increase the length of time involved in completing these trials. It is still worthwhile to consider alternative design options that may be able to reduce sample size.

Combining Randomized and Nonrandomized Data or Trials with Higher Type I Error Rates

Another option is to use nonrandomized data in the design and analysis of randomized trials. Nonrandomized control data from concurrent control subjects could be combined with randomized data, as in a meta-analysis. Historical data could provide a prior estimate for the control success rate that gets updated by prospectively collected data. The benefit of either approach could be to allow a higher likelihood of randomization into the experimental LVAD group.

Finally, another option to complete a premarketing DT study in a tractable period of time is to opt for a smaller randomized trial, and accept a higher-than-conventional type I error rate for statistical tests (e.g., 10% to 20% probability of a type I error). A pivotal factor is the selection of the control group. Given the REMATCH results, a natural choice is to have an available commercial device serve as the control. However, the expected small survival benefit of experimental devices renders a noninferiority design with a broader-than-usual, but clinically reasonable noninferiority margin the only practical design. For example, if the two devices are equally effective with a hypothesized 2-year survival rate of 45%, and we select a type I error of 20% and a noninferiority margin of 15%, then 124 patients would provide 80% power to reject the null hypothesis (if the observed survival in the control arm is 45%, then the lowest observed survival in the experimental arm for a successful trial would be 38%; Fig. 22-3). A lower type I error rate (10%; using the same noninferiority margin of 15%) is achievable by enrolling a slightly larger sample size (n = 146) provided that the experimental device is expected to have a slightly better performance than the control (47.5% vs. 45% 2-year survival). Table 22-3 provides the operating characteristics for

TABLE 22-3	Operating Characteristics of Two Tests of Noninferiority*		
Success Probability for Control Device	Success Probability for Experimental Device	Approximate Probability of Claiming Experimental Device Noninferior	
		Design 1 (N = 124, θ = 0.15, α = 0.20)	Design 2 (N = 146, θ = 0.15, α = 0.10)
0.45	0.25	0.08	0.03
0.45	0.30	0.20	0.10
0.45	0.35	0.39	0.25
0.45	0.40	0.61	0.48
0.45	0.45	0.80	0.71
0.45	0.475	0.87	0.80
0.45	0.50	0.91	0.87
0.45	0.55	0.97	0.96

*Each based on two-sided tests with 80% power.

TABLE 22-4	Destination Therapy Sample Size Estimates under Various Assumptions			
Total Sample Size	Type I Error Level	Noninferiority Margin	2-Year Survival Rate for Control Device	2-Year Survival Rate for Experimental Device
124	.20	.15	0.45	0.45
146	.10	.15	0.45	0.475
146	.10	.125	0.45	0.50
112	.10	.10	0.45	0.55
152	.05	.15	0.45	0.50

both tests. More customary type I error rates (e.g., $\alpha = 5\%$) for a test of noninferiority are possible if the experimental device offers a greater degree of survival improvement. For example, a noninferiority trial with 152 patients would be possible if the experimental device improves 2-year survival to 50% (noninferiority margin 15%; power 80%; $\alpha = 5\%$). Smaller noninferiority margins are also an option if the experimental device improves survival by a small amount compared with the predicate device (Table 22-4).

The level of imprecision of the estimated treatment difference in these types of trials is larger than is customary in pivotal trials. However, this approach provides an advantage over a performance goal–type design in that we obtain an unbiased estimate of treatment effect because of randomization, and can quantify the remaining random variation. If concern remains about an increased type I error rate, one could require evidence of additional endpoints (e.g., device replacement, stroke) demonstrating device effectiveness. For example, one might require demonstrating noninferiority with regard to mortality as described previously, and also require showing superiority on one or more other endpoints with a customary type I error rate. According to Capizzi and Zhang, this approach could maintain the overall type I error rate at 5%, as long as at least one endpoint is significant at the 5% level and the others trend in the same direction and are significant at the 20% level at most.[23] Neuhauser and Steinijans suggested a modification of this approach, essentially arguing for a minor downward adjustment of the alpha level to account for the multiplicity of tests performed.[24]

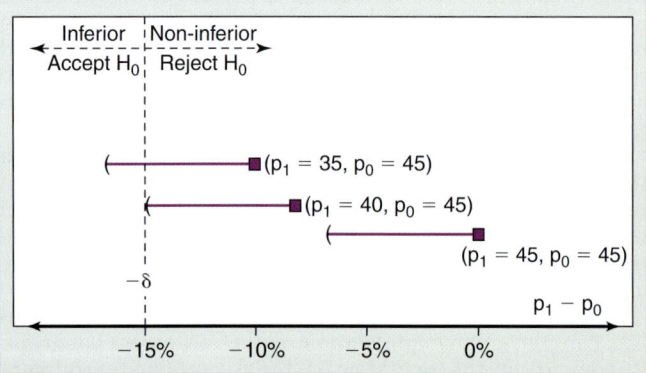

FIGURE 22-3 Illustration of decisions based on results for three different noninferiority trials. In each case, the observed 2-year survival rate for the control arm (p_0) is 45%. The observed 2-year survival rates in the experimental arm (p_1) are 45%, 38%, and 35%.

DESIGNING TRIALS IN LESS SEVERELY ILL PATIENTS WITH HEART FAILURE

The evolution of LVAD therapy and the associated improvements in outcomes have raised an important question for the field: Is the timing right to expand VAD use to patients with less severe heart failure? Or in other words, is there equipoise to conduct a trial in such patients? And if so, what are its design challenges?

Since 2007, there has been considerable interest and debate about a trial of VAD therapy in patients with less severe heart failure. The Heart Failure Society of America (HSFA) and industry both have spearheaded working groups, and the NHLBI-supported Cardiothoracic Surgical Trials Network (CTSN) developed a proof-of-concept trial design in January 2008. The NHLBI subsequently convened a working group in March 2008 to consider such a trial. In July 2009, the NHLBI issued a request for applications for the design and conduct of the REVIVE-IT (Randomized Evaluation of VAD InterVEntion before Inotropic Therapy) Pilot Trial.

Equipoise and Outcome Measures

The answer to whether there is equipoise to conduct a trial like REVIVE-IT depends critically on the survival and quality of life that patients with less severe, NYHA class III heart failure currently experience with standard medical therapy. Class III heart failure subsumes a broad spectrum of patients for whom survival estimates are not precisely known and are often derived from small, selected populations enrolled in larger clinical trials. Risk scores, such as the Heart Failure Survival Score (HFSS) and the Seattle Heart Failure Model (SHFM), are critically important.[25,26] These scores predict mortality based on physiologic variables, but may not include important clinical variables, such as number of recent hospital admissions, which may be an important predictor of mortality. Unfortunately, there is not yet a registry capturing long-term outcomes of medically managed patients that could provide this much-needed information. One group that may be close in its characteristics to the patients that the proposed trial would target is UNOS Status II patients, who have a 1-year survival rate of approximately 75%.

Another critical measure of outcomes for patients receiving standard therapy is their functional status. Consider, for example, the recent HF-ACTION (Heart Failure: A Controlled Trial Investigating Outcomes of Exercise TraiNing) trial.[27] Of patients, 64% were NYHA class II at baseline, 35% were class III, and 1% were class IV. Yet, the mean peak VO_2 for the entire cohort was 14.5 mL/kg/min, and the peak VO_2 for patients with class III heart failure must obviously have been lower. Thus, these data suggest that patients with class III heart failure can be highly functionally impaired.

The equipoise issue, however, depends not only on what outcomes medically managed patients currently experience, but on the outcomes that LVAD therapy may offer these patients. As previously noted for other populations in this chapter, given the invasive nature of LVADs, improvements must be substantial. Outcomes for patients implanted with the HeartMate XVE LVAD as DT improved over time owing to better understanding of patient selection criteria and better patient management.[28] Patients implanted with a DT LVAD during the first 3 years after the approval of the HeartMate XVE for DT, who had an acceptable operative risk according to the DT Risk Score, had a 1-year survival rate of nearly 70%.[20]

Since that time, however, newer continuous-flow devices are continuing to improve the risk–benefit profile of LVAD therapy. The HeartMate II BTT trial and continued-access protocol study showed 85% 6-month and 80% 1-year survival rates.[13] The VentrAssist had 88% 6-month and 85% 1-year survival rates.

Furthermore, both these devices significantly improved patients' quality of life and functional status over baseline, although inferences are limited by the fact that these are unblinded, single-arm studies. These trials also demonstrated that newer devices have improved adverse event profiles, with lower bleeding rates requiring surgery and fewer driveline infections and neurologic events than patients implanted with the HeartMate XVE as BTT therapy. Most important, worldwide experience with patients on these devices for over 2 years suggests that long-term device durability is significantly improved. The results of the HeartMate II DT trial should confirm if the HeartMate II device longevity is better than that of pulsatile LVADs.

Finally, with a reduction in perioperative adverse events, the length of index hospitalization has significantly decreased. In fact, index hospitalization length of stay has been reduced by 50% (from 29 days in REMATCH) to 14 to 16.5 days in experienced centers or with implantation of less sick (INTERMACS profile 6 to 7) patients. With the wide array of rotary pumps in clinical trials, and with newer percutaneously inserted micro-VADS poised to enter clinical trials, this trend is expected to continue.

Thus, many would agree that there is equipoise to explore whether LVAD therapy can provide a substantial improvement in functional capacity, with a modest improvement in survival, compared with contemporary optimal medical management in highly functionally impaired, but not moribund, patients with heart failure.

Characterization of the Patient Population

A critical design issue is defining the specific characteristics of the target population. The CTSN protocol development committee developed the following eligibility criteria: patients would have an left ventricular ejection fraction of less than 35%, NYHA class III or greater for at least 60 days despite optimal medical management, peak VO_2 of at least 12 mL/kg/min, and at least one hospitalization for heart failure in the 6 months before randomization. Selected exclusion criteria include hospitalization for heart failure at the time of randomization and treatment with intravenous inotropic therapy within 30 days before randomization.

Selection of the Primary Endpoint

Another critical design issue is the choice of primary endpoint. There are various options, of which one is disabling stroke–free survival, which is objective, easy to measure, and has precedence as an accepted endpoint in previous LVAD trials. However, such an endpoint fails to capture important aspects of outcomes for patients. Interviews about preferences for VAD therapy were conducted in 105 medically managed patients with heart failure during previous studies. Of those interviewed, 60% considered quality-of-life improvement as important as survival improvement in their decision to opt for an LVAD, and 25% thought quality of life was more important.[29] These observations argue for incorporating functional status into the primary endpoint, and there are two options to do so: the first is by designing a trial with functional status and survival as co-primary endpoints; and the other is to use a composite endpoint of functionally improved survival.

Sample Size Considerations

First we consider the sample sizes associated with stroke-free survival as the primary endpoint. It is important to note that as designed in the CTSN trial, patients in the control group who receive standard medical management, if they deteriorate clinically, can receive a VAD or heart transplant. These patients are not considered treatment failures or crossovers in

TABLE 22-5	Power Analysis for Composite of Functional Status* and Survival		
Control Response (%)	LVAD Response (%)	80% Power	90% Power
10	30	120	160
10	25	200	260
15	30	240	320
15	25	500	670

*As measured by peak VO$_2$.
LVAD, left ventricular assist device.

the analysis. We propose to follow a strict intention-to-treat approach, where essentially the surgical arm receives early LVAD therapy and the medical arm receives late LVAD therapy. We have taken a broad range of assumptions for stroke-free survival at 2 years, ranging from 60% to 70% for the control group and between 70% and 79% for the VAD arm.

The sample sizes for such a trial range from 420 to 6000, and these numbers are based on relatively large relative risk reductions in mortality. Prior experience suggests that enrollment of these numbers of patients in an LVAD randomized trial cannot be completed within a tractable period.

Thus, one may consider a composite of functional status (as measured by peak VO$_2$) and survival. We used a responder analysis approach, with each patient categorized as having responded or not based on reaching a success threshold. Here we define the success threshold as achieving a 20% improvement in peak VO$_2$ over baseline. Obviously, defining a threshold that is clinically meaningful will be critical to the outcome of the trial because it drives the trial's power. Another important analytical challenge is whether one should evaluate functionally improved survival at a fixed time point, which makes the analysis easier. However, if many patients in the control arm eventually receive a VAD, the treatment effect will be attenuated at 2 years. At the same time, providing early and sustained functional status improvement is critical to patients. If that is the case, one should used mixed model approaches to the analysis of the primary endpoint.

Analysis should be geared toward detecting a difference in early and sustained functional improvement between treatments. The sample sizes associated with such a trial are much more feasible, ranging from 120 to 500 patients (Table 22-5).

The timing is right to perform an LVAD trial in patients with less severe heart failure. Yet, uncertainties remain at this time regarding the specific characteristics of the patient population, event rates, and the best approaches to analyzing improvements in functional status. These uncertainties argue for conducting a feasibility trial. The objectives of such a trial would be to (1) provide data on risk-benefit tradeoffs between comparison arms to support the decisions to proceed with a pivotal trial, (2) refine the primary endpoint, (3) more precisely characterize the patient population, and (4) assess the feasibility of enrollment.

CONCLUSION

Left ventricular assist device therapy raises interesting challenges for the design and conduct of efficacy and effectiveness trials. As this chapter highlights, there is a role for both observational studies and randomized trials in evaluating mechanical circulatory assist devices. In the BTT realm, small patient populations have led to single-arm studies based on OPCs. Over time, there has been increased rigor and standardization in the definition of primary endpoints, characterization of the patient population, and definition and adjudication of adverse events. At this point, randomized, controlled trials

remain critical in providing premarketing evidence of efficacy and safety for *major* new devices indicated for DT or novel patient populations, such as those less severely ill with heart failure. Given the limited number of patients being referred for LVAD DT, the field needs to explore ways to decrease the sample size and reduce barriers to enrollment in randomized, controlled trials. This chapter discusses several options, such as using Bayesian statistics, adaptive trial designs, and composite endpoints, and reviews their strengths and limitations. At the same time, it is important to recognize that randomized clinical trials will not yield absolute "yes or no" answers, but, as R. A. Fisher—credited by many as the father of randomized trials—observed, they estimate the effects of interventions and are a means for rigorously specifying uncertainty.

The introduction of INTERMACS, a rigorous registry to collect data on effectiveness and safety of all marketed LVADs, offers substantial promise for improving the clinical development process. Data from this registry can provide an OPC from a well-defined population with standard definitions. It can also provide a concurrent control group, with risk adjustment. In addition, it can make the conduct of randomized trials more efficient by providing a prior estimate of the success distribution in control group (Bayesian analysis), or concurrent control data that can be pooled with randomized data. Finally, a robust postmarketing infrastructure can balance the acceleration of premarketing trials.

To fulfill this promise, it is critical to maximize enrollment into INTERMACS and potentially expand the breadth of its data collection—for example, regarding quality of life and functional status. It is also important to develop a registry for patients with advanced heart failure (non-VAD) to provide data on the control group to expand the use of LVADs to earlier phases of heart failure. Efforts to increase our knowledge about the pathophysiology of heart failure and prognostic factors are essential to ensure that event rates are appropriately adjusted and that trials more accurately target patients. Only after the field has matured in this manner will the balance between the use of randomized, controlled trials and observational studies shift toward nonexperimental methods.

REFERENCES

1. U.S. Food and Drug Administration. *Postmarket Approval Application (PMA) Novacor® LVAS—P980012.* Oakland, CA: Baxter Healthcare Corporation; September 29, 1998; PMA HeartMate® VE LVAS—P920014/S007, September 29, 1998, Thermo Cardiosystems, Inc., Woburn, MA.
2. Rose EA, Gelijns AC, Moskowitz AJ, et al. Long-term mechanical left ventricular assistance for end-stage heart failure. *N Engl J Med.* 2001;345:1435–1443.
3. U.S. Food and Drug Administration. *Postmarket Approval Application (PMA) HeartMate® II LVAS—P060040.* Pleasanton, CA: Thoratec Corporation; April 21, 2008.
4. U.S. Food and Drug Administration. *Postmarket Approval Application (PMA) HeartMate® II LVAS—P060040/S005.* Pleasanton, CA: Thoratec Corporation; January 20, 2010.
5. Deng MC, Edwards LB, Hertz MI, et al. Mechanical Circulatory Support Device Database of the International Society for Heart and Lung Transplantation: third annual report—2005. *J Heart Lung Transplant.* 2005;24:1182–1187.
6. Helman DN, Rose EA. History of mechanical circulatory support. *Prog Cardiovasc Dis.* 2000;43(1):1–4.
7. U.S. Food and Drug Administration. *Postmarket Approval Application (PMA) HeartMate® IP LVAS—P920014.* Woburn, MA: Thermo Cardiosystems, Inc; September 30, 1994.
8. Blackwelder WC. "Proving the null hypothesis" in clinical trials. *Control Clin Trials.* 1982;3:345–353.
9. Kormos RL, Ramasamy N, Sit S. Bridge to transplant experience with the Novacor left ventricular assist system: results of a multicenter US study. *J Heart Lung Transplant.* 1999;18:163 [abstract].
10. Frazier OH, Rose EA, Oz MC, et al. Multicenter clinical evaluation of the HeartMate vented electric left ventricular assist system in patients awaiting heart transplantation. *J Thorac Cardiovasc Surg.* 2001;122:1186–1195.
11. Frazier OH, Rose EA, McCarthy P, et al. Improved mortality and rehabilitation of transplant candidates treated with a long-term implantable left ventricular assist system. *Ann Surg.* 1995;222:327–336.
12. Slaughter M, Tsui S, El-Banayosy A, et al. Results of a multicenter clinical trial with the Thoratec Implantable Ventricular Assist Device. *J Thorac Cardiovasc Surg.* 2007;133:1573–1580.

13. Miller LW, Pagani FD, Russell SD, et al., The HeartMate II Clinical Investigators. Use of a continuous-flow device in patients awaiting heart transplantation. *N Eng J Med.* 2007;357:885–896.

14. Kirklin JK, Naftel DC, Stevenson LW, et al. INTERMACS database for durable devices for circulatory support: first annual report. *J Heart Lung Transplant.* 2008;27:1065–1072.

15. Stevenson LW, Pagani FD, Young JB, et al. INTERMACS profiles of advanced heart failure: the current picture. *J Heart Lung Transplant.* 2009;28:535–541.

16. Kirklin JK, Naftel DC, Kormos RL, et al. Second INTERMACS annual report: more than 1,000 primary left ventricular assist device implants. *J Heart Lung Transplant.* 2010;29:1–10.

17. *Evaluation of the HeartWare Left Ventricular Assist Device for the Treatment of Advanced Heart Failure (ADVANCE) Trial.* Available online at http://clinicaltrials.gov/ ct2/show/NCT00751972?term=HeartWare&rank=1; Last updated January 31, 2011.

18. Park SJ, Tector A, Piccioni W, et al. Left ventricular assist devices as destination therapy: a new look at survival. *J Thorac Cardiovasc Surg.* 2005;129:9–17.

19. Rose EA, Moskowitz AJ, Packer M, et al. The REMATCH trial: rationale, design, and end points. Randomized Evaluation of Mechanical Assistance for the Treatment of Congestive Heart Failure. *Ann Thorac Surg.* 1999;67:723–730.

20. Lietz K, Long JW, Abdalla GK, et al. Outcomes of left ventricular assist device implantation as destination therapy in the post REMATCH era. *Circulation.* 2007;116: 497–505.

21. Parides MK, Moskowitz AJ, Ascheim DD, et al. Progress versus precision: challenges in clinical trial design for left ventricular assist devices. *Ann Thorac Surg.* 2006;82:1140–1146.

22. Slaughter MS, Rogers JG, Milano CA, et al., HeartMate II Investigators. Advanced heart failure treated with continuous-flow left ventricular assist device. *N Engl J Med.* 2009;361:2241–2251.

23. Capizzi T, Zhang J. Testing the hypothesis that matters for multiple primary endpoints. *Drug Info J.* 1996;30:949–956.

24. Neuhauser M, Steinijans VW. The evaluation of multiple clinical endpoints with application to asthma. *Drug Info J.* 1999;33:471–477.

25. Levy WC, Mozaffarian D, Linker DT. The Seattle Heart Failure Model: prediction of survival in heart failure. *Circulation.* 2006;113:1424–1433.

26. Koelling TM, Joseph S, Aaronson KD. Heart failure survival score continues to predict clinical outcomes in patients with heart failure receiving beta-blockers. *J Heart Lung Transplant.* 2004;23:1414–1422.

27. O'Connor CM, Whellan DJ, Lee KL. Efficacy and safety of exercise training in patients with chronic heart failure: HF-ACTION randomized controlled trial. *JAMA.* 2009;301:1439–1450.

28. Long JW, Kfoury AG, Slaughter MS, et al. Long-term destination therapy with the HeartMate XVE left ventricular assist device: improved outcomes since the REMATCH study. *Congest Heart Fail.* 2005;11:133–138.

29. Stewart GC, Brooks K, Pratibhu PP. Thresholds of physical activity and life expectancy for patients considering destination ventricular assist devices. *J Heart Lung Transplant.* 2009;28:863–869.

Role of Government Agencies in Mechanical Circulatory Support — FDA*

Sonna M. Patel-Raman, Eric A. Chen, and Francesca Joseph

510(k) refers to the regulation for premarket notification

513(g) refers to the regulation for a request for device classification

BSA body surface area

CDRH Center for Devices and Radiological Health

CEC Clinical Events Committee

CFR Code of Federal Regulations

CMS Center for Medicaid Services

CU compassionate use

DSMB Data and Safety Monitoring Board

EU emergency use

FDA United States Food and Drug Administration

FD&C Food, Drug, and Cosmetic Act

HDE humanitarian device exemption

HUD humanitarian use device

IDE investigational device exemption

INTERMACS Interagency Registry for Mechanically Assisted Circulatory Support

IRB Institutional Review Board

LVAS left ventricular assist system

MCSD mechanical circulatory support device

NIH National Institutes of Health

NYHA New York Heart Association (classification for heart failure)

OUS outside the United States

Pre-IDE refers to any interaction with FDA prior to regulatory submission requesting action

PMA pre-market approval application

(L) or (R) VAD (left) or (right) ventricular assist device

U.S. FOOD AND DRUG ADMINISTRATION ROLE—MISSION

The Center for Devices and Radiological Health (CDRH) at the U.S. Food and Drug Administration (FDA) was established to promote public health by reviewing and taking appropriate and timely action regarding the marketing applications of regulated medical devices. At the same time, FDA protects public health by ensuring a reasonable assurance of the safety and effectiveness (or probable benefit) of medical devices deemed appropriate for human use.[1]

This chapter reviews the different regulatory applications related to mechanical circulatory support devices (MCSDs) and describes the pathway of obtaining approval to market these devices in the United States. The process for MCSDs typically begins with a clinical study and concludes with marketing approval or clearance. Each category of pre-market regulatory submission is discussed, including investigational device exemption (IDE), premarket approval (PMA), humanitarian device exemption (HDE), and 510(k) applications. Upon obtaining regulatory approval, a postmarket study is often conducted to collect important data on adverse events and real-world use of the device as a condition of approval. As devices are more widely used after approval, we also discuss the importance of reporting of adverse events. The chapter concludes with details of FDA's role in supporting innovative trial design to meet the changing landscape of the field, and a special section addresses regulatory considerations for pediatric MCSDs.

The primary role of the Office of Device Evaluation in CDRH is to review extensive preclinical and clinical data, and make decisions regarding the approval or clearance of medical devices. An MCSD *sponsor* (term used to describe any entity that submits an application for review to the Agency—company, investigator, individual, consultant, etc.) has the responsibility to submit the results of preclinical and clinical (when necessary) evaluations to support either the initiation of a US-based clinical trial or the marketing of a new device in the United States.

The current landscape of MCSDs (as discussed in Chapter 8) constitutes Class III devices and includes approved devices, as well as those under development and in clinical study. The classification determines the amount and type of information needed to support a marketing application. General controls including device registration, good manufacturing practices, and labeling are the expected baseline requirements for all devices. Because MCSDs are designed to support or sustain human life, Class III

---

*This chapter represents the professional opinion of the authors and is not an official document, agency guidance, or policy of the U.S. Government, the Department of Health and Human Services, or the Food and Drug Administration, nor should any official endorsement be inferred.

devices require premarket approval based on evidence that supports a reasonable assurance of safety and effectiveness.

REGULATORY PATHWAY TO APPROVAL/ CLEARANCE

The regulatory pathway to approval of MCSD is a stepwise approach. After receiving preliminary FDA feedback regarding preclinical and clinical testing plans, sponsors submit an IDE for approval to start a clinical study. Following completion of the clinical study, sponsors typically plan to submit a PMA or an HDE for marketing approval of their device.

There are currently two categories of approved use of durable MCSDs: bridge-to-transplant and destination therapy. Bridge-to-transplant (BTT) is a term reserved for patients who are supported with an MCSD until a donor heart is available and they can receive a transplant. Destination therapy (DT) is a term reserved for patients who are supported with a MCSD who have no apparent option of receiving a heart transplant.

Pre-Submission (Also Known as Pre-IDE)

Sponsors are encouraged to interact with the FDA as early as possible to discuss and receive FDA's informal input on preclinical testing as well as feedback to ensure that the proposed clinical protocol and data analysis plan are consistent with FDA's expectations for a well-designed trial. Early interactions, prior to submission of an IDE or marketing application, are referred to as *pre-IDE "submissions or "pre-submissions."* FDA views the pre-IDE interaction as one that can occur at many times during the device development process as well as during the clinical study. Pre-submission interactions are helpful prior to submission of an IDE, prior to major changes in a device or trial design, when planning the submission of a PMA application, or after approval of a PMA when a major device design change or addition of a new indication for use is desired. For example, MCSD sponsors have used the process to obtain feedback on appropriate preclinical bench testing or the adequacy of a statistical analysis plan.

Preclinical Testing

Due to the high risk nature of implantable MCSDs, FDA reviews extensive preclinical bench and animal testing prior to use of the device in a clinical trial in humans. Bench testing provides significant device characterization data while animal data provides a safety profile not achievable on the bench. Both types of testing typically reflect the clinical usage of the device. The preclinical testing requirements typically depend on the proposed indications for use of the MCSD. For example, FDA would expect that for the BTT and DT indications, preclinical testing would need to demonstrate that the device could be performed safely and reliably for at least 6 months and 1 year, respectively, prior to IDE approval. In general, FDA expects testing to continue to failure (at least 1 year for BTT and 2 years for DT) for a marketing application. This type of testing often leads to increased knowledge and understanding of how the devices are functioning for a period of time extending beyond the expected clinical use. Various types of preclinical testing include:
- Animal testing
- Bench reliability and durability
- Biocompatibility
- Computational fluid dynamics
- Device characterization and mechanical testing
- Electrical safety/electromagnetic compatability

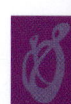

- Human factors
- Packaging and shelf-life testing
- Reliability/durability
- Software
- Sterilization

In general, when conducting any preclinical test, the necessity of the test (e.g., animal evaluations), ultimately depends on how the animal and the testing will inform FDA with regard to device safety and performance.

Investigational Device Exemptions (IDE) Studies

In order to study MCSDs in human subjects in the United States, an approved IDE application is needed in addition to local IRB approval. An FDA-approved IDE allows evaluation of the safety and performance of MCSDs in a clinical trial environment. The required contents of an IDE application are described in detail in 21 CFR 812.20(b), and an FDA guidance document is also available to assist in the preparation of an IDE application.[2] A typical MCSD IDE may include the following types of information:
1. The proposed indications for use (e.g., target population, BTT, DT, failure-to-wean, acute myocardial infarction (MI), patient size or age, length of time on support)
2. Device description (e.g., axial/centrifugal flow, continuous, magnetically levitated/hydrodynamic bearings, etc.)
3. Inclusion/exclusion criteria (e.g., transplant listed/ineligible, NYHA classification, patient size and/or age, etiology of heart failure, etc.)
4. Written protocol describing study methodology including:
   a. Anticipated clinical risk and benefit (e.g., endpoints)
   b. The "control" to which the new treatment is being compared (i.e., the current standard of care treatment for these patients)
   c. Primary and secondary endpoints for study success
   d. Statistical plan (i.e., randomized control group with interim analysis, use of randomized, historical control, INTERMACS as concurrent control, etc.) with prespecified primary and secondary endpoints with mathematical hypotheses
5. Patient informed consent
6. Patient follow-up in tabular format for laboratory visits, procedures, tests, etc.
7. Examples of case (clinical) report forms

In situations where FDA has serious safety questions about the device, concerns with regard to the scientific soundness or validity, or where the investigational plan or report of prior investigations are inadequate, incomplete, or omitted, FDA may choose to disapprove the application. If there are no serious concerns related to these areas, but some minor questions exist (e.g., regarding aspects of the clinical protocol or preclinical data), FDA may grant conditional approval of the IDE application. This allows the manufacturer to begin their clinical trial as long as FDA's remaining questions are adequately addressed in a timely fashion. Once all of FDA's concerns are addressed, an application may receive unconditional approval. IDEs are approved for feasibility and pivotal studies and have been used for various patient populations including BTT and DT, acute MI, failure-to-wean, etc.

Feasibility Study

The FDA may recommend or sponsors may choose to perform a feasibility (or pilot) study prior to the pivotal clinical trial in order to assess the initial device performance in humans as well as to better define the patient population, intended use of the device, and/or appropriate outcome measures. Feasibility studies may employ prespecified endpoints and/or success criteria for such a small study; however, FDA recognizes that they would likely be descriptive in nature. FDA strongly considers these data prior to the start of a pivotal study and reviews it for relevant safety and/or effectiveness signals. FDA typically does not accept feasibility data alone as substantive enough to support a marketing application for MCSDs. In cases where there is historical experience with a particular type of MCSD design and/or performance, it may be appropriate for the sponsor to begin a pivotal study, with the proviso that a report on the first 10 to 15 patients be submitted for FDA review to confirm that no catastrophic safety issues are occurring.

Pivotal Study

Pivotal study data are used to support a marketing application for MCSDs. Some of these populations include the BTT, DT, failure-to-wean, and acute heart failure patients. The statistical plan involves a detailed data analysis that includes primary and secondary endpoints for both safety and effectiveness, in addition to appropriate sample size calculations and mathematic hypotheses. Pivotal trials incorporate endpoints that are clinically relevant to the patient and reflect the intended use of the device, such as mortality and morbidity, rates of adverse events, changes in hemodynamic characteristics, functional assessments, device reliability, etc. Ultimately, the clinical data necessary to support approval of the device may depend on the unique characteristics of the patient population and the expected outcome of the trial.

Design and Protocol Modifications during an Investigational Device Exemption

Design and/or protocol modifications to MCSDs often occur during the course of an IDE as clinical experience leads to improvements in defining the patient population, surgical tools, the device, and/or its accessories. Some changes such as modifications to the device coating, bearings, and/or controller operations require more extensive review but do not require additional clinical data. In some cases, a design modification during the IDE stage may be so significant that collection of additional clinical data will be necessary prior to approval of the modified device in a marketing application.

Compassionate Use

During the course of an IDE, a need arises to implant an MCSD in a particular patient who may not qualify for inclusion in the ongoing IDE study or other approved IDE studies, and cannot receive an FDA-approved device. The compassionate use (CU) provision* allows access for patients who do not meet the requirements for inclusion in an MCSD clinical investigation but for whom the treating physician believes the device may provide a benefit in treating their disease or condition. The compassionate use provision can be used by physicians even if an IDE does not exist. However, physicians are encouraged to apply for an IDE if repeated requests are received for compassionate use of a device. Box 23-1 provides a list of criteria for compassionate use. Compassionate use requests need agreement from the sponsor and approval from the FDA before allowing the treating physician to implant the device in a patient (Fig. 23-1).

---

*http://www.fda.gov/MedicalDevices/DeviceRegulationandGuidance/GuidanceDocuments/ucm080202.htm. Accessed February 1, 2011.

BOX 23-1 Criteria for Compassionate Use

1. A description of the patient's condition and the circumstances necessitating treatment
2. A discussion of why alternative therapies are unsatisfactory and why the probable risk of using the investigational device is no greater than the probable risk from the disease or condition
3. An identification of any deviations in the approved clinical protocol that may be needed in order to treat the patient
4. The patient protection measures that will be followed.
   - An independent assessment by an uninvolved physician
   - Informed consent from patient or legal representative
   - Letter of concurrence from the hospital Institutional Review Board
   - Institutional clearance as specified by their policies
   - Sponsor Authorization; IDE exists.

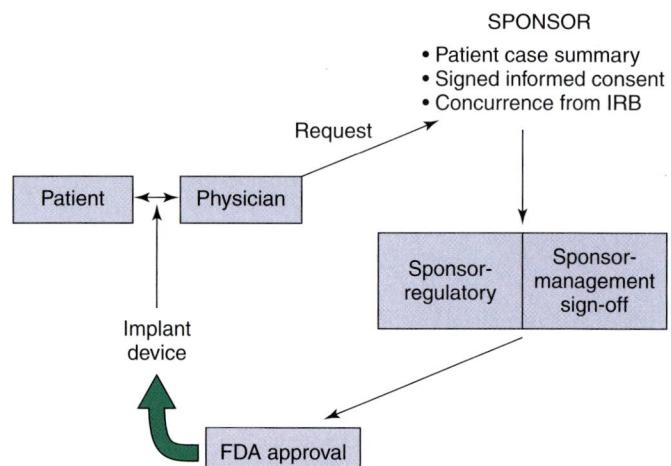

FIGURE 23-1 Logistics of compassionate use. FDA, U.S. Food and Drug Administration; IRB, institutional review board.

Although CU data are not considered as a sole dataset to support an HDE or PMA application, it may still be valuable to the regulatory decision-making process.

Emergency Use

The emergency use provision allows for the use of an MCSD in situations where it is necessary to protect the life or physical well-being of a subject in an emergency. Although prior approval for shipment or emergency use of the investigational device is not required, the use of the MCSD is expected to be reported to FDA. The sponsor should ensure that this report includes documentation confirming that the situation was in fact an emergency and that the patient's protection measures were not violated. Such patient protection procedures include obtaining informed consent from the patient or legal representative, clearance from the institution as specified by their policies, concurrence from the IRB chair, independent assessment from an uninvolved physician, and approval by the trial sponsor.

Outside the United States (OUS) Data and Regulatory Approvals from Other Countries

In some cases, sponsors are interested in collecting OUS data to demonstrate experience with the device, even though it is not a requirement in order to initiate a clinical trial in the US.

Some sponsors utilize OUS data in lieu of conducting a US feasibility study. FDA's acceptance of such clinical data as justification to initiate a pivotal study depends on a number of factors such as experience with the particular MCSD, the number of patients, location of the clinical site(s), use of an identical protocol, similar care of the patients to that in the US, the specific outcome measurements used, and the quality and completeness of patient follow-up. For MCSDs, sponsors have not typically utilized OUS data as part of the pivotal study or as a mechanism to reduce the sample size of a pivotal study. Discussions about the use of OUS data routinely occur during the pre-submission stage and are initiated before non-US clinical studies are performed so as to increase the chance that a similar protocol would be used OUS and that these data would be useful to the FDA in evaluating the device.

In some cases, sponsors with OUS experience often have already obtained international regulatory approval such as a CE mark in Europe. A CE mark is a European certification that a product has met the requirements of and can be sold in the European Union. FDA does not currently recognize foreign regulatory approvals and they are not a requirement for approval of an MCSD. Approval decisions are made independent of a CE mark.[3]

MARKETING APPLICATIONS

FDA reviews the data from the clinical trial to determine if the device performed as intended and the clinical benefits outweigh the risks. Statistical success or failure to meet the primary endpoint does not mandate an approval or disapproval (or clearance) of the marketing application. FDA always reviews the totality of the data to make a determination regarding the risks and benefits of the device, and considers the existing clinical landscape in the context of currently available alternative treatments (including other marketed devices) and how they are being used. There are three types of marketing applications that FDA reviews for medical devices: Premarket Notification 510(k), PMA, and humanitarian device exemption (HDE) applications.

510(k) Pathway

The 510(k) pathway requires comparison between new class II medical devices to a legally marketed predicated device that has already been cleared by the FDA for commercialization. For these applications, the manufacturer must demonstrate that the new medical device is substantially equivalent to another legally marketed device; that is, the new device is at least as safe and effective as the predicate device.[4] Most MCSDs do not qualify for the 510(k) pathway due to the risks associated with the device. Substantial equivalence does not suggest that the new and predicate devices are identical but indicates that the devices are equivalent with respect to the intended use and technologic characteristics (e.g., device design, materials used to develop the device, biocompatibility, mode of therapy, etc.).

Premarket Approval (PMA) Application

Most class III devices follow the PMA pathway, which is considered to be the most stringent because the PMA application must contain sufficient valid scientific evidence to demonstrate a reasonable assurance of safety and effectiveness when the MCSD is used as intended. The application includes information obtained from all prior studies (clinical and nonclinical) such as biocompatibility, device characterization and performance, durability or reliability, sterilization, shelf-life, and if applicable, software, electromagnetic compatibility and electrical safety, and any other relevant bench or animal data. Because of the complexity of MCDS, the applications are often large in volume and require review from experts of varying disciplines. The clinical study reports for MCDS usually include comprehensive, summarized patient level data, the clinical protocols, adverse reactions and complications, any information on procedural or device failures and replacements, and any other clinical data (i.e., foreign clinical data) that have been obtained by the manufacturer.

Humanitarian Device Exemption (HDE)

An HDE application is an option for some Class III MCSDs, which are intended for use in a small population. Before submission of an HDE application, a manufacturer must obtain a humanitarian use device (HUD) designation. To qualify for this designation, a medical device must be intended to benefit patients in the treatment or diagnosis of a disease or condition that affects or is manifested in fewer than 4000 individuals per year in the United States (21 CFR 814.3(n)).

A typical application for HUD designation would include documentation describing the disease or condition, proposed indications for use of the device, the reasons why such a device is needed given the available alternatives, and the population-based estimates to establish that the potential patient population to be treated is fewer than 4000 people per year. One challenging aspect of the HUD application process is when a device is proposed for an indication that represents a subset of a common disease or condition. In these situations, the applicant must demonstrate that the subset is a medically plausible patient population (a regulatory concept that means use of a product precludes its use in the entire disease or condition). In general, the FDA recognizes that multiple MCSDs intended to treat pediatric patients may qualify for HUD designation.

An HDE application is similar in both form and content to the PMA application. The HDE application must provide the same level of assurance of safety as in a PMA, but the HDE is exempt from the requirements to demonstrate a reasonable assurance of effectiveness; rather, the sponsor must demonstrate that the probable benefit of its device outweighs its probable risks. Additionally, the sponsor must demonstrate that no comparable devices are available to treat or diagnose the disease or condition and that they could not otherwise bring the device to market.

Because of the "probable benefit" requirement and limited patient sample size for HDEs, statistically powered clinical trials and robust statistical analyses may not be feasible. In the case of the pediatric MCSD population, FDA recognizes that the small patient population available for an IDE study limits the statistical conclusions that can be drawn from a clinical trial. In some scenarios, particularly for HDE applications, a qualitative evaluation of descriptive statistics may be necessary for understanding that the device demonstrates safety and probable benefit.

Even though a clinical investigation is not an absolute requirement for HDE (as opposed to historical control from the literature or case series), it is rare for the FDA to have approved an HDE without it. The clinical data from a prospective trial provide important information on device performance and specific adverse events that may occur. Furthermore, these data can enable the applicant to better define the intended patient population by assessing patient demographics and refining patient management protocols. Such clinical study data will allow the FDA to develop an informative label for the device that better specifies the patient population and intended use.

Once FDA approves an HDE application, the sponsor is authorized to market the HUD in the United States after IRB

approval has been obtained at each institution for the specific FDA-approved indication.

Advisory Panels

Although an FDA review team consists of multiple experts who are on FDA staffs, the FDA may determine that additional external expertise is necessary to conduct a comprehensive review. A first-of-a-kind device or cutting edge technology different from current therapies (a continuous flow MCSD versus pulsatile), a vulnerable patient population (pediatric patients), significant safety and effectiveness questions, or concerns regarding the conduct of the trial or analysis of the data (significant missing data or failure to achieve a primary endpoint) can result in a decision to seek an Advisory Panel input. Ultimately, the FDA carefully considers the totality of the data including the recommendations from the Panel members' individual comments and discussions in making a decision on approvability.

POSTMARKET

Once devices are approved (through a PMA or HDE application), additional requirements often need to be met in terms of monitoring and evaluation of clinical and device performance in a real-world setting (post-approval study, device modifications, and medical device reporting).

Post-Approval Study

The FDA typically requests that a post-approval study be conducted for MCSDs to allow the FDA and the sponsor to monitor device performance and potential patient- and device-related problems following device approval. This allows the FDA to take appropriate measures if potential risks are identified. Post-approval studies are not used to evaluate unanswered questions regarding safety and effectiveness that need to be addressed during the premarket phase, but can be used to collect data on rarely occurring adverse events. Data collected in such studies is also typically not sufficient to support a new identification for the MCSD. A post-approval study is designed with FDA approval and sponsor input; the FDA expects sponsors will finalize post-market study design prior to receiving marketing approval for their device to ensure that this important data can be collected as quickly as possible. Post-approval studies are beneficial for collecting additional data regarding real-world use, longer-term device reliability, usefulness of training programs, subgroup evaluation within the approved patient population, and evaluation of rare adverse events.

Device and Clinical Modifications after Premarket Approval

The determination of whether additional preclinical or clinical data is necessary for device modification, changes in indications, changes in manufacturing, etc., is dependent on each MCSD and the type of change. Examples of changes requiring clinical data have included modifications for a pump driver to be used outside of the hospital and changes to a valve assembly. Another important change that can often require clinical data is a modification of the indications for use. For example, when a device is approved for BTT patients and the sponsor then wishes to modify the indications to include DT patients, long-term clinical trial data are necessary to demonstrate a reasonable assurance of safety and effectiveness for the new indications. Many types of these changes are submitted via a PMA supplement, but significant modifications to the device or indications for use can result in a new PMA application.

Medical Device Reporting

The purpose of the Medical Device Reporting (MDR) system is to collect reports of adverse events that occur with MCSD after marketing approval. During an IDE trial, patients are closely monitored, and specific follow-up procedures exist to ensure patients receive protocolized care with regard to their MCSD. However, the controlled setting of an IDE does not often exist post-approval. Once an MCSD is approved, the collection of adverse events through MDR can assist in the evaluation of "real-world" use. The FDA is currently collaborating with INTERMACS to ensure that adverse events associated with MCSDs are accurately and efficiently reported. Currently, INTERMACS can notify the FDA and sponsors with an "alert" when an adverse event occurs. In the future, INTERMACS hopes to provide additional information regarding device malfunction in a similar manner.

DESIGN OF BTT AND DT TRIALS

The following sections discuss the development of short- and long-term MCSD trial designs as well as the future of clinical trial designs and how MCSDs will be evaluated.

BTT Trials

Initial BTT trial designs were limited due to small target populations and difficulties in achieving enrollment within a reasonable period of time; the primary endpoint for these trials is survival to transplant. Although this is an objective endpoint, FDA recognized that this approach required long and unpredictable follow-up periods resulting in trials lasting more than 2 to 3 years. The FDA believed that establishing a prospectively identified criterion to define success for bridging patients with cardiac transplantation would facilitate single-arm clinical trials and allow for these life-supporting devices to be made available to the patients that need them. In 2002, after an extensive literature review, six publications were used as the basis for a performance goal of 65% to 70% survival-to–cardiac transplantation rate for approved BTT devices.[5–10] The FDA considered several factors when developing the performance goal, including a well-characterized patient population, extensive history with BTT devices, a well known standard of care, consensus in the clinical community that there is expectation of significant positive results, and sufficient published data to support a robust performance goal (with no specified time point for patient evaluation).

Recognizing the limitations of longer clinical trials, and with the development of new devices, the FDA supported the collection of safety and effectiveness data in a least burdensome manner (i.e., a shorter time frame, easing the burden on sponsors for a lengthy trial). Based on a review of the United Network for Organ Sharing (UNOS) data available to the FDA at the time, it appeared that transplant-eligible patients requiring support could remain on a VAD for up to 6 months or 180 days while waiting for a donor heart.[11] This was the basis for establishment of the endpoint for BTT trials, which was survival to cardiac transplantation or listed for cardiac transplantation (UNOS 1A/1B) at 180 days.

Despite the development of a performance goal in 2002, the FDA also acknowledged the ongoing construction of INTERMACS, which was intended to collect data to facilitate improved patient evaluation, management, and outcomes, while also aiding in device design and improvements.[12] With hundreds of patients regularly being entered into the registry, which opened for enrollment in 2006, the FDA considered the feasibility of using the registry data as a concurrent control.

INTERMACS (see Chapter 24) currently includes data on over 4000 patients with durable MCSDs indicated for BTT and DT, and includes important patient demographic data, patient outcomes, health status, quality of life, and neurologic data.[13]

With an increased use of BTT devices, and more patient data entered into the registry, industry, clinicians, and government agencies have strongly supported the use of a concurrent control group based on many years of experience with BTT clinical studies and a well-characterized patient population.. Additionally, categories for heart failure that clearly define disease severity allow for consistent identification of the BTT patient population[14] (Chapter 24). Currently approved BTT clinical trials are comparing patients receiving the investigational device to a group of similar patients selected from the INTERMACS registry, based on prespecified patient characteristics and demographics.

DT Trial Design

Destination therapy trials involve the studying of a patients ineligible for a heart transplant. The current paradigm for destination therapy involves a randomized, noninferiority comparison of an FDA- approved MCSD to the treatment MCSD, evaluating patients at 2 years. The trial design used for approval of the HeartMate II VAD has served as a model for currently approved DT study designs.[15]

Many external stakeholders have approached the FDA to consider the use of INTERMACS as a concurrent control for the DT population. Although there are indications that the number of patients enrolled in INTERMACS is increasing, the FDA and the medical community remain concerned that the level of characterization and understanding of DT patients in the registry is not sufficient to allow the registry to be used as a concurrent control. As more patients receiving DT devices are entered into the registry and as the clinical community gains more experience with those patients, the FDA believes that a clearer understanding of the patient population will emerge. The FDA intends to continue a periodic review of the available DT data from INTERMACS, as well as discuss its usefulness with the clinical, academic, and industry communities.

BTT versus DT: Is There a Clear Line?

Recognizing the clinical management paradigm shift from clearly identified BTT and DT patients, who are no longer categorized easily in one group or the other, to an evidenced-based categorization of "all-comer," FDA continues to support exploring ways to address this changing practice. Historically, this distinction was created and accepted in the academic and clinical communities to allow sponsors to market their device more quickly. With a shorter endpoint (180 days) for BTT trials, sponsors could complete a trial and submit a PMA within a more reasonable period of time and continue to collect safety and effectiveness data. Currently, patients are remaining on the device for an unpredictable length of time and continue to have improved clinical outcomes per data in INTERMACS. Despite the desire of the clinical community for an "all-comers" trial, FDA believes that trial designs for MCSDs are dictated by important considerations such as a specific target population (i.e., indications for use, inclusion/exclusion criteria), available alternative practices, identification of a control group, criteria for success or failure within the trial, and the anticipated clinical benefit. Nonetheless, FDA would be interested in working with sponsors to design a clinical trial in which the enrollment of patients would be based on severity of heart failure and not whether the patient was specifically listed for transplant or not. The NHLBI-sponsored Randomized Evaluation of VAD InterVEntion before Inotropic Therapy (REVIVE-IT) feasibility clinical study may be the first step in moving toward such a study. The REVIVE-IT study will explore the potential benefit of MCSDs in functionally impaired advanced heart failure patients who have not yet developed serious consequences from their disease.

Limited Number of Control Patients

Another challenge FDA has identified involves consideration of the number of MCSDs in development. Due to the limited number of patients available for study, multiple device trials with the same indications for use conducted at the same time could result in fewer available patients for any individual device in any particular study. FDA believes that for certain patient populations, it may be possible for sponsors to share a "control group." The coordination of this shared group would ultimately be dependent on the sponsors' willingness to collaborate on this effort.

PEDIATRIC MECHANICAL CIRCULATORY SUPPORT DEVICES

Effective pediatric device development continues to be an important initiative for FDA and remains a critical unmet need in the United States as each year thousands of infants die as a result of congenital heart defects and heart disease. The FDA continues to collaborate with external stakeholders through several outreach efforts including workshops and pre-submission meetings to encourage device manufacturers to contact the agency early and often during the development process to ensure that appropriate preclinical testing is performed, thus potentiating progression to a clinical feasibility trial. By the time the clinical phase of testing is reached, the limitations common to pediatric clinical research in general will likely be encountered. Statistically robust study design is challenged by a small sample size and substantial heterogeneity within the population, combined with factors that can impact the interpretability of study results. Enrollment goals may necessitate a large number of enrolling centers that are geographically and clinically (e.g., anticoagulation protocols) diverse, thus contributing to unwanted variability. FDA has discussed the idea of a shared control population depending on the indications for use of each MCSD. Clear study endpoints with prespecified, clinically relevant hypotheses are needed for FDA to make the most appropriate risk-benefit decisions. Furthermore, standardized adverse event definitions across data sources and registries are necessary for meaningful safety comparisons.

Given these challenges, FDA has actively pursued relationships with the pediatric MCSD community to facilitate interactions through various initiatives such as workshops, the Pumps for Kids, Infants, and Neonates (PumpKIN) program, and INTERMACS.

CDRH and Pediatric MCSD Workshops

Recognizing the growing need for MCSDs to treat pediatric patients, FDA convened a workshop in 2006 on the Regulatory Process for Pediatric Mechanical Circulatory Support Devices with NIH/NHLBI, the academic community, and industry in attendance to focus on pediatric ventricular assist device approval.[16–18] This meeting encouraged pediatric device developers to pursue development of their devices and consider that the HDE marketing pathway may be more accessible for making their devices available. In 2007, the Pediatric Medical Device Safety and Improvement Act allowed pediatric devices submitted under an HDE marketing pathway to be sold for profit, further encouraging development in this field.[19]

Neurologic adverse events are one example for which tools and assessments exist, but there are no specific protocols or

standards in place to establish the type and frequency of the tests and the specific age ranges that would benefit from each test. Recognizing this as a critical issue for the study of pediatric VADs, the FDA held a public workshop in 2010 to explore strategies for the standardization of pediatric neurological function and neurocognitive assessments in pediatric MCSDs.[20]

Overall, careful attention to trial design and early consultation with the FDA are excellent strategies to manage potential regulatory hurdles. Through such communication, design of trials for pediatric MCSDs that maximize the likelihood of generating interpretable data can be facilitated most efficiently. Although no single prescriptive approach is likely to be ideal for all of these devices, the interactive process is imperative to efficient device and trial development.

Pumps for Kids, Infants, and Neonates (PumpKIN)

After initial NHLBI support in 2004 that focused on preclinical development for a range of pediatric VADs and similar circulatory support systems, the NIH offered additional support through the Pumps for Kids, Infants, and Neonates (PumpKIN) contract in 2010. This NIH program is discussed in greater detail in Chapter 16. The FDA has collaborated with the NIH on this effort to ensure that contractors are not only meeting requirements of the NIH contract but also developing and designing their pediatric MCSDs to support a future clinical study and marketing application. The required elements of the PumpKIN contract include preclinical tests and analyses, development and documentation of manufacturing processes and procedures, and collaboration to develop an IDE clinical study. The data collected from the clinical studies can then be used to provide the evidence in support of PMA or HDE approval.[21] With the PumpKIN program under way and the pediatric heart failure field continuing to advance, the FDA expects the initiation of multiple clinical trials over the next several years. In support of this program, FDA participates in monthly teleconference with sponsors to provide feedback on regulatory topics such as conducting clinical trials and submitting marketing applications.

INTERMACS—Pediatric

Given that most, if not all, pediatric recipients of novel devices will remain hospitalized throughout the period of mechanical support (at least in the preapproval phase), the "durable" eligibility criterion for INTERMACS is a major limiting factor for pediatric data collection. Although no distinction is made between adult and pediatric patients in INTERMACS, additional data is required for pediatric patients (<22 years of age) and for adult patients with congenital diagnoses. Once a pediatric patient is entered into the registry, the patient remains in pediatric status until the implanted device is explanted. A modified version of the database for pediatrics that would allow for uniform data collection within the framework of consensus definitions (whether as part of IDE studies, emergency or compassionate usage, or during the postapproval period) is gaining support. Further extending the pediatric component of the database to collect data on medical management or ECMO support may also be worthwhile to be used as comparator groups for the evaluation of new devices but remains under discussion.

INTERACTIONS WITH EXTERNAL STAKEHOLDERS

CDRH believes that relationships with external stakeholders and government partners are critical to the success of the MCSD program. CDRH participates in a number of preclinical and clinical initiatives outside of FDA that serve to benefit the research and development of MCSDs.

Engineers in CDRH regularly contribute to the development of MCSD preclinical testing standards led by organizations such as the Association for the Advancement of Medical Instrumentation (AAMI) and the International Organization for Standardization (ISO). Reviewers are also participating in an FDA Critical Path Initiative (CPI) project that specifically focuses on reducing hemolysis and blood damage through improved computational design of MCSDs.[22] Members of the Division of Cardiovascular Devices (DCD) are part of the INTERMACS Operations Committee, working with clinicians as well as organizations such as United Network for Organ Sharing (UNOS), University of Alabama (UAB), NIH, and Centers for Medicare and Medicaid Services (CMS). The committee provides direction, oversight, and approval for the major design features of the registry, as well as other functional components. For example, FDA staff have helped develop standardized adverse event definitions for MCSDs, which will aid in our ability to interpret the data collected. It is the hope of everyone involved with this major enterprise that eventually propensity score analysis can be used to compare investigational device patients to similarly matched control patients who are enrolled in the INTERMACS registry.[23] Finally, acknowledging the challenges of developing and designing pediatric devices, FDA has worked closely with NHLBI and the PumpKIN contractors to provide feedback on the development of devices and related clinical trials. The aforementioned examples are just a few of the outreach opportunities in which FDA participates and illustrates commitment from FDA to advance the field and accomplish its mission.

CONCLUSIONS

FDA's role in the assessment of trial data for MCSDs and approving marketing applications for those that demonstrate a reasonable assurance of safety and effectiveness (or probable benefit) remains challenging due to the constant improvements in MCSD technology, the complexity of the devices, and the changing patient population and management. With thorough preclinical testing, including bench and animal evaluations, and early interaction via the pre-submission pathway, most MCSD study sponsors are able to successfully obtain approval of a clinical trial. Upon completion, the data from the trial have been submitted to FDA for evaluation, and review of these data has led to the approval of several MCSDs that are available on the market today.

Just as the regulatory paradigm has evolved from a BTT performance goal to concurrent controls, the trial designs for DT may also change as more data become available. Ultimately, each indication for use is evaluated in an independent trial that typically considers the clinical risk and benefit, the intended target population, the appropriate comparator group, and the available alternative practices at the time the trial is conducted.

Although each trial ultimately stands on its own, FDA considers the landscape of the field and current medical practices when making regulatory approval decisions. FDA has continued to be actively engaged as the field has evolved and has demonstrated commitment to advancing the field through collaborative programs such as INTERMACS and PumpKIN. FDA has dedicated specific efforts to advancing pediatric MCSD development through stakeholder interactions, including the encouragement of utilization of the HUD/HDE pathway.

FDA remains committed to interacting with all external stakeholders, including industry, clinicians, and government agencies, to ensure that we foster innovation where possible and that safe and effective devices are made available to the patients that need them.

1. Food, Drug & Cosmetic Act, §903(b)(1, 2(C)). http://www.fda.gov/opacom/laws/fdcact/fdctoc.htm; December 31, 2004 Accessed 20.09.09.

2. IDE Guidance Staff. *FDA Guidance Documents.* http://www.fda.gov/cdrh/ode/idepolcy.pdf; January 20, 1998 Accessed December 17.12.08.

3. US Food and Drug Administration. http://www.fda.gov/MedicalDevices/DeviceRegulationandGuidance/HowtoMarketYourDevice/PremarketSubmissions/PremarketApprovalPMA/ucm050503.htm; Accessed 10.10.10.

4. *What Is Substantial Equivalence?* http://www.fda.gov/cdrh/devadvice/314.html#se; Accessed 08.01.09.

5. Frazier OH, Rose EA, Oz MC, et al. Multicenter clinical evaluation of the HeartMate vented electric left ventricular assist system in patients awaiting heart transplantation. *J Thorac Cardiovasc Surg.* 2001;122(6):1186–1195.

6. El-Banayosy A, Korfer R, Arusoglu L, et al. Device and patient management in a bridge-to-transplant setting. *Ann Thorac Surg.* 2001;71(suppl 3):S98–S102.

7. El-Banayosy A, Arusoglu L, Kizner L, et al. Novacor left ventricular assist system versus Heartmate vented electric left ventricular assist system as a long-term mechanical circulatory support device in bridging patients: a prospective study. *J Thorac Cardiovasc Surg.* 2000;119(3):581–587.

8. Di Bella I, Pagani F, Banfi C, et al. Results with the Novacor assist system and evaluation of long-term assistance. *Eur J Cardiothorac Surg.* 2000;18(1):112–116.

9. Minami K, El-Banayosy A, Sezai A, et al. Morbidity and outcome after mechanical ventricular support using Thoratec, Novacor, and HeartMate for bridging to heart transplantation. *Artif Organs.* 2000;24(6):421–426.

10. Farrar DJ, Hill JD, Pennington DG, et al. Preoperative and postoperative comparison of patients with univentricular and biventricular support with the Thoratec ventricular assist device as a bridge to cardiac transplantation. *J Thorac Cardiovasc Surg.* 1997;113(1):202–209.

11. Organ Procurement and Transplantation Network. http://optn.transplant.hrsa.gov; Accessed 09.10.10.

12. Interagency Registry for Mechanically Assisted Circulatory Support. http://www.uab.edu/ctsresearch/intermacs/description.htm; Accessed 31.01.11.

13. Interagency Registry for Mechanically Assisted Circulatory Support. http://www.intermacs.org; Accessed 06.05.10.

14. Chen EA, Patel-Raman SM. *J Cardiovasc Transl Res.* 2011 (in press).

15. *Summary of Safety and Effectiveness Data for the HeartMate II Left Ventricular Assist System.* http://www.accessdata.fda.gov/cdrh_docs/pdf6/P060040S005b.pdf; Accessed 01.08.10.

16. Weber S. Pediatric Circulatory Support Contractors' Meeting: Report of the Clinical Trials Working Group. *ASAIO J.* 2009;55(1):10–12.

17. Pantalos GM. Use of Computer and In Vitro Modeling Techniques during the Development of Pediatric Circulatory Support Devices: National Heart, Lung, and Blood Institute Pediatric Assist Device Contractor's Meeting: Pediatric Modeling Techniques Working Group. *ASAIO J.* 2009;55(1):3–5.

18. United States Department of Health and Human Services. *Notice of public meeting.* Available at http://www.fda.gov/ohrms/dockets/98fr/05-24271.htm; December 20, 2005 Accessed 17.05.10.

19. US Food and Drug Administration. http://www.fda.gov/MedicalDevices/DeviceRegulationandGuidance/GuidanceDocuments/ucm110194.htm#6; Accessed 02.11.10.

20. United States Department of Health and Human Services. *Pediatric Assessments of Neurological and Neurocognitive Function for Cardiovascular Devices Workshop.* Available at: http://www.fda.gov/MedicalDevices/NewsEvents/WorkshopsConferences/ucm199037.htm; March 25, 2010 Accessed 20.05.10.

21. *Pumps for Kids, Infants, and Neonates (PumpKIN).* Available at: https://www.fbo.gov/index?s=opportunity&mode=form&id=3ccf72f3df1cf513cff2a8e24c7755d9&tab=core&_cview=1; Accessed 17.05.10.

22. US Food and Drug Administration. http://www.fda.gov/MedicalDevices/ScienceandResearch/ucm208183.htm; Accessed 10.01.11.

23. Maisel W. *Device Therapy in Heart Failure.* New York: Humana Press; 2010.

INTERMACS (Interagency Registry for Mechanically Assisted Circulatory Support) as a Tool to Track and Advance Clinical Practice

James B. Young and Lynne Warner Stevenson

INTERMACS (Interagency Registry of Mechanically Assisted Circulatory Support) is the largest multicenter scientific compendium of long-term circulatory assist devices used today in patients with advanced heart failure. INTERMACS was created in response to scientific advances in this field over the past several decades. Just over a half century ago Kolf, for the first time, removed the heart of a dog and kept the animal alive with an artificial mechanical circulatory support system entirely implanted in the animal's chest cavity.[1-4] In 1966, DeBakey successfully "bridged" a patient to "recovery" with a pulsatile, pneumatic, paracorporeal left ventricular assist device (LVAD) created and manufactured in his surgical laboratory. The pump was later successfully removed under local anesthesia (Fig. 24-1) and the patient survived, doing well until killed in an autopedestrian accident a year later.

Progress in this remarkable field of biomedical engineering stuttered but advanced, driven by the heady nature of the times. At Rice University in Houston, Texas, on September 12, 1962, John F. Kennedy challenged Americans by stating "we choose to go to the moon in this decade and do the other things, not because they are easy, but because they are hard, because that goal will serve to organize and measure the best of energies and skills ...."[3] The race for outer space and the first moon landing had begun, driven in part by politics and international relations, but also by adventuresome spirit and scientific inquisitiveness. It was believed that anything, particularly from an engineering viewpoint, was possible if the right minds and sufficient financial resources were put behind it. If we could get a man into outer space, particularly on the moon, and back again, surely an artificial heart or ventricular assist device would be a far less challenging goal.[1-3] Lillehei, an acclaimed Minnesota surgeon, noted that "what man can dream, technology can achieve."[5] However, as clinical experiments with mechanical circulatory support (MCS) devices progressed haltingly, Rose, another noted heart surgeon, commented that "biology generally trumped engineering."

However, today, use of MCS devices is common. Indeed, it is a daily event in cardiovascular surgery centers when one counts rudimentary cardiopulmonary bypass machines necessary for "stopped" or "arrested" open heart operations. The remarkable progress in design and development of these machines is a testament to perseverance of a dogged few, the dedication of clinicians and surgeons charged with the care of near dead and dying patients with advanced heart failure, and the bravery of the patients and their families. Figure 24-2 summarizes the current use of MCS devices that ranges from very short-term support during cardiopulmonary bypass procedures to more permanent support of patients not expected to receive heart transplantation.

Although the history and potential future paint a landscape of further innovation and promise for extension of quality life in advanced heart failure, clinical results must be collected and reviewed with care. As exciting as these innovative MCS devices are, they are associated with major morbidity and even mortality, particularly in severely ill, cachectic, and elderly patients who have noncardiac comorbidities in addition to terminal heart failure. In the inexorable accounting of health care resources, the justification for this new technology must include proof of extension not only of survival but also of quality survival.

Clinical trials, particularly large-scale, randomized, controlled, multicenter efforts have become the primary basis of evidence for support and reimbursement of new practices. These endeavors can determine with the greatest degree of certainty the beneficial and adverse impacts of an intervention in a rarefied population of patients selected for purity of disease and willingness to enroll. The rigor of randomization and subsidized data collection can provide the highest standards of unbiased information. However, these experiments are major undertakings even to test a single medication that can be mimicked by a placebo substance in double-blind fashion. Furthermore, testing of surgical interventions in which blinding is not possible for patients or physicians present

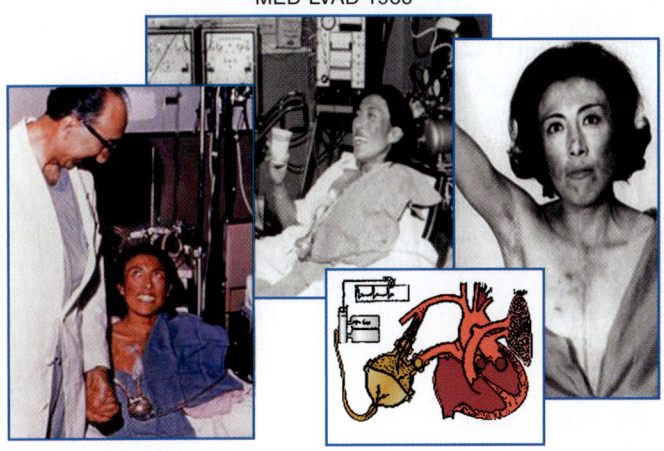

FIGURE 24-1 Device created and manufactured in the surgical laboratory of DeBakey in 1966 that was the first successful left ventricular assist device (LVAD) bridge to recovery. *(Photographs courtesy Dr. DeBakey.)*

CURRENT DURATION OF MECHANICAL CIRCULATORY SUPPORT

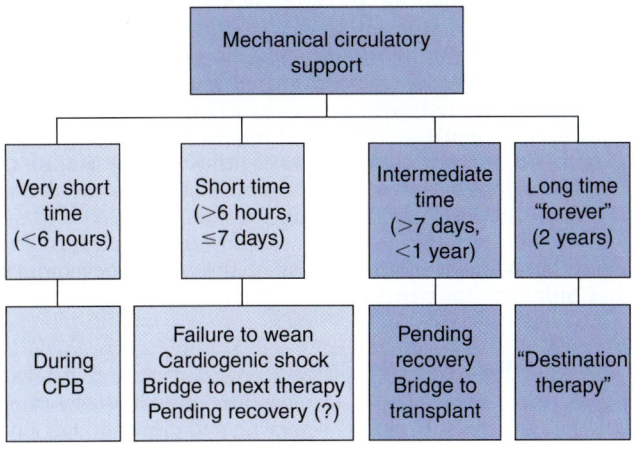

FIGURE 24-2 Mechanical circulatory support (MCS) device use in advanced heart failure. CPB, cardiopulmonary bypass.

daunting and often prohibitive challenges. They are difficult to mount and manage, staggeringly expensive, usually long in duration, and focused on highly selected patient populations that may not reflect clinicians' daily practice. Often clinical trial findings may be obsolete by the time the results are published. One practical option for tracking representative results is the large-scale clinical registry. Most registries have been sponsored by industries interested in the application and outcomes for a single product line, with incentives that influence the collection, censoring, and definitions of outcomes. Registries have often been deservedly criticized for not being sufficiently rigorous to collect and evaluate clinical data adequately. When presented, these data may have been assembled into varied formats, often conflicting, for regulatory, reimbursement, and scientific audiences. In contrast, an independent registry that can collect data for all related devices from all sites for broad use by all individuals and agencies offers a new option for maintaining timely and representative information.

Patients undergoing MCS device insertion with a device approved by the U.S. Food and Drug Administration (FDA) and designed for longer-term support with the capability of hospital discharge with the device in place are the subjects of INTERMACS, regardless of the reason for device insertion.[6]

The sponsoring research agency is the National Heart, Lung and Blood Institute (NHLBI); the regulatory agencies represented are the FDA and Centers for Medicare and Medicaid Services (CMS). Partnership with all involved industry representatives has been vital and collegial. The clinical entities include both academic and community heart failure programs and hospitals. The unprecedented convergence and collaboration of this effort over the past 5 years have helped define and refine the strategies of implantable circulatory support for advanced heart failure and set standards for both device and clinical performance.[6-8] As the field endeavors both to advance and redirect this technology, the registry allows identification of patients likely to enjoy extended quality life-years, patients likely to do well on current medical therapy options, and patients for whom the most appropriate focus may be on enhancing comfort rather than merely prolonging death. Furthermore, INTERMACS is responsive to clinical trial data as they are reported and assists with determining regulatory and reimbursement changes in the mechanical circulatory support field. Some elements of INTERMACS that render it more like a successful large clinical trial than the usual registry include explicit and extensive patient entry and exclusion criteria, ability to ascertain all cases, and standardization of adverse event definitions that are contemporary and meaningful. Perhaps the most significant contribution thus far is the role of INTERMACS to chronicle and accelerate the dramatic shift away from large pulsatile, intracorporeal devices to smaller continuous flow machines that can be inserted and managed with fewer adverse events, better patient acceptability, and longer survival.

INTERMACS ORGANIZATION

Subsequent to the support the National Institutes of Health (NIH) provided to MCS device development, the National Heart, Lung, and Blood Institute (NHLBI) contracted for a national registry, INTERMACS, to track the application and clinical evolution of this emerging technology. The 5-year contract was awarded to the University of Alabama at Birmingham (UAB) and its coprincipal investigators and subcontractors in 2005. A competitive renewal was requested in 2009. The contract renewal request maintained many of the unique features of the existing INTERMACS Registry. As an example, this is a collaborative contract and the "Interagency" component is designed to unite and promote a cooperative partnership among the NHLBI, FDA, and CMS that is linked to a massive effort and contribution of surgeons, heart failure medical experts, nurse coordinators, basics scientists, engineers, and industry stakeholders. It is a remarkable effort and, because of financial constraints, driven in large part by the remarkable academic dedication of hundreds of individuals and institutions around the United States.

Goals of the Registry

The broad goals of INTERMACS are listed in Box 24-1 and include the refinement of patient selection to maximize desirable outcomes with current and new MCS device options. By developing a database with high integrity, accuracy, and reliability, statistical analysis allows creation of post-MCS device outcomes prediction models and this, then, will give clinicians and surgeons the ability to identify predictors of good outcomes, as well as risk factors for adverse events after device implantation. Using this approach can facilitate the creation of guidelines that will improve clinical management by reducing short- and long-term complications. Furthermore, registry data can be used to guide improvements in technology as next-generation devices evolve. Indeed, robust data and its analysis will allow the creation of normative device

CH 24

INTERMACS (Interagency Registry for Mechanically Assisted Circulatory Support) as a Tool to Track and Advance Clinical Practice

BOX 24-1 Goals of INTERMACS (Interagency Registry for Mechanically Assisted Circulatory Support)

- Facilitate the refinement of patient selection to maximize outcomes with current and new device options
- Identify predictors of good outcomes and risk factors for adverse events after device implantation
- Develop consensus "best practice" guidelines to improve clinical management by reducing short-term and long-term complications of MCS device therapy
- Guide clinical application and evolution of next-generation devices
- Use INTERMACS information to guide improvements in technology, particularly as next-generation devices evolve

MCS, mechanical circulatory support.
From INTERMACS Registry; www.INTERMACS.org.

standards and this can give the FDA and device manufacturers methods to analyze performance characteristics of new devices or improvements to existing machines, outside of the randomized controlled trial model. With uniform definitions of adverse events, INTERMACS allows side-by-side comparisons of devices.

Registry Partners

The INTERMACS coalition is diverse, and this is one of the characteristics that make it an unusual effort. The word "Interagency" in the name specifically refers to the partnership of three federal agencies: the NIH, FDA, and CMS. Each brings a different constituency, interest, and mandate to the table. In addition to the federal partners, INTERMACS is strongly aligned with the MCS device industry, hospitals, clinicians, basic scientists, engineers, and several subcontractors. The success of INTERMACS to date is a direct function of the vibrant relationships among the partners who, despite having differing agendas, all strive to meet the key goal of INTERMACS, which is to advance the understanding and application of MCS devices to improve the duration and quality of life in patients with advanced heart failure.

National Institutes of Health Partnership (the Science Partner)

The NIH is the key driving force for INTERMACS as the sponsoring agency and is both the primary partner and the primary regulator of the entire project, which is operated as a contract. The NIH is ultimately responsible for all regulatory, scientific, and operational dimensions. This is one of the few cardiovascular registries that the NIH has funded.

Food and Drug Administration Partnership (the Regulatory Partner)

The FDA serves a crucial role in INTERMACS because of their regulatory procedures for approving new pumps and monitoring approved devices. Their regulatory authority allows them to be the "gatekeeper" for device development. INTERMACS has benefited from close interactions with the FDA, particularly during specification of data elements and the definitions of adverse events used in the registry. As INTERMACS evolved, there were two separate components of FDA interaction. The premarket approval group at the Center for Device and Radiological Health (CDRH) had the goal of creating a registry that would build on previous premarket approval studies of MCS device and help industry by homogenizing the procedures needed for device approval. Also important was the relationship with postmarket approval personnel of the CDRH so that INTERMACS could develop adverse event reporting systems to facilitate the analyses of approved devices. The partnership with the FDA has evolved as INTERMACS has become the ultimate postmarket study tool for approved devices.

Center for Medicare and Medicaid Services Partnership (the Reimbursement Partner)

When INTERMACS began, CMS was reimbursing hospitals for the cost of MCS devices that were implanted as "destination" therapy (DT) (see Fig. 24-2). One of the requirements of this reimbursement was that the data on the implanted patient would be entered into a national database. By the third year of INTERMACS, CMS changed the requirement to explicitly specify INTERMACS as the requisite data repository. CMS also specified that a certified DT center must be a member in good standing within INTERMACS. This partnership with CMS has been critical to enable capture of all DT patients to have as high-quality a database as possible by being a complete representation of this clinical activity.

Industry Partnership (the Device Partner)

Essentially, every company that manufactures approved MCS devices or is in the process of gaining approval for an MCS device has been involved with INTERMACS. The FDA has encouraged companies to work with INTERMACS. Some of these activities fall outside of the strict NIH contract-specified deliverables of INTERMACS but do fall within the goals and academic interests of INTERMACS and have contributed to quality of the database by creating consensus among device developers about patient selection descriptors and adverse event definitions that the FDA endorses as well. One critical element of this relationship has been to have INTERMACS operations informed regularly about the number and locations of device implants. This allows the registry to be proactive in determining whether or not complete ascertainment of subjects has occurred and to account for those missing (most often because of the emergency nature of an implant or inability to obtain informed consent to participate in the registry).

Hospital/Physician/Coordinator Partnerships (the Clinical Partner)

Hospitals that implant MCS devices are critical to the success of INTERMACS. First, the scientific and clinical energy of INTERMACS comes from physicians who care for these heart failure patients and the surgeons who implant the devices. Next, the hospitals, via their coordinators, provide the data that make up the registry. To be an effective and robust high-quality registry, INTERMACS must ascertain all of the MCS devices implanted and benefits from these hospitals reporting data, but the hospitals also benefit from INTERMACS. DT centers must use INTERMACS for data submission in order to be reimbursed. Additionally, hospitals benefit from INTERMACS by being a member of this large MCS device community, which provides many connections to the other hospitals, coordinators, and physicians. Hospitals can submit requests for scientific studies and obtain their own electronic data from INTERMACS. INTERMACS provides a forum, the Coordinators Council, for coordinator feedback and to discuss relevant MCS device topics.

United Network for Organ Sharing

Because the United Network for Organ Sharing (UNOS) coordinates data collection for heart transplantation throughout the United States and is a skilled manager of data repositories, this partnership has been critical to the success of INTERMACS. By recruiting centers performing the vast majority of implantable MCS device procedures and having the ability to link them to heart transplantation, INTERMACS can determine the relationship of this population to heart transplantation. Data entry is made through a Web-based program and protocol. Auditing of INTERMACS centers is done by UNOS on an intermittent and selective basis to ensure data quality. UNOS provides the Data Coordinating Center at the

University of Alabama all data elements for characterization and analysis.

The multiple partners share the common goal of advancing the field of MCS devices for the benefit of the patient, but the goals and agendas of the partners may not be the same or equal. For example, one of the functions of the FDA is to protect the public from unsafe devices, the purpose of the physician is to provide the appropriate treatment for a given patient, the purpose of industry is to produce and market devices, and the NIH has a primarily science-focused agenda. Nonetheless, the organizational structure of this registry is quite distinct and capable of producing a powerful and influential academic and clinical product.

University of Alabama Data Coordinating Center

The University of Alabama Data Coordinating Center (UAB-DCC), under the leadership of its principal investigator, heart surgeon Dr. James Kirklin, and statistician and database expert, Dr. David Naftel, is responsible, with its UAB team, for managing all elements of registry operations, particularly the integration of data collected and collated by UNOS into a cogent academic analysis. This daunting task has been facilitated by an Operations Oversight Committee that has representation from all stakeholders associated with INTERMACS.

COLLECTION OF BASELINE VARIABLES AND ENDPOINTS

Figure 24-3 details the data element organization of INTERMACS. Because it is a registry rather than a clinical trial, with limited numbers of support personnel at participating centers and no financial support provided for data collection, care had to be taken to obtain only critical and essential data. Preimplant variables include baseline patient's characteristics, device and surgical procedure information,[7,8] and heart failure severity classification (patient profile),[9,10] with discrete endpoints including death, heart transplant, device removal, and hospitalizations. Complex endpoints accumulated include adverse events, indices of clinical improvement, quality of life data, and cost information. In addition, a blood and tissue biore-pository has been established for the collection of specimens that will provide valuable future scientific information critical to our understanding of the pathophysiology of advanced heart failure. This compendium of data is robust and gives an accurate picture of the current state of the MCS device art. It allows conclusions to be drawn about different devices, patient management, and surgical procedures, as well as the wisdom of operating on differing patient populations. Development of algorithms to predict outcome in different patients who have disparate clinical characteristics has been done.[11–13]

INTERMACS PATIENT PROFILES

In addition to determining what endpoints were important to address, designing the web-based data collection templates, and defining adverse events,[7,8] an early task for the INTERMACS team was to develop an MCS device patient descriptor that had not been previously used but would better address the patient population trying to be chronicled.[9,10] Both clinical trial data and ordinary practice highlights the deficiencies of using the New York Heart Association (NYHA) functional classification to identify patients who have advanced heart failure that might benefit from various aggressive and radical therapies such as heart transplantation and MCS device insertion. NYHA functional classification of cardiac disease is a tool that has evolved over 75 years but remains subjective and imprecise. To characterize the patient population in INTERMACS better, a descriptive categorization or "profile" of patients was developed, rather than a "progressive" staging system such as the NYHA functional classification. One reason for the difficulty with NYHA classification in this setting is that the vast majority of patients undergoing MCS device insertion are NYHA class IV, which refers to those patients having "symptoms at rest" (Fig. 24-4). The INTERMACS patient profiles include seven categorizations with five of them characterizing patients who are clearly NYHA class IV. The basic problem with NYHA functional classification was recently highlighted by comparison of peak oxygen consumption with investigator-determined NYHA class in the HF-ACTION Trial.[14] In a contemporary heart failure population treated with medical therapy, there was a

CH 24

INTERMACS (Interagency Registry for Mechanically Assisted Circulatory Support) as a Tool to Track and Advance Clinical Practice

BASELINE VARIABLES AND ENDPOINTS

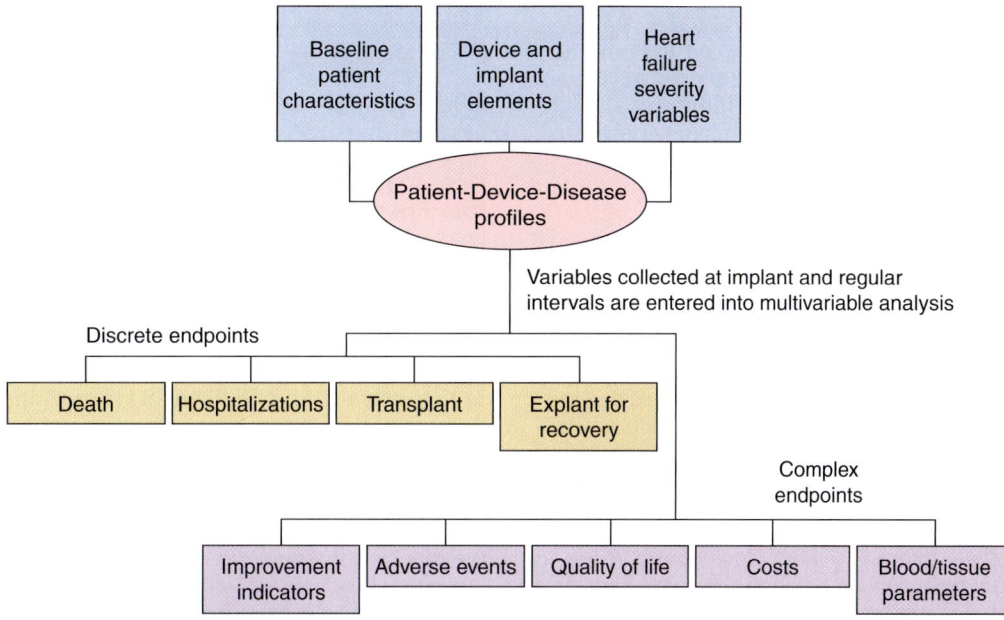

FIGURE 24-3 Baseline variables and endpoints of INTERMACS obtained and analyzed (From INTERMACS Registry; www.INTERMACS.org.)

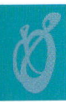

PROFILE-LEVEL	PRIMARY LVADs 12-09	Official shorthand (after Lynne Stevenson)	NYHA CLASS	Modifier option
INTERMACS LEVEL 1	633	"Crash and burn"	IV	
INTERMACS LEVEL 2	841	"Sliding fast" on ino	IV	
INTERMACS LEVEL 3	284	Stable but ino-dependent can be hosp or home	IV ish	*CURRENT VAD INDICATIONS*
INTERMACS LEVEL 4	185	Resting symptoms on oral therapy at home	ambul IV	+FF frequent flyer A for arrhythmia
INTERMACS LEVEL 5		"Housebound", comfortable at rest, symptoms with minimum activity ADL	ambul IV	+FF A
INTERMACS LEVEL 6		"Walking wounded"-ADL possible but meaningful activity limited	IIIB	+FF A
INTERMACS LEVEL 7	(5, 6, 7 = 119)	Advanced Class III	III	A only

FIGURE 24-4 INTERMACS patient profiles. ADL, activities of daily living; LVADs, left ventricular assist devices; NYHA, New York Heart Association.

difference in functional capacity (as adjudicated by peak VO$_2$) between NYHA class II and class III/IV patients, but the dilemma appeared when trying to differentiate among NYHA class III, IIIa ("no dyspnea at rest"), and IIIb ("recent dyspnea at rest"). Also disturbing is that within the classes, contemporary therapies did not affect exercise parameters. Nonetheless, higher NYHA has been consistently associated with poor outcomes in heart failure patients. This creates difficulties when trying to more precisely characterize the very ill patient, such that appropriate risk/benefit decisions can be made when considering MCS device insertion. Far greater descriptive precision is necessary than simply referring to patients as American College of Cardiology (ACC)–American Heart Association (AHA) Stage D, NYHA class IV despite optimal medical therapy. The INTERMACS profiles incorporate both the severity of symptoms and the trajectory of decline over time. For instance, patients who have been ACC-AHA stage D, which is the only stage within which continuous inotropic therapy should be recommended, may improve symptomatically to symptoms consistent with NYHA class III on inotropic therapy, but would still be an INTERMACS profile 3 (see Fig. 24-4).

Figure 24-4 summarizes the INTERMACS patient profiles and relates them to the NYHA classification while using "shorthand jargon" to characterize these individuals better. Profile 1 describes a "critical cardiogenic shock" patient who is "crashing and burning" (well-understood jargon) in which a patient has life-threatening hypotension and rapid-escalating intravenous inotropic support. Profile 2, "progressive decline" or "sliding fast on inotropes," is a patient who has been documented "dependent" on intravenous inotropic agents but nonetheless shows signs of continuous deterioration. Profile 3, "stable but inotrope dependent," describes a patient who is clinically stable on mild to moderate doses of an intravenous inotrope (or has temporary MCS device) and repeated attempts of weaning with documented failures. Profile 4 is a patient with "resting symptoms" who can remain at home on oral therapy but has symptoms of congestion at rest or with minimal activities of daily living. Profile 5, "exertion intoler-

ant" and "housebound," is someone comfortable at rest but unable to engage in any meaningful activity and is largely confined to the home. Profile 6, "exertion limited" or "walking wounded," describes a patient comfortable at rest without evidence of fluid overload who is able to do some activity. Profile 7 characterizes "advanced NYHA III" patients as those who are clinically stable with a reasonable level of comfortable activity despite a history of previous congestion that is not recent.[9,10]

PATIENT ACCRUAL AND EVOLUTION TO CONTINUOUS FLOW MECHANICAL CIRCULATORY SUPPORT DEVICE

Figure 24-5 shows the accrual of MCS device centers (largely heart transplant programs) and patients into the registry beginning in March 2006. There are 113 centers in INTERMACS with 102 actively participating and 101 having entered at least one patient. The average number of patients per center (average/center entering a patient) is 26, with the most active center entering 105 patients to date. Again, to note, for centers to comply with CMS criteria to be reimbursed as a "destination" LVAD implantation program, they must be a participant in good standing with INTERMACS and responsibly report their data. Also important as shown in Figure 24-5 is that in the early era of INTERMACS (years 2 and 3 in Fig. 24-5), there was slow but steady patient accrual that dramatically increased when the HeartMate II device was approved by the FDA mid-year 2008 as a bridge to cardiac transplantation. This rather dramatic change in numbers of patients undergoing MCS device appears constant and is likely driven by the fact that the newer device was a dramatic improvement over previous MCS device choices. Figure 24-6 characterizes this change in the proportion of pulsatile versus nonpulsatile devices being used, with most devices used in the most recent epoch continuous flow machines.

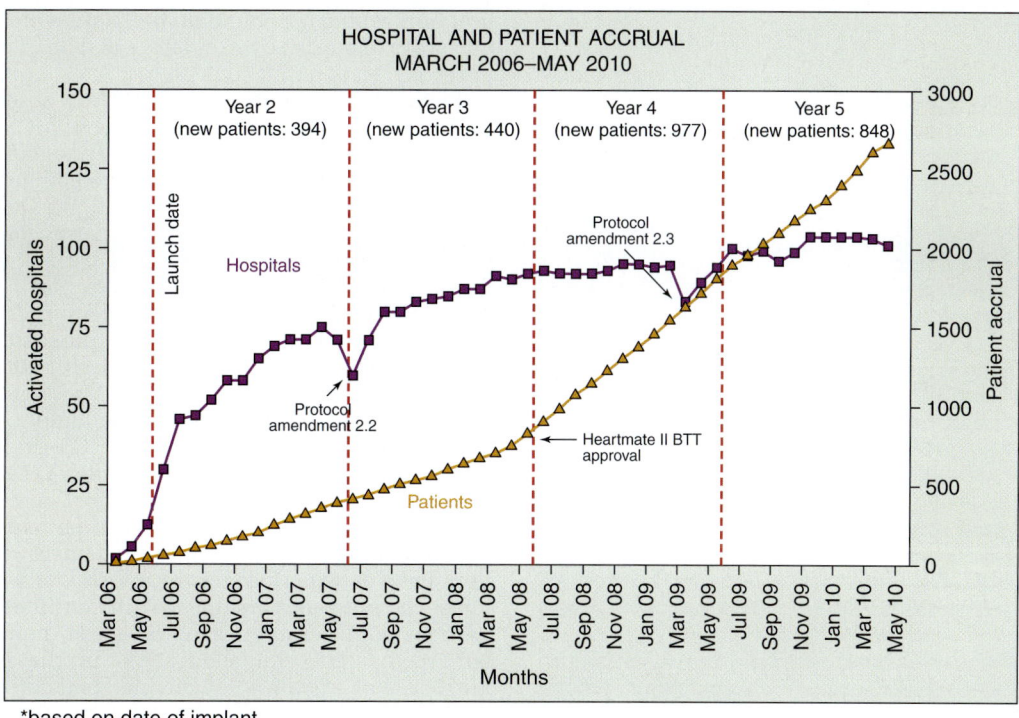

*based on date of implant

FIGURE 24-5 Hospital and patient accrual into INTERMACS. BTT, bridge to transplant. *(From INTERMACS Registry; www.INTERMACS.org.)*

CH 24

INTERMACS (Interagency Registry for Mechanically Assisted Circulatory Support) as a Tool to Track and Advance Clinical Practice

OUTCOMES AFTER MECHANICAL CIRCULATORY SUPPORT DEVICE IMPLANTATION

INTERMACS has shown that survival after MCS device insertion using contemporary pumps is quite reasonable and steadily improving with incremental advances in the devices. Particularly notable are the improved outcomes with an intracorporeal continuous flow system used as an LVAD. Figure 24-7A shows a competing outcomes analysis; at the 6-month follow-up mark, 80% of patients either are alive or have received a heart transplant, and at the 18-month point, 70% have reached this endpoint.[13] Driven by the large number of bridge to transplant patients in INTERMACS, the crossover point for the "alive" and "transplanted" curves is shortly after the 9-month follow-up point. Although the follow-up of continuous-flow devices is shorter because

FIGURE 24-6 Changing proportion of continuous flow mechanical circulatory support devices in INTERMACS. LVADs, left ventricular assist devices. *(From INTERMACS Registry; www.INTERMACS.org.)*

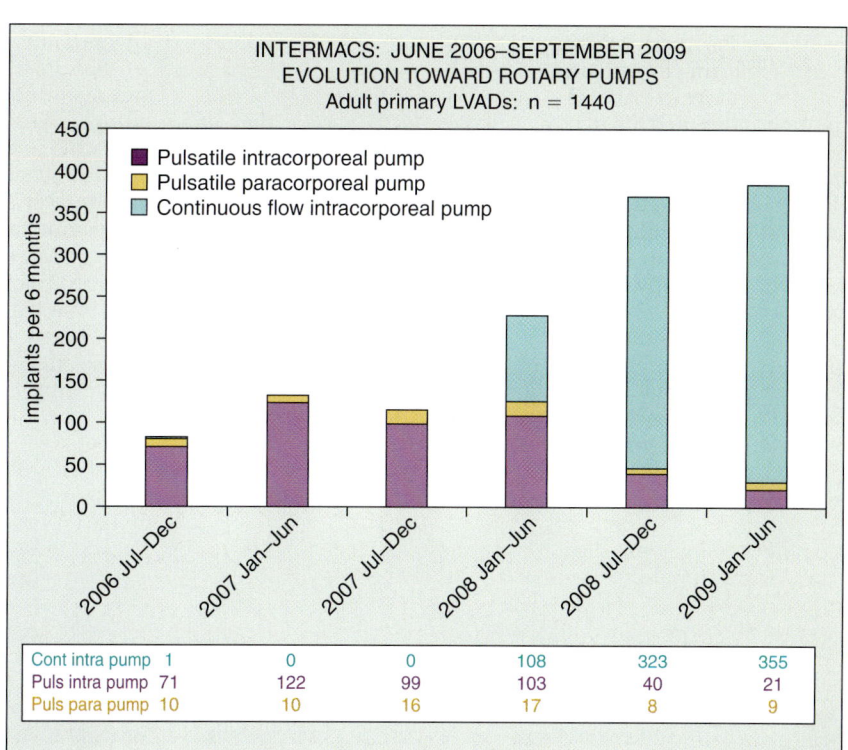

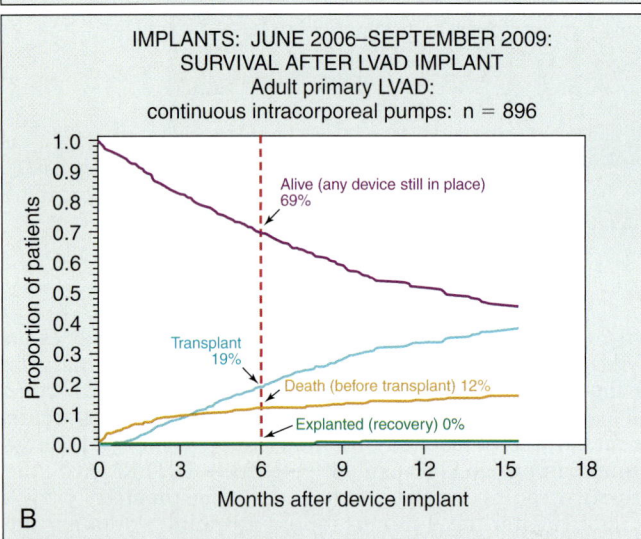

FIGURE 24-7 A, Competing outcomes analysis after placement of an intracorporeal pulsatile left ventricular assist device (LVAD). **B,** Competing outcomes analysis after placement of an intracorporeal continuous flow LVAD. *(From INTERMACS Registry; www.INTERMACS.org.)*

function, enough such that the native heart could carry the entire of burden of circulatory demand (so-called bridge-to-recovery), is rare (about 1%).

Figure 24-8 presents an INTERMACS observation relevant to the profiles of patients at the time of MCS device deployment. There is a highly statistically significant difference between outcomes of patients based on entering profile when overall survival is analyzed. Profile 1 patients (the "crash and burning" group with critical cardiogenic shock) have the worst outcomes while the stable patient who is "inotrope dependent" (Profile 3) appears to have the best survival rate. This is an important observation and suggests that, if possible, it is likely best to move earlier on some patients rather than waiting until they are in dire straits. On the other hand, there are likely too few patients in Profiles 5, 6, and 7 (the "less ill" population) to draw a meaningful conclusion about the selection of these patients for MCS device. This is particularly true of Profile 7, which is the NYHA class III patient population.

Figure 24-9 compares survival of patients with intracorporeal and paracorporeal pulsatile devices with continuous-flow devices when used as an LVAD. As with Figure 24-7, improved outcomes are noted with continuous-flow devices as transplant censored survival at 12 months is close to 90% compared with about 75% in the pulsatile group. Furthermore, patients receiving paracorporeal pulsatile devices have less than a 50% survival at this point (overall comparison $P > .0001$).

Important is the quality of life after MCS device, which can be compromised by many comorbidities that can develop both before and after device insertion.[15] Figure 24-10 shows the impact of MCS device overall in the INTERMACS database when using the EuroQuol-5D instrument to evaluate overall patient "mobility" after device implantation. Because there could be differences between patients on the basis of age, the cohort has been analyzed in groups younger than and older than 60 years. As can be seen, the proportion of patients having "extreme" limitation in mobility dissipates at the 3- and 6-month follow-up points, while disappearing at 12 months. Though the numbers in this analysis are relatively small, the observation is encouraging and suggests that an MCS device can dramatically alter the long-term debility and disability of the patient with very advanced heart failure and favorably affect quality of life.

Table 24-1 details the adverse events tallied in INTERMACS and again compares pulsatile devices with continuous-flow pumps. Numerically, bleeding, infection, respiratory failure, and cardiac arrhythmias were the most common comorbidities seen. Some important and, indeed, rather dramatic differences (all highly statistically significant) between pulsatile and continuous-flow systems include the rate of device

of their later FDA approval, Figure 24-7B shows that at 6 months the likelihood of survival or heart transplant is higher than for pulsatile machines (88% vs. 80%). Another important observation that can be made is that removal of these devices because of adequate recovery of myocardial

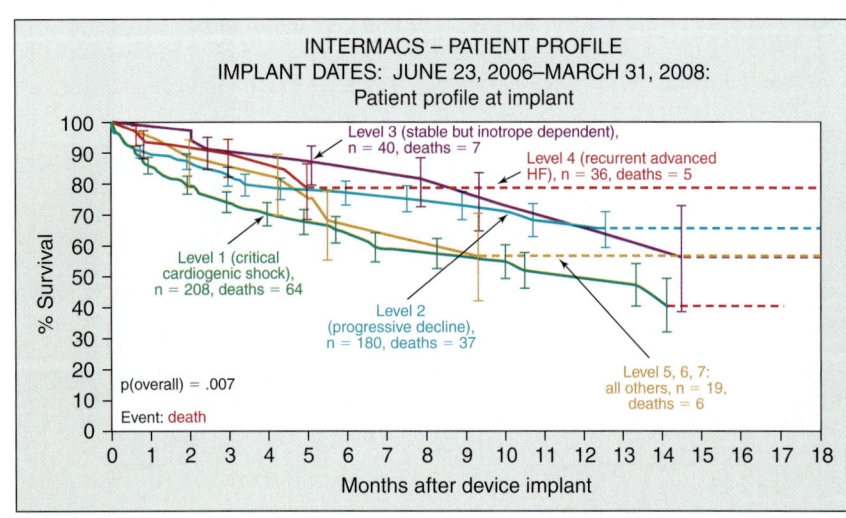

FIGURE 24-8 Survival by INTERMACS patient profiles. HF, heart failure. *(From INTERMACS Registry; www.INTERMACS.org.)*

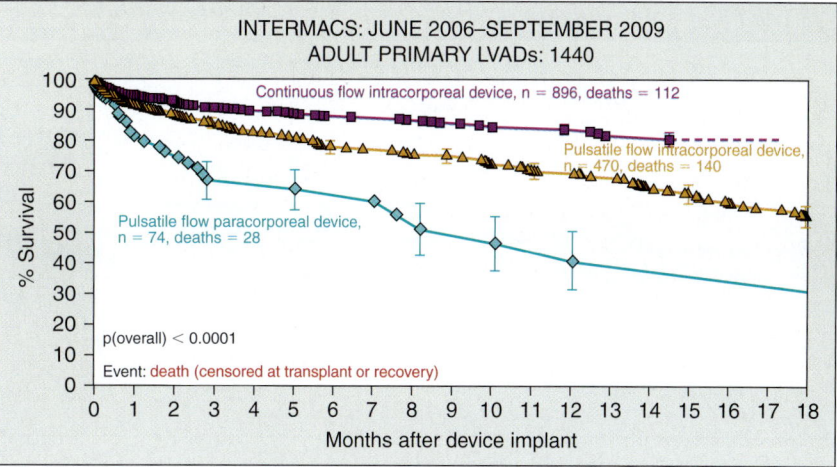

FIGURE 24-9 Survival of pulsatile intracorporeal and paracorporeal devices versus continuous-flow mechanical circulatory support (MCS) devices. LVADs, left ventricular assist devices. *(From INTERMACS Registry; www.INTERMACS.org.)*

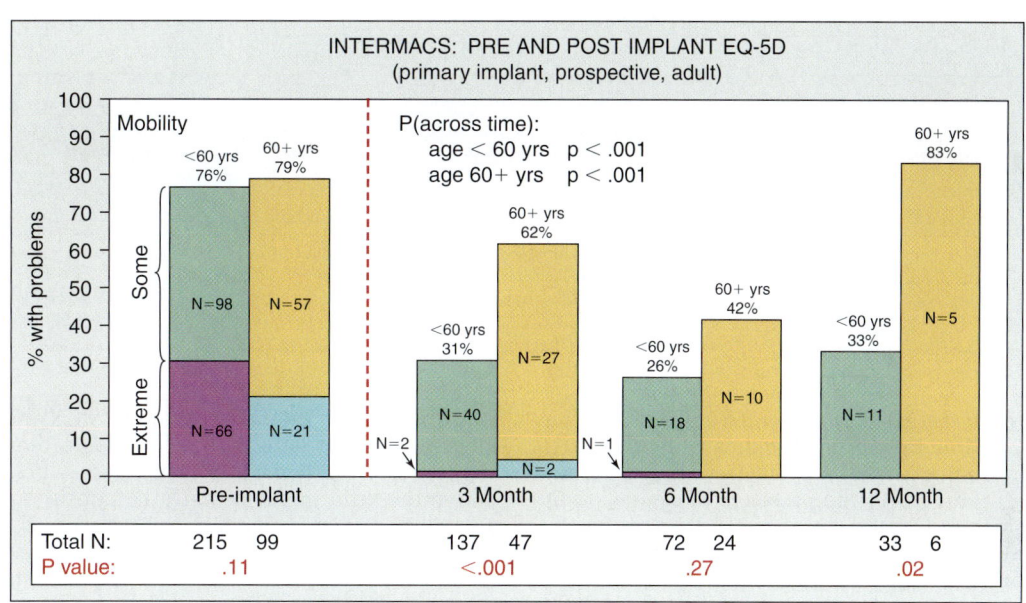

FIGURE 24-10 Quality of life (mobility impairment) after mechanical circulatory support (MCS) device. *(From INTERMACS Registry; www.INTERMACS.org.)*

malfunction (measured as events/100 patient months of follow-up in the first 6 months), which was 2.95 versus 0.82; the incidence of bleeding, 24 versus 17; infection, 28 versus 12; and neurologic dysfunction, 4.33 versus 1.93. Perhaps the fact that not only survival, but also significant adverse event and morbid complication rates are dramatically better with a continuous-flow pump, explains the willingness of clinicians to refer the advanced heart failure patient for MCS device implantation, increasing the number of patients undergoing this life-saving procedure. Clearly, this improvement in technology is a welcome event and the fact that INTERMACS has so nicely demonstrated the change in outcomes and paradigm shift with respect to device choice re-emphasizes the importance of this project.

When cause of death (Table 24-2) was analyzed in the intracorporeal pulsatile and continuous-flow groups, "cardiac failure" was most common. Perhaps this is surprising because MCS devices are supposed to obviate this situation. The reality is, however, that when a patient this ill dies after having gone through a litany of aggressive treatments and suffers many comorbidities, one overarching cause of death is rarely readily identified. Thus while trying to explain the primary cause of death, heart failure is still a substantive culprit. It is worth noting that the relative percentage of this is,

however, less in the continuous-flow group. This is important because, from a theoretic standpoint, there were concerns that continuous-flow devices might actually address the heart failure syndrome worse than pulsatile pumps. In most cases that does not seem to be an issue. Infection, neurologic event, and multiorgan failure round out the list of most common causes of death post MCS device.

PREDICTING SURVIVAL AFTER RECEIVING A MECHANICAL CIRCULATORY SUPPORT DEVICE

An extraordinary value of registry databases that are robust and done well is the ability to use sophisticated mathematic algorithm development to create tools that might help with the prediction of outcomes after certain interventions. INTERMACS has allowed such a tool to be constructed. Under the direction of Naftel at the University of Alabama INTERMACS Data Coordinating Center, preliminary statistic outcome prediction models have been built to achieve this goal. Table 24-3 displays the significant risk factors that were determined for death after MCS device

TABLE 24-1	Adverse Events Noted after Mechanical Circulatory Support Device Implantation*					
	Pulsatile (n = 406)		Continuous (n = 548)		Pulsatile/Continuous	
Adverse Event	Events	Rate	Events	Rate	Ratio	P Value
Device Malfunction	45	2.95	17	0.82	3.60	< .0001
Bleeding	369	24.22	360	17.41	1.39	< .0001
Cardiac/vascular						
Right heart failure	48	3.15	46	2.23	1.41	.05
Myocardial infarction	2	0.13	2	0.10	1.30	.37
Cardiac arrhythmia	154	10.11	218	10.54	0.96	.65
Pericardial drainage	44	2.89	30	1.45	1.99	.003
Hypertension†	75	4.92	17	0.82	6.00	< .0001
Arterial non-CNS thrombosis event	7	0.46	6	0.29	1.59	.21
Venous thrombosis event	38	2.49	32	1.55	1.61	.03
Hemolysis	11	0.72	12	0.58	1.24	.29
Infection	431	28.29	244	11.80	2.40	< .0001
Neurologic dysfunction	66	4.33	40	1.93	2.24	< .0001
Renal dysfunction	63	4.14	45	2.18	1.90	.0007
Hepatic dysfunction	24	1.58	14	0.68	2.32	.009
Respiratory failure	121	7.94	89	4.31	1.84	< .0001
Wound dehiscence	8	0.53	9	0.44	1.20	.34
Psychiatric episode	43	2.82	38	1.84	1.53	.03
Total burden	1549	101.69	1219	58.96	1.72	< .0001

*June 2006 through March 2009. Primary left ventricular assist device implantation for bridge to transplant and bridge to cure (n = 954); adverse event rates (events/100 patient-months) in the first 6 months after implantation.

†With current reporting, identification of hypertension with continuous-flow pumps is unreliable.

CNS, central nervous system.

From INTERMACS Registry; www.INTERMACS.org.

implantation in both the early postoperative phase and the later, longer-term follow-up period. Females, older patients, prior heart surgery, being on dialysis, having a high international normalized ratio (INR), the presence of ascites, high right atrial pressure, and cardiogenic shock all were significant independent predictors of death early postoperatively. During the longer-term follow-up phase, older patients with severe right ventricular dysfunction receiving a pulsatile pump, particularly for DT, had a higher likelihood of dying. Notable was the fact that the most significant hazard for death was use of a pulsatile device (hazard ratio of 3.02, P = 0.001).

Using these data, an algorithm to predict survival in different "modeled" patients is presented. Table 24-4 shows the results for three distinct patients, all male, but being of different ages with varying histories and heart failure findings. Predicted 2-year survival when both a pulsatile and continuous-flow intracorporeal pump is placed can be put into perspective. The predicted survival for patient 1 with, relatively speaking, few adverse findings was 84% for a pulsatile device and 92% for a continuous-flow pump at 2 years compared with patient 3, who had an increased INR, ascites, and was in cardiogenic shock where the predicted survival was 50% and 57%, respectively. It is anticipated that subsequent iterations of this algorithm will be helpful to clinicians as they ponder the relationship of risk to benefit and expected outcomes in a variety of patients being considered as MCS device candidates.

EVOLVING CANDIDATE SELECTION: THE ROLE OF MEDAMACS

The risk prediction models derived from device outcomes have helped to advance the field at the far end of the clinical heart failure spectrum, where patients are assumed to face impending mortality without MCS device. The challenge at that extreme is to differentiate those patients who will do well with devices from those who will not and to determine who might actually be considered "too well" to risk MCS device implantation. However, as devices become more effective for enhancing quality of life and extending survival, earlier implantation may offer benefits to patients for whom some reasonable survival is anticipated even without devices. When the survival and quality of life without devices can no longer be approximated as negligible, they need to be calibrated in contemporary populations on medical therapy for heart failure. The data fields for both baseline and outcome variables in INTERMACS were initially designed to allow comparison with medical treatment outcomes. The renewal of INTERMACS will incorporate a selected study of ambulatory patients followed prospectively on medical therapy at INTERMACS sites. The new dimension provided by MEDAMACS outcome observations is anticipated to provide targets for device outcomes and to guide the extension of mechanical circulatory support into earlier phases of heart failure progression.

SUMMARY

INTERMACS is an example of a successful NIH-funded registry that has chronicled, analyzed, and contributed to the clinical, scientific, and academic medical niche of mechanical circulatory assistance for deathly ill patients with advanced heart failure. With the recent NIH request for proposals for a 5-year extension of the registry contract, even more data and knowledge will accrue that undoubtedly will drive future paradigm shifts in this remarkable field. Though this overview presents some of the more important information gleaned from INTERMACS, much more exists. The public can explore the nuances of this registry further at http://www.intermacs.

TABLE 24-2	Cause of Death after Mechanical Circulatory Support Device Implantation*			
	Continuous/ Intracorporeal		Pulsatile/ Intracorporeal	
Primary Cause of Death	No.	% of 112	No.	% of 140
Cardiac failure	20	17.9	36	25.7
Infection	15	13.4	23	16.4
CNS event	14	12.5	21	15.0
Multiorgan failure	15	13.4	11	7.9
Respiratory failure	7	6.2	6	4.3
Bleeding—other	3	2.7	4	2.9
Gastrointestinal bleeding	1	0.9	1	0.7
Surgical bleeding	5	4.4	4	2.9
Device failure	3	2.7	9	6.4
Renal failure	3	2.7	4	2.9
Hepatic failure	5	4.4	1	0.7
Malignancy	0	0.0	2	1.4
Arterial embolism	0	0.0	1	0.9
Cardiac tamponade	0	0.0	1	0.9
Postexplant failure to recover	0	0.0	1	0.9
Withdrawal of support	6	5.4	3	2.1
Other	15	13.4	12	8.6
Total	112	100.0	140	100.0

*June 2006 through September 2009. Adult primary intracorporeal left ventricular assist devices (*n* = 1366).
CNS, central nervous system.
From INTERMACS Registry; www.INTERMACS.org.

TABLE 24-3	Risk Factors for Death after Mechanical Circulatory Support Device Implantation*			
	Early		Constant	
Risk Factor	Hazard Ratio	P Value	Hazard Ratio	P Value
Female	1.71	.04	—	—
Age (older)	1.14†	.006	1.13†	.008
Previous CABG	2.71	< .0001	—	—
Previous valve surgery	1.99	.01	—	—
Dialysis (current)	2.45	.01	—	—
INR (higher)	1.49‡	.003	—	—
Ascites	2.32	.002	—	—
RVEF: Severe	—	—	2.33	.04
RA pressure (higher)	1.52§	.02	—	—
Cardiogenic shock	1.98	.003	—	—
BTC or DT	—	—	3.00	.01
Pulsatile pump	—	—	3.02	.001

*June 2006 through September 2009. Adult primary intracorporeal left ventricular assist devices (*n* = 1366).
†Hazard ratio denotes the increased risk with a 20-year increase in age.
‡Hazard ratio denotes the increased risk with a 1.0 increase in INR.
§Hazard ratio denotes the increased risk of a 10-unit increase in RA pressure.
BTC, bridge to cure; CABG, coronary artery bypass grafting; DT, destination therapy; INR, international normalized ratio; RA, right atrial; RVEF, right ventricular ejection fraction.
From INTERMACS Registry; www.INTERMACS.org.

CH 24

TABLE 24-4	Hypothetical Patients and Prediction of Outcomes*		
Preimplant	Patient 1	Patient 2	Patient 3
Gender	Male	Male	Male
Age (yr)	50	55	60
History of CABG	No	No	No
History of valve surgery	No	No	No
History of dialysis	No	No	No
INR	1.0	1.5	2.0
Device strategy	BTT	BTT	BTT
Patient profile: Cardiogenic shock	No	No	Yes
RA pressure	12	18	22
RVEF: Severe	No	No	No
Ascites	No	Yes	Yes
Predicted 2-yr survival			
Pulsatile/intracorporeal	84%	74%	50%
Continuous/intracorporeal	92%	82%	57%

*June 2006 through September 2009. Adult primary left ventricular assist device pumps (*n* = 1366).
BTT, bridge to transplant; CABG, coronary artery bypass grafting; INR, international normalized ratio; RA, right atrial; RVEF, right ventricular ejection fraction
From INTERMACS Registry; www.INTERMACS.org.

org on the World Wide Web. The site contains all things INTERMACS including procedure manuals, membership criteria, explanations of devices studied and patients entered, adverse event definitions, data entry forms, and publication and presentation references.

Acknowledgments

The authors would like to acknowledge the contributions of INTERMACS Principal Investigator, James K. Kirklin, M.D.; world-class statistician and database manager, David Naftel, Ph.D.; and their extraordinary support team at the University of Alabama for providing data analysis, statistical consultation, and diagram preparation. Robert Kormos joined Lynne Warner Stevenson as a Co-Principal Investigator and provided crucial energy and emphasis to the development and progress of INTERMACS, particularly as Chair of the Adverse Event Adjudication Committee. Additionally, we would like to thank our National Heart, Lung, and Blood Institute project officers, the FDA, the CMS, and our industry partners, as well as the participating centers with their dedicated nursing coordinators and caregiving staff. Finally, but most importantly, we thank our patients for making INTERMACS such an extraordinary success. Unselfish pursuit of knowledge by so many dedicated individuals to benefit our profession and patients is what INTERMACS has demonstrated.

REFERENCES

1. Kirklin JK, Mehra M, West LJ, eds. *History of International Heart and Lung Transplantation.* Philadelphia: Elsevier; 2010.
2. Copeland JG, Frazier OH, Holman WL. Magic moments in mechanical circulatory support. In: *History of International Heart and Lung Transplantation. ISHLT Monograph Series.* Vol 4. Philadelphia: Elsevier; 2010:111–167.
3. Young JB, Baumgartner WA, Reitz BA, Ohler L. Magic moments in heart transplantation. In: *History of International Heart and Lung Transplantation. ISHLT Monograph Series.* Vol 4. Philadelphia: Elsevier; 2010:45–90.
4. Kirklin JK, Naftel DC. Mechanical circulatory support: a therapy in evolution. *Circulation: Heart Failure.* 2008;1:200–205.
5. Miller GW. *King of Hearts: The Story of the Maverick Who Pioneered Open Heart Surgery.* New York: Crown Publishers; 2000.
6. http://www.intermacs.org.
7. Kirklin JK, Naftel DC, Stevenson LW, et al. INTERMACS: database for durable devices for circulatory support: first annual report. *J Heart Lung Transplant.* 2008;27(10):1065–1072.
8. Kirklin JK, Naftel DC, Kormos RL, et al. Second INTERMACS annual report: more than 1,000 primary left ventricular assist device implants. *J Heart Lung Transplant.* 2010;29(1):1–10.

INTERMACS (Interagency Registry for Mechanically Assisted Circulatory Support) as a Tool to Track and Advance Clinical Practice

9. Warner-Stevenson L, Pagani FD, Young JB, et al. INTERMACS profiles of advanced heart failure: the current picture. *J Heart Lung Transplant*. 2009;28:535–541.

10. Alba AC, Rao V, Ivanov J, et al. Usefulness of the INTERMACS scale to predict outcomes after mechanical assist device implantation. *J Heart Lung Transplant*. 2009;28:827–833.

11. Holman W, Kormos R, Naftel DC, et al. Predictors of death and transplant in patients with a mechanical circulatory support device: a multi-institutional study. *J Heart Lung Transplant*. 2009;28:44–50.

12. Holman W, Pae W, Teutenberg J, et al. INTERMACS: interval analysis of registry data. *J Am Coll Surg*. 2009;28:755–761.

13. Rogers JG, Pagani FD, Kirklin JK, et al. Survival after implant of a left ventricular assist device. Is it the device or is it the patient? *J Heart Lung Transplant*. 2010;29:s40.

14. Russell SD, Saval MA, Robbins JL, et al. New York Heart Association functional class predicts exercise parameters in the current era. *Am Heart J*. 2009;158(1):s24–s30.

15. Grady K, Ulisney K, Kirklin JK, et al. Important improvements in quality of life after MCSD implant: first reports from INTERMACS. *J Heart Lung Transplant*. 2009;28:s207.

CH 24

Reimbursement and Funding Framework for Mechanical Circulatory Support

Robin Roberts Bostic and Tina Ommaya Ivovic

REIMBURSEMENT ANALYSIS: FROM CONCEPT TO COVERAGE

Establishing reimbursement (the ability to be paid) early in product development is essential for patients to have long-term access to any therapy. Although reimbursement is composed of coverage, coding, and payment, coverage is the essential first step that drives subsequent coding and payment. Before any product launch, the analysis of each of these reimbursement drivers is essential to market success. The primary path to payer coverage of a product, procedure, or service occurs when a product is deemed a "reasonable and necessary" medical treatment. Recently, payers are demanding a further level of evidence to show *effectiveness*—does it work in the real world?—and *efficiency*—does it provide a better value? AdvaMed, an industry group representing medical manufacturers, has reported Medicare takes an average of 2 to 5 years to create coverage for a new product with private insurers' timeframes varying widely.[1] The earlier the process is initiated to obtain coverage, the sooner reimbursement will be established. Perhaps most importantly, this 2- to 5-year anticipated time frame for coverage can be reduced if a reimbursement plan is implemented early. When developing a reimbursement plan, the following questions should be asked:

1. Where will this product fit in the larger health care arena?
2. Will this product meet not only the U.S. Food and Drug Administration (FDA) "safe and effective" standards required for regulatory approval but also payers' "reasonable and necessary" and possibly "effective and efficient" requirements?
3. How can the reimbursement adequately cover the cost?

Where Will It Fit?

There are three broad categories in which the technology or procedure could fit:

1. Similar to another product already on the market (a "me, too" device)?
2. An expansion or different use of an existing technology?
   Or is it
3. Truly new and innovative?

Table 25-1 illustrates the reimbursement time implications of "where it fits."

Reimbursement is easiest to obtain with "me, too" products because coverage, coding, and payment have been defined for a similar product. If this is where the product fits, the primary task is to ensure it is identified under the existing technology and grouped with the existing code to trigger appropriate payment.

"Indication expansion" of an existing technology often requires altering coverage, coding, and payment to address the new indication. In this chapter, we focus on coverage expansion for left ventricular assist devices (LVADs) not only as a bridge to heart transplantation (BTT) or as postcardiotomy support but also as long-term, permanent support, known as *destination therapy* (DT). Published studies supporting the proposed expanded indication and revisions of established medical policy are necessary to create additional coverage. Codes may need to be revised including new code descriptions, which can trigger different payment rates.

If the product is a new and innovative technology, while excitement may surround this scientific breakthrough, a new reimbursement structure will need to be constructed and implemented to address coverage, coding, and payment.

Wherever the product "fits," a reasonable timeline for developing and implementing the reimbursement plan must be anticipated. If coverage, coding, and payment already exist for a similar product, 6 to 12 months is currently typical for getting this product positioned within the existing category. To obtain new or modify existing administrative codes used to identify the product or service to payers, whether related to physician procedures (Current Procedural Terminology [CPT]) or to the device itself (Healthcare Common Procedural Coding System [HCPCS]), the process usually takes approximately 1 to

TABLE 25-1 | **Reimbursement Analysis: Implications of Product Fit**

	Similar to Another Product	Expansion of Existing Technology	Truly New and Innovative
Reimbursement components that must be developed	Confirm existing code and inclusion for coverage of this product	Alter coverage, coding, and payment to include this product	Create new coverage, coding, and payment structure for this product
Scientific evidence required	Usually FDA approval with same indications suffice for inclusion in existing coverage	Publication of controlled studies (usually 1-2)	Publication of controlled studies (usually 2-4) and cost-effectiveness data (publications or registry or both) data
Typical time line for components after FDA approval	6 mo to 1 yr	1-2 yr	2-5 yr

FDA, U.S. Food and Drug Administration.

2 years from the product's launch to market entry. For new technologies, historically Medicare has taken 2 to 5 years to create national medical coverage or to substantially expand existing guidelines, and code creation follows along a similar path.

Creating Reimbursement for Left Ventricular Assist Devices for Destination Therapy

LVADs used as DT are an example of expansion of an existing technology, but because of the complexity involved with creating reimbursement, the timeframe is more reflective of the most complicated type, or "innovative therapy" described earlier. In 2002 the REMATCH (Randomized Evaluation of Mechanical Assistance for the Treatment of Congestive Heart Failure) trial had been completed showing efficacy of the device over medical therapy, but there was no payer coverage, no administrative codes, and no payment for devices used for DT.[2] Every reimbursement structure had to be created from influencing Health Technology Assessments (HTAs) for commercial payer coverage and defining a Medicare National Coverage Decision, to clarifying coding in every system including the International Classification of Diseases, 9th Edition, Clinical Modification (ICD-9-CM) codes, Current Procedural Terminology (CPT), and Healthcare Common Procedure Coding System (HCPCS). Payment had to be established under the Medicare inpatient diagnosis-related group (DRG) system and when possible during clinical trials. Allocating reimbursement for physician surgical procedures and replacement of outpatient accessories and supplies required to support the LVAD patient was also necessary. Table 25-2 lists the steps for each provider type.

So how were these roads to reimbursement created? All reimbursement starts with the concept that the technology has to be "reasonable and necessary" to warrant payment. All coverage starts with clinical studies that show clinical benefit to the population treated.

Time Line and Cost to Regulatory and Reimbursement

It took more than 3 decades for the current iterations of ventricular assist devices (VADs) to be available to patients for DT (Fig. 25-1). The company had already invested up to $90 million in product development before approval from the FDA for BTT indication as shown in Table 25-3. These types of costs and the lengthy time frame to obtain reimbursement make market entry almost impossible for many medical devices.

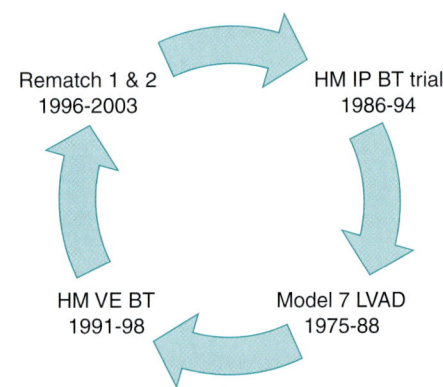

FIGURE 25-1 Evolution of HeartMate coverage over 23 years.

TABLE 25-3 | **Manufacturer Development, Regulatory, and Reimbursement Cost**

Phase 1: Basic technology development	1966-1975	$25 million
Phase 2: Device development	1975-1985	$20 million
Phase 3: Regulatory approval	1985-1994	$42 million
Phase 4: Reimbursement	2000-2003	$3 million
Total		$90 million

TABLE 25-2 | **Pathways of Reimbursement**

	Coverage	Coding	Payment
Inpatient hospital	Medicare National Coverage Determination, influence HTAs for commercial payers	Unique ICD-9-CM procedure code for implant	Appropriate MS-DRG assignment
Physician services	Appropriate National Correct Coding Initiative edits for physician payment	Create CPT codes for surgical procedure and ventricular assist device interrogation	Appropriate RVRBS relative value units assigned to all CPT codes
Replacement accessories and supplies	Coverage policies with replacement intervals for outpatient accessories and supplies	HCPCS codes for outpatient accessories and supplies	Blend manufacturer price with market rate for appropriate HCPCS payments

CPT, Current Procedural Terminology; HCPCS, Healthcare Common Procedural Coding System; HTA, health technology assessment; ICD-9-CM, International Classification of Diseases, 9th Edition, Clinical Modification; MS-DRG, Medical Severity Adjusted Diagnosis Related Group; RVRBS, Relative Value Resource Based System.

History of Mechanical Circulatory Support Reimbursement

Today, VAD therapy is a well-established treatment for end-stage heart failure, with more than 14,000 long-term VAD implants performed in hospitals across the United States since the early 1980s. VADs used for BTT have been covered by Medicare and most other commercial payers for postcardiotomy use since 1993 and for BTT since 1996. In October 2003 the Centers for Medicare and Medicaid Services (CMS) issued a National Coverage Determination (NCD) for VADs used for DT, which was updated in 2007 and again in 2010.[2] A summary of the NCD for DT is provided in Table 25-4. This decision was based on key studies, which showed significant clinical and quality-of-life benefits for end-stage heart failure patients who were implanted with VADs for DT.

In the 1990s, third-party payers were familiar with LVAD technologies but did not have coverage for DT. The device was used solely to assist the left ventricle while patients recovered from heart surgery. In later years, it was used to assist "bridged" patients' failed hearts to cardiac transplant while the patients were on organ waiting lists.

The 2000s saw a different era in LVADs emerge. With a limited number of donor hearts available, LVADs were presented as the solution for end-stage heart failure patients who became refractory to medical management. Thoratec Corporation (Pleasanton, CA), in conjunction with the National Institutes of Health (NIH), conducted a study of LVADs for end-stage heart failure patients ineligible for cardiac transplant, either because of age or other complicating factors, referred to as DT. The FDA provided expedited review of the premarket approval (PMA) application on the basis of the landmark REMATCH trial results and obtained approval in November 2002. Blue Cross Blue Shield conducted its own Technology Evaluation Center (TEC) report on DT and concluded the therapy met its criteria for coverage in October 2002 (Fig. 25-2).[3]

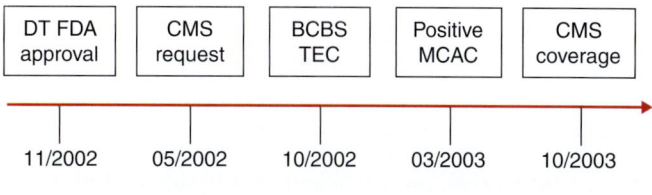

CMS coverage 11 months from FDA approval

FIGURE 25-2 Time line for destination therapy (DT) coverage by payers. VAD, ventricular assist device. BCBS TEC, Blue Cross and Blue Shield Technology Evaluation Center; CMS, Centers for Medicare and Medicaid Services; DT, destination therapy; FDA, Food and Drug Administration; MCAC, Medicare Coverage Advisory Committee.

During 2001 when the REMATCH trial outcomes had been published in the *New England Journal of Medicine,* the company began working with CMS to open a dialogue around the potential for a national coverage decision for DT before FDA approval. Numerous meetings with CMS officials over the next 2 years to establish the clinically appropriate conditions for coverage with the support of multiple clinical societies were held. The technology received Medicare Coverage Advisory Committee (MCAC) endorsement in March 2003. This led to Medicare's decision in October 2003 to establish coverage nationally for a narrow population (limiting the definition of DT to the clinical parameters of the REMATCH trial), and Medicare required certification of centers that would perform these surgeries.[2]

The body of clinical evidence and how it is used significantly affects CMS coverage determinations. The hierarchy of evidence favors randomized, double-blind, placebo-controlled studies published in a peer-reviewed (preferably U.S.) journal. Less attractive are open-label trials in which both patients and physicians know the patient is receiving the product or retrospective studies in which charts are reviewed sometime after a group of patients has received a treatment. Case studies are rarely considered in a technology coverage decision (Fig. 25-3).

In the case of the LVAD, the strength of the published controlled studies supported both CMS and private payers' national DT coverage decisions. With the determination that DT was

TABLE 25-4	Centers for Medicare and Medicaid Services Destination Therapy National Coverage Decision Summary
Patient population	Chronic, end-stage heart failure ineligible for transplant
Background therapy	Failed to respond to optimal medical management (including angiotensin-converting enzyme inhibitor and beta blocker, if tolerated) for 45 of past 60 days or have been balloon pump-dependent for 7 days, or IV inotrope-dependent for 14 days
Duration of medical therapy	45 of past 90 days
Ejection fraction	<25%
Peak VO₂ (mL/kg/min)	<12 unless balloon pump- or inotrope-dependent or physically unable to perform the test
NYHA functional class	IV
Body size (m²)	No criteria
Center requirement	LVAD certified by the Joint Commission member reporting into INTERMACS data registry
Physician requirement	Surgeon with experience of 10 LVAD implants over past 36 months with recent experience in the past 12 months Cardiologist experienced in heart failure

LVAD, left ventricular assist device; NYHA, New York Heart Association.

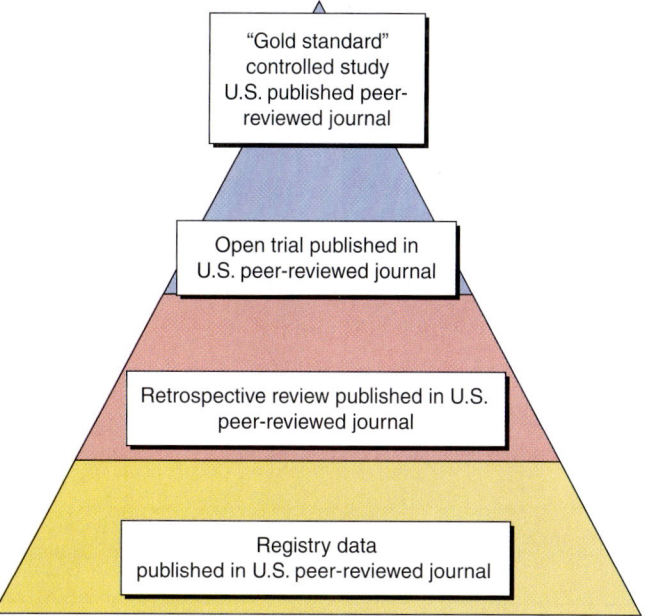

FIGURE 25-3 Hierarchy of clinical evidence.

effective, the question of efficiency or value of the technology in treating end-stage heart failure patients was raised. Determining the cost of a technology is one way of defining value.

Impact of Cost in Coverage Decisions

The coverage analysis of emerging technologies is often difficult before their establishment and refinement. Assessing cost-effectiveness with such therapies involves several factors including determining whether it is safe and effective and establishing its use as reasonable and necessary medical treatment, while reporting clinical benefit along with cost-effectiveness. Applying incremental cost-effective ratios (ICERs) to orphan therapies and therapies directed toward smaller populations' drugs is generally inaccurate and inappropriate. Emerging new technologies are initially costly because of high research and development costs. The costs are higher and more difficult to recoup when the patient population is small, as in the case of orphan therapies and LVADs, which treat select populations. Figure 25-4 shows the cost of other lifesaving therapies as compared with DT.

The overall clinical acceptance of this new therapy led to an immediate review by Blue Cross Blue Shield Association on whether the use of the therapy was a cost-efficient treatment. These initial studies were not cost-effective, with LVAD ICERs as high as $802,700 (BCBS TEC, 2002), which is beyond the considered threshold of $100,000 to $125,000 per quality-adjusted life-year (QALY) gained.[4,5]

Since that time, several studies have evaluated the short- and long-term treatment outcomes and costs associated with LVAD therapy for various indications. Data derived from the REMATCH study, which randomized patients with end-stage HF to either an LVAD or optimal medical therapy, demonstrated an LVAD patient survival rate of 52% at 1 year and 23% at 2 years.[6] The mean initial implantation cost for LVAD was $210,187 ± $193,295.[7]

Russo and colleagues analyzed the mean cost for the care of 52 heart failure patients during their last 2 years of life. The study analyzed data from 52 of the 68 patients in the REMATCH medical therapy arm who were Medicare beneficiaries from the time of their death, retrospectively for the 2 years prior including all inpatient and outpatient services. The mean cost of care of these patients for the last 2 years of their life was more than $160,000 per patient, with 45% of that total, a median of $83,000, spent during the last 6 months

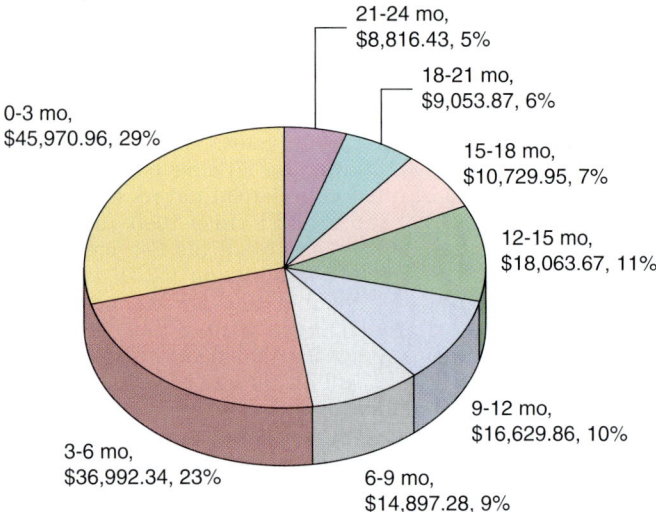

FIGURE 25-5 Cost of medical management of patients with end stage heart failure during last 2 years of life. (From Russo MJ, Gelijns AC, Stevenson LW, et al. *The cost of medical management in advanced heart failure during the final two years of life.* J Card Fail. 2008;14(8):651–658.)

of life.[8] Figure 25-5 breaks down the cost of medical management of heart failure by time frame.

These costs are from the Medicare 1998-2002 database and do not include current treatments for end-stage heart failure such as biventricular pacing or implantable cardiac defibrillators. When compared with other Medicare beneficiaries, these patients consumed 7.2 times more overall cost. Further, when compared with other chronic conditions such as chronic obstructive lung disease, lung cancer, and pancreatic cancer, heart failure care in the last 6 months was two to three times greater than for the other diseases—$83,000 versus $30,000 for the other chronic illnesses as shown in Figure 25-6.

Heart transplantation is a standard form of surgical treatment of end-stage heart failure. Increasing experience with this procedure and advances in immunosuppression were associated with a 45% reduction in cost reported for heart transplantation between 1991 and 1995, shortly after CMS began to cover the procedure. Similarly, a 40% reduction in mechanical support cost was reported over a 3-year period between 2001 and 2004 after this therapy received a positive CMS National Coverage Decision (Fig. 25-7).[9]

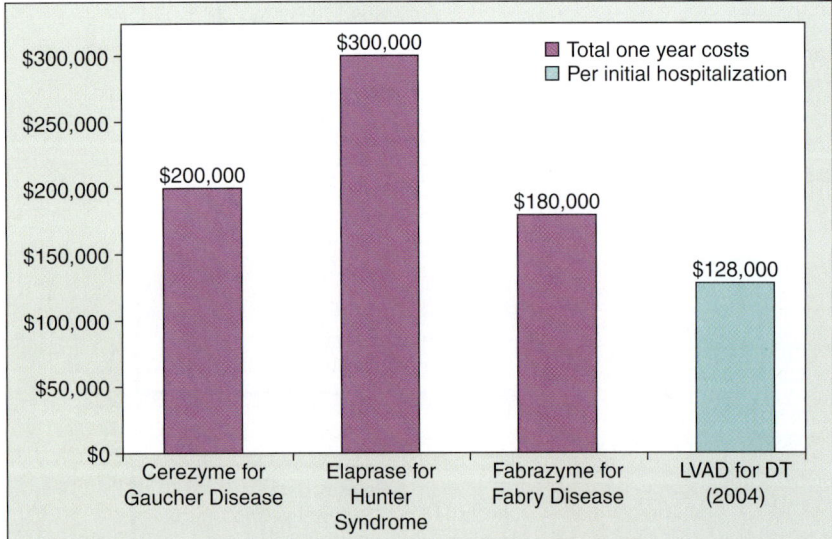

FIGURE 25-4 Cost comparison of lifesaving therapies. DT, destination therapy; LVAD, left ventricular assist device.

- Orphan drug prices from The Boston Globe "It costs how much?" from May 6, 2007 and National Organization for Rare Diseases article "Diseases without clout: So-called 'orphan' illnesses work toward recognition – and funding for drug research" from March 30, 2004.
- Average LVAD hospitalization costs ($128,084) for two of the highest-volume DT-accredited facilities (Miller et al, 2006)

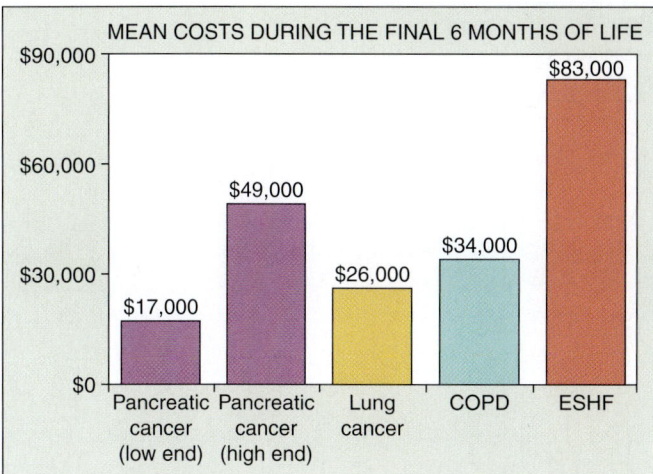

FIGURE 25-6 Cost of terminal disease near end of life. COPD, chronic obstructive pulmonary disease; ESHF, end-stage heart failure.

Clegg reported the cost-effectiveness of DT has greatly decreased, from $802,700 QALY reported by BCBS TEC to $342,573 QALY in 2007.[10] These studies illustrate how the cost-effectiveness of LVAD therapy is trending downward over time (Fig. 25-8).

The survival rate of LVAD patients has increased, and the cost for LVAD implantation has decreased. Use of mechanical circulatory assist devices had increasingly become a surgical treatment option for patients who deteriorate while awaiting heart transplant as well as an alternative to transplant.

Patients implanted with newer-generation LVADs (e.g., continuous-flow pumps) have an improved 1-year survival rate of 68% and a 2-year survival rate of 58% (Fig. 25-9).[11]

It has been reported that the mean cost of implantation was $192,574/patient in the HMII DT trial compared to $389,247 reported during REMATCH (P <.05). The mean post-implant length of hospital stay was shorter in the HMII trial vs. HMVE (27 vs. 44 days, P = .09) In the past 10 years, there has been a 50% reduction in the cost of the initial implant of left ventricular assist devices used for destination therapy.[12] Patient baseline characteristics have not significantly changed suggesting that improved surgical techniques, perioperative management and the continuous-flow devices may be responsible for the observed cost reductions.

Device improvements, reduction in implant cost, increased survival rates, and improved quality of life will ultimately establish the use of LVADs as a cost-effective therapy. Although cost is an important consideration in adoption of a technology and carefully scrutinized globally, in the United States it is not yet a barrier for coverage.

Pathways to Payment

After obtaining national coverage for DT in 2003, it was important to establish adequate payment to cover the cost of the therapy. Historically, hospitals were only reimbursed approximately $35,000 per LVAD implant because there was no specific DRG used to identify the procedure. Table 25-5 shows the DRG assignment and base rate payment over time.

During the coverage process in 2002, 2 years of claims data for DT cases were provided to CMS reflecting the need to increase the inpatient hospital DRG payment. Implanting hospital champions with clinical and cost data worked tirelessly to educate CMS about the clinical benefits and value of the technology. As a result, payment for DT hospitalizations increased over time, culminating in assignment of LVAD procedures to the heart transplant DRG in October 2003. The current average hospital Medicare payment for DT is $196,000 (Fig. 25-10).[13]

Lessons Learned

In the perfect coverage world, steps to reimbursement would seem simple. Manufacturers would initiate randomized, double-blinded, placebo-controlled studies, which report clear statistically significant long-term clinical benefits for patients in need, and simultaneously demonstrate cost-effectiveness to payers such as Medicare. An independent patient registry would follow, monitored by a medical group with no connections to the manufacturer, and ongoing peer-reviewed publications would be produced from this registry.

Many companies designing innovative devices are start-ups with one technology. Financial resources are limited. Meetings with investors seem continuous, with reimbursement an important issue in investors' decisions to provide funding. The need to show some clinical effect early often

FIGURE 25-7 Left ventricular assist device (LVAD) cost trends compared with heart transplant. DT, destination therapy.

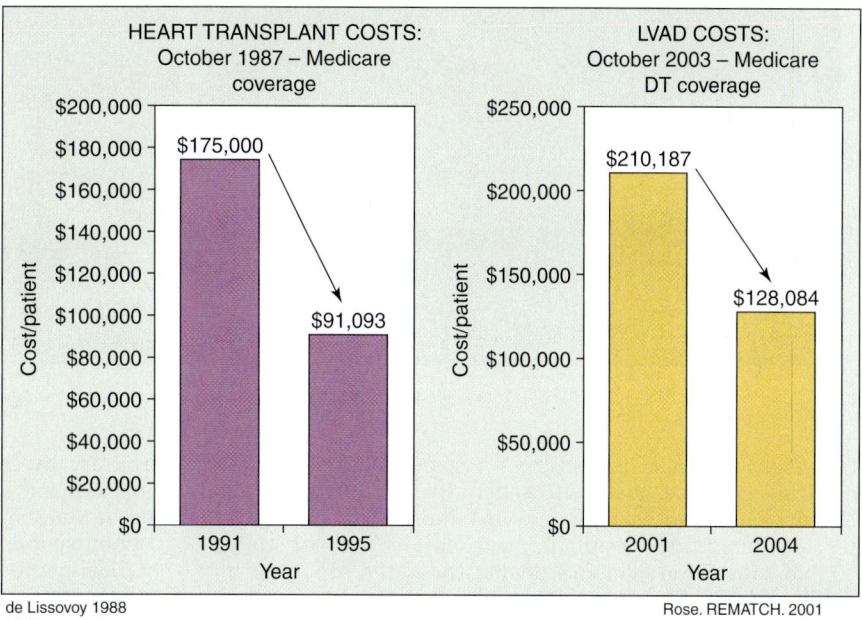

de Lissovoy 1988
NYTimes 1997

Rose. REMATCH. 2001
Miller. Post-REMATCH. 2006

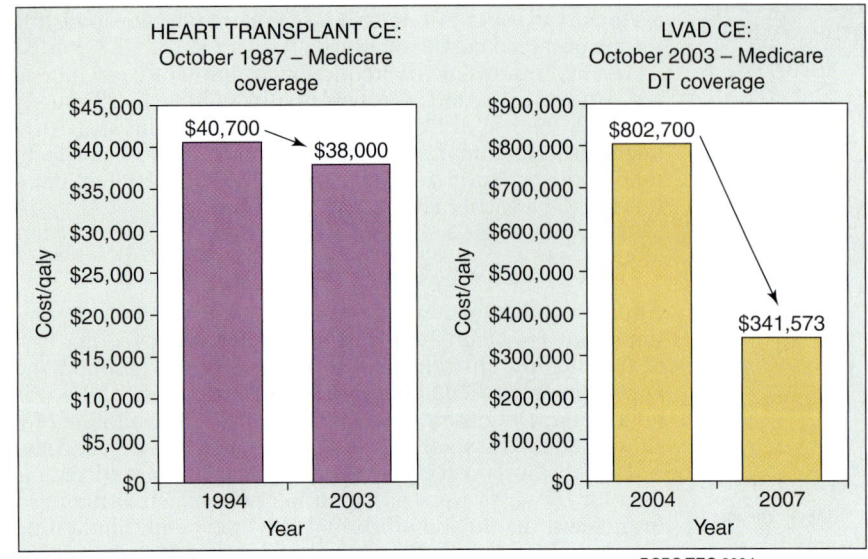

HEART TRANSPLANT CE:
October 1987 – Medicare coverage

LVAD CE:
October 2003 – Medicare DT coverage

FIGURE 25-8 Cost-effectiveness (CE) trends. DT, destination therapy; qaly, quality-adjusted life-year.

JHMC Press release 1994
Ouwens 2003, Dutch study

BCBS TEC 2004
Clegg 2007, UK study, converted

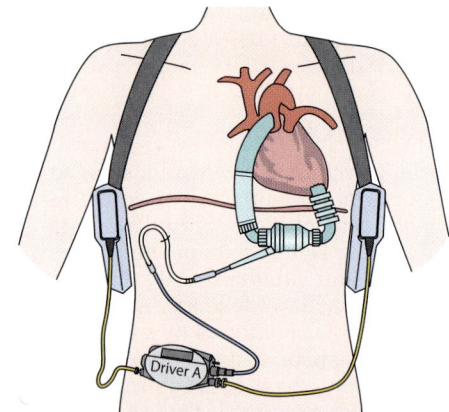

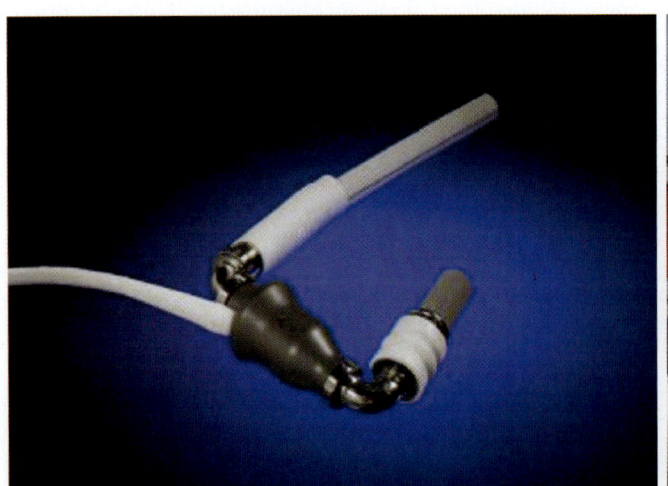

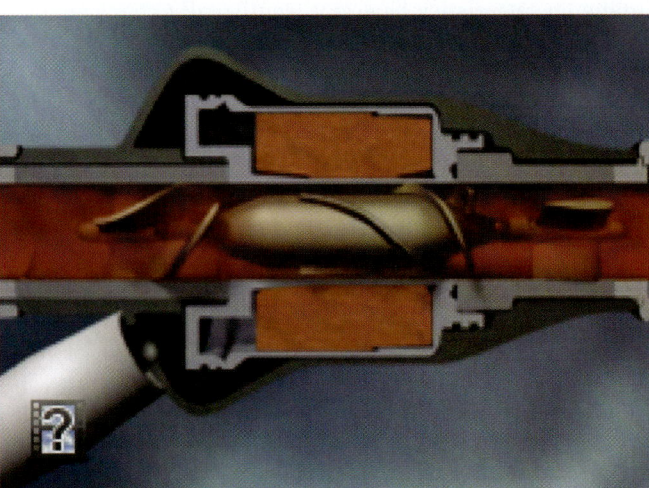

FIGURE 25-9 Continuous flow ventricular assist device (VAD).

outweighs the need to construct a comprehensive body of clinical evidence that will satisfy payers' requirements. Despite early positive trials, payers required additional studies specific to their population or simply additional studies so that substantial evidence demonstrated the benefit of the device. Although such requirements sometimes seem, at best, arbitrary by the payers, identifying the likely payers for a product, and even "partnering" with them in planning studies so the results address their needs, can save years in the reimbursement process.

One method of accelerating market acceptance is to establish reimbursement during clinical trial. Under certain

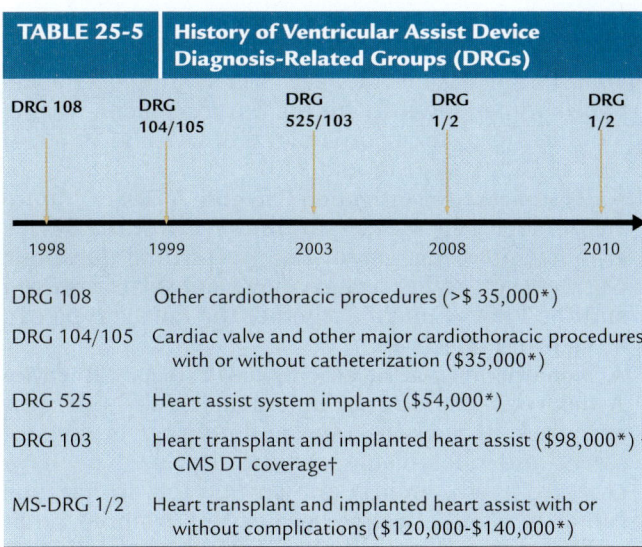

TABLE 25-5 | History of Ventricular Assist Device Diagnosis-Related Groups (DRGs)

DRG 108	DRG 104/105	DRG 525/103	DRG 1/2	DRG 1/2
1998	1999	2003	2008	2010

DRG 108	Other cardiothoracic procedures (>$ 35,000*)
DRG 104/105	Cardiac valve and other major cardiothoracic procedures with or without catheterization ($35,000*)
DRG 525	Heart assist system implants ($54,000*)
DRG 103	Heart transplant and implanted heart assist ($98,000*) + CMS DT coverage†
MS-DRG 1/2	Heart transplant and implanted heart assist with or without complications ($120,000-$140,000*)

*Payment is based on Centers for Medicare and Medicaid Services (CMS) DRG rates across implanting centers in the United States.

†Inpatient hospital payment increased with CMS destination therapy coverage.

Reimbursement can translate to financial viability, which can mean life or death to a technology or a field. During product development, attention to clinical, regulatory, sales, and marketing should be coupled with attention to reimbursement. Almost immediately, a company must start defining who will primarily receive the product and who then will pay for it. In addition, other issues such as who will actually "own" the product (the patient, the payer, the hospital, the physician) and who will do the procedure and in what setting become important in defining a reimbursement plan.

Ideally, reimbursement should be considered before the creation of the first clinical protocol. Attention should be directed to what potential indications are actually being studied and what effects this product will have on the quality of life for particular populations such as Medicare and private payer populations. Once this is determined, meetings with medical directors of the payers who will potentially reimburse for the technology are helpful, if not essential. In preparation for meeting with potential payers, the company should consider how resulting indications benefit this payer's population.

A positive coverage decision also drives the need for a code to identify the product and/or procedures. These codes help to establish payment by Medicare and private payers. However, confirmation of existing codes that can be used for the product can be determined before FDA approval. Applications for new codes usually require 6 months of FDA postmarket approval volume to demonstrate a need for a new code. Companies must also anticipate costs to the health care system because it is increasingly necessary to prove a product is not only clinically beneficial but also cost-effective. Access to billing charges including existing codes can be collected with clinical data during the clinical trial phase by designated data collectors and help clarify whether a modification of a code or creation of a new code will be necessary.

If studies do not support reimbursement, payers may be able to describe what additional information would be important for them to reevaluate the device. Can a small retrospective review study or specific outcome analysis affect their initial decision? A nationally audited registry, maintained by an outside source, may be desirable to them.

In the case of the LVAD, CMS elected to provide "coverage with evidence development" requiring all centers that implant VADs for DT to report specific data into a national registry. With a grant of more than $6 million awarded by the National Heart, Lung and Blood Institute, INTERMACS (Interagency Registry for Mechanically Assisted Circulatory Support) was

circumstances Medicare may provide payment during a clinical trial. CMS uses FDA categorization such as *Experimental/investigational (Category A),* an innovative device, and *Nonexperimental/investigational (Category B),* a device in which the incremental risk is the primary risk in question (i.e., underlying questions of safety and effectiveness of that device type have been resolved) to determine if the therapy should be reimbursed during the study. On the basis of the category determination of the device, CMS will then define if the treatment is reasonable and necessary. Usually with notification from the FDA to CMS with an IDE (investigational device exemption) number, Category B clinical trials can be reimbursed by Medicare. When payment is made, it usually includes routine care services related to a nonexperimental/investigational (Category B) device that is furnished in conjunction with an FDA-approved clinical trial.[14]

Some national payers adhere to CMS guidance in covering certain clinical trials based on category. Often, experimental and investigational (Category A) devices are denied coverage by private payers on the basis of the contract language payers have with their policy holders, which excludes payment for experimental or investigational devices and/or procedures.[15]

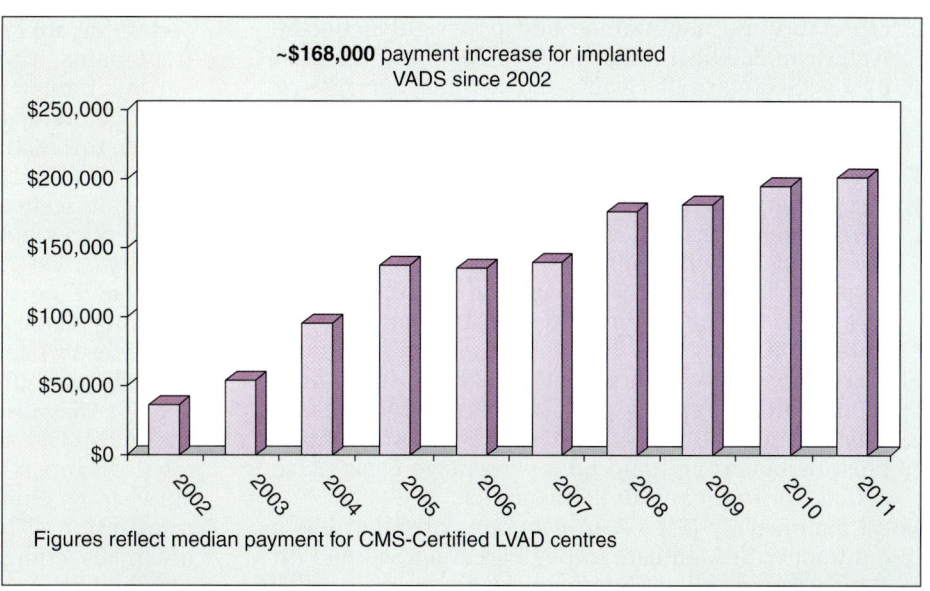

~**$168,000** payment increase for implanted VADS since 2002

Figures reflect median payment for CMS-Certified LVAD centres

FIGURE 25-10 Ventricular assist device (VAD) hospital payments over time. CMS, Centers for Medicare and Medicaid Services; LVAD, left ventricular assist device.

created to meet the reporting requirement established by CMS in collaboration with the FDA, the CMS, and the clinical community[16] (see Chapter 26). Another aspect of the coverage decision was the need for hospitals to become certified in DT by the Joint Commission. Under this program, hospitals are required to demonstrate compliance in three areas:

- Consensus-based national standards
- Effective use of evidence-based clinical practice guidelines to manage and optimize care
- An organized approach to performance measurement and improvement activities[17]

As of 2011, just over 100 facilities were certified to provide DT therapy in the United States.

SUMMARY

The primary components of a reimbursement strategy are (1) obtaining medical coverage, (2) defining coding, and (3) establishing adequate payment. Initial reimbursement efforts focus on coverage by determining where a technology fits, what indications are most appropriate or potentially limit coverage, and what coding modifications will be necessary to obtain payment given the coverage anticipated. After reviewing the clinical study protocols with targeted payers, revisions are often necessary to demonstrate the product is also reasonable and necessary under that payer's criteria, as well as cost-effective. If these topics are addressed, a reimbursement strategy sensitive to the needs of the provider of care, the patient, the payer, and the company can be developed and successfully implemented.

Glossary of Terms

Centers for Medicare & Medicaid Services (CMS) The federal agency that runs the Medicare program. In addition, CMS works with the states to run the Medicaid program. CMS works to make sure that the beneficiaries in these programs are able to get high-quality health care.

Claim A claim is a request for payment for services and benefits you received. Claims are also called bills for all Part A and Part B services billed through fiscal intermediaries. "Claim" is the word used for Part B physician/supplier services billed through the carrier.

Current Procedural Terminology A medical code set of five-character, numeric codes for physician and other services, maintained and copyrighted by the American Medical Association (AMA) and adopted by the Secretary of Health and Human Services as the standard for reporting physician and other services on standard transactions.

Diagnosis-Related Groups (DRGs) A classification system that groups patients according to diagnosis, type of treatment, age, and other relevant criteria. Under the prospective payment system, hospitals are paid a set fee for treating patients in a single DRG category, regardless of the actual cost of care for the individual.

Fee-for-Services Reimbursement method in which each health service is paid on an individual basis. Charges may be paid in full by the insurer but in most instances are paid on a percentage basis. Also called *traditional* or *80/20* insurance.

Fiscal Intermediary (FI) A private company that has a contract with Medicare to pay Part A and some Part B bills. (Also called "Intermediary.")

FDA Investigational Device Exemption (IDE) An FDA-approved IDE application permits a device, which would otherwise be subject to marketing clearance, to be shipped lawfully for the purpose of conducting a clinical trial in accordance with 21 U.S.C. 360j(g) and 21 CFR parts 812 and 813.

FDA Experimental/Investigation Category A Device Innovative device in which "absolute risk" of the device type has not been established (i.e., initial questions of safety and effectiveness have not been resolved and the FDA is unsure whether the device type can be safe and effective).

FDA Nonexperimental/Investigational Category B device A device in which the incremental risk is the primary risk in question (i.e., underlying questions of safety and effectiveness of that device type have been resolved), or it is known that the device type can be safe and effective because, for example, other manufacturers have obtained FDA approval for that device type.

Health Technology Assessment (HTA) Health care technology assessment is a multidisciplinary field of policy analysis. It studies the medical, social, ethical, and economic implications of the development, diffusion, and use of technologies. In support of National Coverage Determinations (NCDs), an HTA often focuses on the safety and efficacy of technologies. Each NCD includes a comprehensive HTA process. For some NCDs, external HTAs are requested through the Agency for Health Research and Quality (AHRQ). For a description of the TA process and guiding principles for selecting which topics are referred for external technology assessment assistance see http://www.cms.gov/medicare-coverage-database/details/medicare-coverage-document-details.aspx?MCDId=7&McdName=Factors+CMS+Considers+in+Commissioning+External+Technology+Assessments&mcdtypename=Guidance+Documents&MCDIndexType=1&bc=BAAIAAAAAAAA&.

Healthcare Common Procedural Coding System (HCPCS) A medical code set that identifies health care procedures, equipment, and supplies for claim submission purposes. It has been selected for use in Health Insurance Portability and Accountability Act transactions. HCPCS Level I contains numeric CPT codes that are maintained by the AMA. HCPCS Level II contains alphanumeric codes used to identify various items and services that are not included in the CPT medical code set. These are maintained by HCFA, the BCBSA, and the HIAA. HCPCS Level III contains alphanumeric codes that are assigned by Medicaid state agencies to identify additional items and services not included in levels I or II. These are usually called "local codes" and must have "W," "X," "Y," or "Z" in the first position. HCPCS Procedure Modifier Codes can be used with all three levels, with the WA to ZY range used for locally assigned procedure modifiers.

ICD-9-CM Diagnosis Code The first of these codes is the ICD-9-CM diagnosis code describing the principal diagnosis (i.e., the condition established after study to be chiefly responsible for causing this hospitalization). The remaining codes are the ICD-9-CM diagnosis codes corresponding to additional conditions that coexisted at the time of admission, or

developed subsequently, and which had an effect on the treatment received or the length of stay.

Incremental Cost-Effectiveness Ratio (ICER) The incremental cost-effectiveness ratio of an intervention in health care is the ratio of the change in costs of a therapeutic intervention (compared with the alternative, such as doing nothing or using the best available alternative treatment) to the change in effects of the intervention.

Interagency Registry for Mechanically Assisted Circulatory Support (INTERMACS) A national registry for patients who are receiving mechanical circulatory support device therapy to treat advanced heart failure.

Joint Commission Disease-Specific Care Certification for Destination Therapy The Joint Commission's Disease-Specific Care Certification Program, launched in 2002, is designed to evaluate clinical programs across the continuum of care.

Medically Necessary Services or supplies that are proper and needed for the diagnosis or treatment of your medical condition; are provided for the diagnosis, direct care, and treatment of your medical condition; meet the standards of good medical practice in the local area; and are not mainly for the convenience of you or your doctor.

Medicare The federal health insurance program for people 65 years of age or older, certain younger people with disabilities, and people with end-stage renal disease (permanent kidney failure with dialysis or a transplant, sometimes called *end-stage renal disease* [ESRD]).

Medicare Coverage Made up of two parts: Hospital Insurance (Part A) and Medical Insurance (Part B). (See Medicare Part A (Hospital Insurance); Medicare Part B (Medical Insurance).)

Medicare Coverage Advisory Committee (MCAC) The MCAC advises CMS on whether specific medical items and services are reasonable and necessary under Medicare law. They perform this task via a careful review and discussion of specific clinical and scientific issues in an open and public forum. The MCAC is advisory in nature, with the final decision on all issues resting with CMS. Accordingly, the advice rendered by the MCAC is most useful when it results from a process of full scientific inquiry and thoughtful discussion, in an open forum, with careful framing of recommendations and clear identification of the basis of those recommendations.

The MCAC is used to supplement internal expertise of CMS and to ensure an unbiased and contemporary consideration of "state of the art" technology and science. Accordingly, MCAC members are valued for their background, education, and expertise in a wide variety of scientific, clinical, and other related fields. In composing the MCAC, CMS was diligent in pursuing ethnic, gender, geographic, and other diverse views and to carefully screen each member to determine potential conflicts of interest.

Medicare Part A (Hospital Insurance) Hospital insurance that pays for inpatient hospital stays, care in a skilled nursing facility, hospice care, and some home health care.

Medicare Part B (Medical Insurance) Medicare medical insurance that helps pay for doctors' services, outpatient hospital care, durable medical equipment, and some medical services that are not covered by Part A.

National Correct Coding Initiative (NCCI) The CMS developed the National Correct Coding Initiative (NCCI) to promote national correct coding methodologies and to control improper coding leading to inappropriate payment in Part B claims.

National Coverage Determinations (NCDs) An NCD sets forth the extent to which Medicare will cover specific services, procedures, or technologies on a national basis. Medicare contractors are required to follow NCDs. If an NCD does not specifically exclude/limit an indication or circumstance, or if the item or service is not mentioned at all in an NCD or in a Medicare manual, it is up to the Medicare contractor to make the coverage decision (see LMRP). Before an NCD takes effect, CMS must first issue a Manual Transmittal, CMS ruling, or Federal Register Notice giving specific directions to claims-processing contractors. That issuance, which includes an effective date and implementation date, is the NCD. If appropriate, the Agency must also change billing and claims processing systems and issue related instructions to allow for payment. The NCD will be published in the Medicare National Coverage Determinations Manual. An NCD becomes effective as of the date listed in the transmittal that announces the manual revision.

National Coverage Analysis (NCA) Decision Memoranda The decision memorandum provides the reasons supporting an NCD and announces CMS' intent to issue an NCD. Prior to any new or modified policy taking effect, CMS must first issue a Manual Transmittal, CMS ruling, or Federal Register Notice, giving specific directions to our claims-processing contractors. That manual transmittal, or other issuance, which includes the effective date, is the actual NCD. If appropriate, the Agency must also change billing and claims processing systems and issue related instructions to allow for payment. The NCD will be published in the Medicare National Coverage Determinations Manual. Policy changes become effective as of the date listed in the Manual Transmittal that announces the National Coverage Determinations Manual revision.

Payer In health care, an entity that assumes the risk of paying for medical treatments. This can be an uninsured patient, a self-insured employer, a health plan, or an HMO.

Performance Measures A gauge used to assess the performance of a process or function of any organization. Quantitative or qualitative measures of the care and services delivered to enrollees (process) or the end result of that care and services (outcomes). Performance measures can be used to assess other aspects of an individual or organization's performance such as access and availability of care, utilization of care, health plan stability, beneficiary characteristics, and other structural and operational aspect of health care services. Performance measures included here may include measures calculated by the state (from encounter data or another data source) or measures submitted by the MCO/PHP.

Physician Services Services provided by an individual licensed under state law to practice medicine or osteopathy. Physician services given while in the hospital that appear on the hospital bill are not included.

Prospective Payment System A method of reimbursement in which Medicare payment is made on the basis of a predetermined, fixed amount. The payment amount for a particular service is derived on the basis of a classification system of that service (e.g., DRGs for inpatient hospital services).

Quality of Life-Year (QALY) A measure of disease burden used in assessing the value for money of a medical intervention. It includes both the quality and the quantity of life lived, based on the number of years of life that would be added by the intervention. Each year in perfect health is assigned the value of 1.0 down to a value of 0.0 for death. If the extra years would not be lived in full health, then the extra life-years are given a value between 0 and 1 to account for this.

Resource-Based Relative Value Scale A scale of national uniform relative values for all physicians' services. Values for each medical procedure are based on the amount of resources required to perform the procedure including physicians' work, practice expenses minus malpractice expenses, and the cost of professional liability insurance. Then the values are weighed against each other to compute relative values.

REFERENCES

1. AdvaMed. www.advamed.com Accessed June 2010.
2. CMS Decision Memo for Ventricular Assist Devices as Destination Therapy (CAG-00119R). www.cms.hhs.gov; Accessed 27.03.07.
3. Blue Cross Blue Shield. www.bcbs.com/tec/; Accessed June 2010.
4. Blue Cross Blue Shield Association Medical Advisory Panel. Special report: cost effectiveness of left ventricular assist devices as destination therapy for end stage heart failure. *Blue Cross Blue Shield Technology Evaluation Center Bulletin.* 2004;19(2):1–29.
5. Lee CP, Chertow GM, Zenios SA. An empiric estimate of the value of life: updating the renal dialysis cost effectiveness standard. *Value Health.* 2009;12(1):80–87.
6. Rose EA, Gelijns AC, Moskowitz AJ, et al. Long-term use of a left ventricular assist device for end-stage heart failure. *N Engl J Med.* 2001;345:1435–1443.
7. Oz MC, Gelijns AC, et al. Left ventricular assist devices as permanent heart failure therapy—the price of progress. *Ann Surg.* 2003;238:577–585.
8. Russo MJ, Gelijns AC, Stevenson LW, et al. The cost of medical management in advanced heart failure during the final two years of life. *J Card Fail.* 2008;14(8):651–658.
9. Miller LW, Nelson KE, Bostic RR, et al. Hospital costs for left ventricular assist devices for destination therapy: lower costs for implantation in the post-REMATCH era. *J Heart Lung Transplant.* 2006;25:77.
10. Clegg A, Scott D, Loveman E, et al. Clinical and cost-effectiveness of left ventricular assist devices as destination therapy for people with end-stage heart failure: a systematic review and economic evaluation. *Int J Technol Assess Health Care.* 2007;23(2):261–268.
11. Slaughter MS, Rogers JG, Milano CA, et al. Advanced heart failure treated with continuous-flow left ventricular assist device. *N Engl J Med.* 2009;361:2241–2251.
12. Slaughter MS, Bostic R, Rogers JG, et al. *Changing costs of mechanical circulatory support: impact of era and device.* The 2010 International Society for Heart & Lung Transplantation Annual Meeting [Abstract].
13. Centers for Medicare and Medicaid Services. *The FY 2010 Hospital Inpatient Prospective Payment System Final Rule.*
14. 60 Federal Registry 48423. Sept. 19 1995.
15. http://www.aetna.com/cpb/medical/data/400_499/0466.html; Accessed June 2010.
16. Interagency Registry for Mechanically Assisted Circulatory Support. http://www.intermacs.org Accessed June 2010.
17. Joint Commission. http://www.jointcommission.org/CertificationPrograms/LeftVentricularAssistDevice//; Accessed June 2010.

CHAPTER **26**

Future of Mechanical Circulatory Support

James F. Antaki and Richard K. Wampler

Current mechanical circulatory support (MCS) devices have made great progress in proving safety, clinical benefit, and durability and appear to be gaining traction in the treatment of congestive heart failure (CHF). However, there have been, and continue to be, significant barriers to widespread clinical use. It has been 30 years since the Office of Technology Assessment report[1] on the cost, risks, and benefits of artificial heart, and we have yet to approach the ambitious goal of 10s to 100s of thousands of artificial heart patients. This chapter aims to address the obvious question, "Why not?" More importantly, it examines the remaining roadblocks so as to propose a course for further exploration and development.

The pace of technology has been one barrier, but it may not be the largest. The initial model, that the surgeon would be the end user, ignored the important role of the cardiologist as the gatekeeper. Consequently, it may be argued that the initial user requirements were flawed from the outset. This would imply that the current technology is, in some ways, a case of an excellent solution to the wrong problem. A look into the future requires first a reflection of the past, specifically to evaluate the limitations of the current technology, the departure from the ideal and potential solutions. Perhaps by assessing any errors of judgment that may have taken place, a more expedient course for future progress may be mapped.

FACTORS INFLUENCING EVOLUTION OF MCS

Despite 5 decades of ardent research and development in the field of MCS, we find great room for improvement. This section examines the current state of the art in terms of its virtues versus weaknesses and costs. We attempt to forecast future trends (or recommend future course) by employing a theory of *directed evolution,* a methodology based on characteristic development patterns that are common in systems that are successful in optimizing their benefit-to-cost ratio.[2] We presume the evolution of MCS obeys a path similar to other medical technologies with extended development histories such as the pacemaker, vascular stent, and insulin pump in which the utility

grows steadily as the adverse costs diminish and thus strives toward "perfection" (Fig. 26-1). In the context of MCS technology, we can also presume that the technology has passed the *tipping point* at which the benefits have begun to outweigh the costs. (It is easy to recall an era in which the opposite was the case.) The ratio of *useful* and *harmful* features in the parlance of directed evolution is termed *ideality.* These concepts are not dissimilar from the regulatory principles involving *efficacy* and *safety.*

Utility Functions

The success of MCS depends on a wide array of factors and influences. This section focuses on the technologic factors but acknowledges the importance of economic and cultural factors as well. The useful functions (or metrics of efficacy) can, and should, be considered from the perspective of multiple stakeholders: those who are affected by this therapy and who are responsible for its adoption and growth. In addition to the surgeon and patient, consideration must be given to the referring physicians, caregivers, payers, and indeed society as a whole. They are listed in Table 26-1 along with the corresponding high-level product requirements. The aggregate of these requirements (or a weighted sum thereof) defines the *optimality* of an MCS technology.

Performance, or efficacy, may be considered in terms of hemodynamic variables (e.g., pressure, flow, pulsatility) but inevitably is driven by the clinical benefit to the patient in terms of improved quality of life, reduced hospitalization, and, potentially, increased survival. For several reasons, there is not agreement on how much circulatory assistance should be provided by a system. One reason is that the labeled flow capacity (liters/minute) of a ventricular assist device (VAD), measured in vitro, may not reflect its performance in the circulation. The wide diversity of patients with respect to size (body surface area), age, and desired level of activity further confounds a definitive relationship between flow rate and clinical benefit. This ill-posed design requirement may therefore explain why there exists such a wide range of hemodynamic specifications among currently

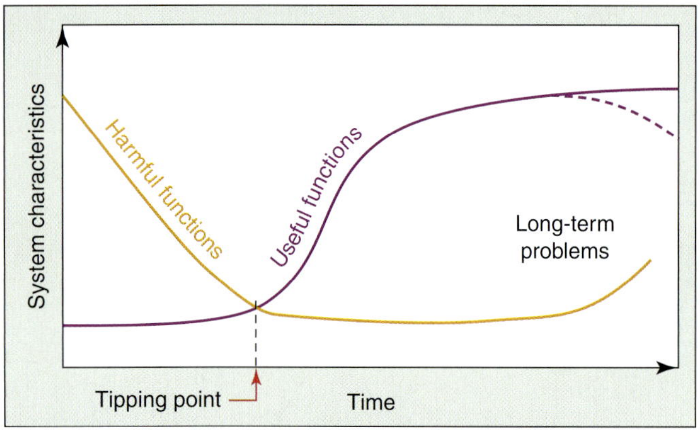

FIGURE 26-1 Pattern of evolution illustrating a successful system, characterized by growth of (perceived) benefits and diminution of costs or adverse effects.

available devices—designed ostensibly for the *same* indication. In addition, it now appears that new indications will necessitate a new generation of pumps that provide significantly less flow capacity. This further obscures our vision toward the *ideal* characteristics of future devices.

The matter of surgical invasiveness also varies depending on perspective. The cardiac surgeon who routinely performs extensive thoracic surgical procedures will have a much more aggressive perception of what constitutes "too much" surgery. The patient has a far lower threshold and obviously would prefer a treatment that avoids surgery altogether. This explains the dramatic increase in angioplasty and stenting versus declining incidence of coronary artery bypass grafting (CABG).

Reliability is a universally desirable quality, for multiple reasons. Consequently, the acceptable incidence of failure (e.g., mean time between failures) may also vary depending on the perspective. The patient who bears the painful consequence of failure once again is most likely to hold the highest standard: zero failure.

Quality of life (QoL) is a design consideration that may have entered into the field of MCS later than others. In the early days of MCS, survival was considered as the primary metric of success. Indeed, even in the present day, it is common to compare efficacy in terms of Kaplan-Meier survival curves.[3–5] Now that less morbidly ill patients are receiving MCS, the importance of QoL and hemodynamic responsiveness has become a greater consideration in deciding on a course of treatment.[6–9] In the words of Robert Jarvik,[10] "If the artificial heart is ever to achieve its objective, it must be more than a pump. It must also be more than functional, reliable and dependable. It must be forgettable."

The financial aspects of MCS are complicated. On one hand, device companies cannot justify the necessary investment in research and development without recouping a significant profit margin. This drives the cost of an average VAD into the many tens of thousands of dollars. On the other hand, the overall costs in terms of quality adjusted life-years (QALYs) severely limit the cost-effectiveness of MCS compared with conventional therapy.[11] If not for the societal, sociologic, and emotional perception of value, it would be difficult to justify the costs on a purely economic basis.[12] Searching far into the future, one may visualize a website where one could purchase a "discount" VAD for perhaps less than $1000, as is now common for automatic external defibrillators.[13] If regulatory restrictions could be dismissed momentarily, the notion of a reconditioned VAD would also make economic sense. Such might be the case in developing countries, for which Qian[14] is striving to develop the "one thousand dollar VAD."

TABLE 26-1	Overarching Design Objectives of Mechanical Circulatory Support with Respect to Multiple Stakeholders Responsible for Its Use						
				Stakeholder			
		Surgeon	Referring Cardiologist	Patient	Caregiver	Industry	Third-Party Payers	Society
REQUIREMENTS	Performance	Restore normal hemodynamics	Restore functional status	Return to normal activity, cognitive function	Minimize care burden, responsibility	Outperform competitors	Decrease hospitalization	Re-enter workforce
	Surgical Invasiveness	Minimal complexity short stay	Minimal surgical risk, complications	Minimal hospital stay; minimal pain	Maximize rehabilitation	Ancillary devices for rapid insertion	Minimal use of expensive resources	—
	Reliability	Avoid reoperation	Optimize long-term outcome	Low tolerance of failure	Minimize adverse complications (e.g., stroke, hemorrhage, infection)	Superior to competitors; minimize liability; warranty?	Avoid costly maintenance, replacement	Maintain functionality
	Quality of Life	At least one functional class improved.	At least one functional class improvement	Forgettable, significant improvement in exercise tolerance	Home-based care	Maximal customer satisfaction	Optimize QALY	Maximize functionality, avoid suffering
	Financial	High payment-to-time ratio	May lose payable procedure	Depends on third-party payers	Profit margin of 5%?	Maximal profit (price/cost)	Cost-effective relative to alternatives	Minimize tax burden
	Other	Routine procedure, no drama	May lose satisfaction, loss to follow-up	Anticoagulants, wound care batteries, etc.	Large support staff for existing devices	Time to market very long	Low readmission rates	—

QALY, quality-adjusted life years.

Cost Functions

Any solution to a problem inevitably begets new problems. Likewise, there are costs associated with MCS that must be weighed against the benefits, some of which are enumerated in Table 26-2. As points of reference, the table juxtaposes related therapies (implanted pacemaker, cardiac transplant), as well as the benchmark of a healthy individual. Standard medical therapy is an obvious benchmark, which has been used in landmark clinical trials such as REMATCH,[15] InTREPID,[16] and various CRT studies.[17] Cardiac transplantation is an important benchmark because it is commonly considered to be the gold-standard or "best" treatment option for patients with end-stage heart failure[18] (see Chapter 6). Minimally invasive VADs such as the Synergy micro pump[19] (CircuLite, Inc., Saddle Brook, NJ) indicate a burgeoning trend in MCS therapy. Finally, implantable pacemakers (and implantable cardioverter-defibrillators [ICDs]) are included to represent an approximation of a nearly ideal outcome.

The associated costs are categorized, in no particular order, in terms of surgical invasiveness, required skilled personnel, risk of adverse events, the encumbrance of external hardware, required maintenance, financial cost, necessity for drugs with associated side effects, and other considerations. For example, the extensive surgery required by most full-sized chronic left ventricular assist devices (LVADs) or biventricular assist devices (BiVADs) is a significant disincentive for the patient. Consider that both the Hemopump and ICDs were heralded by *Discover* magazine as one of the most important inventions of 1988, yet the latter devices have been runaway successes despite modest clinical benefit, whereas the life of the Hemopump was cut short and penetration of MCS has crept along until recently.

This reveals the importance of the complexity of the technology—in terms of required skill and personnel required. It also elucidates the criticality of identifying and considering all who would be end users. The cardiologist serves as the gatekeeper. They are now capable of placing ICDs and CRT devices themselves. Because the risk of device placement is low, it is possible to overlook the somewhat modest clinical benefit the devices provide. Patients also drive this trend because they, understandably, want to avoid a major operation. For example, they are more willing to endure multiple stent procedures rather than undergo a definitive CABG. These realities bode poorly for future growth of the current generation of VADs and further motivate their miniaturization and simplification.

At face value, *adverse events* can refer to additional risks and hazards that are introduced as a result of treatment, or nontreatment. On the other hand, they also reflect the path of inevitable demise. This implies a preferred manner of death—a personal and difficult decision. The patient with end-stage heart failure who is presented the choice of certain imminent death versus a VAD as destination therapy (DT) effectively asked to take an agonizing gamble. Adverse events secondary to the VAD are tantamount to losing positions on this roulette wheel: debilitating stroke, multiorgan failure, pneumonia, septic shock, or in rare cases, pump failure. Clearly, the reduction of these risks afforded by the new MCS technology is most welcome. And future technology must strive to continue this trend.

The matter of external hardware, namely controllers, batteries, and percutaneous cables, is perhaps a secondary consideration. Nevertheless, these do present both an encumbrance and an obligation for vigilant maintenance of these components. They also serve as constant reminders to the patient of their dependency on their VAD for survival and result in numerous readmissions due to minor malfunctions or rapid end of life. Accordingly, future efforts to reduce the bulk and weight, maintenance requirements, and overall user-friendliness would positively affect the *forgettability* factor. The notion of routine maintenance of course also applies to the healthy individual. No technology will completely relieve the individual of maintaining healthy habits and avoiding unhealthy risk factors. However, in the case of MCS and other interventional therapies, the consequences are more imminent.

Financial cost, listed earlier in terms of cost-effectiveness, is also clearly an impediment to widespread use of MCS and has accordingly been the topic of several cost-effectiveness studies. One such recent study by Clegg and colleagues showed that a 50% reduction of overall costs (from approximately $100,000 to $50,000/QALY) could dramatically improve the *cost-effective acceptability.* Nevertheless, the costs are still staggering to most parties involved. They challenge the reimbursement systems to pay, as well as the hospitals to recoup their expenses. It may be said that this financial burden is the elephant in the room. The expectation that chronic VAD therapy will enjoy the same widespread utilization of ICD or CRT technology, in turn, demands that the cost be commensurate (e.g., in the range of $34,000 to $70,200/QALY).[20,21]

For reasons introduced earlier, it is unlikely that the price of the VADs themselves will be significantly reduced in the ensuing 5 to 10 years, unless volume increases dramatically. This leads our attention to the ancillary costs: preparatory assessment, operation, critical care, and long-term medical management. These costs are in turn related to complexity of the technology, and the implementation thereof, which is addressed in a separate section below.

An additional factor that affects quality of life, morbidity, and mortality is the necessity of potent drugs, and their associated side effects, too numerous to list here. Most notably the need for anticoagulants is viewed as a major drawback of any indwelling blood-wetted device. Conversely, the promise of nonthrombogenic surfaces that obviate continuous anticoagulation therapy is often perceived as a decisive factor in selecting one device over another.[22]

A final cost function to be considered with MCS, in some cases, may be the discrediting sociologic response or stigma that it might engender, particularly with younger patients—yet a further reason to make future devices less obtrusive.

In summary, the future of MCS can be determined by the prognosis of the aforementioned costs and benefits.

FUTURE DIRECTIONS

Returning to the theory of Directed Evolution, it can be appreciated by reference to Figure 26-2 that the adoption of a new medical technology (or any complex system) often follows a so-called "S-curve" in which five principle stages of evolution are evident beginning with an initial stage (1) in which the necessary elements for emergence are assembled that give rise to a discovery or invention (2). There is typically a latency period in which the value of the invention is recognized (3), during which there might be limited utilization—analogous to investigational device exemption (IDE) or premarket phase of a new MCS system. Once the value (i.e., safety and efficacy) is demonstrated, an exponential growth in adoption occurs, with commensurate improvement of the technology itself. This growth will rarely continue unabated but will pass an inflection point and ultimately reach a maximum when the resources (or demands) are exhausted (4). A familiar example is the history of cardiac transplantation (Fig. 26-3A).

It is inevitable that a competitive technology or new generation emerges, ultimately supplanting the first system, and reducing the demand/popularity for the old (5). In the context of so-called "first-generation" pulsatile MCS devices, this pattern should be recognizable (Fig. 26-3B). It is likewise reasonable to anticipate that the current generation of MCS devices will, in time, eventually give way to a future, improved technology.

TABLE 26-2 Comparison of Cost Functions Associated with Mechanical Circulatory Support (MCS) versus Related Benchmarks

COST FUNCTIONS	Healthy Individual (=BTR)	Optimal Medical Management	Pacemaker (IAD)	Transplant	MIVAD	Chronic LVAD/BIVAD
Surgical invasiveness	None	None	Catheterization laboratory	Sternotomy	Catheterization laboratory	Sternotomy, thoracotomy
Required personnel	None	Cardiologist/internist	Interventional cardiologist	Cardiac surgery team	Interventional cardiologist/surgeon	Cardiac surgery team MCS coordinators and technicians
Adverse events	None	Hypotension, renal and liver failure	None	Surgical complications, rejection	Thrombosis, bleeding	Thrombosis infection
External bulk	None	None	None	None	Controller, batteries	Controller batteries
Maintenance	Diet, exercise, smoking	Daily medications, regular blood tests (e.g., INR)	Diagnostics, replacement	Antirejection drugs	Charge batteries, exit-site management	Charge batteries exit site management
Financial (5-yr cost)	$0	~$30k*	~$60k†	~$300k‡	$100-250k (est)	~$350k*§
Life expectancy	Normal	25% at 1 yr (class IV)[5]	Near normal	85%-90% (1 yr); 75% (3 yr)	(Unknown)	72% at 18mo[8]
Drugs, side effects	None	Vasoactive antiarrhythmics, diuretics	None	Antirejection	Anticoagulants	Anticoagulants
Other	—	Diminution of function class	—	—	"Stigma"	"Stigma"

*Slaughter MS, Russo MJ, Bostic RB, Rogers J. Cost Effectiveness of Continuous-Flow Left Ventricular Assist Device as Destination Therapy in Advanced Heart Failure. American Heart Association Scientific Sessions, Chicago, Nov 23, 2010. *Circulation.* 122(21_Meeting Abstracts) (suppl 1):A12375.

†Feldman AM, de Lissovoy G, Bristow MR, et al. Cost effectiveness of cardiac resynchronization therapy in the Comparison of Medical Therapy, Pacing, and Defibrillation in Heart Failure (COMPANION) trial. *J Am Coll Cardiol.* 2005;46:2311–2321.

‡Moskowitz AJ, Rose EA, Gelijns AC. The cost of long-term LVAD implantation. *Ann Thorac Surg.* 2001;71(suppl 3):S195–S198.

§Bieniarz MC, Delgado R. The financial burden of destination left ventricular assist device therapy: who and when? *Curr Cardiol Rep.* 2007;9:194–199.

BTR, bridge-to-recovery, implying equivalence of a recovered patient to a healthy individual; INR, international normalized ratio; IVAD, intracorporeal ventricular assist device; MIVAD, minimally invasive ventricular assist devices that do not require thoracic surgery.

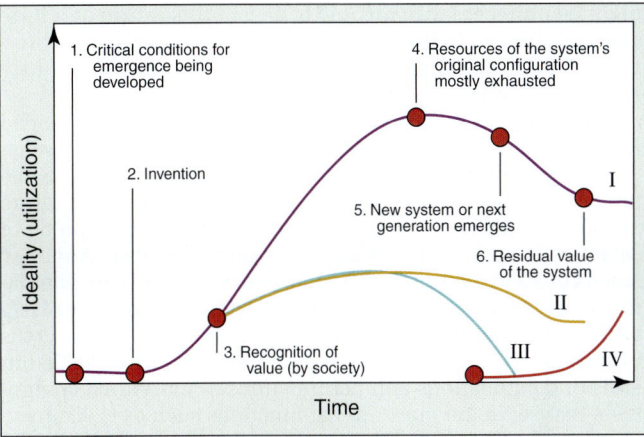

FIGURE 26-2 S-curve illustrating stages of evolution in terms of utilization, success, or ideality. A successful steady-state system is depicted by the *purple line* (I); one in which roadblocks limit maximal utilization is shown by a *gold curve* (II); and a system that fails to thrive is indicated by a *teal line* (III). Curve IV indicates emergence of a new system or next generation as the former declines.

Figure 26-2 also indicates alternative, less desirable paths of evolution (or de-evolution). In cases where critical roadblocks are not surmounted, the maximal utilization can be premature limited (path II). And, of course, some technologies fail to ever gain traction (path III).

An examination of the growth of VAD implants as destination therapy (see Fig. 26-3B) would imply that the current state of the art is approaching point (3) on the S-curve. The future path, however, is indeterminate: Although the community holds optimistic hope that the present course follows Path-I, it is entirely possible that the current technology is actually on Path-II, or possibly awaiting replacement by a next-generation MCS or even alternative therapy (e.g., tissue engineered), represented by Path-IV.

If, indeed, current trends lead to Path-I, then the purpose of this chapter is moot. On the other hand, if some or all the limitations enumerated earlier continue to restrict the full potential of MCS, it may serve us well to consider possible improvements

worth incorporating into the device of the future. Here, various principles of directed evolution may be useful in provoking the imagination. One such principle is *evolution toward increased ideality*. This is the most obvious strategy: to reduce the adverse costs while maintaining or increasing the beneficial effects. It is, however, easier said than done because there are inherent tradeoffs. Reduction of size is desirable from the perspective of anatomic fit; however, this benefit comes at the expense of increased energy losses (e.g., pressure drop in cannulas and anastomoses) or decreased hemocompatibility (e.g., caused by increased impeller speed, decreased pump efficiency, or both).

When such contradictions occur, it often indicates the opportunity for an inventive step. Again, principles of directed evolution may be applied gainfully. One such principle is "separation in space" whereby a component is made small in one region of space, to reap the benefit of smallness, and large in another region, to avoid the associated cost. For example, a small pump may be coupled to large-bore cannulas or tapered cannulas to permit anastomosis to large target vessels while using a small pump. Another recent innovation that illustrates this principle, attributed to Jarvik, is the use of interrupted bearings for a high-speed axial-flow impeller. This invention solved an enduring problem with the biocompatibility of so-called blood-lubricated bearings by solving the following contradiction: Contacting surfaces are necessary to provide support and stability of the impeller, but they create heat and interrupt the passage of blood. The separation principle therefore produced a bearing wherein contacting surfaces were present in localized sectors to provide support, while absent elsewhere to provide washing and cooling.[23]

Another innovative principle is *evolution toward increased involvement of resources*. Application of this principle may suggest harnessing motion, shock, or vibration that is naturally produced by an ambulatory patient, to generate power and extend the life of batteries. An electrical generator incorporated into the shoe[24] or coupled to skeletal muscle[25] has been designed for this purpose.

A third pattern of evolution titled *evolution toward increased dynamism and controllability* states that technologic systems evolve from rigid structures into flexible or adaptive ones. An illustration of this pattern is the development

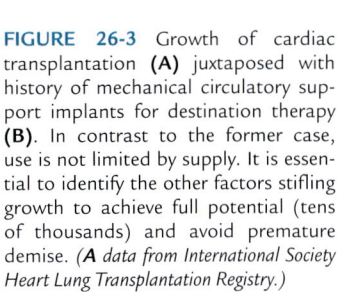

FIGURE 26-3 Growth of cardiac transplantation **(A)** juxtaposed with history of mechanical circulatory support implants for destination therapy **(B)**. In contrast to the former case, use is not limited by supply. It is essential to identify the other factors stifling growth to achieve full potential (tens of thousands) and avoid premature demise. *(A data from International Society Heart Lung Transplantation Registry.)*

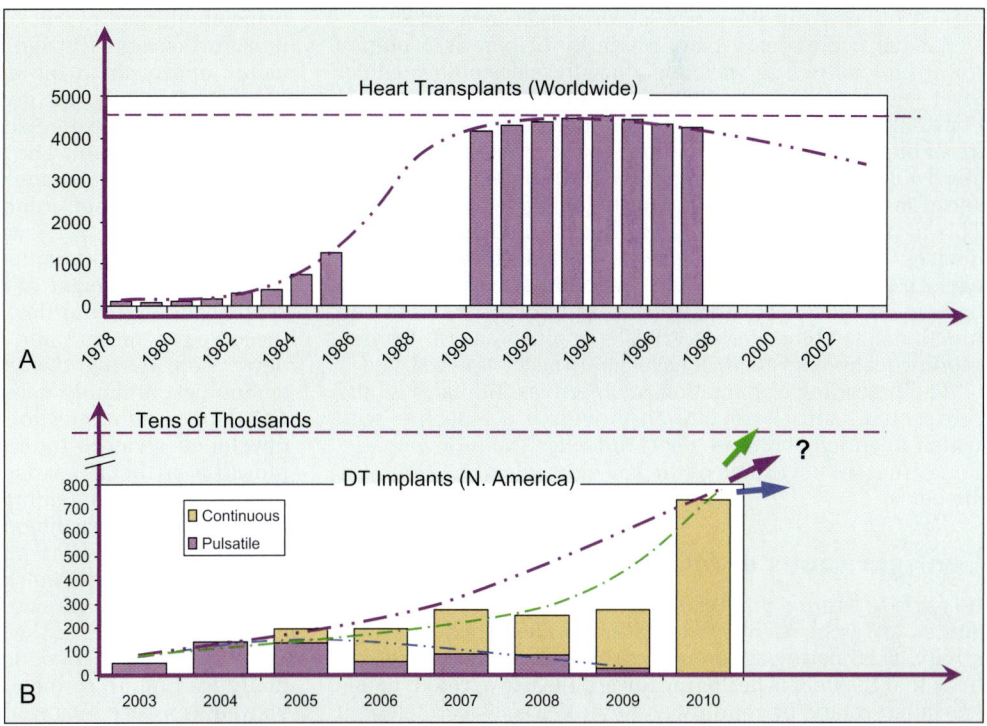

of water turbines such as Kaplan turbines in which the pitch of the blades is adjustable to greatly widen flow range. Following this direction, designers of rotary pumps may be encouraged to consider the possibility of using flexible materials to expand their capacity and capabilities.

Another pattern, *evolution toward increased complexity followed by simplification,* is expressed in the famous quotation of John Norley, "All things are difficult before they are easy." This principle is no better illustrated than by the comparison of today's MCS technology with the pulsatile systems developed through the 1980s and early 1990s, which incorporated implanted controller, battery, compliance chamber and associated refilling port, and transcutaneous energy transmission system coil. Although it might be difficult to imagine how MCS systems could become much simpler than they are today, the same could have been said in the early age of motor vehicles. The 1912 instructional book *Automobile Driving Self-Taught* provided 251 pages describing the procedure for safely and easily operating a vehicle. Chapter 1 begins with inspecting lubricants and grease cups; priming the carburetor; switching on the current; starting the engine; advancing the spark; and adjusting the fuel/air mixture, choke, and throttle.[26] Today's automobiles, although much more complicated in their functionality, are far simpler to operate. When it comes to maintaining the engine, one could say that they are almost forgettable.

To hasten the evolution of MCS, we must ask, "What components or procedures can be combined? simplified? eliminated?" Consider how the Jarvik 2000 eliminated the inflow cannula and associated fluid coupling by employing the housing of the pump itself for insertion into the ventricle.[27] Perhaps ventricular coring may be eliminated altogether (e.g., a transvalvular pump that obviates both apical coring and outflow cannula).[28] The roles of various personnel may also be combined, or eliminated. This leads to a yet further evolutionary principle, *evolution toward decreased human involvement.* Consider joint replacement surgery. In the early days, placement of prostheses was performed crudely and largely freehand. Now there are all varieties of fixtures and robotics to ensure optimal placement. Likewise, it is inevitable that MCS will evolve to rely less on human judgment, perception, and intervention. This will involve incorporation of additional sensors and microprocessors and will require development of new tools. Until recently, the use of sensors has been avoided.

A final evolutionary pattern worthy of note is *evolution toward microlevels.* If we explore length scales of the cellular level, we may discover additional opportunities for innovation. For example, by considering the microhemorrheologic behavior of blood cells within small passages such as the clearance above an impeller blade tip, new ways of increasing impeller speed may be developed without inducing cellular trauma.[29] This in turn could lead to a future generation of much smaller devices. A more timely example is the field of nanotechnology, which promises to produce microminiature sensors, drug delivery devices, actuators/robots, and self-assembling and functionalized biomaterials.[30-33] The applications of this burgeoning technology to MCS have barely been explored.

The preceding examination of objectives, limitations, and prospective paths for evolution provide a perspective with which to anticipate future developments. The following section discusses how some of the key elements of MCS may be affected.

Configurations of MCS Systems

It is safe to assume that the immediate future of MCS will be guided to a great extent by inertia and to a lesser extent by creativity. It is plainly apparent from previous chapters in this book that the field is hastening toward the use of rotodynamic (so-called rotary, or continuous flow) VADs. Nevertheless, it might be unnecessarily myopic to accept this future as a foregone conclusion. In the spirit of preserving a degree of creativity, therefore, it is appropriate to first consider the technology from a panoramic vantage point.

The great variety of MCS devices that have been developed over the decades is an indication of the vastness of the design "space" in which this technology resides. In addition to the numerous devices in clinical use (Chapter 8), the patent literature contains hundreds of inventions claiming to be a blood pump of some sort or another: pulsatile, rotary, and otherwise. And new patents of all varieties steadily continue to appear. This population of devices may be categorized according to taxonomy of features such as pulsatile versus continuous and peristaltic versus rotodynamic. The associated MCS systems can be classified in terms of combinations and permutations of individual components that serve the most critical functions such as (1) connection to the vasculature, (2) means for propulsion of blood, and (3) means for transmitting energy to the implanted hardware. For each function, there may be subfunctions and ultimately a diversity of means for performing these functions. This can be represented concisely through the use of *function-means analysis* and can be depicted schematically in the form of a function-means tree (Fig. 26-4). Designers use such instruments to systematically and exhaustively explore a design space with a wide variety of options. For example, the means of coupling of the device to the body may be accomplished through several approaches: intrathoracic, intra-abdominal, intraventricular, perivascular, intravascular, or extracorporeal. Within the category of intrathoracic, there are options of cannulating the ventricle(s), the atrium(a), or replacing them altogether by anastomosing to the atrial remnants. The former approach implies the form of a VAD, and the latter equates to a total artificial heart.

The most common means of providing pressure and flow is embodied as either a positive-displacement or rotodynamic pump. (For the sake of completeness, one may include alternate approaches such as magnetohydrodynamics, which may also be theoretically possible.[34]) In commercial applications, the type of pump for a given application is dictated by relatively unambiguous rules, governed by the pressure and flow requirements, as well as the availability of power. From an engineer's perspective, it is therefore astonishing that there is such a lack of consensus for the optimal embodiment of mechanical circulatory support devices. It is furthermore intriguing that the pursuit of a rotodynamic approach to the application of circulatory support has lagged many years (decades) behind the large majority of pulsatile, positive-displacement pumps developed through the 1970s to present. The first mention of such a device was made in 1960 by Saxton and Andrews.[35] However, it was not until 1990 that ardent development of a rotary blood pump for chronic MCS was undertaken.[36-40] The success of Wampler's catheter-deployed Hemopump[41] created a tidal wave in development of rotary blood pumps; thus today's centrifugal and axial flow devices are regarded by many as "second-generation" and even "third-generation" technology.[42] Considering the venerable history of rotodynamic technology, arguably dating back to the Renaissance (circa 1475), one might question why such blood pumps were not developed sooner—indeed, *first.* Ironically, developers of pulsatile artificial hearts as early as 1967 had envisioned the use of axial flow pumps to pressurize *hydraulic fluid,* in turn to compress the blood sac.[43] Yet they did consider using the axial pump itself to propel blood.

Psychological inertia could be an explanation. The original notion to replace one positive displacement pump (the heart) with another of the same variety is, after all, intuitive. The ensuing 30 years of development of these devices, eventually leading up to the era of rotodynamic pumps, may be viewed as a very long trial-and-error process. The preceding

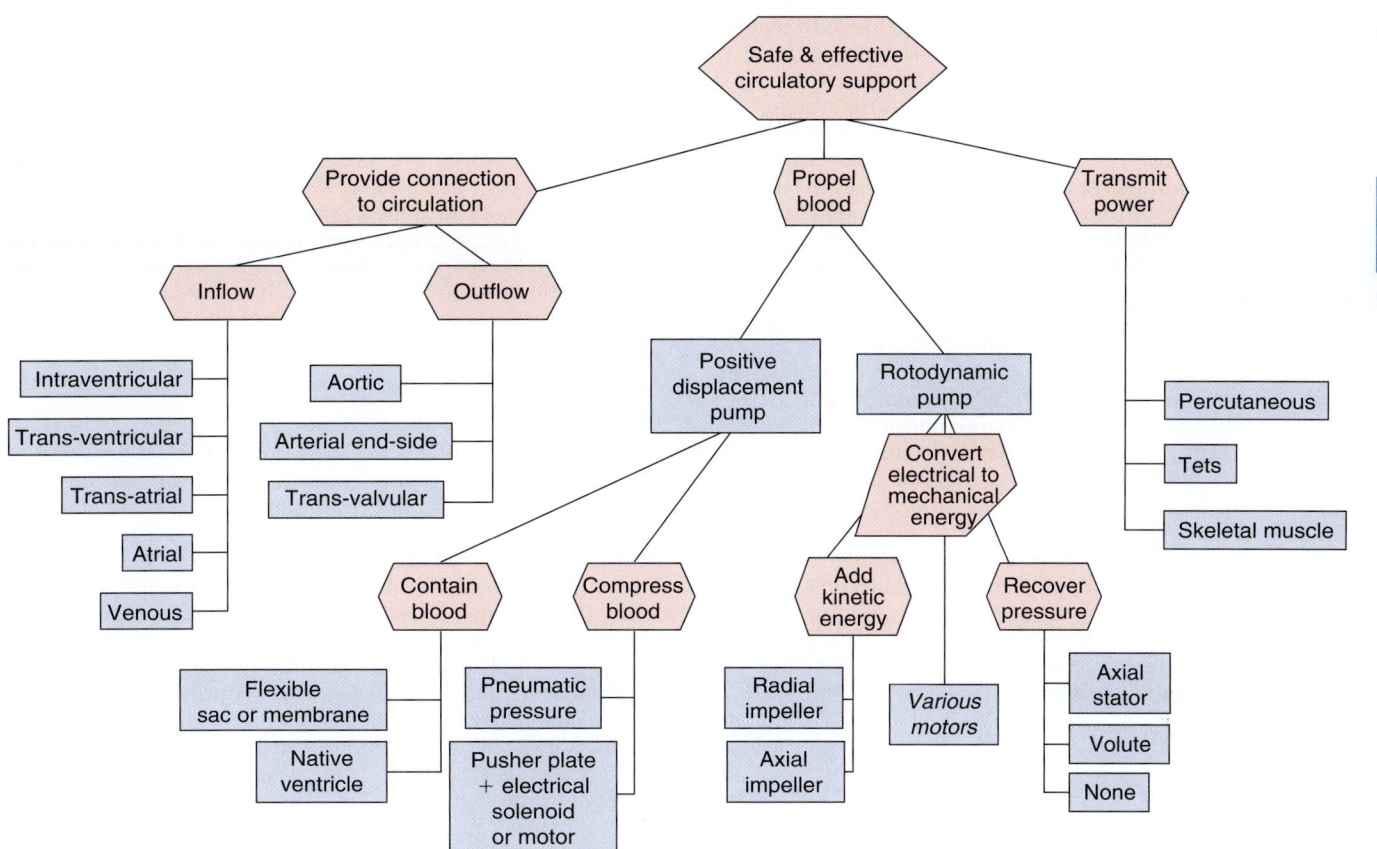

FIGURE 26-4 Partial function-means tree for mechanical circulatory support (MCS). Multiple functions and sub-functions *(hexagons)* are achieved through various choices of means *(rectangles)*. Numerous permutations and combinations of options yield a large variety of design configurations. Tets, transcutaneous energy transfer system

is not intended to negate the certain growth in popularity of the rotary pump, but rather as a disclaimer to acknowledge the fallibility in predicting the future.

Size and Capacity of Implanted Pumps

In many ways the original performance specifications for the total artificial heart and LVAD had been unnecessarily inflated. The requirement for 10 L/min drove devices to larger sizes and greater power consumption, but the clinical value of such high-flow capability has not been realized. For MCDs to become a standard of care in the treatment of CHF, it is necessary to re-evaluate the performance and design specifications on the basis of clinical experience.

Rotary pumps have disproven many of the paradigms that hindered their development in the mid-1980s and clinical acceptance until recently. Specifically, hemolysis has been reduced to astonishingly low levels; patients tolerate, indeed, thrive with profoundly reduced arterial pulsatility. Initial limitations in durability due to shaft sealing have been overcome by successful development of blood-lubricated and hydrodynamic bearings[44] and magnetically suspended rotors[45]. Their small size, potential for high efficiency, and adaptability to minimally invasive methods of insertion will dramatically increase their use in the treatment of CHF.

Widespread acceptance and clinical application will require a device in which the interventional cardiologist can participate (i.e., both personal involvement as a healer and participant in procedures related to device insertion and management). In addition, the target patient population must shift from late-stage IV CHF to less severely ill patients. This is necessary because such patients will have much greater tolerance for device insertion and may well experience greater clinical benefits.[6]

Reduced flow requirements for less severely ill patients will result in smaller pumps that lend themselves to either placement in the pericardial space or for less/minimally invasive placement. Such pumps designed to meet the needs of earlier stages of heart failure could be used in patients who are not candidates for CRT or who do not receive clinical improvement from CRT. The primary endpoints for clinical trials could be hemodynamic improvement, functional improvement, and decreased hospitalization.

There is a growing interest in the use of such devices for use as therapy in CHF of class III early class IV, and there may be a window of opportunity to cause remission or arrest of progress of heart failure in some of these patients. Spence[46] proposed moving in this direction with the Circulite Synergy device, which can be placed through a limited thoracotomy to access left atrial blood and discharge it to an axillary or subclavian artery. However, the present embodiment still requires a surgeon and thoracotomy. Peripheral insertion will be necessary using methods currently employed for percutaneous aortic valve or ASD repair. Possible deployments could include a permanent Hemopump-type device or transvenous delivery with placement of the inflow into the left atria via the atrial septum.

Durability and Longevity

Griffith stated, "When you transplant an older patient, you give him the opportunity to prepare to die. When you transplant a young patient, he does not know whether to prepare to live, or prepare to die." The same could be said of the MCS patient. Therefore as we enter the era of destination therapy, it is essential for these devices to provide virtually "indefinite" durability. It is believed that the emerging generation of magnetically levitated rotary pumps can achieve this goal.[47] However, the current generation of rotary pumps based on blood-lubricated bearings have also demonstrated excellent durability.[48,49] Therefore the longevity of future systems will likely depend on other modes of failure, some not necessarily hardware related. Nevertheless, it is also likely that as the duration of support increases, latent weaknesses are revealed, hopefully leading to improvements in components to make them more rugged: both externally and internally.

Surgical Factors

As described in Chapter 11, the placement of a chronic MCS is a major surgical procedure requiring a highly trained surgical team. The procedure requires a sternotomy or thoracotomy, usually cardiopulmonary bypass and aortic anastomosis and, with many pumps, a subdiaphragmatic pocket or diaphragmatic penetrations. The most significant complications include bleeding, coagulopathy, neurologic abnormalities, multiorgan failure, and sepsis.

For MCS to become a standard of care in the treatment of CHF, the procedure for the placement of a chronic MCS must be simplified and adapted to the setting of nonacademic hospitals. It should parallel the techniques used for the placement of ICDs and CRT devices. Such a user-friendly procedure will require the following changes:

1. Minimal surgical incision such as a limited thoracotomy
2. Ideally, no thoracotomy or sternotomy but rather peripheral placement
3. Ability to place the device without the need for cardiopulmonary bypass
4. Specialized ancillary devices and soft goods to facilitate rapid access and insertion into vascular structures
5. Ideally, no requirement for general anesthesia

Although it may not be possible to implement all of these modifications in all patients, it is important to strive toward simplicity, less or minimally invasive placement, and a significant reduction in mortality and complications when compared with existing devices.

Peripherals Components

Both scientific and patent literature over the past several decades has dedicated a preponderance of attention on the technology of the blood pumps themselves, almost to the exclusion of the so-called *peripheral components*. Yet developers will admit that their attention is often monopolized by what is known in the trade as "the other stuff."[50] Additional elements of the MCS system that are particularly crucial to both safety and efficacy include the cannula, controllers, drivelines, and power sources. Arguably, these have been developed in a somewhat ad-hoc fashion; there has yet to be any standardization. The current state of the art has proven to be "sufficient" but could still enjoy improvement. And now that the most serious risk factors and failure modes of the blood pumps have abated, it is likely that the next phase of evolution will involve more significant improvements to these peripherals.

Features of the external components including their size, durability, ergonomics, and even aesthetics are valid subjects for more concerted attention. Although the sizes of external controllers and batteries have been reduced dramatically since their first-generation predecessors, nevertheless they still present an encumbrance that would be alleviated by further miniaturization. Controllers and drivelines have already undergone environmental testing as a matter of course of validation and verification; however, in the field, clinical engineers, nurses, and patients themselves will admit that these components are exposed to hazards that their developers

never anticipated. Who would have foreseen so many drive lines caught in car doors or cut by scissors or that an external controller would be mistaken by a purse snatcher?[51] With the probable introduction of pediatric blood pumps for toddlers (see Chapter 16), one can only imagine the new failure modes introduced, involving breakfast cereal, melting ice cream, teething marks, and potty training. Consequently, additional failsafe, childproofing, ruggedizing features are likely to appear in future generations. If drivelines are accepted as a necessity of design at present, then some form of protective coating or a tissue-engineered interface will be required to reduce the seemingly inevitable complication of driveline infection (see Chapter 13).

Battery Life

Of all the technologies associated with MCS, battery technology is the one most assuredly to advance in the ensuing years thanks to the mobile phone, laptop, automotive, and gaming industries. The technology has already advanced considerably since the early tetherless VAD systems of the mid-1980s. In fact, the current lithium ion batteries now offer the possibility of carrying a full-day's charge in a rather modest package.[52] Nevertheless, there will always be a demand for smaller batteries, which is at odds with the desire for longer tetherfree operating time, as well as added controller functionalities such as telemetry, which can consume considerable power.

The most dramatic improvements, however, are more likely to occur as a result of improved efficiency rather than battery technology. Consider the effective hemodynamic power required to provide 6 L/min of blood flow at 100 mm Hg, which computes to approximately 1.5 watts. If an MCS system could be 100% efficient in converting electrical energy to hemodynamic energy, this would translate to one D-cell alkaline battery per 12 hours of support. However, when one considers the energy losses caused by inefficiency of the pump and motor, ohmic losses in the driveline, and overhead required by controllers, the actual reported power requirements for portable VADs are in the range of approximately 7 to 12 watts.[53] This translates to 4-7 D-cells, or approximately 0.54 to 0.95 kg of added weight. Of course, partial-support devices would require less power but would not necessarily scale linearly with diminished output because the efficiency of miniature pumps generally decreases with size.[54]

Further reductions of power consumption could potentially render viable the concept of skeletal muscle power, once of great interest in the 1980s-1990s, to either augment battery power or supplant them altogether. Development of skeletal muscle-powered MCS devices continues to the present day[55] and should not be ruled out as a future therapy in the armamentarium.

Transcutaneous Energy Transfer (and Percutaneous Drivelines). The possibility of providing electrical power to implanted MCS through the skin has been considered since the origins of the artificial heart program and by 1984 had even evolved to the point of in-vivo evaluation.[56] The underlying physical principle of operation, electromagnetic induction, has in fact been employed commercially since its discovery in 1831 (independently by Michael Faraday and Joseph Henry). The motivating factors for transcutaneous energy transfer systems are well known: to reduce infection risk and provide completely tether-free support to permit bathing/swimming and facilitate dressing and change of controller, etc. However, their adoption has been stifled, in part by limitations of technology but more so the uncertainty and ambiguity of the tradeoff between benefit and cost. Although early transcutaneous energy transfer systems were considered excessively voluminous, inefficient, and susceptible to misalignment, recent systems have achieved remarkable efficiency, approaching 80%.[57] Contemporaneously, however, the diameter of percutaneous drivelines has become smaller, thereby reducing the risk of infection. Therefore by virtually eliminating one of the most critical needs, we are left with a catalog of costs: added complexity, surgical dissection, risk of misalignment, financial cost, skin erosion, and the need for internal batteries that is offset primarily by the benefit of temporary tether-free operation. Accordingly, the enthusiasm for incorporating this feature into future VADs has diminished and is not likely to be realized in the foreseeable future.

Right Ventricular Assistance. Failure of the right heart is thought to occur in 20% to 50% of patients supported by LVADs alone.[58–60] In the acute, postimplant setting this is often managed with an extracorporeal pump such as the magnetically suspended Centrimag pump. In the majority of cases this temporary measure will be sufficient to support the patient until right ventricular function recovers. In the setting of long-term MCS, an implantable pump is necessary. At this time no dedicated pump for RV assistance is available. However, both the Jarvik 2000 Flowmaker and the Heartware HVAD have been used for biventricular support. At this juncture the clinical experience is limited. The Cleveland Clinic has also begun development of a dedicated right heart device, the DexAid, based on the CorAid technology.[61]

Complete Mechanical Circulatory Support

The original vision for a mechanical circulatory assistance was galvanized by the U.S. government in 1964 with the National Institutes of Health (NIH) initiating research and development for the creation of a total artificial heart. Emphasis and funding were shifted toward left ventricular assistance in response to the substantial technical complexity and challenges of a positive displacement total artificial heart and the preponderance of isolated left ventricular failure in patients with CHF. There is still, however, an unmet need for patients with biventricular failure. Rotary blood pumps could be adapted to full circulatory assistance, for example, with the combination of two separate VADs and fulfill the original vision for a total artificial heart (Fig. 26-5). Several investigators are pursuing rotary blood pump technologies that appear promising for complete mechanical circulatory assistance. Frazier and colleagues[62] have reported early experience explanting the native heart in the bovine and ovine model and replacing it with two commercially available rotary LVADs. To date, the longest survivor has been 48 days; this patient died from tracheostenosis. Hemodynamic parameters, treadmill performance, blood chemistry, and renal and liver function were maintained normal. Flow balance between the right and left heart was stable, despite the absence of autoregulatory or feedback control. Golding and colleagues[63] are developing a coupled biventricular rotary pump that passively controls the flow balance by means of the pressure difference between the right and left atria. Feasibility studies in acute animals have been completed[64] and demonstrate robust control of flow balance over a wide range of physiologic conditions.

Clinical experience with biventricular support with a rotary blood pump is limited to date but encouraging. The Berlin group has reported on eight patients supported with biventricular Heartware LVADs. At the time of publication, six survivors were in rehabilitation in preparation for inclusion to the transplant list.[65] The Jarvik 2000 has been implanted for biventricular support in two patients with survival of 4 and 7 months, ultimately resulting in death due to complications of diabetes and sepsis.

Although counterintuitive, right-sided mechanical circulatory support may not be necessary for full circulatory support in all patients. Quite unexpectedly, there have been reports of hemodynamically stable ventricular fibrillation in patients with an LVAD.[66] Massey, in Rochester, NY, reports on a patient with a "stone" heart that has been supported with a single HeartMate-II as an LVAD.[67] This condition in many ways parallels the Fontan circulation implemented for the treatment of patients with congenital univentricular hearts and suggests the intriguing possibility that patients in CHF with relatively normal pulmonary vascular impedance might be supportable with a single mechanical circulatory device.

Control Algorithms and Related Software. One of the most enduring debates in the rotary MCS community, apart from the importance of pulsatility, is the need for feedback control. At the time the International Society of Rotary Blood Pumps was inaugurated, in 1993, there was but one journal article related to the topic of physiologic control of these devices.[68] The next relevant article to hemodynamic control came 3 years later.[69] Today there is an explosive growth of research into algorithms for providing varying degrees of autoregulation. It would appear that the inflection point on the related S-curve has been reached, which would imply that the ensuing years will lead to some degree of consensus on the subject. As of this juncture in the history of MCS, there endures the belief that these devices do not require any feedback control at all—that they essentially *self-regulate* or *self-balance*.[63] On the other end of the debate, there is a belief that provisions should be incorporated into these systems to compensate for the impairment of autologous regulatory control.[70] Admittedly, the thousands of MCS patients who have been effectively treated to date without feedback control is strong evidence of its dispensability, with respect to the current metrics of efficacy. However, the future expansion of clinical experience, indications, and applications may reveal the potential benefit for MCS devices that respond proactively to changes in preload, afterload, volume status, and possibly adverse events. Furthermore, as interest grows in myocardial recovery and possible weaning from MCS, it is logical to believe in the existence of an optimal level of unloading to promote cardiac rehabilitation: to essentially provide an automated "exercise program" for the recovering ventricle.

Interoperability

Referring to Figure 26-4, it can be appreciated that any type of pump could potentially be coupled with a variety of cannulation schemes, power supplies, controllers, drivelines, etc. For reasons relating to the rigidity of our regulatory process, it is necessary, however, to prearrange these marriages of components early in the development process. To alter the design of a cannula, for example, let alone to adopt a completely different type of cannula, may translate into many months of delay and millions of dollars in development costs. Consequently,

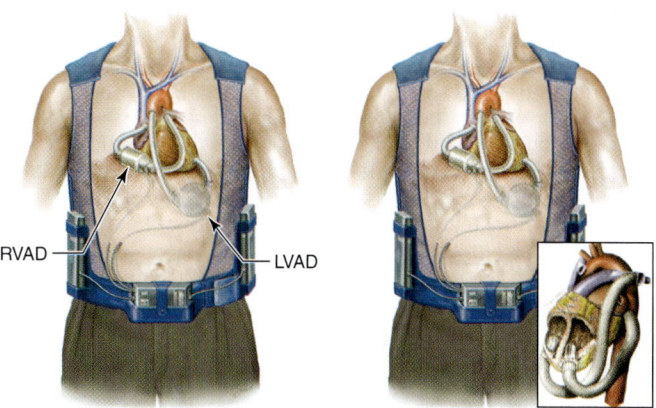

FIGURE 26-5 Biventricular assistance provided by a combination of axial flow and centrifugal ventricular assist devices. LVAD, left ventricular assist device; RVAD, right ventricular assist device. (*Courtesy WorldHeart, Inc; inset courtesy Jarvik Heart, Inc.*)

it is entirely possible that the best cannula becomes coupled to a suboptimal pump. And the decision by a given surgical team to adopt a certain MCS system could ostensibly be made on the basis of a preference of cannulation, at the cost of a less desirable pump. This is unfortunate.

An intriguing, alternative view of the future was recently proposed by Vandenberghe.[71] If future VADs could be made modular, such that specialized developers may focus their strengths on the components they know best, it would become possible to combine a pump from one manufacturer, with a controller of another, a battery of yet another, and so on. This would, of course, require a major paradigm shift in both the corporate and regulatory culture. It would require companies to collaborate. Instead of designing and producing everything in house and being limited by inexperience and a labyrinth of competitor patents, there could be driveline companies, cannula companies, controller companies, and carrying bag companies that work together with all the different pump developers.

Consolidation, Diversification, and Personalization

The preponderance of MCS companies has limited their product line to a solitary device that "fits all." (Berlin Heart is a notable exception.) In aggregate, there are numerous MCS systems, described in Chapter 8, covering a range from small catheter-mounted devices to fully implantable total cardiac replacement systems. Gregoric observed that this variety is necessary to support the vast and complex heart failure population. It is indeed reasonable to believe that there exists a preferred set of product specifications, vis a vis flow capacity, surgical access, feedback control unique to *each* use environment: operating room, inpatient (temporary, cardiogenic shock), and outpatient. The optimum product requirements may likewise depend on the etiology and associated therapeutic goal: acute cardiogenic shock, bridge to decision, bridge to transplant, destination therapy, and bridge to recovery. For certain, no rotary pump is capable of operating efficiently over a multifold range of flow rate such as 1 to 10 L/min. Deviations of 50% from the nominal "best efficiency" point can bear significant consequences with respect to efficiency[54] and hemocompatibility.[72] At the current rate of VAD implantation, the market may not be able to support a great variety of similar products. Hence corporate consolidation is a definite possibility. Conversely, if the market can surmount "point 3" on the S-curve (see Fig. 26-2), there may be opportunities for further diversification and specialization.

Such product diversity, combined with the configurability portrayed earlier, would inevitably offer more *personalized* treatment. It could therefore be envisioned that the selection of pump, cannulas, controller, software, and other peripherals be configured to offer the best outcome for a given patient on the basis of his or her prognosis and personal preferences. In such a scenario, decision support tools would be valuable to help identify the best configuration and course of treatment for an individual.[73]

Beyond the Future: Hybridization

In light of the $3 billion invested annually by the NIH and the National Heart Lung Blood Institute, there is no doubt that new treatments for heart disease will continue to emerge in the years to come. The idea of growing a replacement heart in vitro may seem far-fetched at present, yet the prospect of myocardial tissue regeneration is a realistic possibility in the foreseeable future. Evolving pharmacologic therapy, gene therapy, and other forms of advanced treatments may offer an alternative to patients with currently irreversible heart failure. On the one hand, this would appear to mark the beginning of the end of MCS as destination therapy (point 5

on the S-curve, Fig. 26-2.) Most likely, however, the future success of these treatments will create an *increased* demand for MCS: in the role of bridge to recovery (BTR). The combination of these adjuvant therapies and improved techniques for screening patients may stimulate a new breed of MCS system, specifically configured for this indication. For example, as the heart recovers function, it could be desirable to leave the device in place, rather than exposing the patient to a subsequent invasive procedure. Adaptations of minimally invasive assist devices could fill this role, if provided with a means for completely ligating or otherwise interrupting regurgitant flow (e.g., with the use of a flush-mounted leaflet valve). One device that could be ideally suited for this indication is the Kantrowitz CardioVAD (Cardioplus, formerly L-VAD Technologies).[74] This device features a perivascular balloon pump that is surgically attached to the descending aorta. It therefore offers diastolic augmentation without the need for any blood-wetted biomaterials. Although not currently available clinically, this concept is appealing for temporary, intermittent, partial cardiac support.

Further hybridizations of MCS devices with adjuvant therapy could involve combinations with a drug delivery pump, pacemaker, ICD, or future yet-to-be invented therapeutic device. As stated previously, advanced control algorithms will likely be required to manage the unloading/reloading regimen to optimize myocardial rehabilitation.

Information Management and Connectivity

The technology of telemedicine is not new, per se, although its entry into the MCS arena has lagged behind other medical practices such as emergency medicine and cardiology. More than 13 years ago, Mussivand had envisioned the use of public communication for remote outpatient monitoring.[75] Various prototype systems have been developed, but none to the point of clinical use. To the author's best knowledge, MicroMed Cardiovascular, Inc., in Houston is the only VAD manufacturer actively integrating this technology. They offer a bedside monitoring station, the HeartAttendant, that couples with their HeartAssist 5 VAD to transmit blood flow and related data via secure wireless Internet.

Now that the necessary infrastructure is in place and data security issues have been addressed, it is *inevitable* that all future systems will provide Internet connectivity. In addition to remote data monitoring (e.g., tracking weight for signs of edema/hypovolemia), it is likely that these systems will permit adjustments to be made by the physician, as is done with CRT, etc. Not only is this evolutionary step inevitable, it will be absolutely *essential* for managing the large anticipated volume of outpatients: tracking their condition and responding to their questions. This advance has the potential of reducing the current need for readmission—often based more on the need for more detailed information on the VAD system by clinical teams as opposed to true clinical need.

A related use of the Internet is the development of social networks for communication among patients, their families, caregivers, and tertiary providers. Due to the minimal financial investment and regulatory requirements, this phenomenon is likely to appear on the scene quite rapidly, in the not-too-distant future. It is also possible that countries other than the United States with rapidly growing MCS programs take the lead.[76]

Sundries

Returning to the ideas of interoperability and personalization, it is admitted that the cost may preclude development of interchangeable components such as cannula and controllers, which are life-sustaining U.S. Pharmacopeia Class-III devices. However, a wide-open opportunity exists for enterprising individuals to develop sundry items such as garments, skins, and backpacks for the growing market of destination-therapy MCS patients. Anecdotally, we have learned of patients and their families using needle and thread to make their own modifications to their carrying bags, etc. Vandenberghe has also suggested that a cottage industry that makes customized accessories according to a patient's requirements, akin to support braces, orthoses, and splints, may emerge.[71] Success of such an enterprise could certainly improve the aesthetics of external hardware, as is now being done to prosthetic limbs.[72] Pursuing the same analogy, such a paradigm shift in the treatment of the appearance of external hardware could address the stigma factor that was alluded to previously and potentially contribute to the growth of MCS, particularly destination therapy.

Conclusions and the Ideal Chronic LVAD for 2015

Since the origins of the artificial heart program, there has been persistent optimism that tens to hundreds of thousands of end-stage heart failure patients could be treated with a prosthetic device to replace or augment the function of the heart. This has engendered a myriad of contrivances over the generations to replace or support the human heart. This chapter joins a host of published essays and treatises scattered throughout the literature attempting to forecast the *future* of MCS. The definitive manufactured replacement for the heart that God made has been perpetually just beyond the horizon,[10,77,78] indeed "already here," according to the September 1981 cover of *LIFE* magazine[79]; and again in 2009.[80] The futurists have been consistently wrong, unaware of what they "did not know they did not know."

Today we exercise a modicum of humility, conscious of our relative ignorance. From both an engineering and clinical perspective, acknowledging what we "know we don't know." Therefore this chapter may be considered more of a "wish list" than a prognostication. With this disclaimer, it can be asserted that the following critical milestones must be achieved for MCS to establish itself as a standard of care in the treatment of CHF:

1. Smaller devices adaptable to less and minimally invasive placement must be developed. Ideally, peripheral placement without thoracotomy should be adaptable to any institution performing interventional cardiology procedures.
2. Clinical trials in patients with class III and early class IV CHF need to be completed and demonstrate superior clinical benefit compared with CRT and conventional medical therapy.
3. Mechanisms for managing patients remotely via the Internet need to be implemented.
4. Heart failure and interventional cardiologists need to be major stakeholders in less and minimally invasive devices.

Misplaced hubris notwithstanding, there is today clear evidence of accelerated growth of MCS therapy, indicating we have passed an important milestone on the S-curve of its evolution. Destination therapy is now a reality, as is bridge to recovery. Although it is true that additional technologic advances will be necessary, the likelihood of achieving these goals is better than before, thanks to the accumulated experience of the past decades—both positive and negative—and due to improved, prescriptive design methodologies that reduce the need for blind trial-and-error.[81]

The prognosis for cultural evolution is likewise optimistic due to the rapid dissemination of knowledge through the Internet, increased involvement of the patient in decision making, and of course, clinical success of the current generation of MCS. This positive trend can hopefully be accentuated

through the use of advanced evidence-based practices and the use of decision support systems that can efficiently disseminate accumulated knowledge.[73]

Some of the ambitious predictions presented herein may indeed appear preposterous. On the other hand, history is replete with inventors who were once considered heretics. And innovation is driven by (cautious) optimism: the remedy for psychologic inertia. In the words of the late great Henry Bahnson, former Chair of Surgery at the University of Pittsburgh, "If you did not under estimate the work ahead of you, you'd never embark on any new journey."[82]

REFERENCES

1. Lubeck DP, Bunker JP. The artificial heart: costs, risks, and benefits. In: *NTIS #PB82-239971*:Washington, DC: Office of Technology Assessment; 1982.
2. Zlotin B, Zusman A. *Directed Evolution.* Detroit: Ideation International; 2004.
3. Allan CK, Thiagarajan RR, del Nido PJ, et al. Indication for initiation of mechanical circulatory support impacts survival of infants with shunted single-ventricle circulation supported with extracorporeal membrane oxygenation. *J Thorac Cardiovasc Surg.* 2007;133(3):660–667.
4. Haft JW, Pagani FD, Romano MA, et al. Short- and long-term survival of patients transferred to a tertiary care center on temporary extracorporeal circulatory support. *Ann Thorac Surg.* 2009;88(3):711–717; discussion 7–8.
5. Miller L. The impact of mechanical circulatory support on post-transplant survival a different view. *J Am Coll Cardiol.* 2009;53(3):272–274.
6. Miller LW, Pagani FD, Russell SD, et al. Use of a continuous-flow device in patients awaiting heart transplantation. *N Engl J Med.* 2007;357(9):885–896.
7. Westaby S, Siegenthaler M, Beyersdorf F, et al. Destination therapy with a rotary blood pump and novel power delivery. *Eur J Cardiothorac Surg.* 2010;37(2):350–356.
8. Pagani FD, Miller LW, Russell SD, et al. Extended mechanical circulatory support with a continuous-flow rotary left ventricular assist device. *J Am Coll Cardiol.* 2009;54(4):312–321.
9. Long JW, Kfoury AG, Slaughter MS, et al. Long-term destination therapy with the HeartMate XVE left ventricular assist device: improved outcomes since the REMATCH study. *Congest Heart Fail.* 2005;11(3):133–138.
10. Jarvik RK. The total artificial heart. *Sci Am.* 1981;244(1):74–80.
11. Clegg AJ, Scott DA, Loveman E, et al. The clinical and cost-effectiveness of left ventricular assist devices for end-stage heart failure: a systematic review and economic evaluation. *Health Technol Assess.* 2005;9(45):1–132 iii–iiv.
12. National Heart and Lung Institute. *Artificial Heart Assessment Panel.* The totally implantable artificial heart; economic, ethical, legal, medical, psychiatric [and] social implications; a report. Bethesda: National Institutes of Health; 1973
13. AED Superstore. Accessed at http://www.aedsuperstore.com/; 2010.
14. Qian KX. One thousand dollar assist heart pump for patients from developing countries. *Open Biomed Eng J.* 2007;1:11–12.
15. Rose EA, Moskowitz AJ, Packer M, et al. The REMATCH trial: rationale, design, and end points. Randomized Evaluation of Mechanical Assistance for the Treatment of Congestive Heart Failure. *Ann Thorac Surg.* 1999;67(3):723–730.
16. Rogers JG, Butler J, Lansman SL, et al. Chronic mechanical circulatory support for inotrope-dependent heart failure patients who are not transplant candidates: results of the INTrEPID Trial. *J Am Coll Cardiol.* 2007;50(8):741–747.
17. Young JB, Abraham WT, Smith AL, et al. Combined cardiac resynchronization and implantable cardioversion defibrillation in advanced chronic heart failure: the MIRACLE ICD Trial. *JAMA.* 2003;289(20):2685–2694.
18. Boilson BA, Raichlin E, Park SJ, Kushwaha SS. Device therapy and cardiac transplantation for end-stage heart failure. *Curr Probl Cardiol.* 2010;35(1):8–64.
19. Klotz S, Meyns B, Simon A, et al. Partial mechanical long-term support with the CircuLite Synergy pump as bridge-to-transplant in congestive heart failure. *Thorac Cardiovasc Surg.* 2010;58(suppl 2):S173–S178.
20. Zwanziger J, Hall WJ, Dick AW, et al. The cost effectiveness of implantable cardioverter-defibrillators: results from the Multicenter Automatic Defibrillator Implantation Trial (MADIT)-II. *J Am Coll Cardiol.* 2006;47(11):2310–2318.
21. Sanders GD, Hlatky MA, Owens DK. Cost-effectiveness of implantable cardioverter-defibrillators. *N Engl J Med.* 2005;353(14):1471–1480.
22. Holman WL, Teitel ER, Itescu S. Biologic barriers to mechanical circulatory support. In: Frazier OH, Kirklin JK, eds. *ISHLT Monograft Series.* New York: Elsevier; 2006:9–32.
23. Jarvik R. inventor blood pump bearings with separated contact surfaces: patent. United States Patent 7762941. 2010 7/27/2010.
24. Antaki JF, Bertocci GE, Green EC, et al. A gait-powered autologous battery charging system for artificial organs. *ASAIO J.* 1995;41(3):M588–M595.
25. Trumble D. Potential mechanisms for muscle-powered cardiac support. *Artif Organs.* 2011;35:715–720.
26. Russell T. *Automobile Driving Self-Taught: An Exhaustive Treatise on the Operation, Management, and Care of Motor Cars.* 2nd ed. Chicago: Charles C. Thompson; 1912.
27. Westaby S, Banning AP, Jarvik R, et al. First permanent implant of the Jarvik 2000 Heart. *Lancet.* 2000;356(9233):900–903.
28. Mitamura Y, Nakamura H, Okamoto E, et al. Development of the Valvo pump: an axial flow pump implanted at the heart valve position. *Artif Organs.* 1999;23(6):566–571.
29. Antaki JF, Diao CG, Shu FJ, et al. Microhaemodynamics within the blade tip clearance of a centrifugal turbodynamic blood pump. *Proc Inst Mech Eng [H].* 2008;222(4):573–581.
30. Staples M, Daniel K, Cima MJ, Langer R. Application of micro- and nano-electromechanical devices to drug delivery. *Pharm Res.* 2006;23(5):847–863.

31. Sitti M. Microscale and nanoscale robotics systems. *IEEE Robot Autom Mag.* 2007;14(1):53–60.

32. Cavalcanti A, Shirinzadeh B, Kretly LC. Medical nanorobotics for diabetes control. *Nanomedicine.* 2008;4(2):127–138.

33. Patel GM, Patel GC, Patel RB, et al. Nanorobot: a versatile tool in nanomedicine. *J Drug Target.* 2006;14(2):63–67.

34. Qian KX, Wang SS, Chu SH. A superconductive electromagnetic pump without any mechanical moving parts. *ASAIO J.* 1993;39(3):M649–M653.

35. Saxton G, Andrews C. An ideal pump with hydrodynamic characteristics analogous to the mammalian heart. *Trans Am Soc Artif Intern Organs.* 1960;6:288–289.

36. Antaki JF, Butler KC, Kormos RL, et al. In vivo evaluation of the Nimbus axial flow ventricular assist system. Criteria and methods. *ASAIO J.* 1993;39(3):M231–M236.

37. Butler K, Wampler R, Griffith B, et al. Development of an implantable axial flow LVAS. In: *Int Symposium on Rotary Blood Pumps; 1991.* Vienna; 1991:148–153.

38. Fossum T, Morley D, Benkowski R, et al. Chronic survival of calves implanted with the Debakey ventricular assist device. *Artif Organs.* 1999;23(8):802–806.

39. Macris M, Myers T, Jarvik R. In vivo evaluation of an intraventricular electric axial flow pump for left ventricular assistance. *ASAIO J.* 1994;40:M719–M722.

40. Takeuchi T, Nishimura K, Okabayashi H, et al. Experimental study of mutating centrifugal blood pump in vivo. In: Akutsu T, Koyanagi H, eds. *Artificial Heart & Heart Replacement* (3rd Int Symp Artif Heart Assist Devices). New York: Springer Verlag; 1990:90–93.

41. Wampler R, Moise J, Frazier O, et al. In vivo evaluation of a peripheral vascular access axial flow blood pump. *Trans Am Soc Artif Intern Organs.* 1988;34:450.

42. Olsen DB. The history of continuous-flow blood pumps. *Artif Organs.* 2000;24(6):401–404.

43. Griffith B. Mixed flow electrohydraulic VAD. In: Frank W, Hastings M, Chief, Lowell T, Harmison P, Assistant Chief, eds. *Artificial Heart Program Conference; 1969 June 9-13.* Washington, DC: US Department of Health, Education, and Welfare; 1969.

44. Jarvik RK. System considerations favoring rotary artificial hearts with blood-immersed bearings. *Artif Organs.* 1995;19:565–570.

45. Lewis J, Weibusch B, eds. MagLev pumps sustain the wounded heart. *Design News.* June 5, 2000, pp. 98–103.

46. Spence PA. inventor supplemental heart pump methods and systems for supplementing blood through .... US patent 6,530,876 2003.

47. Hoshi H, Shinshi T, Takatani S. Third-generation blood pumps with mechanical noncontact magnetic bearings. *Artif Organs.* 2006;30(5):324–338.

48. Butler K, Farrar D. No bearing wear detected in explanted clinical Heartmate II LVADs—Implications for long term durability and reliability. *ASAIO J.* 2006;52(2):33A.

49. Westaby S. Destination therapy: time for real progress. *Nat Clin Pract Cardiovasc Med.* 2008;5(8):477–483.

50. Butler KC. Personal communication. New York; c. 1997.

51. Nawrat Z. Review of research in cardiovascular devices. In: Verdonck P, ed. *Advances in Biomedical Engineering.* St. Louis: Elsevier Science; 2008.

52. Rintoul T. Personal communication. 2010.

53. Reul HM, Akdis M. Blood pumps for circulatory support. *Perfusion.* 2000;15(4):295–311.

54. Smith WA, Allaire P, Antaki J, et al. Collected nondimensional performance of rotary dynamic blood pumps. *ASAIO J.* 2004;50(1):25–32.

55. Trumble DR, Magovern JA. A muscle-powered energy delivery system and means for chronic in vivo testing. *J Appl Physiol.* 1999;86(6):2106–2114.

56. Sherman C, Daly BD, Clay W, et al. In vivo evaluations of a transcutaneous energy transmission (TET) system. *Trans Am Soc Artif Intern Organs.* 1984;30:143–147.

57. Rintoul TC, Dolgin A. Thoratec transcutaneous energy transformer system: a review and update. *ASAIO J.* 2004;50(4):397–400.

58. Dang NC, Topkara VK, Mercando M, et al. Right heart failure after left ventricular assist device implantation in patients with chronic congestive heart failure. *J Heart Lung Transplant.* 2006;25(1):1–6.

59. Morgan JA, John R, Lee BJ, et al. Is severe right ventricular failure in left ventricular assist device recipients a risk factor for unsuccessful bridging to transplant and posttransplant mortality? *Ann Thorac Surg.* 2004;77:859–863.

60. Furukawa K, Motomura T, Nosé Y. Right ventricular failure after left ventricular assist device implantation: the need for an implantable right ventricular assist device. *Artif Organs.* 2005;29(5):369–377.

61. Fukamachi K, Ootaki Y, Horvath DJ, et al. Progress in the development of the DexAide right ventricular assist device. *Asaio J.* 2006;52(6):630–633.

62. Frazier OH, Myers TJ, Gregoric I. Biventricular assistance with the Jarvik FlowMaker: a case report. *J Thorac Cardiovasc Surg.* 2004;128(4):625–626.

63. Fukamachi K, Horvath DJ, Massiello AL, et al. An innovative, sensorless, pulsatile, continuous-flow total artificial heart: device design and initial in vitro study. *J Heart Lung Transplant.* 2010;29(1):13–20.

64. Fumoto H, Horvath DJ, Rao S, et al. In vivo acute performance of the Cleveland Clinic self-regulating, continuous-flow total artificial heart. *J Heart Lung Transplant.* 2010;29(1):21–26.

65. Drews T, Krabatsch T, Huebler M, Hetzer R. Paracorporeal biventricular mechanical circulatory support for more than 4 years. *J Heart Lung Transplant.* 2010;29(6):698–699.

66. Frazier OH. *Personal communication.* In; 2010.

67. Massey HT. *Personal communication.* Rochester, NY; 2010 .

68. Schima H, Trubel W, Moritz A, et al. Noninvasive monitoring of rotary blood pumps: necessity, possibilities, and limitations. *Artif Organs.* 1992;16(2):195–202.

69. Konishi H, Antaki JF, Amin DV, et al. Controller for an axial flow blood pump. *Artif Organs.* 1996;20(6):618–620.

70. Antaki JF, Choi S, Amin DV, et al. In search of chronic speed control for rotary pumps. In: Proceedings of *The Waseda International Congress of Modeling and Simulation Technology for Artificial Organs; 1996 August 1-3, 1996.* Tokyo, Japan; 1996.

71. Vandenberghe S. *Personal communication.* Bern, Switzerland; 2010.

72. Wu ZJ, Antaki JF, Burgreen GW, et al. Fluid dynamic characterization of operating conditions for continuous flow blood pumps. *ASAIO J.* 1999;45(5):442–449.

73. Santelices LC, Wang Y, Severyn D, et al. Development of a hybrid decision support model for optimal ventricular assist device weaning. *Ann Thorac Surg.* 2010;90(3):713–720.

74. Jeevanandam V, Jayakar D, Anderson AS, et al. Circulatory assistance with a permanent implantable IABP: initial human experience. *Circulation.* 2002;106(12 suppl 1):I183–I188.

75. Mussivand T, Hum A, Holmes KS, Keon WJ. Wireless monitoring and control for implantable rotary blood pumps. *Artif Organs.* 1997;21(7):661–664.

76. Ono M, Kyo S, Nishimura T, et al. How do we construct an ideal infrastructure for increasing demand of implantable ventricular assist device? *J Card Fail.* 2010;16(9):S144.

77. Watson JT. The present and future of cardiac assist devices. *Artif Organs.* 1985;9(2):138–143.

78. Takatani S. Cardiac prosthesis as an advanced surgical therapy for end-stage cardiac patients: current status and future perspectives. *J Med Dent Sci.* 2000;47(3):151–165.

79. The Artificial Heart Is Here. *Life.* 1981 September.

80. Alba AC, Delgado DH. The future is here: ventricular assist devices for the failing heart. *Exp Rev Cardiovasc Ther.* 2009;7(9):1067–1077.

81. Antaki JF, Ricci MR, Verkaik JE, et al. PediaFlow Maglev ventricular assist device: a prescriptive design approach. *Cardiovasc Eng.* 2010;1(1):104–121.

82. Bahnson HT. *Personal communication.* 1998.

Note: Page numbers followed by *b* indicate boxes, *f* indicate figures, and *t* indicate tables.

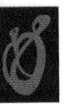

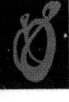